DISASTER MEDICINE

DISASTER MEDICINE

Gregory R. Ciottone, MD, FACEP

Director, International Emergency Medicine Section
Harvard Medical School
Director, Division of Disaster Medicine
Beth Israel Deaconess Medical Center
Boston, Massachusetts

ASSOCIATE EDITORS

Philip D. Anderson, MD

Erik Auf Der Heide, MD

Robert G. Darling, MD

Irving Jacoby, MD

Eric Noji, MD

Selim Suner, MD

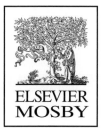

ELSEVIER
MOSBY

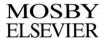

1600 John F. Kennedy Boulevard, Suite 1800
Philadelphia, PA 19103-2899

DISASTER MEDICINE
Third Edition

ISBN-13: 978-0-323–03253-7
ISBN-10: 0-323-03253-2

Copyright © 2006 by Mosby, Inc.

Library of Congress Cataloging-in-Publication Data

Disaster medicine/editor-in-chief, Gregory R. Ciottone; associate editors, Philip D. Anderson ... [et al.];
    section editors, Kathryn Brinsfield ... [et al].–1st ed.
        p.; cm.
    Includes bibliographical references and index.
    ISBN 0-323-03253-2
        1. Disaster medicine. I. Ciottone, Gregory R.
    [DNLM: 1. Disaster Planning-methods. 2. Accidents, Radiation-prevention & control.
    3. Bioterrorism-prevention & control. 4. Emergency Medical Services-methods. 5. Natural Disasters.
    WA 295 D611 2006]
    RC86.7.D56 2006
    362.18-dc22

                                                                            2005047926

Acquisitions Editor: Todd Hummel
Developmental Editor: Martha Limback
Publishing Services Manager: Joan Sinclair
Project Manager: Mary Stermel
Design Direction: Karen O'Keefe Owens
Marketing Manager: Dana Butler

Printed in the United States of America.

Last digit is the print number: 9 8 7 6 5 4 3 2 1

Dedicated to victims and survivors of disasters everywhere and to the medical professionals who care for them.

ASSOCIATE EDITORS

Philip D. Anderson, MD
Assistant Professor in Medicine, Harvard Medical
    School
Director, Division of International Disaster
    and Emergency Medicine
Attending Physician, Department of Emergency
    Medicine
Beth Israel Deaconess Medical Center
Boston, Massachusetts

Erik Auf Der Heide, MD, MPH, FACEP
Medical Officer
Agency for Toxic Substances and Disease Registry
U.S. Department of Health and Human Services
Atlanta, Georgia

Robert G. Darling, MD, FACEP
Captain, Medical Corps, Flight Surgeon, United States
    Navy
Senior Medical Advisor, Navy Medicine Office of
    Homeland Security
Specialty Advisor to the Chief of the Medical Corps for
    Homeland Security

Irving Jacoby, MD
Professor of Medicine & Surgery
University oif California, San Diego, School of Medicine
La Jolla, California
Attending Physician, Department of Emergency
    Medicine
Hospital Medical Director for Emergency Preparedness
    and Response
University of California, San Diego, California

Eric Noji, MD, MPH
Senior Medical Officer
Centers for Disease Control and Prevention
Atlanta, Georgia

Selim Suner, MD, MS, FACEP
Assistant Professor
Department of Emergency Medicine and Surgery
Brown Medical School
Director of Emergency Preparedness and Disaster
    Response
Department of Emergency Medicine
Chairman, Emergency Preparedness Committee
Rhode Island Hospital
Providence, Rhode Island

SECTION EDITORS

KATHRYN BRINSFIELD, MD, MPH, FACEP
Medical Director for Homeland Security
Boston Emergency Medical Services
Assistant Professor, Emergency Medicine and
Environmental Health
Boston University Schools of Medicine and Public
   Health
Boston, Massachusetts

JONATHAN L. BURSTEIN, MD, FACEP
Director, Section of Disaster Medicine
Division of Emergency Medicine
Department of Medicine
Harvard Medical School
Associate Director for Science
Harvard Center for Public Health Preparedness
Harvard School of Public Health
Boston, Massachusetts

JOHN D. CAHILL, MD, DTM
Assistant Professor
Attending Physician in Emergency Medicine and
   Infectious Diseases
St. Luke's/Roosevelt Hospital
New York, New York

EDWARD W. CETARUK, MD
Assistant Clinical Professor of Medicine
University of Colorado Health Sciences Center
Division of Toxicology and Clinical Pharmacology
Toxicology Associates, L.L.C.
Denver, Colorado

FRANCESCO DELLA CORTE, MD
Associate Professor
Chair of Anesthesiology and Intensive Care
Università del Piemonte Orientale
Novara, Italy

ERIC W. DICKSON, MD
Head, Department of Emergency Medicine
University of Iowa Carver College of Medicine
Iowa City, Iowa

ROBERT L. FREITAS, MHA
Program Director for Emergency Medicine
Harvard Medical Faculty Physicians
Boston, Massachusetts

DAVID G. JARRETT, MD, FACEP
Colonel, Medical Corps, Flight Surgeon, U.S. Army
Director, Armed Forces Radiobiology Research Institute
Bethesda, Maryland

MARK E. KEIM, MD
Medical Officer and Team Leader
International Emergency and Refugee Health Branch
National Center of Environmental Health
U.S. Centers for Disease Control and Prevention
Atlanta, Georgia
Clinical Associate Professor
Department of International Health and Development
Tulane University School of Public Health and Tropical
   Medicine
New Orleans, Louisiana
Honorary Faculty
Center for International, Emergency, Disaster and
   Refugee Studies
Johns Hopkins University School of Medicine
Baltimore, Maryland

KATHARYN E. KENNEDY, MD
Assistant Professor of Emergency Medicine
Department of Emergency Medicine
University of Massachusetts Medical School
Director of Emergency Medicine, Marlborough
   Hospital
Worcester, Massachusetts

JAMES M. MADSEN, MD, MPH
Colonel, Medical Corps, Flight Surgeon, U.S. Army
Scientific Advisor, Chemical Casualty Care Division
U.S. Army Medical Research Institute of Chemical
   Defense (USAMRICD)
APG-EA, Maryland
Associate Professor of Preventive Medicine and
   Biometrics, Uniformed Services University (USU)
Assistant Professor of Pathology, of Military and
Emergency Medicine, and of Emerging Infectious
   Diseases, USU
Bethesda, Maryland

KEN MILLER, MD, PHD
Medical Director
Orange County Fire Authority
Irvine, California
Assistant Medical Director
Orange County Healthcare Agency/Emergency Medical
    Services
Santa Ana, California
Medical Team Manager, DHS/FEMA Urban Search &
    Rescue CA Task Force-5
Team Leader, DHS/FEMA/NDMS Disaster Medical
    Assistance Team CA-1
Medical Officer
DHS/FEMA Incident Support Team/Joint Management
    Team
Washington, DC

JERRY L. MOTHERSHEAD, MD, FACEP
Assistant Professor
Uniformed Services University of the Health Sciences
Bethesda, Maryland
Physician Advisor, Medical Readiness and Response
    Group
Battelle Memorial Institute
Columbus, Ohio

ROBERT PARTRIDGE, MD, MPH
Associate Professor of Emergency Medicine
Director, Division of International Emergency
    Medicine
Department of Emergency Medicine
Rhode Island Hospital
Brown Medical School

LEON D. SANCHEZ, MD, MPH
Department of Emergency Medicine
Beth Israel Deaconess Medical Center
Boston, Massachusetts

CHARLES STEWART, MD, FACEP, FAAEM
Colorado Springs, Colorado

GARY M. VILKE, MD, FACEP, FAAEM
Associate Professor of Clinical Medicine
Department of Emergency Medicine
University of California, San Diego Medical Center
Medical Director, San Diego County Emergency Medical
    Services
San Diego, California

ERIC S. WEINSTEIN, MD, FACEP
Medical Director of Emergency Services
Colleton Medical Center
Walterboro South Carolina
Medical University of South Carolina
Charleston, South Carolina
Chair, ACEP Disaster Medicine Section
SC-1 DMAT Emergency Physician

RICHARD D. ZANE, MD
Vice Chair
Department of Emergency Medicine
Brigham and Women's Hospital
Harvard Medical School
Boston, Massachusetts

CONTRIBUTORS

GEORGE A. ALEXANDER, MD
Radiation Research Program
National Cancer Institute
National Institutes of Health
Bethesda, Maryland

ANGELA C. ANDERSON, MD, FAAP
Pediatric Emergency Medicine
Clinical Toxicology and Pharmacology
Hasbro Children's Hospital
Associate Professor of Pediatrics and Emergency
    Medicine
Brown University Medical School
Providence, Rhode Island

ANDREW W. ARTENSTEIN, MD, FACP
Director, Center for Biodefense and Emerging
    Pathogens
Division of Infectious Diseases
Memorial Hospital of Rhode Island
Pawtucket, Rhode Island

KAVITA BABU, MD
Fellow in Toxicology
Department of Emergency Medicine
University of Massachusetts Medical School
Worcester, Massachusetts

FERMIN BARRUETO, JR., MD
Assistant Professor of Surgery/Division of Emergency
    Medicine
University of Maryland Emergency Physicians
Baltimore, Maryland

CARRIE BARTON, MD
Disaster Medicine Research Fellow
Center for Disaster Preparedness
Birmingham, Alabama

BRUCE M. BECKER, MD, MPH
Attending Physician
Department of Emergency Medicine
Rhode Island Hospital/Hasbro Children's Hospital
Associate Professor
Department of Community Health
Brown School of Medicine
Providence, Rhode Island

MATTHEW BERKMAN, MD
Harvard Affiliated Emergency Medicine Residency
    Program
Beth Israel Deaconess Medical Center
Boston, Massachusetts

ANDREW I. BERN, MD, FACEP
Attending Emergency Physician
Delray Medical Center
Delray Beach, Florida
Hollywood Medical Center
Hollywood, Florida

MILANA BOUKHMAN, MD
Instructor of Medicine
Disaster Medicine Fellow
Harvard Medical School
Attending Physician
Emergency Medicine Department
Beth Israel Deaconess Hospital
Boston, Massachusetts

PETER BREWSTER
Education, Training, and Exercise Program Manager
EMSHG
VA Medical Center
Martinsburg, West Virginia

CHURTON BUDD, RN, EMTP
Systems Analyst III
Clinical Informatics
Medical College of Ohio
Toledo, Ohio

JAMES M. BURKE, MD
Staff Physician, Glendale Adventist Medical Center
Glendale, California
Lieutenant Commander, U.S. Naval Reserve
Fleet Hospital
Fort Dix, New Jersey

FREDERICK M. BURKLE, JR., MD, MPH, FAAP, FACEP
Senior Scholar
Scientist and Visiting Professor
The Center for International Emergency, Disaster &
    Refugee Studies (CIERDS)
Johns Hopkins University Medical Institutions
Baltimore, Maryland
Director
CIEDRS Asia-Pacific Branch
Kailu

LYNNE BARKLEY BURNETT, MD
Medical Advisor
Fresno County Sheriff's Department
Vice Chairman, Medical Ethics
Community Medical Centers
Adjunct Professor of Forensic Medicine and Forensic
    Pathology
National University
Adjunct Instructor
EMS Operations and Planning for WMD
Texas, A&M University
Fresno, California

NICHOLAS VINCENT CAGLIUSO, SR., PhD(C), MPH
Emergency Preparedness Analyst
Office of Emergency Management
The Port Authority of New York and New Jersey
Jersey City, New Jersey

JOHN D. CAHILL, MD, DTM
Assistant Professor
Attending Physician in Emergency Medicine and
Infectious Diseases
St. Luke's/Roosevelt Hospital
New York, New York

DUANE C. CANEVA, MD, FACEP
Commander, U.S. Navy
Adjunct Assistant Professor Department
    Military/Emergency Medicine Uniformed Services
    University of the Health Sciences (USUHS)
Bethesda, Maryland

JULIE ANN P. CASANI, MD, MPH
Director
Office of Public Health Preparedness and Response
Maryland Department of Health and Mental Hygiene
Baltimore, Maryland

MARY W. CHAFFEE, SCD(H), MS, RN, CNAA, FAAN
PhD Student, Graduate School of Nursing
Uniformed Services University of the Health
    Sciences
Bethesda, Maryland
Formerly, Director
Navy Medicine Office of Homeland Security
Bureau of Medicine and Surgery
Washington, DC

HENRY C. CHANG, MD
Department of Emergency Medicine
North Shore University Hospital
Manhasset, New York

JAMES C. CHANG, CIH, BS, MS
Emergency Management Coordinator
Duke University Hospital
Durham, North Carolina

ANNA I. CHEH, MD
Harvard Affiliated Emergency Medicine Residency
Beth Israel Deaconess Medical Center
Boston, Massachusetts

ESTHER H. CHEN, MD
Department of Emergency Medicine
University of Pennsylvania Medical Center
Philadelphia, Pennsylvania

TERIGGI J. CICCONE, MD
Chief Resident
Harvard Affiliated Emergency Medicine Residency
    Program
Beth Israel Deaconess Medical Center
Boston, Massachusetts

MARIANNE E. CINAT, MD
UCI Regional Burn Center
University of California Irvine Medical Center
Orange, California

GREGORY R. CIOTTONE, MD, FACEP
Director, International Emergency Medicine Section
Harvard Medical School
Director, Division of Disaster Medicine
Beth Israel Deaconess Medical Center
Boston, Massachusetts

ROBERT A. CIOTTONE, PhD
Clinical Psychologist (ABPP)
Professor of Psychology (Afil.), Clark University
Associate in Psychiatry and Pediatrics
University of Massachusetts Medical School
Worcester, Massachusetts

STEVEN T. COBERY, MD, MC, USNR
Neurosurgery Resident
Brown University Medical School
Rhode Island Hospital
Providence, Rhode Island

JOANNE CONO, MD, SCM
Deputy Associate Director for Science
Coordinating Office for Terrorism Preparedness and
    Emergency Response
Centers for Disease Control and Prevention
Atlanta, Georgia

KELLY J. CORRIGAN, MD, MA
Instructor of Medicine, Harvard Medical School
Attending Physician
Beth Israel Deaconess Medical Center
Boston, Massachusetts

FRANCESCO DELLA CORTE, MD
Associate Professor
Chair of Anesthesiology and Intensive Care
Università del Piemonte Orientale
Novara, Italy

CHRISTO C. COURBAN, MD
Brigham and Women's Hospital
Cambridge Hospital
Harvard Medical School
Boston, Massachusetts

HILARIE CRANMER, MD, MPH
Department of Emergency Medicine
Brigham and Women's Hospital
Boston, Massachusetts

STEPHEN O. CUNNION, MD, MPH, PhD
Department of Emergency Medicine
PENN Travel Medicine
Hospital of the University of Pennsylvania
Philadelphia, Pennsylvania

ROBERT G. DARLING, MD, FACEP
Captain, Medical Corps
Flight Surgeon, U.S. Navy
Senior Medical Advisor
Navy Medicine Office of Homeland Security
Specialty Advisor to the Chief of the Medical Corps for
    Homeland Security
Washington, DC

DAVID DAVIS, MD
Duke University Medical Center
Emergency Medicine
Durham, North Carolina

TIMOTHY DAVIS, MD, MPH
Associate Professor
Emory University School of Medicine
Atlanta, Georgia

JENNIFER E. DELAPENA, MD
Beth Israel Deaconess Medical Center
Boston, Massachusetts

CHAYAN DEY, MD, FACEP
Center for International Emergency, Disaster and
    Refugee Studies
Department of Emergency Medicine
The Johns Hopkins University School of Medicine
Baltimore, Maryland

WILLIAM E. DICKERSON, MD
Colonel, U.S. Air Force, Medical Corps
Head, Military Medicine Department
Armed Forces Radiobiology Research Institute
Bethesda, Maryland

ERIC W. DICKSON, MD, FAAEM
Head, Department of Emergency Medicine
University of Iowa Carver College of Medicine
Iowa City, Iowa

SHARON DILLING
Consultant, University of Medicine and Dentistry of
    New Jersey
Center for BioDefense
Director of Communications
New Jersey Credit Union League
Hightstown, New Jersey

K. SOPHIA DYER, MD
Assistant Professor
Department of Emergency Medicine
Boston University School of Medicine
Attending Physician
Department of Emergency Medicine
Boston Medical Center
Boston, Massachusetts

JASON DYLIK, MD, EMT
Emergency Division, Department of Surgery
Duke University Hospital
Durham, North Carolina

JONATHAN A. EDLOW, MD, FACEP
Vice-Chairman, Department of Emergency Medicine
Beth Israel Deaconess Medical Center
Associate Professor of Medicine, Harvard Medical School
Boston, Massachusetts

MARSHALL EIDENBERG, DO
Chief, Initial Entry Training Division
DCMT Medical Director
Department of Combat Medic Training

KHAMA D. ENNIS-HOLCOMB, MD, MPH
Senior Resident, Department of Emergency Medicine
Brigham & Women's and Massachusetts General Hospital
Boston, Massachusetts

DENIS J. FITZGERALD, MD
Chief Medical Officer
Counter-Narcotics and Terrorism Operational Medical
    Support (CONTOMS) Program
Casualty Care Research Center
Uniformed Services University of the Health Sciences
U.S. Department of Defense
Washington, DC

KERRY FOSHER, BS, BA, MA
New England Center for Emergency Preparedness
Dartmouth Medical School
Lebanon, New Hampshire
Research and Practice Associate
Institute for National Security and Counter-Terrorism
Maxwell School of Citizenship and Public Affairs and
    College of Law
Syracuse University
Syracuse, New York

ROBERT L. FREITAS, MHA
Program Director of Emergency Medicine
Harvard Medical Faculty Physicians
Boston, Massachusetts

RYAN FRIEDBERG, MD
Harvard Affiliated Emergency Medicine Residency
    Program
Beth Israel Deaconess Medical Center
Boston, Massachusetts

FRANKLIN D. FRIEDMAN, MD, MS
Assistant Professor of Emergency Medicine
Tufts University School of Medicine
Director of Emergency Clinical Operations
Tufts-New England Medical Center
Department of Emergency Medicine
Boston, Massachusetts

FREDERICK FUNG, MD, MS
Clinical Professor
Department of Medicine, Division of Occupational
    Medicine
University of California, Irvine
Irvine, California
Medical Director, Occupational Medicine
Sharp Rees-Stealy Medical Centers
Medical Director, Employee Health
Sharp Health Care
San Diego, California

ROBERT D. FURBERG, BS, NREMTP
Paramedic, EMS Education
Parkwood Fire Rescue
Research Triangle Park, North Carolina
Adjunct Instructor, Emergency Health Sciences
Department of Emergency Medicine
The George Washington University
Washington, DC

WADE GAASCH, MD, FAAEM
Assistant Professor
Division of Emergency Medicine
University of Maryland School of Medicine
Director of Pre-Hospital Care
Emergency Medicine
University of Maryland Medical Center
Chief Physician and Medical Director
Baltimore City Fire Department
Baltimore, Maryland

FIONA E. GALLAHUE, MD
Associate Residency Director
Department of Emergency Medicine
New York Methodist Hospital
Brooklyn, New York

LUCILLE GANS, MD
Edmonton, Alberta, Canada

ALESSANDRO GEDDO, MD
Resident in Anaestesiology and ICU
University of Eastern Piedmont
Maggiore della Carità Hospital
Novara, Italy

JAMES GEILING, MD, FACP
Associate Professor of Medicine
Dartmouth Medical School
Assistant Director, New England Center for Emergency
    Preparedness
Dartmouth-Hitchcock Medical Center
Hanover, New Hampshire
Chief, Medical Service
Veterans Affairs Medical Center
White River Junction, Vermont

PAUL GIANNONE, MPHORISE FELLOW
Disaster Planner International Emergency and Refugee
    Health Branch
National Center of Environmental Health
U.S. Centers for Disease Control and Prevention
Atlanta, Georgia

WILLIAM GLUCKMAN, DO, EMT-P, FACEP
Assistant Professor of Surgery New Jersey Medical
    School
Attending Emergency Physician UMDNJ-University
    Hospital, Medical Director, University EMS
Newark, New Jersey

SUSAN E. GORMAN, PHARMD
Associate Director for Science
Strategic National Stockpile Program
Centers for Disease Control and Prevention
Atlanta, Georgia

J. SCOTT GOUDIE, MD
Harvard Affiliated Emergency Medicine Residency
    Program
Beth Israel Deaconess Medical Center
Boston, Massachusetts

ROBERT M. GOUGELET, MD
Assistant Professor Medicine (Emergency Medicine)
Dartmouth Medical School
Medical Director Emergency Response
Dartmouth Hitchcock Medical Center
Lebanon, New Hampshire

MARK A. GRABER, MD
Associate Professor of Emergency Medicine and Family
    Medicine
University of Iowa Carver College of Medicine
Iowa City, Iowa

JILL A. GRANT, MDCPT
San Antonio Uniformed Services Health Education
    Consortium
Emergency Medicine Residency Program
Brooke Army Medical Center
Fort Sam Houston, Texas

MICHAEL I. GREENBERG, MD, MPH
Clinical Professor of Emergency Medicine
Temple University School of Medicine
Professor of Emergency Medicine
Professor of Public Health
Drexel University College of Medicine
Philadelphia, Pennsylvania

P. GREGG GREENOUGH, MD, MPH
Assistant Professor and Co-Director
The Center for International Emergency, Disaster and
    Refugee Studies, Schools of Medicine and Public Health
Johns Hopkins University Medical Institutions
Baltimore, Maryland

SHAMAI A. GROSSMAN, MD, MS, FACEP
Director, The Clinical Decision Unit and Cardiac
    Emergency Center
Department of Emergency Medicine
Beth Israel Deaconess Medical Center
Instructor of Medicine
Harvard Medical School
Boston, Massachusetts

TEE L. GUIDOTTI, MD, MPH
Professor
Chair, Dept. of Environmental and Occupational Health
Director, Division of Occupational Medicine and
    Toxicology (Department of Medicine)
The George Washington University Medical Center
Washington, DC

DEBORAH GUTMAN, MD, MPH
Clinical Assistant Professor
Department of Emergency Medicine
Brown Medical School
Attending Physician
Department of Emergency Medicine
Rhode Island Hospital
Providence, Rhode Island

PINCHAS HALPERN, MD
Director, Emergency Department
Tel Aviv Sourasky Medical Center and the Sackler
    Faculty of Medicine
Tel Aviv University
Tel Aviv, Israel

DAN HANFLING, MD, FACEP
Director, Emergency Management and Disaster
    Medicine
Inova Health System
Falls Church, Virginia
Assistant Clinical Professor of Emergency Medicine
George Washington University
Washington, DC

RACHEL HAROZ, MD
Instructor in Emergency Medicine
Department of Emergency Medicine
Drexel University School of Medicine
Philadelphia, Pennsylvania

BONNIE H. HARTSTEIN, MD
Associate Professor of Pediatrics
Uniformed Services University of Health Sciences
Bethesda, Maryland
Department of Emergency Medicine
Brooke Army Medical Center
Fort Sam Houston, Texas

JOHN L. HICK, MD, FACEP
Assistant Professor of Emergency Medicine
University of Minnesota
Faculty Physician
Hennepin County Medical Center
Minneapolis, Minnesota

STEPHEN F. HOOD, MA
Public Administration/Public Policy Coordinator
The George Washington University
Response to Emergencies and Disasters Institute
Ashburn, Virginia

MICHAEL HOROWITZ, MD
Resident in Emergency Medicine
Department of Emergency Medicine
Drexel University School of Medicine
Philadelphia, Pennsylvania

KURT R. HORST, MD
University of Massachusetts School of Medicine
UMass Memorial Medical Center
Department of Emergency Medicine
Worcester, Massachusetts

HANS R. HOUSE, MD, DTMH
Residency Director
The Iowa Emergency Medicine Residency
Assistant Professor of Emergency Medicine
University of Iowa Carver College of Medicine
Iowa City, Iowa

CURTIS J. HUNTER, MD
Assistant Professor
Military and Emergency Medicine
Uniformed Services University of the Health Sciences
Bethesda, Maryland
Chief, Department of Emergency Medicine
Brooke Army Medical Center
Fort Sam Houston, Texas
Attending Faculty
San Antonio Uniformed Services Health Education
    Consortium Emergency Medicine Residency
San Antonio, Texas

JASON IMPERATO, MD, MBA
Attending Physician
Beth Israel Deaconess Medical Center
Boston, Massachusetts

PIER LUIGI INGRASSIA, MD
Resident in Anaestesiology and ICU
University of Eastern Piedmont
Maggiore della Carità Hospital
Novara, Italy

IRVING JACOBY, MD
Professor of Medicine and Surgery
University of California, San Diego, School of Medicine
La Jolla, California
Attending Physician, Department of Emergency Medicine
Hospital Medical Director for Emergency Preparedness
    and Response
University of California
San Diego, California

THEA JAMES, MD
Clinical Instructor/Attending Physician
Boston University School of Medicine
Boston Medical Center
Boston, Massachusetts

DAVID JASLOW, MD, MPH, EMT-P, FAAEM
Chief, Division of EMS, Operational Public Health and
    Disaster Medicine
Co-Director, Center for Special Operations
Department of Emergency Medicine
Albert Einstein Medical Center
Philadelphia, Pennsylvania

GREGORY D. JAY, MD
Associate Professor of Medicine
Division of Engineering
Brown Medical School
Research Director, Associate Professor of Medicine and
    Emergency Medicine
Department of Emergency Medicine
Rhode Island Hospital
Providence, Rhode Island

MIRIAM JOHN, MD
Resident, Newark Beth Israel Medical Center
Newark, New Jersey

MICHAEL D. JONES, MD
Brooke Army Medical Center
SAUSHEC EM Residency Program
Fort Sam Houston, Texas

JEFFRY L. KASHUK, MD, FACS
Associate Clinical Professor of Surgery
Hahnemann University Hospital
Philadelphia, Pennsylvania

MARK E. KEIM, MD
Medical Officer and Team Leader
International Emergency and Refugee Health Branch
National Center of Environmental Health
U.S. Centers for Disease Control and Prevention
Atlanta, Georgia
Clinical Associate Professor
Department of International Health and Development
Tulane University School of Public Health and Tropical
    Medicine
New Orleans, Louisiana
Honorary Faculty
Center for International, Emergency, Disaster and
    Refugee Studies
Johns Hopkins University School of Medicine
Baltimore, Maryland

KATHARYN E. KENNEDY, MD
Assistant Professor of Emergency Medicine
Department of Emergency Medicine
University of Massachusetts Medical School
Director of Emergency Medicine, Marlborough Hospital
Worcester, Massachusetts

PAUL D. KIM, MD
Associate Director, Operations
The George Washington University
Response to Emergencies and Disasters Institute
Ashburn, Virginia

SYLVIA H. KIM, MD
Harvard Affiliated Emergency Medicine Residency
Beth Israel Deaconess Medical Center
Boston, Massachusetts

LEO KOBAYASHI, MD
University Emergency Medicine Foundation
Department of Emergency Medicine
Brown University
Providence, Rhode Island

LARA K. KULCHYCKI, MD
Harvard Affiliated Emergency Medicine Residency
    Program
Beth Israel Deaconess Medical Center
Boston, Massachusetts

RICK G. KULKARNI, MD
Assistant Professor of Medicine
David Geffen School of Medicine at UCLA
Attending Physician, Director of Informatics
Department of Emergency Medicine
Olive View – UCLA Medical Center
Los Angeles, California

CHRISTOPHER R. LANG, MD
Department of Emergency Medicine
George Washington University
Washington, DC

GREGORY L. LARKIN, MD, MS, MSPH, FACEP
Professor, Department of Surgery
Division of Emergency Medicine
University of Texas
Southwestern Medical Center
Dallas, Texas

THOMAS P. LEBOSQUET III, MD
Resident in Emergency Medicine
Duke University Medical Center
Durham, North Carolina

BRUCE Y. LEE, MD, MBA
Assistant Professor of Medicine
Section of Decision Sciences and Clinical Systems
   Modeling
University of Pittsburgh
Pittsburgh, Pennsylvania

CATHERINE Y. LEE, MPH
Faculty Associate, New York Medical College
Valhalla, New York

DAVID C. LEE, MD
Director of Research
Department of Emergency Medicine
North Shore University Hospital
Manhasset, New York
Clinical Assistant Professor
Department of Emergency Medicine
New York University
New York, New York

JAY LEMERY, MD
Attending Physician, Emergency Medicine
Weill Cornell Medical College
Attending Physician, Emergency Medicine
New York-Presbyterian Hospital
New York, New York

DANIEL L. LEMKIN, MD
Deputy Medical Director, Baltimore City Fire
   Department
EMS Fellow
University of Maryland Baltimore County
Clinical Instructor
Division of Emergency Medicine
University of Maryland School of Medicine
Baltimore, Maryland

JEANETTE A. LINDER, MD
Assistant Professor
Radiation Oncology
University of Maryland Medical Center
Baltimore, Maryland

LAWRENCE S. LINDER, MD, FACEP, FAEM
Director, Emergency Department
Senior Vice President/Chief Medical Officer
Baltimore Washington Medical Center
Glen Burnie, Maryland

SHAN W. LIU, MD
Instructor, Surgery
Harvard Medical School
Faculty, Emergency Medicine
Massachusetts General Hospital
Boston, Massachusetts

CRAIG H. LLEWELLYN, MD
Professor of Medicine and Surgery
Director, Center for Disaster and Humanitarian
Assistance Medicine
Uniformed Services University for the Health Sciences
Bethesda, Maryland

FRANCESCA LOMBARDI, MD
Resident in Anaestesiology and ICU
University of Eastern Piedmont
Maggiore della Carità Hospital
Novara, Italy

HEATHER LONG, MD
Attending Physician
Department of Emergency Medicine
North Shore University Hospital
Manhasset, New York

EDWARD B. LUCCI, MD, FACEPLTC
Chief, Emergency and Operational Medicine
Walter Reed Army Medical Center
Washington, DC

DONALD MACMILLAN, MA, PA, EMT-P
Yale University School of Medicine
Division of EMS
New Haven, Connecticut

LAURA MACNOW, MD
Instructor, Emergency Medicine
Harvard Medical School
Attending Physician
Emergency Department
Beth Israel Deaconess Medical Center
Boston, Massachusetts

JAMES M. MADSEN, MD, MPH
Colonel, Medical Corps, Flight Surgeon, U.S. Army
Scientific Advisor, Chemical Casualty Care Division
U.S. Army Medical Research Institute of Chemical
    Defense (USAMRICD)
APG-EA, Maryland
Associate Professor of Preventive Medicine and
    Biometrics, Uniformed Services University (USU)
Assistant Professor of Pathology, of Military and
    Emergency Medicine, and of Emerging Infectious
    Diseases, USU
Bethesda Maryland

BRIAN J. MAGUIRE, DR.PH, MSA, EMT-P
Associate Director
Department of Emergency Health Services
University of Maryland, Baltimore County
Baltimore, Maryland

JOHN D. MALONE, MD, FACP, FIDSA
Professor of Medicine
Uniformed Services University of the Health Sciences
F. Edward Hebert School of Medicine
Department of Preventive Medicine and Biometrics
Bethesda, Maryland

PAUL M. MANISCALCO, MPA, EMT/P
Deputy Executive Director
Former President, National Association of Emergency
    Medical Technicians
The George Washington University
Response to Emergencies and Disasters Institute
Ashburn, Virginia

DAVID MARCOZZI, MD
Emergency Division, Department of Surgery
Duke University Medical Center
Durham, North Carolina

PIETRO D. MARGHELLA, CFAAMA, FACCP
Commander, Medical Service Corps, U.S. Navy
Adjunct Assistant Professor
Uniformed Services University of the Health Sciences
Washington, DC

JAMES F. MARTIN, MDCPT
San Antonio Uniformed Services Health Education
    Consortium
Emergency Medicine Residency Program
Brooke Army Medical Center
Fort Sam Houston, Texas

JAMES MCKINNELL, MD
Resident Physician, Department of Medicine
Los Angeles County Harbor-UCLA Medical Center
Torrance, California

MICHELLE MCMAHON-DOWNER, MD
Department of Emergency Medicine
Rhode Island Hospital
Brown University School of Medicine
Providence, Rhode Island

C. CRAWFORD MECHEM, MD, FACEP
Associate Professor
Department of Emergency Medicine
University of Pennsylvania Medical Center
EMS Medical Director
City of Philadelphia Fire Department
Philadelphia, Pennsylvania

SUMERU MEHTA, MD, MPH
Staff Physician and Director of Emergency Ultrasound
Department of Emergency Medicine
Brooke Army Medical Center
San Antonio Uniformed Services Health Education
    Consortium
San Antonia, Texas

PATRICIA L. MEINHARDT, MD, MPH, MA
Executive Medical Director
Center for Occupational and Environmental Medicine
Arnot Ogden Medical Center
Elmira, New York

LAURA DIANE MELVILLE, MD
New York Methodist Hospital
Brooklyn, New York

JEFFERY C. METZGER, MD
Emergency Medicine Resident
Duke University Medical Center
Durham Police Department Selective Enforcement Team
Durham, North Carolina

ANGELA M. MILLS, MD
Assistant Professor
Department of Emergency Medicine
University of Pennsylvania Medical Center
Philadelphia, Pennsylvania

ANDREW M. MILSTEN, MD, MS, FACEP
Clinical Assistant Professor
Division of Emergency Medicine
University of Maryland
College Park, Maryland
Assistant Medical Director
Anne Arundel County Fire Department
Medical Director
Expresscare Critical Care Transport and Mass
    Gathering Events
Newsletter Editor, Disaster Medical Section, ACEP

CLIFFORD S. MITCHELL, MS, MD, MPH
Associate Professor of Environmental Health Sciences
Johns Hopkins Bloomberg School of Public Health
Baltimore, Maryland

ELIZABETH L. MITCHELL, MD
Assistant Professor of Emergency Medicine
Boston University School of Medicine
Department of Emergency Medicine
Boston, Massachusetts

DALE M. MOLÉ, DO, FACEP
Captain, Medical Corps, U.S. Navy
Executive Officer, U.S. Naval Hospital
Okinawa, Japan
Assistant Professor of Military and Emergency Medicine
Uniformed Services University of Health Sciences
Bethesda, Maryland

LOUIS N. MOLINO, SR., CET, FF/NREMT-B/FSI/EMSI
WMD EMS Instructor, WMD EMS Program
The Texas A&M University System
Texas Engineering Extension Service
Emergency Services Training Institute
National Emergency Response and Rescue Training Center
College Station, Texas

JOHN MOLONEY, MBBS FANZCA MAIES
Area Medical Coordinator, Medical Displan Victoria
Head, Trauma Anaesthesia
The Alfred
Australia

SEAN MONTGOMERY, MD
Harvard Affiliated Emergency Medicine Residency
Beth Israel Deaconess Medical Center
Boston, Massachusetts

JERRY L. MOTHERSHEAD, MD, FACEP
Assistant Professor
Uniformed Services of the Health Sciences
Bethesda, Maryland
Physician Advisor, Medical Readiness and Response
  Group
Battelle Memorial Institute
Columbus, Ohio

LEWIS S. NELSON, MD
Assistant Professor
Department of Emergency Medicine
New York University School of Medicine
New York, New York
Fellowship Director, Medical Toxicology
New York City Poison Control Center
New York, New York

CONSTANCE G. NICHOLS, MD
Assistant Professor of Emergency Medicine
Department of Emergency Medicine
University of Massachusetts Medical School
Worcester, Massachusetts

PATRICIA A. NOLAN, MD, MPH
Director of Health
Rhode Island Department of Health
Clinical Assistant Professor of Community Health
Brown University
Providence, Rhode Island

DANIEL F. NOLTKAMPER, MD, FACEP
Commander, Medical Corps, U.S. Navy
Emergency Physician, Naval Hospital Camp
  Lejeune
Jacksonville, North Carolina

DZIWE W. NTABA, MD, MPH
Resident in Emergency Medicine
Department of Emergency Medicine
Drexel University School of Medicine
Philadelphia, Pennsylvania

ANDREW S. NUGENT, MD
Vice Chairman, Department of Emergency Medicine
University of Iowa Carver College of Medicine
Iowa City, Iowa

NEILL S. OSTER, MD
Assistant Professor
Emergency Medicine and Attending Physician
Emergency Department, New York Methodist Hospital
New York, New York
Disaster Medicine Consultant to the U.S. Navy
  Medicine Office of Homeland Security
Medical Advisor to the U.S. Department of State's
  Anti-Terrorism Assistance Program

PETER D. PANAGOS, MD
Assistant Professor of Emergency Medicine
Brown Medical School
Attending Physician, Rhode Island Hospital
Providence, Rhode Island

ROBERT PARTRIDGE, MD, MPH, DTM, FACEP
Assistant Professor of Emergency Medicine
Director, Division of International Emergency
  Medicine
Department of Emergency Medicine
Brown Medical School
Rhode Island Hospital
Providence, Rhode Island

NICKI PESIK, MD
Assistant Professor
Department of Emergency Medicine
Emory University and Senior Medical Consultant
Strategic National Stockpile Program
Centers for Disease Control and Prevention
Atlanta, Georgia

JAMES PFAFF, MD, FACEP, FAAEM
Staff Physician, Brooke Army Medical Center
SAUSHEC EM Residency Program
Fort Sam Houston, Texas

WILLIAM PORCARO, MD
Harvard Affiliated Emergency Medicine Residency
  Program
Beth Israel Deaconess Medical Center
Boston, Massachusetts

LAWRENCE PROANO, MD, FACEP
Attending Physician
Brown University Program in Emergency Medicine
Rhode Island Hospital
Providence, Rhode Island

NAJMA RAHMAN-KAHN, MD
Attending, Lutheran Hospital
Brooklyn, New York

VITTORIO J. RAHO, MD
Resident, Harvard Affiliated Emergency Medicine
  Residency Program
Beth Israel Deaconess Medical Center
Boston, Massachusetts

PRASANTHI RAMANUJAM, MBBS
Department of Emergency Medicine
Boston Medical Center
Boston University School of Medicine
Boston, Massachusetts

WENDE R. REENSTRA, MD, PHD
Department of Emergency Medicine
Beth Israel Deaconess Medical Center
Boston, Massachusetts

ANDREW REISNER, MD
Instructor, Harvard Medical School
Massachusetts General Hospital
Emergency Medicine
Boston, Massachusetts

MARK C. RESTUCCIA, MD, FACEP, FAAEM
Assistant Professor of Emergency Medicine
University of Massachusetts Medical School
UMass Memorial Health Care
Worcester, Massachusetts

JAMES MICHAEL RILEY, REMT-P
Senior Security Analyst
Office of Security and Investigations
US Citizenship and Immigration Services
Washington, DC

ALBERT J. ROMANOSKY, MD, PhD
Medical Director
Office of Public Health Preparedness and Response
Maryland Department of Health and Mental Hygiene
Baltimore, Maryland

PETER ROSEN, MD
Senior Lecturer, Department of Medicine
Harvard University School of Medicine,
Attending Physician
Department of Emergency Medicine
Beth Israel/Deaconess Medical Center
Boston, Massachusetts

MARC S. ROSENTHAL, PHD, DO
Assistant Professor of Emergency Medicine
Attending Physician
Research Director/Assistant Residency Director
Wayne State University
Sinai-Grace Hospital Emergency Medicine Residency
  Program
Department of Emergency Medicine Sinai-Grace
  Hospital
Detroit, Michigan

JONATHAN M. RUBIN, MD
Associate Professor of Emergency Medicine
Medical College of Wisconsin
Associate Director of Medical Services
Milwaukee County EMS
Milwaukee, Wisconsin

LEON D. SANCHEZ, MD, MPH
Attending, Emergency Medicine
Clinical Instructor
Emergency Medicine
Harvard Medical School
Beth Israel Deaconess Medical Center
Boston, Massachusetts

DEBRA D. SCHNELLE, MS
Project Staff Associate/Assistant Program Manager
The Research Foundation
The State University of New York
Buffalo, New York

JEREMIAH D. SCHUUR, MD
Chief Resident
Brown University Emergency Medicine
  Residency
Providence, Rhode Island

ERIC M. SERGIENKO, MD
Lieutenant Commander
Bureau of Medicine and Surgery
U.S. Navy
Shoreline, Washington

KINJAL SETHURAMAN, MD, MPH
Albert Einstein University
Emergency Department
Long Island Jewish Medical Center
International Emergency Medicine Fellow
New York

MARC J. SHAPIRO, MD
University Emergency Medicine Foundation
Department of Emergency Medicine
Brown University
Providence, Rhode Island

SAM SHEN, MD, MBA
Attending Physician
St. Luke's Hospital
Southcoast Health System
New Bedford, Massachusetts

SUZANNE M. SHEPHERD, MD, FACEP, DTM&H
Associate Professor
Director, Education and Research
PENN Travel Medicine
Hospital of the University of Pennsylvania
Philadelphia, Pennsylvania

WILLIAM H. SHOFF, MD, DTM&H
Department of Emergency Medicine
PENN Travel Medicine
Hospital of the University of Pennsylvania
Philadelphia, Pennsylvania

SEAN MICHAEL SILER, DO
Captain, U.S. Army, Medical Corps
Senior Resident, San Antonio Uniformed Services
Health Sciences Consortium Emergency Medicine
    Residency
Brooke Army Medical Center
Department of Emergency Medicine
Fort Sam Houston, Texas

ALISON SISITSKY, MD
Harvard Affiliated Emergency Medicine Residency
    Program
Beth Israel Deaconess Medical Center
Boston, Massachusetts

CRAIG SISSON, MD
Rhode Island Hospital
Brown University Emergency Medicine Program
Providence, Rhode Island

PETER B. SMULOWITZ, MD
Harvard Affiliated Emergency Medicine Residency
Beth Israel Deaconess Medical Center
Boston, Massachusetts

JOHN H. SORENSON, PhD
Distinguished Research and Development Staff
Oak Ridge National Laboratory
Oak Ridge, Tennessee

CHARLES STEWART, MD, FACEP, FAAEM
Colorado Springs, Colorado

M. KATHLEEN STEWART, MS
Colorado Springs, Colorado

KENT J. STOCK, DO, MBA, FACP, FAAP
Lowcountry Infectious Diseases, P.A.
Charleston, South Carolina

CAROL SULIS, MD
Associate Professor of Medicine
Boston University School of Medicine
Hospital Epidemiologist
Boston Medical Center
Boston, Massachusetts

NICHOLAS SUTINGCO, MD
Department of Emergency Medicine
Brigham and Women's Hospital
Harvard Medical School
Boston, Massachusetts

NELSON TANG, MD, FACEP
Director, Division of Special Operations
Department of Emergency Medicine
The Johns Hopkins University School of Medicine
Baltimore, Maryland

ELIZABETH TEMIN, MD
Instructor, Emergency Medicine
Boston University School of Medicine
Physician, Emergency Medicine
Boston Medical Center
Boston, Massachusetts

RICHARD A. TEMPEL, MD
Division of Emergency Medicine
Duke University Medical Center
Durham, North Carolina

CRAIG D. THORNE, MD, MPH, FACP, FACOEM
Assistant Professor of Medicine
University of Maryland
Medical Director, Safety and Employee Health
University of Maryland Medical Center
Baltimore, Maryland

JASON A. TRACY, MD
Assistant Residency Director
Beth Israel Deaconess Medical Center
Harvard Affiliated Emergency Medicine Residency
Harvard Medical School
Boston, Massachusetts

STEPHEN J. TRAUB, MD
Co-Director, Division of Toxicology
Department of Emergency Medicine
Beth Israel Deaconess Medical Center
Instructor in Medicine
Harvard Medical School
Boston, Massachusetts

JONATHAN HARRIS VALENTE, MD
Assistant Professor, Brown Medical School
Department of Emergency Medicine
Rhode Island Hospital and Hasbro Children's Hospital
Providence, Rhode Island

VICTORIA M. VANDERKAM, RN, MBA
UCI Regional Burn Center
University of California
Irvine Medical Center
Orange, California

CAROL L. VENABLE, MD
Department of Emergency Medicine
Boston Medical Center
Boston, Massachusetts

FAITH VILAS, PhD, LP
Planetary Astronomy Group
NASA Johnson Space Center
Dallas, Texas

GARY M. VILKE, MD, FACEP, FAAEM
Associate Professor of Clinical Medicine
Department of Emergency Medicine
University of California, San Diego Medical Center
Medical Director, San Diego County Emergency Medical
    Services
San Diego, California

BARBARA VOGT SORENSON, PhD
Senior Research Staff
Oak Ridge National Laboratory
Oak Ridge, Tennessee

SCOTT G. WEINER, MD, MPH
Assistant Professor of Emergency Medicine
Tufts University School of Medicine
Attending Physician
Tufts New England Medical Center
Boston, Massachusetts

ERIC S. WEINSTEIN, MD, FACEP
Medical Director of Emergency Services
Colleton Medical Center
Walterboro, South Carolina
Medical University of South Carolina
Charleston, South Carolina
Chair, ACEP Disaster Medicine Section
SC-1 DMAT Emergency Physician

ROY KARL WERNER, MD, MS
Assistant Professor of Emergency Medicine
University of Iowa Carver College of Medicine
Iowa City, Iowa

SAGE W. WIENER, MD
Assistant Professor
Department of Emergency Medicine
SUNY Downstate Medical Center
Assistant Director of Medical Toxicology
Department of Emergency Medicine
Kings County Hospital/SUNY Downstate Medical
    Center
Brooklyn, New York

ABIGAIL WILLIAMS, RN, JD, MPH
Abigail Williams & Associates, PC
Worcester, Massachusetts

KENNETH A. WILLIAMS, MD
University Emergency Medicine Foundation
Department of Emergency Medicine
Brown University
Providence, Rhode Island

TRACY E. WIMBUSH, MD
Massachusetts General Hospital
Harvard Medical School
Boston, Massachusetts

ROBERT H. WOOLARD, MD
Interim Chairman of the Department of Emergency
    Medicine
Brown Medical School
Rhode Island Hospital
Providence, Rhode Island

KEVIN YESKEY, MD, FACEP
Deputy Director and Associate Professor
Center for Disaster and Humanitarian Assistance
    Medicine
Uniformed Services University of the Health Sciences
Bethesda, Maryland

SANDRA S. YOON, MD
Harvard Affiliated Emergency Medicine Residency
    Program
Beth Israel Deaconess Medical Center
Boston, Massachusetts

PATRICK ZELLEY, MD, MS
Department of Emergency Medicine
Rhode Island Hospital
Brown University School of Medicine
Providence, Rhode Island

FOREWORD

Throughout recorded history, disasters have caused immeasurable amounts of pain and suffering to affected populations. By far, the most common disasters have been natural ones with cataclysmic storms and seismic and volcanic events reeking havoc on the unsuspecting. Recently, however, the news of disaster has also included pre-meditated attacks by the various terror factions around the world. Prior to Sept. 11, 2001, it is not unreasonable to presume that most of us in the United States didn't think long nor hard about terror attacks. We of course were aware of the bad things that were occurring around the world, shook our heads with bafflement at the Sarin attacks in Tokyo, and managed to underestimate and ignore the bombings and terror attacks in our own country, since so few of us were involved. It always seems like an act far out on the bell-shaped curve of sanity.

We couldn't figure out how James Jones could convince a group of people to submit to suicide and murder; we were appalled at the cyanide attacks in the grocery stores; and we came closer to understanding a potential for terror after the bombing in Oklahoma City.

There were of course small numbers of people who were well aware of the potential; tried to prepare themselves and their country, and did attempt to increase education, preparation and awareness for that special kind of disaster.

Although I was personally almost totally ignorant about bioterror, I was asked to chair a committee on Bioterror for the Institute of Medicine. I still don't know why I was invited, but it was a challenging and highly educational experience. I learned at the very least to think about terror in terms of possible responses and needs for education as opposed to putting it aside as a very improbable event that I would never encounter as a citizen, never mind as a physician.[1] What became increasingly obvious after Sept. 11 was the inability to predict the consequences of the attack, and a need to be able to respond with great flexibility and creativity.

In this regard, acts of terrorism, other than the psychological wounding fact that it is deliberate, manmade, and therefore quite unnecessary, is no different than a large unplanned disaster.

We have seen many such incidents around the world and learned a certain amount at how to prepare and how to respond, but we are always struck by the fact that we can't exactly know when or where the next "tragedy" will occur, or just how much damage it will inflict.

Many of the ingredients for both accidental and terrorist events are present in our daily lives, and it doesn't

require much to unleash them. Fortune sometimes plays in our favor, as the time when I was at the University of Chicago. We received a phone call that there had been some kind of industrial accident on the South Side of the city, and that a large cloud of chlorine gas had been released. We had no idea how many victims there would be, or where the victims would be, and we were somewhat frustrated in trying to notify all possible Emergency Departments to enable their response—this despite several years of intensive planning and practice that had followed a train crash of a commuter train on the Illinois Central Railroad.

Fortunately, the prevailing winds that day blew the cloud out over Lake Michigan, and there was not a single victim. It was estimated at the time, however, that if the wind had not been present, or had changed direction from typical, there would have been over 1 million victims.

Similarly, when I was in Denver, there was a cloud of nitric acid released from a train derailment. Again, fortunately, this occurred very early on a Sunday morning. Only 24 hours later, it would have spewed into the traffic rush of early morning workers. This again prevented a horrible disaster, and we had only three victims who were seriously exposed, and about 20 others with very minor exposure.

Thus it doesn't really matter if the disaster is natural or manmade in terms of unpredictability or horrible consequences. It is clear that the best preparation is going to be that of an already developed, practiced, and efficient disaster program. That, of course, doesn't mean that we have such a program in place, nor does it mean that there are not rare diseases, chemicals, or unprecedented event scenarios that we will have to learn about and prepare for.

The following book is a serious attempt to do just that. When I read it, my initial reaction was that perhaps we needed to eliminate some of the terrorism chapters because they were going to suggest methods of attack. I realized then that this is one of the unique characteristics of terror attacks. It is so unthinkable that we begin to think illogically about how to prepare and how to respond.

A later thought, more cynical, was that we are spending too much time and money to prepare for events that will not recur, even if they ever occur in the first place. Finally, some sanity resumed and I realized that the only way to prepare for rare, uncommon, and unrepetitive events is to think about them, to attempt to generalize the problems they cause, and to try to develop a system that can respond to the known but can improvise and also respond to the unknown and not previously experienced as well.

This book is a very good start in doing just that. It may frighten you, as it did me, and perhaps horrify you, especially when you are stimulated into thinking about how

---

[1]IOM report on Bioterror.

many problems you are personally, as well as your system, not publicly prepared to respond and react to, not only from ignorance, but because an efficient system just isn't there.

Whether or not you have a personal role in disaster management in your community, your hospital, or your state, it will be educational and stimulating to be involved in the thinking about, and planning for, how to respond to the unthinkable. Within these pages I believe you will find the descriptions, facts, and creative solutions to many problems you are aware of, as well as many problems you may not have thought about.

All the planning in the world will not prevent tragedy from occurring, whether it is by natural causes or man-made. There is no question, however, that the right system will alleviate the tragedy; will salvage lives and psyches, and will help us to feel less despondent about the world we have forced upon us.

I think you will find this book a good read. Not only is it well written by a series of authors who are very accomplished and experienced in disaster management, but I believe you will find it one of the most thought-provoking books that you have read. I certainly did, and while I still am horrified at the variety and depths of tragedy that we may still have to endure, it left me feeling much less helpless, and finally much less angry about the whole situation.

To plan is to take control; it may be imperfect, but it is significantly better than being a passive victim. Just think how many lives were saved because an alert Emergency Physician was able to think about and diagnose an anthrax victim. Would he have thought about this without Sept. 11, I suspect not, but if only one life is saved by improved education and awareness, this book will have been worth the tremendous amount of work and diligence that went into its preparation.

Peter Rosen, MD
Senior Lecturer Medicine
Harvard University School of Medicine
Attending Physician Emergency Medicine
Beth Israel/Deaconess Medical Center

PREFACE

Walking slowly toward Ground Zero as Commander of one of the first Federal Disaster Medical Assistance Teams into the World Trade Center disaster, I was initially struck by a sense of helplessness at the sight of the devastation. As the plumes of smoke rose from the undulating piles of destruction, we had a sense that the disaster before us was so vast and our task so enormous that we would never be able to mount an effective response. This feeling of helplessness did not abate until we resorted to our training and took up our role in the overall disaster response. We were a cog in a very large machine, placed precisely where we would be supported by the other parts, and function in such a specialized way as to keep the machine running. At that moment of realization, this book was born.

The philosophy behind the writing of this textbook is to bring resources together necessary for the development of a comprehensive understanding of Disaster Medicine and its role in Disaster Management. The release of the book comes soon after Hurricane Katrina has devastated the Gulf Coast of America and approximately 1 year after the horror of the Southeast Asia tsunami. After witnessing the devastation of vast areas around the Indian Ocean, and the destruction of a major U.S. city, it is impossible not to be struck by the destructive powers of such natural events. There is, however, another striking feature about both of these events. Whereas the tsunami struck some of the poorest areas, Katrina struck the most developed and richest country in the world. Regardless of these stark socio-economic contrasts, the destruction to the affected areas was remarkably similar: it was nearly total. Disaster strikes without warning, is indiscriminate in its choice of victims, and has the potential of overcoming even the most prepared of systems. If there is no other justification for a book such as this, it must be said that these recent events demand that we, as healthcare professionals, develop an understanding of the basics of Disaster Medicine and stand ready to integrate into the response system if and when disaster should strike close to home.

This book is designed to serve as both a comprehensive text and a quick resource. Part 1 introduces the many topics of disaster medicine and management with an emphasis on the multiple disciplines that come together in the preparation for and response to such catastrophic events. It is the integration of these various response and preparedness modalities that makes Disaster Medicine such a unique field. This section is meant to be a comprehensive approach to the study of the discipline of Disaster Medicine and should be used by healthcare professionals to develop and expand their knowledge base. The chapters may introduce topics that are unfamiliar to the reader, as most practitioners will not be versed in some of the non-medical subjects discussed. Although much of the information may be very new, it may also be crucial in the unexpected event a disaster strikes nearby.

Part 2 of the book, or the "Event" chapters, introduces the reader to every conceivable disaster scenario, and the management issues surrounding each. This part of the text can be used as both a reference and a real-time consult for each topic. The reader will find very detailed and specific events described in these chapters. Some disaster scenarios discussed have historical precedence whereas others are considered to be at risk for future occurrence. Many describe natural and accidental events while some are dedicated to very specific terrorist attacks. There is no easy way to discuss these topics. In particular, terrorist events may cause a sense of unease as one reads the chapter. The chapters related to terrorism in this section attempt to account for every possible modality terrorist operatives are thought to currently possess or may acquire in the future. In some cases the scenarios may prove true, and in many they may not. It is imperative, however, that all possible modalities of attack be discussed so that if needed, proper preparedness and response can be mounted. The term "attack" has been deliberately used in many of these chapters to emphasize the point that, if these agents and scenarios are purposefully unleashed, it will, in fact, be in the form of an attack. The need for inclusion of such terminology in an academic medical textbook underscores the climate in which this text has been written. After such events as the Sept. 11, 2001 attacks, the elementary school tragedy in Beslan, Russia, and the London bombings of 2005, the clear need for thorough discussion is apparent. Part 2 of this text discusses these scenarios in as complete a way as possible, while respecting the dignity of those afflicted by past events. In a way it is the pain and suffering of both victims and survivors of such events that has contributed most to this text, and it is in celebration of their spirit that it has been written.

Finally, I must mention the outstanding group of editors and contributors you will find within these pages. I went to great lengths to find individuals who are expert in their field, not only because they have studied it, but because they have done it. These are the doers as well as the thinkers. These are the men and women who leave their families when disaster strikes and integrate into the response systems. They are the experts called upon on a regional, national, and international level to prepare for disasters, always learning from the past and planning for the future. This book is more than 2 years in the making, partly because during that time the editors and authors were all too often deployed for lengthy periods into disaster zones around the world. In the study of Disaster Medicine, perhaps like none other, knowledge borne from experience makes for a very robust textbook. You will feel that experience jump from these pages and you will be rewarded by having learned from the best.

Because of the ubiquitous nature of disaster, society is indebted to those who choose to learn and practice this field. As a member of that society, I would like to personally thank you for doing so.

Gregory R. Ciottone, MD, FACEP

CONTENTS

DISASTER MEDICINE

PART I

Overview of Disaster Management

chapter 1

Introduction to Disaster Medicine

Gregory R. Ciottone

Throughout history, emergency medical responders have cared for the victims of disaster. As in other areas of disease and injury, medical personnel assume the responsibility of providing care to patients with illness or injury resulting from the catastrophe. Unlike other areas of medicine, however, the care of casualties from a disaster requires the healthcare provider to integrate into the larger, predominately non-medical multidisciplinary response. This demands a knowledge base far greater than medicine alone. To operate safely and efficiently as part of a coordinated disaster response, either in a hospital or in the field, an understanding of disaster management principles is necessary.

In the mid-1980s, disaster medicine began to evolve from the union of disaster management and emergency medicine. Although Disaster Medicine is not yet an accredited medical subspecialty, those who practice it have been involved in some of the most catastrophic events in human history. Practitioners of present day disaster medicine have responded to the aftermaths of the tsunami in southeast Asia,[1] hurricane Andrew,[2] the Indian earthquake,[3] the Madrid train bombings,[4] and the World Trade Center attack,[5] to name a few. During the past several decades, the first applications of basic disaster medicine principles in real-time events have been carried out, and as demonstrated recently by the 2004 tsunami in southeast Asia, there is sure to be continued need for such applications.

The impetus for this text grew from a realization that, as the specialty of emergency medicine grows, emergency physicians must take ownership of this new field of disaster medicine and ensure it meets the rigorous demands put upon it by the very nature of human disaster. If we are to call ourselves disaster medicine specialists and are to be entrusted by society to respond to the most catastrophic human events, it is imperative that we pursue the highest level of scholarly knowledge in this very dynamic area. Until there is oversight from a certifying board, it is our responsibility to the public we serve to maintain this high level of excellence.

THE DISASTER CYCLE

Because disasters strike without warning in areas often unprepared for such events, it is essential for all emergency services personnel to have a foundation in the practical aspects of disaster preparedness and response. As is discussed in other chapters throughout this text, emergency responders have an integrated role in disaster management. All disasters follow a cyclical pattern known as the *disaster cycle* (Fig. 1-1), which describes four reactionary stages: preparedness, response, recovery, and mitigation/prevention. Emergency medicine specialists have a role in each part of this cycle. As active members of their community, emergency specialists should take part in mitigation and preparedness on the hospital, local, and regional levels. Once disaster strikes, their role continues into the response and recovery phases. By participating in the varied areas of disaster preparation and response, including hazard vulnerability analyses, resource allocation, and creation of disaster legislation, the emergency medicine specialist integrates into the disaster cycle as an active participant. A thorough understanding of the disaster medicine needs of a community allows one to contribute to the overall preparedness and response mission.

NATURAL AND MANMADE DISASTER

Over the course of recorded history, natural disasters have predominated in frequency and magnitude over manmade ones. Some of the earliest disasters have caused enormous numbers of casualties, with resultant disruption of the underlying community infrastructure. *Yersinia pestis* caused the death of countless millions in several epidemics over hundreds of years. The etiological agent of bubonic plague, *Y. pestis* devastated Europe by killing large numbers of people and leaving societal ruin in its wake.[6] As of this writing, there is fear of an impending avian influenza pandemic that may be worldwide in scale.[7] Influenza and severe acute respiratory syndrome (SARS) have proven in recent years that, despite the passage of time and the great advances in medicine, the world continues to be affected by the outbreak of disease. Further, diseases that have been eradicated, such as smallpox, now have the potential of being reintroduced into society, either accidentally from the few remaining research sources in existence or by intentional release. Such an event could be devastating, as the baseline intrinsic immunity

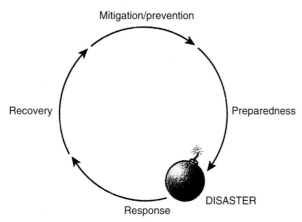

THE DISASTER CYCLE

FIGURE 1–1. The disaster cycle.

the world population had developed during the natural presence of the disease has faded over time, putting much larger numbers of people at risk. Finally, with the advent of the airliner allowing rapid travel to any part of the world, the bloom effect of an outbreak is much harder to predict and control. Disease outbreaks that were previously controlled by natural borders, such as oceans, no longer have those barriers, making the likelihood of worldwide outbreak much greater now than it was hundreds of years ago.

In addition to epidemics, with each passing year natural disasters in the form of earthquakes, floods, and deadly storms batter populations. One need only to remember the destruction in terms of both human life and community resources caused by the Indian Ocean earthquake and subsequent tsunami of 2004 to understand the need for preparedness and response to such natural events. Considering the earthquake that caused the tsunami occurred hours before the devastation, it is difficult to understand how today's advanced society, able to travel far into space among other great achievements, was unable to detect one of the most deadly natural events in recent history. The realization that disaster can strike without warning and inflict casualties on the order of the 2004 tsunami, despite our many technological advances, serves as a warning that mitigation, preparedness, and response to natural disaster must continue to be studied and practiced vigorously.

Today, the possibility of terrorist attack threatens populations across the globe. Both industrialized and developing countries have witnessed some of the most callous and senseless taking of life, for reasons not easily fathomed by civilized people. It is unusual to read a newspaper, listen to radio, or watch television news reports without learning of a terrorist attack in some part of the world. These attacks are so frequent that society has become almost numb to them. Today, an event such as a car bombing may be relegated to a side report on a daily newscast. The commonplace nature of a terrorist attack in modern society ensures it is unquestionably something that will continue long into the future and will very likely escalate in scale and frequency.

The multilayered foundation on which ideological belief evolves into violent attack is beyond the scope of analysis this book ventures to undertake. These ongoing events do demonstrate, however, that the principles studied in the field of disaster medicine must include those that are designed to prepare for and respond to a terrorist attack. Because there are very intelligent minds at work designing systems to bring disaster on others, equally there must be as robust an effort to prepare for and respond to those disasters. Such response involves the deployment of law enforcement, evidence collection, and military personnel and equipment, which are typically not seen in the response to a natural disaster. The integration of these unique assets into the overall response is essential for the success of the mission. The disaster medicine specialist must have a thorough understanding of the role of each.

DEFINING DISASTER

A thorough discussion of disaster preparedness and response must be predicated on a clear definition of what, in fact, constitutes a disaster. Used commonly to describe many different events, disaster is not easily defined. One of the earliest documented testaments to such an event is that of the great flood, reported in several writings, including the *Bible*. This flood is described as covering vast areas of land in the most populated part of the ancient world. Such a flood would have killed millions of people and destroyed vast areas of inhabited land. This surely would fit the definition of a disaster. Similarly, the Indian Ocean tsunami in 2004, killing well over 200,000 people, would also meet the criteria for disaster. However, a 2005 bus crash in the Baharampur district of India that killed 48 people has also been called a disaster. Likewise, the 2003 explosion of the space shuttle Columbia on re-entry into Earth's atmosphere that killed the crew of seven astronauts onboard has often been referred to as the Columbia Disaster in the lay press. How can an event resulting in the loss of seven people be placed in the same category as one that kills hundreds of thousands? Herein lies the paradox of disaster. What is it? Who defines it and by what criteria?

It is difficult to dispute that an event causing thousands of casualties should be considered a disaster, but let's analyze why that is the case. What is it about the sheer number of dead and injured that allows the event to be called a disaster? In terms of medical needs, it is simply because there is no healthcare system on Earth that can handle that number of casualties. Therefore, an event of such magnitude is a disaster because it has overwhelmed the infrastructure of the community in which it occurred. Following this logic, we can then also make the statement that any event that overwhelms existing societal systems is a disaster. This definition is close to the United Nations Disaster Management Training Programme's (UNDMTP) definition of disaster[8]:

A disaster is a serious disruption of the functioning of a society, causing widespread human, material or environmental losses which exceed the ability of the affected society to cope using only its own resources.

A similar definition is used by the World Health Organization (WHO). By applying these definitions, one can understand how an event in a rural area with 10 to 20 casualties may also be considered a disaster because the limited resources in that area may prevent an adequate response without outside assistance.

The widely accepted UNDMTP and WHO definitions of disaster justify describing both the 2004 tsunami and the 2005 bus accident as disasters. But what about the space shuttle Columbia destruction on re-entry? Clearly this definition does not allow one to justify the use of disaster in describing that horrific accident. This brings to light a discrepancy in how disaster specialists and the lay public term events. The Columbia accident, as an example, does not meet any accepted criteria of disaster. It was, however, an exceedingly tragic event, seen by millions on television as it was unfolding. It was tragic by the word's very definition in the *Cambridge Dictionary:* "A very sad event, especially one involving death or suffering." Public perception of such events may cause this misnomer, with a tragic incident being termed a disaster. Much like disaster, tragedy can also have a profound and lasting effect on society, especially a tragedy that is widely viewed through modern media outlets. This text, however, will follow the UNDMTP and WHO definitions when discussing disaster.

DISASTER MEDICINE

Disaster medicine is a discipline resulting from the marriage of emergency medicine and disaster management. The role of medicine, in particular emergency medicine, in disaster response has been clearly defined throughout history. Responsibility for the care of the injured from a disaster has been borne by the emergency specialist. Therefore, disaster medical response, in its many forms, has been around for thousands of years. Whenever a disaster has struck, there has been some degree of a medical response to care for the casualties. In the United States, much of the disaster medical response has followed a military model, with lessons learned through battlefield scenarios during the last two centuries.[9] The military experience has demonstrated how to orchestrate efficient care to mass casualties in austere environments. It does not, however, translate directly into civilian practice. For instance, scenarios encountered on the battlefield with young, fit soldiers injured by trauma are vastly different from those encountered in a rural setting, where an earthquake may inflict casualties on a population with baseline malnutrition or advanced age. With this realization came the need to create disaster medicine as an evolution from the military practice. This recent organization of the medical role in disasters into a more formalized specialty of disaster medicine has enabled practitioners to further define their role in the overall disaster preparedness and response system.

Disaster medicine is truly a systems-oriented specialty. There is no "disaster clinic." There are no practitioners who leave home in the morning intent on seeing disaster patients. Disaster medical care is often thrust upon the practitioner and is not necessarily something that is sought out. The exception to this is the medical specialist who becomes part of organized (usually federal) disaster team, such as a Disaster Medical Assistance team (DMAT). In this case, one may be transported to a disaster site with the intention of treating the victims of a catastrophic event. In all other circumstances, however, the disaster falls on an unsuspecting emergency responder who is forced to abandon his or her normal duties and adopt a role in the overall disaster response.

Unlike the organized disaster team member, if an emergency provider treats casualties from disaster, it will most likely be as a result of a disaster event that has occurred in his or her immediate area. Because of the random nature of disaster, it is not possible to predict who will be put into that role next. Therefore, it is imperative for all who practice in emergency health services to have a working knowledge of the basics of disaster medicine and disaster management. In addition, especially with the recent escalation in perceived and real terrorist threats, there are a host of possible attack scenarios, which may involve exotic chemical, biological, or nuclear agents and modalities. Most clinicians will have a very limited knowledge of many of these agents, so it is therefore important to educate our potential disaster responders on their specifics.

The field of disaster medicine involves the study of subject matter from multiple medical disciplines. Disasters may result in varying injury and disease patterns, depending on the type of event that has occurred. Earthquakes can cause entrapment and resultant crush syndrome; tornadoes may cause penetrating trauma from flying debris; and disease outbreak, either natural or intentional, can result from many different bacteria, viruses, and fungi. Because of the potential variability in casualty scenarios, the disaster medicine specialist must have training in the many injury and illness patterns seen in disaster victims. Even though the expanse of knowledge required is vast, the focus on areas specifically related to disaster medicine allows the science to be manageable. The study of disaster medicine should not be undertaken without prerequisite medical training. A disaster medicine specialist is always a practicing clinician from another field of medicine first and a disaster specialist second. By integrating these many disciplines, one is prepared for the variety of injury and illness patterns that may be faced.

Finally, disaster medicine presents unique ethical situations not seen in other areas of medicine. Disaster medicine is predicated on the principle of providing care to the most victims possible as dictated by the resources available and by patient condition and likelihood of survival. Disaster triage involves assigning patients into treatment categories based on their predicted survivability. This triage process may dictate that the most severely injured patient not be given medical care but rather it be provided to a less critically injured patient.

To the best of his or her ability, the triage officer must make a determination as to whether, in the environment of the specific disaster and the availability of resources, a given patient has a significant probability of survival or does not. If it is the latter, disaster triage principles mandate that care be given to the patient with a higher likelihood of survival. This basic disaster triage principle can have a profound psychological impact on the care provider. As a physician, one is trained to render care to the sick and to not leave the side of a needy patient. To deny care to a critically ill or injured patient can be one of the most anxiety-provoking tasks a disaster medicine specialist performs.

The unique and ever-changing circumstances under which disaster medicine specialists operate mandate the continued evolution and vigorous pursuit of academic excellence in this new specialty. A comprehensive approach that unifies medical principles with a sound understanding of disaster management procedures will yield a well-rounded and better-prepared disaster responder. If emergency medicine providers around the world can develop a basic understanding of the fundamental principles of this specialty, great advances in the systems included in the disaster cycle will surely follow. The more widely dispersed this knowledge becomes, the better prepared we are as a society to respond to the next catastrophic event.

REFERENCES

1. Wattanawaitunechai C, Peacock SJ, Jitpratoom P. Tsunami in Thailand—disaster management in a district hospital. *N Engl J Med.* March 2005;352(10):962-4.
2. Nufer KE, Wilson-Ramirez G. A comparison of patient needs following two hurricanes. *Prehospital Disaster Med.* April-June 2004;19(2):146-9.
3. Jain V, Noponen R, Smith BM. Pediatric surgical emergencies in the setting of a natural disaster: experiences from the 2001 earthquake in Gujarat, India. *J Pediatr Surg.* May 2003;38(5):663-7.
4. Gutierrez de Ceballos JP, Turegano Fuentes F. Casualties treated at the closest hospital in the Madrid, March 11, terrorist bombings. *Crit Care Med.* January 2005;33(1 suppl):S107-12.
5. Simon R, Teperman S. The World Trade Center attack. Lessons for disaster management. *Crit Care.* December 2001;5(6):318-20.
6. Lowell JL, Wagner DM, et al. Identifying sources of human exposure to plague. *J Clin Microbiol.* February 2005;43(2):650-6.
7. Larkin M. Avian flu: sites seek to respond and reassure. *Lancet Infect Dis.* March 2005;5(3):141-2.
8. Disaster Management Training Programme. *Disaster Preparedness Guide.* 2nd ed. Available at: http://www.undmtp.org/english/disaster_preparedness/disaster_preparedness.pdf#xml=http://undmtp.org.master.com/texis/master/search/mysite.txt?q=disaster+preparedness&order=r&id=60413a1214953850&cmd=xml.
9. Dara SI, Ashton RW, et al. Worldwide disaster medical response: an historical perspective. *Crit Care Med.* January 2005;33(1 suppl): S2-6.

chapter 2

Public Health and Disasters

Catherine Y. Lee and James Michael Riley

INTRODUCTION TO PUBLIC HEALTH

As early as 310 BC, a public health philosophy was exhibited by the Romans. They believed that cleanliness would lead to good health and made links between causes of disease and methods of prevention. For example, during this time an association was made between the increased death rate of persons living near swamps and sewage, and as a result the Roman Empire began working on two major public health projects in sanitation control: the building of aqueducts to supply clean water to the city and a sewage system to eliminate waste from the streets. Today, the benefits of public health infrastructure in the United States and abroad continue to strengthen the well-being of society. The impact of interventions has been great. In the past century (1900–1999), the 10 greatest public health achievements have been documented as the following[1]:

1. Vaccination programs, meaning the eradication of smallpox; elimination of poliomyelitis in the Americas; and control of measles, rubella, tetanus, diphtheria, and other diseases around the world
2. Motor-vehicle safety
3. Safer workplaces
4. Control of infectious diseases
5. Decline in deaths from coronary heart disease and stroke
6. Safer and healthier foods
7. Healthier mothers and babies
8. Family planning
9. Fluoridation of drinking water
10. Recognition of tobacco use as a health hazard

Public health is founded on the efforts of a society to protect, promote, and restore the health of its citizens. Public health programs and services emphasize the prevention of disease and administration of health needs to the population as an entity, versus the study and treatment of a single patient, as is found in the discipline of medicine. Today, *public health* is defined as "the science and the art of preventing disease, prolonging life, and promoting physical health and mental health and efficiency through organized community efforts . . . and the development of the social machinery to ensure to every individual in the community a standard of living adequate for the maintenance of health."[2] The mission of public health is to fulfill society's desire to create conditions so that people can be healthy. Public health is divided into the staple pillars of assessment, policy development, and assurance.[3] All three of these pillars are interdependent and cyclical. Two functions address the issues of assessment: (1) monitor health and (2) diagnose and investigate. Under policy development are the functions (1) inform, educate, empower; (2) mobilize community partnerships; and (3) develop policies. The following functions define assurance: (1) link to and/or provide care, (2) ensure a competent workforce, and (3) evaluate.[3]

Like traditional programs in public health, ranging from maternal and reproductive health to injury control and prevention, the public health response to disasters also fulfills the same basic tenets of assessment, policy development, and assurance. This chapter introduces the reader to how public health integrates into disaster preparedness and response systems by highlighting some specific subjects relevant to those tenets. It will cover topics like the public health disaster response cycle, policies in disaster response, the provision of disaster medical services, as well as worker safety and epidemiological/data issues (Figure 1-1).

PUBLIC HEALTH RESPONSE CYCLE

Mitigation is the process of recognizing risks and vulnerabilities and then working to both reduce the vulnerability and strengthen society's ability to withstand an unstoppable event or to reduce the effects from a disaster. Public health seeks to mitigate hazards such as explosions, chemical exposures, natural disasters like floods and earthquakes, and infectious disease, as well as reducing vulnerabilities of the infrastructure such as weak assets, resources, personnel, and science. One form of mitigation may be hardening structures against blast, but also can be the placement of surveillance systems to increase early detection of infectious diseases in a hospital setting, for example. Today, these systems, as well as reporting parameters, are being put into place across the country to both recognize and protect populations from a bioterrorism event. Early warning offers the benefit of a rapid response and reduction in morbidity and mortality.

Preparedness is the process of developing a formal program of response. Preparedness has many components, including: training and staff development; identification and classification of public health resources including personnel, supplies, and facilities; development of standard operating procedures (SOPs), emergency response plans, and communications plans; and pre-placement of key supplies and protective equipment. This phase should also include the participation in table-top and functional exercises. Public health personnel must be integrated and participate with other response agencies during drills and exercises to better familiarize each stakeholder with their respective roles and abilities. In addition, this is the phase in which public health agencies would develop interagency agreements, memoranda of understanding (MOUs), and external support contracts.

The Centers for Disease Control and Prevention (CDC) is one reference source where planners can obtain basic guidelines for disaster preparedness. These include:

1. Form mutual-aid agreements and close relationships with local, regional, state, and federal partners.
2. Conduct a hazard and risk assessment.
3. Conduct a capacity assessment, identifying resources in your system.
4. Obtain those identified resources and surge capacity.
5. Develop plans consistent with other response organizations in your community.
6. Develop surveillance, registries, and data archiving systems.
7. Plan for public affairs and risk communication.
8. Ensure personnel are trained and certified to use personal protective equipment and other health practices.
9. Orientation for volunteers and personnel on procedures, guidelines, and command and management systems.
10. Participate in and conduct exercises.
11. Participate in after-action reviews of exercises and incidents.[4]

Response is the phase in which each agency and section with responsibility to respond activates its emergency response plan to the specific threat or situation and can incorporate local, regional, and federal response. For example, in response to a biologic or chemical terrorist event, public health agencies would respond by conducting site surveys, recommending public safety measures and communicating risk, providing epidemiologic investigations, providing medical treatment of prophylaxis for those exposed, and initiating disease prevention and environmental decontamination measures.[5]

RECOVERY

Public health agencies must identify what resources may be available to assist in restoring the operation as well as address other physically and emotionally affected populations. Public health recovery operations are multidisciplinary and involve multiple sectors of society (law enforcement, military, public policy, public works), and they vary depending on the extent of the disaster's societal impact. Furthermore, recovery efforts comprise several components, some of which are Search and Rescue (SAR) in the case of an earthquake, bombing, or landslide; reinstitution of medical services if clinics and hospitals are destroyed; and establishment of corrupted lifelines like sanitation, electricity, and water. Those affected by the horrendous Tsunami disaster—that killed hundreds of thousands in Indonesia, Thailand, India, and so many other nations—demonstrated the international public health relief operation: an extreme example of multilateral, global relief spanning commercial and government sectors. The recovery from this disaster is ongoing and likely will last several years.

DISASTER POLICY

For weeks after the 2004 tsunami, survivors on makeshift rafts were miraculously saved and brought back to shore. At the same time, the United States faced its own disasters. Thirteen people were trapped and 6 died from

---

 LOCAL PUBLIC HEALTH RESPONSE TO THE WORST TERRORIST ATTACK IN U.S. HISTORY

On Sept. 11, 2001, two commercial jets that were hijacked by terrorists crashed into the two towers of the World Trade Center in New York City. Within 90 minutes, both 110-story towers had collapsed. The New York State Department of Health (NYS DOH) had pre-established Emergency Operations Center committees that came together and began working within 30 minutes of the attack. NYS DOH nursing staff assisted in triaging and treating injured persons at an emergency triage center. In collaboration with the American Red Cross, the DOH also provided nursing staff for emergency shelters that housed displaced residents. Within the disaster site and surrounding commu-

nity, DOH performed environmental monitoring. With losses in power and water as well as having tons of airborne contaminants in the area, DOH had its hands full with monitoring both the general public and emergency responders in addition to performing its daily activities. The DOH regularly sent faxes, e-mail alerts, and press releases containing urgent public health information and/or concerns to local hospitals and physicians. The DOH designed and implemented a rescue and recovery worker-safety plan. Additionally, the DOH initiated four disease and injury surveillance systems after the disaster, with assistance from the CDC.

mudslides in La Conchita, California; and a train disaster in Graniteville, South Carolina released concentrated chlorine fumes, leading to 9 deaths and 250 hospitalizations. Finally, in the fall of 2005 Hurricane Katrina devastated the Gulf coast of the United States, resulting in the flooding and complete evacuation of New Orleans. Although these disasters are not on the same scale in terms of death, injury, social loss, and destruction as the tsunami, they still maintain criteria that classify them as disasters.

What determines whether an event is treated as a federal disaster? Locally, only the governor of a state or his or her appointee can declare a federal disaster through coordination with the Federal Emergency Management Agency (FEMA) regional director through the Federal Response Plan (FRP), under the Stafford Disaster Relief and Emergency Assistance Act.[7] The FRP under the Stafford Act is an interagency plan that outlines the delivery of federal resources to state and local governments when a disaster overwhelms the region's ability to respond self-sufficiently. When state or local resources are insufficient to respond to and recover from a disaster, the presidential declaration sets forth long-term federal disaster recovery programs.[7] The Stafford Disaster Relief and Emergency Assistant Act's definition of a major disaster is stated in the following[7]:

> Any natural catastrophe (including any hurricane, tornado, storm, high water, wind-driven water, tidal wave, tsunami, earthquake, volcanic eruption, landslide, mudslide, snowstorm, or drought), or, regardless of cause, any fire, flood, or explosion in any part of the United States, which in the determination of the President causes damage of sufficient severity and magnitude to warrant major disaster assistance under this Act to supplement the efforts and available resources of states, local governments, and disaster relief organizations in alleviating the damage, loss, hardship, or suffering caused thereby.

A major disaster declaration makes available all federal disaster relief assistance to affected communities. This can include repair, replacement, and reconstruction of public and nonprofit facilities; cash grants for personal victim needs; temporary housing vouchers or replacement accommodations; and unemployment assistance.[8]

Following the Sept. 11 attacks in 2001, the President declared the Homeland Security Presidential Directive (HSPD)-5, in which he called for the development of a new National Response Plan (NRP) "to align Federal coordination structures, capabilities, and resources into a unified, all-discipline, and all-hazards approach to domestic incident management."[6] The premise of this robust plan is to standardize and make seamless the manner of operations for all levels of disaster response from local to federal, as well as private and public, agencies. The NRP will establish a national framework, standardizing aspects of coordination, communications, incident management, and information sharing, as well as streamline disaster policy directives and protocols. Upon full implementation of the NRP, it will supersede the Initial National Response Plan (INRP), the Federal Response Plan (FRP), the U.S. Governmental Interagency Domestic Terrorism Concept of Operations Plan (CONPLAN), and Federal Radiological Emergency Response Plan (FRERP).

The NRP also provides for guidance to initiate long-term community recovery and mitigation.[6]

When the NRP is fully implemented, the Secretary of Homeland Security will declare "incidents of national significance." The drafted NRP in December 2004 outlined four criteria that constitute an "Incident of National Significance":

1. A federal department or agency acting under its own authority has requested the assistance of the Secretary of Homeland Security.
2. State and local resources and authorities are overwhelmed and federal assistance has been requested by the state and local authorities.
3. More than one federal department or agency has become substantially involved in responding to an incident.
4. The Secretary of Homeland Security has been directed to assume responsibility for managing a domestic incident by the President.[6]

One specific support function most applicable to public health is called the Emergency Support Function #8 —Public Health and Medical Services, or ESF-8. ESF-8 provides supplemental assistance to State, local, and tribal governments in identifying and meeting the public health and medical needs of victims of an Incident of National Significance. This support is categorized in the following core functional areas:

- Assessment of public health/medical needs (including behavioral health)
- Public health surveillance
- Medical care personnel, and
- Medical equipment and supplies.[6]

The NRP stipulates that the coordinator and the primary agency is the Department of Health and Human Services.

OPERATING PUBLIC HEALTH

The American Public Health Association (APHA) provides principles to guide public health's response toward terrorism.[11] From a list of 12 principles, the following seven are of specific interest to this chapter:

1. Strengthen the **public health infrastructure** (which includes workforce, laboratory, and information systems) and other components of the public health system (including education, research, and the faith community) to increase the ability to identify, respond to, and prevent problems of public health importance, including the health aspects of terrorist attacks.
2. Ensure the availability of and accessibility to **health care, including medications and vaccines,** for individuals exposed, infected, made ill, or injured in terrorist attacks.
3. **Educate and inform health professionals** and the public to better identify, respond to, and prevent the health consequences of terrorism and promote the visibility and availability of health professionals in the communities that they serve.

4. Address **mental health needs** of populations that are directly or indirectly affected by terrorism.
5. Ensure the protection of the **environment**, food and water supply, and health and safety of **rescue and recovery workers**.
6. Ensure clarification of the roles, relationships, and responsibilities among public health agencies, **law enforcement, and first responders**.
7. Build and sustain the public health capacity to develop **systems to collect data** about the health and mental health consequences of terrorism and other disasters on victims, responders, and communities and develop uniform definitions and standardized data classifications systems of death and injury resulting from terrorism and other disasters.

This chapter introduces basic concepts, discussions, and recommendations regarding the following key issues arising from these selected APHA principles: (1) public health infrastructure; (2) medical services, including the distribution of drugs and supplies; (3) education, training, and communications; (4) environmental health and precautions; (5) mental health; (6) worker safety and first responders; and (7) data collection and analysis.

PUBLIC HEALTH INFRASTRUCTURE

Formal public health programs in the United States have existed for well over 200 years. For example, the origins of the U.S. Public Health Service (USPHS) (initially known as the Marine Hospital Service) may be traced to the passage of an act in 1798 that provided for the care and relief of sick and injured merchant seamen. After its inception and over the next 200 years, the Marine Hospital Service was restructured to provide a much wider variety of essential services.

Today's USPHS is recognized worldwide. Working alongside its other federal partners and state agencies, including the DHHS (and its agencies, such as the CDC, the Food and Drug Administration [FDA]), and the U.S. Department of Agriculture (USDA), the USPHS continues to be an active partner in the nationwide system of public health at the federal level and to influence public health on a national scale. The USPHS has, until recently, provided active support and direction to the NDMS (now directly under FEMA). The USPHS continues to respond to and support operations as a partner of NDMS, providing expertise in several areas.

The U.S. public health system encompasses a broad integration of commercial, public, government, and nongovernment entities. It is as diverse as the very population it serves. It includes government public health agencies operating on federal, regional, state, and local levels; healthcare delivery infrastructure, such as hospitals and clinics; public health and health science academic institutions; community entities, such as schools, organizations, and religious congregations; commercial businesses; and the media.[3] Public health is also augmented by its partnerships and increasing collaboration with expert military health institutions, such as the U.S. Army Medical Research Institute of Infectious Diseases

(USAMRIID) and other defense agencies; national institutions such as the National Institute for Allergy and Infectious Disease (NIAID), under the National Institutes of Health (NIH); law enforcement and emergency responder communities on federal (Federal Bureau of Investigation) and local levels; and the medicolegal community, which is composed of national medical examiners offices and forensic scientists.

Public health response is not centralized (for better or worse) and incorporates multiple government agencies, ranging from those involved in research and development (e.g., Bioshield at DHHS) to victim assistance (e.g., NDMS at DHS). Bioterrorist response, for example, involves an enormous breadth of players and their respective functions.[9] The DHHS alone elicits responses from its agencies: the Agency for Healthcare Research and Quality (AHRQ), CDC, FDA, NIH, and Office of Emergency Preparedness (OEP). Other departments that participate in public health include the USDA, including its Animal and Plant Health Inspection Service (APHIS), Agricultural Research Service (ARS), Food Safety Inspection Service (FSIS), and Office of Crisis Planning and Management (OCPM); agencies under the Department of Commerce (DOC), including the National Institute of Standards and Technology (NIST); agencies under the DOD, including the Defense Advanced Research Projects Agency (DARPA), Joint Task Force for Civil Support (JTFCS), National Guard, and U.S. Army; the Department of Energy (DOE); the Department of Justice (DOJ), including the Federal Bureau of Investigation (FBI) and the Office of Justice Programs (OJP); agencies under the Department of the Transportation (DOT), including the U.S. Coast Guard (USCG); agencies under the Department of Treasury (Treasury), including the U.S. Secret Service (USSS); the VA; the Environmental Protection Agency (EPA); and FEMA.[9]

Different agencies function to deliver services to varying target audiences. For example, the target audiences of the CDC are state and local health agencies. In terms of activities, the CDC provides grants, technical support, and performance standards to support preparedness and response planning for bioterrorism; chemical and radiological incidents; natural disasters; and terrorist incidents, such as explosions, that may yield significant physical trauma.[9] The OEP enhances medical response capabilities, such as early identification of a biologic incident, mass prophylaxis, mass casualty care, and mass fatality management.[9] Its target audiences are local jurisdictions, including fire and police departments, emergency medical services (EMS), hospitals, and public health agencies.[9] The DOJ helps states develop strategic plans and funds training, the obtaining of equipment, and the planning of drills and exercises for fire, law enforcement, emergency medical and hazardous response (HazMat) teams, hospitals, and public health departments.[9] FEMA supports state emergency management agencies by providing grant assistance to sustain local-consequence management planning, training, and exercises for all disasters, including biological incidents.[9] For example, FEMA, with the U.S. Army, conducts the Chemical Stockpile Emergency Preparedness Program (CSEPP) and the Radiological Emergency Preparedness (REP) program.[12] The goal of CSEPP is to improve preparedness in the event of an accident involving U.S. stockpiles of obsolete chemical munitions.[12] The REP carries out exercises to ensure that residents living around nuclear power plants are safe and prepared in case of a disaster.

In the event of a disaster, responders on the front line will be public health officials, health care workers (physicians, nurses, other medical professionals), public works personnel, firefighters, EMS personnel, and law enforcement officers.[9] The core public health component will involve local public health departments, which have been described as ". . . the critical components of the public health system that directly deliver public health services to citizens."[13] A public health department is an administrative and/or service unit of local or state government that is staffed with a median of 20 people, varying between 1 and sometimes more than 20,000, with an average of 72 full-time workers.[13] Local public health departments provide services ranging from immunizations to food and milk inspections.[13] Most departments conduct childhood and adult immunizations, communicable disease control practices, epidemiology and surveillance, community assessment, and sexually transmitted disease counseling.[13] Some others have injury control programs, solid waste management, and comprehensive primary care services.[13]

Health departments will likely not be the lead agency in a disaster and therefore must work closely with other organizations and fall into the incident command during an emergency.[9] Health departments and all emergency response agencies should establish, in the planning phase, mutual aid agreements and close working relationships with key partners in their region.

Partners include emergency management agencies (EMAs); EMS; medical and behavioral healthcare providers; fire departments; law enforcement; local emergency planning committees; state, regional, and tribal public health response coordinators; neighboring health jurisdictions; humanitarian and volunteer organizations; private businesses; and academic institutions, such as schools of public health and medicine.[9] For example, between August and September 2004, four hurricanes (Charley, Frances, Ivan, and Jeanne) ripped through Florida, ravaging hundreds of thousands of homes; displacing huge populations; and prompting the aid of 5000 FEMA workers in 15 states and 3800 National Guard members who provided security, directed traffic, and distributed supplies.[14] Additionally, more than 140,000 volunteers spanning state and national volunteer organizations, such as the Red Cross and faith-based groups, arrived in Florida to lend help, ranging from preparing meals to removing trees.[15] Further, the U.S. Public Health Services works alongside its other federal partners and state agencies, including the DHHS and its agencies, the CDC, and the FDA, as well as the USDA. They continue to be an active partner in the nationwide system of public health at the federal level in order to influence public health on a national scale. The USPHS has until recently provided active support and direction to the National Disaster Medical System (now directly under FEMA) in the Department of Homeland Security. They continue to respond and support operations as a partner of NDMS, providing expertise in several areas.

Medical Services

A biologic attack could result in the infection thousands of people without any indication in the first few hours of how many people are infected.[16] For example, one hypothetical scenario depicted a national and global spread of smallpox, resulting in 15,000 cases and 2000 deaths.[17] It is therefore recommended to provide mass prophylaxis to the population—the use of antibiotics being the primary key to survival for most people.[16] Some believe that vaccines are not the first line of defense against biological threats but can be used for control of a smallpox epidemic, prophylaxis against anthrax in combination with antibiotics, control of global pandemic infections, and pre-exposure prophylaxis for high-risk workers in laboratory and health care environments.[18]

Because most public health departments, hospitals, and local institutions lack the amount of drugs needed for a national emergency, federal medical resources are available through the Strategic National Stockpile (SNS), formerly named the National Pharmaceutical Stockpile (NPS). After institution of the Homeland Security Act of 2002, the DHS and CDC began to jointly manage the SNS, with the DHS defining the goals and performance requirements of the program and being responsible for administering the actual deployment of the 12-hour push package.[19] The cache of medical supplies includes antibiotics, chemical antidotes, antitoxins, life support medications, intravenous administration and airway maintenance supplies, and medical/surgical items that can be delivered in the event of a national emergency within 12 hours to strategically designated warehouses across the United States and its territories.[19] The SNS is not meant to be a first response tool but rather to augment and restock existing state and local health agencies' medical supplies. The SNS program conducts quarterly quality assurance checks, rotates materials, performs a full annual inventory of all package items, and regularly inspects environmental conditions, security, and overall package maintenance.[19] Deployment of the SNS is made when the state governor's office directly requests assets from the CDC or DHS.[19]

Once the SNS cache has been delivered, several key steps must be taken to effectively use it: officially receive the supplies and unload them; have adequate personnel for packaging, distributing, dispensing, tracking, and storing the supplies; have the local public health department assign dosages; and provide communication and security.[16]

There are additional public health issues beyond these logistics that should be taken into account when distributing mass prophylaxis to the public. They include dividing the population into groups who require medication first, a step that is politically sensitive and should be decided before a biologic attack happens.[16] Also, public health personnel should be ready to distribute clear agent-specific and drug information, to make available multilingual staff and handouts, to handle the needs of special populations, to provide personal protective equipment

(PPE) for people at staffing and dispensing centers, and to provide security in case of crowd panic.[16]

Disasters cause various patterns of injury and disease, ranging from blast injuries by a terrorist bombing to ventilatory failure from the chemical release of a nerve agent. As a result, responses significantly vary in terms of how widespread the response is (local to international), which personnel are used to respond, the duration of the response, and what medical management must be used to treat those affected or exposed.

For example, some infectious diseases require a larger response, for which the help of national and sometimes international partners and resources is needed to identify the agent, conduct surveillance, report, and treat the range of people who may be infected. Such responses may vary in location and size. However, natural disasters, such as hurricanes, call for a different type of medical response altogether, in which medical problems seem to arise out of environmental hazards resulting from the natural disaster's aftermath. For instance, injuries and deaths occur because victims fail to evacuate and take shelter, do not take precautions in securing property, and do not follow guidelines for food and water safety or injury prevention during the recovery phase.[20] Injuries from a hurricane can result from near-drowning; electrocution; lacerations from flying debris; blunt trauma or bone fractures from falling trees and other heavy objects; stress-related disorders; heart attacks; gastrointestinal, respiratory, vector-borne, and skin diseases; toxic poisoning; fires; bites from displaced wild animals, such as animals and snakes; and even improper use of mechanical equipment, such as chain saws and power tools.[20]

Chemical and radiological incidents have more specific medical issues, including the recognition of patterns of injury, prophylaxis, and antidotes. Managing a volume of exposed patients in a limited healthcare environment can be challenging and can include issues of decontamination; on-site prehospital management; transportation; the use of PPE; and treatment of patterns of injury specifically associated with chemical and radiological sequelae, such as skin lesions, blisters and burns, nervous system disorders, inhalational injuries, and acute radiation syndrome. Some disasters fall into less specific points for medical management due to the nature of the event.

Consider the blackout on Aug. 14, 2003, in the Northeastern United States and Southeastern Canada (Ottawa and Toronto) that affected 50 million people and a total of 240,00 square kilometers in areas including New York, New Jersey, Vermont, Michigan, Ohio, Pennsylvania, Connecticut, and Massachusetts.[21] The blackout, suspected to have been caused by a downed 340,000-volt power grid, caused the shutdown of 21 power plants across the nation.[22] The blackout affected all electrical functions, shutting down computers, trapping passengers in high-rise elevators, stalling subways, and disrupting airport control and landing procedures, hospital activities, food refrigeration, traffic operations, and most channels of communication. Facilities with backup generators were able to continue operations, but only sparingly. In the United States, three people died as a result of the blackout and one firefighter was injured. In Ottawa, a teenager died from fire-related injuries and another person died after being hit by a car. In New York during the 30-hour period of no electricity, 3000 fires were reported, mainly from people using candles, and EMS personnel responded to 80,000 calls to 911, double the average.[22]

On the other hand, finite, sudden disasters causing immediate injury and mortality (such as terrorist bombings, transportation disasters, and building collapses) require a more robust response capacity at a local and perhaps regional level. This differs from the national and sometimes international assistance required after large-scale natural disasters that affect vast regions of terrain, as was seen in the case of the 2004 tsunami disaster, as well as in several instances of floods, hurricanes, and even complex humanitarian emergencies overseas. In the case of an explosion, trauma systems must be equipped and ready to accept incoming patients, manage the bulk of patients with minor wounds who will flood the nearest hospital, and prepare for possibly unexpected rates of casualty flow. Physicians should be prepared to treat hundreds of trauma patients, which may be complicated by loss of utilities, difficulty in reaching hospitals, or possible damage to hospital facilities.[23] The physically injured from high-energy disasters, such as earthquakes, tornadoes, or explosions, will most likely be treated at regional trauma centers for severe injuries. In the United States, there are 600 regional trauma centers.[24] They coordinate EMS, including paramedics and air medical transport. A regional trauma center is composed of paramedics and emergency medical technicians (EMTs) who transport injured victims to trauma teams that include a trauma surgeon, emergency physician, several trauma nurses, and specialized personnel. Up to 16 physicians in various specialties, from neurosurgery to obstetrics, comprise a trauma team ready to receive injured patients in the operating room and critical care unit.[24]

For disease outbreaks, the provision of medical services and public health capabilities is considerably great and involves a large network of local to sometimes international response. When severe acute respiratory syndrome (SARS) made its way onto the global front as a highly threatening disease in November 2002, it crippled the Asian healthcare system and brought to light serious questions about the U.S. public health system's ability to respond to a similar crisis at home. SARS had the greatest impact on Asian countries, with 7782 cases and 729 deaths, challenging Asian healthcare systems, adversely affecting Asian economies, and testing the effectiveness of international health codes.[25] SARS is part of the coronavirus family. Within 2 to 10 days after infection, the affected person can develop symptoms including cough, fever, and body aches that are indiscriminate from other respiratory illnesses, appearing as an atypical pneumonia.[25] The fatality rate from SARS is 11% and can be greater than 50% for people older than 65.[25] SARS is a person-to-person transmitted disease that is acquired primarily through direct and indirect contact with respiratory secretions and/or contaminated objects.

An international outbreak of SARS took place from February through deep into the spring of 2003. When an infected physician who treated SARS patients in China stayed at a hotel in Hong Kong on travel, those who resided at the hotel acquired the disease and subsequently departed to Vietnam, Singapore, and Toronto, Canada, seeding secondary outbreaks.[25] Cases spread from Asia to 26 countries, and at is peak in May 2003, hundreds of cases of SARS were being reported each week.

To prevent and control the spread of SARS, public health efforts of case identification and contact tracing, transmission control, and exposure management were utilized. *Case identification and contact tracing* is "defining what symptoms, laboratory results, and medical histories constitute a positive case in a patient and tracing and tracking individuals who may have been exposed to these patients."[25] *Transmission control* is "controlling the transmission of disease-producing microorganisms through use of proper hand hygiene and personal protective equipment, such as masks, gowns, and gloves."[25] *Exposure management* separates those infected from noninfected individuals through the use of quarantine, which restricts movement of those who are not ill but were exposed to the disease agent and are potentially infectious.[25]

EDUCATION, TRAINING, AND COMMUNICATIONS

Tabletop exercises are one form of disaster planning education. Participants of a tabletop exercise are broad and may include government officials (mayors, city council members, risk manager), public works/utilities personnel (water superintendent, gas company representative), law enforcement (police chief, sheriff), community services (Red Cross representative), emergency management (emergency program manager, National Guard representative), fire department representatives (fire chief, dispatcher), emergency medical/health personnel (emergency medical coordinator, public health official), and public information officers.[12] The tabletop exercise, which commonly includes senior-level officials, prompts participants to discuss how their respective agencies or units might react to a specific set of scenarios, emphasizing higher-level policy and procedural issues.[12] Unlike full-scale exercises or field exercise drills, such as a hospital disaster simulation in which operations are evaluated on scene and equipment is deployed, tabletop exercises do not involve management of equipment or personnel, but are rather classroom-type exercises held in a classroom setting.[12]

Full-scale exercises engage tactics, techniques, and procedures that could be used in an actual incident and are designed to be realistic.[12] In May 2000, May 2003, and most recently May 2005, FEMA led three exercises called the Top Officials (TOPOFF1, TOPOFF2, and TOPOFF3), which were large-scale, "no-notice" field drills involving federal, state, and local agencies. TOPOFF1 in 2000 was jointly led by FEMA and DOJ and was conducted in three cities: a biological weapons incident in Denver, Colo., a chemical incident in Portsmouth, N.H., and a mass casualty radiological incident in the Washington, D.C. region.[12] In 2003, the TOPOFF2 4-day drill involved a Radiological Dispersal Device (RDD), or "dirty bomb," release in Seattle, Washington, and a biologic incident involving *Yersinia pestis*, or Pneumonic Plague, in Chicago.[26] TOPOFF3 was the largest U.S. counter-terrorism exercise to date. It exceeded 10,000 players, and involved 275 federal, state, local, and private organizations, as well as international partners Canada and the United Kingdom, with 13 countries sending representative observers. The exercise simulated a chemical release attack in New London, Connecticut, and a biologic attack in New Jersey.

Physicians and other healthcare providers are oftentimes on the front line when detecting a disease outbreak and play a primary role in early detection of the disease:

> "Health-care providers should be alert to illness patterns and diagnostic clues that might indicate an unusual infectious disease outbreak associated with intentional release of a biologic agent and should report any clusters or findings to their local or state health department. . . ."[23,27]

Physicians and other healthcare providers are recommended to maintain a high level of suspicion for rare disease, ascertain thorough patient histories, and evaluate occupational and environmental exposures.[28] The CDC indicates the following three signs of a possible intentional biological release, emphasizing physicians should stay alert for the following[27]:

1. An unusual temporal or geographic clustering of illness (e.g., persons who attended the same public event or gathering) or patients presenting with clinical signs and symptoms that suggest an infectious disease outbreak

2. An unusual age distribution for common diseases

3. A large number of cases of acute flaccid paralysis with prominent bulbar palsies, suggestive of a release of *botulinum* toxin

Most of the knowledge base and skills needed to treat patients after a terrorist or nonterrorist disaster involves an extension of everyday tools that physicians already possess.[23] What is necessary is to "fill in the blanks," as proposed by the American Medical Association.[23] This may include symptoms to become familiar with for early recognition of an unusual infection, guidelines to manage chemical- and radiation-contaminated patients, and protocols to triage and treat acute trauma patients after an explosion. To this extent, professional organizations and societies have become involved in the development of education on disasters and terrorism, and a great degree of seminars, distance learning programs, books, periodicals, web sites, and self-study material have been organized to educate healthcare providers.[23] Such steps have been taken not only in physician communities but also in nursing, physician assistant, and technician communities through the same routes of education and training. Notable experts have commented that public health Internet sites, such as the CDC's bioterrorism web page, have kept the public informed and have helped keep physicians aware of the latest developments and recommendations in bioterrorism.[28]

In times of disaster, there is an essential need to communicate certain health matters to the public. Public health officials often gain and transmit information from a range of various sectors[20]:

- The public (most importantly)
- Hospitals and their emergency departments
- Community providers
- Social service agencies
- First responders, such as fire, police, and EMS
- National Guard representatives
- Local and regional laboratories
- Policy makers, such as public officials, mayors, and governors
- Traditional partners, including the American Red Cross and the public works system

Through communication with the media, public health agencies can set up a network, delivering health reports regularly so that the general public can receive important updates and educational messages.[20] These messages must be factual and credible to the public and delivered through advance protocols, in which a single public information officer has been appointed to deliver the information.[20] Some likely public health information might include food and water safety, injury prevention measures, and warnings that, for example, increase timely evacuation from hurricanes and shelter against tornadoes.[20] Also, information should contain facts about the expected hazards (natural, man-made, or technological disaster), safety precautions, and requirements for evacuation or shelter-in-place.[20] All messages should be clear (messages in writing should be understood and bilingual, if needed) and concise; technical information should be translated into simple language for a general audience. Importantly, the sender of information should verify that the transmitted message has been received and understood by the intended audience. When the public heeds the actions and recommendations made by public health officials, those messages have been adequately delivered to the audiences.[20] Experts emphasize that warning messages should not be withheld until the last minute. This has been documented to happen out of fear that panic will overwhelm the public and lead to more deaths and injuries than the actual disaster.[20]

Internally among public health systems and partners, secure and redundant lines of communication should be set up during a disaster. These include computers with a CD drive, e-mail capability, continuous online Internet access, and security software to protect sensitive data from intruders.[20] Fixed facilities such as hospitals and health departments should have a standby source of power to operate electrical and communication systems in case a disaster strikes the main source.[20] Communication equipment that has been used for public health response includes radio equipment, such as two-way radios, pagers, broadcast radios, televisions, and satellites; wire lines, such as telephones, facsimile machines,

and computer modems; and a combination of both radio and wire lines, including cellular and satellite telephones.[20] However, it is important to realize that in times of disaster, routine communications like these may not be readily available, especially to the public and private sectors. Such was the case in the London Bombings on July 7, 2005, when private businesses found it nearly impossible to access e-mails or make mobile phone calls, as cellular networks were congested from a surge in traffic.

ENVIRONMENTAL HEALTH AND PRECAUTIONS

Environmental health precautions after a disaster will decrease illness, injury, and death. The risks of infection increase in the days after a disaster due to disrupted water supplies and the problem of sanitation control. These include maintaining water and food safety, proper sanitation and waste disposal, and the control of vector populations.[20] The environmental health priorities of most heath departments include the following[29]:

1. Ensuring an adequate supply of safe drinking water
2. Providing food protection measures
3. Ensuring basic sanitation services
4. Promoting personal hygiene
5. Assisting the efforts of first responders by providing health risk consultations or advising on exposure pathways
6. Providing information to emergency managers to help assess the scale of the emergency to ensure an effective response

Landesman[20] recommends a three-tiered approach to reduce exposure to environmental hazards:

1. Measures of control that involve preventing the hazard in question from being released or occurring; controlling its transport; and keeping people from being exposed, such as cleaning, treating, and collecting clean water
2. Establishing multiple barriers, meaning setting up redundant obstacles to separate unsanitary conditions from human contact that can sometimes be a matter of public works engineering
3. Distance between hazards and populations

Quantitative analyses must be used in a survey fashion to identify existing disposal facilities and procedures in a community; to determine how to deliver sanitation coverage; and to distribute safe drinking water and establish water consumption rates. Consumption of and contact with contaminated water supplies from run-off sewage and disrupted sewage systems can lead to fecal-oral diseases such as cholera, typhoid fever, hepatitis A, and shigella.[20] Public health notices to boil water, avoid certain foods that may have spoiled, and that provide locations of potable water are key to environmental safety. Improper food storage, for example, is often associated with *Bacillus cereus*, *Clostridium perfringens*, *Salmonella*, *Staphylococcus aureus*, and group A *Streptococcus*.[20] Sufficient shelter must take into account weather conditions during the disaster, such as warm or cool climates. Insufficient housing can expose people to environmental conditions that make them susceptible to frostbite, hypothermia, heat stroke, and dehydration.[20] Especially important to take into account are educational messages and warnings about carbon monoxide poisoning and untrained use of mechanical power generators. Pest control to reduce infestation of rat and mosquito populations is also important.

MENTAL HEALTH

Several studies describe, characterize, and propose interventions for mental health issues encountered after a disaster. Experts note the wide range of questionnaires, surveys, interviews, and psychiatric classification systems used to document postdisaster psychological sequelae and note the difficulty in cross-comparison and generalization of these findings toward many disasters.[29] Although the disaster community agrees that effects of mental health require more investigation, they also agree that "the worst scars in disasters are psychological and social scars."[30] Mental health issues stemming from disasters are becoming increasingly integrated into postdisaster assessment, with more emphasis on mental health being an urgent aspect of public health relief.

The mental health community stresses that providers and disaster relief personnel need to have a meaningful understanding of the psychological and social needs of victims in a disaster.[30] Disasters can provoke specific emotional reactions that take on a variety of different psychological responses, affecting primary victims (those directly involved in the disaster) and secondary victims (such as relatives, co-workers, and schoolmates). Other people who can experience mental health issues include onlookers, rescuers, body handlers, health personnel, evacuees, and refugees.[30] It is important to realize that most adults and children will experience normal stress reactions for several days after a disaster (Box 2-1).[31] One should note that normal stress reactions can also spawn personal introspection, growth, and resilience.

The three forms of mental health problems that may follow a disaster are acute stress reactions, posttraumatic stress disorders (PTSDs), and adjustment disorders or enduring personality change.[30] Acute reactions are characterized by absence of emotion; lack of response to external stimuli; total inhibition or outward activity and random movements; persons being stunned or shocked; and psychosomatic symptoms such as tremor, palpitations, hyperventilation, nausea, and vomiting.[30] *PTSD is defined as*[32]:

> An anxiety disorder (and diagnostic construct used in the *Diagnostic and Statistical Manual of Mental Disorders-IV*) that can develop after exposure to a terrifying event, or ordeal in which grave physical harm occurred or was threatened. The criteria for PTSD require:

BOX 2-1 NORMAL STRESS REACTIONS AFTER A DISASTER

Temporary emotional reactions
    Shock
    Fear
    Grief
    Anger
    Hopelessness
    Emotional numbness
Cognitive reactions
    Confusion
    Disorientation
    Worry
    Memory loss
    Unwanted memories
Physical reactions
    Tension
    Fatigue
    Difficulty with sleeping
    Change in appetite and sex drive
    Interpersonal reactions to relationships at work and school or within a marriage or family (these may be characterized by distrust, irritability, isolation, judgmental attitude, and being distant)

A. Exposure to a traumatic event
B. Reexperiencing of the event
C. Persistent avoidance of stimuli associated with the trauma
D. Persistent increased arousal
E. Duration of B, C, D of more than one month
F. Clinically significant distress or impairment

One of three survivors experiences severe stress that can lead to PTSD, anxiety disorders, or depression. Severe reactions possibly leading to PTSD include dissociation, intrusive reexperiencing (nightmares), extreme attempts to avoid disturbing memories (substance use), extreme emotional numbing, hyperarousal (panic attacks, rage), severe anxiety (extreme helplessness, compulsions, or obsessions), and severe depression. The mental health ramifications are possibly greater for those who witness or are involved with certain experiences from a disaster. Some examples include loss of loved ones; life-threatening danger or physical harm (especially to children); exposure to gruesome death, bodily injury, or dead and maimed bodies; extreme environmental or human violence and destruction; and loss of home.[31] Inherently, specific individuals might have a typically higher risk of severe stress and lasting PTSD, such as those with a history of exposure to other traumas, chronic medical illness and psychological disorders, chronic poverty, and recent emotional strain.[31] On the other hand, the National Center for PTSD states that some factors might be protective, including social support, higher income and education, successful mastery of past disasters and traumatic events, reduction of exposure to trauma, and provision of regular and factual information about the emergency.

At a recent national workshop on mental health and disasters, experts recommended some early intervention actions.[32] *Early intervention* is defined as[32]:

The provision of psychological help to victims and survivors within the first month after a critical incident, traumatic event, emergency, or disaster aimed at reducing the severity or duration of event-related distress. For mental health service providers, this may involve psychological first aid, needs assessment, consultation, fostering resilience and natural supports, and triage, as well as psychological and medical treatment.

Interventions include provision of the following:

1. Basic needs
2. Psychological first aid
3. Needs assessment
4. Rescue and recovery environment observation
5. Outreach and information dissemination
6. Technical assistance, consultation, and training
7. Fostering resilience and recovery
8. Triage
9. Treatment

In regard to training, there are specific issues to consider when conducting mental health studies in foreign nations. International authors agree that a definite level of cultural social awareness, support for indigenous and local authorities, multi-integration into capacity and infrastructure rebuilding, understanding of the political dynamic (especially in regions where there is conflict), and assessment of mental health based on scientific and clinical knowledge are imperative from an ethical standpoint and will increase the success of the program.[33]

WORKER SAFETY AND FIRST RESPONDERS

In the United States, there are more than 1 million firefighters, with about 75% of those on a volunteer-basis; 556,000 full-time law enforcement personnel at police departments; 291,000 full-time sheriff's personnel; and more than 155,000 nationally registered EMTs.[34] These first responders are faced with dual functions: report the first observations about the environment and its risks and simultaneously carry out prehospital tasks. Because the disaster scene is dynamic, with active primary and secondary hazards, emergency responders must characterize the site, where oftentimes the evidence of the causative agent is not yet determined and therefore situational awareness is imperative. This poses emotional, mental, and physical challenges where dangers are likely to arise.

Disasters present emergency responders with primary hazards stemming from the actual causative agent. For example, the release or spillage of a chemical can cause toxic injury, whether it is by a physical asphyxiant (e.g., hypoxemia from inert gas in an enclosed space such as a silo), respiratory irritant (e.g., pulmonary damage and inflammatory response from chlorine or phosgene), or systemic toxicants (e.g., upper airway or alveolar injury or skin or neurological damage from organophosphates, volatile hydrocarbons, or hydrogen cyanide).

Emergency first responders are also jeopardized by secondary risks on site. These hazards can take the shape of several types of environmental risks. For example, rescue personnel can be in danger of confronting hazards from disasters such as riots, explosions and fires, road accidents, farm accidents, factory accidents, and railroad disasters.[35] Consider a scenario in which an overturned tanker truck has caused a major road accident; emergency personnel are likely to confront vehicle fires, fuel explosions, the instability of overturned vehicles and truck loads and cargo, the dangers of traffic control and safety, and exposure to release of toxic and dangerous chemicals. Explosions present the first responder with the potential of building collapse, secondary explosions, and toxic smoke release hazards.

First responders are trained to use PPE for a chemical, biological, or radiological event, either intentional or unintentional (as is the case with an industrial accident). Toxic agents can be "invisible" to the senses, and the quantity, type, and time of exposure are not easily known. The National Institute of Justice (NIJ) states: "The purpose of personal protective clothing and equipment is to shield or isolate individuals from the chemical, physical, and biological hazards that may be encountered during hazardous materials operations."[36] PPE consists of a wardrobe of clothing and gear that allows the responder to confront and thwart exposure and to function normally. NIJ categorizes PPE into the three following basic categories[36]:

- Respiratory equipment (e.g., air purifying respirators and supplied air respirators)
- Protective garments (e.g., encapsulated suits, coveralls, and overgarments)
- Other protective apparel (e.g., protective hoods, boots, and gloves)

The NIJ *Guide for the Selection of Personal Protective Equipment for Emergency First Responders* is a good resource for more thorough and detailed information on PPE.[36]

As the National Institute for Safety and Health points out, large incidents (such as the terrorist attack on the World Trade Center), unlike smaller-scale disasters (such as localized traffic accidents and explosions), pose serious challenges that make it more difficult to protect the responder from injury, illness, and death. Large-scale disasters can do the following[37]:

- Affect, injure, or kill large numbers of people
- Cover large geographical areas
- Require prolonged response operations
- Involve multiple, highly varied hazards
- Require a wide range of capabilities and resources not routinely maintained by local response organizations
- Attract a sizable influx of independent ("convergent") volunteers and supplies
- Damage vital transportation, communications, and public works infrastructures
- Directly affect the operational capacity of responder organizations

Therefore, responder safety also requires human resource management, in which thoughtful planning can help one to operate in a chaotic, multiagency environment. This includes charting out the chronology of the response (short-term and extended); setting reasonable and efficient work shifts to prevent the exhaustion of personnel; controlling the perimeter and scene to manage convergent volunteers; inventorying and providing access to PPE and resources; and developing highly skilled "disaster safety managers" who possess experience, knowledge, and tactical skills to respond to hazards on site.[37] Importantly, and not often considered to be a life-saving function, is the need to manage health and disaster information flooding the scene. This includes the delivery and sharing of critical information among multiple agencies of all types and levels in addition to making sense of overabundant information. This information can include reports of the changing conditions of the disaster scene; data on the number of available workers and their respective health conditions; and standard data on the number, type, and availability of PPE and important resources.[38]

DATA COLLECTION AND ANALYSIS

Public health detection and analysis follow key functional areas that involve the development and use of surveillance systems, analysis via algorithms and statistical methods, and investigation of disease and injury with great emphasis on critical agents.[5] Biological agents of highest concern, as categorized by the CDC, are *B. anthracis* (anthrax), *Y. pestis* (plague), variola major (smallpox), *C. botulinum* toxin (botulism), *Francisella tularensis* (tularemia), filoviruses (Ebola hemorrhagic fever, Marburg hemorrhagic fever), and arenaviruses (Lassa [Lassa fever], Junin [Argentine hemorrhagic fever], and related viruses).[27]

Epidemiology in bioterrorist incidents is not too different from standard epidemiological investigations.[39] First, laboratory and clinical findings are used to confirm that an outbreak has occurred, using case definitions to determine the number of cases and attack rate. To characterize unusual levels of activity, the attack rate for the disease in question is compared against that of previous years to measure deviation from the norm. The outbreak can then be characterized in terms of time, place, and person, lending crucial data to determine the origin of the disease.[39] By analyzing data of cases over time, an epidemic curve can be calculated that will allow for differentiation between an outbreak and normal pattern of disease.[39] However, if an intentional release of a biological agent is suspected, time is of the essence, and as previously emphasized, early detection is key. Therefore, the development of surveillance systems, including syndromic surveillance systems and real-time computer models, are being developed. Surveillance "concentrates on the incidence, prevalence, and severity of illness or injury due to ecological changes, changes in endemic levels of disease, population displacement, loss of usual source of health care, overcrowding, breakdowns in sanitation, disruption of public utilities, monitors increases in communicable diseases, including vector-borne, waterborne, and person-to-person transmission" and ultimately helps one to determine an association between exposure and outcome, whether that outcome includes specific injuries, illnesses, or death.[20] In setting up a surveillance system, managers should consider using existing systems, such as those used to track reportable diseases, or developing temporary systems to track specific injuries and illnesses before, during, or after the disaster.[20] Primary and secondary sources of data need to be identified and can vary from patient medical records (primary) to victim surveys and interviews (secondary). Primary data collection methods are direct observations or surveys, and secondary methods are interviews with key informants or review of existing records.[20]

Data sets can be obtained from numerous places, including state hospitalization data, hospitals and clinics, private providers, insurance companies, temporary shelters, first responders, and mobile health clinics.[20] Increasingly, nontraditional data sources such as worker sick days from employer records are being used to screen for disease outbreaks. Next, case definitions need to be developed for uniformity of reporting outcomes. Finally, appropriate analytical methods should be used and can include descriptive measures, geographical analysis of spread, rates of disease or death, or an analysis over time measuring total numbers of cases and rates of appearance.[20] It is also important to remember that in a disaster situation, rigorous epidemiological approaches may not be time-conducive and that there will be an immediate need to quickly collect key, important data that may be perishable as time goes on and populations change in exposure and impact to the hazard. As a result, disaster situations invoke the use of "quick and dirty" data collection, "quick" being simple and flexible and "dirty" being that some quantitative data are rough estimates gathered to answer immediate questions.[18]

Increasingly, for bioterrorism purposes, health departments are developing and testing syndromic surveillance systems. *Syndromic surveillance* is "an investigational approach where health department staff, assisted by automated data acquisition and generation of statistical alarms, monitor disease indicators continually (real-time) or at least daily (near real-time) to detect outbreaks of diseases earlier and more completely than would otherwise be possible with traditional public health methods (e.g., by reportable disease surveillance or telephone consultation)." Syndromic surveillance uses nontraditional data sources, or those other than laboratory data. These data reflect events "that precede clinical diagnosis, such as emergency department chief complaints, clinical impressions on ambulance run sheets, prescriptions filled, retail drug and product purchases, school or work absenteeism, and constellations of medical signs and symptoms in persons seen in various clinical settings."[40]

PUBLIC HEALTH ASSESSMENT

CDC deployed field teams to New York City emergency departments on Sept. 14, 2001, to conduct surveillance for possible covert biological releases. For the first two weeks, epidemic intelligence service officers (EISOs) staffed 15 hospitals for 24 hours and then provided 18-hour coverage at 12 hospitals for the remaining 30-day surveillance period. The teams entered data on-site and reported data to the New York City departments of Health and Mental Health each morning and followed up on significant cases. Between Sept. 13 and Oct. 12, 68,546 emergency department visits were recorded, with trauma as the highest syndrome-to-none-ratio (SNR) found (18.6%), followed by exacerbation of a chronic respiratory condition (7.6%). Diarrhea/gastroenteritis (4.4%) and upper and lower respiratory infections (4.2%) were also reported. Children younger than 15 years presented most often with respiratory syndrome complaints (67%) and rash syndromes (59%). Those between 25 and 64 years old made up 80% of inhalational visits and 75% of anxiety visits. Analyses were also specifically conducted for home postal codes within a two-mile radius of the World Trade Center and revealed that persons in the two-mile radius were no more likely to have a syndrome of bioterrorism interest than those who were outside of that proximity. However, the study found that people in close proximity to the towers on Sept. 11 were 61.5 times more likely to visit the emergency department for smoke/dust inhalation complaints than people from other areas. Overall, no health data to support a bioterrorist release were found.[41]

CONCLUSION

Historically, promoting and managing the health of a society have shown to increase the welfare of the community. This discipline, called public health, is a broad one, encompassing multiple sectors of the community and professional fields; government and nongovernment agencies; and local, regional, federal, and sometimes international institutions. Collectively, these groups respond to disasters to study, reduce, and develop ways to mitigate adverse health effects in the future. This chapter has summarized phases of the disaster cycle, the players involved, and the basic policy of disaster declaration and response. Additionally, we have reviewed components of public health infrastructure, provision of medical services, education and communications in disasters, mental health issues, worker safety, and finally the value and techniques of data collection and analysis.

It is recommended that the newcomer to public health and disaster medicine review the many references in this chapter and refer to resources on the Internet. Importantly, responders should be proactive and become trained, well-informed, experienced providers and openly disseminate factual knowledge to the community and their peers. This is the beginning to a more efficient, life-saving public health response to disasters.

REFERENCES

1. Ten Great Public Health Achievements—United States, 1900-1999. *MMWR.* April 1999;48(12):241-3. Available at: http://www.cdc.gov/mmwr/preview/mmwrhtml/00056796.htm.
2. Gostin LO. Public health law, ethics, and human rights: mapping the issues. Available at: http://www.publichealthlaw.net/Reader/ch1/ch1.htm.
3. Institute of Medicine, Committee on the Future of Public Health. *The Future of Public Health.* Washington, DC: National Academy Press; 1988.
4. Centers for Disease Control and Prevention. Public health emergency response guide for state, local, and tribal public health directors. Version 1.0. Available at: http://www.bt.cdc.gov.
5. Biological and chemical terrorism: strategic plan for preparedness and response: recommendations of the CDC Strategic Planning Workgroup. *MMWR.* April 2000;49(RR-04):1-14.
6. National Emergency Management Association. National response plan—initial draft. Available at: http://www.nemaweb.org/docs/national_response_plan.pdf.
7. National Governors Association. *A Governor's Guide to Emergency Management. Volume One: Natural Disasters.* Washington, DC: National Governors Association; 2001.
8. Bea K. *Federal Disaster Policies After Terrorists Strike: Issues and Options for Congress.* American National Government and Finance Division; 2002.
9. US General Accounting Office. *Bioterrorism: Public Health and Medical Preparedness.* Testimony Before the Subcommittee on Public Health, Committee on Health, Education, Labor, and Pensions. Washington, DC: US General Accounting Office; 2001. Available at: http://www.gao.gov/new.items/d02141t.pdf.
10. US Department of Homeland Security. Initial national response plan fact sheet. Available at: http://www.dhs.gov/dhspublic/display?content=1936.
11. American Public Health Association. One year after the terrorist attacks: is public health prepared? A report card from the American Public Health Association. Available at: http://www.apha.org/united/reportcardfile.htm#back1.
12. US General Accounting Office. *Combating Terrorism: FEMA Continues to Make Progress in Coordinating Preparedness and Response.* Washington, DC: US General Accounting Office; 2001. Available at: http://www.gao.gov/new.items/d0115.pdf.
13. National Association of County and City Health Officials. *Preliminary Results from the 1997 Profile of U.S. Local Health Departments.* Washington, DC: National Association of County and City Health Officials; 1998. Available at: http://www.edgewood.army.mil/downloads/reports/comp_mass_casualty_care.pdf.
14. Landesman LY. *Public Health Management of Disasters, the Practice Guide.* Washington, DC: American Public Health Association; 2001.
15. CBS News. Floridians seek relief. Available at: http://www.cbsnews.com/stories/2004/09/28/national/main646024.shtml.
16. Community Outreach, Mass Prophylaxis: a mass casualty care strategy for biological terrorism incidents, June 2001.
17. O'Toole T. Smallpox: an attack scenario. *Emerg Infect Dis.* 1999;5:540-6.
18. Russell PK. Vaccines in civilian defense against bioterrorism. *Emerg Infect Dis.* July-August 1999;5(4):531-3.
19. Centers for Disease Control and Prevention. Strategic National Stockpile. Available at http://www.bt.cdc.gov/stockpile.
20. Federal Emergency Management Agency. Thousands of volunteers help Floridians recover. Available at: http://www.fema.gov/news/newsrelease.fema?id=15437.
21. GlobalSecurity.org. Great Northeast power blackout of 2003. Available at: http://www.globalsecurity.org/eye/blackout_2003.htm.
22. CNN.com. Power returns to most areas hit by blackout, U.S.-Canadian task force charged with investigating outage. Available at: http://www.cnn.com/2003/US/08/15/power.outage.
23. American Medical Association. Featured CSA report: Medical preparedness for terrorism and other disasters. Available at: http://www.ama-assn.org/ama/pub/category/print/14313.html.
24. National Foundation for Trauma Care. U.S. trauma center crisis: lost in the scramble for terror resources. Available at: http://www.traumacare.com/NFTC_CrisisReport_May04.pdf.

25. US General Accounting Office. *SARS Outbreak: Improvements to Public Health Capacity Are Needed for Responding to Bioterrorism and Emerging Infectious Diseases.* Washington, DC: US General Accounting Office; 2003. Available at: http://www.gao.gov/new.items/d03769t.pdf.

26. US Department of Homeland Security. Top Officials (TOPOFF) Exercise Series: TOPOFF2. After action summary report for public release. Available at: http://www.dhs.gov/interweb/assetlibrary/T2_Report_Final_Public.doc.

27. Recognition of illness associated with the intentional release of a biologic agent. *MMWR.* Oct 2001;50(41):893-7.

28. Lane HC, Fauci AS. Bioterrorism on the home front: a new challenge for American medicine. *JAMA.* 2001;286:2595-7.

29. North CS, Kawasaki A, Spitznagel EL, Hong BA. The course of PTSD, major depression, substance abuse, and somatization after a natural disaster. *J Nerv Ment Dis.* December 2004;192(12):823-9.

30. Dubouloz M. Mental health. In: de Boer J, Dubouloz M, eds. *Handbook of Disaster Medicine.* Netherlands: Van der Wees Publishers; 2000.

31. US Department of Veteran Affairs, National Center for PTSD. Available at: http://www.ncptsd.va.gov.

32. National Institute of Mental Health. *Mental Health and Mass Violence: Evidence-Based Early Psychological Intervention for Victims/Survivors of Mass Violence. A Workshop to Reach Consensus on Best Practices.* Washington, DC: US Government Printing Office; 2002. NIH Publication No. 02-5138. Available at: http://www.nimh.nih.gov/healthinformation/massviolence_intervention.cfm.

33. Weine S, Danieli Y, Silove D, Van Ommeren M, et al. Guidelines for international training in mental health and psychosocial interventions for trauma exposed populations in clinical and community settings. *Psychiatry.* Summer 2002;65(2):156-64.

34. US Department of Homeland Security. About first responders. Available at: http://www.dhs.gov/dhspublic/display?theme=63&content=237.

35. Badiali S. Pre-hospital care. In: de Boer J, Dubouloz M, eds. *Handbook of Disaster Medicine.* Netherlands: Van der Wees Publishers; 2000.

36. National Institute of Justice. Guide for the selection of personal protective equipment for emergency first responders. NIJ Guide 102-00 (Volumes I, IIa, IIb, and IIc.) Available at: http://www.ojp.usdoj. gov/nij/pubs-sum/191518.htm.

37. Centers for Disease Control and Prevention. Protecting emergency responders, volume 3. Available at: http://www.cdc.gov/niosh/docs/2004-144.

38. RAND. Protecting emergency responders: lessons learned from terrorist attacks. Available at: http://www.rand.org/publications/CF/CF176.

39. Pavlin J. Epidemiology of bioterrorism. *Emerg Infect Dis.* July-August 1999;5(4):528-30.

40. Centers for Disease Col and Prevention. Draft framework for evaluating syndromic surveillance systems for bioterrorism preparedness. Available at: AU: ?

41. Syndromic surveillance for bioterrorism following the attacks on the World Trade Center—New York City, 2001. *MMWR.* September 2002;51(special issue): 13-15. Available at: http://www.cdc.gov/mmwr/preview/mmwrhtml/mm51SPa5.htm.

chapter 3

The Role of Emergency Medical Services (EMS) in Disaster

Robert D. Furberg and David E. Marcozzi

The role of emergency medical services (EMS) systems in disaster management is to provide effective, responsible prehospital care; however, multiple considerations must be made long before the first EMS unit arrives on scene. Disaster management may be examined in the following four phases[1]:

1. Prevention and planning
2. Preparedness
3. Response
4. Recovery/analysis

The process of prevention and planning uses an effective application of the hazard vulnerability analysis (HVA) concepts discussed briefly later in this chapter and in more detail in Chapter 17. The HVA establishes the probability of risk and identifies key components of an operative response plan. Measures to reduce potential loss of life and property may be achieved through the combined effort among members of the jurisdiction's local emergency planning committee (LEPC) and other participants in incident response.

Preparatory functions of management personnel must occur to ensure that responders, emergency managers, and citizens are adequately informed of and trained on appropriate operational expectations.

During the response phase, public safety personnel must implement the Incident Command System early and effectively. Once operating within the paradigm, responders assume the specific tasks required to mitigate the incident. Triage, treatment, and transport are the highest priorities for most paramedics and emergency medical personnel. Specialized medical units with the necessary training and equipment may assume additional duties as directed by the incident commander.

Initial and long-term recovery efforts are directed toward the reconstruction and rehabilitation of infrastructure and the community. EMS systems usually do not serve a primary role in recovery, but this final phase of management is critical for system reassessment and improvement. Analysis of specific methodologies used during incident management, including the efficacy of triage and predictive outcome assessments, are useful to the global community.[2]

After their inception on the battlefield, modern civilian EMS systems have found themselves using many of the same techniques, under similar conditions, as the pioneers of the field when managing disasters domestically. Modern EMS systems are capable of moderating the daily burden of emergencies; however, disaster operations often require emergency services to assume a different perspective to ensure effective resolution of significant incidents. This chapter details the operational adjustments that have been designed to optimize the role of EMS in disaster management.[3]

HISTORICAL PERSPECTIVE

EMS is a product of war. From the first organized use of ambulances on the battlefields of Crimea to the birth of the modern field medic in the jungles of Vietnam, the history of EMS is undeniably blood-tinged with rich militaristic tradition.

Baron Dominique-Jean Larrey, Napoleon's surgeon-in-chief, is largely credited with placing the first ambulance in service more than 150 years ago during the Crimean War. Larry, well-versed in the critical nature of traumatic injuries, initiated the use of covered, horse-drawn carts to expedite the movement of injured soldiers to treatment areas. This improvement drastically reduced the number of ineffective combat troops recovered from battle.

During the Civil War, Clara Barton coordinated and rendered emergency care to wounded infantry. After serving as the superintendent of Union nurses, she crusaded tirelessly for medical relief of sick and wounded soldiers. Barton established the Red Cross within the United States, serving as the organization's first president. During her tenure, she directed relief work for disasters such as famines, floods, pestilence, and earthquakes in the United States and throughout the world.

With the improvement of military technology, casualties increased. As a consequence, soldiers received greater training in the management and transport of injured infantry during World War I. Aeromedical transport systems were established during World War II and refined during the Korean conflict.[4]

The corpsman of Vietnam most closely resembles the paramedic of today. Personnel were well trained in a variety of increasingly advanced interventions. Care was often rendered in extreme environments to multiple patients at once. The military demonstrated a profound effect on battlefield mortality rates with the aggressive application of early advanced intervention and expeditious transport via helicopter from the front lines of engagement to definitive care installations. The evolution of trauma care in military medicine proved to be the major factor in a progressive decrease in casualties among compromised soldiers. Casualty rates were reduced from 8% in World War I to 4.5% in WWII to 2.5% in the Korean War to less than 2% during the Vietnam conflict.[5] Despite aggressive engineering feats that mechanized warfare and drastically increased the power of ordnance, the medical experience gained from the two World Wars and multiple international conflicts resulted in fewer soldiers killed in combat. The shift from empiricism to the practice of evidence-based medicine and the provision of acute care in the field made armed conflict much more survivable. The immense benefits of rapid, advanced field stabilization and swift transport to definitive care facilities realized by the armed services would soon become the expectation of politicians and civilians alike in the United States.

After the advances made in trauma care on the battlefield, researchers in the United States during the early 1960s found that an infantry soldier in Vietnam had a statistically greater chance of survival than the average citizen involved in a motor vehicle collision on any of the nation's highways. This disparity prompted two significant legislative acts in 1966. First, the National Academy of Sciences-National Research Council (NAS-NRC) published *Accidental Death and Disability: The Neglected Disease of Modern Society*. This white paper put forth 11 recommendations to improve care for injured persons. Recommendations included the creation of various standards within EMS, including training, public safety infrastructure, and the creation of "... a single nationwide number to summon an ambulance." The second bill prepared by Congress was the Highway Safety Act of 1966. This act mandated the creation of the U.S. Department of Transportation (USDOT) and the National Highway Traffic Safety Administration (NHTSA). Both entities provided legislative authority and financial assistance to EMS systems in the United States. Between 1968 and 1972, approximately $142 million was distributed among states to develop and assess the first advanced life support programs.

Initial training centered on the kinematics of trauma, stabilization, and provision of appropriate transport to definitive care facilities. Over the last three decades, EMS systems in the United States have established their own niche within the public safety sector. Paramedics have become increasingly autonomous as a result of the steadily expanding complexity of medical conditions and treatment options. In addition to these advancements, EMS systems have remained a reliable resource on the "domestic battleground," where individuals in need of assistance may exceed available resources. To ensure that an EMS system is used most effectively in large-scale incidents, a specific, highly organized structure was developed.

However, before that structure was established, major incidents in the civilian sector routinely required the response of several agencies. Effective management was often confounded by multiple entities performing independently of one another without adequate interaction or communication. A significant example of how impaired communications can poorly affect the outcome of event mitigation can be demonstrated by what occurred after the attack on the World Trade Center on Sept. 11, 2001. New York City's Office of Emergency Management (OEM) assumed its current form in 1996 and was headquartered at 7 World Trade Center.[6,7] Communications from OEM were based off an antenna atop 1 World Trade Center. Less than nine hours after the first strike, 7 World Trade Center collapsed, significantly impairing coordinative abilities among EMS, the New York Police Department, and the Fire Department of New York. Responders lacked the common resource to communicate reliably among these agencies due to the lack of radio frequency interoperability. Additionally, triage and transport of patients were adversely affected by the lack of coordinated communications with local and regional hospitals in the New York City metropolitan area.[8-9]

During the early 1970s, fire administrators in California developed the Incident Command System (ICS) to manage rapidly moving wildfires and operational deficits that were previously encountered. Specific complications cited before the creation of the ICS included "too many people reporting to one supervisor; different emergency response organizational structures; lack of reliable incident information; inadequate and incompatible communications; lack of structure for coordinated planning among agencies; unclear lines of authority; terminology differences among agencies; and unclear or unspecified incident objectives." In 1980, federal officials developed a national program called the National Interagency Incident Management System (NIIMS) based on the original ICS construct. The inherent flexibility of the ICS to accommodate issues of incident size and utilization of available resources has allowed the system to be used to mitigate both minor crises and major disasters exacted by nature and humans alike. As public safety personnel developed familiarity with the ICS, the federal government identified the need for the development of a body of government to establish standards of practice within increasingly complex applications of disaster management. In response to the increasing threat of terror attacks and the need to ensure a more cohesive response to large-scale incidents, federal guidelines were created to establish the role of EMS.[10,11]

In 1998, Congress issued a report underscoring concern regarding "... the real and potentially catastrophic effects of a chemical or biological act of terrorism." Legislators indicated that although the federal government is integral in the prevention and secondary response to such incidents, state and local public safety personnel who respond initially require additional assistance. The Appropriations Act (Public Law 105-119) authorized the U.S. attorney general to aid state and local responders in acquiring specialized training and equipment to "... safely respond to and manage terrorist incidents involving weapons of mass destruction (WMD)."

The U.S. attorney general delegated authority to the Office of Justice Programs (OJP) on April 30, 1998, to develop and administer training and equipment assistance programs for state and local emergency response agencies. To accomplish this mission, the Office for Domestic Preparedness (ODP) was established to develop and administer a national domestic preparedness program.

On Oct. 8, 2001, by executive order, the Office of Homeland Security and the Homeland Security Council were established. The functions of the newly created offices included incident management and oversight of preparation, response, and recovery after terrorist incidents. The Homeland Security Act of 2002 formally established the Department of Homeland Security (DHS). In the most significant federal restructuring since the 1960s, the newly anointed DHS has been placed in command of 22 government agencies, including the Federal Emergency Management Agency.[12]

CURRENT PRACTICE

The role of EMS in the disaster management paradigm incorporates the four-phase approach of prevention and planning, preparedness, response, and recovery/analysis. These key phases have defined the mitigation of crises of all sizes since their inception in the early 1970s. After the establishment of the DHS and ODP, both agencies issued guidelines for municipal, state, and federal responders within public safety. These guidelines, in conjunction with the serial reassessment of current practice methodologies, allow responders to ensure that the most appropriate management strategies have been selected for a given situation. Adhering to the use of this construct allows EMS systems to optimize their ability to react to disaster.[13,14]

The prevention and planning phase includes the identification of specific hazards, threat assessments to life and property, and preemptive steps to minimize potential losses. Measures to reduce potential loss of life and property are commonly referred to as *disaster mitigation*. Mitigation measures may include public awareness campaigns, LEPC involvement, and legislative action.

Preparedness encompasses the training and education of both public safety personnel and members of the community. The DHS has specified the ODP as the lead agency for directing domestic preparedness efforts and creating standards for the implementation of response plans. Under executive order, the National Disaster Medical System (NDMS) was formed in 1983. With cooperation between local communities and the federal government, Disaster Medical Assistance Team (DMAT) and International Medical and Surgical Response Team (IMSuRT) resources have developed throughout the nation. These deployable teams are designed to be a rapid-response element to supplement local medical care until contract resources or federal assistance can be mobilized. The responsibility of DMATs may include triaging patients, providing high-quality medical care despite the challenging environment found within disaster scenes, and assisting with patient evacuation. EMS personnel who participate in operations involving a DMAT deployment often are used in more of a primary care role rather than their typical emergency response capacity. The development of a strong relationship among primary care facilities, providers, and EMS systems regionally during the planning phase of action may significantly improve the transition of EMS personnel into this role. The NDMS also ensures that teams are equipped to sustain operations for 72 hours without additional resources. This dramatic difference underscores the disparity between routine and extended operations. Typically, EMS systems and personnel may be equipped or prepared to function for 24 to 48 hours; however, major disaster scenes are rarely mitigated completely without a more significant time commitment.[15-17]

On Aug. 1, 2002, the ODP released its *Emergency Responder Guidelines* to assist agencies in establishing a baseline understanding of the training necessary to safely and effectively respond to incidents involving the use of WMD. Designed and compiled as a resource, the guidelines present advice of experts from the private and public sectors. The guidelines were prepared with assistance from key federal agencies involved with first-responder training and incorporated existing codes and standards established by the National Fire Protection Agency and the U.S. Occupational Safety and Health Administration. The guidelines provide an integrated compilation of baseline knowledge, skills, and responder capabilities for use as a reference by providers as well as course developers and trainers to underscore the importance of interoperable response strategies. The *Emergency Responder Guidelines* specify training objectives and establish the baseline level of operational knowledge of three distinct levels of responsibility— awareness, performance, and management—required of specific response disciplines (Table 3-1). Training is based on a provider's level of experience and operational accountability with the three levels of responsibility. Commonalities among specific response disciplines (e.g., law enforcement, fire, EMS) illustrate areas in which common training and understanding can be established to ensure a more cohesive operational response.[18,19]

Awareness-level guidelines pertain to law enforcement officers, firefighters, and basic level emergency medical technicians. At a minimum, response personnel within this category are expected to be among the first to encounter an incident. Once management operations are under way, awareness-level personnel assume a more supportive role. These providers are responsible for recognition and referral after encountering a hazardous environment. The training objectives establish a basic understanding of operational actions, including notification of need for additional specialized resources, maintenance of scene control, and demonstrated competence of self-protection measures.

Performance-level guidelines apply primarily to advanced level providers on scene, including paramedics and firefighters involved in rescue or fire suppression operations or a hazardous materials event. Depending on the various ICS assignments in use during a given incident, the performance-level providers must efficiently multitask their primary responsibilities with additional

TABLE 3-1 LEVELS OF RESPONSIBILITY

AWARENESS	PERFORMANCE	MANAGEMENT
Recognize hazardous materials (HazMat) incidents.	Have successfully completed proper training at awareness and performance levels.	Have successfully completed proper training in awareness, performance, and management levels.
Know protocols used to detect WMD agents or materials.	Know ICS and UCS, and assist with implementation as needed.	Know and follow ICS and UCS procedures. Understand how the systems are implemented and integrated.
Know and follow self-protection measures for WMD and HazMat events.	Know and follow self-protection measures and rescue and evacuation procedures.	Know and follow protocols to provide emergency medical treatment to persons involved in the event.
Know procedures for protecting a potential crime scene.	Know and follow procedures for working at the scene of a potential WMD event.	Know and follow self-protection measures.
Know and follow agency's or organization's scene security and control procedures for WMD and HAZMAT events.		Know plans and assets available for transporting the victims of events to primary care facilities.
Possess and know how to properly use equipment to contact higher authorities to request additional assistance or emergency response personnel.		Know and follow procedures for protecting a potential crime scene.
		Know and follow department procedures for medical monitoring of response personnel involved.

Adapted from Office for Domestic Preparedness. *Emergency Response Guidelines. August 1, 2003.*

assignments from their commander. As a consequence, performance-level personnel require a strong working knowledge of the ICS and the ability to follow the Unified Command System (UCS). The provider must be able to follow procedures for the integration and implementation of each system and know how the two structures can be used to manage the incident. Procedures include establishing adequate communication capabilities to manage the incident; securing triage, treatment, and transport areas; and coordinating multiple responding agencies. The performance-level responder must also demonstrate competence in self-protection measures, rescue and decontamination operations, and evacuation procedures for managing victims.

Planning-level and management-level providers are typically service administrators, supervisors, and emergency management officials. Those who operate within these guidelines must first complete both awareness-level and performance-level objectives. Individuals responsible for training at this level will be a part of the leadership and management of subordinate emergency medical personnel during the response operation. Objectives include planning before the incident as well as managing resources used to conduct the event. Leadership personnel must also be capable of overseeing medical surveillance of subordinates.

In accordance with the preparatory phase, the ODP offers multiple training opportunities for responders at all levels. To enhance the capacity of local and state agencies, the ODP's Equipment Grant Program provides funds to 50 states, the District of Columbia, the Commonwealth of Puerto Rico, American Samoa, the Commonwealth of Northern Mariana Islands (CNMI), Guam, and the U.S. Virgin Islands.[20]

The priority among EMS responders must be rendering responsible prehospital care. To enable this goal, responders must first integrate an ICS into their response plan to allow for effective management of an incident.

During the response phase, multiple responders and agencies must be coordinated to operate effectively. Civilian responses routinely incorporate the responsibility of several different specialties, such as fire and rescue, EMS, and law enforcement, beneath a single commander. As the scale of an incident grows, the command structure must expand to meet the increasingly diverse needs to provide effective management. With large-scale incidents, the underlying organizational construct becomes even more critical as coordination extends to incorporate local, state, and federal resource allocation.

All responders on scene must be familiar with the structure and function of the ICS and UCS. The ICS enables integrated communication by establishing a manageable span of control. Beneath a single incident commander (IC), subordinate commanders exercise their own span of control among context-specific divisions. The overall structure of the system describes four divisions beneath the IC, including operations, planning, logistics, and finance. With each application of the ICS, commanders may elect how to delegate these various designations among responders. The benefits of operating within the ICS structure are apparent. First, the role of every responder on scene is clearly defined by the commander. Leadership responsibilities are delegated, optimizing the ability of each officer to complete very specific tasks. Ability to ensure the fulfillment of every critical intervention is simplified.

As local responders arrive, an initial ICS system is established to manage resources. Upon the arrival of additional local, state, federal, and private-party personnel, the ICS structure may be modified to accommodate the expanding operation. The purpose and function of the UCS is to allow for expansion of the initial ICS structure. When operating within a large-scale incident, the UCS allows for the unification of multiple ICs. The IC is responsible for overall management of the incident and directs incident activities, including development and implementation of overall objectives and strategies as well as the ordering and releasing of resources. Members of the UCS work together to develop a common set of incident objectives, produce strategies, share information, maximize the use of available resources, and enhance the efficiency of the individual response organizations.

The final phase of disaster management is the process of recovery/analysis. Initial recovery is the method by which an affected community is assisted in regaining a proper level of functioning after an incident. Long-term recovery addresses community-specific deficits of reconstruction and rehabilitation. The roles of EMS systems in these direct recovery processes are usually limited; however, systems must address their own logistical and psychological recovery so that they can return to a proper level of functioning after an incident. Specifically, equipment must be accounted for and repaired if necessary and disposable supplies must be replaced and organized. A critical function of recovery within an EMS system must also account for responder well-being. Critical incident stress debriefing (CISD) or jurisdictional peer-moderated counseling may accommodate the personal recovery necessary to resume normal operations. Alternatively, this phase affords the EMS system the opportunity to engage in critical analysis of its own performance during the incident. The opportunity to engage in self-assessment is critical in identifying system weaknesses that may be targeted in future improvements as well as create the forum for commending personal actions that had a positive influence on the outcome of an incident. On completion, this analysis offers evidence that may be used to support the use of specific methodologies.[20-23]

Although also considered an element of preparation, exercise planning and evaluation programs provide valuable data for review. The ODP's Homeland Security Exercise and Evaluation Program provides state and national opportunities for evaluating response methodologies. For example, the ODP conducted the Top Officials (TOPOFF 2) exercise May 12-16, 2003. The event was the largest of its kind, involving 25 federal, state, and local agencies and departments and the Canadian government to test domestic incident management. The exercise simulated the detonation of a radiological dispersal device in Seattle, Wash., and the release of the pneumonic plague in several Chicago metropolitan areas. There was also significant pre-exercise intelligence play, a simulated cyber-attack, and credible mock terrorism threats against other locations. After the completion of the exercise, significant discussion was initiated to critique the response. After extensive review, DHS provided a detailed after-incident report for public release on Dec. 19, 2003.

The "T2 After Action Summary Report" cited multiple topics of interest following analysis. Critical shortcomings were noted within the Homeland Security Advisory System. Participating jurisdictions failed to agree on reaction to the elevation of the nation's threat condition to "red/severe" for the first time; declarations of "disaster" and "emergency" by officials revealed confusion among interagency responders. During the exercise, DHS used the newly developed role of principal federal official (PFO) in an effort to create a single position of accountability to bridge federal and local governments. Evaluators observed integration of the PFO within ICS/UCS paradigms. In addition, logistically complex prophylaxis distribution from the Strategic National Stockpile was evaluated. Challenges associated with resource allocation, communications, and information-sharing during the mock public health emergency illustrated the need for improvements within the participating municipal systems. Operationally, balancing the safety of first responders and the rescue of victims by conducting a detailed risk-benefit analysis was deficient among participants functioning at the planning/management level.

Analysis of significant incidents worldwide may also offer some compelling data. Modeling triage methods based on the predictive value of anatomical scoring systems has revealed evidence-based, outcome-driven improvements in field triage and resource allocation. Significant analysis of the outcome among blunt and penetrating trauma patients provided the framework for the Sacco Triage Method. Support for improvements in the management of disaster result only from effective analysis. Due to the globalization of healthcare and mitigation, the resulting data from events worldwide must be delivered in a useful format. Application of the Utstein template may be useful to ensure international value of data by standardizing terminology and significance. Originally created to classify data used to determine cardiac arrest survival rates and allow for international comparison of statistically similar events, the Utstein method has been applied to disaster outcome in recent years. Applying sound epidemiological methods to postincident management is critical to the reduction of empiricism within disaster medicine methodology.[24]

PITFALLS

The role of EMS systems in a disaster is to provide responsible prehospital care to victims. To facilitate this objective effectively, EMS personnel must use the ICS/UCS and effective triage methodology. Multiple, universal shortcomings must be addressed even before responders find themselves on the scene of a major incident. Systems easily succumb to inadequacies in the prevention/preparation phase despite the widespread availability of federal training resources and funding. Specifically, failure to provide appropriate HVA, inexperience among responders in the application of ICS, and shortsighted planning on the part of management-level personnel allow for massive deficits in domestic response.

HVA describes the process by which potential events are scrutinized using three categories: probability, risk, and preparedness. Probability is determined by analyzing the known direct risk, relevant historical data, and any additional pertinent statistics. The risk assessment defines potential totals among lives, property, financial, and legal stature. Finally, preparedness integrates the overall value of probability and risk into a cohesive plan that dictates training requirements, contingency plans, and resource allocation. On completion, the HVA allows managers to consider common elements within preparedness procedures. These priorities are then used to direct a coordinated and integrated effort among all necessary participants within incident management, affording an ease of transition into the ICS/USC paradigm. Widespread failure to adequately address HVA has direct implications on the effective establishment of ICS/USC during the initial response phase of an incident.

Improper or inadequate training in the use of the approved ICS structure may further complicate an incident during the initial response phase. Failure to acknowledge the importance of a properly functioning leadership model can quickly overwhelm the entire operation. It is critical for responders to understand that implementation of a dynamic command structure, which can expand as needed and easily integrate multiple responding agencies, may precede actual patient care. As a part of the initial assessment by the IC, a detailed risk-benefit analysis must be confirmed to ensure environmental suitability for rescue efforts to even begin. Providers are easily overwhelmed when inadequate resources impair their ability to provide emergency care to those in need. The greater critical failure in this example becomes clear as direct threats to rescuers greatly impede the success of an entire incident. Fortunately, all EMS personnel are taught the basic concepts of ICS in every initial certification course in the United States. It is imperative that agencies recognize the importance of establishing an ICS, whenever reasonable, to maximize exposure and operational familiarity among all responders. As a matter of practical familiarity, services should mandate the use of an ICS at every opportunity. The benefit to personnel at the awareness and performance levels becomes clear. As these providers gain real-time experience with the implementation of the ICS structure, delegation among divisions, and transition of command, they become more reliable with the application of the ICS concept. With repeated use, the responders use the techniques with more certainty, regardless of incident size.

Planning and preparation phase failure is extremely common and evident more so in stationary healthcare facilities. Although EMS systems have used proactive measures to ensure preparedness, many are wholly unprepared for significant events within their jurisdiction. Probability is a significant factor within the HVA process previously detailed. Minimal preparation in light of minimal risk is appropriate; however, systems must ensure that all potential incidents are adequately addressed. Despite a decreased risk within a single response area, managers must consider all aspects of mutual aid agreements, neighboring HVA results, preparation phase actions, and cohesive integration of multiple adjacent agencies. Recognizing the

failure to address critical aspects of local and regional planning/preparation efforts and effective program integration, while costly, is better managed during a jurisdiction's preincident phase rather than after the event.

REFERENCES

1. de Boer J. Order in chaos: modeling medical management in disasters. *Eur J Emerg Med.* 1999;6(2):141-8.
2. Abrahams J. Disaster management in Australia: the national emergency management system. *Emerg Med (Fremantle).* 2001;13(2): 165-73.
3. Pozner CN, Zane R, Nelson SL, Levine M. International EMS systems: the United States: past, present, and future. *Resuscitation.* 2004;60(3):239-44.
4. Sanders MJ. *Mosby's Paramedic Textbook.* Revised 2nd ed. St. Louis: Mosby; 2001:2-13.
5. Committee on Trauma and Committee on Shock, Division of Medical Sciences, National Academy of Sciences, National Research Council. *Accidental Death and Disability: The Neglected Disease of Modern Society.* Washington DC: National Academy of Sciences; 1966.
6. New York City Office of Emergency Management. Available at: http://www.ci.nyc.ny.us/html/oem/.
7. New York State Emergency Management Office. Available at: http://www.nysemo.state.ny.us/.
8. Simon R, Teperman S. The World Trade Center attack: lessons for disaster management. *Critical Care.* 2001;5:318-20.
8a. Asaeda G. The day that the START triage system came to a STOP: observations from the World Trade Center disaster. *Acad Emerg Med.* 2002;9(3):255-6.
9. US Department of Labor, Occupational Safety and Health Administration. Incident Command System eTool. Available at: http://www.osha.gov/SLTC/etools/ics/nrs.html.
10. National Interagency Management System. Available at: http://www.niims.net/.
11. US Department of Homeland Security. Available at: http://www.dhs.gov/dhspublic/.
12. Cuny FC. Principles of disaster management lesson 1: introduction. *Prehospital Disaster Med.* 1998;13(1):88-92.
13. Becker B. Disaster management: problems and solutions. *RI Med J.* 1991;74(8):383-9.
14. Alson RA, Alexander D, Leonard RD, Stringer LW. Analysis of medical treatment at a field hospital following hurricane Andrew. *Ann Emerg Med.* 1994;22(11):726-30.
15. Roth PB, Gaffney JK. The Federal Response Plan and Disaster Medical Assistance Teams in domestic disasters. *Emerg Med Clin North Am.* 1996;14:371-82.
16. US Department of Homeland Security, National Disaster Medical System. Available at: http://www.ndms.dhhs.gov/.
17. US Department of Homeland Security. Initial National Response Plan. Available at: http://www.dhs.gov/interweb/assetlibrary/Initial_NRP_100903.pdf.
18. Office of Domestic Preparedness. *Emergency Responder Guidelines.* Washington DC; 2002.
19. US Department of Homeland Security, Federal Emergency Management Agency. Available at: http://www.fema.gov/.
20. Weddle M, Prado-Monje H. Utilization of military support in the response to hurricane Marilyn: implications for future military-civilian cooperation. *Prehospital Disaster Med.* 1999;14(2):81-6.
21. Holsenbeck LS. Joint Task Force Andrew: the 44th Medical Brigade mental health staff officer's after action review. *Mil Med.* 1994;159(3):186-91.
22. Johnson WP, Lanza CV. After hurricane Andrew. An EMS perspective. *Prehospital Disaster Med.* 1993;8(2):169-71.
23. Branas CC, Sing RD, Perron AD. A case series analysis of mass casualty incidents. *Prehospital Emerg Care.* 2000;4(4):299-304.
24. Task Force on Quality Control of Disaster Management. Health disaster management: guidelines for evaluation and research in the Utstein style. Volume 1. *Prehospital Disaster Med.* 2003;1(suppl 3)17:1-177.

chapter 4

Role of Emergency Medicine in Disaster Management

Andrew I. Bern

To understand the role of emergency medicine in disaster management, one needs to understand the development and evolution of the specialty of emergency medicine, disaster medicine and disaster medical services, emergency medical services (EMS), emergency management, public health, and legislative interventions by government and nongovernment entities during the last 50 years (Table 4-1). This chapter highlights historical events that helped mold the current practice of disaster management and shines light on areas that need improvement.

Although disasters have global importance, there are differences in the approach to disaster management in the United States when compared with the rest of the world. This may, in part, be due to the nature of historical disasters in the United States. In the area of lives lost in the United States before 1987, for example, Quarantelli[1] identified only six disasters with deaths exceeding 1000 individuals. These disasters occurred between 1865 and 1928 and included two hurricanes, two fires (one on board a steamship), a flood, and an explosion on board a steamship.[1] The loss of life in the United States is contrasted by disaster events that have occurred in the rest of the world. The 1917 influenza pandemic resulted in 20 million deaths worldwide. The Soviet Union famine in 1932 left 5 million dead. A 1931 flood in the Republic of China resulted in the death of 3.7 million. A Nov. 13, 1985, volcanic eruption in Colombia resulted in the death of 21,800.[2] Flash floods killed approximately 2000 people in Mapou, Haiti.[3] More recently, more than 200,000 were killed in the tsunami of southeast Asia in December 2004.

Death tolls alone do not tell the whole story. Hurricane Andrew, which battered the United States from Aug. 14 to 27, 1992, was the costliest natural disaster in U.S. history. Total costs for both Florida and Louisiana equaled $26 billion. The cost was also felt in the homes and businesses destroyed and the population left homeless in south Florida (between "150,000 to 250,000 people were left homeless with approximately 600,000 homes and businesses destroyed or severely impaired" by the effects of Andrew).[4] Hurricane Andrew was a category four storm on the Saffir-Simpson Hurricane Scale, with sustained winds of 145 mph and gusts of up to 175 mph.[4] These numbers may be dwarfed by the total cost from damage caused by Hurricane Katrina striking the Gulf Coast of the United States in 2005.

Frequently, in nondeveloped or developing countries or those in the midst of conflicts and wars, the civilian population faces complex humanitarian emergencies. These events are multifaceted, of long duration, often involve large geographical areas, and are associated with famine and difficulty in providing or finding shelter. Many of these complex humanitarian emergencies include public health emergencies, with infectious disease outbreaks and loss of infrastructure. They often involve social, psychological, and political problems that have required the assistance of the world community— most often the United Nations, the International Committee of the Red Cross, and the interventions of multiple countries and other nongovernment groups.[5-11]

Although there is a significant amount of social science and engineering research reported by the Disaster Research Center (Newark, Del.) and the Natural Hazards Center (Boulder, Colo.), there are few centers in pursuit of clinical, bench, or even "evidence based" research that supports how disaster medicine and emergency management are practiced.

HISTORICAL PERSPECTIVE

Those who cannot remember the past are condemned to repeat it.

George Santayana

The history of mankind's fears and struggles with disasters and their aftermaths are as old as recorded history and man's fear of death. In ancient times, pagan belief was that sacrifice, including human sacrifice, would appease their deities and avert their disasters, such as an erupting volcano, climatic catastrophes, and war. Recurrent fires and floods gave rise to systematic attempts to cope with these events. After a fire destroyed almost one quarter of Rome in 6 AD, Roman Emperor Augustus created the Corps of Vigiles. This was the first recorded professionally trained and equipped fire service.[12] Early fire mitigation and recovery programs, as

TABLE 4-1 TIMELINE OF DEVELOPMENTAL/SENTINEL EVENTS

YEAR	EVENT
6 AD	The Corps of Vigiles—first professional fire service established
13th century	England: Fire protection insurance becomes available
1666	Great Fire of 1666 in London—changes that took place after this disaster resulted in the model of today's fire service
1798	Marine Hospital Service created (later to become the Public Health Service)
1917	Influenza pandemic
1931	Flood in China
1932	Famine in Soviet Union
1953	U.S. Department of Health, Education, and Welfare (cabinet level)
1954	Volcanic eruption in Colombia
1966	*Accidental Death and Disability* report by the National Academy of Sciences/National Research Council
1968	Foundation of American College of Emergency Physicians (ACEP) established
1973	Emergency medical services created
1979	Federal Emergency Management Agency formed
	FIRESCOPE and Incident Command started
	Public Health Service is moved to Department of Health and Human Services
1983	Critical incident stress debriefing begins
1988	ACEP forms Section of Disaster Medicine
1991	National Fire Protection Association begins standard development
1992	Hurricane Andrew
1993	World Trade Center attack
1995	Oklahoma City bombing
1999	Federal Response Plan
2000	Disaster Mitigation Act of 2000
2001	Joint Commission on Accreditation of Healthcare Organizations standards for preparedness change
	Sept. 11 attacks at the World Trade Center, Pentagon, and in Pennsylvania
	Anthrax attacks
2002	Passage of the Homeland Security Act
2003	Homeland Security Presidential Directive/HSPD-5 calls for a National Incident Management System (NIMS) and a National Response Plan (NRP)
	Department of Homeland Security established
2004 (November)	States must file to qualify for predisaster hazard mitigation funds—threat assessments completed

well as building regulations and fire protection insurance, began to appear in England in the 13th century.[12] Today's fire service is modeled after changes that were implemented after the "Great Fire of 1666 in London, which left 200,000 homeless and burned out the heart of the city."[12] As evidenced in the *Bible,* mitigation principles were practiced by Noah when he constructed the ark. The first recorded mitigation project to prevent flooding occurred when Amenemhet II (pharaoh, 12th dynasty) created an "irrigation canal and a dam with sluice gates."[12]

The Exodus story, in the Old Testament, refers to the 10 plagues (disasters) brought down on Egypt to persuade the pharaoh to let the Israelites leave. As man's weapons have evolved from stones, to knives, to spears, to the use of explosives, guns, chemical, biological, and nuclear agents, so has the ability to medically cope with these consequences and minimize the impact of these events. We can trace and credit the modern approaches of today's triage to concepts first introduced during the Napoleonic wars by Baron Dominique-Jean Larrey in the 18th century. The triage concept was simple— sort the patients by the severity of their injury and treat and stabilize the most critically injured first. In following this practice, the greatest good could be delivered to the greatest number of casualties. Surgical techniques and rapid frontline interventions were used during the Civil War. The concept of rapid evacuation after initial treatment to an advanced treatment facility demon-strated a significant reduction in mortality during the Korean and Vietnam wars when compared with World War II. In 1966, a report was released by the National Academy of Sciences/National Research Council, *Accidental Death and Disability: The Neglected Disease of Modern Society*. The report called for applying these military lessons learned to civilian society. Ultimately, it gave rise to what is currently thought of as EMS in 1973.

Emergency Medicine

In the early 1960s, a patient's personal physician or a physician from the hospital medical staff, who was on rotation for the day, provided medical care for patients who showed up in the "emergency room." The first full-time providers of care exclusively in the "emergency room" began appearing in 1965. In 1968, the American College of Emergency Physicians (ACEP) was established in Lansing, Mich. Its mission was to educate physicians in this new practice environment (i.e., emergency medicine) and to improve the quality of care to these patients. ACEP did this by developing and periodically revising a "core content of Emergency Medicine"[13] and by creating the American Board of Emergency Medicine in 1976, resulting in approval from the American Board of Medical Specialties for a modified conjoint board in 1979 and primary specialty board in 1989 (with emergency medicine becoming the 23rd medical specialty). ACEP also developed training through residencies in emergency medicine (with the first graduate in 1970), educational conferences, and a research agenda to further define and develop the specialty.

Disaster Medicine and Disaster Medical Services

By 1976, the ACEP published *The Role of Emergency Physicians in Mass Casualty/Disaster Management*.[14] This policy was later approved (1985), reaffirmed (1997), and revised and expanded (2000).[15] (See Box 4-1 for the full policy statement.) In this policy, "ACEP believes that emergency physicians should assume a primary role in the medical aspects of disaster planning, management, and patient care." It also calls for emergency physicians to participate in "local, regional, and national disaster networks." The University Association of Emergency Medicine echoed the calls for training in disaster medicine and further called for the development of fellowship training in disaster medicine.[16] The ACEP also was an advocate for emergency physician participation in the "development of comprehensive plans developed by communities" to cope with disasters and of the National Disaster Medical System through disaster medical assistance team (DMAT) participation (1985, revised 1999).[15] The ACEP Section of Disaster Medicine was formed in 1988. Through continued involvement and advocacy of disaster medicine, section members are participating on many levels: participation in DMATs, research and writing, educational conferences, and hospital and community disaster and emergency management.

Emergency Medical Services

Today, EMS and disaster medical services are linked through the first responder (emergency medical technician EMT, paramedic, firefighter, law enforcement representative, nurse, and emergency physician).[17] Whether it is a fire, transportation, or hazardous materials incident, it is the first responders from the local EMS unit who determine whether adequate resources are available to address the incident. These first responders also are in a position to determine whether there are any injured people who need to be triaged, stabilized, and transported to a definitive medical facility. This unity of purpose was not always so. Disaster management developed from a civil defense model after World War II, with a focus on mitigation and preparedness. EMS developed from an applied military model, with a focus on response. EMS (as an outgrowth of its relationship with fire services) was the first to adopt the Incident Command System.[18]

Emergency Management

The Federal Emergency Management Agency (FEMA) can trace its beginnings to the Congressional Act of 1803. In this first federal disaster legislation, "assistance was provided to a New Hampshire town after an extensive fire."[19] Emergency management concepts developed from a civil defense model ("duck and cover") to "protect" against a nuclear attack in the 1950s.

BOX 4-1 ACEP POLICY STATEMENT—DISASTER MEDICAL SERVICES

"The American College of Emergency Physicians (ACEP) believes that emergency physicians should assume a primary role in the medical aspects of disaster planning, management, and patient care. Because the provision of effective disaster medical services requires prior training or experience, emergency physicians should pursue training that will enable them to fulfill this responsibility.

A medical disaster occurs when the destructive effects of natural or man-made forces overwhelm the ability of a given area or community to meet the demand for health care.

Disaster planning, testing, and response are multidisciplinary activities that require cooperative interaction. Each agency or individual contributes unique capabilities, perspectives, and experiences. Within this context, emergency physicians share the responsibility for ensuring an effective and well-integrated disaster response.

Emergency medical services and disaster medical services share the goal of optimal acute health care; however, in achieving that goal, the two systems use different approaches. Emergency medical services routinely direct maximal resources to a small number of individuals, while disaster medical services are designed to direct limited resources to the greatest number of individuals. Disasters involving the intentional or accidental release of biological, chemical, radiological, or nuclear agents present an extremely difficult community planning and response challenge. In addition, they may produce a far greater number of secondary casualties and deaths than conventional disasters. Because the medical control of emergency medical services is within the domain of emergency medicine, it remains the responsibility of emergency physicians to provide both direct patient care and medical control of out-of-hospital emergency medical services during disasters.

Improvement of established disaster management methods requires the integration of data from research and experience. Emergency physicians must use their skills in organization, education, and research to incorporate these improvements as new concepts and technologies emerge.

Where local, regional, and national disaster networks exist, emergency physicians should participate in strengthening them. Where they are not yet functional, emergency physicians should assist in planning and implementing them.

This policy statement was prepared by the Emergency Medical Services Committee. It was approved by the ACEP Board of Directors June 2000. It replaces one with the same title originally approved by the ACEP Board of Directors June 1985 and reaffirmed by the ACEP Board of Directors March 1997."

Reproduced with permission from American College of Emergency Physicians. Disaster medical services. *Ann Emerg Med.* August 2001;38:198-9.

Four significant hurricanes and two earthquakes in the 1960s and 1970s illustrated the need for national coordination and financial resources, which were beyond the capability of the local communities affected.

These disasters also moved the national mindset from civil defense to natural disasters. The National Emergency Management Association was established in 1974, consisting of state directors of emergency services and emergency management. In 1979, President Carter created FEMA by executive order (Executive Order 12148). To more effectively perform its function as an all-hazards emergency management program, multiple existing agencies were consolidated into FEMA. They included the Federal Insurance Administration, the National Fire Prevention and Control Administration, the National Weather Service Community Preparedness Program, the Federal Preparedness Agency of the General Services Administration, and the Federal Disaster Assistance Administration activities from Housing and Urban Development. In addition, civil defense responsibilities were transferred from the Department of Defense's Defense Civil Preparedness Agency.[19]

FEMA, like many in the field of emergency management, began to think in terms of the following four unique phases of a disaster incident:

- Mitigation
- Preparedness
- Response
- Recovery

Mitigation involves actions that could prevent a disaster or minimize its consequences. Lessons learned from the 1994 Northridge, Calif., earthquake affected building codes, engineering standards, and where structures were built.[20] In a similar way, mitigation actions for a hurricane would include preplanned evacuation routes, building codes, warning systems, and recommendations for family hurricane supplies. *Preparedness* and *planning* include taking steps to avoid or minimize the consequences of a threat through probability assessment, currently described as a "hazard vulnerability assessment (HVA)."[21] An example would include a community or hospital disaster response plan based on threat assessments.[26,27] *Response* includes all activities involved in bringing resources (supplies, personnel, and coordination) to an incident to minimize health consequences of the affected population and, where appropriate, providing security, rescue, triage, stabilization, and transportation to safety and definitive care. The involvement of government and private organizations to provide interventions is not only associated with response, but also with the fourth phase, recovery. *Recovery* includes actions needed to return the community to normal operations. Recovery may take weeks and months, or in the case of hurricane Andrew, more than a decade. In some cases, the community may never recover from a disaster incident.

In 1982, the International City Management Association conducted a national survey. Its finding was that "20% of local governments did not have a formal disaster plan."[12,22] Almost a decade later, hospitals were not any better prepared. "According to the Joint Commission on Accreditation of Healthcare Organizations (JCAHO, 1990), only 21% of surveyed hospitals meet their requirements for disaster preparedness."[23] In 2002, the Homeland Security Act was passed, and in 2003 the Department of Homeland Security was created. FEMA was transferred to the Department of Homeland Security, and the National Disaster Medical System was placed under FEMA's operational control.[24] Homeland Security Presidential Directive/HSPD-5 established a "single, comprehensive National Incident Management System."[25] The primary focus was to establish a national standard and improve interoperability between all involved agencies and organizations. This new standard replaces the National Fire Incident Command System.

CURRENT PRACTICE

Disaster management is a multidisciplinary practice that involves many professional disciplines. The complexities of this interdependent approach can be appreciated by reviewing the Federal Response Plan (1999). In this plan, Emergency Support Functions (ESFs) are categorized into the following 12 areas:

- Transportation
- Communications
- Public works and engineering
- Firefighting
- Information and planning
- Mass care
- Resource support
- Health and medical services
- Urban search and rescue
- Food
- Energy
- Emergency medicine (which functions within health and medical services in this plan)

The role of emergency medicine in disaster management can be viewed as one of three: a traditional role, an activist leadership role, or the role of a system integrator. Figure 4-1 identifies nine potential interactions within the system. At the core is the emergency physician-patient relationship (Fig. 4-1, *1*). When a disaster strikes locally, every emergency physician will find the need to assume roles identified as *2* through *5* in Fig. 4-1, even if he has no experience in disaster medicine. The on-duty emergency physician will need to provide leadership to his department, hospital, EMS, and community. The emergency physician's duties will depend on specific "job actions" defined through the hospital's Incident Command System (a standard required by JCAHO)[30] and the disaster plan implemented by the hospital. One model is the Hospital Emergency Incident Command System.[31] The roles identified as *1* through *5* in Fig. 4-1 are part of the local hospital response to any given all-hazards event. This is known as a level one local response. Level two and three responses (see Fig. 4-1) refer to the involvement of state and federal resources for incidents that are beyond the capability of the local or regional disaster response. The state and federal resources brought into play and the timeline involved define levels. A central theme in the mitigation, planning, response, and recovery preparations will be the self-reliance of the community for the initial 2 to 3 days, at minimum, after an event.

Current practice is also influenced by JCAHO standards that are used in hospital disaster management;

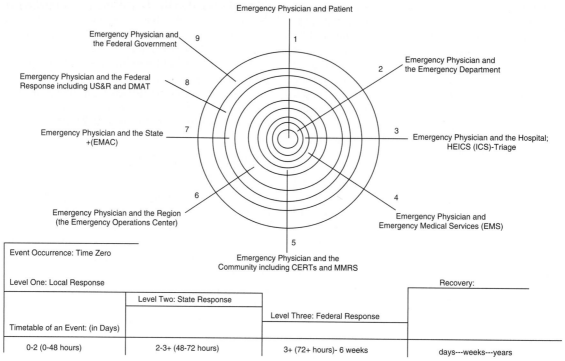

FIGURE 4–1. Rings of engagement: The different roles of the emergency physician in disaster medicine.

principles common to disaster incidents; and future directions, such as the movement to national standards and training.[28-30]

General Concepts and Definitions

Many of these are covered more extensively in other chapters of this textbook.

National Incident Management System

The National Incident Management System (NIMS) is a national best practice for incident management required by Homeland Security Presidential Directive/HSPD-5, "Management of Domestic Incidents."[25] The directive is to be implemented by fiscal year 2005 as a precondition for eligibility for federal preparedness assistance to state, local, tribal, or local organizations in their mitigation, preparedness, response, or recovery efforts. NIMS evolved from FIRESCOPE,[18] the Incident Command System developed by fire services when battling the California wildfires in the late 1980s and which later grew into the National Fire Incident Command System.

National Fire Protection Association 1600

The National Fire Protection Association (NFPA) published *NFPA 1600: Standard on Disaster/ Emergency Management and Business Continuity Programs 2004 Edition,*[32] a national best-practice, terminology, and reference resource developed through a consensus between public and private organizations. It is the culmination of work begun in 1991 by the Disaster Management Committee established by the NFPA

Standards Council. It was approved January 2004 as an American National Standard.

Convergence

Convergence is a behavior associated with the movement of people toward or away from a disaster event. It includes the unplanned arrival of individuals, including healthcare providers, who want to become involved in the rescue process. It also includes individuals from the impact zone of the disaster who find their own way, outside of the EMS system, to healthcare providers.

Mutual Aid

Mutual aid is used in the context of organized, preplanned coordination and use of resources from adjacent or remote organizations through the use of memoranda of understanding or contracts. An Emergency Management Assistance Compact (EMAC) is an example of shared resources between states.

Special Response Teams

Special response teams include community emergency response teams (CERTs), DMATs, urban search and rescue (US&R) teams, the Metropolitan Medical Response System, the National Response Team (NRT) for releases of oil and nonradiological hazardous substances, and other specialized teams. These resources are accessed through federal channels (taking up to 72 hours for implementation on-site), with the exception of the Metropolitan Medical Response System that is locally controlled and organized and the EMAC teams that are state controlled.

National Pharmaceutical Stockpile

The National Pharmaceutical Stockpile program is part of a level III federal response to provide pharmaceutical support to a medical disaster event.

Joint Commission on Accreditation of Healthcare Organizations

Eight months before the Sept. 11, 2001, World Trade Center disaster, JCAHO published a revision to its Environment of Care Standards (Box 4-2). One month after the disaster, on Oct. 10, 2001, JCAHO President Dennis O'Leary, MD, delivered testimony before Congress, stating: "Some people believe that the healthcare delivery system—if faced with a bioterrorism event—will somehow be able to accommodate the thousands of ill, injured, and worried well who will seek healthcare in that situation. The unfortunate truth is that we have much to do before such a belief can be fulfilled."

Current JCAHO standards encourage a comprehensive emergency management and "all-hazards" approach in which both internal and external threats are considered. The example of the Houston floods that caused the evacuation of Memorial Hermann Healthcare and Memorial Hermann Children's Hospital in the summer of 2001 lead to further changes in JCAHO standards that addressed emergency/disaster hospital privileging. The (ACEP) published a policy statement recommending the steps necessary to comply with these standards.[33]

BOX 4-2   SUMMARY OF REVISED JCAHO STANDARDS

January 2001—Significant Changes
1. Shifting attitudes and practices from Emergency Preparedness to Emergency Management (mitigation, preparedness and planning, response, and recovery).
2. "All Hazards" assessment of threat using a Hazards Vulnerability Analysis (HVA) approach to include consideration of NBCEI (Nuclear, Biologic, Chemical, Explosive, and Incendiary) as well as natural and man-made events.
3. Healthcare organization Command and Control—an example, HEICS (Hospital Incident Command System). The purpose of which is to improve interoperability between organizations using a common system. This will include defining criteria for plan activation.
4. Community-wide practice drill with all departments within the hospital organization participating in a live simulation. The prime goal of the drill is evaluate all elements of the written plan and test the interoperability of the response structure, communication capabilities, coordination, and command and control.
5. Off site capacity/treatment is to be developed to include capability for decontamination and potential isolation and treatment of contagious patients and delivery of healthcare in home and at alternative sites.
6. Healthcare organization's integration with public health to include bi-directional surveillance communication, reporting, vaccination and treatment programs.

Principles Common to Disaster Incidents

It had been said that the best way to combat the fear of the unknown or unexpected is to understand it and anticipate it through study, characterization, and shining the light of preparation. We do not fear what we expect and understand. This is the driving force behind the various systems that are used to describe disaster events. Disaster category, class, and type demonstrate one means of classification. Time course of the event is another. A tornado strikes suddenly with little warning. A hurricane usually can be tracked with warning and preparation times of up to 72 hours. Following the rising tide, historical occurrences, monitoring riverbanks, or tracking precipitation can sometimes be used to predict floods. Multiple areas of destruction that take place over a large geographical area define some disasters. The Haddon matrix plots factors and elements such as the prodrome; impact; and recovery against human, structure, physical environment, and socioeconomic conditions in an attempt to better anticipate needs for preparation, response, recovery, and resource allocation.[34]

Many of the principles associated with the four phases of disaster management—mitigation, preplanning and preparedness, response, and recovery—have been discussed (Table 4-2). Special treatment considerations and skills are associated with particular events. They include, but are not limited to, decontamination; treatment of blast injuries, crush and compartment syndrome, radiation exposure, shock, infectious disease, and injuries resulting from nuclear, biological, or chemical events; mass care; and humanitarian complex disasters. A seven-step process has been developed and is used in critical incident stress debriefing (a systematic program for psychological support developed by Dr. Mitchell in 1983 for first responders or affected members of the event).[35]

Future Directions

The implementation of standard terminology and processes,[32] education and training,[36-39] coordination of the federal response through the Department of Homeland Security,[24] establishment of the National Response Plan,[40] adoption of the NIMS,[25] standardization of a pharmaceutical stockpile, standardization of training and equipment for specialty response teams such as DMATs, focused research through dedicated centers, and increased coordination and communication between interdisciplinary public and private organizations[32] will lead to improved and enhanced capabilities in the area of emergency management.

PITFALLS

Today, our communities face increasing threats while after-action reports continue to recognize problems in 10 major areas (Box 4-3). These problems were evidenced in the results of the report from the National Commission on Terrorist Attacks upon the United States (also known as the 9-11 Commission), as documented by the *New York Times*. The lives of many of the first responders were lost due to problems identified in the report, including

TABLE 4-2 DISASTER PRINCIPLES ASSOCIATED WITH THE FOUR PHASES OF EMERGENCY MANAGEMENT

Mitigation	Threat assessments should include: ■ Hazard vulnerability assessment (HVA) ■ Historical events of high probability ■ Findings of agencies such as the National Oceanic and Atmospheric Administration
Preparedness	Take corrective and protective actions based on information learned during mitigation. Execute mutual-aid plans and memorandum of understanding.
Response	Out of hospital: ■ Impact-notification-verification-first responder actions, including establishing command and control—an Incident Command System (ICS). ■ Identification of hot, warm, and cold zones and a security perimeter. ■ Begin triage, stabilization, and documentation. ■ Transport to secondary assessment areas or definitive care within the healthcare organization with adequate communication. In hospital: ■ Implement the Hospital Emergency Incident Command System ■ Continue triage, stabilization, and treatment or discharge within the healthcare organization ■ Conduct appropriate documentation and communication with patients, family, media, and the community Other: ■ Activate and involve community organizations and public health.
Recovery	Interdisciplinary response that involves multiple organizations returning to normal operations Critical incident stress debriefing of first responders and community members

inadequate communication, inadequate coordination between police and fire rescue units with a history of jurisdictional battles (turf wars), and a lack of a functional, unified command.[41] Air traffic controllers suffered "maddening miscommunications, mangled coordination, and broken chains of command. They (were) improvising a defense for a disaster for which they had never trained . . . ."[42]

Another problem area, as described Auf der Heide in 1989[1] based on the study by Quarantelli of 29 disasters in the 1970s, is maldistribution of patients among potential receiving hospitals. Auf der Heide reported that "in 75% of cases studied, a majority of the casualties were sent to the closest hospital. In 46% of the cases, more than three-fourths of the casualties were sent to the nearest hospital. Only in about half of the disasters did a simple majority of the hospitals in the area receive even one casualty."[1] Causalty distribution during the Sept. 11 events underwent

BOX 4-3 CHRONIC PROBLEMS: THE 10 C'S

1. Charge: who is in charge (operational control)?
   a. Who has the authority to activate and deactivate the plan?
2. Command and control: the Incident Command System—lack of implementation (chain of command)
3. Communication
4. Coordination
5. Convergence (either the movement of unsolicited volunteers toward the disaster scene or the movement of event individuals outside of the EMS system toward a healthcare organization [hospital])
6. Contamination and decontamination
7. Capacity and surge capacity issues
8. Cooperation (between community and healthcare organizations)
9. Chaos and confusion with the failure or compromise of a system
10. Critical incident stress debriefing (providing necessary psychological support to first responders and individuals affected by the event)

these same problems. Most hospitals in a wide area had activated their disaster plans and were waiting for an influx of patients that never came. At the same time, the closest hospital to the World Trade Center site received more than 600 patients in the first day. The Greater New York Hospital Association, however, reported that "after the attacks, 7300 patients were seen at more than 100 hospitals scattered throughout the metropolitan region."[43] This continues to point out both the lack of adequate plans for patient distribution on a regional basis and the challenge of appropriately capturing disaster epidemiology directly related to the disaster event as opposed to routine patient flow.

Preparation through the drilling requirements outlined by JCAHO is quite minimal when compared with the drilling practices elsewhere, such as Israel, where, as often as monthly, hospitals are tested without prior notification at up to 20% of their licensed bed capacity. In the United States, realistic drills and exercises have been cost-prohibitive as hospitals and communities have attempted to fulfill an underfunded mandate from organizations such as JCAHO.[43-45]

There are multiple triage systems currently in use without uniform standards or agreement as to a single tool that provides accurate triage and identification of critical injury for all patients in all situations.[36,37,39]

Advancement of disaster medicine as a multidisciplinary professional specialty will require well-funded and organized research and the development of core content and competencies for its practitioners.[46] The United States after Sept. 11, 2001, has been in a crisis mode, catching up and plugging the holes.[24,47] More than 20 pieces of significant legislation have been passed.[48] Recognition that national standards, training, exercising, and equipment have not been adequately funded in the past is supported by a report by the Council on Foreign Relations, chaired by Sen. Warren B. Rudman. The report, *Emergency Responders: Drastically Underfunded, Dangerously Unprepared,* details how bad the underfunding is. The monetary needs just for emergency responders in all jurisdictions (local, state, and federal) could equal $201.4 billion over 5 years.[49]

This is the current situation, which provides an opportunity for emergency physicians as they seek to define their role and the role of emergency medicine in disaster management.

REFERENCES

1. Auf der Heide E. *Disaster Response: The Principles of Preparation and Coordination*. St. Louis: Mosby; 1989.
2. The Disaster Center. The most deadly 100 natural disasters of the 20th century. Available at: http://www.disastercenter.com/disaster/TOP100K.html.
3. Weiner T. Floods bring more suffering to a battered Haitian town. *The New York Times*. May 29, 2004.
4. Hurricaneville. The story of hurricane Andrew. Available at: http://www.hurricaneville.com/andrew.html.
5. Burkle FMJ. Complex humanitarian emergencies. In: Hogan DE, Burstein JL, eds. *Disaster Medicine*. Philadelphia: Lippincott Williams & Wilkins; 2002:431.
6. Sharp TW, Burkle FM Jr, Vaughn AF, Chotani R, Brennan RJ. Challenges and opportunities for humanitarian relief in Afghanistan. *Clin Infect Dis*. 2002;34(suppl 5):S215-28.
7. Spiegel PB, Burkle FM Jr, Dey CC, Salama P. Developing public health indicators in complex emergency response. *Prehospital Disaster Med*. 2001;16(4):281-5.
8. Sharp TW, Wightman JM, Davis MJ, Sherman SS, Burkle FM Jr. Military assistance in complex emergencies: what have we learned since the Kurdish relief effort? *Prehospital Disaster Med*. 2001;16(4):197-208.
9. Burkle FM Jr. Complex emergencies: an introduction. *Prehospital Disaster Med*. 2001;16(4):182-3.
10. VanRooyen MJ, Eliades MJ, Grabowski JG, et al. Medical relief personnel in complex emergencies: perceptions of effectiveness in the former Yugoslavia. *Prehospital Disaster Med*. 2001;16(3):145-9.
11. Burkle FM Jr, Hayden R. The concept of assisted management of large-scale disasters by horizontal organizations. *Prehospital Disaster Med*. 2001;16(3):128-37.
12. Quarantelli EL. *Disaster Planning, Emergency Management, and Civil Protection: The Historical Development and Current Characteristics of Organized Efforts to Prevent and To Respond To Disasters*. [Preliminary report.] Newark, DE: Disaster Research Center; 1995. Available at: http://www.udel.edu/DRC/preliminary/227.pdf.
13. Allison EJ, Aghababian RV, Barsan WG, et al. Core content for emergency medicine. *Ann Emerg Med*. 1997;29(6):791-811.
14. The role of the emergency physician in mass casualty/disaster management. ACEP position paper. *JACEP*. 1976;5(11):901-2.
15. Skiendzielewski JJ. American College of Emergency Physicians Policy Compendium 2003. 2003:21-2.
16. Disaster medicine: current assessment and blueprint for the future. SAEM Disaster Medicine White Paper Subcommittee. *Acad Emerg Med*. 1995;2(12):1068-76.
17. Bern AI. Disaster medical services. In: Roush WR, Aranosian R, Blair T, et al, eds. *Principles of EMS System: A Comprehensive Text for Physicians*. Dallas: American College of Emergency Physicians; 1989:77-93.
18. Irwin RL. The Incident Command System. In: Auf der Heide E, ed. *Disaster Response: Principles of Preparation and Coordination*. St. Louis: Mosby; 1989.
19. Federal Emergency Management Agency. FEMA history. Available at: http://www.fema.gov/about/history.shtm.
20. Berman MA, Lazar EJ. Hospital emergency preparedness—lessons learned since Northridge. *New Engl J Med*. 2003;348(14):1307-8.
21. Joint Commission on Accreditation of Healthcare Organizations. *Guide to Emergency Management Planning in Health Care*. Oakbrook Terrace, IL: Joint Commission Resources, Inc; 2002.
22. International City Management Association. *Emergency Management, Baseline Data Reports V*. Vol. 15. Washington, DC: International City Management Association; 1983.
23. *Community Medical Disaster Planning and Evaluation Guide*. 1st ed. Dallas: American College of Emergency Physicians; 1995. Community Medical Disaster Planning and Evaluation Guide.
24. Noji EK. Creating a health care agenda for the Department of Homeland Security. *Manag Care*. 2003;12(suppl 11):7-12.
25. The White House. Homeland Security Presidential Directive/HSPD-5. Management of Domestic Incidents. Available at: http://www.whitehouse.gov/news/releases/2003/02/20030228-9.html.
26. Terrorism preparedness in state health departments—United States, 2001-2003. *Morb Mortal Wkly Rep*. 2003;52(43):1051-3.
27. Barbera JA, Macintyre AG. The reality of the modern bioterrorism response. *Lancet*. December 2002;360 Suppl:s33-4.
28. General Accounting Office. *Bioterrorism: Public Health Response to Anthrax Incidents of 2001*. October 15, 2003. GAO-04-152. Available at: http://www.gao.gov/new.items/d04152.pdf.
29. Mothershead JL, Tonat K, Koenig KL. Bioterrorism preparedness. III: state and federal programs and response. *Emerg Med Clin North Am*. 2002;20(2):477-500.
30. Joint Commission on Accreditation of Healthcare Organizations. *2003 Hospital Accreditation Standards. Accreditation Policies, Standards, Intent Statements*. Oakbrook Terrace, IL: Joint Commission Resources, Inc; 2003.
31. California Emergency Medical Services Authority. Hospital Emergency Incident Command System (HEICS III) Update Project. Available at: http://www.emsa.ca.gov/Dms2/download.htm.
32. National Fire Protection Association. *NFPA 1600: Standard on Disaster/Emergency Management and Business Continuity Programs 2004 Edition*. Available at: http://www.nfpa.org/PDF/nfpa1600.pdf?src=nfpa.
33. Hospital disaster privileging. *Ann Emerg Med*. 2003;42(4):607-8.
34. Noji E, Siverston K. Injury prevention in natural disasters. A theoretical framework. *Disasters*. 1987;11:290-6.
35. Mitchell JT. When disaster strikes . . . the critical incident stress debriefing process. *JEMS*. 1983;8(1):36-9.
36. Kennedy K, Aghababian RV, Gans L, Lewis CP. Triage: techniques and applications in decision making. *Ann Emerg Med*. 1996;28(2):136-44.
37. National Disaster Life Support Education Consortium. *Basic Disaster Life Support*. 2nd draft ed. National Disaster Life Support Education Consortium; 2003.
38. Waeckerle JF, Seamans S, Whiteside M, et al. Executive summary: developing objectives, content, and competencies for the training of emergency medical technicians, emergency physicians, and emergency nurses to care for casualties resulting from nuclear, biological, or chemical (NBC) incidents. *Ann Emerg Med*. 2001;37(6):587-601.
39. Garner A, Lee A, Harrison K, Schultz CH. Comparative analysis of multiple-casualty incident triage algorithms. *Ann Emerg Med*. 2001;38(5):541-8.
40. US Department of Homeland Security. Initial National Response Plan fact sheet. Available at: http://www.dhs.gov/dhspublic/display?content=1936.
41. Smith D. Save the rescuers from one another. *The New York Times*. May 18, 2004.
42. Schmitt E, Lichtblau E. To the minute, panel paints a grim portrait of day's terror. *The New York Times*. June 18, 2004.
43. Greater New York Hospital Association. Hospital expenditures for emergency preparedness. February 2003. Available at: http://www.gnyha.org/pubinfo/200302_Emergency_Prep_Exp.pdf.
44. Bern AI. Question arises as to who pays for disaster drills under DRGs. *Emerg Dep News*. 1984;6(8):5, 11.
45. Bern AI, Galloway E, Krohmer JR, Gamm SR, Roth RM. Financial implications of disaster preparedness: a cost analysis of an area-wide community-based mass casualty/disaster incident (UAEM, abstract #28). *Ann Emerg Med*. 1984;13(5):389.
46. Waeckerle JF, Lillibridge SR, Burkle FM Jr, Noji EK. Disaster medicine: challenges for today. *Ann Emerg Med*. 1994;23(4):715-8.
47. Koenig KL. Homeland security and public health: role of the Department of Veterans Affairs, the U.S. Department of Homeland Security, and implications for the public health community. *Prehospital Disaster Med*. 2003;18(4):1-7.
48. Rubin CB. *Emergency Management in the 21st Century: Dealing with Al Qaeda, Tom Ridge, and Julie Gerberding*. [Working paper 108.] Boulder: Natural Hazards Center, University of Colorado; May 5, 2004.
49. Rudman WB, Clarke RA, Metzl JF. *Emergency Responders: Drastically Underfunded, Dangerously Unprepared. Report of an Independent Task Force Sponsored by the Council on Foreign Relations*. 2003.
50. American College of Emergency Physicians. Disaster medical services. *Ann Emerg Med*. August 2001;38;198-9.

chapter 5

The Role of Hospitals in Disaster

Mary W. Chaffee and Neill S. Oster

INTRODUCTION

When the first rain began to fall in Houston, Texas, in June 2001, did hospital staff know they would soon be providing care for hundreds of patients without electrical power or running water in flooded hospital buildings?

On April 19, 1995, did the emergency department staff arriving for the day shift at 13 Oklahoma City hospitals know that a former soldier was driving a rented van filled with 4000 pounds of ammonium nitrate toward the Murrah Federal Building and that they would soon be faced with 324 bombing victims?

In 1984, did restaurant patrons in Wasco County, Ore., have any idea, as they selected food from salad bars, that they would soon be evaluated in hospitals for profuse, watery diarrhea from intentional food contamination by a religious cult?

In March 2003, did the 11 Toronto healthcare workers who were caring for patients with respiratory symptoms know they would soon become infected with severe acute respiratory syndrome (SARS)?

We can be quite certain that none of them knew. The capricious nature of disaster implies victims and responders are generally caught unaware.

But we do *know* some things. We *know* there will be hurricanes, typhoons, tornadoes, earthquakes, mudslides, fires, and blizzards this year. We *know* people will pick up firearms, make bombs, and inflict pain and suffering on others. We *know* there will be casualties from train accidents, cars crumpled in chain reactions, building collapses, and explosions. We *know* infectious diseases will do what they do best: spread, sicken, and kill. We *know* terrorists have not given up their violent assaults. We *know* there will be mental health symptoms in accident survivors and the caregivers who respond to their needs.

It is the *hospital*, at the heart of the health system, that will receive the injured, infected, bleeding, broken, and terrified from these events. We *know* the victims will seek life-saving care, comfort, and relief at hospitals, but many U.S. hospitals continue to prepare for disaster as though it will not happen to them.

Hospital Capacity in the United States

There are more than 5700 hospitals in the United States that form a diverse patchwork of healthcare services.

U.S. hospitals vary greatly by geographic location (urban, suburban, and rural); financial and management structure (for profit, not-for-profit, private, public); type of care (general medical services or specialty care, such as psychiatric or pediatric); and government affiliation (Department of Defense, Veterans Health Administration, or Public Health Service). Any of these hospitals may be called on to respond to the next disaster or may be the victim of a disaster. Many experts believe that these hospitals are not adequately prepared to respond effectively (Table 5-1).

HISTORICAL PERSPECTIVE

The Role of the Hospital in Society

The hospital was of little significance in American healthcare before the Civil War. Only 178 hospitals existed in 1873 when the first survey was conducted—a time when no proper gentleman or lady would venture into a hospital by choice.[1] The murky medical practices of the 1800s offered little that couldn't be found in homes, and physicians had little in their armamentarium to change the course of disease and injury. However, discovery and scientific advance changed that. Effective anesthesia, surgical antisepsis, antibiotics, the x-ray, and other advances turned the hospital into a place of comfort, hope, and healing. The 20th-century hospital became a sophisticated financial institution, the core of medical education, and the site of dazzling technological display. Medical advances offered aid not only to the chronically ill but offered hope to those who suffered acute trauma or medical or psychiatric emergency.

The Effect of Disaster on Hospitals

Past events illuminate the variety and complexity of demands placed on a hospital in a disaster:

- *Hurricane Katrina*. The flooding in the wake of Hurricane Katrina in 2005 left hospitals in greater New Orleans, Louisiana, and Mississippi in crisis. Patients and staff were trapped in facilities without essential services, resulting in the largest mass hospital evacuation in U.S. history.

TABLE 5-1 SNAPSHOT OF 2005 U.S. HOSPITAL CAPACITY*

Total U.S. Hospitals	5764
U.S. community hospitals	4845
U.S. federal government hospitals	239
Institutional hospitals (e.g., prisons, colleges)	23
Nonfederal psychiatric hospitals	477
Nonfederal long-term–care hospitals	180
Total staffed U.S. hospital beds	965,256
Staffed community hospital beds	813,307

*Source: American Hospital Association. Hospital statistics, 2005 edition. Available at: www.hospitalconnect.com/aha/resource_center/fastfacts/fast_facts_us_hospitals.html.

- *Floods caused by tropical storm Allison in Houston, Texas.* In June 2001, 3 feet of rain from tropical storm Allison fell in the Houston area, causing the flooding and complete disruption of services at the University of Texas Health Science Center and its clinical affiliate hospitals. One of the hospitals, Memorial Hermann Hospital, experienced failure of every hospital system. The main and emergency power generators and communications system failed and personnel could not come, go, or be reached. The water supply failed, and the sewer system stopped functioning. The vertical evacuation of 570 patients was conducted, and the hospital was closed for 38 days. The storm flooded an area not considered to be at risk.[2]
- *The Northridge, Calif., earthquake.* An earthquake struck Northridge on Jan. 17, 1994, damaging a number of area hospitals. Six hospitals evacuated patients immediately: four of these evacuated all inpatients, and two evacuated some. Five of the facilities evacuated the most severely ill first, but the sixth, fearing imminent structural collapse, evacuated the healthiest patients first to permit the evacuation of the largest number of patients in the shortest period. That facility moved 334 patients from buildings to open areas in two hours. All hospitals used improvised transport devices, including backboards, blankets, and mattresses.[3]
- *The 2001 World Trade Center bombing.* Bellevue Hospital, a level-1 trauma center in New York City, is approximately three miles from the World Trade Center. Ninety patients presented within the first five hours after the incident; a total of 194 were triaged and treated within the first 24 hours. Despite best efforts, the hospital lost track of patients, ran out of supplies, and struggled with coordination of physicians to ensure rest and safety.[4] New York University Downtown Hospital, a few blocks from the disaster, received 350 patients within the first two hours of the World Trade Center attacks. Many patients arrived on foot.[5] St. Vincent's Catholic Medical Center executed its disaster plan within minutes of the bombing, as they had done during the 1993 World Trade Center bombing. On Sept. 11, 2001, St. Vincent's Hospital treated nearly 800 victims. Because St. Vincent's shared water lines with the World Trade Center and telecommunications lines were routed through the World Trade Center, function of these systems was affected. Crisis counseling, pastoral care, and mental health services were immediately made available for victims, families, rescue workers, and staff.[6]
- *The Oklahoma City Bombing.* After the explosion of a bomb at the Murrah Federal Building, 168 were killed and 700 were injured—388 with acute injuries. The first patients arrived in emergency departments within 15 minutes, and the hospitals within 1.5 miles of the blast site received the greatest number of victims.[7]
- *The Rhode Island nightclub fire.* On Feb. 20, 2003, fire erupted in a crowded nightclub in West Warwick, R.I. Almost 100 were killed immediately, and nearly 200 were injured. Kent County Hospital, a 350-bed community hospital 2 miles from the site of the fire, received 40 victims within an hour; 25 were rapidly intubated. The hospital ran out of critical supplies and ventilators and struggled with supporting family members, poor communications from the scene, and pain management.[8] Ultimately, 16 hospitals in Rhode Island and Massachusetts received 196 burn victims; this included the Shriners Hospital for Children, which received and treated 16 adult victims.[9]

The potential impact of disaster is staggering. The release of 40 tons of methyl isocyanate from the Union Carbide factory in Bhopal, India, in December 1984 exposed more than 500,000 to the deadly gas and killed about 6000 in the first week after the release. In September 1987, workers scavenging a dismantled cancer clinic in Goiania, Brazil, took home a source containing cesium-137. They sold it to a junkman who showed the glowing item to friends and neighbors. Once radiation exposure victims presented to hospitals, and the release became well known, hospitals were overwhelmed. Although 250 were actually exposed and 28 showed signs of radiation sickness, 112,800 people were evaluated. When the Aum Shinri Kyo cult placed sarin on five trains in the Tokyo subway system on March 20, 1995, 4000 people made their own way to hospitals, 641 were transported by authorities, and 245 hospital staff and rescue personnel were contaminated due to poor or nonexistent decontamination procedures.[10]

Evolving Perspective on the Health System Role in Disasters

On Sept. 11, 2001, when U.S. hospitals and healthcare professionals were confronted with the worst attack on American soil, and again during the anthrax attacks along the Eastern Seaboard, individuals and organizations responded heroically. A powerful change in thinking, also called a *paradigm shift,* occurred after the terror attacks: the health system came to be viewed as a foundation of national security. Another perspective has changed as well. In the event of a disaster, Emergency Medical Services (EMS), police, and fire have long been recognized as first responders. However, just recently, hospitals also have been designated as first responders—and first receivers.

The value of the hospital in national security has been increased, and hospitals are recognized as safe havens in communities, the public expects hospitals to be prepared to care for their needs, and the hospital is now recognized as a first responder in emergencies. However, hospitals remain significantly underprepared to respond as effectively as the public expects. Most importantly, preparedness is at direct odds with productivity. Daily operating requirements stretch most hospitals' resources. Allocating funds to improve emergency response capabilities that may never be used could be viewed as foolhardy. Community integration is now seen as necessary, but hospitals (other than those in networks or that are government facilities) have had few reasons to build healthy relationships with other hospitals in their communities. To meet the needs of communities in a disaster, business competitors must work as partners.

Public Expectations

Hospitals play a vital role in the health, social structure, and economic life of a community. Patients expect hospitals, and health system workers, to be available to provide care for them in all circumstances. A level of preparedness that was viewed as adequate in the past is no longer seen as acceptable. To be more highly prepared and to be able to respond effectively, hospitals must make substantial investment in equipment, training, facilities improvements, and supplies.[11] Hospitals depend on public trust; poor performance during a disaster could be financially crippling to a facility. Rubin[12] writes that hospitals are expected to handle whatever they receive and do it right the first time.

CURRENT PRACTICE

Sources of Hospital Vulnerability

Hospitals are vulnerable to the stresses of disaster responses due to a number of inherent characteristics:

- *Complexity of services:* Hospitals are facilities that provide healthcare but must also function as laundromats, hotels, office buildings, laboratories, restaurants, and warehouses.
- *Dependence on lifelines:* Hospitals are completely dependent on basic public services: water, sewer, power, medical gases, communications, fuel, and waste collection.
- *Hazardous materials:* The hospital environment contains toxic agents and poisonous liquids and gases.
- *Dangerous objects:* Heavy medical equipment, storage shelves, and supplies can fall or shift during an event such as an earthquake.[13]

Forces Influencing Preparedness

Multiple forces have placed hospitals in a precarious preparedness posture. The capacity of the health system has been scaled down to a bare minimum to cut operating costs. Emergency departments are crowded with the uninsured and the underinsured who have no other access to care. The nursing workforce has withered, and physicians have left practice due to uncontrolled liability insurance costs.

Surge Capacity

Many hospitals determine their surge capacity by the number of patients they could comfortably care for using standard spaces, quality care standards, and additional teams of personnel to help. In reality, a disaster is not going to comply with the limits of hospital capacity. If 300 bombing victims arrive at a 50-bed community hospital, spaces will need to be converted and used that planners may have never imagined, such as chapels, hallways, and offices. Nurses accustomed to a certain nurse-to-patient ratio may find the ratio in a disaster much higher and have to adapt practice accordingly. Surge capacity must not be viewed only as the number of beds or spaces that can be allotted to care for patients, but it must include all supporting hospital services that are involved in patient care.

Critical Elements in Hospital Preparedness

If hospital services fail during a disaster, the hospital fails the population depending on it. The population includes not just the victims of the disaster, but the others presenting for needed care—women preparing to give birth, patients with chronic disease exacerbation, and children with lacerations that need sutures. A vital hospital emergency management program acts as an insurance policy that increases the chances of continued operations under difficult circumstances. An effective hospital emergency management program guides the development and execution of activities that mitigate, prepare for, respond to, and recover from incidents that disrupt the normal provision of care.[14] The program should include the following components:

- *Emergency manager:* The emergency manager is the primary point of leadership in the development, improvement, exercise, and execution of the hospital's emergency management plan.
- *Emergency management plan:* The plan identifies the hospital's response to internal and external emergencies. Deliberate (advance) planning permits the development of strategies while the organization is not under pressure to react.
- *Executive leadership:* Hospital executive leadership charts the course for an organization. A hospital that lacks executive leadership committed to emergency preparedness will be significantly hampered in its efforts.
- *Strategic planning:* The hospital's strategic plan is the blueprint that guides all efforts to achieve its mission. It is critical that emergency management and preparedness efforts are woven into strategic planning.
- *Emergency management committee:* Extremely broad membership is desired to ensure all hospital

operations that will be stressed in a disaster are integrated and well prepared.

- *Hazard vulnerability analysis (HVA):* The HVA is a tool used to assess the risks in a specific environment. The emergency management plan can be tailored to address the hazards most likely to affect hospital operations.
- *Vulnerability analysis:* Every aspect of hospital operations that will be depended on in a disaster should be assessed to determine whether there are weaknesses present that fail when stressed. Hospitals in the U.S. Navy Medical Department and a number of civilian hospitals in New York have had their level of preparedness assessed using the Hospital Emergency Analysis Tool (HEAT). The HEAT examines more than 230 factors that contribute to effective emergency preparedness and response. After the systematic analysis by a team of experts, the hospital receives an after-action report that documents strengths and weaknesses and permits the development of a strategic plan to improve preparedness.[15]
- *Staff training, exercise, and continuous improvement:* The Joint Commission on Accreditation of Healthcare Organizations requires hospital staff members involved in the execution of the emergency management plan to receive orientation and education relative to their role in an emergency. Exercise of the emergency plan is also required. Lessons learned should be integrated into plans to continuously revise them.

Hospital Preparedness Philosophy

A commitment to the following philosophies will enhance hospital emergency preparedness:

- *Imagine the unimaginable:* When flood waters rise in a community, when a tornado touches down and demolishes an elementary school, when a disgruntled hospital employee opens fire with an automatic weapon in the emergency department, when a passing train derails and spills toxic chemicals, or when a wildfire closes in, it is too late to update an old plan, train staff to respond effectively, check phone numbers, and stock disaster supplies. Disaster complacency—believing a problem won't happen to you or your hospital—is a significant threat to effective planning and response.
- *Protect the staff:* Only a true obsession with self-protection will ensure that staff members are not injured or become ill during disaster response. Adequate stockpiles of gloves, masks, and other equipment must be available, along with training and leadership commitment to self-protection policies.
- *Build in redundancy:* Expect the primary plan to fail and build in alternatives to every emergency measure.
- *Rely on standard procedures whenever possible:* People perform best in unusual situations when they perform activities that closely mirror what they do under normal conditions.
- *Maintain records:* Patient care records are critical to obtaining reimbursement for disaster care provided.

- *Plan to degrade services:* Normal levels of services cannot be maintained during disaster response. Identify services, such as elective surgery, that can be temporarily curtailed or minimized so that personnel and resources can be reassigned.

The Federal Role in Hospital Emergency Preparedness and Response

The federal government has implemented programs to augment local and state capabilities when they are overwhelmed.

The National Disaster Medical System

The United States has a well-established emergency medical safety net: the National Disaster Medical System (NDMS). The NDMS has two primary capabilities designed to enhance disaster medical response. The first is specialized disaster response teams who augment the medical emergency response at the site of disaster. The second NDMS capability is a plan to share the inpatient bed capacity of the civilian and federal health systems in the event either system is overwhelmed with patients requiring inpatient care.

NDMS federal coordinating centers (FCCs) play a regional role in maintaining a supply of NDMS hospital members and providing training and exercises. When the NDMS is activated, FCCs coordinate patient reception and distribution of patients being evacuated.

Hospitals enter into a voluntary agreement to participate in the NDMS. They must be accredited and generally have more than 100 beds. The agreement commits a hospital to provide a certain number of acute care beds to NDMS patients; however, it is recognized that hospitals may or may not be able to provide the agreed-upon number of beds. Hospitals that receive NDMS patients are reimbursed for care by the federal government.[16]

The Strategic National Stockpile

The Strategic National Stockpile (SNS) was established in 1999 as the National Pharmaceutical Stockpile. It is now managed by the U.S. Department of Homeland Security and serves as a national repository of antibiotics, chemical antidotes, antitoxins, intravenous therapy, airway management equipment, and medical/surgical items. The stockpile is designed to supplement local agencies that are overwhelmed by a health emergency.

The Noble Training Center

The Noble Training Center in Anniston, Ala., (on the site of the former Fort McClellan army base) is the only hospital facility in the United States that trains health-care professionals in disaster preparedness and response. The Department of Homeland Security operates the Noble Training Center, which offers a variety of training programs, including one for hospital leadership. More information is available online at: http://training.fema.gov/emiweb/ntc/.

Even though the federal government has many emergency response assets that can help in the response to an emergency, experience has shown that hospitals must be prepared to be self-sufficient for 24 to 72 hours after an event.[14]

Critical Elements in Hospital Disaster Preparedness

A comprehensive hospital emergency management program must address a number of critical elements to adequately protect patients and staff and permit the facility to continue to operate. These are discussed in the following.

Incident Command

Just as one team leader is necessary for a controlled response to a cardiac arrest, an organized approach is essential to a successful hospital-wide emergency response. The Hospital Emergency Incident Command System (HEICS) is designed to provide that coordination. Developed and tested in Orange County, Calif., in 1992, it provides structure to response. HEICS uses:

- A reproducible, predictable chain of command
- A flexible organizational design that can be scaled to the scope of the problem
- Checklists for each position to simplify response and carefully define each task
- A common language that permits communication with outside agencies

Emergency Operations Center (EOC)

The EOC will serve as the command post for operations during an emergency response. It should be fully operational and integrated into local and county emergency operations (Box 5-1).

Exercises, Drills, and Training

Hospital disaster drills have often been treated as annoyances and are planned in ways to render them futile. Exercises are generally announced (unlike actual events), planned during regular business hours, and rarely include all hospital operations that will be affected by an actual event. Hospitals are encouraged to drill individual units—frequently and during nights and weekends—and then build up to full, functional exercises involving management of moulaged "casualties." Community participation is critical to identify elements that work or that need fine-tuning. Only through exercise will the plan be adequately stressed so that failure points are identified.

Essential Services and Facilities Engineering

The facility's structural integrity and essential services are an often overlooked part of preparedness. In 2003 a

---

BOX 5-1 RECOMMENDED EQUIPMENT AND SUPPLIES FOR A HOSPITAL EOC

Location
- Secure interior space; windows not desirable
- Alternative, equipped space in distant part of complex or building in the event the primary EOC is damaged or disabled

Equipment
- Incident command gear to identify EOC staff (vests, ball caps)
- Computers with Internet access
- Dedicated telephone lines
- Communications-on-wheels (COWS)
- Two-way communications (400 MHz, 800 MHz)
- Fax
- Television with cable access
- Refrigerator
- Radio
- Bull horns
- Barrier tape
- Flashlights and batteries
- Back-up power generator
- Chalk board, dry-erase board, or other means of communicating to EOC team member

Information
- Hospital emergency management plan
- Reference materials (emergency response, clinical references, hazardous materials)
- Emergency reference contact numbers/e-mail addresses/fax numbers for local emergency response agencies (police, fire, emergency medical services, office of emergency management, department of health)
- Emergency contact information for national resources, including Centers for Disease Control and Prevention (CDC), Radiation Emergency Assistance Center/Training Site (REAC/TS), Agency for Toxic Substances and Disease Registry (ATSDR), Environmental Protection Agency (EPA), and National Response Center
- Staff notification information (phone contact numbers)
- Memoranda of understanding/agreement (MOU/MOA) with agencies and vendors
- Local and regional maps that include utility stations, hyperbaric capability, emergency medical services, police departments, fire stations, burn units, and other critical infrastructure

---

major power blackout in the northeastern United States and Canada demonstrated the impact of the loss electrical services. It is recommended that every hospital:

- Possess emergency power generating capacity for 3 to 4 days' duration
- Perform annual load testing on the generator(s)
- Maintain the water supply and an alternative water supply in secure areas in sufficient quantity to support all services (sanitation, hygiene, laundry) for 3 to 4 days
- Maintain medical gases in a secure location and have a 3- to 4-day supply for the hospital
- Configure the heating-ventilation-air conditioning

(HVAC) system so that it can be shut down and, ideally, so that specific zones can be manipulated to control airflow in the building in case of contamination

- Maintain a fuel source for full-load demand for 3 to 4 days' duration
- Develop a plan for the management and disposal of increased volumes of contaminated waste

Physical Security

Maintaining the physical security of the structure is important on a daily basis but becomes more of a challenge during a disaster. To ensure that the environment remains safe, egress must be controlled. Additional elements of the physical security plan should include the following:

- A security force with full-time security responsibilities; the force should have undergone criminal background checks and professional law enforcement training.
- All entrances and exits should be controlled, monitored, and capable of being locked.
- The hospital should be able to perform perimeter security protection ("lockdown") within minutes of notification.
- Hospital staff should be trained and drilled on the performance of lockdown.
- Hospital leadership should know what triggers the execution of a lockdown procedure.
- A plan should exist for supplementing security staff in a disaster.

Situation Report (Rapid Needs Assessment)

It is critical that a hospital be able to rapidly assess the impact of a disaster on its operations and communicate the status to leadership in a situation report (often referred to as a "sitrep"), or a rapid needs assessment (RAN). The assessment should, at a minimum, include the following:

- The extent and magnitude of the disaster and the scope and nature of casualties
- The status of operations and any disrupted critical services
- The impact of disruptions on operations and the ability to sustain operations[17]

Staff Notification

Hospital staff must be able to receive timely and accurate notifications in a disaster, including when and where to report and for how long and other essential information. Contact information for all staff members must be continuously updated and tested. Additionally, the facility must be able to receive warnings and notifications from external agencies and be able to send warnings.

Triage System

Triage is performed daily in emergency departments, where the most critical are treated first. But during a dis-

aster, triage procedures must adapt to become like what is used on the battlefield, where the greatest good is offered to the greatest number. Multiple disaster triage systems exist, including START (simple triage and rapid treatment), ID-ME (immediate, delayed, minimal, expectant), and MASS (move, assess, sort, and send). It is important that a hospital use a system that is consistent with what is being used by services delivering patients to the facility. Whatever system is selected, there must be predisaster training and exercises.

Alternative Triage Area

When casualties present to an emergency department in numbers that overwhelm the facility, an alternative area must be available to manage overflow. The alternative triage area should be lit so that it can be used at night, weatherproofed, and temperature-controlled.

Risk Communications and Media Management Plan

A plan for working with the media will be needed. It is not recommended that media personnel be permitted access to a hospital during a disaster, but rather be provided regular, factual updates on activities and the status of the facility at a predetermined meeting place. Risk communications involve using credible experts to deliver carefully worded messages to communicate most effectively in a high-stress, low-trust environment, such as a disaster. Preparing hospital leaders in risk communications principles will ensure that they are able to communicate effectively to the public via the media.

Disaster Mental Health Services

There is conflicting evidence about the value of certain types of mental health services in the wake of disaster, but it is clear that every disaster creates emotional trauma victims. Primary victims are those who have been directly affected by the disaster. Secondary victims are rescue workers in whom symptoms develop, and tertiary victims are relatives, friends, and others who have been affected. The critical incident disrupts a victim's sense of control as daily life is abruptly changed.[18] Hospitals must plan for providing mental health services to disaster victims but must also consider the needs—acute and long-term—of the hospital staff who attempt to respond to an overwhelming event. It is recommended that hospitals have trained crisis intervention teams that are well integrated into the emergency management plan.

Evidence and Crime Scene Management

In the event of an intentional act that results in mass casualties, not only must a hospital care for the victims, but it has a critical role in bringing perpetrators to justice. Hospital staff members require training in proper management of potential evidence—in both collection and preservation. Evidence collection containers, including 50-gallon drums for patient decontamination run-off, should be available as well as bags to preserve other types of evidence. Law enforcement agencies and forensic departments can provide training and guidance. Staff members should be familiar with and follow procedures for maintaining chain of custody for evidence that is collected during patient care activities.

Food Services

A disaster will place significant demands on the food service system of a hospital. The adequacy of food supplies for patients and staff should be evaluated. Because a hospital may need to be self-sufficient for several days in a disaster, a 3- to 4-day supply of food products is advisable. Food service personnel should be included in disaster exercises.

Role of Volunteers

Volunteers may or may not be of assistance, depending on their relationship with the hospital and their background. A volunteer pool that consists of individuals who serve regularly at the facility, are familiar with standard procedures, and participate in exercises can add valuable manpower to a disaster response effort. On the other hand, disasters will draw volunteers who wish to assist, a phenomenon known as "convergent volunteerism," in which unexpected and uninvited healthcare workers arrive and wish to render assistance at a large-scale incident.[19] These "freelancers" may cause problems or may even be impostors.

Disaster Supplies

Despite "just-in-time" supply schedules and empty warehouses, hospitals should maintain dedicated disaster supplies and arrangements for rapid resupply in the event of a disaster. Disaster response will rapidly deplete critical supplies—administrative as well as clinical. Conducting realistic exercises will help with the determination of the adequacy of stock and can be done without opening actual supplies so they can be restocked. Disaster supplies can be rotated into the daily-use stream to ensure stock does not expire.

PITFALLS

Experience with disasters has demonstrated a number of predictable pitfalls that occur in hospital disaster response.

Distribution of Casualties

Because immediate on-scene control of a disaster is chaotic and communication is often problematic, patients will present to the closest hospital available. This often leaves other nearby facilities with capacity and personnel that go unused.

Personal Protective Equipment

Hospital personnel must be experts in protecting themselves, or they will become part of the problem and further stress the facility. Some controversy exists over the level of protection needed in certain environments, but it is clear that masks (N95) and gloves (latex or nonlatex) will prevent transmission of biological agents.

Communications

Communications failure has often been identified as a predictable failure in disaster response. Hospitals need to examine both internal communications systems (with staff and patients) and with external agencies. Multiple layers of redundancy are essential to deal with expected failures and include the use of 800-mHz radios, dedicated trunk lines in the emergency operations center, two-way communications for hospital units and essential personnel, communications-on-wheels (COWS), and access to amateur radio (Ham) operators. The last resort is using runners who carry messages.

Emergency Patient Decontamination

Hospitals must be able to identify and decontaminate patients who have been exposed to radiation or a compound that poses a threat to the patient's health and the safety of the facility. If the hospital depends on an external agency or has decontamination equipment that requires time to set up, an immediate alternative must be in place, such as a hose and hose bib outside of the emergency department. Consideration should be given to patient privacy, managing patient valuables and clothes, and handling weapons brought into the hospital. A trained, exercised, and well-equipped team will be the foundation of successful efforts.

Child Care

Hospitals will benefit from having a plan to care for children and other dependents of staff. In a disaster, staff will be called on to work extended hours, and usual family care arrangements may be unavailable.

Patient Admission, Identification, and Tracking

The creation of emergency patient admission packs that are maintained with disaster equipment will facilitate the admission of a large number of patients. If an automated patient tracking system is used, a back-up manual system should be available. All systems should be able to manage unidentified (John and Jane Doe) patients.

Mass Fatalities

Many hospitals have wholly inadequate or nonexistent plans to manage mass fatalities. Morgue space is generally limited in most facilities, so additional surge capacity must be identified in advance. Arrangements for refrigerated storage trucks, refrigerator space, and other alternatives, including ice rinks, should be addressed with socially sensitive plans. Complex cultural and religious issues may come into play in the event that there are contaminated remains and should be examined in advance.

Disaster Pharmaceuticals

Emergency drugs must be available at the point of care. Often they are secured in pharmacy departments or warehouses, resulting in precious minutes of life-saving time being lost as personnel try to locate and obtain critical medications. In addition to drugs needed to respond quickly to nerve agents and other emergency situations, stockpiles of antibiotics should be maintained to provide prophylaxis to patients and staff.

CONCLUSION

In a disaster, patients converge on the place they know they can obtain care—the hospital—and they arrive using any means possible. Furthermore, with the victims of disaster, come their families, loved ones, and the media—all who have very important needs that must be addressed. Hospitals can no longer approach disaster planning with a minimalist attitude that relies heavily on luck and belief that it will be someplace else that gets hit by the disaster.

The hospital that received the most patients from the Rhode Island nightclub fire got lucky—the victims began arriving during a change of shift so there were two shifts of nursing staff available. However, the hospital also attributes its effective response to having drilled critical departments and procedures.

Emergency planning is the backbone of preparedness, but events will occur in each disaster that demand creative responses under pressure. This ability to respond flexibly is known as *planned innovation.* Good plans will use general "all hazards" templates for disaster management but will permit independent initiative and a tailored response to a specific situation.[20]

The U.S. health system appears to be emerging from the dark ages of emergency planning. A minimalist attitude of preparedness was acceptable in the past despite the regular occurrence of natural disasters. The threat of terrorism and the resulting health system impact have stimulated investment in research, a resurgence of disaster training in nursing and medical schools, and visionary projects such as ER One. ER One is a national prototype for a next-generation emergency department. Located in Washington, D.C., it is developing new approaches to the medical consequences of terrorist attacks, natural disasters, and emerging illnesses. More information is available online at: http://er1.org.

The next phase of hospital emergency management will be a renaissance if creative planning prevails over naysayers, if resources are applied to priority preparedness activities, and if healthcare leaders are committed to ensuring that all who depend on hospitals will receive the care they need in a disaster (Box 5-2).

BOX 5-2 HOSPITAL PREPAREDNESS AND RESPONSE RESOURCES

- Auf der Heide E. **Principles of hospital disaster planning.** In: Hogan DE, Burstein JL, eds. *Disaster Medicine.* Philadelphia: Lippincott Williams and Wilkins; 2002:57-89.
- **National Advisory Committee on Children and Terrorism.** Recommendations to the Secretary, U.S. Department of Health and Human Services. (Includes recommendations on prehospital and hospital care.) Available at: http://www.bt.cdc.gov/children/word/working/Recommend.doc.
- **Preparing for the Psychological Consequences of Terrorism—A Public Health Strategy.** This 2003 publication of the National Academies of Science includes an examination of current infrastructure and response strategies. Available at: http://search.nap.edu/books/0309089530/html/.
- Joint Commission on Accreditation of Healthcare Organizations. **Guide to Emergency Management Planning in Health Care.** Oakbrook Terrace, IL: Joint Commission Resources; 2002.
- **Rocky Mountain Regional Care Model for Bioterrorist Events.** Available at: www.ahrq.gov/research/altsites.htm.
- **The Hospital Emergency Incident Command System.** Available at: http://www.heics.com/.
- **The American Academy of Experts in Traumatic Stress.** Available at: http://www.aaets.org/.
- **The International Critical Incident Stress Foundation, Inc.** Available at: http://www.icisf.org/.

REFERENCES

1. Rosenberg CE. *The Care of Strangers—The Rise of America's Hospital System.* Baltimore: The Johns Hopkins University Press; 1987:5.
2. Nates JL. Combined external and internal hospital disaster: impact and response in a Houston trauma center intensive care unit. *Crit Care Med.* 2004;32:686-90.
3. Schultz CH, Koenig KL, Lewis RJ. Implications of hospital evacuation after the Northridge, California, earthquake. *N Engl J Med.* 2003;348:1349-55.
4. Wolinsky PR, Tejwani NC, Testa NN, et al. Lessons learned from the activation of a disaster plan: 9/11. *J Bone Joint Surg Am.* 2003; 85:1844-6.
5. Cushman JG, Pachter NL, Beaton HL. Two New York City hospitals' surgical response to the September 11, 2001 terrorist attack in New York City. *J Trauma.* 2003;54:147-55.
6. Feeney J, Parekh N, Blumenthal J, et al. September 11, 2001: a test of preparedness and spirit. *Bull Am Coll Surg.* 2002;87:12-17.
7. Hogan DE, Waeckerle JF, Dire DJ, et al. Emergency department impact of the Oklahoma City terrorist bombing. *Ann Emerg Med.* 1999;34:160-7.
8. Dacey MJ. Tragedy and response—the Rhode Island nightclub fire. *N Engl J Med.* 2003;349:1990-2.
9. Gutman D, Biffl WL, Suner S, et al. The Station Nightclub fire and disaster preparedness in Rhode Island. *Med Health R I.* 2003;86:344-6.
10. Sullivan DK. Mass decontamination: why re-invent the wheel? *J Emerg Mgmt.* 2001; 2:52-4.
11. Healthcare Association of New York State. *Meeting New Challenges and Fulfilling the Public Trust: Resources Needed for Hospital Emergency Preparedness.* New York: Healthcare Association of New York State; 2001:1-4.
12. Rubin JN. Recurring pitfalls in hospital preparedness and response. *J Homeland Security.* January 2004;1-15. Available at: http://www.homelandsecurity.org/journal/articles/rubin.html.
13. Pan American Health Organization. *Principles of Disaster Mitigation in Health Facilities.* Washington, DC: Pan American Health Organization; 2000:7-25.
14. Joint Commission on Accreditation of Healthcare Organizations. *Health Care at the Crossroads—Strategies for Creating and*

Sustaining Community-wide Emergency Preparedness Systems.
Oakbrook Terrace, IL: Joint Commission on Accreditation of
Healthcare Organizations; 2003:11.

15. Chaffee MW, Miranda SM, Padula R, et al. DVATEX: Navy Medicine's
pioneering approach to improving hospital emergency preparedness. *J Emerg Mgmt.* 2004;2:35-40.

16. US Department of Homeland Security. National Disaster Medical
System. Available at: http://oep-ndms.dhhs.gov/dmat_faq.html.

17. Briggs SM, Brinsfield KH. *Advanced Disaster Medical Response—
Manual for Providers.* Boston: Harvard Medical International
Trauma and Disaster Institute; 2003:27-33.

18. Oster NS, Doyle CJ. Critical incident stress. In: Hogan DE, Burstein
JL, eds. *Disaster Medicine.* Philadelphia: Lippincott Williams and
Wilkins; 2002:41-6.

19. Cone DC, Weir SD, Bogucki S. Convergent volunteerism. *Ann
Emerg Med.* 2003;41:457-62.

20. Gabriel EJ. Making room for outside the box thinking in emergency management and preparedness. *Jt Com J Qual Saf.*
2003;29:319-20.

chapter 6

Complex Emergencies

Frederick M. Burkle, Jr. and P. Gregg Greenough

Since the end of the Cold War, 95% of all major conflicts have been internal nation-state wars. These are commonly referred to as *complex emergencies (CEs)* because of the myriad political, sociocultural, and economic factors that provoke them.

Zwi and Ugalde[1] defined CEs as "situations in which the capacity to sustain livelihood and life are threatened primarily by political factors and, in particular, by high levels of violence." National disruption resulting from conflict and war has occurred this last decade in nation-states such as Liberia, Somalia, Rwanda, Angola, the former Yugoslavia, the province of Kosovo, East Timor, and Iraq. Unfortunately, CEs represent catastrophic public health emergencies that often develop into a continuum of protracted social conflict.

MAJOR CHARACTERISTICS

The defining characteristics of CEs include the following:

- CEs have existed for many years; however, during the last two decades, they have become the most common type of human-generated disasters.[2] Currently there are 35 countries at risk of serious conflict, 11 of which are near collapse. Primarily because of unresolved war and conflict, worldwide hunger has climbed 18%, leaving more than 850 million people without food for basic health.[3] Conflict has degraded the agricultural and public health infrastructures during the past decade, directly increasing the toll of civilian morbidity and mortality.
- CE victims commonly suffer from social, economic, and gender inequities; poverty; injustices; cultural and religious persecutions; ignorance; racism; oppression; religious fundamentalism; and other lethal factors that contribute to internal strife among varied ethnic, tribal, and religious groups. All adversely affect the public health and the access to and availability of healthcare.
- The majority of victims are civilians, with mortality and morbidity largely among vulnerable and unprotected children, women, the elderly, and the disabled. During the Cold War, one-half of all conflict-related deaths were among civilians. Civilians in CEs account

for 90% of all war-related deaths, and more children than soldiers, about 2 million through 1993, have died as a result of internal civil strife.[4] Genocide and other wanton violations of the Geneva Conventions have contributed to the high violence rates directed at civilians.

- There is a linear relationship between mortality of children younger than 5 years (per 1000) and the percentage of nations engaged in armed conflict. The worst conditions and highest mortality rates are recorded among orphaned and unaccompanied children who frequently fall through the cracks of the humanitarian response effort and who require parental or surrogate adults for the distribution of critical aid. In large, rapidly forming refugee camps, the most vulnerable can easily be lost among the masses and go unrecognized by those operating fledgling humanitarian relief efforts.
- CEs must be understood and managed in the context of politics. Intervention, relief, success, and failure of CEs are dependent on politics and outside military actions to end, or at least contain, the violence. During the 1990s, the world community, with varying success, responded to the more publicized CEs (Iraqi Kurds fleeing the Saddam regime to northern Iraq, severe hunger in rebel-ravaged Somalia, the ethnic and religious cleansing in the Balkans, and the political plight of East Timor). However, outside assistance has been limited or avoided in other conflicts (mass slaughter in Rwanda and the Democratic Republic of the Congo and the unrelenting conflict in Sudan). With minority and ethnic groups at risk of extinction, the customs, skills, and the very foundations of health and public health refinements that have defined their cultures have ceased to exist.
- Healthcare professionals face major challenges just to decrease the immediate mortality and morbidity resulting from communicable disease, trauma, and the dire health consequences of infrastructure losses in water, sanitation, shelter, and food.
- The targeting of healthcare providers and medical neutrality is a consistent feature of CEs. Hospitals are predictably the first to be destroyed and the last to be rehabilitated.[5] Therapeutic feeding centers for starving infants and primary health centers are commonly

destroyed and looted, and female and child patients are slain in their beds. Warring factions have purposely politicized health and with it have summarily executed or detained physicians and nurses to foment fear. As political violence increases, access and availability to healthcare diminishes.[1]

HISTORICAL PERSPECTIVE

A wealth of evidence has accumulated for more than 25 years on the massive effect of war on health. Field epidemiological research has defined the health and public health characteristics of CEs.[6] Data have further demonstrated a consistent negative association between violent conflict and health outcome indicators (life expectancy, infant mortality rates, and immunization rates).[1,7] Additional studies have confirmed the negative impact of landmines and sanctions on the health of children and that government instability and societal decline are the complex catalysts whereby controls on tuberculosis, malaria, and human immunodeficiency virus (HIV) become unchecked. Between 1990 and 1995, the disease burden of war equaled that of homicide and suicide when measured in disability adjusted life years (DALYs). Further, data analyses now suggest a trend in which the ranking of lives lost from the total consequences of war and conflict would move from the top 20 causes of disability, where it is now, to the top 10 by the year 2010.[8]

Populations suffer both direct and indirect effects of conflict. Direct effects include injuries, deaths and disabilities, human rights and international humanitarian law abuses, and psychological stress. Indirect effects actually contribute to the majority of mortality and morbidity due to population displacement, disruption of food supplies, and destroyed health facilities and public health infrastructure. At least three epidemiological models exist that may guide the current practice of the humanitarian response effort.

EPIDEMIOLOGICAL MODELS

Developing Country Model

The health profile of countries in Africa and Asia during the acute phase of a conflict or war is usually identified by moderate or severe malnutrition, outbreaks of communicable diseases, or often both. The most common CEs of the past two decades have involved famine and forced migration in developing countries. Since the 1980s, few famines have occurred that were not human induced, and many famines catalyzed the onset of CEs.[4]

The most severe consequences of population displacement have occurred during the acute phase, when relief efforts have not yet begun or are still in the early stages.[6] Refugees (populations that cross borders) and internally displaced populations have experienced high mortality rates during the period immediately after their migration. Internally displaced populations do not enjoy the immediate protections against persecution and human rights abuse under international law that are afforded to refugees by the UNHCR (United Nations High Commissioner for Refugees). Internally displaced populations must fend for themselves without benefit of basic healthcare services, food, water, or sanitation. Stripped from their supportive infrastructure, refugees suffer mortality rates that are 7 to 10 times higher than those for the baseline indigenous populations. In the refugee camps at Goma, Congo, the crude mortality rates exceeded 60 times those of the baseline population.[9]

The health consequences are both directly and indirectly related to the conflict itself.[4] Three-fourths of all epidemics of the last decade took place in CEs. Epidemiological indicators show high crude mortality rates and, if disaggregated, demonstrate the vulnerability among the populations as to age (children younger than 5 years and the elderly) and gender (women and female-headed households). For instance, high case fatality rates were common among malnourished children in Somalia, with measles contributing to between 50% and 81% of deaths.[4,10,11]

Developed Country Model

Countries such as Iraq, the former Yugoslavia, Macedonia, and Kosovo had relatively healthy populations with demographic profiles similar to those of Western countries before the onset of internal conflict. In these places, the few epidemics and low prevalence of malnutrition among children and infants were superseded by undernutrition and chronic diseases among the elderly who could not flee the conflict or were unable to access healthcare. In these settings, war-related trauma from advanced weaponry contributed to the primary cause of mortality. Children, adolescents, and pregnant women were specific targets in Yugoslavia, with more than 3000 children killed by snipers alone. Rape and traumatic exposures commonly contributed to psychological morbidity.[12]

Chronic or Smoldering Country Model

Both Haiti and Sudan have unique problems related to long-standing conflict and unrest that prevent progress in health, healthcare delivery and access, disease prevention, and education. Except for high rates of HIV/AIDS, Haiti's health profile in disease is representative of one that was last seen in the United States in the early 1900s. Massive deforestation has led to severe environmental collapse that has contributed inextricably to chronic health and infrastructure loss.[13,14] Haiti is representative of a smoldering country model that is suffering both an acute emergency situation as well as ongoing severe development problems. It is a dilemma to know where the assistance should be placed to do the most good. Some would rightly argue that without attention first to critical development priorities, acute emergency situations will continue to worsen. Sudan has experienced war since 1955, and as such, its children grow up chronically malnourished and know only a culture of violence with little access to healthcare and education. Reproductive health is an unknown luxury, and most healthcare must be imported.

EVOLUTION OF INTERVENTION

Pugh[15] describes evolutionary phases of intervention seen during the 1990s. Initially, humanitarian assistance was believed to be all that was needed to meet the demands of what were considered temporary post-Cold War conflicts. By the mid-1990s, it was clear that CEs were more dangerous, longer lasting, and complex than first thought.

The humanitarian response was first dominated by international relief organizations, which based their presence on neutrality and impartiality protected under international treaties and covenants such as the Geneva Conventions. If and when military forces became involved, they did so under the rubric of ensuring relief security, which in places such as Somalia had been severely compromised by undisciplined rebel groups who had no knowledge about protections afforded to relief workers under the Geneva Conventions.

Intervention, relief, and the successes and failures of CE interventions depend on politics and the political action of many countries, agencies, and organizations. For both the United Nations (UN) and Western powers, political action is translated as "military action." In the early 1990s, the UN response consisted of deploying peacekeeping forces under Chapter VI of the UN Charter to help quell the conflict and provide some semblance of security for the intervening UN agencies and international relief organizations (IROs). These loosely defined civil-military relationships over time proved problematic. Many in the humanitarian community considered military involvement dangerous and unnecessary because a foreign, primarily Western, military presence threatened the neutral status of *all* expatriate workers. In these civil-military "interventions" both sides were ambivalent about their roles, cooperation, and under what security criteria the military should leave (the so-called exit strategy or end state that is constantly debated within the humanitarian and military-political communities).

It was soon recognized that sustained development and long-term improvements would never occur without a political solution. The "humanitarian imperative" that drove the initial relief assistance was threatened by naysayers and others who strongly believed that assistance without a clear political road map to mitigate the causes of the conflict was self-defeating. By the mid-1990s, studies exposed a parallel crisis in humanitarian protection. The humanitarian community was not protecting those that needed protection. The relief agencies, called on to implement assistance programs, were inconsistent and lacked professionalism. In addition, despite growing needs worldwide for intervention, both donors and governments were allocating less and less to fund the needed resources. The frustration during the 1990s was characterized over time by healthcare providers meeting the challenge to save lives, only to find the situation sliding back into crisis.[15]

By the turn of the century, studies revealed alarming data on mortality from intentional violence and banditry against humanitarian relief agencies and peacekeeping forces. One study[16] found that 68%, or 253 deaths, of 375 deaths among staff of certain relief agencies and UN peacekeeping forces between 1985 and 1998 were a result of intentional violence. Of 52 deaths among staff for the International Committee of the Red Cross (ICRC) and the International Federation of Red Cross and Red Crescent societies, 77% were a result of intentional violence.[16]

These events contributed to the decision to replace UN peacekeeping forces with peace enforcement troops. The peacekeeping forces had been deployed by the Security Council under UN Charter Chapter VI, which lacked the military resources and legal mandate to quell the violence. With the new method, under Chapter VII, peace enforcement troops have the resources to cease the violence required to protect civilians before a peace agreement is in place. This process of moving from peacekeeping to peace enforcement was slow, taking three years and 33 new Security Council resolutions to complete. All UN military interventions have been authorized under Chapter VII since its inception.[17]

Encouragingly, relief organizations found common ground for collaboration and cooperation in projects, programs, education, training, and decision-making. This common ground catalyzed the relationship between health and human rights and the defining of the "rights discourse," which declares that victims have the *right* to humanitarian assistance and that nongovernment organizations (NGOs) and UN agencies have the *duty* to provide assistance. This common ground process also spurred the argument for a consistent framework of standards of care and benchmarks for professionalism within the ranks of the relief community.

In the midst of the chaos of CEs, healthcare professionals have taken on roles, other than that of providers, to negotiate and mediate with and cajole the warring factions to spare the health infrastructure from total annihilation. In doing so, negotiation and mediation with warring factions and rogue regimes have become increasingly necessary to maintain viable health programs threatened by political violence. This increasing presence of healthcare providers in the "political process" as decision-makers in conflict resolution is not always a comfortable role. Rather, these interventions could be fraught with personal risks and seeming violations of an organization's impartiality and neutrality strictly defined under existing covenants. In taking on these roles, healthcare providers have been instrumental in developing unique solutions through negotiating "immunization days" with rebel groups and delineating "tranquility zones," where vulnerable groups are isolated from the surrounding fighting.

CURRENT PRACTICE

Multinational Model Response

It is not uncommon for NGOs and other relief organizations to be established in a country in conflict long before the violence garners the attention of the international community. The larger multinational humanitarian response begins with a decision by the international community to intervene, usually because of increasing violence and the migration of refugees across the borders into neighboring nations. This process comes after weeks and often months of debate within the UN Security Council before a resolution is passed that directs the scope of the humanitarian assistance and defines the actors who will participate. Since the major reason for intervention is to cease the violence that leads to health consequences, a UN resolution will first define the requirements of peace enforcement troops authorized under Chapter VII of the UN Charter. These peace-enforcement troops are needed to end the violence and abuses of international law and human rights, to provide a protective environment that allows for assistance to decrease mortality and morbidity, and to ensure a secure environment in which IROs can function. Diplomatic assets are used to develop peace accords and agreements that must be in place before the peace enforcement troops are redeployed and replaced by UN peacekeeping forces, who function to maintain the peace (under Chapter VI of the UN Charter).

Humanitarian assistance usually comes from assets contributed by the UN Office of the Coordinator for Humanitarian Assistance (OCHA) and UN agencies such as the World Food Program (WFP), World Health Organization (WHO), and the UN Children's Fund (UNICEF); the Red Cross Movement; NGOs; and donor agencies that primarily represent industrialized nations' governments, such as the U.S. Agency for International Development (USAID), the Canadian International Development Agency (CIDA), and Japan International Cooperation Agency (JICA).

The multiagency response to CEs grew rapidly in the decade of the 1990s. NGOs assumed increasingly more responsibilities for governments and international organizations by implementing major relief and assistance programs for vulnerable civilian refugees and displaced populations. In 1991, NGOs numbered 28 in northern Iraq; by 1995 in Haiti, there were more than 710 NGOs.

Health Assessment

The humanitarian community (international organizations, NGOs, private government organizations, and peacekeeping militaries) has a professional obligation to base assistance on the best evidence available.[18] This supposition is the cornerstone of the concept of evidence-based healthcare.

The need and demand for healthcare in CEs increases at a rate determined, in part, by the rate at which public health infrastructure is destroyed and the moral integrity of governance disappears. Initially, healthcare needs may be greater than the rate at which resources are being made available.[19] Historically, response activities in CEs have often been ineffective because of the poor quality of information available as well as the manner in which an assessment was conducted. Assessment and assistance are often hampered by organizational problems and lack of personnel, medical records, and financial resources.[20] Epidemiological methods established for situations in which there are restricted resources use a simpler method of statistical analysis, which is known as a *rapid assessment*[20] and is sometimes referred to as

a "quick and dirty" assessment.[21] The initial assessment by an experienced interdisciplinary team must be carried out as soon as it is clear that an emergency exists.

During the decade of the 1990s, both health and nutritional assessments, despite being performed rapidly and under difficult situations and restraints, gained a reputation for quality. With critical advances in indicator identification, epidemiological analysis, data retrieval technologies, and education and training of relief personnel, health and nutritional assessments have continued to improve as an art and science.

Data collection commences before the field assessment and originates from existing country profiles, maps, census data, previous demographic and health surveys, early warning system tools, and previous or ongoing in-country assessments.[22] Additional data may come from over-flights and satellite imagery; these are especially useful in tracking refugee migration. Background health information is gleaned from previous reports inherent to organizations such as WHO, the Disaster Epidemiology Research Center in Belgium, the European Expert Group in Practical Epidemiology (EpiCentre), and the Centers for Disease Control and Prevention's (CDC) *Mortality and Morbidity Weekly Report (MMWR)* publications. This information includes, but is not restricted to, baseline data on the following[4,23-25]:

- Endemic diseases
- Mortality rates
- Morbidity-incidence rates
- Nutritional status
- Sources of healthcare
- Impact of disruption of health services

Assessment documents are available that provide detailed checklists, information on the principles of an assessment, planning techniques, methods, and forms.

Use of an evidence-based approach makes it possible for decision-makers (policy, operational, and field level) to differentiate the needs of the population, the resources available, and the costs of any decision. An evidence-based approach helps one to differentiate between what is supported by evidence and that which is made on an unsubstantiated assertion. Health assessments today are expected to be reliable and valid and, as such, are inextricably linked to the analysis of specific performance and outcome indicators, region- and disaster-specific epidemiological studies, and measures of effectiveness.[26] Assessment in one form or another never stops.[25,27*]

The assessment tool used can vary depending on the phase of the CE. The rapid health assessment of a CE concentrates on the needs of relief managers and decision-makers to obtain timely and accurate data necessary to rationally allocate available resources according to the emergency situation. Rapid assessment stimulates the development of more organized and focused surveys and the longer-lasting surveillance system, as well as a

---

*A full account of the assessment process can be found in: Burkle FM. Evidence-based health assessment process in complex emergencies. In: Cahill KM, ed. *Emergency Relief Operations.* New York: Fordham University Press and The Center for International Health and Cooperation; 2003.

health information system (HIS). The HIS facilitates the collection of demographic and vital statistics data, administration of a disease surveillance system, regular monitoring of hospital and clinic discharge diagnoses, and investigation of disease outbreaks.[28] How rapidly an HIS can be implemented is often used as a measure of efficiency and effectiveness of the relief effort.

During the early 1990s, response initiatives suffered because of poor and inconsistent humanitarian response and lack of assessment standardization. By the late 1990s, WHO rapid assessment protocols[23] and the Humanitarian Charter and Minimum Standards (SPHERE Project) provided the needed standardization guidelines to assess and assist in water supply and sanitation, nutrition, food aid, shelter and site planning, and health services.[24] The Sphere Project's Humanitarian Charter describes the core principles that govern humanitarian action and defines the legal responsibilities of states and parties in conflict to guarantee the right to assistance and protection.[13] When states are unable to respond to a CE, they are obliged to allow the intervention of humanitarian organizations, which in itself begins with an assessment.

The concept of *excess deaths* is a critical epidemiological tool, especially in areas where there is conflict and where population movements are high. In war-affected areas of the eastern Democratic Republic of Congo (largely inaccessible to aid organizations and assessments because of insecurity),[29] the ongoing fighting drove hundreds of thousands of internally displaced people into forests, jungles, and other remote areas where they had no food, medicine, or shelter. Health systems and basic environmental public health infrastructure were destroyed. An epidemiological assessment was conducted, at considerable risk to the assessment team, of 11 mortality surveys in five provinces throughout eastern Congo. Results determined that over a 32-month period, approximately 2.5 million excess deaths (deaths greater than expected during the period studied) had occurred due to the conflict in that country. Previous reports had documented that approximately 100,000 people had died as a result of war.[29] The assessment revealed that the war casualties were not limited to victims of violence, but rather that 90% of the deaths were attributed to infectious diseases (e.g., malaria, diarrheal diseases) and other nonviolent causes (e.g., malnutrition) directly or indirectly related to the environmental disruptions. The destruction of the region's health infrastructure and lack of regional security meant that the vast majority of the population had minimal access to medical and public health services, making them more prone to disease. In addition, this assessment provided the only evidence that a humanitarian crisis of "staggering proportions" existed.[29] The assessment demonstrated the critical importance of how an epidemiological approach to an assessment can be used to document the denial of human rights associated with a lack of access to medical care, basic public health, and environmental services. Even though the study lacked the empirical scrutiny guaranteed with exact numbers, the assessment did reveal that a massive international response was indicated.

Health Interventions

All health and nonhealth interventions that support public health needs in CEs are determined by rapid assessments, focused surveys, and surveillance. Poor surveillance design, at all three levels (rapid assessment, surveys, and surveillance) will lead to a predictable resurgence of disease and public health disruption. If survey indicators and surveillance methodologies are incomplete or inaccurate, the ability to monitor the sensitive relationships between health, nutrition and environmental indicators, endemic disease, injury prevention (e.g., landmine injuries), and gender- and age-specific vulnerabilities will be lacking.

The goal of any health intervention is to minimize mortality and morbidity. Endemic disease control, especially in a developing country model, is always a priority. All children in developing countries in conflict should receive measles vaccine and vitamin A supplementation to mitigate the complication rate of measles and other infectious diseases, such as diarrheal and respiratory diseases. Malaria, HIV, and sexually transmitted diseases (STDs) also take a severe toll. Once humanitarian assistance reaches these populations, during the acute phase (first 4 to 6 weeks), the mortality and morbidity rates should decline. Priorities in camps shift to maintaining the public health protective infrastructures in water and sanitation, food, and shelter; ensuring security and fuel; and rebuilding the basic public health system. Abuses against women and failures in reproductive health have led to high rates of STDs and pregnancy in refugee camps. WHO Emergency Health Kits, which include safe birthing and surgical supplies to care for a population of 10,000 for approximately three months, can provide immediate assistance in CEs.[30]

Food Programs

Food programs must ensure proper nutrition for the general displaced population as well as therapeutic or supplemental feedings for the acutely malnourished. These programs also should address micronutrient deficiencies as well as give special attention to the nutrition needs of those with HIV/AIDS or tuberculosis. Emphasis must be placed on maternal and child health, reproductive health, and the protection of those with disabilities and injuries. Attacks on infant feeding centers occurred with regularity in Sudan, Mozambique, Ethiopia, Somalia, Angola, and Liberia, and the diversion of food by warring factions became commonplace.

Protein energy malnutrition (PEM) has three components: malnutrition, micronutrient deficiency diseases (especially those related to a lack of vitamins A, C, B_6 and zinc), and secondary infections. The term *PEM* is often used instead of *kwashiorkor* or *marasmus* to define the state of illness. Indeed, many cases are mixed in their presentation (marasmus-kwashiorkor) and difficult to clinically distinguish. Nutritional assessments are performed with population convenience samples, in which new arrivals to the refugee camps are screened, and through cluster sample surveys. The malnutrition rate of children younger than 5 years ranks just below crude mortality rates as the most specific indicator of a population's health.[9,18,25,31] The malnutrition rate also determines the urgency for food ration delivery and requirements for supplementary feedings and therapeutic feeding centers. Some interventions are now so routine that they no longer require an assessment before implementation in the acute phase of CEs. Most demonstrable is the provision of vitamin A supplementation and measles vaccine in refugee populations in developing countries. Studies from the early 1990s on CEs have shown that vitamin A reduces mortality and morbidity in malnourished children, especially those with measles (active, susceptible, and exposed) and other respiratory illnesses. Indeed, vitamin A supplementation reduces all-cause mortality in children.[32] By the time measles becomes identified in a population-dense camp environment, the mortality and morbidity may already be out of control. Based on this evidence, it has become protocol to provide all children between 1 and 6 years old, at the time of registration into the camp, both measles vaccine and vitamin A supplementation. This being the case, the initial assessment focuses on identifying the population in need of services and in ensuring continuing monitoring through program outcome surveys and surveillance. Relief programs emphasize a primary health care approach, focusing on oral rehydration, feeding centers, immunization, promoting involvement by the refugee community in the provision of health services, and stressing effective coordination of programs and information sharing among the NGOs that deal directly with the recipients of care.[33]

Medical Personnel

Medical and nursing assets that are needed most under the developing country model are personnel from public health, preventive medicine and infectious disease, primary care, obstetrics and gynecology, family practice, and emergency medicine.[34] For CEs in developed country, the desired expatriate medical and nursing care includes surgery, anesthesia, and emergency medicine.[34] Chronic and smoldering countries with CEs require a public health focus; however, it is critical to provide healthcare personnel based on the assessment of need to restore both the curative as well as the preventive public health core of the society. This assessment usually reflects the objectives of individual projects and programs. Typically, assistance agencies use trained personnel from relief, development, and advocacy groups.

UNILATERAL MODEL RESPONSE

In the 2003 war with Iraq, the United States and its coalition partners chose a unilateral approach that did not adhere to Chapter VII of the UN Charter. This approach was based on the assumption that this was first a war that would be short with no major humanitarian crisis occurring. Internal U.S. governmental changes also occurred. Under presidential directive, the Department of Defense (DoD) assumed the lead for humanitarian assistance, a position traditionally played by the U.S.

State Department and USAID's Office of Foreign Disaster Assistance (OFDA). Planning for relief, recovery, and reconstruction was placed under the DoD's newly formed Office of Reconstruction and Humanitarian Assistance (ORHA), later renamed the Coalition Provisional Authority (CPA).

Initially, because it was determind by the DoD that there would be little need for humanitarian assistance, the UN agencies and major NGOs had a minimal role in the planning and received little funding support from the United States. Many, including UNHCR, WHO, and ICRC, had expended their reserve funds in limited preparations.

However, international studies published since the end of the Persian Gulf War suggested that civilian health was substantially worse and that specific humanitarian outcomes might occur. Specifically, since 1990 some indicators demonstrated a progressive decline, whereas others reached a nadir in the mid-1990s before the Oil-for-Food and Oil-for-Medicine programs allowed Iraq to import and distribute food, medication, and health supplies and equipment. Infant mortality rates (deaths in children younger than 12 months per 1000 live births) increased from 47.1 to 108 during the period from 1994 to 1999. During the same time, mortality rates for children younger than 5 years increased from 56 to 131 (per 1000 live births). Acute malnutrition increased from 3.6% in 1991 to 11% in 1996. However, the rate of acute malnutrition decreased to 4% in 2002 because of the coordinated work of Iraqis with UNICEF, WHO, the Red Cross Movement, and several major international NGOs. Increases were seen in reported cases of tuberculosis, cholera, typhoid fever, amoebic dysentery, giardiasis, leishmaniasis, and malaria. It was not known whether this represented a true increase or was the result of better surveillance and record keeping.[35-39]

As a contingency, the main relief resources warehoused by the humanitarian organizations included nationally and regionally prepositioned WHO emergency health, surgical, and safe birthing kits; tents; blankets; water bladders; and high-protein food baskets.[30]

Many NGOs chose not to work with the military-dominated relief effort. The ICRC was the only humanitarian organization functioning during the war, with specific responsibilities mandated under the Geneva Conventions to mitigate civilian casualties and provide repair to vital infrastructure destroyed during the hostilities. Iraqi national staff previously trained by WHO and UNICEF provided a functional semblance of outbreak control, basic healthcare, and repair of water and sanitation infrastructure.

Unfortunately, widespread looting and trashing of public health facilities and hospitals caused a collapse of the health system. The U.S. and coalition militaries, due to flawed planning, were unprepared and undermanned for the security and recovery needs required under international law as an occupying power. In general, health consequences were similar to those found in the developed country model, where trauma and unattended chronic diseases in the elderly predominate. In time, the United States actively requested and supported the return of UN agencies; however, security continued to be the overriding concern that prevented the rapid return of essential services.

Whether this unilateral approach to conflict and war will represent a new model for dealing with CEs has yet to be determined.

Even with the paucity of NGOs serving in Iraq and Afghanistan, there were more fatal attacks reported among humanitarian aid workers in both countries in 2003 than in any prior year. Of the 76 humanitarian workers killed in 2003, 43 were victims of "terrorist-style or terrorist affiliated attacks." The majority of victims in both countries were local staff employed by NGOs.[40]

PITFALLS

Problems persist. The world humanitarian community lacks a concerted approach to meeting the needs that occur during CEs. Reforms are needed in the UN and its agencies. NGOs are nonhomogeneous organizations; their proliferation during the past decade has made coordination in the field of operations difficult. Major inconsistencies of Sphere standards occur: the use of basic indicators such as mortality rates in evaluating and monitoring programs are often improperly interpreted or neglected.

Whatever the epidemiological model, the larger humanitarian community has found itself often unprepared and at times overwhelmed with the demands for assistance. Wanton violations of the Geneva Conventions and international humanitarian law make it increasingly difficult for relief workers to maintain security for their programs and projects. The recent trend since the Balkan Wars—to militarize and politicize humanitarian assistance—has made it almost impossible for relief organizations to maintain neutrality and impartiality.

Although both the multilateral and unilateral approaches have desperate flaws that need immediate reform, humanitarian assistance will always require an integrated, international approach with lateral integration, communication, and information sharing of multisector and multiagency participants. This cannot be accomplished without coordinating with the leadership of UN agencies and IROs.

The urbanization of populations in warfare has caused humanitarian assistance to move from traditional rural to urban settings. Almost two-thirds of African populations are now living in urban settings with tenuous social and physical protections. Ninety-five percent of the Iraqi population lives in cities where public health infrastructure disrepair and lack of security are major impediments to recovery and reconstruction. Currently, the humanitarian community is unprepared to defend the collapse of urban public health, especially when the environment remains insecure.

Training for work in a CE is essential before deployment. To be both successful and safe, health providers need to expand their knowledge base to include issues of integrated management, transportation, logistics, communications, negotiations and mediation, security, and international humanitarian law. Despite growing trends toward the professionalization of and educating and training the humanitarian community in the late 1990s, the career requirements for training and education have not kept up with demands.

REFERENCES

1. Zwi A, Ugalde A. Political violence in the Third World: a public health issue. *Health Policy Plan.* 1991;6:203-17.
2. Burkle FM. Lessons learnt and future expectations of complex emergencies. *BMJ.* 1999;319:422-6.
3. International Crisis Group. Crisis Watch. Available at: http://www. crisisgroup.org/home/index.cfm?id=1200&l=1.
4. Toole MJ, Waldman RJ. Refugees and displaced persons: war, hunger and public health. *JAMA.* 1993;270:600-5.
5. Coupland RM. Epidemiological approach to surgical management of the casualties of war. *BMJ.* 1994;308:1693-7.
6. Burkholder BT, Toole MJ. Evolution of complex emergencies. *Lancet.* 1995;17(3):187-201.
7. Spiegal P, Burkle FM, Dey CC, Salama P. Developing public health indicators in complex emergency response. *Prehospital Disaster Med.* 2001;16(4):281-5.
8. Michaud CM, Murray CJL, Bloom BR. Burden of disease: implications for future research. *JAMA.* 2001;285:535-9.
9. Davis AP. Targeting the vulnerable in emergency situations: who is vulnerable? *Lancet.* September 1996;348:868-71.
10. Moore PS, Marfin AA, Quenemoen LE, et al. Mortality rates in displaced and resident populations of central Somalia during 1992 famine. *Lancet.* April 1993;341(8850):935-8.
11. Toole MJ. Mass population displacement. A global public health challenge. *Infect Dis Clin North Am.* June 1995;9(2):353-66.
12. Spiegel PB, Salama P. War and mortality in Kosovo, 1998-99: an epidemiological testimony. *Lancet.* 2000;357(9257):2204-9.
13. Deforestation rates for Haiti: forest cover statistics for 2000. Available at: http://rainforests.mongabay.com/deforestation/2000/Haiti.htm.
14. Bradshaw AL. *International Environmental Security: The Regional Dimensions.* Carlisle Barracks, PA: Center for Strategic Leadership; 1998.
15. Pugh M. Military intervention and humanitarian actions: trends and issues. *Disasters.* 1998;22(4):339-51.
16. Sheik M, Guitierrez I, Bolton P, et al. Deaths among humanitarian workers. *BMJ.* July 2000;321:166-8.
17. Burkle FM. Complex emergencies and military capabilities. In: Maley W, Sampford C, Thakur R, eds. *From Civil Strife to Civil Society: Civil and Military Responsibilities in Disrupted States.* Tokyo and New York: United Nations University Press; 2002:68-80.
18. Davidoff F. In the teeth of the evidence: the curious case of evidence-based medicine. *Mt Sinai J Med.* 1999;66:75-83.
19. Desendos JC, Michel D, Tholly F, et al. Mortality trends among refugees in Honduras, 1984-1987. *Int J Epidemiol.* 1990;19(2):367-73.
20. Margolis RA, Franklin RR, Bertrand WF, et al. Rapid post-disaster community needs assessment: a case study of Guatemala after the civil strife of 1979-1983. *Disasters.* 1987;13(4):287-99.
21. Gregg MB. *Field Epidemiology.* Oxford, UK: Oxford University Press; 1996.
22. United Nations High Commissioner for Refugees. *Handbook for Emergencies.* 2nd ed. Geneva: United Nations High Commissioner for Refugees; 2002:40-60.
23. World Health Organization. *Rapid Health Assessment Protocols for Emergencies.* Geneva: World Health Organization; 1999.
24. Sphere Project. *Humanitarian Charter and Minimum Standards in Disaster Response.* 2nd ed. Oxford, UK: Oxfam Publishing; 2003.
25. Hakewill PA, Moren A. Monitoring and evaluation of relief programs. *Tropical Doctor.* 1991;21(suppl 1):24-8.
26. Burkle FM, McGrady KAW, Newett SL, et al. Complex emergencies: III. Measures of effectiveness. *Prehospital Disaster Med.* 1995;10(1):48-56.
27. Burkle FM. Evidence-based health assessment process in complex emergencies. In: Cahill JM, ed. *Emergency Relief Operations.* New York: Fordham University Press and the Center for International Health and Cooperation; 2003:55-79.

28. Elias CJ, Alexander BH, Soky T. Infectious disease control in a long-term refugee camp: the role of epidemiologic surveillance and investigation. *Am J Public Health.* July 1990;80(7):824-8.

29. Roberts L. *Mortality in Eastern Democratic Republic of Congo: Results from Eleven Mortality Surveys.* Final draft. New York: Health Unit, International Rescue Committee; May 2001.

30. World Health Organization. The new emergency health kit: 1998. Available at: http://www.who.int/medicines/library/par/new-emergency-health-kit/nehk98_en.pdf.

31. Anker M. Epidemiological and statistical methods for rapid assessment: introduction. *World Health Stat Q.* 1991;44(3):94-7.

32. Glaziou PT, Mackerras EM. Vitamin A supplementation in infectious diseases: a meta-analysis. *BMJ.* 1993;306:366-70.

33. Organization for Economic Cooperation and Development. *Evaluation and Aid Effectiveness: Guidance for Evaluating Humanitarian Assistance in Complex Emergencies.* London: Development Assistance Committee/Overseas Development Institute; 1999:13-14.

34. Van Rooyen MJ, Eliades MJ, Grabowski JG, Stress ME, Juric J, Burkle FM. Medical relief personnel in complex emergencies: perceptions of effectiveness in the former Yugoslavia. *Prehospital Disaster Med.* July-September 2001;16(3):145-9.

35. UNICEF, Ministry of Health Iraq. *Child and Maternal Mortality Survey 1999: Preliminary Report.* New York: UNICEF and Ministry of Health Iraq; 1999.

36. International Study Team. Health and welfare in Iraq after the Gulf Crisis: an in-depth assessment, 1991. Available at: http://www.warchild.ca/docs/ist_1991_iraq_report.pdf.

37. UNICEF, Central Statistical Office, Ministry of Health Iraq. *Multiple Indicator Cluster Sample (MICS-1996).* Baghdad: UNICEF, Central Statistical Office, and Ministry of Health Iraq; 1996.

38. UNICEF, Ministry of Health Iraq. *Integrated Nutritional Status Survey of Under Five Years and Breastfeeding/Complementary Feeding Practices of Under Two Years in S/C Iraq.* New York and Baghdad: UNICEF and Ministry of Health Iraq; 2002.

39. World Health Organization. *Communicable Disease Profile—Iraq.* Geneva: World Health Organization; 2003.

40. King DJ. The year of living dangerously: Attacks on humanitarian aid workers in 2003. [Special posting.] Washington DC: Humanitarian Information Unit, Washington DC: US State Department; March 29, 2004.

chapter 7

Children and Disaster

Bruce M. Becker

Children, along with the elderly and pregnant women, are the most vulnerable populations in disasters. Physiologically and psychologically they are less fit than adults are to survive the acute, subacute, and chronic stresses imposed by a disaster. The younger the child, the more vulnerable he or she is. Children depend on their parents or guardians for food, clothing, shelter, hygiene, sanitation, water, medical care, and general personal safety. Regardless of the type of disaster, inevitably a certain percentage of surviving children will be separated from one or both of their parents or guardians, sometimes forever. Without the appropriate stewardship of adults, the hazards imposed on children by the disaster situation are multiplied. Children are more likely than others to suffer from malnutrition in the predisaster period and, therefore, are more sensitive to decreased food availability after a disaster when the incidence of protein energy malnutrition and micronutrient deficiencies increases. Children are also more likely to suffer closed head injury during a disaster due to their body proportions. In addition, they are more vulnerable to the risks of dehydration and respiratory insufficiency from acute infection or hypothermia if rendered homeless in the wake of the vast structural destruction that follows many natural and manmade disasters. Disruption of the social fabric of their lives can lead to long-term depression, posttraumatic stress disorder (PTSD), interruption of normal growth and development, and lifelong disability. Sadly, orphaned children are also potential victims of unscrupulous adults who may seek to exploit them in as slave workers, sex workers, or combatants in civil war and rebellion. Children fare as badly or worse than their adult counterparts during and after a disaster because of their unique physical and psychological vulnerability, with age inversely related to increased morbidity and mortality. Disaster planning modules in the past have given children short shrift, with small and inadequate chapters devoted to their needs. Clearly an entire text could be written about the proper medical and psychological care of children in disasters. This chapter will serve as an introduction and overview. References and additional readings are included at the end of the chapter for the interested reader.

Disaster response planners must consider the unique characteristics and needs of children when designing, preparing, implementing, and assessing any disaster relief intervention. This chapter focuses on and highlights the particular needs of children in disasters. It provides a historical perspective; focuses on current practice; highlights pitfalls; and provides references and additional readings. It is important to note that most medium- to large-scale natural or manmade disasters destroy the homes and social structures of the families of children. The children and their parents or guardians, if they survive, then become displaced populations or refugees. Therefore, it is impossible to discuss the disaster response issues for children without focusing on the medical aspects of children as refugees or displaced populations, as well. This chapter considers both of these issues, which represent a continuum of medical and psychological challenges for children. Acute medical care must be provided in the immediate wake of the disaster (assuming that there is a discrete chronological impact), and then subacute and chronic care must be provided to locally or distantly displaced or refugee populations of children who were forced out of their domestic environment as a result of the disaster itself.

HISTORICAL PERSPECTIVE

In the past, the international community's response to disaster was very disorganized, poorly monitored, and inefficient, focusing on capital investment, structural replacement, and trans-shipment of large amounts of materials such as medical supplies and equipment, clothing, canned food, and tentage. Much of this material was outdated, culturally unacceptable, untranslated, misunderstood, shoddy, and of little use to the affected population, particularly children because almost none of it was pediatric-specific. The cost of transporting, sorting, storing, and distributing these disaster relief materials was quite high, diverting resources that could have been better used in other ways. Moreover, there were unintended negative outcomes resulting from improper use of pharmaceutical agents and equipment by personnel untrained in their use. These historical problems associated with disaster relief were magnified when children were considered. Using the example of the emergency medical services (EMS) system in the United States, it was only in the very recent past that EMS began to treat children differently than adults in the prehospital setting. This change came about because most of the equipment, medications, and training were completely irrelevant to the care of most children and, therefore, children were not receiving an adequate, medically appropriate, evidence-based approach to prehospital medical care. In the same vein, the disorganized and rarely assessed response to disaster relief that existed before the mid-1980s completely disregarded the separate and even more important medical and psychological needs of children affected by disasters. This was especially tragic because almost half of the population of most developing countries is younger than 15 years, and the most medically devastating natural and manmade disasters typically occur in developing countries. The level of human devastation is a direct result of inadequate intrinsic infrastructure, severely compromised vulnerable populations before the disaster, and inadequate local and nationwide resources to provide acute and long-term responses to the disaster.

Even though many healthcare practitioners were eager to "do something" before there was a change in focus on children affected by disaster, few had experience and almost none was trained specifically in pediatric disaster medicine. Preliminary need assessments were not performed, planning was haphazard, and outcomes research was nonexistent. Reportage ruled. In the 1980s, primary healthcare, which was just beginning to be applied to healthcare development projects in developing countries, began to be applied to refugee and disaster medicine. Concepts of immunization; nutrition; oral rehydration therapy; cooperation and collaboration with the affected populations; involvement of the local ministry of health; collaboration between local and international nongovernment organizations; appropriate information gathering, including postimpact (but preresponse) assessment; and outcome assessment were becoming more commonplace. This conceptual and process approach to disaster and refugee medical relief has demonstrated increased effectiveness. Despite the increase in the number of articles and texts addressing these concepts and processes, there remains a paucity of information and research in this field, specifically information and research directed toward the treatment of children in disaster, complex emergency, and refugee situations. This is unfortunate because its quite clear that children make up the highest mortality rates in disaster situations, and those rates are highest for children younger than 5 years.[1,2]

There are many specific examples of the high mortality rates among children in the disaster literature. In Thailand, Sudan, and Somalia in the 1980s, children younger than 5 years were twice as likely as the rest of the population to die during forced transmigration or in the early days of arrival to a refugee camp, with accrued mortality rates exceeding 105/1000 per month.[1] To provide some perspective, the rate of 90/1000 per month must be compared with a baseline crude mortality rate in the country before disaster of 1-2/1000 per month, an increase of almost 4500%. Among Ethiopians displaced to Sudan in the mid-1980s, the overall mortality rate was 27/1000 per month, but the mortality rate among children younger than 5 years was 65/1000 per month.[3]

In the mid-1990s, among Nicaraguan and Honduran children displaced to refugee camps because of the Contra war, babies represented 42% of all deaths and children younger than 5 years represented 54% of all deaths.[4] During the famine of 1992 in Somalia, the death rate for displaced children was 74%.[5] During the civil unrest in Rwanda in 1996, displaced Tutsi children represented 54% of all deaths among refugees in camps in Goma, Zaire.[6] The accrued mortality rate for children younger than 5 years in the Zaire refugee camps averaged 36/1000 per month, 15 to 18 times greater than their baseline mortality rates.

It is clear from these examples that the highest mortality rates among populations who are suffering as a result of natural or manmade disasters and who are also generally displaced or become refugees are children and that the youngest children have the highest mortality rates. These mortality rates reflect tremendous suffering and waste of human capital; they represent the most specific indicators available in the acute and chronic situations of the underlying health status of the population but are likely to be underestimated. The rates are underestimated due to recall bias, the failure to report perinatal deaths in many cultures, and the political forces that inflate denominators (baseline population for increased aid) and deflate numerators (decreased deaths, which represents better health and relief service).

Why are children dying? The common reported causes of death of children caught up in natural and man-made disasters involving civil unrest or war and transmigration to refugee camps include acute respiratory infection, measles, malaria, severe malnutrition, diarrheal disease, injury (gunshots, mines and shrapnel, contusions), and burns.[2] There is little evidence in the current medical literature that improved response to disaster, complex emergency, and refugee crises has changed either the causes of childhood death or, in many situations, the death rates themselves. Clearly, better approaches to the assessment and treatment of children in disaster situations are needed if great improvements are to be made on these distressing mortality rates.

CURRENT PRACTICE

Appropriate disaster intervention aimed at decreasing the morbidity and mortality of children requires proper predisaster preparation, training, and equipment; prompt and appropriate assessment of the disaster situation; rapid intervention appropriate to the specific disaster and the particular health and psychological needs of the children affected; and short- and long-term intervention strategies. During a disaster, implementation of sustainable programs that address the acute, subacute, and chronic predictable problems of children associated with different forms of disaster and complex emergencies is also important.

During the last few decades, disaster medical relief activities have been more scrupulously reviewed, and sufficient data have been gathered and analyzed to allow planners to appropriately train and prepare disaster intervention teams to respond to most types of disaster and complex emergencies that may arise in the world. Some of that data have focused on the needs of children. There are six major pillars that support the foundation of disaster response, particularly as it relates to the care of children: water, sanitation, nutrition, shelter, medical response and treatments, and psychological support. If any of these pillars or supporting columns is inadequately addressed, the protective edifice that the disaster response team or organization is trying to build to help the affected populations will collapse. The following sections briefly address these subject areas from the perspective of children and disaster.

Water

Water is essential for life. Most manmade or natural disasters and complex emergencies interrupt the clean water supply to a population. Earthquakes may destroy wells, urban water lines, and water treatment systems. Hurricanes and tsunamis introduce fecal material, toxic chemicals, and salt water to standing water sources and wells. Combatants in war and civil unrest often destroy water sources as strategic acts of war. The minimum personal water requirement is 10 L per day. It is not acceptable to assume that children require less. Fifteen to twenty liters per person per day is needed for drinking, cooking, and personal hygiene. Twenty to thirty liters per person per day is required for children being fed in collective feeding centers that address the needs of children who are undernourished or malnourished. Hospitals require 40 to 60 L per person per day. Water must be accessible; wells must be within a reasonable distance. Family members must have containers to transport and store water. In most cultures, women, mothers, or older female children are responsible for collecting and managing water. A mother's time spent on water is diverted from other aspects of caring for her children. It is also important to note that contamination of water sources by human contact, especially by the small hands of children reaching through large openings into jars and bottles, is a major concern for the spread of fecal-orally transmitted pathogens such as shigellosis, cholera, and typhoid, which are key sources of mortality for those same children.

Gastroenteritis followed by dehydration may be the leading causes of death in children younger than 5 years in disaster situations. The so-called dirty hands diseases, which include diarrheal dysentery, cholera, typhoid, hepatitis A, polio, and helminthiasis, are prominently prevalent in baseline pediatric populations in developing countries and are transmitted as a result of poor hygiene and a lack of adequate clean water and soap. Providing soap and educating the population about appropriate handwashing before meals and after defecation can have a profound effect on the incidence and new cases of diarrheal disease. Soap distributed to refugees from Mozambique decreased the incidence of diarrhea in children by almost 30%.[7] Water containers with covers or small spouts provided to the same population of refugees led to a 30% reduction in diarrheal disease in children younger than 5 years.[8]

Some members of the disaster response team should have training and experience in the assessment of the water supply and water treatment as well as simple interventions directed at keeping the water supply safe and available to mothers and children. Short-term rapid interventions may involve the provision of a mobile water supply or the installation of temporary filtration systems. Long-term interventions include the drilling of deep or artesian wells that are protected from contamination by fenced wellheads. Soap-and-water carrying devices can decrease the incidence of waterborne and potentially fatal gastrointestinal illness.

Sanitation

The lack of sanitation is a very important problem on-site during and after disasters and complex emergencies. Sewage lines and sewage treatment are disrupted by most natural and manmade disasters. Many countries do not have any toilets, underground sewage, or sewage treatment in rural districts. Children are particularly vulnerable to fecal-oral pathogens. In a Kurdish refugee population in 1991, children younger than 5 years had mortality rates of 15/1000 per month, and more than three quarters of those cases were a result of diarrheal disease associated with malnutrition.[9]

Disaster response teams should be prepared to understand the implications of poor sanitation after a disaster. They should have an ability to assess the sanitation needs of the disaster-struck population and the cultural and sociological parameters of defecation in the affected population. In many developing countries, it is uncommon for children younger than 3 years to wear diapers or other coverings. Defecation takes place randomly throughout populated areas, facilitating the spread of fecal pathogens. It is common for mothers to place children with diarrhea over their legs to defecate, thereby facilitating fecal contamination of the mother and other siblings. Defecation fields, trenches, and pit latrines all provide protection from fecal pathogens; however, responders must consider traditional methods and habits of defecation as well as religious, cultural, and social mores concerning defecation and joint use of facilities across gender and age. These problems are more easily solved in the developed world, where individual toilets are widely accepted but just not functional after disruption by the forces of natural and manmade disasters. Decisions must be made and solutions implemented rapidly because large populations separated from free access to toilets will find other means and sites of relief that are fraught with the potential for spreading epidemics.

Cholera is a common and deadly postdisaster disease. Risk factors include poor sanitation and a lack of soap and clean water. There is a direct relationship between the incidence of cholera in a family and the number of children younger than 5 years in that household.[10] Mortality as a result of cholera is greatest in children younger than 4 years, with a relative risk of 4.5 when compared with older children and adults.[11] Most deaths among these young children occur within 24 hours of diagnosis and hospital admission.

Nutrition

Protein energy malnutrition (PEM) is highly prevalent in children who have suffered a natural or manmade disaster and is a major contributor to death in these children. The case fatality rate (CFR) for most infectious diseases, including measles, malaria, diarrhea, and acute respiratory infection, increases dramatically in children who are also afflicted by PEM. Children who are 0-5 years old are at greatest risk.[12] Even mild to moderate undernutrition can be a significant contributor to the death of children in complex emergencies or disasters.[13,14] PEM in children after a disaster often is a result of an exacerbation of underlying famine conditions that existed in that population before the disaster. Such postdisaster famine conditions can be predicted based on an understanding of the socioeconomic condition of the population before the event. Pre-existing conditions that will evolve into famine include widespread poverty; intractable death; underemployment; and a high prevalence of malnutrition, with a moderate to large percentage of the pediatric population who were routinely underfed and were experiencing hunger and starvation. Unfortunately, this is not an unusual condition in many developing countries in the world today. The prevalence of PEM is directly proportional to the crude mortality rate in the underlying population of children. PEM in less than 5% of the children's population is associated with a crude mortality rate of less than 0.9 deaths/1000 per month. Conversely, a prevalence of PEM exceeding 40% in the underlying pediatric population generally is reflected in a crude mortality rate of 30–40/1000 per month, an increase of more than 4000%.

A disaster assessment team arriving on-site should be prepared to evaluate the pediatric population's nutritional status. Nutritional assessments of children in these situations focus on changes in the child's weight in relation to his or her height (weight for height [WFH]). Weight and height are easily, quickly, and accurately measured in sample populations of children. Weight is more sensitive than height to sudden changes in food availability. WFH measurements are also appropriate for assessing the effectiveness of feeding programs. Height-for-age (HFA) measurements reflect more chronic nutritional deficiency, and an abnormal HFA is referred to as *stunting*. Both WFH and HFA measurements are compared with established normal values for the particular population being evaluated (a reference population), and the results are reported as Z scores. Z scores are the number of standard deviations (SD) the patient falls above or below the median when compared with the reference population.

In well-nourished populations, less than 3% of children younger than 5 years have WFH Z scores of less than –2, or 2 SD below the median. In countries where children normally experience some degree of undernutrition, up to 5% of those younger than 5 years have WFH Z scores

of less than –2. A nutritional emergency exists if more than 8% of the WFH Z scores among these very young children are less than –2. The prevalence of moderate to severe PEM in a random sample of children younger than 5 years is a strong indicator of this condition in the underlying population. Causes of death of children with severe PEM include dehydration, infection, hypothermia, cardiac failure, and severe anemia. Acute respiratory infection, urinary tract infection, measles, diarrhea (either infectious or malabsorbed), malaria, skin infections, and sepsis are more common and more fatal in children with PEM. Clinical symptoms such as fever and pain may be masked. For example, measles in children with PEM can have a CFR of up to 30% (a <5% CFR is seen in well-fed, healthy children). Infections should always be suspected in children with PEM and treated aggressively.

Thermoregulation is impaired in children with PEM; therefore, extra blankets and co-sleeping with the mother should be encouraged, and these children should not be bathed. PEM also results in limited glucose stores and impaired gluconeogenesis. Hypoglycemia often accompanies infection. Congestive heart failure (CHF) can be seen secondary to fluid overload that may occur in the process of rehydrating children with gastroenteritis and dehydration. CHF may also result from severe anemia with high output failure, electrolyte disturbances, wet beriberi from thiamine deficiency, or cardiac muscle atrophy associated with prolonged protein deprivation. Mild to moderate anemia is very well tolerated in these children; they should not be given transfusions because these will often result in CHF from fluid overload. The diagnosis of dehydration can be complicated because these children are often edematous from hypoproteinemia. They can be limp, apathetic, or even unconscious. The high prevalence of PEM and the increased incidence of infectious disease explain much of the excess mortality seen in children after disaster, particularly if they become displaced or refugees.

Micronutrient deficiencies, including iron, vitamin A, vitamin C, niacin, and thiamine, are often seen in refugee or displaced children after disasters or complex emergencies. These children may have anemia, scurvy, pellagra, or beriberi. Nutritional deficiencies can persist in chronically displaced children.[15,16] More than two-thirds of children in a Palestinian refugee camp were found to be anemic.[17]

If initial assessment of the underlying population of children affected by the disaster or complex emergency reveals a substantial prevalence of PEM, the relief team should initiate supplemental or therapeutic feeding programs as quickly as possible. Supplemental feeding programs are conducted in the outpatient setting and generally are made available for children whose Z scores are between –2 and –3. Children up to 12 years old may be included, as well as pregnant or lactating women. These programs generally provide an additional 500 calories and 15 g of protein a day in addition to the ordinary rations provided by relief agencies. Supplemental feeding programs either can prepare the food on-site and have the child consume it in a community center or can distribute dry rations to the mother. There are major social and cultural issues that will impinge on the effectiveness of these approaches. Supplemental feeding programs that distribute wet rations require preparation and distribution at a particular site and intensive administration by the organization. In addition, there is a time cost to mothers who must bring the children there and feed them on-site. Furthermore, children with PEM will be concentrated in one area, increasing the risk for spreading communicable disease. However, a smaller population can be treated with this type of distribution program. Nevertheless, by providing wet feedings on-site, it is clear that the child will receive the supplements. When dry rations are distributed to the mother, the family is responsible for providing clean utensils, having firewood, and doing the cooking. It is likely that some of the rations may be taken from the mother by other family members or sold by the mother to purchase additional items for the family. Cultural constraints often dictate the distribution of food in families, with fathers getting the most, then the male children, who are followed by female children and mothers. This may affect the distribution of supplemental dry rations to malnourished children. Children younger than 5 years with Z scores of less than –3 and/or edema should be enrolled in therapeutic inpatient feeding programs. These children are given 100 calories and 1 to 2 g of protein per kilogram per day in the first week and then 200 calories and 2 to 3 g of protein per kilogram per day until their Z scores are greater than –2.

Shelter

Natural and manmade disasters often destroy homes and lead to widespread homelessness of families. Lack of shelter has a tremendously pejorative effect on children, irrespective of the climate in which the disaster occurs. The disaster medical response team must consider emergency shelter as part of the intervention.

Poorly planned and designed shelters or groups of shelters create one of the most pathogenic environments possible for children and families. Overcrowding and poor hygiene inevitably lead to epidemics of infectious disease. Environmental factors such as exposure, vectors, and lack of privacy exacerbate the psychological distress of children and adults and can lead to subsequent depression and PTSD. It is very difficult to predict the longevity of homelessness among the affected population. For instance, some Palestinians have been in refugee camps since the mid-1940s.

Considerations for preplanning individual and group shelters at disaster sites include security and protection. Many complex emergencies involve some degree of civil unrest, and combatants from both sides are often displaced and share living spaces. This can result in internal turmoil within the encampment. Clearly, this has implications for children; they need to be protected from any incipient violence. Easy access to a reasonable supply of clean water is essential to preserve health in children. Environmental health risks must be considered, including stagnant open water and swamps. In addition, open cooking fires present considerable health hazards to children. Burns from these fires are one of the more common pediatric injuries treated by medical teams in these situations.

Replacement of infrastructure can be quite important in restoring some social order to the lives of children after disaster. These structures may include playgrounds, schools, and health and nutritional facilities.

Medical Response and Treatments

Upon reaching the impact site, the disaster response team should initiate a rapid health assessment of the children present to determine an appropriate strategic plan for intervention. Team members should determine the major health and nutritional needs of the affected children and create an ongoing health and nutritional surveillance system. They should assess the local response capacity of the underlying population. They also should determine the total number of affected children as well as an age/gender breakdown and average family or household size. This can be accomplished by convenience sampling. It is important to obtain background health information as well, including an understanding of what the main health problems of children in the region were before the disaster; previous sources of healthcare; important health beliefs; the traditions of parents; the social structure of families, including decision-making pathways within the family; and the strength and coverage of public health programs at the impact site, including immunization rates for various childhood illnesses. The assessment team should determine available food supplies and sources and the logistics needed and opportunities to institute feeding programs, if necessary. Environmental conditions need to be assessed, including climate, geography, availability of materials in the field for shelter and fuel, existing shelter and sanitation arrangements, and water. The response team should use existing facilities first whenever possible. Temporary health facilities created by the response team should have a water supply, refrigeration, heat (in a cold climate), windows with screens (in a hot climate), a generator, vaccine and vaccination equipment, including materials to maintain a cold change and supplies of essential drugs and medical disposables and nondisposables. The medication and equipment should be appropriate for children, including, if possible, items such as Broselow tapes with accompanying medical packs containing sized airway and intravenous equipment as well as standard drugs for resuscitation. Local medical personnel should be included in the relief efforts at the earliest possible stage because of their experience and familiarity with the language, culture, and sociological background of the children, as well as their familiarity with the country and intrinsic health resources. The disaster medical response team should bring in preprinted health records for children. It is likely that health records and vaccination forms will have been destroyed by the disaster and, therefore, will need to be re-created on durable materials that can be maintained long after the team has left the area.

Particular types of disasters and complex emergencies are associated with particular health problems in children. These have been reviewed elsewhere in this text in the disaster-specific chapters; therefore, they will not be covered in great detail here. However, volcanic eruptions, for example, produce smoke and ash, precipitating acute respiratory illness, asthma exacerbations in patients with chronic asthma whose controller medications have been destroyed, and acute incidents of new asthma and reactive airway disease. Medical response teams should have adequate beta agonists for metered dose inhalers and nebulizer administration as well as steroids and oxygen. Earthquakes are commonly associated with head injuries, orthopedic injuries, and crush syndrome in children; fortunately, crush syndrome has been reported far less commonly in children than in adults. Earthquakes are typically also associated with burns because of electrical fires and disruption of natural gas lines, stoves, and heating units. The team should carry proper burn care supplies and identify a referral destination with burn care capability that is outside of the impact zone. Tsunamis, hurricanes, and floods massively contaminate water supply with fecal pathogens; gastroenteritis and dehydration are very common in children in these settings, as seen with the 2004 tsunami in southeast Asia. The team should have adequate water filtration, purification, and transportation supplies; oral rehydration therapy (ORT); and intravenous equipment in children's sizes, as well as experience in starting pediatric intravenous lines.

Measles has been identified as a leading contributor to mortality in children who are displaced after disaster. Measles vaccination campaigns should be assigned the highest priority by response teams when predisaster vaccination coverage has been poor or is unknown. Vaccination coverage of 80% is considered adequate to induce herd immunity in regular populations but may be inadequate in displaced populations of children, where 100% coverage should be sought. In populations of children where the crude mortality rate exceeds 1/10,000 per day or 3/1000 per month, all children from 6 months to 15 years old should be immunized. Vaccination should be given the highest priority for children with PEM or other underlying medical problems, including infectious disease. PEM, fever, acute respiratory illness, diarrhea, human immunodeficiency virus (HIV), tuberculosis, and acute measles are not contraindications to vaccination. The only contraindication is pregnancy. Vitamin A deficiency increases the CFR of measles; therefore, vitamin A should be administered to all children as part of the nutrition program early on in a disaster response, especially if there has been population displacement. Measles vaccination requires constant refrigeration of the vaccine and appropriate quantities of sterile vaccination disposables.

Diarrheal disease has a high prevalence and high mortality rate in children younger than 5 years in disasters, especially if the water supply has been compromised. Prevention is as important as treatment: establish an adequate supply of clean water situated close to each family unit, distribute soap, and encourage handwashing. The disaster response team should address sanitation as well, providing latrines as quickly as possible at the disaster site. The mainstay of treatment for diarrheal disease in children is ORT. Children younger than 2 years should be provided with 50 to 100 mL of ORT per stool. Children older than 2 years should be provided with 100 to 200 mL per stool. Feedings should be continued throughout the diarrheal episode. Severe dehydration (≥10%), especially resulting from cholera infection, should be treated with intravenous fluids, 70 to 100 mL per kilogram. However, nasogastric tube hydration can be very effective and is more resource-efficient than intravenous therapy; it should only be abandoned if persistent vomiting renders it ineffective. In children with PEM, ORT and intravenous hydration should be carried out carefully to avoid CHF.

If possible, laboratory testing for *Vibrio cholerae, Salmonella,* and *Shigella* should be carried out, with appropriate antibiosis in response to diagnosis. Children with bloody diarrhea and fever should be treated with antibiotics regardless of the presence of laboratory facilities. Surveillance is very important in managing an outbreak of diarrhea in a population of children after disaster or complex emergency. Surveillance should include case definitions, number and severity of cases, type of diarrhea by pathogen, age-specific and diarrhea-specific mortality, and demographics of the affected population. Cholera epidemics should be identified early on to institute appropriate preventive health measures, including distributing water and soap, reheating leftover food, banning the consumption of fish from contaminated waters, and temporarily separating family members to prevent the spread of infections. Surprisingly, cholera is one of the few infectious agents that can be spread by handling corpses.

Acute respiratory infection may be the leading cause of death in displaced populations of children younger than 5 years. Children with acute respiratory infection who are febrile and younger than 5 should be treated with antibiotics, according to World Health Organization protocol.

If a disaster or complex emergency occurs in a tropical or semitropical environment, malaria becomes a significant risk to children. It contributes to mortality in 25% of children who are infected. Malaria is especially concerning when displaced populations travel from an area of low endemicity to an area of high endemicity because the former lacks appropriate immune response. Patterns of resistance geographically should govern treatment choices. Prevention is very important. Disaster medical relief teams should identify and attempt to decrease the opportunities for mosquito reproduction, particularly in standing water. Permethrin-treated netting, blankets, tents, and clothing are more cost-effective and much cheaper than medical treatments for malaria.

Reproductive health and sexually transmitted diseases are often ignored in disaster response activities. This oversight may be acceptable in the immediate aftermath of a disaster when the saving of lives and rebuilding of essential health infrastructure dominate responders' focus. Nevertheless, in the subacute and chronic phases, with there is disruption of the family unit and social fabric coupled with PTSD and deteriorating socioeconomic conditions, these issues take on a larger significance. Sexual and gender-based violence is common in displaced populations, and this violence is often directed at children because they are more vulnerable. Single mothers trying to feed their children, adolescent girls and boys, and orphaned children of all ages can be ensnared in the sex trade. Universal and free condom distribution and education should be widely available as well as emergency postcoital contraception.

Disaster relief workers should practice universal precautions and should be aware of the prevalence of HIV and AIDS in the indigenous population of the country in which they are working. Medical, dental, and surgical material should be disinfected and sterilized. Use of injections and injectables should be limited. Blood transfusions should be carried out rarely or never, especially if shoddily tested local blood is being used for transfusion as opposed to emergency supplies brought in by the disaster response team. The team must dispose of medical waste and sharp instruments. Many developing countries reuse sharps after minimal or no sterilization procedures, thus promulgating bloodborne pathogens. The disaster response team also should bring postexposure prophylaxis for themselves in case of needle stick or other exposure.

Psychological Support

Disasters and complex emergencies impose a tremendous amount of psychological stress on children. Children who are victims of disaster or complex emergencies are often overwhelmed by anxiety and fear, including fear of death, injury, being separated from their families, or being orphaned. These children may often display regressive or aggressive behavior, depression, and even suicidal behaviors. Many children who were exposed to a 1999 earthquake in Athens demonstrated anxiety or PTSD. There was a direct relationship between the prevalence of these problems and the child's proximity to the epicenter of the earthquake, as well as female gender and their sense of exposure to threat.[18] There is a direct relationship between the parents' response to disaster and the subsequent effects on their children. After an earthquake in Bolu, Turkey, researchers found that the severity of PTSD in children was mainly affected by the presence of PTSD and depression in their father. Fathers who had experienced the disaster and who became more irritable and detached because of these symptoms affected their children more significantly.[19] The prevalence of depression after the Athens earthquake was high, with 78% of children who had experienced the disaster exhibiting severe to moderate PTSD symptoms. Severe to moderate symptoms of PTSD in these children were also associated with high depression scores.[18] A concerning prevalence of depression, PTSD, and anxiety in children was also found in Japan after the Hanshin earthquake.[20]

Several researchers have reported an increase in the incidence of child abuse after natural disasters. Researchers in the United States studying the effects of the Loma Prieta earthquake in California and hurricane Andrew in Florida concluded that most of the evidence presented indicated that child abuse escalates after major disasters.[21] Researchers in North Carolina found that the incidence of inflicted traumatic brain injury in children increased most in counties affected by hurricane Floyd. This increase in incidence returned to baseline levels 6 months after the impact of the disaster.[22]

It is clear that both children and parents are affected psychologically by disasters; moreover, the effect on parents can have a domino-like or ricochet effect on their children. The earlier that disaster medical response teams initiate psychological counseling for the child victims of disaster, the more likely they are to circumvent the long-term development of disabling morbidity, including PTSD, anxiety, depression, and suicidal behavior. Restoring "normalizing" social structures, such as schools, playgrounds, and community centers, as well as basic human services—shelter, water, sanitation, food, and clothing—can be as effective as formal counseling in ameliorating the psychologically devastating effects of disaster.

There are also several psychosocial concomitances of disaster and complex emergencies that must be considered when focusing response on children. Disasters in which there are many adult deaths result in widespread orphaning of children. Identification and database services need to be set up soon after the medical response team arrives to try to pair children who are separated from their parents back with their parents or with other appropriate family members or relatives. These orphaned children are especially vulnerable to abuse from adults who may draw them into sexual slavery or forced work situations. In countries with ongoing civil unrest or conflict, children as young as 10 years old who are orphaned or separated from their parents are often drafted into rebel armies and trained to carry out armed warfare. The long-term disturbing psychological effects of these activities can only be presumed.

PITFALLS

1. Appropriate care for children who are victims of disasters and complex emergencies requires proper preparation of the disaster medical response team and an early on-site needs assessment that is specially geared to children before the disaster medical response is launched.
2. Appropriate equipment and training geared specifically toward the treatment of children are a necessity for any disaster medical response team hoping to provide appropriate care for children on-site after a disaster or complex emergency.
3. The basic primary healthcare components normally considered in adult disaster medical relief are equally important in providing relief to children, with the focus on providing water, food, clothing, sanitation, shelter, treatment of injuries and illnesses, and psychological counseling.
4. PEM is a huge problem in children after disasters or complex emergencies because in many countries where these events occur, the children have a prevalence of undernutrition or malnutrition. Rapid nutritional assessment and the provision of therapeutic or supplemental feeding can have a huge effect on decreasing pediatric morbidity and mortality.

5. Effective and rapid immunization programs, especially those focusing on measles, can have a large impact on children in the aftermath of disaster, particularly if the baseline immunization rates in the population were inadequate.

6. Clean water and appropriate sanitation are the two most important interventions in the prevention of epidemics of potentially fatal gastrointestinal infectious diseases in children, who are more prone to fecal-oral transmission of pathogens.

7. Psychosocial issues must be addressed early in a disaster medical response to prevent long-term debilitating PTSD and depression in children.

REFERENCES

1. Toole MJ, Waldman RJ. Prevention of excess mortality in refugee and displaced populations in developing countries. *JAMA.* 1990;263:3296-3302.

2. Toole MJ, Waldman RJ. The public health aspects of complex emergencies and refugee situations. *Annu Rev Public Health.* 1997;18:283-312.

3. Shears P, Berry AM, Murphy R, Nabil MA. Epidemiological assessment of the health and nutrition of Ethiopian refugees in emergency care in Sudan, 1985. *BMJ.* 1987;295:314-18.

4. Desenclos JC, Michel D, Tholly F, Magdi I, Pecoul B, Desve G. Mortality trends among refugees in Honduras, 1984-1987. *Int J Epidemiol.* 1990;19:367-73.

5. Moore PS, Marfin AA, Quenemoen LE, et al. Mortality rate in displaced and resident population of central Somalia during 1992 famine. *Lancet.* 1993;341:935-8.

6. Nabeth P, Vasset B, Derin P, Doppler B, Tectonidis M. Health situations of refugees in eastern Zaire. *Lancet* 1997;349:1031-2.

7. Peterson EA, Roberts L, Toole MJ, Peterson DE. The effect of soap distribution on diarrhea: Nyamithuthu Refugee Camp. *Int J Epidemiol.* 1998;27:520-4.

8. Roberts L, Chartier Y, Chartier O, et al. Keeping clean water clean in a Malawi refugee camp: a randomized intervention trial. *Bull World Health Organ.* 2001;79:280-7.

9. Yip R, Sharp TW. Acute malnutrition and childhood mortality related to diarrhea: lessons from the 1991 Kurdish refugee crisis. *JAMA.* 1993;270:587-90.

10. Hatch DL, Waldman RJ, Lungu GW, Piri C. Epidemic cholera during refugee resettlement in Malawi. *Int J Epidemiol.* 1994;23:1292-9.

11. Swerdlow DL, Malenga G, Begkoyian G, et al. Epidemic power among refugees in Malawi, Africa: treatment and transmission. *Epidemiol Infect.* 1997;118:207-14.

12. Mason KB. Lessons on nutrition of displaced people. *J Nutrition.* 2002;132:2096F-103S.

13. Rice AL, Sacco L, Hyder A, Black RE. Malnutrition as an underlying cause of childhood death associated with infectious disease in developing countries. *Bull World Health Organ.* 2000;78:1207-21.

14. Pelletier DL, Frongillo EA Jr, Shroeder DT, Habicht JP. The effects of malnutrition on child mortality in developing countries. *Bull World Health Organ.* 1995;73:443-8.

15. Prinzo ZW, de Benoist B. Meeting the challenges of micronutrient deficiencies in emergency-affected populations. *Proc Nutr Soc.* 2002;61:251-7.

16. Toole MJ. Micronutrient deficiency in refugees. *Lancet.* 1992;339:1214-16.

17. Hassan K, Sullivan KM, Yip R, Woodruff BA. Factors associated with anemia in refugee children. *J Nutrition.* 1997;127:2194-8.

18. Groome D, Soureti A. Post-traumatic stress disorder and anxiety symptoms in children exposed to the 1999 Greek earthquake. *Br J Psychol.* August 2004;95:(Pt 3):387-97.

19. Kilic EZ, Ozguven HD, Sayil I. The psychological effects of parental mental health on children experiencing disaster: the experience of Bolu earthquake in Turkey. *Fam Process.* Winter 2003;42(4):485-95.

20. Kitayama S, Okada Y, Takumi T, Takada S, Inagaki Y, Nakamura H. Psychological and physical reactions on children after the Hanshin-Awaji earthquake disaster. *Kobe J Med Sci.* October 2000;46(5):189-200.

21. Curtis T, Miller BC, Berry EH. Changes in forced incidents of child abuse following natural disasters. *Child Abuse Negl.* September 2000;24(9):1151-62.

22. Keenan HT, Marshall SW, Nocera MA, Runyan DK. Increased incidence of inflicted traumatic brain injury in children after a natural disaster. *Am J Prev Med.* April 2004;26(3):189-93.

ADDITIONAL READINGS

1. *Clinical Guidelines.* 4th ed. Medecins Sans Frontieres; 1999.

2. *Refugee Health: An Approach to Emergency Situations.* Medecins Sans Frontieres; 1997.

3. Mandalakas A, Torjesen K, Olness K, eds. *Helping the Children: A Practical Handbook for Complex Humanitarian Emergencies.* Kenyon, MN: Health Frontiers; 1999.

4. Sphere Project. Humanitarian Charter and Minimum Standards in Disaster Response. Available at: http://www.sphereproject.org/.

5. Mears S, Chowdhury S. *Health Care for Refugees and Displaced People.* Oxford, UK: Oxfam; 2001.

chapter 8

Psychological Impact of Disaster

Tracy E. Wimbush and Christo C. Courban

The psychological impact of disaster is often immeasurable. Whereas the physical injuries caused by disaster can be visualized, it is much more difficult to identify the psychological trauma that many experience as a result of a disaster event. Though most people who are exposed to even worse traumatic stressors will recover with minimal intervention, all agree that there is no such thing as "no response" when discussing emotional reactions to disaster.

HISTORICAL PERSPECTIVE

Traditionally, disaster medicine has focused solely on the medical and surgical needs of individuals, and little effort was made to meet the emotional and psychological needs of disaster victims and workers. The psychological aspects of traumatizing events such as natural disasters, war, accidents, and terrorism have been a focus in psychiatry for many years, and early reports of psychological trauma after railway accidents occur in the literature as early as 1866.[1] In recent years, those interested in disaster management have given increased attention to the psychological consequences of disaster. As a result, the body of evidence identifying those at risk, documenting signs of emotional trauma, and supporting interventions after disaster has grown significantly.

Although it was not until 1980 that the *Diagnostic and Statistical Manual of Mental Disorders,* edition 3 *(DSM-III),* first codified one of the most devastating psychological outcomes of disaster—posttraumatic stress disorder (PTSD)—many experts believe this disorder existed hundreds of years earlier and suggest that the elements of the disorder can be identified in Homer's *Iliad.* Others argue that psychological responses to disaster are culture-bound. Supporting this notion is a study by Jones and colleagues,[2] who reviewed war pension files of 1856 disabled veterans. They found that those disabled from conditions thought to be similar, if not the same, as PTSD, such as shell shock and disordered action of the heart, did not meet the criteria for PTSD. Interestingly, nearly all of the disabled veterans lacked evidence of "flashbacks." *Flashbacks,* a term used to describe persistent re-experiencing of the event, is a criterion required for the diagnosis of PTSD. Some experts argue that flashbacks are a culturally based phenomenon that became prominent within the latter 20th century when cinema became popular. The suggestion that psychological response to traumatic events such as disaster evolves with culture points to the need for culturally sensitive and up-to-date psychological interventions.

CURRENT PRACTICE

Before determining what interventions are needed after a disaster event, it is important to understand the phases of mental health disturbances after disaster. Researchers describe multiple phases of response. Burkle[3] summarizes three main phases. Phase one is the preimpact phase. This phase occurs before the event takes place; the stressor of this phase is worry. Response to this stress ranges but normally includes denial and anxiety. The second phase is the impact phase, in which the disaster is actively occurring. Our knowledge of expected reactions during the impact phase of disaster is credited to the early work of Tyhurst and Glass from the 1950s. They reported that a small percentage of individuals (12%-25%) remain calm and high functioning, whereas an equal percentage demonstrate disorganization, confusion, and other serious coping difficulty. The majority of individuals during the impact phase are found to temporarily have a blunted response, demonstrate a lack of emotion, and evidence bewilderment. During the aftermath phase, also called the recoil or postimpact phase, emotional reactions vary widely and range from relief at personal survival to survivor guilt, feelings of self-consciousness, emotional lability, and numbness.[3]

Victims of disaster can be classified into three groups. Primary casualties suffer physical injury and acute psychological sequela as a consequence or may experience psychological harm alone. Secondary casualties include affected relatives and friends of primary casualties and witnesses of the event who were not directly affected. Tertiary victims are rescue workers and healthcare providers.[3,4]

BOX 8-1 COMMON RESPONSES TO DISASTER

Apathy
Anxiety
Denial
Helplessness
Inappropriate joking
Insomnia
Mild confusion
Mood swings
Overinvolvement in survival activities
Restlessness
Terror

BOX 8-3 DIAGNOSTIC CRITERIA FOR PTSD

Exposure to a traumatic event
Event is persistently re-experienced (flashbacks)
Avoidance of stimuli associated with the trauma and
   numbing of general responsiveness
Demonstration of increased arousal
Symptoms last at least 1 month and cause significant
   impairment or stress

Identifying a pathological posttraumatic reaction early is crucial, with many studies showing that early interventions and treatment lead to better outcomes.[3,4] Triage classifications of disaster rarely screen for or include those at high risk for psychological trauma, thus leading to a substantial delay in detection of this pathologic condition. Many triage algorithms for primary, secondary, and tertiary casualties in disaster exist in the neuropsychiatric literature.[4] Triage classification should be sensitive and inclusive. Once primary triage identifies the potential need for assistance, mental health teams can further triage and determine the need for and timeliness of treatment.

There is a spectrum of psychopathology associated with trauma. Victim responses vary, and one victim may manifest a wide range of illness. Most victims manifest only mild symptoms that often resolve without intervention. A list of common symptoms is found in Box 8-1.[1] Providers should be cautioned against classifying severe reactions as a "natural" response to a disaster event because this may prevent early intervention.[3] A list of commonly associated psychopathological features related to trauma is provided in Box 8-2. PTSD is by far the most notable psychological consequence of trauma (Box 8-3). However, providers are cautioned not to ignore other potentially treatable pathological features, such as major depression or anxiety disorders, in efforts to diagnose PTSD.[5]

PTSD is diagnosed in persons exposed to an extreme stressor or traumatic event who manifest the following three groups of symptoms:

1. Re-experiencing of the event, or "flashbacks"
2. Avoidance of any stimuli that reminds the victim of the event and a decreased ability to feel emotion (also known as "numbing")
3. Hyperarousal, which is characterized by increased startle response, anxiety, and irritability

BOX 8-2 PSYCHOPATHOLOGY ASSOCIATED WITH TRAUMATIC EVENTS

TSD
Substance abuse
Anxiety disorders
Depressi

Symptoms must be present for a least 1 month at the time of diagnosis.[6,7] PTSD is the fourth most common psychiatric disorder in the United States.[8] Several risk factors for the development of severe PTSD have been identified. They include serious physical injury, persistent anger, witnessing the death or injury of others, dissociation, poor social support, and intense exposure to the traumatic event.[9] PTSD may be acute or chronic. If symptoms persist for more than 3 months, chronic PTSD is diagnosed.[6,7]

Davidson[9] divides prevention of PTSD into three methods: primary (preventing exposure), secondary (preventing the development of symptoms immediately after traumatic exposure), and tertiary (preventing the worsening of PTSD). Although preventing exposure to trauma is ideal, circumstance rarely allows this. Efforts aimed at secondary treatments suggest that targeting central nervous system disturbances with medications, such as hydrocortisone and propranolol, within weeks of the event may prevent the development of PTSD symptoms.[9] Tertiary treatments often consist of counseling and prescribing medications. Initial counseling can often be done by nonspecialists and should emphasize education and convey feelings of safety and support. When greater assistance is needed, research suggests that exposure therapy, cognitive therapy, and interpersonal therapies may be effective.[8] Effective medications include selective serotonin-reuptake inhibitors (SSRIs), tricyclic antidepressants (TCAs), and monoamine oxidase inhibitors (MAOIs) and anticonvulsants.[6,8] A list of effective medications and their target symptoms is provided in Box 8-4. It should be

BOX 8-4 MEDICATIONS USED FOR TREATMENT OF PTSD

SSRIs (shown to be effective on all three symptom clusters)
Sertraline (Zoloft)
Paroxetine (Paxil)
MAOIs (shown to be effective in all three symptoms but used with caution due to potential for adverse interaction with alcohol)
Phenelzine
Brofaromine

TCAs (especially helpful with intrusive symptoms)
Amitriptyline
Imipramine

Anticonvulsants
Lamotrigine

Benzodiazepines are rarely indicated and should be used with caution.

noted that many experts caution against the use of benzodiazepines in patients with PTSD.[6,8]

Another secondary PTSD prevention method includes critical incident stress management (CISM). The most commonly used element of CISM is critical incident stress debriefing (CISD). CISD, developed by Mitchell in 1988, is commonly used as an intervention after an unusually traumatizing event. It is primarily aimed at rescue workers and other tertiary victims, including nurses, physicians, and even 911 dispatchers but has recently been widely applied to groups ranging from financial workers after bank robberies to prisoners after the murder of a fellow inmate.[10,11] Even though there are many variations of CISD, a debriefing is generally a group session facilitated by a mental health professional and a group member who was not part of the traumatizing event. During the session, participants recount their experiences and express fears and concerns while facilitators acknowledge victim experiences and discuss coping strategies. The goal of CISD is to normalize the crisis experience, prevent the development of poor coping mechanisms, and assess the need for follow-up.[6,12,13]

Pioneers of CISM, Everly and Mitchell, point out that CISM, or variations of it, have gained great popularity and are becoming a "standard of care" in many industries.[19] Examples of industries that use their crisis management technique include the U.S. Air Force; the Bureau of Alcohol, Tobacco, and Firearms; the Australian Army; and the Massachusetts Department of Mental Health.

Although CISM, specifically CISD, is generally accepted, opinions differ regarding its effectiveness.[12-16] Wessely and Deahl[14] comment: "The effectiveness of psychological debriefing and other early interventions remains one of the most contentious areas of mental health research." Research findings often contradict each other, and many point out the lack of randomized controlled studies in the literature.[14,17] In a meta-analysis of single-session debriefing after psychological trauma, Van Emmerik and colleagues[18] found that CISD did not improve natural recovery after psychological trauma. Weiss and colleagues[5] conducted a survey of 46 acknowledged international experts on mental health and disaster management and found that psychological debriefing immediately after disaster, while valued by some, was mostly viewed as useless and even potentially harmful. Others point out that the positive effects of CISD are more probable and that harmful effects are reduced when the facilitators avoid common mistakes, such as failure to have an adequate number of and properly trained mental health providers, allowing breaks in confidentiality, allowing CISD to turn into psychotherapy sessions, lack of a CISD strategy team, and a general lack of understanding of the CISM process.[6,12]

Realizing the confusion surrounding the use of CISD and CISM in general, Everly and Mitchell recently clarified terminology and provided updated information on the use of CISM.[19] They explain that CISD refers to one debriefing session of CISM. The session generally lasts 1.5 to 3 hours and is recommended 2 to 14 days after a critical incident. They caution that in cases of mass disaster, CISD is not recommended until 3 weeks after the event. Even though CISD is often used alone, Mitchell contends that it was never intended to be a stand-alone intervention or a replacement for psychotherapy. Rather, CISD is intended to be a single component in the CISM system. There are eight core components of the CISM system. These components are listed in Box 8-5, and each is briefly described in the remainder of this section.

The first component of CISM is precrisis intervention. The goal of this component is to identify those at risk of psychological trauma/crisis and to provide information to them. It also consists of stress management education, stress resistance training, and crisis mitigation for team members and management.

The second component of CISM consists of crisis intervention programs. Examples include demobilization, staff consultation, and crisis management briefings (CMBs). The goal of these sessions is to allow for psychological decompression and provide opportunity for stress management. Decompressions are intended for emergency medical services personnel and should occur immediately after a shift when there has been exposure to a critical event. Staff consultation is intended to provide advice for command staff. Examples of staff advisement recipients include disaster response team leaders, nursing supervisors, and fire captains. CMBs are similar to decompressions but are intended for use with civilians. Examples of groups needing a CMB might include teachers after a particularly violent school event or store workers after a robbery.

The third component of CISM is defusing. The goal of defusing is to allow for symptom mitigation and to give opportunity for closure. It also serves as an opportunity to triage those needing greater assistance. Defusing is a small-group discussion held within 12 hours of the critical incident in which group members are encouraged to discuss events that have just occurred. Defusing has three phases: (1) introduction of the debriefing team, (2) exploration of the experience, and (3) providing information about expected emotions and availability of resources.

The fourth component of CISM is the aforementioned CISD. As intended by Mitchell, it is a seven-phase small-group discussion:

1. Phase one is *introduction* of the team.
2. Phase two is a *fact phase,* in which members describe their role in the event.
3. Phase three is the *thought phase,* when participants explore their thoughts that occurred during the event.

BOX 8-5 CORE COMPONENTS OF CISM

Preincident preparation
Crisis intervention programs
Demobilization, staff consultations, and/or crisis management briefings

Defusing
CISD
Individual crisis intervention
Pastoral crisis intervention
Family CISM and/or organizational consultation
Follow-up/referral

4. Phase four, the *reaction phase*, allows individuals to express their emotional reactions or feelings.
5. The *symptoms phase*, in which participants explore the physical, emotional, and behavior symptoms since the event, is the fifth phase.
6. The sixth phase is a *teaching phase*. During this phase the debriefing team helps to normalize participants' feelings and provides information about expected reactions.
7. The seventh phase is the *re-entry phase*, in which the meeting is summarized and questions are answered.

CISD typically takes two hours and should occur 1 to 14 days after the crisis. However, it should be delayed further in the setting of mass disasters. As with defusing sessions, its goal is also to allow for symptom mitigation, closure, and triage. Again, in its original form, it is not intended as a stand-alone intervention.

Other components of CISM, such as individual crisis intervention, pastoral crisis intervention, and family/organizational CISM, should be available on an as-needed basis. Follow-up/referral is key, and the CISM leader must make an effort to maintain relationships with their community providers to make the referral and follow-up processes function seamlessly.[19]

PITFALLS

Although clear benefits of CISM are still debatable according to the research, there are definite pitfalls to avoid when dealing with the psychological impact of disasters:

- Failure to recognize that everyone has some type of emotional response to disaster and providing support only to those exhibiting the most obvious or dysfunctional responses
- Evaluation and treatment of medical and surgical injuries without acknowledging the psychological ramifications of a disaster event
- Failing to recognize early warning signs of poor emotional coping; CISM is often an afterthought to the initial response
- Using CISD as a stand-alone intervention rather than as a single element of the CISM plan
- Having poorly trained or untrained individuals lead CISM efforts

REFERENCES

1. Lamprecht F, Sack M. Posttraumatic stress disorder revisited. *Psychosom Med.* 2002;64:222-37.
2. Jones E, Vermaas RB, McCartney, H et al. Flashbacks and post-traumatic stress disorder: the genesis of a 20th-century diagnosis. *Br J Psychiatry.* 2003;182:158-63.
3. Burkle FM. Acute-phase mental health consequences of disaster: implication for triage and emergency medicine services. *Ann Emerg Med.* 1996;28:119-28.
4. Burkle FM. Triage of disaster-related neuropsychiatric casualties, in psychiatric aspects of emergency medicine. *Emerg Med Clin North Am.* 1991;9:87-105.
5. Weiss M, Saraceno B, Saxena S, van Ommeren M. Mental health in the aftermath of disasters: consensus and controversy. *J Nerv Ment Dis.* 2003;191:611-15.
6. Hageman I, Andersen HS, Jorgensen MB. Post-traumatic stress disorder: a review of psychobiology and pharmacotherapy. *Acta Psychiatr Scand.* 2001;104:411-22.
7. American Psychiatric Association. *Diagnostic and Statistical Manual-IV-TR.* Washington DC: American Psychiatric Association; 2000.
8. Yehuda R. Current concepts: post-traumatic stress disorder. *N Engl J Med.* 2002;364:108-14.
9. Davidson JRT. Surviving disaster: what comes after the trauma. *Br J Psychiatry.* 2002;181:366-8.
10. Simms-Ellis R, Madill A. Financial services employees' experience of peer-led and clinician-led critical incident stress debriefing following armed robberies. *Int J Emerg Ment Health.* 2001;3:219-28.
11. Stoll B, Edwards LA. Critical incident stress management with inmates: an atypical application. *Int J Emerg Ment Health.* 2001;3:245-7.
12. Hammond J, Brooks J. The World Trade Center attack: helping the helpers: the role of critical incident stress management. *Crit Care.* 2001;5:315-17.
13. Dyregrov A. Helpful and hurtful aspects of psychological debriefing groups. *Int J Emerg Ment Health.* 1999;1:175-181.
14. Wessely S, Deahl M. Psychological debriefing is a waste of time. *Br J Psychiatry.* 2003;183:12-14.
15. Everly GS, Boyle SH. Critical incident stress debriefing (CISD): a meta-analysis. *Int J Emerg Ment Health.* 1999;1:165-8.
16. Bledsoe BE. Critical incident stress management (CISM): benefit or risk for emergency services. *Prehosp Emerg Care.* 2003;7:272-9.
17. Everly GS, Flannery RB, Eyler VA. Critical incident stress management (CISM): a statistical review of the literature. *Psychiatr Q.* 2002;73:171-82.
18. Van Emmerik A, Kamphuis J, Hulsbosch A, Emmelkamp P: Singles session debriefing after psychological trauma: a meta-analysis. *Lancet.* 2002;260:766-71.
19. Everly GS, Mitchell JT. The debriefing "controversy" and crisis intervention: a review of lexical and substantive issues. *Int J Emerg Ment Health.* 2000;2:211-225.

chapter 9

Ethical Issues in the Provision of Emergency Medical Care in Multiple Casualty Incidents and Disasters

Pinchas Halpern and Gregory L. Larkin

Disasters and multiple casualty incidents (MCIs) affect every corner of the globe. Although natural disasters and wars have plagued humanity for thousands of years, man-made MCIs comprise a relatively new and growing threat with which medicine must contend—even in peacetime. Citizens of all nations have increasingly encountered MCIs that, without warning, can instantly overwhelm the capacity of both prehospital and hospital-based systems, imposing significant clinical, organizational, and even ethical challenges. Disasters and MCIs introduce unique moral, triage, resource allocation, and public health issues. The disaster paradigm demands rapid reorganization of medical systems and, in tandem, a recalibration of familiar ethical and moral codes that govern providers during times of stability. Many of the most crucial moral dilemmas can be anticipated, however, and policies can be developed in advance that clearly delineate the duties and priorities for medical support personnel during MCIs and disasters. Prospective ethical deliberation, advance austerity planning, and prophylaxis policy can streamline moral medical decision-making and ensure optimal service delivery downstream to both individual patients and the public at large.

The chronology of preparedness for MCIs and disasters involves three stages: (1) pre-event, (2) event, and (3) postevent. Each stage may be addressed by different medical caregivers, and each poses somewhat different management, clinical, and ethical dilemmas. Major dilemmas within the context of these three timed stages include adequate preparation for eventualities, scene triage and transport, duty to treat, scope of practice off site, stewardship of resources, and ethical long-term goals of fairness in matters of rehabilitation. This chapter will focus mainly on overarching ethical challenges and event-based dilemmas that face emergency medical services (EMS) and emergency medicine (EM) providers in the throes of MCIs and disasters.

HISTORICAL PERSPECTIVE

Over the years, sets of ethical rules have been developed to guide medical personnel in their work, but they usually do not address MCIs and disasters, thereby creating potential uncertainty. Many of the accepted practices have little scientific basis and therefore compel physicians to use common sense. However, common sense may sometimes contradict generally accepted ethical guidelines or leave physicians no choice but to apply some intuitively created adaptation of the ordinary ethical rules to a situation that was not considered when the rules were originally formulated.

In the following are some examples of sets of ethical rules composed throughout history, according to which medical personnel are expected to practice. The Hippocratic oath[1] has been taken by newly appointed physicians in the West for centuries. Inspired by the Pythagoreans, this classic treatise dictates that the physician must be ready and willing to assist a patient with any medical problem under any circumstances, without any economic or other stipulation:"The regimen I adopt shall be for the benefit of the patient according to my ability and judgment and not for their hurt or for any wrong. . . . Whatsoever house I enter, there will I go for the benefit of the sick refraining from all wrongdoing or corruption."

The Geneva Conventions[2] are also concerned with the obligation of integrity and respect of the physician toward the practice of medicine. They regard the patient's health as being the first priority for the physician, who is mandated to use the power of medicine for the general good and maintain good relationships with his or her colleagues, while forbidding any kind of discrimination among patients.

Basic Principles

Borrowing from Beachamp and Childress's concepts of ethical principlism, Priel and Dolev[3] define four principles on which routine medical ethics are based:

1. **Beneficence:** This important Judeo-Christian concept enjoins medical staff members to do their best to optimize outcomes and prolong the life of the patient/victim.
2. **Nonmaleficence:** This is the classic notion of *primum non nocere,* or "the first thing (is) to do no harm." This is the ordering principle of most emergency medical ethics.
3. **Respect for autonomy:** The medical staff must engage in full disclosure with patients and honor their own informed decisions regarding their own medical care.
4. **Justice:** The resources and means of medical personnel must be equitably distributed among all victims.

These four principles are not absolute, and shifting circumstances may dictate their reordering or prioritization. They may even contradict each other. For example, a surgeon's desire to do good for a patient through an operative procedure may also cause the patient some short-term discomfort or even harm from complications. Therefore, providing both beneficent and nonmaleficent care can create a conflict of principles, whereupon the clinician must choose one principle over another.

Medical Organizations

Many medical organizations have developed ethical codes, but few have specifically addressed the issue of MCIs and disasters. The World Medical Association (WMA) code of ethics has a specific section on disaster care.[4] The code of ethics of the American College of Emergency Physicians (ACEP) specifically addresses situations in which "the resources of a health care facility are overwhelmed by epidemic illness, mass casualty, or the victims of a natural or manmade disaster" and states that it is the duty of the emergency physician to "focus health care resources on those patients most likely to benefit and who have a reasonable probability of survival."[5] The American Academy of Emergency Medicine's code of ethics does not address disaster/MCI situations.[6] The ethics code of the American College of Physicians does not contain specific mention of the care of victims of disasters or MCIs,[7] whereas that of the American Medical Association (AMA) states in its ethics code as follows: ". . . physicians and other health professionals should be knowledgeable of ethical and legal issues and disaster response. These include: (a) their professional responsibility to treat victims (including those with potentially contagious conditions); (b) their rights and responsibilities to protect themselves from harm; (c) issues surrounding their responsibilities and rights as volunteers, and (d) associated liability issues."[8] Since studies have demonstrated the poor state of preparedness of medical professionals for disasters and MCIs, such as in the event of bioterrorism,[9] the AMA code also states that ". . . a social obligation for physician response can be defined, then certainly a derivative obligation can be placed on the profession—an obligation to insure that its members are prepared . . . to effectively respond. This obligation of the profession must be not only clearly defined but expeditiously met."

The European Society of Emergency Medicine (EuSEM) has no explicit code of ethics. The World Association for Disaster and Emergency Medicine's Health Disaster Management (WADEM) states[10]:

> Triage . . . means that scarce resources will be used to provide the maximum benefit to the population at large, even if it means that single victims who might have been saved under other circumstances are sacrificed for the greater good. However, when the triage concept is expanded into other management areas, the concept becomes more difficult to accept. For example, should limited water resources be distributed in a manner so as to provide the minimum amounts needed to sustain life to only a part of the population, and accept the high probability that the rest will die of thirst? Or should 1 litre (less than the critical threshold) be distributed to everybody, well aware that then everybody will succumb, but at a later stage in the disaster? Since ethics, as such, are not natural laws, but human 'inventions', how is what decided deemed to be ethically correct?

The ethical principles of the Israeli Medical Association (IMA) state: "In an emergency, the physician may act according to his best judgment, thus effectively absolving the physician of requirements such as informed consent, privacy, the patient's right to choose a caregiver and provision of information."[11] U.S. common law does not impose any duty to render aid or assistance to a person in need, even if one could do so with no risk to oneself. However, experts point out that health providers could be required to provide care in the event of an emergency through licensure requirements.[12] In addition, even though individual physicians do not have a duty to provide care, hospitals and other institutions sometimes do, particularly for emergent situations. The current legal establishment, including the requirements of the Americans with Disabilities Act, seeks to expose physicians while still encouraging them to act. The system provides weak incentives to be a hero. So far, only the Model State Emergency Health Powers Act (MSEHPA) has systematically addressed the duty to care issue.[13] Even though the MSEHPA is not law, it does serve to offer guidance to state legislators and may influence what types of laws and schemes will be enacted. For example, MSEHPA would allow states to *require* healthcare providers to provide care in the event of emergencies. The duty does vary with risk, since a scheme that would overburden healthcare providers would be unacceptable.[12] Israeli common law (1988) states that "it is the duty of a person to assist another person. . . in immediate severe danger to his life. . . when he can do so without endangering himself or other."

The International Red Cross and Red Crescent Movement's code of conduct in disaster relief states: "Aid is given regardless of the race, creed or nationality of the recipients and without adverse distinction of any kind. . . . Aid priorities are calculated on the basis of need alone. . . . We hold ourselves accountable to both those we seek to assist and those from whom we accept resources."[14] The ethics code of Magen David Adom

(MDA), the Israeli national EMS organization, includes the following text regarding disaster and MCI: ". . . to treat victims by priorities set according to medical criteria, without any other considerations such as age, sex, religion, nationality, social or economic status. . . caregivers will, as a rule, attempt to save the largest number of victims possible, even at the possible detriment of the chances of saving an individual victim. . . to treat victims while guarding the victims' and the caregivers' safety as well as possible. Determining the correct balance between risk to victim and risk to caregiver is the responsibility of the caregiver and the event commander's." (Personal communication, Pinchas Halpern, MD.) The ethical code of the Israeli Army Medical Corps assumes that the operational protocols governing the administration of medical care in the field cover potential ethical dilemmas and does not deal with the issue specifically.

MCI AND ETHICAL ISSUES ARISING FROM IT

All the ethical codes presented here demonstrate a continuity of principles involving patient-caregiver relationships as well as physician-system relationships. Thus, according to these more classic codes, the physician must be professionally and logistically prepared to manage disasters and do what is best for the patient, including doing everything in his or her power to save the patient's life. The physician should not discriminate among patients but treat them with a uniform, balanced, and just approach. The physician ought to share his or her decision-making with patients and provide them with truthful information about treatment and prognosis, except when sharing information is expected to cause any delay in or otherwise negatively affect patient care. How an MCI changes the order of these principles and relative contribution of each level of obligation is discussed next.

MCI is defined as a state in which there is an imbalance between the numbers or types of injured who need medical care and the medical ability of the emergency systems to deliver *optimal* care to each individual. Disasters may be defined as MCIs that involve significant disruption of the infrastructure (human, logistic, or medical) of the region/nation coping with the event (e.g., natural disaster, war). The effects of disasters, such as famine and epidemics, may be prolonged and result in an extended need for medical care, with a more complex interaction between purely medical and logistic support (e.g., water and food supplies, shelter). In an MCI or a disaster, some of the ethical principles previously mentioned may not be realistically applicable and therefore raise some interesting ethical issues:

- *Beneficence:* If the physician were to act according to this principle of maximizing the good, he or she would be expected to spend an inordinate amount of time on only one or a few patients and would essentially fail to fulfill his or her ethical obligations toward the rest of the patients who require care. Should the caregiver then focus treatment on one person, or partially take care of a maximum number of patients, or perhaps only take care of patients for whom it is cost-effective to intervene, thereby only partly fulfilling the beneficence principle?

- *Distinction without discrimination (nondiscrimination):* It is generally agreed on that patients must not be discriminated against with regard to receiving medical care and the allocation of resources. This issue takes on greater significance during an MCI since it is, by definition, a situation in which there are not enough resources relative to patient requirements. Discrimination among patients must occur, but on what basis should this be done and in a way that does not introduce any form of unfair or improper discrimination? Should medical treatment be administered according to the criterion of severity of injury or according to the patient's age/social status/benefit to society, ethnic group, etc.? Decision rules that optimize outcomes for all concerned in disasters have not been validated. If the decision was made to deliver medical assistance according to the criterion of injury severity, would it be appropriate to favor patients who are injured severely and whose lives can most likely be saved if they receive immediate care, or would it be better to favor potentially fatally injured patients whose odds of survival are low but who may have a remote chance at survival? This question of treatment priorities is one of the most difficult ethical issues during an MCI.

- *Nonmaleficence:* Due to the nature of an MCI, caregivers may be forced into making critical decisions regarding treatment and evacuation of individual casualties based on superficial evaluation and without the guidance of diagnostic techniques that are normally available in modern medical practice. In addition, caregivers may be under special duress due to personal risk or discomfort. As a result, errors may occur in the diagnosis (e.g., undertriage or overtriage), which may harm certain patients. Should providers in MCIs be liable for these harms, and does the liability of a volunteer differ from that of a nonvolunteer?

- *Patient autonomy and right to information:* During an MCI, this principle may need to be subjugated due to the overarching need for expediency in administering care because medical personnel may not have enough time to share decisions regarding treatment with the patient. Professional and policy considerations regarding the type of injury or available hospital facilities will dictate where the patient will be evacuated, even against a patient's wishes or best interest from other perspectives (e.g., closeness to home). When a person refuses to receive medical care, the medical personnel will have no time to decide whether the person is rational, thus raising the question whether coercion or force should ever be used to administer medical care during an MCI. Also, how and to what extent should the patient's requests to choose a hospital or to be evacuated with relatives be considered? Should more time be devoted to every patient to explain to him or her the medical care that will be given? Should the explanations be foregone to care for more patients faster and more efficiently?

- *Staff safety:* There are situations in which the cause of danger has not yet been neutralized (e.g., rescue of wounded persons from a collapsing building; terrorist activity in which there might be an additional explosive charge; care of a chemically, radiologically, or biologically contaminated patient). How should medical personnel behave in such cases? Should they administer care while risking their personal safety, or should they wait until the cause of danger is eliminated? How much personal risk is acceptable? Should medical personnel be compelled to receive vaccination for potential bioterrorism weapons (e.g., smallpox) before or even after an event has occurred? Should nonvaccinated personnel be forced to treat contagious patients even though these physicians had previously refused (or were unable) to receive the vaccine? Which medical personnel should receive limited prophylactic antibiotics in case of an attack with anthrax? Should physicians be forced to respond to a call to manage a chemical incident even though their hospital may not be completely prepared for the event and personal protection equipment may be suboptimal or lacking?
- *Use of nonstandard or investigational procedures and drugs:* Advancement of medical knowledge is based on experimentation. For example, many new MCI triage methodologies have been proposed by public and private sources. How should they be tested? Should physicians accept grants or other inducements to study an unproven technology in a personal experience with an MCI? Experimenting in a disaster/MCI situation produces specific ethical issues not usually addressed during Institutional Review Board processes, and there are few contemporary guidelines.

The unique reality during an MCI creates difficult ethical issues arising from the fact that life is often threatened at an alarming rate; in the heat of a novel disaster, old platitudes and even widely accepted medical ethical codes may no longer apply in their original form.

CURRENT PRACTICE

Real-Time Ethics During MCIs and Disasters

Triage

Some authors agree with the ethics of utility and would counsel medical personnel to reduce morbidity and mortality as much as possible during an MCI.[15] The concept of utility attempts to maximize the general good and may seem to be at variance with the traditionally accepted principle of doing the utmost for the individual patient, even when ignoring some patients may raise the level of the cumulative benefit. During an MCI, providers must be prudent stewards of the limited resources entrusted to them. It would, therefore, be wrong for a clinician to devote his or her energies to

only one patient since, by doing so, the odds of survival for other casualties may be unfairly limited. In an MCI, equitable sharing of resources based on need may eclipse the first-come, first-served practice of routine operations in peacetime.

Assuming that a utilitarian sharing of resources is an appropriate paradigm shift for an MCI, there is still a need to set treatment priorities. Fortunately, there is broad agreement on which victims a clinician should approach first. Those with a lethal injury or in a perimorbid status will be managed expectantly, whereas those with serious but nonlethal injuries are often given high priority. The literature offers a number of suggestions to determine the order of treatment, but studies have documented the high rate of overtriage and undertriage in MCI situations.[16,17] Before we accept this evolution in attitude, it behooves us to consider other potential ways of setting treatment priorities in an MCI:

1. *Randomly choosing the order of patients to treat:* This position is based on the concept that every person has an equal right to receive medical treatment and, as such, it affords every casualty an equal chance to be chosen via random selection. The problem is that it does not allow every person an equal right to survive: caregivers may invest their time in treating individuals whose lives are not at risk while the other untreated patients may die. This approach is not consistent with the principle of reducing the mortality in as many cases as possible or with the principle of fair and just distribution, which correlates the extent to which a person needs treatment with the extent to which he or she is actually treated.

2. *Choosing according to "first-come, first-served":* This model may appear fair and, like the previous method, may connote a certain randomness. It may, however, portend greater casualties over time, and it is also inconsistent with the principle of equitable distribution of resources based on need. Also, rules set according to the sequence when casualties arrive on site—thereby determining who will be "first"—seem unacceptably arbitrary.

3. *No treatment to anybody:* Team members are not capable of making a decision of whom to treat first; therefore, they prefer not to administer any treatment until sufficient personnel reach the scene so that all patients can be treated equally. This theoretical solution contradicts the principles of beneficence and nonmaleficence. Withholding time-sensitive benefits and causing harm are both antithetical to the clinician's ethical duty.

4. *Using nonmedical standards (e.g., gender, age, profession, social status, contribution to society, ethnic origin):* In times of national crises or war, saving a president or a general may have collateral benefits for the good of the nation-state, and it seems natural to first help a wounded child or an esteemed public personality. However, given that all people have equal rights to live regardless of status, age, gender, origin, creed, or disability, physicians must not discriminate against patients who have legitimate needs for care. Ideological issues must not eclipse the humanistic priorities embodied in ethical rules.[18,19]

5. *Urgency of need:* The priority of treatment is determined according to the severity of the injury and the likelihood of benefit from care. The World Medical Federation has suggested the following scale of priorities:

- *First priority:* victims whose lives are at risk and can be saved by an urgent medical treatment
- *Second priority:* victims whose lives are not at immediate risk but who need immediate medical treatment
- *Third priority:* victims whose treatment may be delayed for an extended period
- *Fourth priority:* victims who suffer from emotional reaction to the event
- *Fifth priority:* victims who are too severely injured to be rescued

Such a scale of priorities may be considered immoral at first glance, like "abandoning a victim in the field."[15] However, herein is the major difference between an MCI and a routine event. The exigency of an MCI dictates the rule of reduction of morbidity and mortality as well as significant suffering in as many cases as possible. Adhering to this rule means preferring several severely injured victims who might be rescued over a near-fatally injured person who has only a slim chance of survival. Healthcare does not have to be equally distributed; it has to be *equitably* distributed, with each victim receiving care according to medical need. This system determines treatment priorities at the scene, but it is also valid in determining the priority of evacuation to hospitals.

Based on these two principles—reduction of mortality and permanent morbidity in as many cases as possible and giving priority of treatment according the severity of injury—a working scheme has been in place for years in all EMS/EM protocols for MCI triage. Triage is from the French word *trier*, "to sort," and sorting patients according to need is critical to "determining the order of priorities to medical treatment, based upon prognostic observations and evaluation."[15,17] Triage is performed at the scene in parallel (observing the entire scene simultaneously) and in tandem at the medical facility (triaging patients as they arrive). In practice, scene triage implies that before medical treatment begins, medical personnel will scan the scene and sort the victims into various categories according to the severity of their injury. Medical personnel begin treatment and evacuation only after the evaluation of all the wounded and consideration of extant resources have been completed. This brief planning stage is not "wasted" since it allows the medical personnel to evaluate the situation and determine who needs them most. The evacuation of victims from an MCI scene will take place according to the principle of the severity of injury. First to be evacuated will be unstable victims— those who suffer from a severe breathing disorder, an uncompensated situation of trauma, or a deteriorating state of consciousness. Following will be the stable but urgent victims, and lastly will come nonurgent cases. Often, the priority of evacuation is not identical to the priority of treatment (e.g., a patient with a pneumothorax needs extremely urgent treatment; however, once

treated on-scene, he or she is no longer defined as requiring urgent evacuation).[20] Both treatment and triage during an MCI must be orchestrated by well-trained and experienced disaster medical personnel. Minimizing the number of undertriage and overtriage situations will maximize goods and minimize harms. Triage must take into account patients who arrive at hospitals, patients already there, patients expected to arrive, and the resources available to them all on a dynamic, minute-by-minute basis.

Patient Autonomy

A recent medical newsletter opined: "In a massive epidemic, such *niceties* as patient autonomy, detailed record keeping, personalized care . . ." will be sacrificed.[21] Indeed, the principle of respect for patient autonomy may be overruled in certain disaster situations if it contradicts the main objective of providing the most good to the greatest number of victims.[22] This is not to say, of course, that respecting patient autonomy is not terribly important; rather, all attempts should be made to listen to the patient's specific medical wishes when possible, even though there will be little time. Specific wishes may be respected when they do not contradict the benefit of the majority of casualties and/or the operational requirements and protocols in force during the event. An exception to this rule may be the attempt to evacuate small children together with a parent or relative.

Personal Security of Medical Personnel During an MCI

Medical personnel work in cooperation with additional emergency authorities, such as the police and security forces. Scene safety includes not only the site of the event, but also the care sites. Thus, hospitals may be damaged and rendered unsafe by natural disasters. Hospitals have come under attack in battle zones, and water and food contamination endangers medical personnel as well as the populace. Terrorists have targeted hospitals, and chemical and biological agents pose grave risks to medical personnel both on-site and in care facilities. Balancing personnel safety and casualty needs is usually an ad-hoc decision to be made on-site by the medical commander in consultation with security and other rescue force commanders. Principles, however, must be set a priori. The principle of utility (i.e., maintaining the safety and thus functionality of medical forces who are usually not trained rescuers or fighters) must be balanced with the duty of the medical personnel to offer time-sensitive care as soon as practical. Noteworthily, the Israeli National EMS, MDA, forbids its thousands of underage volunteers to enter the scene of a disaster, but many have still participated in MCI care by functioning on the periphery of the site in areas declared safe by scene commanders. In this way, medical service is given to the victims while minimizing risk to the medical personnel. Having said that, 12 EMS personnel were injured and two killed in the line of duty in MCIs in Israel between September 2000 and September 2003.

Bioterrorism and Epidemics

Despite the 2002 anthrax attacks in the United States and the SARS mini-epidemic of 2003, no modern nation has had to deal with large-scale epidemics with modern means. Even though there is lack of experience and evidence-based information, it is important to at least mention the ethical issues likely to arise from such a situation, which presumably would have a potentially huge impact on a society and its medical system. An abbreviated listing includes:

1. The intrinsic dialectics between the good of society and that of the individual, as evidenced by the questions of whether to limit an individual's movement or his or her autonomy to decide whether to receive a vaccine or care versus society's need to isolate the contagious sick and to treat a contagious individual, perhaps by force
2. The application of experimental treatments during the epidemic, in lieu of existing therapy (pure research) or when other viable therapies are lacking
3. The responsibility of society toward those suffering side-effects of coercive (or even voluntary) therapies, medical personnel family members who contract a disease, affected caregivers, etc.
4. Forcing physicians to receive prophylactic antibiotics or vaccines
5. The right of physicians to refuse to care for contagious patients if these physicians refused (or were unable to or were not offered) vaccines/prophylactic treatment
6. Forcing physicians to remain in the hospital for extended periods to minimize disease transmission
7. Allocating scarce resources to the public versus medical/rescue personnel or politicians/defense forces, etc.
8. Forcing patients to seek care at community clinics by denying access to hospitals
9. Disseminating classified research information to the civilian sector
10. Withholding or modifying information to preserve public order and compliance
11. Manufacturing scarce medications in infringement of patent rights
12. Forcing private companies to produce needed medications
13. Forcing hospitals to take in contagious patients even though it will likely affect their income by turning away other patients
14. Permitting the government to take over stocks of vital supplies from private companies
15. Administering needed therapy to nonmentally competent, institutionalized patients; prison inmates; etc.

Natural Disasters

The deaths of patients in hospitals submerged by floodwater in New Orleans, LA, by Hurricane Katrina in 2005 have highlighted the issue of physician responsibility to his or her patients in times of extreme natural disasters. The physician faces at least three dilemmas under such circumstances: (1) balancing personal, family, and colleague safety with the duty to ensure patient safety and ongoing medical care, (2) providing adequate or at least life-saving care under conditions of severe infrastructure disruption, and (3) the responsibility to mitigate the consequences of disasters by adequate prior preparation for such emergencies. The most acute problem seems to be the immediate or even slightly delayed malfunction of life-sustaining equipment, such as ventilator shut-off due to lack of electrical power or oxygen, or dialysis machine dysfunction due to lack of electricity and dialysate. The lack of air-conditioning, degradation or destruction of stores of medicines, death, incapacitation or desertion of staff, destruction of all or parts of the medical facility, etc., may create an environment that renders the provision of adequate medical care impossible or tenuous.

What is, then, the duty of the physician under such circumstances? It seems futile to provide advice such as "patients first" or "save yourself and/or your loved ones first." It is the physician's duty to do his utmost, under the specific circumstances, to save the patient's life or prevent irreversible injury or organ damage. It seems reasonable to demand that any decision to withhold life- and limb-saving care should be taken only after due deliberation, discussion with peers and superiors, and, whenever feasible, documentation. Admittedly, sometimes the relevant time frame is extremely short (e.g., avalanche, tsunami), in which case it would seem that it is the physician's duty to save as many patients as is compatible with saving his own life. Finally, it is the duty of physicians (and managers, of course) to prepare the medical facility for disasters by appropriate planning, equipping, and staff training, in order to minimize or obviate some or all of these problems. Such mitigation activity is taken, by definition, prior to the event, and is therefore done under less or no time constraints. This makes the physician's duty in this respect much more binding, and any failure to fulfill it much less pardonable.

PITFALLS

The number and complexity of potential dilemmas are too numerous to address in their entirety in this chapter. Moreover, it is both impossible and unnecessary to have a policy for every situation that arises. Technical confusion, professional paralysis, and emotional numbing can seriously impair provider response, and even the classic codes of ethics fall short of a formulaic "one-size-fits-all" approach to moral challenges during mass casualty events.

Specific obstacles may be encountered before an event, during the event, and after the event. Professional ennui and lack of preparedness may be encountered at the individual and system levels. Ethical pitfalls during the event include all of those previously discussed regarding triage, resource allocation, safety, and fairness, as well as duty to care issues when the only contract is of the unwritten, Lockean, social contract variety. In the wake of an event, there are opportunities for fame and fortune and the chance to change practice.

However, there are overarching virtues and vices that can help or hinder a properly ethical MCI response, respectively. Virtues inform a wide variety of behaviors well beyond the reach of most ethics codes, principles, and policies. Around 330 BCE, Aristotle made virtues the basis for all ethics and discussed in his famous *Nicomachean Ethics* that the exercise of virtue was properly the middle ground or "golden mean" between deficiency and excess. Courage, for example, is vital for a healthcare provider to respond bravely to dangerous disasters and MCI situations. Ill-tempered or overexuberant foolhardiness to rush into a contaminated area without proper personal protection equipment when the equipment is available is not considered courage; it is merely foolishness. At the other extreme of this spectrum is the frightened provider who is afraid to act, immobilized by fear. Courage is a willingness to respond in the throes of danger, and it demands that we bravely treat both the perpetrators and the victims of MCIs and have the inner fortitude to take a stand for moral principles when it is difficult or unpopular to do so. Saying "no" to esteemed members of society, family, and friends for the greater good; allowing expectant patients to die under austere conditions; enforcing quarantine and reporting provisions with friends and colleagues; willingly responding to the call for help without fear of malpractice threats, infectious disease exposure, or economic risk are all examples of courage in action.

Justice is vital to promote fairness and the proper allocation of scarce resources according to need. Justice also enjoins providers to adhere to the mandate of the World Medical Association's Declaration of Geneva to treat patients regardless of "age, disease or disability, creed, ethnic origin, gender, nationality, political affiliation, race, sexual orientation or social standing."[4]

Similarly, prudence, or sound judgment, is the practical wisdom required to weigh competing interests and apply technical and moral facts to particular scenarios. Determining who to triage, refer, transport, and decontaminate all require prudential wisdom.

Stewardship is similar to prudence because it requires common sense in using scarce resources. This has application to everyday health resource distribution, but it is especially important under the resource and time limitations of a disaster to use personnel and equipment optimally.

Vigilance was perhaps the virtue most evidently lacking on Sept. 11, 2001. Around-the-clock guardianship does not relax on nights, weekends, and holidays. Surveillance activities and MCI preparedness plans mandate an ever-ready, argus-eyed vanguard of medical personnel who are prepared and able to respond before they are ever activated in the field. "Closing the stables after the horses are free" is a meaningless gesture—too little, too late.

Although the foregoing discussion may readily suggest that prudence, courage, justice, stewardship, and vigilance are central for responding to and being prepared for disasters and MCIs, their opposites—impulsivity, cowardice, prejudice, profligacy, and procrastination—are dangerous pitfalls to avoid. As Thomas Aquinas pointed out many centuries ago, for every virtue there is an antagonistic vice that hinders its expression. One way to avoid these vices is to prospectively draft policies and procedures that define role expectations that virtuous persons would manifest.

SOLUTIONS

Virtue, or character, is an important antidote to the many pitfalls and vices. The following principles for administering medical assistance amplify the core virtues of justice, prudence, courage, stewardship, and vigilance and take into account the tripartite obligations of medical professionals to patients, the profession, and the society in an MCI.

1. It is the ethical as well as the professional duty of society and the medical establishment to provide the infrastructure and timely local means to healthcare to minimize the disparity between demands and capabilities, thereby minimizing the number of casualties receiving suboptimal care, even in an MCI. At the same time, providers have parallel obligations to prudently manage and distribute scarce medical resources to avoid waste and to maximize the benefits for all victims.

2. It is essential to be prepared for a designated role in an MCI by continued study, drills, vigilance, and training, even in the face of financial and organizational constraints.

3. The principles of utility and justice mandate that care be distributed equitably and in a manner that maximizes survival and minimizes suffering for the greatest number of victims. Therefore, triage must be carried out fairly and without bias toward individual patients regardless of gender, age, race, creed, ethnicity, or role in the conflict. Medical and operational consideration should be the only factors determining the priority of care. The identity of the victim should play no role in decision-making, except in very extreme situations and those to be determined by policy set forth before the event.

4. Caregivers have a duty to treat MCI victims even in the face of personal danger. Balancing the needs of patients with the right of the caregiver to personal safety should be discussed and spelled out by the authorities before the event. Keep patients, other providers, and oneself safe to the extent that it is compatible with timely and efficient care of the majority of victims. Administer maximal amounts of medical care compatible with the operational limitations. At the very least, strive to minimize suffering.

5. Respect for patient autonomy, dignity, and right to privacy and to information are important even in an MCI. However, these rights may be subordinate to the exigencies of the situation when expeditious care for all patients is the first consideration.

6. Guard the identity, privacy, and confidentiality of victims of an MCI.

7. Work cooperatively with others who care for and about MCI victims and safeguard the public health.

8. Honor your profession by serving in an MCI without self-concern or demands for compensation or remuneration for service. Avoid opportunism and the lures of fame and fortune.

CONCLUSIONS

MCIs and disasters introduce numerous ethical challenges in triage, resource allocation, and patient care at the microlevel (patient care), mesolevel (professional principles), and macrolevel (societal). Prospective consideration of these challenges, disaster drills, and development of ethical MCI policies and protocols can help medical personnel function in a manner compatible with most of the basic ethical principles that guide medicine. To guarantee widespread commitment, ethical MCI policies and procedures must be drafted in advance with the input of both medical leadership and the people delivering actual care in the field. The realities of MCI are difficult to comprehend for anybody who has not "been there"; thus, learning from the experience of those who have been personally involved in MCI and disaster care can benefit medical professionals in all parts of the world who are only now preparing for their first MCI.

REFERENCES

1. Zuger A, Miles SH. Physicians, AIDS, and occupational risk. Historic traditions and ethical obligations. *JAMA*. October 1987;258(14): 1924-8.
2. United Nations High Commissioner for Refugees. Geneva Convention relative to the Treatment of Prisoners of War. Available at: http://www.unhchr.ch/html/menu3/b/91.htm.
3. Priel I, Dolev E. [Ethical considerations in mass casualty situation.] *Harefuah*. July 2001;140(7):574-7, 680.
4. World Medical Association. Medical ethics in the event of disasters. *Bull Med Ethics*. October 1994;102:9-11.
5. Larkin GL, Moskop J, Derse A, Iserson K. Ethics manual of the American College of Emergency Physicians. Available at: http://www.acponline.org/ethics/ethicman.htm.
6. American Academy of Emergency Medicine. Code of ethics. Available at: http://www.aaem.org/codeofethics/index.shtml.
7. Ethics manual. Fourth edition. American College of Physicians. *Ann Intern Med*. 1998:128(7):576-94.
8. American Medical Association. Code of medical ethics. H-130.946 AMA Leadership in the Medical Response to Terrorism and Other Disasters. Available at: http://www.ama-assn.org/apps/pf_new/pf_online?f_n=resultLink&doc=policyfiles/HnE/H-130.946.HTM&s_t=disaster&catg=AMA/HnE&catg=AMA/BnGnC&catg=AMA/DIR&&nth=1& &st_p=0&nth=3&, last accessed July 2, 2005.
9. Alexander GC, Wynia MK. Ready and willing? Physicians' sense of preparedness for bioterrorism. *Health Affairs*. 2003;22:189-97.
10. World Association for Disaster and Emergency Medicine. Health Disaster Management: Guidelines for Evaluation and Research in the Utstein Style. Available at: http://wadem.medicine.wisc.edu/Ch9.htm.
11. Israeli Medical Association. Available at: http://www.ima.org.il/EN/.
12. Garland B. Bioethics and bioterrorism. *J Philosophy Sci Law*. March 2002;Volume 2. Available at: http://www.psljournal.com/archives/newsedit/bioethics_bioterrorism.cfm.
13. The Center for Law and the Public's Health at Georgetown and Johns Hopkins universities. The Model State Emergency Health Powers Act. Available at: http://www.publichealthlaw.net/MSEHPA/MSEHPA2.pdf.
14. International Federation of Red Cross and Red Crescent Societies. Humanitarian ethics in disaster and war. Available at: http://www.ifrc.org/publicat/wdr2003/chapter1.asp.
15. Trotter G. Of terrorism and healthcare: jolting the old habits. *Camb Q Healthc Ethics*. Fall 2002;11(4):411-14.
16. Kilner T. Triage decisions of prehospital emergency health care providers, using a multiple casualty scenario paper exercise. *Emerg Med J*. July 2002;19(4):348-53.
17. Hirshberg A, Holcomb JB, Mattox KL. Hospital trauma care in multiple-casualty incidents: a critical view. *Ann Emerg Med*. June 2001; 37(6):647-52.
18. Resnik DB, DeVille KA. Bioterrorism and patient rights: 'compulsory licensure' and the case of Cipro. *Am J Bioeth*. Summer 2002;2(3): 29-39.
19. Raymond NA. Medical neutrality: another casualty of the intifada. *J Ambul Care Manage*. October 2002;25(4):71-3.
20. Parmet WE. After September 11: rethinking public health federalism. *J Law Med Ethics*. Summer 2002;30(2):201-11.
21. *Ramifications* [Newsletter of the Richmond Academy of Medicine]. December 2001;13(17):19. Available at: http://www.msv.org/public/articles/Ramifications_December_01.pdf.
22. Wynia MK, Gostin L. Medicine. The bioterrorist threat and access to health care. *Science*. May 2002;296(5573):1613.

chapter 10

Liability Issues in Emergency Response

Abigail Williams

Emergency response to a potential or actual catastrophic event has become more frequent and is now performed by a greater variety of organizations, including those whose sole mission is to respond to disasters and others who perform a variety of services, including disaster response. In the past, response from the Salvation Army and Red Cross to disasters and other large-scale events was common, anticipated, and accepted by the public. During the past 10 to 20 years, however, a greater number of more diverse agencies have routinely become involved in emergency response. In large measure, the plethora of media coverage has taught the public to expect that when an emergency situation occurs, the response will be professional, efficient, effective, and capable.

What has caused this enhancement of emergency response to occur? A number of factors have emerged, including, but not limited to, a quasi-government hierarchy that developed in part from the Civil Defense network of the 1960s. Local jurisdictions have emergency managers and emergency planning groups that may have staff and resources capable of emergency tracking, incident awareness, and rapid scene response. This structure builds both horizontally and vertically to include mutual aid from neighboring jurisdictions and from county, state, regional, and federal levels. This traditional structure is best represented at the primary level by local responders in law enforcement, fire, and emergency medical services (EMS). The Federal Emergency Management Agency (FEMA), as well as a variety of federal subteams, represent the next level of responders.[1] However, if the event involves an epidemic illness or chemical exposure, agencies such as the Centers for Disease Control and Prevention (CDC) and the Occupational Safety and Health Administration (OSHA), may respond. If there is a transportation incident, the National Transportation Safety Board (NTSB) and the Department of Transportation (DOT) may become involved. Where there is a terrorist event or crime involved in a disaster, the Federal Bureau of Investigation (FBI) and other law enforcement agencies, such as the Central Intelligence Agency (CIA) and the Bureau of Alcohol, Tobacco and Firearms (ATF), will also be part of the response and de facto command structure.

Parallel to this government response structure are other local and regional responders. Each of these agencies, although acknowledging the incorporation of the Incident Command System (ICS) into its overall operations, has different command structures. These agencies may include search and rescue teams; critical incident debriefing teams; canine search resources; regional air medical (helicopter) programs; various utility and construction assets; supply and logistics resources; religious organizations; and other agencies, whether volunteer or paid or trained or untrained. Incident command, although implemented by a number of agencies, has been used throughout the United States in an inconsistent manner and is almost always cited in the after-action reports of emergency responses and drills as one of the processes that failed.[2-8] In one of the most well-critiqued and available after-action reports from the 1993 World Trade Center bombing, the problems with the incident command structure and multijurisdictional and interagency response and communications were well documented.[9] In the investigation of the Columbine High School shooting, it was noted in the section on "lessons learned" that: "Fire department communications were severely stressed at this operation . . . . Department communications capabilities must be established so that they can handle the largest of emergencies that could occur in their jurisdiction . . . . Our standard portable radio, tactical frequency was overloaded and ineffective. The same problems were encountered with the command channels."[10]

Because of the lay publicity of these human resources and assets, response, in any perceived or real emergency situation, has become a public expectation in the United States. As a result of this expectation, the focus is now increasingly being placed on the timeliness and adequacy of that response. This paradigm shift in the public perception is reflected in great measure by a recent federal court decision involving the emergency response to the Columbine shooting. In the investigation of the Columbine High School shooting, it was found that standard fire department communication modalities were overwhelmed and therefore became ineffective.

The implication of that federal case for emergency responders is that they will now be held to a reasonable standard of care in the implementation and utilization of ICS. Any failure to act reasonably in the implementation of ICS may now result in responders being held liable for any injuries that are caused to victims under certain circumstances. The almost blanket protection that government and municipal responders have relied on, which traditionally has been provided by the Good Samaritan and other qualified immunity statutes, has been eroded, and the right to reasonable emergency response under certain circumstances has been strengthened. The overall impact, theoretically, will be one of heightened awareness of the obligations of emergency responders during a response. However, the *Sanders* decision, on which this chapter is partly based, thus far has been unrecognized as having this effect on the emergency response system.[11]

HISTORICAL PERSPECTIVE

The threat of malpractice litigation against EMS in relation to disaster response is almost nonexistent. There are no reported cases of successful lawsuits against disaster response providers for negligently providing medical care. However, questions regarding the adequacy of patient care and provider safety during a disaster response remain the topic of much controversy. The topic is most commonly raised in a number of specific situations:

- The first situation is one in which a responder becomes injured or dies during a response to a disaster. Such could have been the case when a young nurse, Linda Anderson, died while entering an unsecured area and attempted a rescue at the Oklahoma City bombing of the Murrah Federal Building.[12]
- The second situation is when a person believes that his or her civil liberties are being violated as a result of forced decontamination, quarantine, immunization, or isolation.
- The third situation is when the responder becomes injured due to the negligence of a third party.[13]
- The fourth situation is when a live victim is not cared for either properly or timely and dies from nonmortal injuries.[11] While attempting to evacuate students during the Columbine shooting, Dave Sanders, a teacher at Columbine High School was shot. Repeated calls to 911 were met with the response that help would come in 10 minutes. Unfortunately, no help came from noon until nearly 4 PM, when David Sanders died.[11]

Typically, victims injured in a disaster commonly sue the agency responsible for the accident, which causes such disasters to draw attorneys as well as rescuers. At some point, attorneys are going to look not only at the primary cause of the victim's injury (e.g., the plane crash, train crash, building collapse, or bombing), but they also will consider any secondary injury sources. The key, therefore, is to enhance the coordination and quality of care provided by the emergency responders in response to a disaster and to ensure that all applicable laws, regulations, and standards of care are met.

ABOUT THE LAW

Although coordinated and dedicated emergency response systems are a fairly recent development in the delivery of healthcare, it is important to recognize that the laws that govern the legal liability of these services are far from new. In fact, these laws and rules come from a progressive development of case law, statutory laws, and regulations promulgated over centuries. The rules of law that apply to emergency responders, therefore, are a composite of traditional general rules, transportation law, and rules flavored with recent federal mandates. Understanding the source of the rules and the applications that have arisen over the years is essential to a consideration of legal liability and distinctions that have arisen for emergence response application.

Sources of the Law

The federal constitution and each state's constitution are the foundation of all laws and individual rights in the United States. These documents create legislatures that write laws, courts that interpret the laws, juries that determine facts, rights that the government must protect, and the executive divisions of governments that enforce the laws as interpreted by the courts. In the past half century, a new source of law has emerged— administrative regulations, which blur the distinction between the legislative and executive branches of government as it applies to the emergency responder liability discussion. However, constitutionally protected rights have seldom been used beyond whether a jury trial must be provided to determine a malpractice claim. That changes somewhat when one considers the need for governmental infringement of an individual's constitutionally protected rights, i.e., martial law, forced isolation, forced quarantine, and decontamination in certain circumstances during a disaster. The dominant source of law in the medical field has been the court system, specifically with its decisions on interpersonal rights and responsibilities and the jury system driving the price of liability. To a limited degree, legislatures have attempted to reform the court systems and limit liability in malpractice cases, but at the same time, increasing volumes of regulations create new standards that may become the basis for claims of malpractice liability.

Court Concepts

The courts of this country function on a number of basic principles, which are essential to understand in a discussion of legal liability for emergency responders and emergency care providers.

Venue

Most negligence cases are based on state standards and tried in state courts, unless a case involves "diversity of citizenship" (residents or services of different states involved), constitutional issues, or a claim arising out of the alleged actions of a federal employee. State law determines the rights of parties to the case, the procedures they must follow, and the damages (money) or limits to damages they may recover.

State courts are typically organized according to county. Juries are normally selected from the community where the case is filed (venue). This is usually the county where the medical care occurred, but technicalities may result in a pitched legal battle over where the case must be tried to control which judge will preside over the case or the type of community from which the jury members will be selected. The venue for filing a case is often very important to the outcome or size, if any, of the verdict. In emergency response situations, the location of the care might involve more than one state or county and that may further expand the possibilities of where the case may be tried.

Case Law

Courts are expected to follow established precedent to the extent that it fits the case before that particular court. This is called *stare decisis*. The process of following these prior decisions is often referred to as "common law," or "case law."

The Role of the Court

The U.S. legal system is based on a respect of the roles of the various government branches. The legislature makes the laws, and the courts are to apply the laws as written. If an ambiguity exists in the language of the law, the courts are to interpret what the law means. Courts, however, have become more active in creating new rules and interpretations by distorting or expanding the language of the legislature, depending on the view of the critic.

A Hierarchy of Authority Exists

Not all sources of law are equal. There is a definite hierarchy of authority based on the source of the law being applied and the court system applying it. In most judicial systems, the highest court, usually the U.S. Supreme Court, issues decisions that control all of the lower appellate and trial courts in the system. The decisions of a state supreme court only control the courts of that state; decisions in other states may be influential, but they are not binding on another state. State appellate court decisions are generally binding only on trial courts within the subdivision controlled by the appellate court rendering the decision. Local level courts may have rules that regulate the procedures in the courts of that county. The decisions of a trial judge, however, only bind the litigants in the individual case. In the federal court system, the same hierarchy exists and the binding effect of the ruling is generally confined to the same federal structure, which is much like the state system. One exception is when the ruling provides an interpretation on the U.S. Constitution, and such a ruling typically is controlling at the federal and state levels. A similar exception would be in a case in which a federal law "pre-empts" or overrides state law. The federal court decision would control the federal courts below it and the state courts within its geographic, jurisdictional area. A different exception would apply in the event that a state is a party to the lawsuit before the federal court. A ruling by the federal court would control the specific state involved in the case.

Role of the Trial Judge

The role of the trial judge is to rule on the law, the process, and the evidence in a case. The trial judge controls what issues are allowed to be presented by ruling on the legal sufficiency of various elements of court documents. The judge also controls what items of information the parties can have access to through the process of "discovery."

During trial, the judge serves as the referee to ensure that both sides follow the rules of courtroom decorum. In addition, the judge rules on motions and objections that determine what evidence is presented and how it is presented. These rulings on evidence often have a profound influence on the ultimate outcome of a case. At the conclusion of the presentation of evidence and after attorneys for both sides have presented closing arguments, the judge gives a verbal "charge" to the jury. This is a reading of the written instructions that jury members will use while deliberating the verdict. The outcome of many cases hangs on the precise wording of these instructions.

After the verdict is given, the trial judge may rule on motions for a new trial or to overturn the verdict of the jury. These post-trial motions are usually in preparation for an appeal to a higher court. Once an appeal is filed, the trial judge loses jurisdiction over the case unless the higher court returns the case with instructions or rulings.

The Role of the Jury

Most states in the United States and all federal courts allow either side of a negligence case to request a jury trial. The number of jurors may vary by locality or jurisdiction. Different courts follow different procedures for selecting jury members from the pool of potential jurors. The cost and complexity of a case increase dramatically when a case is tried before a jury rather than having the case tried before a judge without a jury (bench trial), but the overwhelming majority of negligence cases are jury cases.

The jury members sit through the trial, listen to the witnesses' testimony, view the physical evidence, consider the arguments of all the attorneys, and are charged to follow the law given to them in the judge's instructions. The jury must reach its decision in any case based on what facts it finds to be true by a preponderance of the evidence. This means that the jury must be convinced that a given fact is more likely true than untrue, or just beyond 50% probability. The jury is considered the "conscience" of the court system. It is charged with the duty to render its decision based on the facts, evidence, and law presented to it, without allowing sympathy or prejudice to interfere with the process.

Standard of Care

Often, the most significant fact that the jury must determine is whether the emergency responder's care in the case was within the "standard of care." This essentially is a determination of whether the emergency responder "negligently injured" another person(s) in some way, as claimed in the lawsuit.

A standard of care may be created by a law, regulation, case law, or testimony on the standards observed by emergency responders of the same type. For example, alleged failure to appropriately use the ICS formed the basis of a lawsuit against municipal emergency responders to the Columbine shooting. Generally, to prove negligence, an expert of the same responder specialty must testify that the care provided did not meet the "standard of care" expected in similar circumstances. The "standard of care" definition varies by state, but in concept, it is the minimally acceptable level of competency and care expected of a responder of the same type acting in the same circumstances.

Although the court often makes legal rulings on issues that may affect what facts go to the jury, we will consider the concept of liability for negligence claims as presented in the following, based on four factual elements that the jury generally determines:

1. **Duty:** Did the emergency responder establish a relationship with the patient that created a duty?
2. **Breach:** Did the emergency responder fail to effectuate that duty in a manner that fell below the standard of care of the specialty or profession?
3. **Injury:** Did the action or inaction of the emergency responder that failed to meet the standard of care cause a legally recognized injury (physical, psychological, property damage, or damage to another legal right), worsen the injury, cause or increase expense, or (in some states) reduce the chances for a favorable outcome? Was there a logical connection between the failure to meet the standard of care and the resulting injury?
4. **Damages:** What award of money will compensate the victim for the injury or losses suffered and reasonably likely suffer in the future? This typically includes medical expenses, hospitalization, home care, loss of wages, and pain and suffering sustained.

This issue of standard of care will reappear frequently throughout the following discussions of emergency response liability.

BASIC CONCEPTS OF LAW THAT APPLY TO EMERGENCY RESPONSE

First and foremost in any healthcare-related law is the concept of patient choice as a fundamental right. The competent, unimpaired adult has the right to choose (or refuse) whatever medical treatment he or she will receive, even if that choice might otherwise seem illogical or may result in death. Persons who are unable to consent due to injury or medical condition, intoxication, mental illness, or legal incompetence are presumed to consent to care reasonably necessary under the concept of "implied" consent. In an emergency, the "emergency exception" allows care, rescue, and decontamination to be provided without obtaining consent. This issue

becomes important when one considers that in the event of nuclear, radiological, chemical, or biological contamination, people will be required to be decontaminated, isolated, and possibly quarantined for a period. For public health and safety reasons, they will not have the option of refusing such care. Even though some organizations recognize the right of an individual to refuse care under emergency circumstances, the majority of emergency response organizations advise that no person who has been contaminated should leave an area without being decontaminated, unless that person is critically injured and transported to a hospital for emergency medical care and subsequent decontamination. This raises one of two options. The first is to allow the person to remain in the contaminated area at his or her own peril, which the person will unlikely agree to do. The second is to decontaminate the person against his or her will, which may lead to various claims of restraint, battery, false imprisonment, etc. It is critical to emphasize that the response to allegations of criminal or constitutional violations, arising out of the involuntary treatment of an individual, is for the purpose of mass decontamination, isolation, and quarantine in a contamination incident and to prevent the spread of the contaminant and thus avoid a significant public health disaster. In such cases, the rights of the individual are superseded by the obligation to the rights of the many.

Consent may be legally obtained from a competent, unimpaired adult for his or her own care; however, issues frequently revolve around who may consent when a minor is involved. For the purposes of this chapter, the emergency exception to the requirement of consent will always apply and rescue care and other emergency response services must be provided with or without formal consent and may even be provided in the presence of an expressed refusal.

REGULATORY VIOLATIONS

The rules that apply to regulatory violations and their effect on liability vary from state to state. In some states, when regulatory violations occur and harm results, normal medical malpractice may be established without resorting to experts to establish the standard of care. This approach is called a "per se" standard—the violation is automatically conclusive proof of negligence. Other states use a "prima facie" rule that shifts the burden to the defendant to prove that the violation of the regulation was not negligence. In either case, however, there must be resulting harm to the patient for liability to exist.

Not every violation of regulations would result in liability. If the maintenance regulations were not being properly complied with, it would not be grounds for a negligence claim, but it may form the basis for a criminal or administrative complaint. In the absence of explicit intent of the legislature or government agency to create a safety standard or the absence of prior court rulings on the issue, it is up to the injured party to prove to a judge that the regulation is a safety standard that should be applied to create liability.

WHEN CIVIL LEGAL LIABILITY ATTACHES

The question that commonly follows a description of this concurrent and overlapping medical response is, "When does *legal* liability attach—or detach?"

The answer to that question is: Legal liability flows to any identifiable person for emergency response. Even though U.S. citizens may assume that during a disaster emergency, response services will provide competent and trained scene stabilization, search and rescue, medical care, and transport services, these are not articulated constitutional rights. Nevertheless, persons who are called on to respond to disasters or who may volunteer to do so must understand how to provide safe and effective care and not succumb to the mantra that "there are no rules in a disaster." Although unpredictability is characteristic of disasters, many types of disasters recur with regularity, resulting in a body of research, called *disaster epidemiology*. Disaster epidemiology allows for retrospective data collection and analysis of similar types of disasters and prospective consideration of the best practices in similar types of disaster management.[14]

The analysis that a Colorado court went through regarding the Columbine shooting case in determining whether any liability attached to the actions of the Jefferson County Sheriff's department articulates the basis of the nonconstitutionally based quasi-establishment of a "right" to emergency response in a disaster.[11] The court noted that central to the question of liability of responders (in this case municipal) is the primary consideration of whether there is a recognized "right" on the part of any particular individual to emergency response. The court reviewed the traditional legal test by which a right is determined by first determining whether there was a "generally applicable right protected under the Fourteenth Amendment of the U.S. Constitution." The Fourteenth Amendment states in part that[15]:

> Every person who, under color of any statute, ordinance, regulation, custom, or usage, of any State ... subjects, or causes to be subjected, any citizen of the United States ... to the deprivation of any rights, privileges, or immunities secured by the Constitution and laws, shall be liable to the party injured in an action at law, suit in equity, or other proper proceeding for redress.

Accordingly, the *Sanders* court reasoned that this section, enacted in its original form in 1871, was "specifically drafted to provide a method for an individual to seek redress of violations of their rights so protected under the Fourteenth Amendment by any person or group of people who act on behalf of the state."[11] The court acknowledged that the framers of this amendment apparently contemplated it to provide a method of redress under specific circumstances, those being the willful, knowing, or purposeful deprivation of life, liberty, or property by state action. It has been held by most courts and was articulated by the *Sanders* court that "the Fourteenth Amendment does not specifically serve to transform tortuous conduct into a constitutional violation."[16] Instead, the *Sanders* court noted that the Fourteenth Amendment does somewhat serve to protect citizens from the "arbitrary, abusive, or oppressive use" of

government (state, local, or municipal) power.[15] This basic principle articulated by the *Sanders* court when defining the basis for the right to assistance in an emergency was that the Fourteenth Amendment does not confer an "affirmative right to governmental aid, even where such aid may be necessary to secure life, liberty, or property interests of which the government itself may not deprive the individual."[17] As a result, the court noted that any specific individual has no affirmative constitutionally based right to emergency response under ordinary circumstances.[11] Thus, in the general sense, no one person can in an ordinary circumstance sue a government or municipal responder (or private responder) for injuries that occur as a result of a rescue, failure to rescue, or other emergency response activity, providing that the actions taken were in accordance with the identified standard of care.

Specifically, the *Sanders* court in its decision announced that even the U.S. Supreme Court has held that the due process clause of the Fourteenth Amendment "does not impose a Constitutional duty upon a state to protect individuals from violence, fire, or other need for emergency medical response."[17] Relying on previous decisions from other courts, both state and federal, the *Sanders* court stated that the due process clause actually "serves as a limitation on the state's power to act, not as a guarantee of certain minimal levels of competent or effective safety and security."[11] Again, as noted in this case, the court relied on prior decisions but had also accepted exceptions to the general rule of "no duty," which creates some concern for emergency responders.[18] The court relied on the recognition of the "special relationship doctrine" and the "state created or enhanced danger doctrine," discussed in the following section, as potential vehicles for affording redress to an individual who has sustained an otherwise compensable injury as a result of actions or inactions of emergency response personnel.[11]

NATURE OF THE LEGAL OBLIGATION OF RESPONDERS TO AN EMERGENCY

The Special Relationship Doctrine

The "special relationship doctrine" adopted by the courts is well established and universally accepted. This doctrine only applies in situations where the state, municipal, or other government agency imposes limitations on an individual's "freedom to act on his own behalf and therefore protect himself from harm."[11] Examples of this limitation occur in cases such as the institutionalization of a psychiatric patient; restraint of movement, such as when one is in handcuffs or restrained for his or her protection for the purposes of medical treatment during necessary transport; or during periods of incarceration (isolation and quarantine).[19] Thus the court notes: "it is the governmental restriction of freedom that triggers the exception to the Fourteenth Amendment right, and not the creation of a Constitutional right to the protection in and of itself."[20] The courts have noted that over the years there has been much wrestling with the definition and interpretation of specifically what level of restraint, "similar" to incarceration or institutionalization, is sufficient to give rise to a state's duty to protect a specific individual. Most jurisdictions, such as the Federal Tenth Circuit in Colorado, have adopted the requirement that an injured party must show involuntary restraint by a government official to establish a duty to protect under the special relationship theory.[21] As a nonprivate sector (municipal) emergency responder or as a private responder acting under the direction of a government agency, liability will attach once some form of involuntary restraint occurs, such as isolation, quarantine, forced decontamination, perimeter shutdown, or forced sequestration during an emergency. If, as an emergency responder, one decides to restrain an individual or group of individuals, that responder or responder group is then reasonably responsible for the individual's or group's protection.

Thus the *Sanders* court acknowledges that the "special relationship theory" exception, when taken a step further, would logically result in the acknowledgment that "inaction by the state or state-directed entity absent involuntary restraint even in the face of a known danger is not enough to trigger a Constitutionally based 'duty to protect.'"[11] That is, of course, unless the state or state-directed entity has a custodial, restrictive, or other special relationship with the person who claims lack of protection resulting in an injury. The courts have uniformly taken the position, as noted in the *Sanders* case, that any affirmative duty to protect an individual must arise from the limitation of movement that is imposed on the individual's freedom to act on his or her own behalf. It is not simply the responder's knowledge of the individual's actual or potential predicament that controls, but rather it is a "restraint" or limitation on movement that controls. Moreover, it is accepted that an emergency responder's knowledge of the risk of harm to another is not relevant to the determination of whether a special relationship between the parties in fact existed. Even under circumstances in which the emergency responder can reasonably foresee a reasonable likelihood of harm from inaction, "an affirmative duty to protect is not created unless or until the injured party can prove that a custodial relationship limiting his or her ability of self-protection did in fact exist."[22]

State Created or Enhanced Danger Doctrine

The second exception to the general rule that the government entity has no duty to protect any individual citizen from private violence is the "state created" or "enhanced danger doctrine."[11] Courts across the country have considered the question of just what state conduct "creates or enhances" danger sufficient to establish a duty to protect.[23] Some courts have decided, for example, police officers who engage in a high-speed car chase resulting in injuries to a bicyclist, motorist, or pedestrian could be legally responsible for creating a special danger faced by the injured party. Clearly the door has been left open for government liability where the state creates a dangerous situation or renders citizens more vulnerable to danger.[24] It is therefore accepted that the environment

created by state actors must actually be dangerous; they must actually know it is dangerous; and to be liable, they must have used their authority to create an opportunity that would not have otherwise existed. "If the danger to the plaintiff existed prior to the state's intervention, then even if the state put the plaintiff back in that same danger, the state would not be liable because it could not have created a danger that already existed."[11] If the alleged injured party fails to prove some form of affirmative action by the defendants that created or increased the danger to the individual victim, courts have universally dismissed the plaintiffs' complaints.[18] Under the Uhlrig test, to determine whether a government entity has created or enhanced a danger for the injured party, the following must be proved[18]:

1. Whether the injured party was a member of a limited and specifically definable group
2. Whether the emergency responder's conduct put the plaintiff at substantial risk of serious, immediate, and proximate harm
3. Whether the risk to the injured party was obvious or known
4. Whether the emergency responder acted recklessly in conscious disregard of that risk
5. If such conduct, when viewed in total, "shocks the conscience" of federal judges

An injured person must also show that the state entity and the individual emergency responder created the danger or increased the danger in some way.

LEGAL PROTECTION FOR EMERGENCY RESPONDERS: CURRENT PRACTICE

Volunteer Protection Act

In 1997, President Clinton signed into law the Volunteer Protection Act of 1997 (VPA) in an effort to provide some immunity from liability for claims that are made against volunteers who are providing services under the auspices of not-for-profit organizations.[25] This law preempts any state laws "to the extent that such laws are inconsistent with the Act" so that any state that chooses to have a law that is more protective than the VPA may, but any state that offers less protection is preempted by the VPA. The VPA does require, however, that some provisions be written into state law, including the requirement that the not-for-profit entity has risk management procedures in place and a provision for vicarious liability of the not-for-profit organization for the acts of a volunteer. Essentially what the VPA serves to do is to provide a qualified immunity for volunteers who are providing services for a not-for-profit organization under certain circumstances. To claim the benefit of this qualified immunity, the following circumstances must exist. The VPA provides immunity from lawsuits filed against a not-for-profit organization's volunteer when the claim is one of carelessness or traditional negligence. It is critical to note that the act does not provide immunity to the organization itself. The law only protects individuals who are acting in a volunteer capacity on behalf of a not-for-profit entity and preempts state laws that might hold a volunteer personally liable. The VPA only applies to uncompensated volunteers who provide services to appropriately designated 501(c)(3) and 501(c)(4) not-for-profit organizations. The immunity is a qualified immunity and protects the volunteer only against claims of ordinary negligence and not against claims of gross negligence; willful, wanton, reckless, behavior; or criminal misconduct. Any conduct that is intentional, conscious, or demonstrates a flagrant indifference to the rights or safety of the individual harmed is not covered by the VPA.

The VPA includes a provision that, if taken advantage of, ensures that innocent third parties hurt by the carelessness of not-for-profit organization volunteers will be adequately compensated for their injuries while, at the same time, providing personal immunity to such volunteers. This part of the act allows a state to require that a charitable organization "provide a financially secure source of recovery for individuals who suffer harm as a result of actions taken by a volunteer on behalf of the organization" before its volunteers gain immunity under the act. A general liability policy with adequate limits would be considered a financially secure source of recovery.

Qualified Immunity Statutes

At the core of qualified immunity is objective reasonableness. As long as the actions of the emergency responder, viewed from the perspective of the responder at the time and under the same or similar circumstances, can be determined to be within the range of reasonableness, then no liability will attach. Federal disaster medical assistance teams (DMATs) also have government immunity because when they are deployed and are providing care in a disaster environment, they are considered to be federal entities employed by the federal government for the specific purpose of an identified emergency response. Some argue that Good Samaritan and other immunity statutes provide blanket protection for the "best they can do under the circumstances" medical care in these emergency or disaster situations and therefore promote volunteerism during times of great need. Many questions have been raised, however, regarding the adequacy of such protection and immunity when disaster response is an expected, trained for, and perhaps even specialized, aspect of emergency response. Although it has been convincingly argued that the Good Samaritan and other immunity statutes and laws, as they are applied in disaster response, are of significant benefit, it is interesting to note that there are no studies to date that prove the theory: It is the threat of liability that prevents volunteers from acting. The other side to this blanket protection is that it can serve to open the door for substandard practice during a disaster response because there is no fear of legal repercussion for failure to act in a reasonable manner. Government responders, such as municipal fire, police, and EMS, have a number of limits on their legal liability. For one, there is no recognized right to an emergency response, and thus if no response occurs, there is no liability. The Federal Tort Claims Act (FTCA)[26] allows the federal government to be

held liable for the negligent acts of its employees, providing that the care that is in dispute is performed within the course and scope of their duties. This is in contrast to the general rule that the federal government has absolute immunity from liability. Thus, under the FTCA, the federal government can be held liable in the same circumstances as a private person in accordance with the law in the jurisdiction where the care occurred. The FTCA does limit the type and amount of damages that can be recovered under its umbrella and sets up some procedural hurdles for bringing claims. It should also be noted that there are exceptions to the waiver of immunity that is addressed in the FTCA. There is a specific prohibition against bringing any claims for damages that are caused by the imposition of quarantine, based on acts or omissions during the execution of a statute or regulation, provided that there was an exercise of due care or discretionary function. Other federal acts that address immunity for emergency management and consequence management are the Robert T. Stafford Disaster Relief and Emergency Assistance Act and the Homeland Security Act.[27] Even though these statutes serve to protect the government and responders from liability, a showing of recklessness, negligence, or bad faith may pierce them. The Military Claims Act serves to compensate for personal injury or death resulting from military service. This act covers claims that are brought for negligent acts or omissions against a federal employee who is acting within the scope of his or her duty and claims that are based on noncombatant activities of the military, such as training exercises. Similar types of immunity statutes exist on state and municipal levels.

The basic principles of qualified immunity, as previously noted, are well settled, and the purpose of an immunity statute is to limit the deleterious effects that the risks of civil liability would otherwise have on government operations at all levels.[28] It has been well settled by the courts that discretionary decisions such as emergency management and response by government agents inevitably influence the lives of private individuals, sometimes with harmful effects despite the best of intentions and rigorous attention to practice.[11] Moreover, decisions made in an emergency are understandably and to some extent inescapably imperfect.[11] In the context of emergency management, decisions must be made in an atmosphere of great stress, haste, and uncertainty. Holding emergency responders liable in hindsight for every injurious consequence of their actions would only have a chilling effect on the functions of emergency response. Qualified immunity thus allows state, municipal, and federal emergency responders the freedom to exercise fair judgment, protecting "all but the plainly incompetent or those who knowingly violate the law."[31] In summary, although there seems to be growing potential for liability, there are only limited circumstances under which a government, municipal, or private emergency (in some states) responder may be held individually liable for negligence that results in injury to another. To prove negligence, there must either be a "state created danger," a "special relationship," or conduct so negligent that it constitutes willful, reckless conduct that triggers such a duty of response.

PITFALLS

1. Assuming that there are no rules in a disaster
2. Failing to plan for emergency response to a disaster
3. Assuming that one cannot be sued because of Good Samaritan or other qualified immunity statutes
4. Acting outside the scope of one's license or certification
5. Failing to make a change in response to identified problems
6. Failing to critique each response and identify opportunities for improvement
7. Treating "lessons learned" in any given emergency response or drill as an oxymoron
8. Failing to adopt and practice an integrated ICS

REFERENCES

1. Federal Emergency Management Agency. Terrorism training resources. Available at: http://training.fema.gov.
2. Reinvestigation into the death of Daniel Rohrbough at Columbine High School on April 20, 1999, Executive Summary. Available at: http://news.findlaw.com/hdocs/docs/columbine/columbine41702 shrfrpt.pdf.
3. Kallson G. Collapse of Coalinga. *J Emerg Serv*. 1983;8(7):26-7.
4. Kems DE. EMS response to a major aircraft incident in Sioux City, Iowa. *Prehospital Disaster Med*. 1990;5(2):159-66.
5. Morris GP. The Kenner air disaster. A 727 falls into a New Orleans suburb. *J Emerg Med Serv*. 1982;7(9):58-65.
6. Nordberg M. United Flight 232: the story behind the rescue. *Emerg Med Serv*. 1989;18(10):15, 22-31.
7. Okumura T, Takasu N, Ishimatsu S, et al. 1996 Report on 640 victims of the Tokyo subway sarin attack. *Ann Emerg Med*. 1996;28(2):129-35.
8. National Transportation Safety Board. *Collision of Two Canadian National/Illinois Central Railway Trains Near Clarkston, Michigan*. Washington, DC: U.S. Government Printing Office; 2002. NTSB Publication No. PB2002-916304.
9. Federal Emergency Management Agency, US Fire Administration, National Fire Data Center. The World Trade Center Bombing: Report and Analysis. Available at: *http://www.usfa.fema.gov/downloads/pdf/publications/tr-076.pdf*.
10. El Paso County Sheriff's Office. Reinvestigation into the death of Daniel Rohrbough at Columbine High School on April 20, 1999, Executive Summary. Available at: http://news.findlaw.com/hdocs/docs/columbine/columbine41702shrfrpt.pdf.
11. *Angela Sanders, et al., v The Board of County Commissioners of the County of Jefferson Colorado, et al,*. 192 F Supp 2d 1094.
12. CBS News. Victims of the Murrah Building Bombing. Rebecca Needham Anderson. Available at: http://www.cbsnews.com/stories/2000/04/14/national/main184045.shtml.
13. Worcester Cold Storage firemen sue the building owner. Available at: http://www.firehouse.com/worcester/26_APsuit.html.
14. Auf der Heide E. *Resource Management in Disaster Response*. St. Louis: Mosby; 1989.
15. Fourteenth Amendment, 42 USC 1983.
16. *Daniels v Williams*, 474 US 327, 331 (1986).
17. *DeShaney*, 489 US 196.
18. *Uhlrig v Harder*, 64 F3d 567 (1995).
19. *City of Revere v Mass General Hosp.*, 463 US 239 (1983).
20. *Youngblood v Romero*, 457 U.S. 307 (1982).
21. *Leibson*, 73 F3d 276.
22. *Reed v Gardner*, 986 F2d 1122.
23. *Medina v City and County of Denver*, 960 F2d 1493.
24. *L.W. V. Grubbs*, 974 F2d 119.
25. Pub L No. 105-19 (Volunteer Protection Act).
26. Biotech.law.lsu.edu/cases/immunity/ftca.hat
27. US Department of Homeland Security. Available at: http://www.dhs.gov/dhspublic/.
28. *Harlow v Fitzgerald*, 457 US 800

chapter 11

Disaster Response in the United States

Jerry L. Mothershead

Response to emergencies and disasters for the protection of life, health, safety, and the preservation of property is a government responsibility. In the United States, governors, not the president, are primarily responsible for the health and welfare of their respective citizens and possess broad "police powers" that include the various legal authorities to order evacuations, commandeer private property, require quarantine, and take other actions to protect public safety.[1] Emergency response is carried out by local government entities within defined jurisdictions (e.g., towns, cities, counties). State governments coordinate needs identified by local governments with resources available either at the state or federal level.

In this chapter, the evolution of emergency and disaster management in the United States is discussed and an overview of disaster response as currently practiced in this country is provided.

HISTORICAL PERSPECTIVE

The Early Years: 1776–1945

The first recorded involvement of the federal government in disaster response dates to 1803, when the state of New Hampshire requested funding assistance after a series of devastating fires.

During the ensuing 150 years, response to major emergencies and disasters by government entities above the local level can only be characterized as reactive. Typically, a significant event would occur, outside resources would arrive from neighboring communities, and the event would be contained. Recovery operations were often slow, prompting requests to state governments for economic assistance. Only when the state was unable or unwilling to assist these local communities would the federal government become involved. At that point, federal legislation was usually required to authorize the expenditure of supplemental funds to assist the state and community involved.

Certain disasters occurred with greater frequency than others, and when the frequency and severity became significant enough to draw national attention, Congress would establish an office or agency to address these types of events. Thus, during the first half of the 20th century, the Reconstruction Finance Corporation was established to make disaster loans after certain types of disasters. The Bureau of Public Roads provided funding for transportation infrastructure damage. The Flood Control Act, which gave the U.S. Army Corps of Engineers greater authority to implement flood control projects, was also passed. This uncontrolled and disorganized approach remained in effect until after World War II.[2]

Civil Defense Era: 1945–1974

The development of modern emergency management began in the 1950s with the passage of two pieces of federal legislation: (1) the Civil Defense Act, aimed at funding initiatives that prepared for civil defense against enemy attack (shelter programs, packaged disaster hospitals) and (2) the Disaster Relief Act, which provided funds to state and local governments for rebuilding damage to public infrastructure.[3]

During the 1950s and much of the 1960s, civil defense from enemy attack was the federal government's priority, particularly the threat from nuclear attack that the Cuban Missile Crisis exemplified in 1961. At the same time, state and local governments were contending with significant natural disasters, such as the Alaskan earthquake (1964) and Hurricanes Betsy (1965) and Camille (1969). Federal funding for civil defense greatly outweighed that provided for natural disasters, and federal requirements prohibited the use of civil defense funds for preparedness to natural disasters.

At about this time, research and guidelines for disaster response started to appear. Severe wildland fires in southern California in the early 1970s gave rise to the congressional-funded project, Firefighting Resources Organized for Potential Emergencies (FIRESCOPE), which developed the Incident Management System (IMS) concept. The first standards for disaster management were authored by the National Fire Protection Association (NFPA) and were aimed at healthcare facility preparedness (J. Kerr, personal communication, Ottawa, Canada, 2000).

The "first assessment" of disaster research occurred in 1975 and summarized the findings of the disaster research community.[4]

Coordinating State and Federal Response: 1974–2001

Throughout the 1970s, the National Governor's Association (NGA) called for streamlining the fragmentation of federal civil defense and disaster assistance programs. In 1974, Congress passed the Robert T. Stafford Disaster Relief and Emergency Assistance Act, which unified federal funding of civil defense and disaster assistance programs.[5] In 1979, President Carter established the Federal Emergency Management Agency (FEMA) to serve as the overall executive branch coordination agency for disaster response.[6] Parallel efforts at the state level resulted in the establishment of either a state Emergency Management Agency or offices with similar coordination functions.

The creation of FEMA and promulgation of various executive orders during the 1970s and 1980s improved overall federal response, but in general, authorities and responsibilities remained confusing and, on occasion, contentious. In an attempt to resolve many of these conflicts and promote a coordinated approach to disaster response, the Federal Response Plan (FRP) was developed to serve as the principal organizational guide for defining the roles and responsibilities of 26 federal member agencies and the American Red Cross, which are in charge of delivering emergency assistance during major crises.[7] Although revised several times, the FRP did not solve all response and coordination problems and, in reaction to various disasters, additional federal plans were developed, including the Federal Radiological Emergency Response Plan (FRERP) and the National Oil and Hazardous Substances Pollution Contingency Plan, more commonly referred to as the National Contingency Plan (NCP).

Problems other than coordination continued. One example was the often significant delay in the arrival of state and federal response resources. The NGA successfully lobbied Congress to enact the Emergency Management Assistance Compact (EMAC)[8] legislation, the first significant alteration to model state Civil Defense legislation passed in the 1950s. This legislation established a template for state-to-state resource sharing during disaster response.

Thus, by the turn of the century, the framework existed at the state and federal levels for coordinated response and recovery operations to disasters caused by nature or as the result of technological mishaps. Unfortunately, a new threat loomed that would again result in a major revision of the approach to disaster management.

New Millennium, New Threats: Post-2001

Terrorism arrived in the United States in the 1990s, with the first attack on the World Trade Center in 1993, followed by the bombing of the Murrah Federal Building in Oklahoma City in 1995. Internationally, terrorist organizations were growing in numbers, and terrorist acts were becoming more lethal. In addition to conventional weapons, these organizations were using chemical, biological, and radiological agents to cause greater harm and were turning these threats against civilians as well as the political or industrial figures attacked in the past. The Aum Shinri Kyo religious sect used the nerve agent sarin unsuccessfully against several magistrates in Japan in 1994 and in the following year successfully attacked passengers in a Tokyo subway station. U.S. interests were increasingly under attack overseas, evidenced by dual embassy bombings in Africa in 1998, which were followed by the maritime attack on the destroyer *USS Cole*.

These events drew the attention of both the executive and legislative branches of the federal government. Under the Clinton administration (1992-2000), there was a promulgation of a series of executive orders, referred to as Presidential Decision Directives (PDDs), and the enactment of federal statutes to increase the defensive posture of and to protect the United States and its citizens against terrorist attacks. A number of new offices and programs were established in federal agencies, including in the departments of Justice, Health and Human Services, and Defense. The most significant legislation was the Defense Against Weapons of Mass Destruction Act,[9] commonly referred to as the Nunn-Lugar-Domenici legislation. One of the Act's many purposes was to provide resources for equipment and the training of local response personnel for mitigating a weapons of mass destruction (WMD) incident.

These initiatives, while significant, proved insufficient to prevent the terrorist attacks that totally destroyed the World Trade Center in New York, significantly damaged the Pentagon, and resulted in nearly 3000 deaths on Sept. 11, 2001. One month later, weaponized *Bacillus anthracis* (anthrax) spores were distributed through the U.S. mail system, resulting in 11 deaths and another 11 infected persons. In combination, these events have resulted in some of the greatest restructuring of the federal government since its inception.

CURRENT CONCEPTS OF DISASTER RESPONSE

The terrorist events of 2001 sent shock waves throughout the U.S. government. New legislation was introduced in the first three months after the attacks that surpassed all antiterrorism legislation of the previous decade. President Bush, who had been recently elected, issued and continues to issue new and revised executive orders, now termed Homeland Security Presidential Directives, that call for changes in executive branch agencies to meet the current threat against terrorism. Funding to fight the "global war on terrorism" at home and abroad increased by a full order of magnitude and does not include the expenditures to fight the wars in Afghanistan and Iraq.

To best understand the emergency management system in the United States, it is important to first realize that all levels of government have certain roles and responsibilities in mitigation, preparedness, response, and recovery and that various government entities have different functions in preparedness and response.

Regardless of the government level, however, the designated emergency management agency is responsible for day-to-day coordination of mitigation and preparedness activities involving agencies and organizations at that level and for synchronization of these agencies during response and recovery phases. The designated emergency management agency also serves as the focal point for hierarchical coordination between local, state, and federal response agencies.

Local Level Emergency Management

Because there are subordinate jurisdictions within each state that are usually established by geographic boundaries, local emergency management may occur at the city, township, borough, county, or (in some states) parish level. To a great extent, the attention given to emergency and disaster preparedness and response will be dictated by the overall population within the jurisdiction, actual or perceived threats to the area, and population concentration. Ultimately, however, emergency management comes down to funding.

Regardless of the type of jurisdiction, an executive/managerial official will be in charge of emergency management operations. This official may be the community safety official, the fire chief, or the police chief. It is this individual's responsibility to form a multicratic organizational model within the community that brings together the disparate response and recovery organizations, including entities such as hazardous materials teams; fire services; law enforcement agencies; city, county, or district health departments; and public works departments.

State Level Emergency Management

All 50 states and the six territories have emergency management agencies that fall under the executive branch of the state government. In most cases, these agencies are either independent entities or increasingly are incorporated into the agency responsible for the state's National Guard. State Emergency Management Agencies (SEMAs) are responsible for standards, training, and oversight of emergency management organizations at lower jurisdictional levels; coordination with other state level agencies and organizations in their preparedness and planning activities; and the administration and distribution of state or federal funds earmarked for emergency management. In some states, disaster-related organizations, such as the state emergency medical services (EMS) office, are part of the SEMA, but this subordinate organization is by no means uniform across the states.

During response and recovery operations, SEMAs usually provide overall operations and support at state level emergency operations centers, provide liaison personnel to federal coordinating officers (the on-scene federal emergency manager), receive requests for assistance from local EMAs, and provide state level resources (both personnel and material) and expertise to local emergency managers.

In addition to its own resources, a state could request outside assistance from other states that are an EMAC signatory. Although, initially, few states signed on to this agreement, in the wake of the terrorist attacks of 2001, almost all states and territories have now signed this legislation. Under an EMAC, a requesting state may ask for resources and personnel from a signatory state. If available, the assisting state will provide those resources, with the understanding that the requesting state will provide appropriate legal coverage from assisting personnel and will reimburse the assisting state for resources used. Depending on the actual wording and annexes of individual EMACs, such resources could include the National Guard or medical personnel who are not state employees.

Finally, a number of states, particularly in the Northeast, have signed international EMACs with provinces in Canada to allow resource sharing across the border.

Federal Level Emergency Management

With the rare exception of a disaster that meets the criteria of a national security event, coordinated federal response to disasters usually does not occur unless the governor of the affected state requests a presidential declaration of a national disaster, which then must be approved. However, each federal agency that could be involved in disaster response is still able to exercise its autonomy and respond directly to a request for assistance outside this coordinated federal response. For example, the Environmental Protection Agency could provide expert assistance during clean-up operations from an oil spill that did not meet national emergency thresholds. Similarly, the Centers for Disease Control and Prevention could mobilize one of its Epidemiological Investigative Service teams to assist in the evaluation and containment of a contagious disease outbreak. Under these circumstances, however, the funding stream to reimburse the agencies would fall outside that which is established for presidential declarations and may have to be through either state or agency resources.

Department of Homeland Security

Because of its pivotal role in overall federal level emergency management, one must understand the current organization and functions of the Department of Homeland Security (DHS). DHS initially was authorized to serve an advisory role to the president; however, a shift toward the concept of "Homeland Security" evolved, and through Congressional efforts DHS became the federal entity focused exclusively on this issue. In November 2002, the president signed into law H.R. 5005,[10] the Homeland Security Act of 2002, which established the DHS[11] as a cabinet level executive agency. DHS consolidated 22 agencies and 180,000 employees, unifying many federal functions into a single agency dedicated to protecting America. Agencies under the DHS include the newly created Transportation Security Administration, the U.S. Coast Guard, and FEMA. FEMA's traditional role as the lead coordinating agency for all disaster response in the United States continues, but under the oversight of DHS. The secretary of DHS was given extraordinary powers, including the authorization to initiate a federal response under the Stafford Act without prior consultation with the president under certain exigencies.

DHS is organized around four principal functional directorates and a supporting, management directorate:

- The science and technology directorate coordinates the department's efforts in research and development, including preparing for and responding to the full range of terrorist threats involving WMD.
- The information analysis and infrastructure protection directorate assesses intelligence information concerning threats to the homeland, issues warnings, and takes appropriate preventive and protective action.
- The border and transportation security directorate is responsible for maintaining the security of borders and transportation systems and is home to agencies such as the Transportation Security Administration, the former U.S. Customs Service, the border security functions of the former Immigration and Naturalization Service, Animal and Plant Health Inspection Service, and the Federal Law Enforcement Training Center.
- The emergency preparedness and response directorate ensures that the United States is prepared for and able to recover from terrorist attacks and natural or technological disasters. FEMA was incorporated into this directorate in 2003, but retains its name and, to a certain degree, its autonomy, especially during response operations.

All responses to disasters and emergencies that reach the threshold for a presidential declaration of a national disaster fall under the coordination purview of DHS. Under these circumstances, FEMA is the operational arm of DHS in executing response and recovery initiatives and does so within the framework of two recently promulgated documents, the National Response Plan (NRP) and the National Incident Management System (NIMS).

National Response Plan. On Feb. 28, 2003, the president issued Homeland Security Presidential Directive #5[12] to enhance the ability of the United States to manage domestic incidents. To implement this directive, the secretary of DHS directed that a single, integrated federal Emergency Operations Plan (EOP) be developed. This NRP[13] parallels the earlier NRP in format and links the following hazard-specific EOPs:

- FRP[14]
- U.S. Government Interagency Domestic Terrorism Concept of Operations Plan[15]
- FRERP[16]
- Mass migration response plans
- National Contingency Plan[17]

Under the NRP, FEMA serves as the overall coordinator for federal support. However, under the NRP construct, support is considered to fall within 15 different Emergency Support Functions (ESFs), which are listed in Table 11-1. Because resources and expertise in these various functions may exist within multiple federal agencies, each ESF response is coordinated by an ESF coordinating agency; a primary agency, which is usually the same as the coordinating agency; and a number of secondary (supporting) agencies.

TABLE 11-1   EMERGENCY SUPPORT FUNCTIONS

ESF NO.	FUNCTIONAL AREA
1	Transportation
2	Communications
3	Public works/engineering
4	Firefighting
5	Emergency management
6	Mass care, housing
7	Resource support
8	Public health and medical services
9	Urban search and rescue
10	Oil and hazardous materials
11	Agriculture and natural resources
12	Energy
13	Public safety and security
14	Recovery and mitigation
15	External communications

In the event of a national disaster, various emergency operations centers and oversight and policy entities will be activated at the headquarters level, not only of the DHS but of other federal agencies. The principal headquarters office responsible for interacting with state/local operations managers is the Regional Response Coordination Center (RRCC). At the local/regional level, the principal coordinating office is now termed the Joint Field Office (JFO). The JFO provides a local coordination of federal, state, local, tribal, nongovernment, and private-sector response organizations, and, in addition to federal, defense, and state field officers, is staffed by representatives from appropriate ESF coordinating agencies and other state representatives.

National Incident Management System. Homeland Security Presidential Directive #5 (an executive order) called for the creation of a standardized incident management system to facilitate interoperability and integration among the many federal, state, and local response organizations. NIMS[18] provides a standardized system for implementing the NRP. NIMS provides a consistent yet flexible nationwide framework within which local, state, and federal levels of governments and the private sector can work effectively and efficiently to be aware of, prepare for, prevent, respond to, and recover from domestic incidents, regardless of their cause, size, or complexity. NIMS is mandated for use by all agencies in the executive branch of the federal government. Although not mandatory for use by the states and local jurisdictions, federal funding for disaster and homeland security initiatives is directly tied with these jurisdictions' use of the NIMS in preparation, planning, and response.

SUMMARY

Emergency management has evolved over the past 200 years. With the creation of DHS as an authoritative central executive agency for oversight of all federal emergency management activities, a level of cooperation and collaboration never before achieved is a possibility. At the same time, refinements of and support for emergency management initiatives at the state and local levels offer the promise of better hierarchical integration during response and recovery.

Although some standards exist for emergency management, many more meaningful and measurable standards are needed. Education and training, although improved, still have not reached all levels of emergency management to the degree desired. Many communities still are short of critical supplies and resources, and certain problems, such as mass care issues and environmental recovery and surety operations, have not been resolved.

Nonetheless, great strides have been made, especially in the last few years, and have established a framework by which further improvements are indeed possible.

REFERENCES

1. Pine J. *A Review of State Emergency Management Statutes.* Washington, DC: Federal Emergency Management Agency; 1989:8.
2. Federal Emergency Management Agency. FEMA history. Available at: http://www.fema.gov/about/history.shtm.
3. LaValla P, Stoffel R. Blueprint for Community Emergency Management: A Text for Managing Emergency Operations. Olympia, WA: Emergency Response Institute; 1983.
4. White GF, Haas JE. *Assessment of Research on Natural Hazards,* Cambridge: MIT Press, 1975.
5. Robert T. Stafford Disaster Relief and Emergency Assistance Act, as amended by Pub L No. 106-390, October 30, 2000. Available at http://www.fema.gov/library/stafact.shtm.
6. Drabek T. The evolution of emergency management. In Drabek T, Hoetmer G, eds. *Principles and Practices for Local Government.* Washington, DC: International City Management Association; 1991:17.
7. Federal Emergency Management Agency. *Federal Response Plan.* Washington, DC: Government Printing Office; Document 9230.1-PL: Supersedes FEMA 229 (April 1992).
8. National Emergency Management Association. Emergency Management Assistance Compact. Available at: http://www.emacweb.org/.
9. Pub L No. 104-201 (Defense Against Weapons of Mass Destruction Act of 1996).
10. U.S. Citizenship and Immigration Services. HR 5005 Homeland Security Act of 2002. Available at: http://uscis.gov/graphics/hr5005.pdf.
11. U.S. Department of Homeland Security. The Department of Homeland Security. Available at: http://www.dhs.gov/interweb/assetlibrary/book.pdf.
12. The White House. Homeland Security Presidential Directive/HSPD-5. Available at: http://www.dhs.gov/dhspublic/display?theme=42&content=496.
13. U.S. Department of Homeland Security. Initial National Response Plan fact sheet. Available at: http://www.dhs.gov/dhspublic/display?theme=43&content=1936.
14. U.S. Department of Homeland Security. Emergencies and disasters: planning and prevention: National Response Plan. Available at: http://www.fema.gov/rrr/frp/.
15. Federal Emergency Management Agency. U.S. Government Interagency Domestic Terrorism Concept of Operations Plan. Available at: http://fema.gov/pdf/rrr/conplan/conplan.pdf.
16. U.S. Department of Homeland Security. Federal Radiological Emergency Response Plan (FRERP)—Operational Plan. Available at: http://www.fas.org/nuke/guide/usa/doctrine/national/frerp.htm.
17. Environmental Protection Agency. National Contingency Plan overview. Available at: http://www.epa.gov/oilspill/ncpover.htm.
18. U.S. Department of Homeland Security. National Incident Management System. Available at: http://www.dhs.gov/dhspublic/display?theme=51&content=3423.

Local Disaster Response

Jerry L. Mothershead

All disasters are local. Regardless of type, magnitude, or progression, disasters affect communities; therefore, community responders will be the first on-scene and will remain for recovery operations well after supporting resources and organizations have departed.

Depending on the type of disaster, various government, public, and private organizations responsible for public safety, public security, and infrastructure maintenance will be tasked to save lives, preserve property, and identify and rebuild essential services for the population served. Prioritizing and coordinating these missions will require collaboration, cooperation, and understanding on the part of the leadership and membership of these response and recovery organizations.

In general, these services are organized in the United States within a jurisdictional framework, and overall coordination falls to the governing entities within these jurisdictions. Unfortunately, these government systems are not identically established throughout America. The general framework usually involves metropolitan areas (e.g., cities, towns) within a county, which is within a state organization. However, many "states" are in fact commonwealths, counties may be supplanted by parishes, and some states recognize townships or independent cities not subordinate to surrounding counties.

Thus, no single description of local response can be provided that is applicable to all localities. Rather, this chapter will address functional entities and notional organizational structures, processes, and responsibilities; concepts, rather than specifics, will be emphasized.

LOCAL GOVERNANCE

Protection, prevention, and response to emergencies and disasters are well-recognized government responsibilities. Depending on a number of factors, local jurisdictions either have systems in place for emergency response or band together with neighboring communities to provide overall emergency management to a large constituency. Certainly, jurisdictions with substantial populations tend to establish discrete offices, referred to herein as *emergency management offices,* to provide coordination for prevention, mitigation, planning, and response functions.

However, even in those discrete functional areas, there might be multiple government entities involved. Law enforcement is but one example. Cities usually have a discrete police department, with the chief of police reporting to the city governing entity (e.g., mayor, city council). However, if that city is within a recognized county, certain law enforcement responsibilities, even within city limits, may fall to the county sheriff's office, and state police might be tasked with other or overlapping duties. The city might also harbor a local Federal Bureau of Investigation (FBI) office with federal law enforcement and investigatory responsibilities, and should that community include ports of ingress, other federal law enforcement entities, such as Customs and Border Protection, and U.S. Citizenship and Immigration Services, may have certain authorities within the jurisdiction.

Responsibilities become even more confusing when applied to public health and medical services. All states have a division or department of public health that usually falls within the executive branch of the state government. A public health infrastructure, which may contain regional, county, district, and city public health offices, may exist. Members of the public health organization are state employees. Medical care, on the other hand, may fall within the responsibilities of a variety of organizations. There are very few public health hospitals left in America, and most inpatient care is provided through private, for profit and not-for-profit, hospitals that do not limit their services to discrete jurisdictional boundaries. Physician offices and independent clinics outside of any one hospital's organization are common in all communities. Increasingly, freestanding laboratories, other diagnostic centers, and other healthcare services also exist that are not part of larger healthcare systems, but they do form part of the healthcare network. Emergency medical services (EMS) (emergency ambulance services) may be provided by fire services, discrete government entities, hospitals, or contracted providers, and multiple EMS providers may support individual or multiple jurisdictions. EMS (and fire services) may be paid, career agencies, volunteer groups, or composites. Statewide, EMS may fall within the public health department, Emergency Management Agency, or another state organizational construct.

Under the paradigm of the National Response Plan (NRP), there are 15 essential functions that potentially

TABLE 12-1 COMMUNITY ESSENTIAL FUNCTIONS

FUNCTION	RESPONSIBLE ORGANIZATIONS
Transportation	Public works department
Communications	
Public works	Public works department
Firefighting	Fire and emergency services department
Emergency management	Local emergency management agency
Mass care	
Resource support	Various
Public health and medical	Jurisdiction's public health department
Urban search and rescue	Fire and emergency services department
Oil spills and hazardous materials	Fire and emergency services department
Agriculture and natural resources	
Energy	
Public safety and security	Jurisdiction's law enforcement organization
Recovery and mitigation	Various
External communications	Area emergency warning agency

NOTE: Blanks in the table indicate that the function is not typically a responsibility of a local jurisdictional office or entity or is not provided by government.

are required in the event of a disaster.[1] In the case of federal support, a discrete federal agency or organization has been identified as the primary coordinating entity for providing this functional support to state and local government. (Note that several states have additional, state-level essential functions.) These 15 essential functions, with the usual local entity responsible for their provision, are outlined in Table 12-1. What is most important is not the specific organization, since this may vary with the jurisdiction, but that, at the local level, some organization or entity has been assigned the principal coordinating responsibility and has the necessary resources (material, manpower, and economic) to provide for the reestablishment and maintenance of these services under emergency conditions or has the processes and framework to request, acquire, and incorporate outside resources into this functional organization.

Perusal of Table 12-1 will make it clear that not only are multiple, disparate local government agencies and organizations crucial to emergency management, but that participation may be necessary with nongovernment and industry organizations if the response is to be fully effective. Power, light, and natural gas resources and services are provided almost exclusively by private corporations. Crucial communications with the public will entail cooperation by local news media organizations and telecommunications corporations.

SUPPORTING ORGANIZATIONS AND CAPABILITIES

It is thus imperative that a full accounting of all local resources be considered during preparation and planning for emergency response. The most common forum in which this occurs is through Local Emergency Planning Committees (LEPCs). LEPCs and State Emergency Response Commissions (SERCs) are mandated by the Emergency Planning and Community Right to Know Act.[2]

The act requires each state to set up an SERC.[3] The 50 states and the U.S. territories and possessions have established these commissions. Indian tribes have the option to function as an independent SERC or as part of the state SERC in which the tribe is located.

In some states, the SERCs have been formed from existing organizations, such as state environmental, emergency management, transportation, or public health agencies. In others, they are new organizations with representatives from public agencies and departments and various private groups and associations. Duties of SERCs include:

- Establishing local emergency planning districts
- Coordinating activities of the LEPCs
- Reviewing local emergency response plans
- Monitoring legislation and information management concerning hazardous materials
- Maintaining situational awareness of locations of all major quantities of defined toxic industrial materials
- Establishing procedures for receiving and processing public requests for information collected under the Emergency Planning and Community Right to Know Act
- Taking civil action against facility owners or operators who fail to comply with reporting requirements

LEPCs normally include elected officials and representatives of law enforcement, civil defense, fire services, EMS, public health, local transportation agencies, communications and media organizations, facilities involved with the handling of toxic industrial materials, and the medical community.[4] Others from the public at large may also be included. The primary responsibility of an LEPC is to plan, prepare for, and respond to chemical emergencies. LEPCs must identify and locate all hazardous materials; develop procedures for immediate response to a chemical accident; establish ways to notify the public about actions they must take; coordinate with corporations and plants that harbor toxic industrial materials; and schedule and test response plans. An LEPC also receives emergency releases and hazardous chemical inventory information submitted by local facilities and must make this information available to the public. An LEPC serves as a focal point in the community for information and discussions about hazardous substances, emergency planning, and health and environmental risks.

LOCAL RESOURCES

One of the many goals of the Metropolitan Medical Response System (MMRS) Program is to try to coalesce all potential response capabilities into collaborative functional areas.[5] In the case of health and medical support, this extends far beyond the traditional boundaries of EMS, hospital-based care, and local jurisdiction public health. Under the MMRS paradigm, one or multiple jurisdictions should join together to optimize the use of resources along a more regional approach, to the benefit of all. The ability of all functional elements of response to surge capabilities and capacity in reaction to an emergency cannot be overemphasized. Failure of complementary surge in even one sector can result in bottlenecks and lack of optimal response across the spectrum.[6]

In addition to traditional entities and organizations, there is a wealth of additional resources that could be brought to bear in the event of a public health emergency or other disaster with significant health effects. These range from private organizations, corporations, and other business ventures through the recruitment of appropriate volunteers, either from volunteer organizations or the public at large. A partial listing of these other medical or paramedical resources is included in Table 12-2. What is important in local planning is the recruiting, training, and cataloging of all potential participatory organizations, entities, and individuals; cooperative planning on best use of these resources; and training of these individuals and organizations to produce a cohesive response organization. Convergent volunteerism is an important adjunct to area emergency managers, but planning for utilization of these resources is a necessity for optimal use.[7]

One organization of particular note is the National Voluntary Organizations Active in Disaster (NVOAD).[8] NVOAD coordinates efforts by many organizations responding to disaster. These organizations provide more effective service with less duplication by getting together before disasters strike. This cooperative effort has proven to be the most effective way for a wide variety of volunteers and organizations to work together in a disaster.

An initiative recently sponsored by the U.S. Department of Health and Human Services (DHHS), through the Office of the Surgeon General, is the Medical Reserve Corps (MRC).[9] The mission of the MRC program is to establish teams of local volunteer medical and public health professionals who can contribute their skills and expertise throughout the year as well as during times of crisis. The MRC program office functions as a clearinghouse for community information and "best practices."

MRC units are made of locally based medical and public health volunteers who can assist their communities during emergencies, such as an influenza epidemic, a chemical spill, or an act of terrorism. MRC units are community-based and function as a specialized component of Citizen Corps, a national network of volunteers dedicated to making sure their families, homes, and communities are safe from terrorism, crime, and disasters of all kinds. Citizen Corps, AmeriCorps, Senior Corps, and the Peace Corps are all part of the USA Freedom Corps, which promotes volunteerism and service throughout the United States.

LOCAL RESPONSE CONCEPTS OF OPERATIONS

Since no two disasters are identical, the actual concepts of operations during response will vary depending on the actual circumstances. There are, however, some basic concepts that will affect operations that should be well appreciated by emergency managers and planners.

Community Warning

The ability of the community to be prepared for the disaster is predicated on adequate forewarning of the impending event. Unfortunately, many disasters do not lend themselves to early detection by any form of sensor, or analysis has not reached the point that actions may be appropriately taken. It is well documented in the literature that "false" warnings actually impede future community actions, a classic example of "the boy crying wolf" once too often.

Most warnings are issued by government agencies. Most dissemination and distribution systems are owned and operated by private companies, and effective public-private partnerships are required. Great strides are taking place in threat detection and warning communications technology. Warnings are becoming much more useful to society as lead time and reliability are improved.

To be effective, warnings should reach, in a timely fashion, every person at risk and *only* persons at risk, no matter what they are doing or where they are located. There is a window of opportunity to capture peoples' attention and encourage appropriate action. Appropriate response to warning is most likely to occur when people have been educated about the hazard and have developed a plan of action well before the warning. Warnings must be issued in ways that are understood by the many different people within our diverse society. A single, consistent, easily understood terminology should be used, which may need to be conveyed multilingually in certain communities. If warnings that are not followed by the anticipated event are inconvenient, people are likely to disable the warning device.

Examples of failed or ineffective warnings include:

TABLE 12-2 SOURCES OF MEDICAL RESOURCES IN A COMMUNITY

EMS/Transportation
Ambulance companies
Hospital ambulances
Military field ambulances
Air ambulance services
School buses
Transit services
Taxi services

Diagnostic Services
Freestanding laboratories
Diagnostic centers
Dialysis units

Inpatient Facilities
Nursing homes
Rehabilitation centers
Addiction treatment centers
Hotels
Gymnasiums

Outpatient Facilities
Physician offices
Physical therapy centers
Urgent care clinics
Dental offices

Logistics
Pharmacies
Medical supply centers
Department stores
Furniture stores

Allied Heath Personnel
Veterinarians
Medical students
Nursing students
Allied health training centers
Medical explorer units
School/occupational health nurses

- Alabama, March 27, 1994: A tornado killed 20 worshipers at a church service. A warning had been issued 12 minutes before the tornado struck the church. Although it was broadcast over the electronic media, the warning was not received by anyone in or near the church.
- Florida, Feb. 22-23, 1998: Tornadoes killed 42. The National Weather Service issued 14 tornado warnings. The warnings were not widely received because people were asleep.

A variety of warning devices needs to be used to reach people according to the activity in which they are engaged. Effective warning systems should also have redundancy. On May 31, 1998, a tornado in South Dakota killed six. Sirens failed because the storm had knocked out power.

Response Scene Operations

The immediate concern of response organizations is the preservation of life. This not only includes actions directed at victims of the disaster—search and rescue, extrication, triage, scene treatment, transportation, and definitive treatment and rehabilitation—but also at preventing further risks to the community through containment of the disaster.

The disaster *must* be contained. This is relatively easy to envision in the case of a spreading hazardous materials incident, but the concept applies to *any* disaster. Containment can be both geographic (erecting levees for flood protection) or can be internal to the disaster area; for example, frequent sequelae of certain disasters are rioting and looting or vandalism. These types of actions actually represent secondary or compound disasters. In the case of a progressive infectious disease outbreak (e.g., one caused by a contagious agent—measles, influenza, or smallpox), containment of disease spread is the principal goal of public health. Failure to contain the disaster early on will result in significantly greater losses, whether economic or lives.

All the actions one would think of to rescue and treat individuals directly affected by the disaster must take priority over salvage and property protection operations. Sequentially, these actions include:

- **Search and rescue:** In a hazardous materials (HazMat) environment, up to an hour may pass before HazMat teams even enter the "hot zone." Thus, those minimally injured may self-extract and seek treatment well before those most severely injured, resulting in a bimodal presentation to area hospitals.
- **Triage of victims:** This may have to be done at multiple stages of the operations. Classic triage is based on trauma, and this form of triage may not be the best for victims of chemical or biological incidents.
- **Decontamination, especially in known HazMat incidents:** A study[10] conducted several years ago revealed that only 18% of victims of HazMat incidents who were treated at hospitals underwent decontamination before arrival. In the 1995 sarin attack in

Tokyo, nearly 600 patients arrived at St. Luke's Hospital within the first 45 minutes of the incident. None had been decontaminated (fortunately most did not require this). Still, a number of hospital personnel developed nerve agent exposure symptoms from treating and evaluating the victims.

- **On-scene treatment of victims:** The majority of injured victims do not stay at the scene long enough to receive prehospital triage and treatment. Those who remain on the scene are usually the most severely injured and are unable to escape the scene before the arrival of rescue assets. Also of interest, however, is that several studies have recently called into question the efficacy of victims waiting for responders.[11] In one study, the morbidity and mortality of those who waited for EMS agencies was significantly higher than for those who were transported to community hospitals by the most expeditious method available.
- **Transportation of victims:** This is also more complicated in a disaster situation. Although the nearest hospital might be the best equipped, if it has already been overwhelmed by the arrival of other critically ill victims, EMS will need to invoke "first wave" protocols.[12] This occurs when the most critically ill patients are distributed among potential receiving hospitals with little regard of proximity.
- **Re-triage of victims and receiving fixed-site medical treatment facilities:** Procedures and policies must be in place to handle this sudden surge of victims while still tending to already anticipated patients not involved in the mass casualty incident.

First responders will be overwhelmed in a true mass casualty incident. Most first responders and EMS personnel have been trained in the simple triage and rapid treatment (START) algorithm.[13] This algorithm, which assesses mental status, respiratory effort, and peripheral perfusion, can be performed in as little as 30 seconds and allows only minimal treatment—reposition of the head to decrease airway resistance and bandaging of gross hemorrhage.

Ambulance and vehicle control at the scene are important considerations. In the Avianca plane crash on Long Island in 1979, so many rescue vehicles arrived unsolicited that departing vehicles could not get on the one-lane road that provided the sole ground access to the scene. All arriving vehicles should be sent to staging areas out of the way, with at least one staff member remaining with the vehicle at all times.

Contaminated vehicles pose a risk to both patients and staff as a result of residual contamination or from offgassing from patients in the confined treatment compartment. In general, patients whose conditions are stable should undergo full decontamination at the scene before transportation. Patients whose conditions are unstable may undergo gross decontamination, which may entail removal of clothing only, and be placed in nonporous patient wraps for transport. Once a vehicle is used for a potentially contaminated patient, it should be considered contaminated until fully cleaned inside and out.

Receiving Facility Considerations

Receiving facilities must have capabilities to decontaminate potential patients and should have sufficient space to maintain these patients for a period, even if the patients are to be eventually transferred elsewhere.

First-wave protocols should be developed in communities with multiple hospitals. A first-wave protocol matches hospital resources with total victim requirements. It does a victim little good to be taken to a facility already overrun with critical patients merely because it is the nearest hospital, while other facilities that are slightly farther away remain empty. Distribution of victims throughout the entire hospital "system" will do the most good for the most number of patients, and this may be considered a form of transportation triage.

During planning, treatment facilities must determine how to rapidly expand their services for a surge of patients. This entails increasing staff through recall, expedient credentialing of volunteers, canceling elective procedures, and premature discharge of patients whose conditions are stable. It also means that additional bed space be made available by using, for example, cots, litters, cafeterias, other open spaces, and same day surgery clinics. Although historically few hospitals have suffered supply shortages in disasters in the United States, some caches should be available to handle the disaster until outside resources arrive.

Above all, facilities must be protected. If a facility becomes contaminated, it threatens this entire function. Facilities should have methods for expedient collective protection and must have security personnel available for access control.

Public Welfare Issues

In a disaster that involves large geographic areas, people will be displaced. Depending on the location, the socioeconomic status of the community, the type of disaster, and adequacy of the warning (that was heeded by the population), this may or may not be a problem.

- **Shelter:** The majority of evacuees on the East Coast as the result of hurricane warnings generally travel inland and stay with friends or relatives over a larger geographic area where the impact of this surge population is not felt as greatly. Still, those who have not evacuated, or those without family support, may be forced into shelters.
- **Healthcare:** It must be remembered that a displaced population has additional needs due to the recent stressors, but individuals within this cohort may also have special needs in and of themselves—especially if residents of nursing homes or rehabilitation centers or significant numbers of chronically ill patients are part of the displaced population.
- **Family assistance programs:** These programs become important very early in a disaster. People from outside the region want to know that their loved ones are safe. Families get separated during the disaster, and relocation is an important issue. Bereavement

programs for survivors must be ready to implement during this period.

ISSUES IN LOCAL RESPONSE

There are a number of cross-cutting issues or functions that affect all phases of emergency response. These include:

- The establishment and manning of emergency operations centers and command posts.
- Effective unified or incident command systems operations.
- Intra-agency and interagency communications.
- Effective resource management, both material resources and manpower.
- The ability of different sectors of the response to rapidly and seamlessly integrate with outside agencies, whether locally through memoranda of understanding or through activation of state or federal emergency response plans.
- The media, who will arrive almost immediately and demand information (effective media relations will pay off during after-action reviews; at the same time, the public will want information and may need both information and direction).
- In the event of a disaster caused by criminal or terrorist acts, forensic issues will be important as crime scene investigators and consequence management agencies work together.
- Legal issues are always present, ranging from the application of Occupational Safety and Health Administration standards to liability issues.
- Finally, depending on the particular disaster and the community's response to it, there may be issues of crowd control, vandalism protection, and other law enforcement agency functions beyond crime scene investigation.

SUMMARY

Local response to disasters is where the rubber meets the road. Effective planning, preparation, and response entail identification and cataloging of all available resources, education and training of personnel from disparate organizations, and a response structure that allows seamless integration of these assets.

REFERENCES

1. U.S. Department of Homeland Security. National Response Plan. Available at: http://www.dhs.gov/dhspublic/interapp/editorial/editorial_0566.xml.
2. U.S. Environmental Protection Agency. Emergency Planning and Community Right to Know Act, 42 USC 11001 et seq. 1986. http://www.epa.gov/region5/defs/html/epcia.htm.
3. State Emergency Response Commission. Available at: http://www.lepcinfoexchange.com/sercpages.html.
4. U.S. Environmental Protection Agency. Local Emergency Planning Committee (LEPC) Database. Available at: http://www.epa.gov/ceppo/lepclist.htm.

5. Metropolitan Medical Response System. Available at: https://www.mmrs.fema.gov/default.aspx.

6. Hick JL, Hanfling D, Burstein JL, et al. Health care facility and community strategies for patient care surge capacity. *Ann Emerg Med.* September 2004;44(3):253-61.

7. Cone DC, Weir SD, Bogucki S. Convergent volunteerism. *Ann Emerg Med.* December 2003;42(6):847.

8. National Voluntary Organizations Active in Disaster. Available at: http://www.nvoad.org/.

9. Medical Reserve Corps. Available at: http://www.medicalreservecorps.gov/.

10. Okumura T, Ninomiya N, Ohta M. The chemical disaster response system in Japan. *Prehospital Disaster Med.* July-September 2003;18(3):189-92.

11. Demetriades D, Chan L, Cornwell E, et al. Paramedic vs private transportation of trauma patients. Effect on outcome. *Arch Surg.* February 1996;131(2):133-8.

12. Auf der Heide E. *Disaster Response: Principles of Preparation and Coordination.* St. Louis: Mosby; 1989.

13. Bozeman WP. Mass casualty incident triage. *Ann Emerg Med.* April 2003;41(4):582-3.

chapter 13

Disaster Planning: State Programs and Response

Esther H. Chen, Bruce Y. Lee, and Jerry L. Mothershead

State disaster management has changed dramatically in the past 15 years. State administrations have emerged from the shadow of the federal government to develop their own disaster response systems and become the umbrella agencies that protect their citizens from disasters. Because the state can exercise its authority over community disaster control programs and can mobilize federal resources, it has become a focal point in disaster planning and relief. After the attacks on the World Trade Center and the Pentagon on Sept. 11, 2001, preparedness against terrorism became another important focus of state governments. Nonetheless, comprehensive, all-hazards emergency management continues to be the principal goal of state emergency response agencies. This chapter discusses a typical state's emergency management organization, reviews pertinent state laws, and highlights a few specific policy changes of the post-Sept. 11 era.

HISTORICAL PERSPECTIVE

Before World War II, most states did not have well-organized disaster response organizations or systems and relied primarily on fragmented federal programs for postdisaster assistance. Between World War II and the 1970s, the establishment of several federal agencies, such as the Communicable Disease Center (forerunner to the Centers for Disease Control and Prevention) in 1946 and the Department of Health, Education, and Welfare in 1953; the passage of federal laws to deal with civil unrest in the 1960s; and airplane hijackings in the 1970s improved communications among the different states and encouraged slightly more uniformity among state disaster programs.[1] In 1974, the National Emergency Management Association was formed to share common state experiences in dealing with natural disasters and provide interstate assistance.[2] However, disaster management remained fragmented until 1979, when President Carter established the Federal Emergency Management Agency (FEMA) to consolidate federal response and coordinate local, state, and national disaster preparedness and mitigation efforts.[3-5] In 1986, the Emergency Planning and Community Right to Know Act (EPCRA) mandated states to develop their own emergency management agencies (EMAs) or commissions to plan for and respond to state and local disasters.[6,7] State and community governments now share the responsibility of protecting the citizens within their own jurisdictions. Currently, all 50 states and U.S. territories have EMAs, and 23 states have followed the federal lead and have established state departments of Homeland Security.[7-9]

CURRENT PRACTICE

Emergency Management Infrastructure

Emergency Management Agency

A state's EMA is responsible for coordinating state disaster response, supporting county and local governments in predisaster planning and postdisaster relief, and accessing external aid. A typical EMA consists of several state and local agencies and is headed by a director who reports to the state governor (Table 13-1). The governor is the chief constitutional officer authorized to declare a "state of emergency," mobilize state and local agencies to provide assistance, and temporarily suspend statutes or orders that would obstruct actions during a state disaster. Some states have more disaster-related resources, and many have established extensive emergency management commissions.[10]

The EMA is also responsible for the state's Emergency Operations Plan (EOP), which facilitates timely and algorithmic response to specific disasters.[11] A state's EOP typically has three major components: a tactical plan assigning specific response tasks, an action plan to deploy resources, and a long-range needs and resources plan.

Elements of emergency preparedness common to all states' emergency management programs include:

1. **Communications:** This includes response personnel notification and maintaining and testing statewide communications architectures.
2. **Hazard awareness:** Information about natural disasters is provided to educate the public on safety and simple prevention measures. Some states also publish information on hazard mitigation.[5,12]

TABLE 13-1 EMERGENCY MANAGEMENT COUNCIL

PARTICIPANT	DESCRIPTION
Governor	Chief executive officer: Declares disaster emergencies, directs all state and local agencies to provide assistance, and temporarily suspends any statute or order that would delay action during a state disaster emergency
Director	Coordinates the state's disaster management activities in coordination with the directors of other state agencies
State Agency Officials	Adjutant general
	Commissioner, State Police
	Attorney general
	State fire commissioner
	Director, Emergency Services Agency
	Secretary of Health
	Secretary of Environmental Protection
	Secretary of Transportation
	Secretary of Agriculture
	Secretary of Public Welfare
	Secretary of Labor and Industry

3. **Disaster preparedness:** A two-tiered approach to community preparedness is used. At the local level, state funds are provided to establish temporary shelters, develop appropriate disposal for hazardous materials, and organize emergency response protocols. Information is provided to the general public on evacuation procedures, disaster supply kits, and family emergency planning. Several states have even developed resources for children.[13,14]

4. **Training and exercises:** Professional development for emergency response and administrative personnel and technical training are provided, often in conjunction with courses developed by FEMA.[11,12] At the community level, disaster drills and exercises are also offered.

5. **Threat alerts:** The EMA provides daily advisories and warnings on natural and technological threats. More specific information on potential disasters is provided to emergency managers.

6. **Emergency resources:** The EMA maintains a current compendium of available emergency management resources.

7. **Regional planning:** Local and community governments have their own EOPs and can use state resources to disseminate public safety information, schedule training exercises, and periodically assess the hazard risks of their community.

A representative from the state EMA is normally the chief operations officer for the state Emergency Operations Center and is responsible for coordinating all state responses in the event of actual statewide disasters.

State Emergency Response Commission

Mandated by the EPCRA, the State Emergency Response Commission (SERC) consists of the EMA director, directors of state agencies (e.g., Department of Health, Department of Transportation, Department of Food and Agriculture), and representatives of Local Emergency Planning Committees (LEPCs). SERC responsibilities include establishing and supervising LEPCs, providing the public with hazardous materials information, and reviewing state and local emergency response plans.

Department of Homeland Security

Since the development of the federal Department of Homeland Security (DHS), 23 states have separated state homeland security from the jurisdiction of the EMA. The state DHS director reports directly to the governor; coordinates state and local resources devoted to terrorism detection, prevention, response, and recovery; and has full authority to use all available state and local agencies for public safety. Other state programs include:

1. **State security plan:** All states have security plans that provide the framework to enhance their ability to protect their citizens from terrorism. This includes a counterterrorism system, distributing funds to local and state agencies dedicated to public safety, and a tactical response strategy.

2. **Security grant funding:** States can distribute federal funds to enhance all programs dedicated to terrorism preparedness and training.

3. **Citizen preparedness:** Information is provided to the public about preparing for a potential terrorist act and to educate citizens about potential chemical, biological and radiological exposures.

4. **Training:** Training programs are offered on community and state levels. Emergency medical teams are trained to recognize biological, chemical, and radiological exposures and respond to mass casualty events.

Keeping state EMAs and DHSs separate has its advantages. Two separate, smaller, leaner organizations can focus on their respective areas and build the necessary expertise more efficiently than a single large organization burdened by a wider variety of responsibilities. Having two separate but similar organizations also means that backup resources are available should one organization be unable to fulfill its duties. Separate organizations with different organizational cultures and personnel can also offer different perspectives on the same problem.

Conversely, there are disadvantages. Two different organizations may mean redundant services and personnel, significantly increasing costs. Also, communication, which is crucial to any emergency management infrastructure,[15] may be hindered by bureaucratic and administrative barriers separating the two. Moreover, it is not always clear which problems fall under whose jurisdiction, especially when it cannot readily be determined whether bioterrorism, natural disasters, or both are responsible. Additionally, differing protocols and philosophies can cause conflict and confusion.

National Guard

The state National Guard, supervised by the Adjutant General and composed of both the Air National Guard and the Army National Guard, was established in colonial times to protect citizens during war and to provide assistance during emergencies. It has dual state and federal responsibilities.[16] Its mission under state law is to protect life, restore property, and preserve peace and public safety. When not under federal control, Guard personnel may be deployed by the governor for emergency management.[17,18] The National Guard offers additional personnel, federal training, and federal resources. However, relying on the National Guard has its potential perils. The National Guard's other responsibilities, especially during wartime, may limit its availability. Even when Guard personnel are available, it takes time for them to assemble and respond. Moreover, during peaceful times, the state may have little experience working with the National Guard, which may prevent the state from efficiently using it when crises arise. Guard personnel would have to work with unfamiliar state and local personnel and resources. Additionally, competing responsibilities and a shortage of career advancement opportunities may be hindering the National Guard's ability to recruit and retain adequately specialized personnel.[19]

Department of Health

Each state has a Department of Health (DOH) whose mission includes providing public health surveillance and response to a medical incident or public health threat. The DOH usually has jurisdiction over the following state agencies and programs:

1. **Emergency medical services (EMS):** Local EMS systems provide first responders to disasters. Funding is provided toward responder training, equipping vehicles for catastrophic casualty events, and coordinating regional and interstate EMS systems when local resources are overwhelmed.
2. **Community health districts:** Programs supported include reporting and detecting communicable diseases, providing immunizations, and promoting public and environmental health in the community. Health center personnel are educated on recognizing and containing bioterrorism agents and diseases.
3. **Public health surveillance:** The DOH is responsible for public health disease surveillance (including those due to bioterrorism) and interfacing with appropriate federal agencies.
4. **Environmental health epidemiology:** Responsibilities include surveillance of environmental toxins and chemical and physical agents as well as biomonitoring.
5. **Hospital organizations:** During an emergency, the DOH has the authority to mobilize medical personnel and acquire pharmaceutical and medical supplies from hospitals. It also provides coordination between emergency management and medical organizations.
6. **Strategic National Stockpile:** The state DOH is responsible for oversight and coordination of public mass prophylaxis and vaccination campaigns in the event of a bioterrorist attack or other public health emergency.

EMS Agency

The state EMS agency oversees the statewide EMS system to ensure timely and appropriate prehospital care. It is also responsible for managing the state's emergency prehospital response to disasters and for providing funds to support disaster preparedness. This agency has several specific roles and responsibilities:

1. **EMS systems development:** The agency is responsible for assessing and improving the multiple regional and local EMS systems based on community needs, providing resources for developing new EMS systems, developing standards for EMS systems statewide, and reviewing local EMS plans.
2. **Trauma systems development:** The agency sets state trauma systems standards. It also evaluates trauma systems in accordance with changing needs of the community, designates trauma centers, and reviews the major trauma registry for continuous quality improvement.
3. **Education and training:** Standards for all aspects of out-of-hospital care systems are established by the state agency. The state agency also reviews the course curricula for regional EMS providers, develops a statewide EMS communications plan, and sets the standards for first aid training programs.
4. **Disaster preparedness and response:** A state's EMS agency is responsible for developing or assisting local health agencies in the establishment of emergency response plans, forming and coordinating a statewide mutual aid system, and testing these protocols through drills and exercises.
5. **Public education and information:** Information about the EMS system is distributed to promote public awareness of its role in the community.

State Hospital Organizations

Hospitals, health systems, and continuing care providers in each state have formed a collective association with the purpose to improve the healthcare delivery in their communities, provide access to healthcare for their citizens, and improve laws and regulations. The organization represents its members to state and federal governments and national organizations on issues of public health policy, promotes professional development for healthcare personnel and leaders, and facilitates communication among its members. Furthermore, it coordinates disaster preparedness in the hospitals and develops guidelines, including those pertinent to disaster preparedness.

State Legislation

Disaster Response

Numerous federal and state statutes, executive directives, and regulations that address terrorism, homeland security, and consequence management have been enacted since 2001, but the first comprehensive approach to federal disaster assistance was enacted in

1974 with the passage of the Robert T. Stafford Disaster Relief and Emergency Assistance Act.[20] One operational component of the Stafford Act is the Federal Response Plan,[21,22] which, in December 2004, evolved into the National Response Plan.[23] Federal resources that may be deployed include damage assessment, medical personnel and equipment, and emergency communications. The Stafford Act and the EPCRA form the backbone of federal policy on disaster assistance and are discussed in other chapters of this textbook.

Around the time the EPCRA was passed, each state also passed its own Emergency Services Act, which confers emergency powers to the governor, assigns functions to state agencies during emergencies, and authorizes the mobilization of all local and state resources toward disaster management. Through this and other legislation, the governor is usually authorized to create or suspend any statute during a state emergency, procure all state and local resources needed during a disaster, mobilize the National Guard and private personnel if necessary, and use news wire services if other communication methods are unavailable.

Since most states lack the resources to respond to a major catastrophe on their own, Congress passed the Emergency Management Assistance Compact (EMAC) in 1996 to enable states to assist each other during any disaster.[24] Any EMAC state can request personnel (including from the National Guard) and material resources from another state for any emergency. The requesting state is responsible for the legal liability of all out-of-state personnel and costs incurred. Any EMAC state can refuse another state's request. As of May 2005, 48 states (excluding California and Hawaii) had signed this agreement.

Public Health Emergency Response

Federal legislation delineates federal and state public health responsibilities. The U.S. Department of Health and Human Services (DHHS) is responsible for controlling contagious diseases threatening U.S. borders, conducting disease surveillance and biomedical research, and providing medical assistance during disasters. After 2001, following the lead of the DHHS, most states established Public Health Agency offices that are specifically responsible for public health emergency preparedness and response programs. Under the Public Health Services Act, state and local DOHs may be requested to assist in the quarantine of communicable diseases, are required to train their personnel for health-related activities, and can request temporary aid from the DHHS during health emergencies.[25]

Although most states had existing public health and disaster-related laws and regulations sufficient to cover most exigencies, after the anthrax incidents in the fall of 2001, a systematic review of those codes was conducted, deficiencies were identified, and the Model State Emergency Health Powers Act (MSEHP) was prepared for the Centers for Disease Control and Prevention.[26,27]

A "model act" is one that states look to as they consider their own legislation. Many states have incorporated many of the MSEHP provisions into law. The MSEHP is designed to facilitate the early detection of and response to a health emergency, and, among other requirements, grants extraordinary powers to an adoptive state executive branch in the event of a defined public health emergency.

Comprehensive State Disaster Response

Idaho's response to potential anthrax exposures in October 2001 illustrates how local, state, and federal resources may be coordinated during a major disaster. The crisis began when Idaho's Emergency Medical Services Communication Center received an exponential increase in the number of calls for suspicious powdery substances and other hazardous materials. The majority of these calls were from local law enforcement officers, who serve as on-scene commanders during hazardous materials investigations. The communications center then informed, per protocol, the governor, EMA director, and state public health, law enforcement, and hazardous materials officials at the state EMA to determine the best management strategy. Those officials alerted the state laboratory representatives that they would be receiving samples for testing, distributed public health guidelines for healthcare providers to district health departments and hospitals, and contacted the Federal Bureau of Investigation to deal with the few associated mail threats. The Centers for Disease Control and Prevention provided protocols for 11 additional laboratories whose personnel had to be trained in test procedures because the state laboratory staff was quickly overwhelmed.[28] If in-state resources were inadequate to handle the disaster, such as after the events of Sept. 11, the governor could have elicited the aid of laboratories, healthcare providers, and law enforcement or military personnel from neighboring states.

SUMMARY

States play a key role in coordinating local and federal responses to natural and manmade disasters. Many states, by themselves, lack the resources to cope with large-scale disasters and therefore must enlist the aid of other states through the EMAC or federal government. The events of Sept. 11, 2001, have prompted significant improvement in states' ability to handle terrorist attacks, and as a consequence, state government agencies are now better able to respond to all potential disasters. Future directions to optimize emergency management include establishing standards for disaster management and planning on state and local levels, enhancing communications between emergency responders, improving threat detection and identification through technological advances, and modifying existing emergency response capabilities to meet the challenges of emerging threats.

REFERENCES

1. Mothershead JL, Tonat K, Koenig KL. Bioterrorism preparedness. III: state and federal programs and response. *Emerg Med Clin North Am*. May 2002;20(2):477-500.
2. National Emergency Management Association. Available at: http://www.nemaweb.org.
3. Federal Emergency Management Agency. Emergency health and medical occupations: final rule. *Fed Regist*. February 1980;45(28):8600-2.
4. Disaster assistance: reorganization and revision of regulations—Federal Emergency Management Agency. Proposed rule. *Fed Regist*. November 1979;44(213):63058-71.
5. Implementation of state assistance program for training and education in emergency management—Federal Emergency Management Agency. Final rule. *Fed Regist*. January 1981;46(3):1270-3.
6. Chaff L, Blevins-Doll C. Community right-to-know. *J Healthc Prot Manage*. Spring 1990;6(2):27-35.
7. Biological and chemical terrorism: strategic plan for preparedness and response. Recommendations of the CDC Strategic Planning Workgroup. *MMWR Recomm Rep*. April 2000;49(RR-4):1-14.
8. US Department of Homeland Security. State homeland security and emergency services. Available at: http://www.dhs.gov/dhspublic/interapp/editorial/editorial_0306.xml.
9. Snyder JA, Baren JM, Ryan SD, Chew JL, Seidel JS. Emergency medical service system development: results of the statewide emergency medical service Technical Assessment Program. *Ann Emerg Med*. June 1995;25(6):768-75.
10. Mignone AT Jr, Davidson R. Public health response actions and the use of emergency operations centers. *Prehospital Disaster Med*. July-September 2003;18(3):217-19.
11. *State and Local Guide (SLG) 101: Guide for All-Hazard Emergency Operations Planning*. Washington, DC: Federal Emergency Management Agency; 1996.
12. Jardine C, Hrudey S, Shortreed J, et al. Risk management frameworks for human health and environmental risks. *J Toxicol Environ Health B Crit Rev*. November-December 2003;6(6):569-720.
13. Hohenhaus SM. Pediatric emergency preparedness in schools: a report from the 2001 Southeastern Regional EMSC annual meeting. *J Emerg Nurs*. August 2001;27(4):353-6.
14. Sapien RE, Allen A. Emergency preparation in schools: a snapshot of a rural state. *Pediatr Emerg Care*. October 2001;17(5):329-33.
15. Laxminarayan S, Kun L. The many facets of homeland security. *IEEE Eng Med Biol Mag*. January-February 2004;23(1):19-29.
16. Lalich RA. The role of state government, local government, and nongovernmental organizations in medical innovative readiness training. *Mil Med*. May 2002;167(5):367-9.
17. Likos AM, Neville J, Gaydos JC. Influenza outbreak and response preparedness in the Air National Guard. *Mil Med*. November 2002;167(11):929-33.
18. Zarychta WA. National Guard Civil Support Teams. Responding to weapons of mass destruction. *Emerg Med Serv*. March 2003;32(3):63-5.
19. Gebicke M. *Combating Terrorism: Use of National Guard Response Teams Is Unclear*. Washington, DC: US General Accounting Office; May 1999.
20. USC 5121. Available at: http://www4.law.cornell.edu/uscode/42/5121.html.
21. Becker SM. Are the psychosocial aspects of weapons of mass destruction incidents addressed in the Federal Response Plan: summary of an expert panel. *Mil Med*. December 2001;166(12 suppl):66-8.
22. Roth PB, Gaffney JK. The Federal Response Plan and disaster medical assistance teams in domestic disasters. *Emerg Med Clin North Am*. May 1996;14(2):371-82.
23. Couig MP, Martinelli A, Lavin RP. The National Response Plan: Health and Human Services the Lead for Emergency Support Function #8. *Disaster Manag Response*. Apr–Jun 2005;3(2):34–40.
24. Pub L No. 104-321 (Granting the Consent of Congress to the Emergency Management Assistance Compact). Available at: http://thomas.loc.gov/cgi-bin/bdquery/z?d104:HJ00193:TOM:/bss/d104query.html.
25. Reich DS. Modernizing local responses to public health emergencies: bioterrorism, epidemics, and the model state emergency health powers act. *J Contemp Health Law Policy*. Spring 2003;19(2):379-414.
26. Bayer R, Colgrove J. Bioterrorism, public health, and the law. *Health Aff (Millwood)*. November-December 2002;21(6):98-101.
27. Gostin LO, Sapsin JW, Teret SP, et al. The Model State Emergency Health Powers Act: planning for and response to bioterrorism and naturally occurring infectious diseases. *JAMA*. August 2002;288(5):622-8.
28. Tengelsen L, Hudson R, Barnes S, Hahn C. Coordinated response to reports of possible anthrax contamination, Idaho, 2001. *Emerg Infect Dis*. October 2002;8(10):1093-5.

chapter 14

Selected Federal Disaster Response Agencies and Capabilities

Jerry L. Mothershead, Kevin Yeskey, and Peter Brewster

Chapter 11 provides a historical accounting of the evolution of emergency management in America and the basic framework for current concepts of operations. This chapter discusses selected federal response organizations and agencies, supporting programs for state and local emergency managers, and response capabilities. With the near-exponential growth in disaster management capabilities and initiatives that has occurred since the terrorist attacks of 2001, it would be impossible to discuss all of the many federal capabilities to any significant degree. Thus, this chapter focuses on the agencies of principal interest to public health, medical emergency managers, and healthcare professionals.

A more detailed presentation of current concepts of federal operations is provided as well as a discussion of some of the more significant issues and challenges facing the federal sector in responding to disasters or catastrophic emergencies of any type.

PRINCIPAL FEDERAL AGENCIES

Although virtually all of the federal executive branch agencies have capabilities and expertise that could be brought to bear in a disaster to save lives, reduce pain and suffering, and otherwise mitigate the impact of these events on the human condition, five stand out as supporting programs that provide the most direct support in this endeavor:

- U.S. Department of Homeland Security (DHS)
- U.S. Health and Human Services (DHHS)
- U.S. Department of Defense (DoD)
- Department of Veteran's Affairs (DVA)
- American Red Cross (ARC)

Department of Homeland Security

The organizational structure and overarching functions of DHS are described in Chapter 11. Among the many provisions of the Homeland Security Act of 2002, three important programs were transferred from DHHS to DHS: the National Disaster Medical System (NDMS), the Strategic National Stockpile (SNS) program, and the Metropolitan Medical Response System (MMRS).[1] Additionally, although it maintained many of its autonomous functions, the Federal Emergency Management Agency (FEMA) was transferred into the Emergency Preparedness and Response Directorate of DHS in 2003.

National Disaster Medical System

NDMS is a public/private partnership between DHS/ FEMA, DHHS, DoD, DVA, and civilian hospitals and health professionals. NDMS serves two primary functions: it is a backup to military healthcare operations in the event of overwhelming combat casualties, and it provides federal healthcare support to casualties resulting from disasters in the United States and its territories.[2] Originally established by memorandum of understanding in 1984, NDMS was codified into law in 2002. There are three components to NDMS: (1) on-site healthcare operations, (2) medical evacuation, (3) and definitive care. NDMS may be activated as the result of a presidential declaration of a national emergency. It may also be activated at the direction of the secretaries of DHS, DHHS, or DoD.

On-site healthcare operations are provided principally through the mobilization of disaster medical assistance teams, or DMATs. There are 85 teams, of which approximately 24 are considered operational at any given time. The number and capability of DMATs are evolving continually as new teams are being formed and established teams are augmenting their capabilities. Most teams are composed of more than 100 physicians, nurses, and allied healthcare personnel who are sworn in as temporary federal employees and who volunteer their time to prepare and train for emergency operations. In the event of activation, they become federal assets, with attendant liability protection. The majority of DMATs provide general clinical operations in disaster areas, either on-scene or as augmentation staff to local hospitals. A number of specialty teams exist, including burn, pediatric, crush injury, and mental health teams. Four disaster veterinary assistance teams (DVATs) and 10 disaster mortuary operations response teams (DMORTs) are also components of NDMS. One DMORT is specially trained in the handling of contaminated or contagious remains. There are also three larger national medical response teams/weapons of mass destruction teams (NRMT) located in North Carolina, Colorado, and California. These teams are specially equipped and trained to assist local emergency response organizations in the event of terrorist events involving chemical, biological, or radiological substances. Finally, a newly developed Family Assistance Core Group has been incorporated into NDMS. When deployed, DMATs are self-sustaining for three days and are supported by management support units (MSUs) for resupply.

Medical evacuation operations are coordinated by the DoD.[3] Medical regulation is managed by the Global Patient Movement Requirements Center (GPMRC) at Scott Air Force Base, Ill. This is the same system used to evacuate military casualties in peacetime or during combat operations worldwide. Actual medical evacuation occurs primarily through the use of fixed-wing U.S. Air Force assets, such as the C-141 Starlifter and the C-17 Globemaster III (each of which can accommodate in excess of 50 litter patients), under the auspices of the commander of the U.S. Transportation Command. Nontraditional air evacuation platforms or ground conveyances can also be used, as required. Most DMAT members have training in basic fixed-wing and helicopter operations as they pertain to the evacuation of patients.

Definitive care is provided by the 1800 hospitals that have voluntarily agreed to support NDMS operations. In all, approximately 100,000 beds (including the staff to support them) could be made available throughout the United States. Cooperating hospitals are coordinated through regional federal coordinating centers (FCCs), which are managed by the VHA or the military services hospitals.[4]

Strategic National Stockpile (SNS)

The SNS, originally authorized by Congress in 1998, has as its goal the rapid mobilization and provision of pharmaceuticals and other medical supplies to areas affected by public health emergencies or disasters of any cause. The SNS program has a number of elements, including scientific review, education, training, and technical and logistical support. The primary material components of the SNS are the 12-hour push packages and vendor managed inventory (VMI) supplies.[5]

Twelve push packages, preconfigured and under environmental and security safeguards, are strategically placed throughout the United States and can be deployed to arrive at the nearest suitable airfield to a disaster within 12 hours of release by either the secretary of DHS or DHHS. Push packages are large caches, requiring more than 5000 square feet of storage space, that may be transported by air or ground conveyance. Supplies include antibiotics, antiviral agents, and airway and intravenous supplies. Ventilators, stored separately, may be shipped as needed. Vaccines, also stored separately, may be shipped with or without the entire cache. In 2003, regionally placed chemical agent antidotes were established under the CHEMPACK program to provide for more timely arrival.

If specific supplies are known to be needed in advance of push package shipment, these may be obtained through VMI stocks, which are maintained by pharmaceutical or medical supply corporations that have contracts with the federal government. VMIs were designed, however, to be follow-on packages of specifically needed supplies to arrive 24 to 36 hours after the push packages.

All states are required to develop and exercise plans for the request, acquisition, storage, staging, distribution, and dispensing of SNS caches to prophylaxis or vaccination centers or area hospitals. Caches will be accompanied by a small team of medical logisticians referred to as technical assistance response units (TARUs).

Metropolitan Medical Response System.

In 1997, DHHS established the Metropolitan Medical Strike Teams (now the Metropolitan Medical Response System [MMRS]) to integrate the various, disparate response functions. Although designed principally to enhance preparedness for chemical or biological terrorist attacks, MMRS can be used effectively in all types of disasters. The MMRS program provides technical assistance and funding to large metropolitan areas to establish enhanced capabilities within existing systems. Grants are linked to compliance with a series of specific measurable objectives. Originally designed to focus on the largest 120 communities in the United States, the program has been expanded with the goal of establishing MMRS presence in 200 metropolitan areas.[6]

Department of Health and Human Services

DHHS is the federal agency that has the responsibility of protecting the health of the nation and providing essential services to all U.S. citizens. DHHS has an annual budget of $502 billion (2003 fiscal year) and employs more than 65,000 personnel.[7] DHHS administers more than 300 programs in 11 operating divisions and is the parent organization for the Commissioned Corps (CC) of the U.S. Public Health Service (USPHS).

DHHS has a long history of providing disaster response and preparedness activities domestically and internationally.[8] DHHS is the lead federal agency for coordinating the federal health and medical response services (Emergency Support Function #8), as described in the National Response Plan (NRP) (Box 14-1).[9] DHHS is a partner in the NDMS. The Public Health Threats and Emergencies Act of 2002 authorizes the DHHS secretary to take appropriate actions if a public health emergency is determined to exist and to establish a Public Health Emergency Fund.[10] Other statutes authorize the U.S. Surgeon General to make and enforce regulations to "prevent the introduction, transmission, or spread of communicable diseases from foreign countries into States or possessions, or from one State or possession into any other State of possession."[11]

DHHS disaster response and preparedness activities are conducted in the Operating Divisions and the USPHS CC.

BOX 14-1 EMERGENCY SUPPORT FUNCTION #8: PUBLIC HEALTH AND MEDICAL SERVICES

1. Assessment of health/medical needs
2. Surveillance of healthcare issues
3. Acquisition and distribution of medical care personnel
4. Acquisition and distribution of health/medical equipment and supplies
5. Patient evacuation
6. In-hospital care
7. Food/drug/medical device safety
8. Worker health/safety
9. Radiological monitoring
10. Chemical monitoring
11. Biological monitoring
12. Mental health assessment
13. Development and dissemination of public health information
14. Vector control
15. Water safety; wastewater and solid waste disposal
16. Victim identification/mortuary services

Coordination is performed at the assistant secretary level within DHHS. DHHS also convenes the National Science Advisory Board for Biosecurity, which guides the development of systems for biosecurity research peer review, guidelines for identification and conduct of research that might require security surveillance, professional code of conduct for scientists and laboratory workers, and materials to educate the research community about biosecurity.

Office of the Assistant Secretary for Public Health Emergency Preparedness (ASPHEP)

This office provides (1) interface between agencies within DHHS and other federal departments, agencies, and offices and (2) interface between DHHS and state and local entities responsible for public health and emergency preparedness. The ASPHEP ensures that health and medical vulnerabilities are identified and prioritized within the DHHS; that DHHS preparedness programs are coordinated and integrated with other federal programs; and that response activities are coordinated within DHHS and integrated with other federal, state, and local response.[12] ASPHEP manages a state-of-the-art command center for the DHHS secretary. This facility serves as the information management and communications hub for DHHS agencies and is the primary point of contact for other federal agencies. The command center is staffed around the clock, daily. The office also maintains a scientific group that oversees the development and procurement of all SNS medical countermeasures.

ASPHEP works with state and local officials to enhance health and medical preparedness and coordinates various federally funded preparedness activities. DHHS has established guidelines, benchmarks, and competencies to serve as markers of preparedness.

APSHEP has personnel who are deployed to the field during responses. The team, known as the Secretary's Emergency Response Team (SERT), deploys to the DHHS regional office (although they can deploy to more forward positions) and serves as an advisory team to the secretary, through the ASPHEP. DHHS uses its regional offices and regional health administrators as the primary response coordinators of field operations. SERT members and regional response personnel can also serve as Emergency Support Function #8 liaisons at the state operations center, DHS disaster field office, or DHS regional office.

Agency for Healthcare Research and Quality (AHRQ)

AHRQ's mission is to improve the quality, safety, efficiency, and effectiveness of healthcare by sponsoring, conducting, and disseminating research that relates to the aforementioned mission.[13] AHRQ has a number of disaster-related functions within DHHS, with an emphasis on bioterrorism (BT)-related issues. The organization has funded BT-related research, conducted a variety of audio conferences for clinical providers, issued evidence-based practice reports, and distributed issue briefs based on the audio conferences. AHRQ also provides technical support to ASPHEP during responses.

Centers for Disease Control and Prevention (CDC)

The CDC is the world's foremost public health organization, and it has had significant experience in responding to disasters and public health emergencies globally.[14] It also has a major role in disaster response mitigation through its leadership in disease prevention activities. CDC is the national leader in the areas of epidemic outbreak response, disease surveillance, environmental health, public health laboratory readiness, and public communications. In conjunction with the Agency for Toxic Substance and Disease Registry, the CDC serves as the DHHS lead for infectious disease response, chemical/hazardous materials exposure, vector control, radiological monitoring, and public (risk) communications. Additionally, the CDC has the lead scientific responsibility for the SNS.

CDC epidemiologists and other response team personnel deploy in support of public health incidents. These personnel perform case investigations and contact tracing, assist with surveillance, and serve as technical advisors for issues such as vector control. CDC laboratories can perform specialized assays to identify biological and chemical agents from clinical and, in some cases, environmental specimens. CDC also manages the Laboratory Response Network (LRN) for BT and a national network of public health laboratories, each capable of performing sophisticated testing of infectious agents. Participants in the LRN program receive training, protocols, supplies, and a secure reporting system.

Public communications can occur through a variety of CDC venues. The *Morbidity and Mortality Monthly Report (MMWR)* has long been recognized as a periodical that serves to notify and update professionals about public health investigations and incidents. CDC also developed two other lines of communication. The Health Alert Network (HAN) and the Epidemiologic Exchange (Epi-X) were developed as web-based communications networks. HAN is used to distribute information through a widespread open network. Epi-X is more secure and is directed to epidemiologists and other public health professionals at the federal, state, and local levels. CDC also conducts provider training through on-site courses and teleconferences.

CDC maintains a state-of-the-art emergency operations center that serves as the information-gathering center for the agency and maintains 24-hour, daily access for local, state, and federal agencies.

Food and Drug Administration (FDA)

The FDA's stated public health mission is "assuring the safety, efficacy, and security of human and veterinary drugs, biological products, medical devices, our nation's food supply, cosmetics, and products that emit radiation."[15] The FDA regulates the safety of biologics (including the blood supply), cosmetics, drugs (prescription and over-the-counter), foods (except meat and dairy products), medical devices, radiation-emitting electronic products, and veterinary products. The FDA also has the responsibility for animal health, as it relates to food safety and security.

The FDA has investigated foodborne outbreaks and medication tampering and has supported DHHS response to domestic disasters. In recent years, the FDA has played a major role in the preparedness activities against terrorism and has organized several new offices to facilitate its activities. The Office of Crisis Management (OCM) coordinates FDA emergency response activities. The Office of Emergency Operations within OCM coordinates FDA field and headquarters activities and maintains the FDA emergency operations center.

The FDA maintains expertise to assist in areas of food safety, including the production, processing, storage, and holding of domestic and imported foods. It has worked with other federal agencies to implement a national laboratory network capable of responding to a food security incident. FDA uses field personnel to perform food import examinations at approximately 90 U.S. ports. FDA collaborates with U.S. blood banks to ensure the continuous supply of safe blood. It also works with other DHHS agencies and the pharmaceutical industry to help guide the development of new medical countermeasures for BT. Recent new regulations have facilitated the FDA approval process for new products and medical countermeasures. The FDA works with other federal agencies in developing guidance for using these countermeasures in special populations or when there is no FDA-approved product or no approved indication for a marketed product; devices under investigational new drug (IND); and investigational device exemption (IDE) applications. The FDA works with other federal agencies in developing guidance for countermeasure use in special populations or when there is no FDA-approved product or no approved indication for a marketed product.

Health Resources and Services Administration (HRSA)

HRSA's involvement in disaster response has largely been the issuance of grants to improve hospital BT preparedness. HRSA grants have provided funding through state health departments to address surge capacity, communications, decontamination, and exercises related to hospital operations.[16]

The Federal Occupational Health office is a component of HRSA that provides clinical services, environmental health services, and employee assistance programs for federal workers. Personnel from this organization have provided postdisaster clinical and counseling services to federal employees at disaster field offices, regional offices, and headquarters.

Indian Health Service (IHS)

The IHS has provided leadership in addressing disasters affecting the health and medical systems directly associated with tribal nations and reservations.[17] In the Hantavirus outbreak on the Navajo reservation, IHS medical personnel were active participants in the response. (Hantavirus disease was virtually unknown in the Americas until 1993, when a physician at IHS in New Mexico reported that two previously healthy young people had died from acute respiratory failure.)[17a] Tribal leaders and medical personnel have been actively engaged with their state counterparts in preparing for BT. The IHS Office of Surveillance was established in 2002 to address public health needs associated with disease outbreaks and BT. IHS personnel have also been deployed to domestic events.

National Institutes of Health (NIH)

NIH's role in the nation's health response system has been parsed out to a variety of its 27 institutes and centers. The NIH mission relates to the stewardship of medical and behavioral research.[18] Its National Institute of Mental Health supports research in the area of response to trauma and violence.[19] The National Institute of Environmental Health Sciences supports research directed at the health consequences of environmental toxins.[20] NIH also supports and performs research that enhances the understanding of the basic biology and mechanisms of immunological response to particular biological agents. The National Institute of Allergy and Infectious Diseases (NIAID) has the NIH lead on many of these activities and receives substantial funding within DHHS to accelerate development of new and improved vaccines, diagnostic tools, and therapies against potential agents of BT.[21] NIH has also been dedicated to the expansion of the medical countermeasures for biological agents of terrorism. NIAID has created the Office of Biodefense Research and the Biodefense Clinical Research Branch in the Office of Clinical Research. In addition to the research activities, NIH sponsors regional centers for biodefense research and biocontainment laboratories.

Substance Abuse and Mental Health Services Administration (SAMHSA)

SAMHSA provides the coordination of federal mental health services for the government. SAMHSA assists in the assessment of mental health needs and the identification of mental health services that can be provided to those affected by disasters. SAMHSA provides grants to states that assist in training mental health counselors and enhancing mental health response capacity.[21] It also produces publications related to planning and preparedness and the mental health impact of disasters as well as training manuals for mental health responders. SAMHSA maintains a technical assistance center that can be accessed by responders.

Commissioned Corps of the U.S. Public Health Service

Headed by the U.S. Surgeon General, the CC consists of more than 6000 commissioned officers who have degrees in health- and medical-related professions.[22] CC officers are distributed among all of the DHHS Operating Divisions and can be assigned to other federal agencies. The CC serves as the healthcare corps for the U.S. Coast Guard. CC personnel have responded internationally to a full spectrum of disasters. Two specific units merit discussion: the USPHS DMAT and the CC Readiness Force (CCRF). The USPHS DMAT has been the prototype for all subsequent DMATs and has been one of the most deployed federal medical response units to domestic disasters. The CCRF, consisting entirely of USPHS officers, is a readily deployable force of more than 3000 that can be sent into a variety of health and medical emergencies.[23] CCRF personnel receive training similar to that of the NDMS response teams and must meet additional requirements beyond those of other USPHS officers. Deployed CCRF personnel must rely on the host organization to provide food, shelter, water, sanitation, local transportation, and communications.

Department of Veterans Affairs

The DVA is a cabinet-level agency with three primary divisions: Veterans Benefits Administration, National Cemetery System, and the Veterans Health Administration (VHA). VHA is the largest healthcare system in the United States. Within its 21 Veterans Integrated Service Networks (VISNs) are more than 150 hospitals, 800 clinics, and 400 additional facilities, such as counseling centers. VHA employs more than 15,000 physicians and nearly 200,000 other healthcare professionals. VHA principally exists to provide medical care to military veterans. It also has important roles in medical research and the education of the healthcare workforce.

Its fourth mission is that of emergency management.[24] In that capacity is supports medical operations as a backup for DoD (through the Integrated Continental United States Medical Operations Plan), as a supporting agency under the NRP, as a partner to the NDMS, and for continuity of governmental operations functions. VHA also has a unique role in fielding emergency medical response teams for radiological emergencies.

Interagency coordination and policy matters related to emergency management and response reside at the secretary level, but day-to-day management and oversight comes from the Emergency Management Strategic Healthcare Group (EMSHG). EMSHG is headquartered in Martinsburg, W.Va., and it has a peripheral staff composed of three district and 37 area emergency managers. These peripheral staff members coordinate all emergency management activities within the VISNs and subordinate facilities.

VHA personnel have deployed to the vast majority of national disasters in the last decade, including the response to the New York City terrorist attack of 2001. These personnel have also provided support to National Security Special Events (NSSE), such as presidential inaugurations and the Olympic Games.[25]

Executive order 12657 places an additional responsibility on the VHA to provide medical response to incidents involving radiological emergencies.[26] VHA has the 25-member Medical Emergency Radiological Response Team (MERRT), which can arrive at the site of a radiological emergency and is self-sustaining. As such, it is not a first response organization, but rather it provides supplemental medical care at hospitals and technical assistance and guidance in decontamination and monitoring. When MERRT is deployed, it is considered a federal resource.

Several VISNs also have developed 80-member, multidisciplinary Emergency Medical Response Teams (EMRTs), which are not self-sustaining and are not considered federal resources. These teams were developed primarily to provide augmentation capabilities within the VISN area of responsibility. They could, however, be used in response to a remote national disaster under other deployment venues.

A current initiative within VHA is the population of the Disaster Emergency Medical Personnel System (DEMPS) database. DEMPS is a voluntary enrollment of full-time VHA employees who have agreed to deploy if requested to a disaster site to augment capabilities. This program is in its infancy as of this writing.

VHA also has a role in federal disaster cache management. In addition to its role as logistical manager of SNS caches, VHA maintains caches for its facilities' use, and by extension, these could be used in community-wide disasters. It also maintains caches for NSSE events as well as a stockpile for response involving disasters that would affect the U.S. Congress.

VHA probably has its greatest role in local emergency management. VHA operates the majority of the NDMS FCCs. Additionally, VHA hospitals are charged with assisting local community healthcare resources in their preparedness and planning. Finally, as part of the community healthcare network, VHA resources would be automatically drawn into the response to a local disaster, such as what occurred in Houston, Texas, in 2000, when VHA facilities accepted transferred patients from area civilian hospitals incapacitated as the result of flooding.

Department of Defense

The DoD is identified as a support agency for nearly all of the 15 Emergency Support Functions identified in the NRP. Its component services have large amounts of material and personnel resources that could be brought to bear in response to a disaster, anywhere in the world. The Army Civil Affairs branch (primarily found in the Reserves component) even has expertise in governmental function reestablishment. In addition to the active duty component, DoD can call on Reserve forces of all the services, and, under certain circumstances, can federalize Army and Air Force National Guard personnel as part of its military response. To chronicle all of the many assets would far exceed the scope of this chapter.

DoD support to federal, state, or local emergency managers is governed by a number of statutes and executive orders, collectively referred to as "Military Support to Civil Authorities" (MSCA).[27] General guidance for the use of MSCA includes the following:

- Civil resources are applied first.
- DoD resources are provided only when requirements are beyond the capabilities of civil authorities.
- Specialized DoD capabilities requested for MSCA are used efficiently.
- Military operations other than MSCA will have priority over MSCA.
- National Guard forces that are not in federal service have primary responsibility for providing military assistance to state and local government agencies in civil emergencies.
- DoD and the military services will not procure or maintain any supplies, material, or equipment exclusively for providing MSCA.
- In general, DoD resources will not be used for law enforcement or intelligence-gathering functions.

Imminently serious conditions resulting from any civil emergency or attack may require immediate action by military commanders to save lives, prevent human suffering, or mitigate great property damage. When such conditions exist and time does not permit prior approval from higher headquarters, local military commanders are authorized to take necessary action to respond to requests of civil authorities. This is commonly referred to as "Immediate Response."

Under the MSCA doctrine, and in line with the NRP, requests for military support are submitted by lead federal agencies (LFAs) through FEMA to the Joint Director of Military Support (JDOMS) on the Joint Chiefs of Staff. The JDOMS has the authority to task Unified Combatant Commanders, services, and defense agencies to provide MSCA support for presidentially declared disasters and emergencies. The JDOMS validates requests for military assistance from LFAs, and plans, coordinates, and executes DoD civil support activities. The JDOMS controls a joint staff to conduct operations during declared disasters.

Operationally, MSCA is directed through the U.S. Northern Command (USNORTHCOM) in Colorado Springs, Colo., through an operational Joint Task Force-Consequence Management (JTF-CM).[28] The two continental armies of the United States (First Army and Fifth Army) have response task forces that can deploy to the vicinity of the disaster and assume operational control over all military forces assigned to the response. In addition, USNORTHCOM has a standing task force, the Joint Task Force-Civil Support (JTF-CS), that was established specifically for the homeland defense mission.

DoD resources fall into two broad categories: (1) mass resources that can augment similar capabilities in the other federal agencies and (2) unique resources that can provide expertise and technical assistance. Mass resources of interest to civilian medical planners would include:

- More than 75 military hospitals and more than 100,000 public health and healthcare professionals
- Deployable medical platforms, ranging in size from the U.S. Air Force's air transportable Expeditionary Medical Support (which can be expanded up to 25 beds each) to the two U.S. Navy 1000-bed hospital ships
- Significant air assets that can be used to evacuate casualties, as described in the section on the NDMS
- Caches of pharmaceuticals and medical supplies, referred to as wartime stocks; these would only be mobilized for MSCA missions in the most unusual circumstances
- Specialized resources[29] that may be brought to bear in the event of an overwhelming disaster:
  - Deployable public health laboratories
  - Specially trained response teams, such as the U.S. Army Chemical and Biological Special Medical Augmentation Response Teams (C/B-SMART), the U.S. Navy Special Psychiatric Intervention Teams (SPRINTs), or the U.S. Air Force Radiation Assessment Teams (AFRATs)
  - Reach-back expertise capabilities through the U.S. Army Medical Research Institute of Infectious Disease (USAMRIID) and the Medical Research Institute for Chemical Defense (USAMRICD), the Armed Forces Radiobiological Research Institute (AFRRI), or the Armed Forces Institute of Pathology (AFIP)

Other specialized capabilities exist within the DoD due to its combat mission. For example, the Technical Escort Unit (TEU), which is trained and equipped to handle extreme hazardous materials and radiation sources, forms the nidus of the much larger Guardian Brigade, which has specific homeland defense functions. The U.S. Marine Corps includes the Chemical and Biological Immediate Response Force (CBIRF), a 350-member rapid response unit trained to work in hazardous environment operations, including patient extrication, decontamination, and emergency stabilization and treatment.

American Red Cross

Chartered by Congress in 1905, the Red Cross[30] has as its mission to ". . . carry on a system of national and international relief in time of peace and apply the same in mitigating the sufferings caused by pestilence, famine, fire, floods, and other great national calamities, and to devise and carry on measures for preventing the same." Each year, the ARC responds to more than 60,000 disasters of various sizes and complexities. ARC is the LFA for the Mass Care Emergency Support Function of the NRP and has supporting roles in the Public Health and Medical Services Emergency Support Function.

ARC provides shelter, food, and health and mental health services to address basic human needs. Family and individual assistance is also given to those affected by disaster to enable them to resume their normal daily activities independently. ARC also feeds emergency workers, handles inquiries from concerned family members outside of the disaster area, provides blood and blood products to disaster victims, and helps those affected by disaster to access other available resources.

ISSUES IN FEDERAL RESPONSE TO DISASTERS

With its many resources and vast expertise, the U.S. government has the capabilities and capacities to effectively respond to virtually all but the most cataclysmic disasters imaginable. There are, however, a number of issues that remain unresolved. Some of these include:

- **Response time:** Identifying, activating, and mobilizing these resources may take considerable time, and local response agencies should not anticipate significant federal support to be on-site and fully operational for 24 to 48 hours, especially at remote locations or those whose transportation infrastructures (airfields, railways, or highways) have been compromised due to the disaster.
- **Identification of appropriate resources:** In general, federal resources have been designed for primary functions other than disaster response and relief. As a consequence, no two response teams are identical in capabilities. Requests for federal resources must be in the form of a capabilities request, as opposed to a platform, and identifying specific agency resources to meet those requested needs may slow response. Resource typing, which is currently under way through the National Incident Management System (NIMS) construct, could address this issue.
- **Command and control:** With the exception of forensic and other law enforcement functions in the case of a terrorist event, federal resources are to augment state and local authorities. With numerous response organizations from all levels of government, each operating by its own protocols and procedures, collaboration and integration during high-tempo operations may at times be problematic. Again, NIMS was designed to alleviate some of the previous problems with command and control.

SUMMARY

The U.S. government, through its many federal agencies, has a wealth of capabilities and capacity to respond to natural, technological, or terrorist-induced disasters. These resources may be accessed through a process to respond at the request of local or state civil authorities. Challenges continue to exist in command and control, coordination, and access of these resources in a timely manner.

REFERENCES

1. U.S. Citizenship and Immigration Services. H.R. 5005, Homeland Security Act of 2002. Available at: http://uscis.gov/graphics/homeland.htm.
2. U.S. Department of Homeland Security. National Disaster Medical System. Available at: http://ndms.dhhs.gov/.
3. Defense Technical Information Center. Department of Defense Directive 6000.12. Health Services Operations and Readiness. Available at: http://www.dtic.mil/whs/directives/corres/pdf/d600012wch1_042996/d600012p.pdf.
4. U.S. Department of Homeland Security. National Disaster Medical System. Federal coordinating centers. Available at: http://oep-ndms.dhhs.gov/fcc.html.
5. Centers for Disease Control and Prevention. Strategic National Stockpile. Available at: http://www.bt.cdc.gov/stockpile/.
6. Federal Emergency Management Agency. Metropolitan Medical Response System. Available at: http://mmrs.fema.gov/.
7. U.S. Department of Health and Human Services. Available at: www.os.dhhs.gov.
8. Roth P, Gaffney J. The federal response plan and disaster medical assistance teams in domestic disasters. *Emerg Med Clin North Am*. May 1996;14(2):371-82.
9. Federal Emergency Management Agency. Department of Homeland Security National Response Plan, 2005. Washington DC: Government Printing Office.
10. Pub L No. 106-505 (The Public Health Threats and Emergencies Act of 2002).
11. USC 42 (The Public Health and Welfare Act, January 2003).
12. Pub L No. 107-188 (The Public Health Security and Bioterrorism Preparedness and Response Act of 2002).
13. Agency for Healthcare Research and Quality. Available at: http://www.ahrq.gov.
14. Centers for Disease Control and Prevention. Available at: http://www.cdc.gov/.
15. U.S. Food and Drug Administration. Available at: http://www.fda.gov/.
16. Health Resources and Services Administration. Available at: http://www.hrsa.gov/.
17. U.S. Department of Health and Human Services. Indian Health Service. Available at: http://www.ihs.gov/.
17a. Health and Human Resources. Available at: http://www.hhs.gov/asl/testify/t990629c.html.
18. U.S. Department of Health and Human Services. National Institutes of Health. Available at: http://www.nih.gov/.
19. National Institute of Mental Health. Available at: http://www.nimh.nih.gov/.
20. National Institutes of Health. National Institute of Environmental Health Sciences. Available at: http://www.niehs.nih.gov/.
21. U.S. Department of Health and Human Services Administration. Substance Abuse and Mental Health Services Administration. Available at: http://www.samhsa.gov/index.aspx.
22. Mullan F. *Plagues and Politics: The Story of the United States Public Health Service*. New York: Basic Books; 1989.
23. U.S. Department of Health and Human Services. Office of Public Health Emergency Preparedness. Available at: http://www.hhs.gov/ophep/.
24. Koenig KL. Homeland security and public health: role of the Department of Veterans Affairs, the U.S. Department of Homeland Security, and implications for the public health community. *Prehospital Disaster Med*. October-December 2003;18(4): 327–33.
25. Hodgson MJ, Bierenbaum A, Mather S, et al. Emergency management program operational responses to weapons of mass destruction: Veterans Health Administration, 2001-2004. *Am J Ind Med*. November 2004;46(5):446-52.
26. Federal Emergency Management Agency. Executive Order 12657: Federal Emergency Management Agency Assistance in Emergency Preparedness Planning at Commercial Nuclear Power Plants. Available at: http://www.fema.gov/library/eo.shtm.
27. Defense Technical Information Center. Department of Defense Directive 3025.15. Military Assistance to Civil Authorities. Available at: http://www.dtic.mil/whs/directives/corres/pdf/d302515_021897/d302515p.pdf.
28. U.S. Northern Command. Available at: http://www.northcom.mil/.
29. Joint Publication 3-41 "Joint Doctrine for Chemical, Biological, Radiological, Nuclear, and High Yield Explosive Consequence Management" (draft document) February 2005. Available at: http://www.dtic.mil/doctrine/publications_status_operations.htm.
30. American Red Cross. Available at: http://www.redcross.org/.

chapter 15

International Disaster Response

Dan Hanfling, Craig H. Llewellyn, and Frederick M. Burkle, Jr.

Global disasters—natural, technological, and terrorist-related—occur almost daily, resulting in significant human, economic, and environmental consequences. Recent disasters have highlighted the need for the United States to be able to provide rapid, responsive, and sustainable disaster relief in the international setting. During the past quarter century, earthquakes alone have caused more than 1 million deaths worldwide.[1] In just the past 5 years, three catastrophic earthquakes occurred in Izmit, Turkey (17,118 deaths; more than 50,000 injured); Gujarat, India (20,000 deaths; more than 167,000 injured); and Bam, Iran (43,200 deaths; more than 30,000 injured).[2] In December 2004, the cataclysmic tsunami that swept across Southern Asia killed an estimated 200,000 to 300,000 people and displaced more than 1.1 million people. Moreover, since the end of the Cold War, the world has witnessed an increase in the number of complex emergencies (CEs). These may be defined as intrastate conflicts resulting from administrative, economic, political, and social decay and are marked by intense violence, often pitting cultural, ethnic, or religious groups against one another.[3] More than two decades of ongoing armed conflict in the Islamic state of Afghanistan recently culminated in military intervention by the United States and Great Britain in the war on terrorism. More than 5 million Afghans live as refugees or internally displaced persons and are greatly in need of the basic minimum resources necessary to maintain health and well being.[4] At its worst, the genocidal spasms of violence in Bosnia-Herzegovina (1992-93), Rwanda (1994), and Chechnya (1994 to present) and the recent crisis in Darfur, Sudan, represent the embodiment of the need for rapid, coordinated, international disaster response. In the current crisis in Sudan, hundreds of thousands of refugees, with limited access to international assistance, are at risk of dying as a result of the political upheaval, severe drought and famine, and sluggish international intervention.[5]

Beyond death and destruction lie families in ruin; communities torn asunder; and basic social, economic, and medical needs left unmet. Into such voids created by CEs, there quickly mobilizes an international disaster response capability composed of government, nongovernment, and international agencies and military elements. The goals of such efforts include the provision of adequate food, clean water, shelter, sanitation, and basic medical care. Such basic care may be augmented by specialized response capability, such as search and rescue,[6] surgical response,[7] or public health technical assistance.[8,9] The intent of this chapter is to briefly review the components of an international disaster response mounted by the U.S. government (USG) in conjunction with the United Nations (UN), UN agencies, the Red Cross, nongovernment organizations (NGOs), and other providers of humanitarian assistance (HA).

CURRENT PRACTICE

U.S. Government's Role in Response to International Disasters

Under Section 491 of the Foreign Assistance Act of 1961, the USG is provided the flexible authority that permits the U.S. Agency for International Development (USAID) to respond to the needs of disaster victims upon an official state-to-state request initiated by the country seeking assistance. The U.S. president designates the USAID administrator as the special coordinator for international disaster assistance. The Bureau for Democracy, Conflict and Humanitarian Assistance (DCHA) and its Office of Foreign Disaster Assistance (OFDA) are chiefly responsible for the coordination and implementation of all official USG disaster assistance efforts.

OFDA's mandate is to "save lives, alleviate suffering, and reduce the economic impact of disasters." This is primarily accomplished in coordination with the government of the affected country, other donor governments, international organizations, UN relief agencies, private voluntary organizations (PVOs), and NGOs. The initial responsibility for disaster relief rests squarely with the government of the affected country. OFDA only responds when the United States and the affected country declare a disaster using the following criteria. First, the magnitude of the disaster exceeds the affected country's capacity to respond. Second, the affected country has requested or will accept U.S. government assistance and such assistance is deemed to be in the interest of the USG.[10]

After the official declaration of disaster and request for USG assistance, OFDA has a discretionary fund of up to $50,000 that can be made immediately available to meet initial relief needs. The use of this Disaster Assistance Authority is intended solely to initiate assistance efforts. OFDA has several options beyond the provision of monetary assistance. With the approval of the affected country's government, the U.S. Embassy may request that OFDA deploy one or more regional advisors or an assessment team to the disaster site or send a disaster assistance response team (DART) to provide direct coordination in the management of USG assistance (Boxes 15-1 and 15-2).

OFDA has regional advisors attached to USAID missions throughout the world, specifically covering the Europe/Middle East, Asia/Pacific, and Latin America/Caribbean regions. These disaster relief experts can draw on public and private sector resources to respond within 24 hours of a disaster event worldwide. Fairfax County, Va., and Los Angeles County, Calif., have specialized teams experienced in search and rescue, medical assessment and response, operational leadership, and logistical support available to OFDA. Fairfax County Virginia International Search and Rescue Team 1 (referred to as Virginia Task Force 1 in the Federal Emergency Management Agency National Urban Search and Rescue Response System) deployed to the embassy bombings in Nairobi, Kenya (1998), and to the earthquakes in Mexico City, Mexico (1985); Manila, Philippines (1990); Izmit, Turkey (1999); Duzce, Turkey (1999); Touliu, Taiwan (1999); and Bam, Iran (2004).

Especially in the case of response to collapsed structures resulting from a significant seismic event or a terrorist attack, members of the assessment team and DART are often drawn from the ranks of one of the two international search and rescue assets. An assessment team composed of key participants—such as search and rescue, medical, logistics, and technical experts, including a structural engineer—deploy as soon as possible to provide initial on-scene evaluation of the scope and scale of the disaster event. The search-and-rescue team may

follow, depending on Department of Defense (DoD) airlift support. The search and rescue team is composed of more than 70 members; deploys with more than 58,000 pounds of equipment, including food and water; and can maintain self-sufficiency in an austere environment for 7 to 10 days. In the response to the Izmit, Turkey, earthquake the Fairfax County team conducted reconnaissance in an area that was more than 11 square miles, evaluated more than 70 potential rescue sites, averaged approximately 27 worksites per day, and completed four successful live rescues and more than 40 body recoveries.[11]

OFDA is not the only office within the USG that provides humanitarian assistance to foreign nations. The Food For Peace Program (FFP), also administered under the direction of USAID, is responsible for coordinating the government's foreign food aid programs, which are authorized under U.S. Public Law 480, Titles I and III. These programs are provided as bilateral grant programs to countries in need of food aid assistance. On the other hand, Title II emergency food aid programs are targeted specifically for populations suffering from "food insecurity as a result of natural disasters, civil conflicts or other crises."[12] Title II programs are provided without request for repayment. Much of this food aid is also coordinated with the U.S. Department of Agriculture (USDA), which works closely with FFP in allocating surplus commodities to developing countries, under Section 416(b) of the Agricultural Act of 1949. This law ensures that the United States helps support emergency feeding programs, especially those related to events of natural consequence, such as drought, and those resulting from the onset of civil strife.

The U.S. Department of State (DOS) also plays a significant role in international disaster response. Whereas OFDA primarily responds to the needs of internally displaced persons (IDPs), the DOS retains chief responsibility for the care and support of refugee populations (those that cross state boundaries) on behalf of the USG. The Bureau of Population, Refugees and Migration (PRM) administers multilateral grants to international relief organizations, such as those operating under the umbrella of the UN. These grants may be requested in response to refugee emergency appeals. In addition, DOS/PRM regularly contribute to the program budgets of relief organizations.

In response to attacks directed against U.S. embassies in Nairobi, Kenya, and Dar es Salaam, Tanzania, in August 1998[2,13] and in large part because of the disorganized local response to these events and the absence of trusted medical and surgical capabilities, DOS elected to support the development of an International Medical Surgical Response Team (IMSuRT). Under any disaster circumstances, the already fragile medical infrastructure in developing nations is strained beyond capacity and capability, ultimately resulting in the inadequate delivery of healthcare to those in need. IMSuRT deployed to Guam in 2002 after the landfall of the devastating supertyphoon Pongsona to support the delivery of healthcare services on the island and in 2003 was sent to Micronesia in the West Pacific Ocean, again after the effects of a natural disaster. IMSuRT was most recently deployed in the aftermath of the Bam, Iran, earthquake in January 2004.[7]

With respect to international response as a result of terrorist activity, the Presidential Decision Directives (PDDs) issued in 1995 (PDD 39) and 1998 (PDD 62) clearly outline the mechanics of response to terrorist threat or use of weapons of mass destruction in the United States or against U.S. interests abroad. These executive orders clearly reaffirm that DOS is the lead federal agency for foreign consequence management and specify that DOS is responsible for leading and managing the Foreign Emergency Support Team (FEST) and the Consequence Management Response Team (CMRT). The creation of the Department of Homeland Security (DHS) has necessitated a wholesale revision of the domestic response to disaster. However, the newly drafted National Response Plan (NRP) clearly specifies that "the Secretary of State remains responsible for coordinating international prevention, preparedness, response and recovery activities relating to domestic incidents, and for the protection of U.S. citizens and U.S. interests overseas."[14]

The DoD assumes a significant responsibility for providing international disaster assistance. Since the end of the Cold War, there has been increasing involvement of military assets in missions directly related to peacekeeping, disaster response, and humanitarian assistance (Table 15-1). Within DoD, the Office of Peacekeeping and Humanitarian Affairs (PK/HA) has the chief responsibility to work with USAID and DOS as specified by the Denton Amendment, which allows the U.S. military to airlift or transport by sea privately donated humanitarian relief commodities on a space-available basis to countries affected by disasters. Some of the capabilities and strengths the military can bring to HA and disaster relief operations include logistical support and heavy lift operations, security, establishment of a communications infrastructure, additional manpower, and the overlay of command and control.

Military operations in support of diplomatic efforts are usually one of two types. "Peacekeeping" missions are undertaken with the consent of all major parties to a dispute. They are designed to monitor and facilitate the implementation of specific agreements, such as a cease-fire or a truce. Their intent is to encourage the continued negotiation, mediation, arbitration, and judicial review required to reach a lasting political settlement. When deployed under a UN mandate, this operation may be referred to as a "Chapter VI operation," referring to Chapter VI of the UN Charter, titled "Pacific Settlement of Disputes." A mission that involves the threat or application of military force to achieve compliance with resolutions or sanctions designed to restore peaceful relations between nations may be referred to as a "Chapter VII operation," referring to Chapter VII of the UN Charter, titled "Action with Respect to Threats to the Peace, Breaches of the Peace, and Acts of Aggression." Both types of mission profiles often will involve disaster relief activities. However, the military leadership will remain very cognizant of the risk of sustaining "mission creep," in which the military operation ultimately takes on a broader role or assumes responsibility for elements of the event that initially were not planned.

A command and control element established specifically for such missions, known as a Joint Task Force (JTF), will commonly accompany any large-scale military participation to improve field coordination and integration of the multiple military services involved. In turn, the JTF will often establish the Civil Military Operations Center (CMOC) to coordinate and facilitate humanitarian operations of the United States and any multinational force with those of international and local relief agencies and with the recognized authorities of the affected country. The CMOC may request USAID DART advisors to join the CMOC staff to assist in screening and validating requests for military support from the relief community. DART representatives, who often have previously established relationships with key elements of the international disaster response community, can also assist the military leadership in understanding the capabilities, levels of expertise, and operational methods of the involved relief organizations. DART representatives can also advise and educate the responding relief agencies about the capabilities, operational methods, and priorities of the U.S. military.

Military commanders may elect to establish a Humanitarian Assistance Coordination Center (HACC) to focus specifically on coordination of HA needs. This is done when the CMOC takes on the expanded role of developing other civilian-military initiatives, particularly those related to infrastructure development and the reinstitution of civil authority, such as is the current situation in postwar Iraq. On a related point, the National Security

TABLE 15-1 DoD MISSIONS IN HUMANITARIAN ASSISTANCE OPERATIONS

Northern Iraq	1991-1996
Former Yugoslavia (including Bosnia)	1992-1998
Somalia famine relief	1992
Rwanda refugee crisis	1994
Hurricane Mitch	1998
Kosovo	1999-2000
Venezuela floods	1999
Mozambique floods	2000
Afghanistan	2001-present
Iraq	2003-present
South Asia tsunami	2005

Council (NSC), which serves as the principal forum for national security and foreign policy matters, including those related to humanitarian issues, may play a role in influencing international disaster response. Finally, when needed, the U.S. Geological Survey, the Centers for Disease Control and Prevention, the U.S. Forest Service, and the Environmental Protection Agency all provide technical assistance in response to disasters and potential hazards overseas.

International Organizations and their Role in International Disaster Response

Since its inception, the United Nations has played an important role in the response to and coordination of international disaster relief efforts. Historically, a number of UN agencies have had responsibilities in ensuring coordination among responding nations and NGOs. These have included the United Nations Development Program (UNDP), United Nations High Commissioner for Refugees (UNHCR), United Nations Children's Fund (UNICEF), Food and Agriculture Organization (FAO), World Food Program (WFP), and World Health Organization (WHO). Each of these agencies was created under separate international treaties, is overseen by separate mechanisms of governance, and is funded predominantly by bilateral donor contributions separate from the UN budget. A result of this fractured organizational approach, often compounded by the exigencies of international political "power plays," has been an uneven and sometimes unhelpful UN presence in the response to disaster events and CEs.

In 1991, the UN General Assembly passed UN Resolution 46/182 calling for the improvement and strengthening of humanitarian assistance.[15] This resolution mandated the identification of the UN Emergency Relief Coordinator and resulted in the creation of the Department of Humanitarian Affairs, which in 1998 became the UN Office for the Coordination of Humanitarian Affairs (OCHA). OCHA coordinates response to humanitarian crises, serves as an advocate for HA, and promotes the development of policy supportive of this mission. This includes the facilitation of the relationship between humanitarian and military components participating in a relief operation. OCHA carries out its responsibilities, in part, by providing oversight to the UN Disaster Assessment and Coordination (UNDAC) teams and the International Search and Rescue Advisory Group (INSARAG). UNDAC teams are composed of a mix of international disaster management experts who can be deployed immediately after a disaster event to conduct a rapid assessment of priority needs. This group is expressly focused on providing support to host government authorities and to the UN Resident Coordinator to facilitate international disaster relief coordination. In earthquake responses, the UNDAC is used to coordinate international search and rescue operations. Often, the first international search and rescue team to arrive in-country establishes the On-Site Operations Coordination Center (OSOCC).

With regard to health and medical issues arising from sudden or slow-onset disaster events, WHO has the chief responsibility as the UN's lead technical agency. WHO is mandated by its constitution to "furnish appropriate technical assistance, and in emergency, the necessary aid upon the request or acceptance of Governments."[16] Along with its regional offices, including the Pan American Health Organization (PAHO), WHO is structured to deliver technical advisory support to national and local authorities, the donor community, and international NGOs. It has an operational role in defining public health priorities and plans of action.

Of all the international organizations involved in humanitarian assistance and disaster response, the International Committee of the Red Cross (ICRC) remains the oldest; largest; and, with its "red cross" symbol, the most universally recognized. It is a Swiss-based organization with a mandate under the internationally accepted Geneva Conventions to act as a neutral intermediary to protect victims of conflict, and by extension, support victims of disaster. It remains separate from all other international humanitarian organizations and NGOs and is neutral with regard to politics, religion, and ideology. The International Federation of Red Cross and Red Crescent Societies (IFRC), also Swiss-based, serves as the umbrella organization for all Red Cross and Red Crescent Societies throughout the world. It comprises 178 member societies, with a secretariat in Geneva, and more than 60 delegations that help coordinate relief efforts in response to natural disasters and assist with refugee populations in flight from areas of conflict. It must be noted that the American Red Cross (ARC), although not a USG agency or organization, is not neutral and is not a member of the IFRC.

Finally, and perhaps most importantly, at least with regard to the overall burden of responsibility assumed for disaster response and HA in CEs, are the PVOs and NGOs. PVOs are private, not-for-profit HA organizations that are involved in economic development and relief activities. These organizations are registered with USAID and are equivalent to NGOs, which is the term normally used by non-U.S. organizations. With an increasing emphasis on the provision of emergency aid, government agencies, the UN, and private donors increasingly rely on NGOs to distribute the bulk of humanitarian aid going to victims of disaster. More than 90% of all relief assistance coordinated by the UN is implemented through NGOs.[17] Well-known groups that specifically address health and medical needs include Medecins sans Frontieres (MSF) ("Doctors without Borders"), the International Medical Committee (IMC), and the International Rescue Committee (IRC). MSF was formed in the late 1960s in direct response to the inept and uncoordinated efforts at providing relief to the Nigerian region of Biafra, which was beset by civil strife, leading to severe disease and starvation. MSF was the first of a number of organizations to take an "activist approach" to providing disaster relief, and it remains an important participant in the international arena. However, the increasing use of military support for humanitarian operations creates a unique conflict for many international relief organizations. Because they are protected in their humanitarian work by international law—provided they maintain humanitarian principles of impartiality, neutrality, and universality—many NGOs will not work with the military of any nation.

Partly in reaction to the increasing reliance on military support for humanitarian response, a multilateral group comprised of members of national and international NGOs, the Red Cross Movement, UN Agencies, and the academic community developed the Sphere Project in 1997. This work was focused on the development of "minimum standards" in six critical areas: water supply and sanitation, nutrition, food aid, shelter and health services, and food security. These minimum standards and an accompanying Handbook are based on two fundamental philosophical beliefs. The first is that "all possible steps should be taken to alleviate human suffering arising out of calamity and conflict." The second is that "those affected by disaster have a right to life with dignity and therefore a right to assistance."[19]

PITFALLS

Many misperceptions exist concerning the form, content, and mission of responders to disaster events in the international community (Box 15-3). These may result in the import and distribution of too many relief items. This, in turn, may trigger a cascade of unintended consequences. For example, the snack biscuits delivered to the Kosovo IDP settlement camps in 1998 were not popular among the camp residents. They were not eaten and were discarded, subsequently introducing rodent and snake vectors into the camp.[18] It is also critically important to recognize the importance of strengthening local capabilities, particularly those in the health and medical sector, in a proactive manner before disaster strikes.[20,21]

The most egregious mistakes made include those that result in a wholly inappropriate response effort. These may be marked by an obvious lack of responsiveness to local needs (e.g., the establishment of mass vaccination clinics in place of improving sanitary conditions after a natural disaster). Another example would be the employment of expatriate staff when local skills could have been equally successful. At their worst, response efforts may become a burden to the host government of the affected country. An example would be the deployment of expensive field hospitals that arrive long after the last survivors are rescued from the precipitating event and then depart after a week or two in-country without confirming the re-establishment of the indigenous healthcare delivery sector. In the rush to provide visible action to satisfy the international public, more pragmatic and, ultimately, more useful approaches may be abandoned.

There are a number of barriers that impair the execution of successful disaster response efforts relief. A recent IFRC evaluation of existing international disaster response laws cites the following challenges to response organizations. There is an inconsistency of access to disaster-affected populations. Furthermore, some of these impediments are the result of delays, inefficiencies, and inconsistencies in the facilitation of disaster response by state authorities. In certain instances, this may be due to an under-resourced host government infrastructure being overwhelmed by the impact of the disaster. On the other hand, this may also occur as part of an intended manipulation of the international relief community for political or financial gain.[22]

BOX 15-3 MYTHS REGARDING INTERNATIONAL DISASTER RESPONSE

Perception:	Large numbers of foreign medical volunteers are needed.
Reality:	Local populations are usually able to manage immediate lifesaving needs. Only medical personnel with skills not available in the affected country may be needed.
Perception:	All forms of urgently delivered international assistance are needed.
Reality:	Any hasty response not based on a needs-assessment only contributes to the chaos of the event. In many instances, the disaster victims or their local governments or support agencies meet most immediate needs.
Perception:	Epidemics of disease inevitably occur after every disaster event.
Reality:	Epidemics do not spontaneously occur after a disaster. Dead bodies do not pose a threat to trigger the outbreak of infectious disease. The key elements contributory to preventing such an outbreak are improving sanitary conditions and educating the affected population.
Perception:	Food aid is always required after a natural disaster.
Reality:	Food aid is not usually required because natural disasters rarely cause loss of crops.
Perception:	Victims of disaster always need clothing.
Reality:	Used clothing is almost never needed and is often culturally inappropriate.
Perception:	Locating victims of disaster in temporary settlements, including the use of tents for shelter, represents the best means of managing the loss of domicile.
Reality:	Funds spent for the purchase of tents are better applied to the purchase of building materials, tools, and other construction-related support in the affected country.
Perception:	Things are back to normal within a few weeks after a disaster event.
Reality:	The effects of a disaster last a long time. Disaster-affected countries deplete much of their financial and material resources in the immediate postdisaster phase. Successful relief programs gear their operations to the fact that international interest wanes as needs and shortages become more pressing.

Adapted from Noji E. The nature of disaster: general characteristics and public health effects. In: Noji E, ed. *The Public Health Consequences of Disasters*, Oxford: Oxford University Press; 1997:17-18.

In addition, there is often a lack of coordination within and between national and international disaster response entities. In part, this may result from the absence of "institutional memory" as individual participants involved in the disaster response change. As a consequence, large bureaucratic organizations repeat mistakes made in previous response efforts, or worse yet, do not account for the variations in the approach given the organization's mission. A tragic example of this occurred recently during U.S. military operations in Afghanistan. Human daily rations (HDR) are a high-protein, 2000-calorie ration that were introduced in 1993 for use by the DoD in humanitarian relief efforts. They are designed to be acceptable by all ethnic and religious groups and are meant to be used as a stopgap feeding asset until the arrival of other foods chosen to meet specific or multiple nutritional deficiencies. The HDRs, placed in highly visible yellow packages, were dropped in Afghanistan at the same time that the DoD was dropping yellow painted cluster bombs. Although this had occurred previously during U.S. military actions in Kosovo, the institutional knowledge of this "work issue" was lost due to military rotations from operational forces.[18]

Difficulties are also encountered in the coordination of responsibilities at the disaster site. Standardized protocols that govern such coordination do not exist. A "lack of hand-over planning, incomplete and absent documentation, non-overlap of individual successive job holders, poor communication with beneficiaries, (and a) misunderstanding of expectations" contribute to such problems.[23] Difficulties such as these may be due as much to the barriers existing within the NGO community as they are to the need to improve and strengthen coordination by the appropriate international partners, such as OCHA and other key response agencies in the international arena.

CONCLUSION

The response to international disaster events and humanitarian crises by the USG is an important manifestation of its role in global affairs. Even though such efforts usually reflect the dire need for assistance and support on the part of the affected country, it must be recognized that there are instances in which such participation may appear to be a veiled attempt at influencing foreign governments. The major USG participants, including USAID, DOS, and DOD, must work closely together. They must also work in tandem with the key international organizations involved in disaster response, including key UN agencies, the ICRC, and the many NGOs and PVOs that comprise the backbone of the response community.

REFERENCES

1. Noji E. Earthquakes. In: Noji E, ed. *The Public Health Consequences of Disasters*. Oxford: Oxford University Press; 1997:135-78.
2. US Geological Survey. Earthquake Hazards Program. Available at: http://neic.usgs.gov/neis/eqlists/eqsmajr.html.
3. Burkle FM. Lessons learnt and future expectations of complex emergencies. *BMJ*. 1999;319:422-6.
4. Sharp TW, Burkle FM, Vaughn AF, et al. Challenges and opportunities for humanitarian relief in Afghanistan. *Clin Infect Dis*. 2002;34:S215-28.
5. Time for action on Sudan. *The New York Times*. [Editorial]. June 18, 2004;A26.
6. Macintyre AG, Weir S, Barbera JA. The international search and rescue response to the US Embassy bombing in Kenya: the medical team experience. *Prehospital Disaster Med*. 1999;14(4):215-21.
7. Schnitzer JJ, Briggs SM. Earthquake relief—the U.S. medical response in Bam, Iran. *NEJM*. March 2004;350(12):1174-6.
8. Keim ME, Rhyne GJ. The CDC Pacific Emergency Health Initiative: a pilot study of emergency preparedness in Oceania. *Emerg Med (Fremantle)*. June 2001;13(2):143-4.
9. Keim ME. History of the Pacific Emergency Health Initiative. *Pac Health Dialog*. March 2002;9(1):146-9.
10. US Agency for International Development, Bureau for Humanitarian Response, Office of Foreign Disaster Assistance. Field Operations Guide for Disaster Assessment and Response. Policy Guidelines. August 1998:xix. Available at: http://www.usaid.gov/our_work/humanitarian_assistance/disaster_assistance/resources/pdf/fog_v3.pdf.
11. Fairfax County Urban Search and Rescue, Izmit, Turkey Earthquake Response After Action Report, August 1999.
12. 2002 USAID Annual Report. Available at: http://www.usaid.gov/our_work/humanitarian_assistance/disaster_assistance/publications/#annual_reports.
13. Clack ZA, Keim ME, Macintyre AG, Yeskey K. Emergency health and risk management in sub-saharan Africa: a lesson from the embassy bombings in Tanzania and Kenya. *Prehospital Disaster Med*. April-June 2002;17(2):59-66.
14. National Response Plan, Draft No. 2, U.S. Department of Homeland Security, p. 21, April 28, 2004. Available at: www.dhs.gov.
15. UN General Assembly. Resolution 46/182. December 1991. Available at: www.un.org/documents/ga/res/46/a46r182.htm.
16. World Health Organization. Handbook for Emergency Field Operations. Available at: http://www.who.int/hac/techguidance/tools/7661.pdf.
17. Burkle FM Jr. Complex humanitarian emergencies. In: Hogan DE, Burstein JL, eds. *Disaster Med*. Philadelphia: Lippincott Williams & Wilkins; 2002:49.
18. Disaster Assessment and Response Team orientation training. Lecture presentation at: USAID Office of Foreign Disaster Assistance. July 2003; Arlington, VA. 2004 Sphere Handbook. Available at: www.sphereproject.org/handbook/hdbkpdf/hdbk_ann.pdf.
19. 2004 Sphere Handbook. Available at: www.sphereproject.org/handbook/hdbkpdf/hdbk_ann.pdf.
20. VanRooyen MJ, Eliades MJ, Grabowski JG, et al. Medical relief personnel in complex emergencies: perceptions of effectiveness in the former Yugoslavia *Prehospital Disaster Med*. July-September 2001;16(3):145-9.
21. Hsu EB, Ma M, Lin FY, et al. Emergency medical assistance team response following Taiwan Chi-Chi earthquake. *Prehospital Disaster Med*. January-March 2002;17(1):17-22.
22. International Federation of Red Cross and Red Crescent Societies. International Disaster Response Laws (IDRL) Project report 2002-2003. Presented at: 28th International Conference of the Red Cross and Red Crescent Societies—"Protecting Human Dignity"; December 2-6, 2003; Geneva. Available at: http://www.icrc.org/web/eng/siteeng0.nsf/iwpList189/B38EC5E7ECBC52F9C1256E6D00364BF5.
23. Bradt DA, Drummond CM. From complex emergencies to terrorism—new tools for health-sector coordination in conflict-associated disasters. *Prehospital Disaster Med*. 2003;18(3):263-71.

chapter 16

Disaster/Emergency Management Programs

Peter Brewster

The public health and medical sector is a crucial element of emergency management. Emergency management is the discipline and profession of applying science, technology, planning, and management to deal with extreme events that can injure or kill large numbers of people, do extensive damage to property and disrupt community life.[1] This chapter describes many of the government and other public agency programs that assist this sector.

EMERGENCY MANAGEMENT (EM) CONCEPTS, PRINCIPLES, AND SYSTEMS

The creation of the Federal Emergency Management Agency (FEMA) in 1980 brought with it a new federal focus on all hazards. FEMA was transferred to the U.S. Department of Homeland Security (DHS) as part of the Homeland Security Act of 2002; however, even before this transfer, FEMA sponsored many educational programs and concepts applicable to the public health and medical sector. These programs, available on-site, through distance learning courses or self-study, focus on the following concepts.

Comprehensive Emergency Management

Comprehensive emergency management (CEM) addresses all hazards through the following four phases of activity:

- **Mitigation:** Examples of activities that occur within the mitigation phase include conducting an analysis of potential hazards, threats, and events; the negative effects these hazards may have on populations, infrastructure, and the operational capabilities of response organizations; and planning the structural and non-structural actions to reduce or eliminate these effects.
- **Preparedness:** Preparedness activities include identification of physical, human, and informational resources needed to offset losses or damage to infrastructure or operating systems. Available resources are maintained and inventoried, and for those not on hand, arrangements for obtaining them are pre-planned. Public education about hazards and family preparedness are components of preparedness activities, as are training and exercises for organizations with emergency responsibilities.
- **Response:** The response phase begins with incident recognition and generally transitions into the recovery phase once ongoing negative effects of the incident have been stopped. Key response activities include situation assessment, warning and notifications, coordinating with other agencies, setting objectives and priorities, and assigning resources to work on disaster-related problems.
- **Recovery:** Recovery activities begin with determining the operational status of priority community systems and working toward their reestablishment and making disaster assistance services available (financial and mental health services). Final components of the recovery phase are the identifying "lessons learned" and making revisions to future mitigation, preparedness, response, and recovery activities.

Integrated Emergency Management System

To implement CEM, FEMA developed the Integrated Emergency Management System (IEMS). IEMS consists of three fundamental parts: (1) a set of program development steps tied to the four phases of CEM, (2) a philosophy of inclusiveness (those groups that will respond to disasters are brought into the planning process), and (3) a method of organization around functions generic to all disasters, not around specific hazards, agencies, or people.

Incident Command System

As IEMS taught planners to think along functional lines in the early 1980s, the Incident Command (Management) System (ICS) was unveiled. ICS was part of a larger National Interagency Incident Management System (NIIMS) that included standardized training, qualifications and certification, supporting publications, and technologies.[1a] The "system" of incident command/management is described in detail elsewhere in this text. The ICS concept formed the backbone of National Incident Management System (NIMS) concepts. The Hospital Emergency Incident Command System (HEICS), developed in San Mateo County, Calif., is a specific adaptation of the ICS system to fixed-site healthcare facilities.

Standardized Emergency Management System

Because the ICS was so successful as a management system for field response, the state of California extended its components, principles, and organizational structure into a statewide model that consisted of five response levels: field response, local government, operational area (county), mutual aid region, and state. The Standardized Emergency Management System (SEMS) was made mandatory for all public sector agencies with emergency responsibilities.[2] SEMS was aimed at solving interagency coordination problems that occurred in and between Emergency Operating Centers (EOCs) at the various response levels.

Disaster Research

Use of disaster research has improved the effectiveness of the emergency management field(s). Sociological studies and reports on human behavior in disasters have identified the "myths" perpetuated by the media (looting, helpless disaster victims, and so on); pushed the profession away from a hazards focus to a generic focus on functions; and brought gender, ethnic, and special population issues to the forefront. Environmental and physical scientists have made advances in land use policies, structural designs and building codes, and monitoring and warning systems that have improved safety.

FEDERAL PROGRAMS

Cities Readiness Initiative

The Metropolitan Medical Response System programs have been discussed in previous chapters. Twenty cities and the National Capital Region/District of Columbia have been identified to participate in this pilot program, based on demographic characteristics and location. The purpose of the Cities Readiness Initiative (CRI) is to assist these localities in increasing their capacity to receive and disburse medications and medical supplies from the Strategic National Stockpile. One particular focus is on the development of unified, intergovernmental (local, state, and federal) operations plans, training, and exercises.

Bioterrorism Preparedness Program

The U.S. Department of Health and Human Services (DHHS) initiated a multiyear program aimed at upgrading the preparedness of the nation's public health and healthcare systems to respond to bioterrorism, other outbreaks of infectious disease, and other public health threats and emergencies.[3] The Centers for Disease Control and Prevention (CDC), Health Resources Services Administration (HRSA), and Agency for Healthcare Research and Quality (AHRQ) have combined forces to ensure the most effective use of resources.

The umbrella structure for the program concentrates on the following "focus areas:"

- Preparedness planning and readiness assessment
- Surveillance and epidemiology capacity
- Laboratory capacity—biological agents
- Laboratory capacity—chemical agents
- Health alert network/communications and information technology
- Communication of health risks and health information dissemination
- Education and training (criteria included below)
- Cross-cutting initiatives (integration point for the National Disaster Medical System and Metropolitan Medical Response System programs as well as smallpox preparedness and mental health services)

As part of this program, HRSA administers a grant program aimed at increasing the surge capacity of America's hospitals.[4] Until now, the healthcare industry has not received significant financial support for emergency preparedness activities. These funds along with grant guidance, existing hospital preparedness standards, and training available through AHRQ and other sources will help to ensure a more effective nationwide emergency management capability.

Domestic Preparedness Program

The Department of Justice's Office of Justice Programs, in conjunction with the National Domestic Preparedness Program, funds the purchase of specialized equipment for fire, emergency medical, and hazardous materials response services and law enforcement agencies. The purpose of these funds is to enhance the capabilities of jurisdictions to respond to acts of terrorism involving chemical and biological agents and radiological, nuclear, and explosive devices. Early grants paid for a needs assessment, which formed the basis of statewide strategy—a "roadmap" identifying where grant funds would be targeted.

The Homeland Security Act of 2002 transferred the Domestic Preparedness Program to the DHS. DHS's Office for Domestic Preparedness (ODP) is the primary agency at the federal level for managing the preparedness of the United States for acts of terrorism. ODP responsibilities include coordinating federal preparedness efforts; working with all state, local, tribal, parish, and private sector emergency response entities designated to combat terrorism; and providing support for training, exercises, and equipment.[5] ODP administers a number of grant programs, exercises, training, and technical assistance services to support state and local emergency responders.

Military Medical Educational Resources

Research and development centers within the Department of Defense (DoD), specifically the U.S. Army Soldier and Biological Chemical Command (SBCCOM),[6] U.S. Army Medical Research Institute of Infectious Diseases (USAMRIID),[7] and U.S. Army Medical Research Institute of Chemical Defense (USAMRICD),[8] remain the preeminent authorities and sources for chemical, biological, radiologic/nuclear, and explosive agent countermeasures. These agencies also offer educational programs to the civilian sector.

UNIVERSITY PROGRAMS

Disaster Research Centers

The Disaster Research Center (DRC) was established at Ohio State University in 1960 and moved to its current location at the University of Delaware in 1985.[9] DRC directors and staff are some of the best-known sociologists in the field, contributing to practitioners' knowledge of how individuals, family units, organizations, communities, and society as a whole behave when faced with emergency situations. The Natural Hazards Research and Information Applications Center ("Hazards Center") at the University of Colorado in Boulder has been at the forefront of establishing effective linkages between the disaster research community, policy makers, and practitioners.[10] The Hazards Center provides a clearinghouse function for disaster research centers from around the world.

Emergency Management Degree Programs

The University of North Texas offered the first four-year degree program in emergency management before the 1990s. Through FEMA's Higher Education Project, many state and private colleges and universities offer a full range of degree programs based on the sample course modules that FEMA has produced.[11] Although hazards have increasingly been added to the curricula of schools of geography, land use planning, public health, and nursing, medical school curricula are lacking sufficient knowledge matter in emergency preparedness to provide a uniform baseline for physicians.

STANDARDS

ASTM 1288 and E54 Committee on Homeland Security

The American Society for Testing and Materials (ASTM) is one of the largest organizations that develop voluntary standards through objective, consensus processes. ASTM 1288, Standard Guide for Planning for and Response to a Multiple Casualty Incident, elucidates emergency medical service and hospital coordination and operations issues.[12] The ASTM Committee E54[13] on Homeland Security is developing standards and guidance in the following homeland security applications: protecting borders, ports,

and transportation systems; advancing and harnessing science and technology; protecting the nation's infrastructure; and preparing for and responding to national emergencies. Seven subcommittees focus on the following areas: chemical, biological, radiological, nuclear, and explosive (CBRNE) sensors and detectors; training and procedures; decontamination; personal protective equipment (PPE); building and infrastructure protection; security controls; and threat and vulnerability assessment.

NFPA 99, 1600

The National Fire Protection Association (NFPA) is another global developer of consensus standards. The NFPA standards process involves technical committee product requests for proposals from members of the committee and the public, review of proposals and voting by the committee, development of draft standards, request for public comment, final review of comments, and voting by the committee to arrive at a final draft of a standard every five years.

The original emergency preparedness standard for hospitals was drafted by an NFPA Technical Committee in 1975 (NFPA 99), and it remains a leading reference to this day.[14] In the early 1990s, federal, state, and local government and private sector emergency planners began developing recommended practices for disaster/emergency management and business continuity programs (NFPA 1600). NFPA 1600 has been the framework for the state and local Capability Assessment for Readiness (CAR) (1997) and the Emergency Management Accreditation Program (EMAP) (2000).[15] In 2004, NFPA 1600 was recognized as the nation's preparedness standard by the National Commission on Terrorist Attacks Upon the United States (also known as the 9-11 Commission).[16,17]

Joint Commission on Accreditation of Healthcare Organizations Environment of Care Standards

The Joint Commission on Accreditation of Healthcare Organizations (JCAHO) is the leading developer of standards for the healthcare industry in the United States. Without JCAHO accreditation (for those organizations using JCAHO standards), healthcare organizations cannot receive reimbursement for services under Medicare and Medicaid. The Environment of Care (EC) standards are designed to support a safe environment for patient care and consist of safety, hazardous materials and wastes, fire safety, medical equipment, utility systems, security, and emergency management. The JCAHO emergency management standards (EC 4) reflect the core concerns of mainstream emergency management agencies with those of the healthcare industry.[18]

SUMMARY

The management of routine, daily emergencies in the United States is handled at the local level by law enforcement, fire, rescue, hazardous materials, and emergency medical service providers. When disasters occur, many other organizations may also get involved.[19]

Emergency managers work to improve the ability of individuals and groups to solve the problems created during emergencies and disasters. The problem-solving capacity is enhanced by creating structures and procedures that can collect, organize, and allocate information and resources; identify problems; determine objectives and priorities; and assign available resources. These arrangements are built through a regular process in which various agencies interact to identify hazards, develop plans and training programs, establish communications and support facilities, and practice through drills and exercises.[20]

REFERENCES

1. Hoetner G. Introduction. *Emergency Management: Principles and Practices for Local Government*. Washington, D.C.: International City Management Association, 1991: xiii.
1a. National Interagency Incident Management System. Incident Command System. Available at: http://www.fs.fed.us/fire/operations/niims.shtml.
2. State of California, Governor's Office of Emergency Services. Standardized Emergency Management System (SEMS) guidelines. Available at: http://www.oes.ca.gov/Operational/OESHome.nsf/0d737f261e76eeb588256b27007ac5ff/b49435352108954488256c2a0071e038?OpenDocument.
3. Centers for Disease Control and Prevention. Continuation guidance for cooperative agreement on public health preparedness and response for bioterrorism—budget year five. Available at: http://www.bt.cdc.gov/planning/continuationguidance/index.asp.
4. Health Resources and Services Administration. Bioterrorism Hospital Preparedness Program. Available at: http://www.hrsa.gov/bioterrorism/index.htm.
5. US Department of Homeland Security, Department of Justice, Office for Domestic Preparedness. Available at: http://www.ojp.usdoj.gov/odp/.
6. U.S. Army Soldier and Biological Chemical Command (SBCCOM). Available at: http//www.hld.sbccom.army.mil/ip/detectors.
7. U.S. Army Medical Research Institute of Infectious Diseases (USAMRIID). Available at: http://www.usamriid.army.mil/index.htm.
8. U.S. Army Medical Research Institute of Chemical Defense (USAMRICD). Available at: http>//chemdef.apgea.army.mil/.
9. University of Delaware, Disaster Research Center. Disaster data. Available at: http://www.udel.edu/DRC/disdat/busbib.html.
10. University of Colorado, Natural Hazards Center. Available at: http://www.colorado.edu/hazards.
11. Emergency Management Institute. FEMA's EMI Higher Education Project. Available at: http://training.fema.gov/emiweb/edu/.
12. American Society for Testing and Materials. F1288-90(2003) Standard Guide for Planning for and Response to a Multiple Casualty Incident Available at: http://www.astm.org/cgi-bin/SoftCart.exe/DATABASE.CART/REDLINE_PAGES/F1288.htm?L+mystore+qjcg0290+1089149374.
13. American Society for Testing and Materials. Committee E54 on Homeland Security Applications. Available at: http://www.astm.org/cgi-bin/SoftCart.exe/COMMIT/COMMITTEE/E54.htm?L+mystore+qjcg0290+1089168340.
14. National Fire Protection Association. Hospital requirements. In: *NFPA 99: Standard for Health Care Facilities, 2002 ed.* Quincy, MA: National Fire Protection Association; 2002.
15. Federal Emergency Management Agency. Capability Assessment for Readiness (CAR). Available at: http://www.fema.gov/pdf/rrr/car.pdf.
16. National Emergency Management Association, Emergency Management Assistance Compact. Available at: http://www.emacweb.org/emac/index.cfm?CFID=5327&CFTOKEN=28115803.
17. National Emergency Management Association, Council of State Governments. Available at: http://www.csg.org/CSG/default.htm.
18. Joint Commission on Accreditation of Healthcare Organizations. Emergency Management Standards—EC.1.4 and EC.2.9.1. Available at: http://www.jcrinc.com/subscribers/perspectives.asp?durki=2914&site=10&return=2897.
19. Drabek T. *Strategies for Coordinating Disaster Responses*. Boulder: Institute of Behavioral Studies, University of Colorado; 2003:42. Monograph 61.
20. Dynes RR. Community emergency planning: false assumptions and inappropriate analogies. *Int J Mass Emerg Disasters*. 1994;12:141-58.

chapter 17

Community Hazard Vulnerability Assessment

James C. Chang

The community hazard vulnerability assessment (HVA) is the systematic examination of the multitude of hazards, their individual probabilities, and consequences that may be encountered in the community. This assessment requires an in-depth knowledge of the community and is typically performed by a multidisciplinary team. The HVA is often used as the basis for the community's emergency management program.

Like the hospital-based HVA presented in Chapter 18, the community HVA helps emergency planners define the universe of potential threats that the community may face. As with the hospital-based example, community leaders face the same challenges of budgeting, limited resources, and selection of hazards on which to focus their resources. Unlike the hospital-based HVA, however, the scope and performance of a community HVA are often beyond the direct control (and sometimes, influence) of hospital-based planners and are conducted by local emergency management officials.

For a healthcare facility to develop a successful emergency preparedness program and meet its obligations to provide care to the members of the community, it must engage with community planners and response agencies, since healthcare facilities are integral components of the community.

HISTORICAL PERSPECTIVE

To understand where the practice of HVA arose, one must look at the short, fragmented history of emergency management in the United States.

After a devastating fire in Portsmouth, N.H., that overwhelmed both local and state resources in 1803, the U.S. Congress established the precedent for federal aid that is in place today by passing legislation allowing federal resources to be used to support state and local governments. Congress passed 128 other similar pieces of ad hoc legislation in support of victims of the 1906 San Francisco earthquake and other major disasters between 1803 and 1950.[1]

In 1916, civil defense programs were born when Congress enacted the U.S. Army Appropriations Act.

This act established the Council of National Defense (CND) with subordinate state and local defense councils in response to a perceived enemy threat. Much of the interest in civil defense ceased with the end of World War I.

After a brief hiatus, federal agencies were given the authority to respond to specific disasters. In 1933, the Reconstruction Finance Corporation was given the authority to fund the repair and/or reconstruction of public facilities damaged by earthquakes. In 1934, the Bureau of Public Roads was given the authority to provide grants to repair federal-aid highways and bridges damaged by natural events (i.e., primarily floods). A noteworthy change in the approach from response to proactiveness (preparedness) occurred with the Flood Control Act of 1936. This act allowed the U.S. Army Corps of Engineers to proactively construct dams, dikes, and levees to reduce local vulnerability to floods.[1]

Continuing in the track of responding to actual or perceived emergencies, in 1941 the CND was dissolved and the Office of Civil Defense was established. As with the CND, the focus of the Office of Civil Defense was the establishment of protective services programs oriented toward a specific (i.e., enemy) threat. These activities included the establishment of the Civil Defense Corps, which coordinated the activities of approximately 10 million volunteers and 44 state and 1000 local councils. The Office of Civil Defense was abolished with the end of World War II.[1]

The Federal Civil Defense Administration (FCDA) was established by President Truman in 1949 in response to increasing Cold War concerns. The Federal Civil Defense Act of 1950 was quickly passed to give the FCDA the authority and resources to begin planning and coordination activities. One of the most noteworthy successes of the FCDA and its new director, Val Peterson, was the idea that civil defense activities such as disaster planning had a peacetime value. Meanwhile, Congress continued to reinforce the role of the federal government in responding to (but not preparing for) disasters with the Federal Disaster Act of 1950. This act, intended for "getting assistance to rebuild the streets and farm-to-market highways and roads,"[1] was viewed by many as Congress's establishing the legal basis for a continuing federal role in disaster relief.[1] Subsequent acts, including the Disaster Relief Acts of 1970 and 1974, reinforced the federal government's role in disaster relief.

In 1972, the Office of Civil Defense, which had been reestablished in 1961, was renamed the Defense Civil Preparedness Agency. Increasing international tensions and growing stockpiles of nuclear weapons gave rise to the concept of Crisis Relocation Planning (CRP). The premise behind CRP was the dispersal of the populace from high-risk areas in times of heightened international tensions; in essence, this was an extension of existing hurricane evacuation programs that many coastal areas had successfully developed. In 1974, Congress passed the Disaster Relief Act of 1974 that specifically authorized the federal government to assist in disaster preparedness activities.

Difficulties in implementing CRP and the resulting frustrations experienced by federal, state, and local emergency planners led to a study and report by the National Governor's Association (NGA) in 1978 calling for a coordinated federal policy and approach to emergency planning. The NGA report introduced the concept of comprehensive emergency management (CEM), which is the cornerstone for emergency management today. In response to the NGA report and pressure from the constituency, President Jimmy Carter established the Federal Emergency Management Agency (FEMA) in 1979 to pull together many fragmented federal programs and implement a CEM program.

The new agency, under Director Louis Giuffrida, adopted a position calling for an enhanced civil defense program with an improved ability to deal with natural disasters and other large-scale domestic emergencies. In response to continued skepticism and outright resistance to CRP, the new agency abandoned CRP in favor of CEM. Under CEM, instead of focusing on specific scenarios and their consequences (e.g., nuclear attack, earthquake, or flood), local and state agencies were now encouraged to ask the following:

- What hazards confront our community?
- What resources are available? What needed resources are not available? Over what period of time could local government reasonably acquire these resources?
- What mitigating actions could be taken to reduce future vulnerabilities?

These questions are integral to an Integrated Emergency Management System (IEMS) approach; IEMS is the tool under which FEMA implements CEM. Under IEMS, emergency managers perform systematic assessments of both hazards and response capabilities. Gaps are identified, and then multiyear remediation plans, along with hazard mitigation and recovery plans, are created to address these gaps. Implicit in the use of IEMS is the change from a reactionary to a proactive approach to emergency management. This planning approach facilitates the transition from a hazard-specific to an all-hazards approach to emergency management.[1]

CURRENT PRACTICE

To properly plan for emergencies in the community, it is necessary to identify the list of potential hazards, their probability or relative risk, and their consequences. This HVA helps the planning team decide what hazards merit special attention, what actions must be planned for, and what resources are likely to be needed.

To better describe the community HVA process, it will be broken down into the following actions:

- HVA team membership
- Hazard identification
- Hazard profiling (probability and consequences)

HVA Team Membership[2]

A team approach should be considered for both the HVA and the development of the final Emergency Operations Plan for many reasons, including:

- To share (synergistic) expertise
- To develop and foster teamwork and working relationships
- To ensure that a holistic view of hazards is taken
- To create a sense of ownership and buy-in from all parties

The constituency of the teams will differ depending on their stated purpose (e.g., HVA versus plans development). Prospective members of the HVA team may include representatives from:

- Emergency Management Agency
- Community leadership (e.g., city manager, county executive)
- Each community public safety agency (law enforcement—police department, sheriff's office; fire department; emergency medical services [EMS])
- Hospitals and other community healthcare facilities
- Public health agencies (local health department)
- Planning departments or agencies
- Public works
- Local Emergency Planning Committee (LEPC)
- Professional groups (e.g., Certified Hazardous Materials Managers, American Society of Safety Engineers)
- Special hazards occupancies or operations (e.g., military bases, industrial complexes, dams, nuclear power plants)
- Major business entities
- Other emergency management planners (e.g., from local, county, regional, or state agencies or private industry)

Hazard Identification

Hazard identification is the exercise of identifying what kinds of emergencies have occurred or could occur within the jurisdiction. For assessment purposes, it may be helpful to divide emergencies into the following categories:

- **Naturally derived emergencies:** (e.g., floods, hurricanes, tornadoes, winter storms)
- **Technologically derived emergencies:** (e.g., power or utility failures, hazardous materials releases, computing systems failures)
- **Manmade emergencies:** (e.g., attacks involving weapons of mass destruction)

A partial listing of potential emergencies is provided in Box 17-1. This listing is not all inclusive, and care must be taken to ensure that hazards are not inappropriately excluded or omitted when assembling the community's overall list of potential hazards.[2] It is also important to note that hazards may arise from differing sources (e.g., epidemics may be naturally occurring or the result of bioterrorism). Finally, hazards and emergencies may be linked together. For example, a hurricane may generate flooding, mudslides, and loss of utilities.

There are many potential sources of information to support the hazard identification effort, including[3]:

- Experiences of planning team members
- Experiences of utilities or other major business entities in the community
- Local and/or state Emergency Management Agency records
- Local emergency response agency records
- Newspaper or other historical archives
- Experiences of similar or adjacent communities
- Hazard information maps compiled by FEMA and state emergency management agencies, the U.S. Geological Survey (USGS) and state geological surveys, the National Weather Service (NWS), and the Federal Insurance Administration (National Flood Insurance Program)

BOX 17-1 LIST OF POTENTIAL EMERGENCIES

Naturally Derived

Avalanche
Drought
Earthquake
Epidemic
Flood
Hurricane (cyclone, typhoon)
Landslide
Mudslide
Severe thunderstorm
Temperature extremes
Subsidence
Tornado
Tsunami
Volcanic eruption
Wildfire
Windstorm
Winter storm (blizzard, ice storm)

Technologically Derived

Airplane crash
Dam failure
Hazardous materials release
Hog or other animal farm waste containment failure
Information technology system failure
Power failure
Radiological release
Train derailment
Urban conflagration
Utility interruption (natural gas, water, sewer, telephone, data)
Water supply contamination

Manmade

Civil disturbance
Mass casualty events
Terrorism (chemical, biological, radiological, nuclear, or high-yield explosive [CBRNE])

- Maps of 10- and 50-mile emergency planning zones (EPZs) around nuclear power plants
- Maps of hazardous materials sites prepared by the LEPC
- Risk management plan submittals by users of extremely hazardous substances
- Local American Red Cross or other disaster relief agency records
- Results of any federal, state, or private hazard analyses
- Local or state historical society or area universities (e.g., departments of history, sociology, geography, engineering)
- Professional or business associations (e.g., insurers, engineers, and builders)
- Engineering assessments (e.g., reliability studies, mean time between failure studies)
- Longtime community residents

Hazard Profiling (Probability and Consequences)

Once the list of possible hazards has been assembled, the next action is to profile or characterize each hazard for probability and effect or consequence.

Probability

This is an assessment of the likelihood of the hazard or emergency occurring and is often described as improbable, low, medium, or high. Other related factors that may be helpful in assessing or describing probability include[4]:

- **Frequency of occurrence:** The more frequent the occurrence, the higher the likelihood.
- **Location of the hazardous event and the region affected:** Events that occur within or proximal to the community are more likely to affect the community, whereas events that occur at some distance may be less likely to affect the community.
- **Seasonal (or other cyclical) variations:** Events that occur with some regularity may be presumed to be more probable. Commonplace examples include the occurrence of "influenza season" each fall through winter and drought and/or floods (location-dependent) associated with El Niño.

Some hazards, such as civil disorder and terrorism, are by their nature highly unpredictable and may be difficult to properly assign a probability level.

Consequences

This is the effect of the hazard on the community and may be categorized into human, property, and business. Examples of each category include, but are not limited to:

- **Human impact**
  - Injuries
  - Illnesses
  - Fatalities
  - Psychological impact

- **Property damage**
  - Damage to or loss of use of buildings, structures, or domiciles
  - Damage to or loss of use of infrastructure (e.g., roadways, utility distribution systems)
- **Business loss**
  - Business interruption (including recordkeeping issues arising from loss of records, inability to access, compromise of integrity)
  - Unanticipated costs
  - Loss of revenue (from all causes such as loss of tourism, sales tax revenue, and fees for services)
  - Decline in property values
  - Adverse publicity
  - Fines, penalties, and legal costs

The degree of impact may be expressed qualitatively as nonexistent, low, medium, high, or catastrophic, or it may be expressed quantitatively as a numerical score. As a consideration, the HVA team may wish to add greater weight to hazards that occur without warning (e.g., tornado strike).

SUMMARY

The end goal of a community HVA should be a listing of hazards facing the community. Depending on the needs of the emergency management or lead planning agency, this listing may or may not be prioritized. An example of Durham County's (N.C.) HVA, excerpted from the county's 2001 Emergency Operations Plan, is presented in Box 17-2.[5]

As mentioned earlier in this chapter, the HVA is the foundation for the community's integrated emergency management activities, such as creation of plans, preparedness activities, hazard mitigation programs, and recovery plan development.

BOX 17-2   EXAMPLE OF DURHAM COUNTY'S HVA PLAN

Durham County is exposed to many hazards, all of which have the potential to disrupt the community, cause damage, and create casualties. Potential hazards (natural, technological, and national security) are:
a.   Major Fires
b.   Floods/Dam Failure
c.   Tornadoes/Severe Thunderstorms
d.   Severe Winter Storms
e.   Hurricanes
f.   Power Failure
g.   Drought
h.   Earthquake
i.   Mass Casualty/Fatality
j.   Hazardous Material
k.   Fixed Nuclear Facility (Ingestion pathway)
l.   National Security Emergency
m.   Civil Disorder
n.   Sabotage/Terrorism
o.   Aircraft Crash (Civilian/Military)
p.   Severe Bridge Damage
q.   Public Utility Damage (Phone, Electricity, Water, Sewer, etc.)

Threat Assessments

A subset of the community HVA that is receiving increased emphasis is the terrorism-specific vulnerability assessment (or threat assessment) tool.

Although a threat assessment appears similar to a community HVA in format and process, the threat assessment differs in several ways. For example, the threat assessment focuses only on the effects of malicious activities or persons on the community (versus all hazards). More sophisticated threat assessments actually look at the consequences of these malicious acts on specific targets, such as infrastructure, critical function areas, symbolic targets, or even special events (e.g., concerts). Threat assessments also are typically performed by law enforcement officials (versus a multidisciplinary team).

An excellent discussion of the terrorism vulnerability assessment process is provided in *Risk Management Series: Reference Manual to Mitigate Potential Terrorist Attacks Against Buildings*.[6] Other good examples of terrorism threat assessments are the North Carolina Department of Agriculture & Consumer Services' Terrorism Threat Vulnerability Self Assessment Tool[7] and the Pennsylvania Municipal Police Officer's Education and Training Commission's Vulnerability Assessment Worksheet.[8]

CONCLUSION

The HVA is a critical step for any community's emergency management activities. It is the HVA that methodically defines the scope and breadth of hazards that may be encountered in the community. Under CEM, hazards identified (and prioritized) by the HVA team will be addressed through a variety of means, including the development of emergency operations and response plans, hazard mitigation programs, and preparedness efforts such as training and drills. Although it is not possible to plan or prepare for every conceivable emergency, the HVA can ensure that plans are developed to deal with higher probability hazards or those with more significant consequences.

A special type of HVA, the threat assessment, focuses on the threat from terrorism or other malicious acts. There are even more specialized versions of these threat assessments that focus on specific utilities, industries, or operations. For example, RAM-W (or Risk Assessment Methodology—Water) is a threat assessment tool developed by Sandia Laboratories that focuses on the terrorism threat to potable water treatment plants.[9]

Healthcare facilities can both contribute to and benefit from the community HVA effort. Hospital administrators and experts may provide expertise to community emergency managers on issues such as mass casualty management, infectious disease consequences, and surge management. At the same time, the community HVA may be used as a basis for external hazards in the healthcare facility's own HVA. For example, if the community HVA identifies mass casualties arising from a hazardous materials event as a probability, this should be reflected in the healthcare facility's HVA. Ultimately, it should be the goal of both community and healthcare facility emergency planners to have a coordinated response to all likely hazards.

REFERENCES

1. Federal Emergency Management Agency. State and Local Guide (SLG) 101: Guide for All-Hazards Emergency Operations Planning. Chapter 2: The Planning Process. Available at: http://www.fema.gov/pdf/rrr/2-ch.pdf.
2. Drabek T. The evolution of emergency management. In: Drabek TE, Hoetmer GJ, eds. *Emergency Management: Principles and Practice for Local Government*. Washington, DC: International City Management Association; 1991:6-8, 10-13, 17-18.
3. The National Lessons Learned & Best Practices Information Network. Emergency Management Programs for Healthcare Facilities: Hazard Vulnerability Analysis: Comparing and Prioritizing Risks. Available at: https://www.llis.dhs.gov/frontpage.cfm.
4. Mitigation and hazard management. In: Drabek TE, Hoetmer GJ, eds. *Emergency Management: Principles and Practice for Local Government*. Washington, DC: International City Management Association; 1991:140-2.
5. Basic Plan. In: *Durham/Durham County Emergency Operations Plan*. Durham, NC: Durham County Emergency Management Agency; 2001:BP-2.
6. Federal Emergency Management Agency. *Risk Management Series: Reference Manual to Mitigate Potential Terrorist Attacks Against Buildings*. FEMA publication 426. Washington, DC: Government Printing Office; December 2003. Available at: http://www.fema.gov/pdf/fima/426/fema426.pdf.
7. North Carolina Department of Agriculture & Consumer Services. Terrorism Threat Vulnerability Self Assessment Tool. Available at: http://www.ncagr.com/BioTerror_Assessment.htm.
8. Municipal Police Officers' Education and Training Commission. Vulnerability Assessment Worksheet. Available at: www.mpoetc.state.pa.us/mpotrs/cwp/view.asp?a-1133&q-441444
9. Sandia National Laboratories Security Risk Assessment Methodologies Overview. Available at: http://www.sandia.gov/ram/RAM%20Overview%20%20Pres%20 rev1.pdf.

chapter 18

Health Care Facility Hazard and Vulnerability Analysis

James C. Chang, William Gluckman, and Eric S. Weinstein

In 1988 Jan deBoer and colleagues[1] published the first attempt to mathematically score and classify a disaster to be used prospectively during the management of the calamity. A disaster was defined as "a destructive event that caused so many casualties that extraordinary mobilization of medical services was necessary."[1] In the proposed Medical Severity Index of Disasters, the parameters needed to quantify a disaster were the casualty load (number of casualties), the severity of incident (severity of injuries sustained), and the capacity of medical services.[1] Seventeen years later, the importance of determining the impact of a disaster on a healthcare facility (HCF) has heightened because HCFs have become industrial leaders in the community and therefore must be able to swiftly return to normal business functioning. Individual healthcare providers are acutely aware of the business side of their practice while at the bedside, but they are not cognizant of the ramifications that a disruption of normal HCF operations would have on the community. Business and industry emergency management principles for HCFs to accommodate the clinical impact of a disaster are discussed in this chapter.

Disasters are events that cause significant enough damage to disrupt the normal activities or function of a community and overwhelm the local resources. What may be an easily handled event in a large urban city may be a disaster for a rural town. Although disasters are not predictable with any great accuracy, many consequences of disasters can be anticipated as part of a comprehensive emergency management plan that includes a hazard and vulnerability analysis (HVA). The HVA will help HCFs plan for these events and allow them to continue operating while assessing structural and operational damage, acquiring needed essentials, and protecting staff and patients. Much can be learned from business and industry with respect to preparedness.

Although not a new concept in business and industry, an HVA is a component in the development of a hospital disaster plan, as recognized since 2001 by the Joint Commission on Accreditation of Healthcare Organizations (JCAHO). The emergency management standard (EC.4.1) requires hospitals to identify specific procedures in response to a variety of disasters based on an HVA performed by the organization.[2] The HVA will assist in the mitigation and preparedness of the HCF to respond to and then recover from a disaster. A hazard can be any threat that could cause injury; fatality; property, infrastructure, or environmental damage; or impair operations. An HVA is a tool used by emergency management to screen for risk and plan for strategic use of potentially limited resources.

HISTORICAL PERSPECTIVE

Many events have affected HCFs in the past. The future is certain to exhibit challenges as we move into a more technologically advanced society challenged by geopolitical terrorist threats. Hospitals inherently have to be prepared for emergencies. Preparation traditionally was based on informal HVAs and largely dependent on perceived issues. For example, hospitals in northern climates typically planned for adverse winter weather related issues; hospitals in the South planned for hurricanes; and hospitals in Southern California planned for forest and wild land fires and earthquakes. Failure to consider all hazards when developing the facility emergency response plan was a flaw in the informal approach.

Hazard identification relies on the collection of potential emergencies that the HCF or operation could anticipate encountering. This list may be assembled by cause, by location, or by a combination of both criteria. Causes may be divided into the following categories for assessment purposes: naturally derived emergencies, technologically derived emergencies, and manmade emergencies (Box 18-1).

HCFs experience two types of disasters: (1) those internal to the HCF, isolated to the confines of the HCF physical plant, and (2) those occurring external to the HCF that produce direct effects (casualties) and indirect effects (e.g., loss of electricity, supply due to damaged roads). The more common internal disasters are similar to those encountered by business and industry and until recently were not formally considered in an HVA. Milsten's[3] exhaustive review of direct and indirect disasters that hospitals faced from 1977 to March 1997 showed that external and internal disasters are not mutually exclusive.

BOX 18-1 HAZARD IDENTIFICATION

BOX 18-1 HAZARD IDENTIFICATION—cont'd

Natural Events

Drought
Earthquake
Flood
Hurricane (cyclone, typhoon)
Landslide
Severe thunderstorm
Temperature extremes
Tidal wave
Tornado
Wildland fires
Windstorm
Snow/ice storms/blizzard
Volcanic ash
Meteor crashes
Infestation

Technological Events

Aircraft crash
    Medical evacuation helicopter
    Other aviation crash
Loss of medical gases
    Air
    Oxygen
    Nitrogen
    Nitrous oxide
Electrical/power shortage or failure
    Loss of backup generator(s)
Fire: chemical, paper, wood, other
Computer network disruption or loss
Loss of fire alarm, smoke detection
Loss of steam
Food contamination
Pneumatic tube disruption or loss
Food supply interruption
Loss or leak of potable water
Fixed facilities incidents
Loss of suction/vacuum
Loss of fuel oil supply or delivery
Elevator service disruption or loss
Hazardous material release
Structural failure
Natural gas/pipeline disruption
    Noxious fumes
Sewer failure
HVAC failure
    Loss of equipment requiring cooling
    Patient/staff at risk
    Loss of instrumentation (thermostat control/regulation)
Supply chain interruption
Labor dispute
Shortage of labor
Communication failure
    Paging: internal, external
    Emergency medical services or other radio
    Internal HCF telephone
    External telephone
    Cellular phone
    Satellite
Transportation disruption
    Labor dispute
    Roadway/highway incident/blockage

Human Events: With or Without Political, Terrorist, or Criminal Intent

    Mass casualty incidents
    Trauma
    Civil disturbance
    CBRNE*
    Infectious disease
    Foodborne illness

Abduction (infant, child, or adult)
Armed or threatening intruder
Bomb threat
Civil disorder
Forensic admissions
Hostage situation
Violent labor action
VIP visitor
Workplace violence

*Chemical, biological, radiological, nuclear, or high-yield explosive.

This chapter focuses on the HVA for events specific for internal disasters or those that directly occur within the confines of the HCF or indirectly affect the HCF due to consequences of the disaster.

CURRENT PRACTICE

Successful mitigation efforts and effective response plans are based on the best possible knowledge of the HCF's vulnerability in terms of deficiencies in its capacity to provide services, physical weaknesses, and organizational shortcomings in responding to emergencies. The HVA should also highlight and identify strengths within personnel, processes, plans, and other attributes. Past successes during disasters should be revisited to learn best practices, even if these occurred spontaneously due to inventiveness, teamwork, and a strong spirit to succeed.

All HVAs have some degree of subjectivity in their findings because many assumptions are made with regard to the perceived risk and even the level of preparedness if hard data are not available. Use of a multidisciplinary team should be encouraged to ensure a holistic characterization of each hazard and to help minimize the inherent subjectivity of the analysis and skewed or erroneous results. The team should be led by someone familiar with the HVA process and consist of representatives from at least the following areas within the HCF:

- Emergency management
- Security/safety
- Facilities (e.g., engineering, maintenance, information technology, telecommunications)
- Operations (e.g., nursing, medical staff, laboratory, radiology)
- Ancillary services (e.g., materials, food, housekeeping or environmental services)
- Administration
- Finance/business

Community representatives, such as the local emergency manager, fire official, police official, and city manager, can also provide valuable input. Additional members, including the hospital administrator-at-large may be beneficial as long as the group size remains manageable and consensus is achievable within a reasonable amount of time.

Regularly scheduled meetings with a defined agenda and other business-related models will assist the completion and maintenance of the assignment of the HVA team.

Most HVA tools come preloaded with a listing of likely hazards that the developer believes the average HCF could face. It is important that the HVA team begin by reviewing the listing of hazards in the HVA tool to ensure that it is applicable to the facility(s) and comprehensive. The HVA tool should address all possible events regardless of their likelihood. The first step is to "brainstorm" and determine all possible hazards, which can be accomplished with assistance from the county Local Emergency Planning Committee (LEPC) in conjunction with the Office of Emergency Management for both the county and state. The hazards are then classified into categories, as described in Box 18-1.

Risk, or impact, relates to the threat a particular hazard has with respect to the human impact: safety of people (patients and staff); property impact: structure(s) and property; and business impact: the ability to continue operations. Each risk can be assigned a numerical value to allow for a comparison or relative risk. The three types of impacts are averaged, and a score is assigned for each category. This will be important in the overall assessment.

Examples of each category include but are not limited to:[4]

- **Human Impact**
  - Potential for injury or death to staff members
  - Potential for injury or death to visitors
  - Potential for injury, death, or adverse outcomes to patients
- **Property Impact**
  - Damage to the facility (up to and including loss of the facility)
  - Loss of use of the facility
  - Loss of or damage to equipment and/or supplies
  - Costs associated with replacement/repair of the facility, equipment, or services
- **Business Impact**
  - Business interruption
  - Unanticipated costs
  - Loss of revenue (from all causes)
  - Recordkeeping issues (e.g., loss of records, inability to access, compromise of integrity)
  - Employees unable or unwilling to report for work
  - Patients unable to reach the facility
  - Damage to reputation
  - Fines, penalties, and legal costs
  - Future insurance premium increases

The degree of risk may be expressed as a numerical score or verbally with use of terms such as *nonexistent, low, medium, high,* and *catastrophic.* As a consideration, the HVA team may wish to add greater weight to hazards that occur without warning (e.g., tornado strike).

Probability relates to how likely an event is to occur at the facility or affect the facility, based on proximity. This, too, can be assigned a numerical value and is best determined from historical data (e.g., a scale of 1 to 5, with 1 representing a low probability of occurrence and 5 a very high probability of occurrence). Looking back at historical data is critical in making an "educated guess" about the future. This is an assessment of the likelihood of a hazard or emergency occurring and is often described as *improbable, low, medium,* or *high.* Other related factors that may be helpful in assessing or describing probability include the following[5]:

Frequency of occurrence: Obviously, the more frequent the occurrence, the higher the likelihood.
Location of the hazardous event and the region affected: Events that occur proximal to the healthcare facility are more likely to directly (or indirectly) affect the facility, whereas events that occur at some distance may be less likely to affect the HCF.
Seasonal (or other cyclic) variations: Events that occur with some regularity may be presumed to be more probable. Commonplace examples include the occurrence of "influenza season" each fall through the winter and drought and/or floods (location-dependent) associated with El Niño.

Where possible, probability should be based on objective data such as historical archives to learn of local disasters. Equipment failure rates or mean time between failure data should be available to the HVA team. Even maintenance records and expected length of service of equipment may lead to objective data that influence an HVA. Often, however, probability assessments are colored by the prior experiences of HVA team members and recent organizational memory.

Facility preparedness may be expressed explicitly in a separate category or integrated with another element (probability or risk). Intuitively, if the facility is well prepared to deal with an emergency, the impact of the emergency should be lessened. The presence of a preparedness component aids in tracking the organization's preparedness efforts and is a means to decrement HVA scores as preparedness levels increase. Preparedness also should be reported to help determine the need for improvement in areas that have high risk and/or probability. Preparedness may be assigned a numerical value, or it simply may be a listing of what, if any, plans currently exist to address that particular event. It may also represent *resources* and the amount of them available (e.g., a lot, little, or none); resources can be subdivided into internal and external resources. The average of these two is the numerical value for preparedness.

Adding the numerical values of these three components (risk, probability, and preparedness) provides a value. Graphically looking at probability versus impact (Fig. 18-1), one would expect higher sums for those events that fall in the high probability–high impact areas and lower values for those events in the low probability–low impact areas.

For maximum benefit, the HVA should generate a prioritized listing of hazards with sufficient detail to characterize each one. To do this, a means to grade or rank each hazard, vulnerability, risk (consequence), and preparedness level should be considered. This characterization may be qualitative or quantitative; each approach has pros and cons.

Qualitative assessments may be simpler and faster to perform; however, these are often more difficult to fully

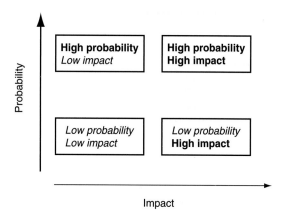

High probability
Low impact

High probability
High impact

Low probability
Low impact

Low probability
High impact

Probability

Impact

FIGURE 18–1. Probability versus impact.

implement in the end. A qualitative analysis may be as simple as having HVA members team rank-order a listing of potential hazards based on their subjective judgment. A slightly more involved approach to qualitative assessment is found in the HVA model provided by the Emergency Management Strategic Healthcare Group (EMSHG) of the Veterans Health Administration. This model uses a scoring system from 0 (not applicable) to 3 (high) for probability and risk (consequence). Any hazard with a score of 2 or greater in either category requires action.[6] Qualitative HVA models often generate little differentiation between hazards and tend to group all hazards into one category (such as "high") or another. These models have little flexibility in implementation and do not help the organization when it is time to determine organizational priorities for emergency planning and/or allocation of resources.

Quantitative assessments can be used to provide additional flexibility in implementation by enhancing the differences between each hazard. Depending on the HVA tool chosen, the scores for each hazard may be the sum or product of probability, risk, and preparedness scores or may be derived from more complex weighting schemes. For example, the HVA model used by Duke University Hospital (Durham, N.C.) takes the sum of the products of the probability of a hazard multiplied by the risk to people, property, and business, and then multiplies the resulting product by a facility preparedness score.

Σ (Probability of Each Event × Risk of Each Event) × Facility Preparedness Score = Weighted Score of Event

See Table 18-1 for an example of the Duke University Hospital HVA.

The end result of the Duke University Hospital and similar quantitative HVA models is weighted scores that address the probability, consequences, and preparedness level of each hazard. The weighted score of the event is then used to order its priority for emergency planning purposes. An institution may choose to address potential emergencies beginning with the highest-scoring event and progress down the list until all potential events are addressed. A variation of this theme may be to address the top five (or other number) high-scoring

events in year one, and presuming completion of planning, preparedness, and/or mitigation activities, address the next five-highest scoring events in year two and so on. A third alternative may be to establish a predefined threshold level; any hazard scenario exceeding this threshold value would require some type of action (i.e., planning, preparedness, mitigation).

Some more sophisticated HVA tools, such as the one developed by the Kaiser Permanente healthcare system, take the quantitative approach one step further by generating scores (percentages) and a graphical/visual output product.[7]

The HVA is the foundation for the organization's emergency management program. It is therefore advantageous to expend the effort and resources to ensure that the job is done properly. The assessors should begin by developing a list of potential emergencies that the organization may face and then characterize each hazard as to its probability and consequence. An automated HVA tool is a significant time saver both as a means to test different scenarios for each hazard and as a documentation aid. Often a quick review of actual disasters, internal and external, that the HCF faced over the past 5 to 10 years is sufficient to commence action by the HVA team.

A systematic and consistent approach is needed. The team leader should ensure that all team members have equal input into the process.

The end product of the HVA should be a prioritized, all-encompassing, objective (to the extent possible) assessment of the possible, potential, or historical internal and external indirect events that may affect the HCF. The HVA produced is the foundation of the HCF's emergency management program. It is used as the basis for planning and budgeting for hazard mitigation, preparedness, and response efforts within the institution. It should be intuitive that emergencies with the highest scores or ranks should be addressed first and lesser items handled as time and funding permit.

An annual review and revalidation of the HVA should be performed to ensure that changes to the operating environment of the facility are assessed for their impact on the facility's emergency management program. Another reason for periodically reassessing the HVA is to reflect the benefit of hazard mitigation and preparedness activities. For example, as hospital preparedness activities reduce the risk (and consequences) of an emergency, such as a power failure, the item may be moved down on the list of priorities and other more pressing items may be moved up.

As a final consideration, the HVA work product (including drafts and working papers) should be considered a sensitive document and protected to the same degree as a patient record or a peer review, quality assurance/improvement, or sensitive business document. Remember that the HVA details the organization's vulnerabilities, and depending on the format used and level of supporting documentation maintained, may describe how the facility will respond to an emergency. In the wrong hands, this information may actually increase a facility's vulnerability to attack, and for this reason, it should not be freely disseminated (e.g., placed on the Internet). Contact the Interagency OPSEC Support Staff

TABLE 18-1 SAMPLE HVA

TYPE OF EMERGENCY	PROBABILITY RATING	HUMAN IMPACT	PROPERTY IMPACT	BUSINESS IMPACT	IMPACT RATING	INTERNAL RESOURCES	EXTERNAL RESOURCES	RESOURCE RATING	TOTAL*	EMERGENCY PLANS IN PLACE?
	High Low	High Impact		Low Impact		Few Resources	Many Resources			
Score	5 ⟵⟶ 1	5 ⟵⟶ 1				5 ⟵⟶ 1				
Technological Events										
Electrical failure	3	1	3	1	1.7	2	2	2.0	6.7	
Transportation failure	2	1	1	2	1.3	3	2	2.5	5.8	
Fuel shortage	2	1	1	1	1.0	1	1	1.0	4.0	
Natural gas failure	2	1	1	1	1.0	2	1	1.5	4.5	
Water failure/ contamination	3	1	1	1	1.0	3	3	3.0	7.0	
Sewer failure	2	1	1	1	1.0	3	3	3.0	6.0	
Steam failure	2	1	1	1	1.0	3	3	3.0	6.0	
Fire alarm failure	3	1	1	1	1.0	3	1	2.0	6.0	
Communications failure	5	3	3	3	3.0	2	2	2.0	10.0	
Medical gas failure	2	2	1	1	1.3	2	2	2.0	5.3	
Medical vacuum failure	2	3	1	1	1.7	2	2	2.0	5.7	
HVAC failure	3	2	1	2	1.7	2	2	2.0	6.7	
Information systems failure	3	3	3	3	3.0	2	2	2.0	8.0	
Fire, internal	4	4	4	4	4.0	2	1	1.5	9.5	
Hazardous materials exposure, internal	4	2	1	2	1.7	3	1	2.0	7.7	
Unavailability of supplies	3	1	1	2	1.3	2	2	2.0	6.3	
Structural damage	2	2	2	2	2.0	4	2	3.0	7.0	
Natural Events										
Hurricane	3	3	3	4	3.3	2	2	2.0	8.3	
Tornado	2	1	3	2	2.0	2	2	2.0	6.0	
Severe thunderstorms	4	2	2	2	2.0	2	2	2.0	8.0	
Snow fall	5	2	1	3	2.0	2	2	2.0	9.0	
Ice storm	4	3	2	3	2.7	2	2	2.0	8.7	
Earthquake	2	1	3	1	1.7	2	2	2.0	5.7	
Tidal wave	1	1	2	1	1.3	2	2	2.0	4.3	
Temperature extremes	4	2	1	1	1.3	1	1	1.0	6.3	
Drought	3	2	2	2	2.0	2	2	2.0	7.0	
Flood, external	2	3	2	3	2.7	2	2	2.0	6.7	
Wild fire	2	1	1	1	1.0	1	1	1.0	4.0	
Landslide	1	1	1	1	1.0	1	1	1.0	3.0	
Volcano	1	1	1	1	1.0	1	1	1.0	3.0	
Epidemic	3	2	1	4	2.3	2	2	2.0	7.3	
Human Events										
Mass casualty incident (trauma)	5	4	1	4	3.0	3	3	3.0	11.0	

Continued

TABLE 18-1 SAMPLE HVA—cont'd

TYPE OF EMERGENCY	PROBABILITY RATING	HUMAN IMPACT	PROPERTY IMPACT	BUSINESS IMPACT	IMPACT RATING	INTERNAL RESOURCES	EXTERNAL RESOURCES	RESOURCE RATING	TOTAL*	EMERGENCY PLANS IN PLACE?
Mass casualty incident (medical)	5	4	1	4	3.0	3	3	3.0	11.0	
Mass casualty incident (hazardous materials)	4	3	1	4	2.7	3	3	3.0	9.7	
Terrorism, chemical	5	5	1	5	3.7	3	3	3.0	11.7	
Terrorism, biological	5	5	1	5	3.7	3	3	3.0	11.7	
Terrorism, nuclear	5	5	3	5	4.3	3	3	3.0	12.3	
Accidental, chemical	4	5	1	5	3.7	3	3	3.0	10.7	
Accidental, biological	1	5	1	5	3.7	3	3	3.0	7.7	
Accidental, nuclear	1	5	3	5	4.3	3	3	3.0	8.3	
VIP situation	3	1	1	1	1.0	2	2	2.0	6.0	
Infant abduction	2	4	1	3	2.7	2	2	2.0	6.7	
Hostage situation	3	3	1	3	2.3	3	2	2.5	7.8	
Civil disturbance	5	2	2	3	2.3	2	2	2.0	9.3	
Labor action	3	1	1	3	1.7	2	2	2.0	6.7	
Forensic admission	4	1	1	1	1.0	2	2	2.0	7.0	
Bomb threat	5	2	1	2	1.7	2	2	2.0	8.7	

Total* is the sum of the probability, impact rating, and resource rating.

(IOSS) (www.ioss.gov) for operational security program development guidance, training courses, and consultative support.[8]

PITFALLS

A typical pitfall is underestimating the time required to develop an HVA and not allowing sufficient time to adequately complete the evaluation. In a large facility in a complex urban environment, an HVA may be a multiday process. A related pitfall is the gradual decline in interest as the evaluation progresses; the amount of time spent on each topic is typically directly related to how long the team has been working. Most assessments begin with an extremely thorough discussion of hazards and decline rapidly to more cursory examinations as the day progresses.

It is sometimes necessary to reiterate the sole purpose of the HVA—that is, the development of a prioritized listing of hazards to be addressed in the hospital's emergency planning process. It is not uncommon for representatives of a particular service or group to consider any mention of a hazard in their area as a personal affront. Care should be taken to ensure that this bias does not cause hazards to be arbitrarily dismissed with an "it'll never happen here" attitude.

HVAs are important in a well-designed disaster plan and thus need to be updated on a regular basis.

Geographic and industrial changes will affect a hospital and need to be considered. The establishment of a new chemical company in town, for instance, may make a significant change in an institution's assessment of hazardous materials threat.

Another problem, sometimes referred to as the "paper plan syndrome," gives the illusion of true preparedness simply because a written document exists. "Disaster planning is an illusion unless: It is based on valid assumptions about human behavior, incorporates an inter-organizational perspective, is tied to resources, and is known and accepted by the participants."[9]

CONCLUSION

In today's resource-constrained healthcare environment, it is not realistic to plan for every conceivable hazard or eventuality that may befall the institution. Healthcare administrators need to allocate their limited resources to ensure that likely scenarios are addressed promptly, whereas the "one-in-a-million" occurrences may be held in abeyance until some later date. The HVA is a tool for HCF administrators to systematically assess and characterize the plethora of hazards that their facility may face. Failure to exercise due diligence when conducting the HVA may have adverse consequences, ranging from professional embarrassment on the part of the emergency management coordinator to loss of life, business interruption, damage to reputation, and litigation from inadequate emergency planning. Proper use of the HVA helps minimize these risks.

REFERENCES

1. deBoer J, Brismar B, Eldar R, et al. The medical severity index of disasters. *J Emerg Med.* 1989;7:269-73.
2. Joint Commission on Accreditation of Healthcare Organizations. Available at: http://www.jcaho.org/.
3. Milsten A. Hospital responses to acute-onset disasters: a review. *Prehospital Disaster Med.* 2000;15(1):32-45.
4. The National Lessons Learned & Best Practices Information Network. Emergency Management Programs for Healthcare Facilities: Hazard Vulnerability Analysis: Comparing and Prioritizing Risks. Available at: https://www.llis.dhs.gov/frontpage.cfm.
5. The National Lessons Learned & Best Practices Information Network. Emergency Management Programs for Healthcare Facilities: Hazard Vulnerability Analysis: Identifying Potential Disasters and Probability. Available at: https://www.llis.dhs.gov/frontpage.cfm.
6. Emergency Management Strategic Healthcare Group, Veterans Health Administration. Section 3.10.3-Hazard Vulnerability Analysis (HVA) Instructions. Available at: http://www1.va.gov/emshg/apps/emp/emp/hva_instructions.htm.
7. California Emergency Medical Services Authority. Kaiser Permanente Medical Center Hazard and Vulnerability Analysis. Available at: http://www.emsa.ca.gov/dms2/kp_hva.xls.
8. Interagency OPSEC Support Staff. Available at: http://www.ioss.gov/.
9. Auf der Heide E. Disaster Response: Principles of Preparation and Coordination. Chapter 3. Available at: http://orgmail2.coe-dmha.org/dr/DisasterResponse.nsf/section/03?opendocument.

chapter 19

Public Information Management

Sharon Dilling, William Gluckman, Marc S. Rosenthal, and Eric S. Weinstein

In the chaos and craziness that ensues during or immediately after a disaster, whether it is a suspected contagious disease, an earthquake, or the explosion of a dirty bomb, there will be two constants: (1) the public will demand information about what is happening and (2) the media will be at the scene trying to tell them. Ever since images from Vietnam broadcast live into the living rooms of millions of Americans, the public has come to see breaking news coverage not only as a given, but as their *right*. The thirst for information grows with every passing minute, fueled by the ever-increasing competition within the media for advertising, sponsorship, and viewers. All of this factors heavily into disaster response. Balancing emergency care for the sick or injured with the need to disseminate accurate public information is always a challenge. Emergency responders would never think of treating a patient without having the proper medical training. Training for disaster communication is also highly important—preparation is the key. Understanding what types of information the public and the media will want and need will help mitigate the effects of the disaster, win the confidence of the media, and reassure the public. Information presented in a clear and truthful manner within a reasonable amount of time will further its effectiveness.

MEDIA HISTORY

The development of the printing press in the 15th century allowed inexpensively produced newspapers and books to spread information to large numbers of people.[1] When Marconi sent a wireless message in 1896, radio came alive, allowing electronic communication during World War I.[2] The newsreel brought edited pictures of World War II to moviegoers, albeit somewhat delayed. In the 1950s the "American dream" turned out to be a television as the centerpiece of every living room. By the 1960s, nearly all of America tuned in to watch the son of President John Fitzgerald Kennedy salute the flag-draped coffin of his father. Walter Cronkite became "the most trusted man in America." And, of course, there was the Vietnam War. Television coverage has arguably changed the course of history by providing a window into the harsh realities of war that had never been seen before by most of America.

By the late 20th century, new media outlets developed, offering 24-hour-a-day news coverage, as cable television proliferated America. A few years later, as a new millennium approached, the Internet and e-mail revolutionized communication, allowing information to travel rapidly right to the desktop. This, coupled with the competitive news business, created even more demand by both the public and the media for up-to-the-minute communication. This urgency for information has surpassed accuracy and even, in some cases, reason. In 1994, millions tuned in to watch a white Ford Bronco with O.J. Simpson inside drive down a freeway. And then there was Sept. 11, 2001. The television images could not be edited to shelter viewers. They unfolded in real time, with real heartache. The world watched again and again with the hope of somehow hitting the pause button to allow the victims an additional moment or two of peaceful existence. Viewers tuned in for days, hoping to see people emerge alive from the burning rubble. News coverage was 24 hours a day for almost two weeks. Regular programming was preempted, and viewers struggled to come to terms with what had happened. As sad as it was, this horrific tragedy is a good example of what is expected of emergency response and public information.

MEDIA AND DISASTERS

The medical management of disasters, both small and large, requires a multifaceted response to ensure timely evacuation, assessment, treatment, and recovery. This response, usually based on the Incident Command System (ICS), requires the appointment of an incident commander, a logistics chief, and others. One important and often overlooked component of the ICS and disaster management in general is an area defined as *public information management*. The ability to provide appropriate, timely information can significantly affect the disaster response.

The components of public information management include not only the release of information to prepare rescue workers and volunteers, but the dynamic ongoing release of information to the media and the incorporation of the media within the response mission. Effective interaction with the media can improve the accurate distribution of information that ultimately aids the response, while at the same time satisfying the needs of the media to "get the story." This applies not only to hospitals or other institutions providing support in a disaster, but also to the rapid response elements (e.g., police, fire, and emergency medical services [EMS]) and to intermediate response organizations, such as the National Disaster Medical System's disaster medical assistance teams, the U.S. Department of Health and Human Services' Medical Reserve Corps, and the Federal Emergency Management Agency, to name a few.

During a disaster, potentially significant amounts of information should be communicated to the region affected to achieve a good response. This information provides the basis for management of the disaster as well as development of the public trust in the responsible agencies. For example, if a government frequently notifies the population of potential storms and their need to evacuate immediately, and subsequently, each storm causes insignificant damage, the population will learn to not trust the local government. If a category 5 hurricane then heads to this same region, the population may not heed requests to evacuate because they have been misled many times before and may not believe the local government or disaster coordinators. However, if the local government warns residents of only potentially dangerous storms and only requests evacuation for events that most likely will cause significant damage and injuries, while providing the details behind its decisions, the population will more likely respond to an evacuation request and, therefore, injuries and loss of life will be reduced. Obviously, the decision to warn or request evacuations is not just dependent on actual risks, but also on potential legal action or bad publicity should the disaster be worse than expected.

Further, immediately after an event, those who evacuated or had interests in the area will want to access the affected area to find family members, recover personal items, and assess the damage so that they may start to rebuild or repair. They will depend on information provided by functioning public communications systems. If this recovery action by those affected is not coordinated in a timely manner, people returning to the affected area can hamper appropriate response efforts and hinder response communications. For example, cellular phone towers may become overloaded with users and, therefore, important phone calls are not able to be placed. Providing re-entry instructions contained in the evacuation order and subsequent evacuation instructions is the best strategy. Phone numbers, radio stations, Web sites, and other means to provide timely and accurate information to those returning to an evacuated area will reduce anxiety, potential traffic jams, and the overuse of the limited resources of response agencies that will have to divert their focus to communication to an uninformed population searching for information. Finally, information about sources of food, potable water, medical care, cash, shelters and housing, fuel, and available government assistance needs to be communicated to the residents returning to the affected area.

Effective management of information can help minimize property loss and reduce the chance of injuries, even deaths, but also can improve the effectiveness of response teams. To do this, methods need to be developed to communicate information to the population from one reliable, consistent source. Disasters do not just include the typical natural occurrence (e.g., flooding, hurricane, tornado) or manmade acts (e.g., industrial accident or terrorism) but also include loss of infrastructure (e.g., computer information systems, power grids, potable water, sewers, job action). Even though a disaster may not result in any injuries or fatalities, the fact that "something" went wrong brings the problem into the public eye. In such cases, the news media become interested and so do the government and public. The handling of the incident by the "offending" corporation or entity (1) can provide for a good public relations (PR) review and minimize the PR effect of the disaster, or (2) if poor PR ensues, can make the disaster more significant and potentially harm the corporation.

CURRENT PRACTICES

When a disaster strikes, media flood into the area. Be prepared to share your space. As word of the planes crashing into the two World Trade Center towers and the Pentagon spread, firefighters, police, and rescuers rushed to the scene. Not far behind were reporters, photographers, and camera crews. Tune into the local television station near where a hurricane is headed and undoubtedly reporters donning bright yellow rain slickers will be broadcasting from an evacuated beachfront while waves crash around them and lightning lights up the seas. Turn on the radio to hear broadcasters coughing out their report as the smoke of a nearby wildfire burns brush just steps away. Pick up a newspaper to learn how a reporter interviewed a family as they crouched in a storm cellar with a tornado blowing overhead.

Accepting media presence at events is important. Reporters will not go away, so it is best to help them find their way to a place that is close enough to the action to satisfy their needs, yet far enough away to prevent them from broadening the crisis by becoming a victim, or worse, placing emergency personnel at risk. When the media shift into crisis mode, they will broadcast whatever information they have in the order in which they receive it.[3] Providing factual information to the media will allow one to effectively control the information instead of the information being in control. Reporters may or may not have time to verify the information, but they would rather report something than have nothing to report. If they have nothing to report, they probably will speculate. When the *New York Post* went to press with its July 6, 2004, headline, "Kerry's Choice," they declared Dick Gephardt as presidential candidate John Kerry's running mate. Kerry announced his choice of John Edwards for vice president that same morning. The debacle mirrored the infamous 1948 *Chicago Daily Tribune* headline, "Dewey Defeats Truman." In the Gephardt case, the already tarnished reputation of the *Post* took a hit, and the Kerry campaign benefited from the exposure.[4] Although a mistake by the media can hardly be deemed a crisis, it clearly illustrates the pressure that time and competition weigh on the media. In most instances, it is best to offer some information, even a small amount, to the media as long as it is correct.

Provide the media with factual information as soon as possible; even small or minor details or known truths can be helpful. The first source often becomes the most credible. Also, remember to demonstrate empathy when providing information.[5] In the immediate aftermath of the destruction of the World Trade Center towers, New York City Mayor Rudy Giuliani spoke to the people of New York and the nation. He provided very little new information, but he told what he knew and demonstrated empathy—that he was grieving, too. "The number of casualties," he said, "will be more than any of us can bear."[6] This was not an unknown fact, and it most certainly was not a new piece of information. Giuliani had never been known for his compassion, and his behavior after the World Trade Center disaster was a turning point in his career, making him arguably the most popular mayor in the city's history.

Be honest. The truth almost always comes out anyway. There are numerous instances throughout history in which an initially dishonest action was forgiven by the public after the truth was told. If one shares inaccurate information and later the information is determined to be false, all credibility will be lost.

Time and space in the media are money. When a newspaper is put together, the first pieces to go in are the advertisements. Articles fill in the spaces around them. Space is at a premium. Select words wisely. Studies have shown that the average level of reading comprehension is at grade 6. If the message is targeted to a sixth-grader, the majority of the population will understand it; however, keep the audience in mind and adjust accordingly. For television, the rule of 27/9/3 is extremely helpful. Developed by Dr. Vincent Covello of the Center for Risk Communication, this rule suggests keeping messages to 27 words, 9 seconds, and 3 ideas or concepts for maximum comprehension.[7]

Media may not always be a friend, but they do not have to be an enemy.[3] The media have a job to do, just like those who respond to a disaster. The media may play an essential role in communicating to the public during a disaster situation by offering evacuation routes, safety tips, or other important advice. Keeping the media up-to-date in an emergency is essential and should not be overlooked. Failure to provide frequent updates may result in the media using any means to get closer to the scene to get the information firsthand or going to possibly less-reliable sources. Make the media a friend, and let them relay the information you provide, as opposed to what someone else provides.

"Hope for the best but prepare for the worst" is a very applicable cliché concerning the need to have prepared public information systems in place before a disaster. Current practice for emergency preparation is to plan and drill response. This should always include testing the public information component.[8]

Medical/EMS/Fire Models

Disasters occur frequently, ranging from bus accidents with 10 to 20 injured persons, to hazardous material events requiring local evacuation, to regional incidents such as hurricanes. In all of these cases, the local community or larger region enters a disaster mode as the resources needed are greater than one segment can provide. EMS must redirect ambulances and rescue vehicles, hospital emergency departments must prepare for casualties, and government provides resources for scene control and forensic investigation, with preservation of evidence balanced with response and recovery. All of this must occur while the daily standard delivery of healthcare and maintenance of law and order are maintained and the community infrastructure is preserved. The totality of the response is dependent on the size of the disaster and the numbers affected with the dynamic match of available resources, supplies, and the specific demands.

Many events happen simultaneously during the early stages of a disaster response: EMS/fire/police personnel are dispatched to the event and use an incident management system. Bystanders render aid, or as the word spreads, people arrive who may be able to help, but more than likely, they are not suitable responders. Plans should be made for this convergent volunteerism because it cannot be avoided (this is explored in other chapters of this text).[9] Local emergency management representatives should work with local media to prevent a situation in which the media take it upon themselves to call emergency responders for help before the responders get direction from their office. If the media are asked to communicate a call for help, specific emergency personnel, upon arrival to the disaster scene, can then be directed to a gathering place and then directed to their duty station. Management of volunteers can consume precious resources away from critical aspects of a timely response. By reporting certain types of information, the media can fulfill an important role in assisting healthcare providers travel to their workplace, ensuring that any response teams are directed to their prearranged muster stations, and helping in prevention of injuries to unnecessary volunteers. The media responding to an event must also be directed to a location that enables them to accurately report while being kept safe.

In addition, it must be recognized that each response unit from various government and nongovernment agencies will have differing perspectives based on their interpretation of the dynamics of the event guiding their management or role. Unfortunately, all these views can diverge and provide a confusing and inconsistent picture of events, simply due to each unit's perspective and underlying knowledge base. Caution must follow because each unit or members of each unit may be approached separately by members of the media and innocently provide inconsistent information. This can lead to misperception and loss of public trust. Further, if such misperception is acted upon by members of the command and control system, this may lead to disruption of the disaster response. Such misinformation may be a direct consequence of the real-time reporting that often occurs around disaster scenes. With media at the scene reporting in real time but missing vital elements or reporting unsubstantiated information, decisions can be rendered that can interfere with the dynamic response and recovery or divert resources, triggered by political expediency or a microphone held in someone's face under bright lights.

Effect of Media Reports

A new area of media interaction related to disaster medicine is how the public responds to news reports and images that have the potential to induce posttraumatic stress disorder (PTSD).[10] It has been reported that there is increased incidence of PTSD with intense coverage of an event, especially one associated with many images. This was reported to be especially true with the pediatric population.[11] The authors believe that intense exposure to significant events, such as the World Trade Center disaster, is associated with psychopathology.[12]

Media Communication

Several studies have looked at the public's response to uncertainty. These results can have implications on how the public will respond to media communications. One study found that a majority of respondents prefer ranges of risk estimates because they believe that these ranges makes the government look more honest. However, about half just want to know whether an area is safe or unsafe. Finally, disagreement among scientists about risk, even if a majority has one opinion, tends to result in the public assuming the worst. The implications of this reinforce the need for one spokesperson for a disaster response.[13] Other studies looking at risk communication have provided goals for risk communication that could also apply to disaster communication, especially before the event. These are building trust, raising awareness, education, agreement, and motivating action. Before a hurricane or another major disaster, the development of these goals will help foster action by the community. The media become the vehicle for the communication of these goals and needs to work with the public information officer (PIO) and responsible organization to develop them.[14]

Detroit Free Press Example

The media are also concerned with safety and minimizing interference with the relief effort. The *Detroit Free Press* requests that their reporters and photographers work as teams. These teams are allowed to do whatever is needed to get a story as long as they feel comfortable or safe, obviously a very large leeway for the reporter. The teams are expected to be as inconspicuous as possible and to identify themselves to responsible agencies, including the police, to reduce potential problems. Reporters and their editors want to publish information that they believe is accurate, timely, and has been verified with multiple sources, if possible. They prefer to verify information with at least two, but preferably three, sources. In addition, they have deadlines that must be met. Finally, these teams are willing to help responsible agencies to disseminate information as long as they have access (T. Fladung, managing editor, *Detroit Free Press*, private communication, 2004).

Lessons from Recent Disasters

Multiple disasters have occurred within the last 10 to 15 years that provide a glimpse into the *do's* and *don'ts* of public information management. These events have stemmed from airplane and train disasters, earthquakes, and terrorist actions. In each case, lessons learned have improved disaster response and have shown the importance of public information management.

Tokyo Sarin Attack, 1995

On March 20, 1995, Tokyo experienced a nerve gas poisoning attack with sarin. The first patient from this attack arrived at the hospital before ambulances began delivering patients. Approximately 2.5 hours after the event, the first press conference was held at one hospital, and the first televised news announcement was made 3 hours after the attack. At this point, most patients had reported to a local medical facility. In addition, there was no initial report to the population from an official source until after all patients had left the scene. In this case, the media notification and distribution of information from an official were late, but the information after the initial conference was consistent.[15]

Oklahoma City Bombing, 1995

On April 19, 1995, a terrorist action caused an explosion that destroyed the Murrah Federal Building in Oklahoma City. The blast was felt by many in the local area and was reported by news networks very quickly. The local emergency departments (EDs) immediately became fully staffed; many medical personnel immediately offered their services to local EDs, and as the departments became staffed, personnel decided to go directly to the explosion site and provide freelance medical care and rescue efforts. In addition to the local response, the local media, without notification or request, directed those with medical training to go to the federal building to provide care. This resulted in more than 300 volunteers at the site. Even though volunteers provided evacuation assistance, the site was unsafe and the responders did not have protective gear; as a result, one volunteer died from falling debris.[16]

Some of the lessons learned from this disaster included how to request that additional healthcare providers go to their respective facilities and how to prevent untrained and superfluous volunteers from converging on the scene. If the need for additional support arises at the incident location, the incident management commander can request this through emergency management channels. The media can then receive a specific request for specific volunteers to be directed to a gathering, muster, or staging area for credentialing, briefing, equipping, and transportation assignments. The receiving medical facilities can then, either by direct communication or preexisting disaster protocols, have their requests met through proper channels and be prepared for the additional healthcare professionals, limiting resources dedicated to incorporate them into the existing staff. The media should be informed early in a disaster of set expectations of their role, any boundaries placed on them, and how they could potentially hinder the response and recovery. This partnership should be communicated to the public to build public trust. In addition, if the incident management team does not want bystanders because of safety concerns, this should also be conveyed to the media so that they might communicate this information to the public.

PITFALLS OF MANAGING PUBLIC INFORMATION

Managing the flow of information in a crisis or disaster is no small task. There are, however, 10 common pitfalls to be avoided.

Failing to Bring in Experts

Emergency responders are supposed to respond to emergencies: physicians are supposed to take care of sick or injured patients, search and rescue teams are called in to look for trapped individuals, and firefighters battle fires. When a disaster occurs, be it large or small, an expert who can speak about it effectively should be summoned.

This is not to say that a firefighter is not the best spokesperson at the scene; it means that anyone speaking to the media, or formally to the public, should have some basic public information officer training.[3] In a large-scale disaster, it is strongly recommend to have a designated key spokesperson. There are training programs available through the Centers for Disease Control and Prevention, the Federal Emergency Management Agency, and a number of private companies that specialize in crisis and risk communication.

Avoid Using Complex Language or Jargon[17]

In a crisis situation, the listening skills of people involved are highly challenged. They often do not hear correctly, are overcome with emotion, and are experiencing high anxiety. Additionally, audiences in a crisis may vary in their level of education and comprehension. A best practice guideline is to target communications to the reading level of a sixth-grader.[17] Try to keep information clear, succinct, and to the point. Do not use acronyms or abbreviations because they may confuse the public.

Avoid Arguing, Fighting, or Losing Your Temper

Disasters by nature are stressful. It is difficult to remain calm when dealing with situations that involve extensive loss of life or property. Often, disaster workers go without proper rest for long periods, and it is easy for tempers to flare. When speaking to the public or a reporter, remaining calm is the key. Do not be afraid to politely end a conversation if it becomes heated or uncomfortable. Reporters almost always win an argument; they have the editor on their side. Offer a succinct and truthful

response for best results, and stay on your message.[8] Repeat your main idea as many times as necessary. Do not deviate from your main message or key points.

Do Not Predict

Often, questions about what will happen next will be asked after a crisis. Unless one arrives on-scene with a working crystal ball, these kinds of questions should not be answered. No one can predict the future. Reassure the public that every effort is being made to mitigate the crisis or that the best possible care is being offered.[18]

It Is OK to Say, "I Don't Know"

Do not answer a question that you are not qualified to answer. In fact, when offering information to the public, be prepared to repeat the information you do know several times in several different ways. Admitting you are not qualified to answer a specific question and suggesting someone who can may even add to your credibility.[7]

Failing to Show Empathy

Empathy or sensitivity is essential in disaster communication. Whereas many first responders or healthcare providers often emotionally detach themselves from a crisis situation, public information officers cannot. The most effective communicator is one who cares.[7]

Lying, Clouding the Truth, or Covering Up

History has shown us, from Watergate to the Monica Lewinsky scandal to the legal woes of Martha Stewart, that it is often not the initial incident that is the problem, but rather the cover-up. Never cover up or hide information. In this day and age of e-mail, cellular phones, and up-to-the-minute communication, the information is almost always going to get out. Of course, discretion and good judgment are factors, but avoid lying or blatant cover-ups.

Not Responding Quickly

Slow and steady do not win the race in a disaster response, be it rescuing the injured or communicating the issues.[18] Respond quickly and thoughtfully. Also, be sure to be accurate and truthful.

Not Responding at All

The infamous words "no comment" bring chills to experienced PIOs everywhere. There is almost always something better to say than "no comment." Some suggestions include, "I don't know," or "I'll get back to you with an answer to that question." The main thing to remember when tempted to respond with "no comment" is that this refrain instantly makes the speaker sound as if something is being hidden or there is something dishonest about what is happening. Always remember what can be commented on and offer that instead, even if it does not answer what the reporter asked.

Failing to Practice Emergency Communications

Schools practice fire drills. Communities practice evacuations. Hospitals drill for emergency response. Communications should be an essential part of any drill. Practice is the key to success when a real disaster hits. Allow the information officer to participate in scheduled exercises, and ask local media to attend. Work with them in advance so that they may provide a more realistic scenario with the stresses that come along with the reporting of a major event.[8]

The key to managing public information is to be prepared, respond quickly with accurate information, and show empathy.

CONCLUSION

Good disaster management provides for a mass communication system with appropriate information. The goal of this system is to establish relationships between the response agencies, the media, and the public. A major underpinning for success is accurate and timely information to the public.[19] The media can be a friend or foe. Mutual respect for each other will generally result in better cooperation and a smoother interaction. The provision of timely and accurate information will help keep reporters from searching for unreliable facts. The media most likely will not be the cause of any panic. Any panic by the population will be based on the incident, not the reporting of it.[20] It is recommended for organizations that may have to deal with the media to have a media policy in place before an event. In addition, a representative or PIO is needed on-site. The media also do not just want facts, but human interest stories. Establish procedures to allow responders to tell their story: highlight outstanding efforts or acts of heroism and then notify the media.[21] PIOs should consider predeveloped news release forms and develop a contact list for the area and a list of "experts" to call on to explain the situation to the public and reporters.[22] Even though the media can be intrusive, they also can disseminate accurate information as well as advice or warnings.[23] Recommend that the media assist in providing accurate information to the public. Before events, have the media participate in disaster drills and network with organization leaders for disaster events.[24]

REFERENCES

1. McLuhan M. *The Gutenberg Galaxy.* Toronto: University of Toronto Press; 1962.
2. Weightman G. *Signor Marconi's Magic Box: The Most Remarkable Invention of the 19th Century and the Amateur Inventor Whose Genius Sparked a Revolution.* New York: DeCapo Press; 2003.
3. Society for Healthcare Strategy and Market Development. *Crisis Communications in Healthcare: Managing Difficult Times Effectively.* Chicago: 2002.
4. Colford P. Another Post Exclusive. *New York Daily News.* July 7, 2004.
5. Emergency Management Laboratory of the Oak Ridge Institute for Science and Education. *Emergency Public Information Pocket Guide.* Oak Ridge, TN; May, 2001.
6. Pooley E. Time Magazine Person of the Year 2001: Mayor of the World. *Time Magazine.* Dec. 31, 2001.
7. Covello VT. *Risk Communication.* New York: Center for Risk Communication/Consortium for Risk and Crisis Communication Slides; 2004.
8. Reynolds B, Hunter-Galdo J, Sokler L. *Crisis and Emergency Risk Communication.* Atlanta: Centers for Disease Control and Prevention; 2002.
9. Cone DC, Weir SD, Bogucki S. Convergent volunteerism. *Ann Emerg Med.* 2003;41:457-62.
10. Njenga FD, Nyamai C, Kigamwa P. Terrorist bombing at the USA embassy in Nairobi: the media response. *East African Med.* 2003;80(3):159-64.
11. Pfefferbaum B, Seale TW, Brandt EN Jr, et al. Media exposure in children one hundred miles from a terrorist bombing. *Ann Clin Psychiatry.* 2003;15(1):1-8.
12. J Ahern, Galea S, Resnick H, et al. Television images and psychological symptoms after the September 11 terrorist attacks. *Psychiatry.* 2002;65(4):289-300.
13. Johnson BB. Further notes on public response to uncertainty in risks and science. *Risk Analysis.* 2003;23(4):781-9.
14. Bier VM. On the state of the art: risk communication to the public. *Reliability Engineering System Safety.* 2001;71:139-50.
15. Okumura T, Suzuki K, Fukuda A, et al. The Tokyo subway sarin attack: disaster management, part 2: hospital response. *Acad Emerg Med.* 1998;5:618-24.
16. Maningas PA, Robison M, Mallonee S. The EMS response to the Oklahoma City Bombing. *Prehospital Disaster Med.* 1997;12(2):9-14.
17. Covello VT. Best practices in public health risk and crisis communication. *J Health Communication.* 2003;8:5-8.
18. Sandman PM. Anthrax, Bioterrorism, and Risk Communication: Guidelines for Action. Presented at: Centers for Disease Control and Prevention; November 20, 2001; Atlanta.
19. Quarantelli EL. Ten criteria for evaluating the management of community disasters. *Disasters.* 1997;21(1):39-56.
20. Garrett L. Understanding media's response to epidemics. *Public Health Reports.* 2001;116(suppl 2):87-91.
21. Anzur T. How to talk to the media: televised coverage of public health issues in a disaster. *Prehospital Disaster Med.* 2000;15(4)196-8.
22. Allison EJ. Media relations at major response situations. *JEMS.* December 1984; 39-42.
23. Auf der Heide E, Lafond R, et al. Theme 1. Disaster coordination and management: summary and action plans. *Prehospital Disaster Med.* 2001;16(1)22-5.
24. Schultz CH, Mothershead JL, Field M. Bioterrorism preparedness I: the emergency department and hospital. *Emerg Med Clin North Am.* 2002;20:437-55.

SUGGESTED READING

1. Covello VT. Message Mapping, Risk Communication, and Bio-terrorism. Presented at: World Health Organization Workshop on Bio-terrorism and Risk Communication; October 1, 2002; Geneva, Switzerland.

chapter 20

Informatics and Telecommunications in Disaster

Churton Budd

The United States and many other countries are facing the threat of a number of new crises as the result of terrorist activities. Behind them looms the ever-present danger of a natural disaster, such as an earthquake, fire, or hurricane, and manmade or technological disasters, such as a transportation accident or loss of an electrical grid. All of these incidents generate strong demands on the collection, analysis, coordination, distribution, and interpretation of many types of health and preparedness information. Along with the increasing risk of bioterrorism, there is a greater requirement and stronger emphasis on the use of sophisticated information-gathering tools and information technologies to accomplish. These tools are necessary to manage the complex surveillance needs and the data analysis necessary to spot trends and make early identification of outbreaks, as well as allow for rapid communication of health information, mitigation strategies, and treatment modalities to healthcare workers in the field.

Fortunately, many of those involved in emergency management have begun to embrace technology, and consequently, many vendors have recognized the need to produce hardware and software to meet the needs of disaster responders. Various tools have been used to help mitigate, prepare for, and respond to disasters. One of the more difficult issues during a response to a disaster is the inability to communicate. The breakdown of communications has been a recognized effect of almost every major response to a disaster. Communications issues occur at some level in almost every disaster response, no matter how large or small. As the disaster community has experienced these failing communications systems, it has found strategies to improve the systems or replace them with methods that work. Over time, the ability to accumulate, analyze, and disseminate disaster preparedness and response information has improved. Largely, this is due to advances in information technology that have taken place during the past half century.

HISTORICAL PERSPECTIVE[1]

The disaster response community got off to a slow start with embracing information technology; however, this technology is rapidly gaining momentum. In the past, before the 1980s, computer systems were primarily used in the business, banking, and scientific communities. For the most part, anything close to emergency or disaster planning use of these systems was limited to the Department of Defense and large commercial research firms who did operation planning and simulation, or occasionally, epidemiological or sociological studies.

During the 1980s, the desktop, or personal computer (PC), was introduced. Data could be stored on a disk that was easily carried in a briefcase. By the mid-1980s, disaster responders could enter data into a computer so that documents could be produced, spreadsheets updated, and commodities and resources tracked, sometimes even in the field. During the late 1980s, the Internet began to gain popularity and became more in the reach of the average person. The precursors to the Internet—BITNET and ARPANET—transformed into the World Wide Web, and at that time the average citizen began getting a dial-up Internet connection via CompuServe or America Online. Online resources at major centers of learning began to accumulate databases related to disaster management and planning. People could exchange files and documents via e-mail or by way of a number of sites that acted as file repositories, called FTP sites (for file transfer protocol—the methodology of transferring binary and text files from one computer to another). Special software programs called "gophers" (short for "go for this and that") cataloged these file repositories and allowed a person to search for them by keyword. These programs were the precursor to the big search engines such as Yahoo and Google.

Applications such as CAMEO (computer-aided management of emergency operations) were developed in 1988 by the National Oceanic and Atmospheric Administration. CAMEO is used to assist first responders with easy access to response information. It provides a tool to enter local information and develop incident scenarios. It contains mapping, an air dispersal model, chemical databases, and other tools to help display to the emergency responder critical information in a timely fashion. Hazardous materials information and material safety data sheets (MSDS) became available on CD-ROM.

Other databases also became available on CD-ROM to allow the responder access to a library of information while at the disaster site. About this time, the Centers for Disease Control and Prevention (CDC) released Epi Info (www.cdc.gov/epiinfo). Using this software, an epidemiologist or public health professional could develop a questionnaire or form, customize the data entry process, and enter and analyze data. Epi Info can be used to produce epidemiological statistics, tables, graphs, and maps.

Specialized computer mapping software called geospatial information systems (GIS) integrates data with map information. Because disasters are usually spatial events, GIS can assist in all phases of disaster management. It is often easier for disaster planners to see a map of the disaster to assist in plan development. A map will show the scope of the disaster, where damage is greatest or has the greatest impact, what property or lives are at risk, and what resources are available and where are they needed. Disaster managers, using GIS to graphically display critical information that is location-based, can quickly map the disaster scene, establish priorities, and develop action plans.

In the 1990s, information exchange improved exponentially. List servers on the Internet allowed emergency managers, disaster responders, and medical providers the ability to discuss disaster response in an informal setting. It was not uncommon to see a post to a list server from a responder actually at the site of the disaster. Lessons learned could be immediately disseminated throughout the disaster response community. Agencies such as the Federal Emergency Management Agency, the Natural Hazards Center at the University of Colorado, and the CDC all began to publish large amounts of public information about disasters on their Web sites. The use of satellite telephone systems and cellular phone–based data networks allowed those with a laptop to stay connected in the field and collect and transmit a large amount of information to other responders and to their response agencies.

Today, it is hard to find someone in the disaster response field that has not used e-mail or some type of computer resource to do his or her job. It appears that the use of information technology is reducing operational costs and increasing productivity, although this is difficult to quantify because information technology is still growing so rapidly. Portable computers have now decreased in size to as small as a handheld personal digital assistant (PDA). The cellular phone and PDA have merged into a communications/information device. Although still falling behind that of the corporate sector, information technology training for disaster response and management personnel is beginning to be a job requirement. Electronic commerce is allowing disaster responders to achieve real-time procurement and payment for relief supplies. Broadband and wireless networks can be set up rapidly and cheaply to allow for access to vast informational resources. The public has become far better educated, and they seek information on their own healthcare; manage their finances online; and now are able to research, mitigate, and prepare for disasters using the many publicly available resources on the Internet.

What does the future hold for informatics in disaster management? It is hard to tell because information technology in general continues to develop so quickly. It is more than likely that the disaster responder will one day use a wearable computer with a small flexible screen. It is also probable that voice and data technologies will continue to merge so that interaction with digital devices can be accomplished by voice command. Storage devices will continue to become smaller so that victims of a disaster may have their entire financial records, health records, and other personal information archived on a chip they carry in their pocket, which will allow them to save this important personal information from being destroyed by a disaster. Real-time monitoring and surveillance will assist the disaster responder to become aware of an impending disaster sooner. The ability to monitor patient flow, track resources, and perform real-time mapping and visualization of the disaster scene will allow planners and managers to "roll with the punches" during a disaster and modify the response effectively. It is likely that information technology will continue to be a stronger and stronger tool for disaster response personnel.

CURRENT PRACTICE

To help understand how informatics and telecommunications can assist during disasters, various tools and elements of informatics and communications that are currently being used by disaster managers and responders are discussed. Some of these tools are used in the preparation and mitigation stage, and some are used during the response phase. Some tools can be used in all phases of the disaster cycle.

Computer Devices

One can quickly realize that the computer has revolutionized many aspects of our lives. Some people are so dependent on e-mail for doing their daily work that when the corporate e-mail system goes down, they find it hard to conduct business. The same is true for researchers using the Internet and the vast amount of knowledge on the World Wide Web to do their research—when it is inaccessible, they almost feel withdrawal symptoms. There are many types of computer devices available to a disaster manager or responder—everything from corporate mainframes to wearable personal computers.

The Laptop

Probably the most commonly used device other than the desktop PC is the laptop. As technology improves, the speed and power of laptops are becoming close to that of a desktop. Because memory and storage are cheap, the average laptop has a larger hard drive than it did just a few years ago. Many of the applications written for the desktop are also used on the laptop, so many laptops have memory equivalent to that of the desktop. New chipsets and microprocessors use lower power and run cooler, allowing for longer running time on batteries. Some laptops are even fanless, greatly improving battery life. Laptops are getting thinner, and many of them are bundled with all the accoutrements such as wide theater-like screens, DVD players, CD burners, and high-speed connections for peripheral devices such as fire wire and universal serial bus (USB) connectors. Most new laptops also include wireless access technologies, such as Bluetooth and WiFi. With a docking station and external keyboard, mouse, and monitor, many people are finding that they can use their laptop docked at their desk and then pop it out and take it when they travel. This takes the place of a desktop computer and provides the user all the amenities of the office or home while out in the field. See Box 20-1 for tips on traveling with a laptop.

The Tablet PC

Similar to a laptop is a specialized portable computer called a tablet PC. Only recently on the market but finding rapid popularity, these devices use primarily a pen input for data entry. Tablet PCs are finding a niche in vertical markets such as healthcare and on the warehouse floor. They can be extremely useful for filling out forms such as a medical record or a field survey at a disaster site that can be plugged into a GIS for mapping. Tablet PCs usually have equivalent performance to that of a laptop, with the added convenience of usually a

BOX 20-1 CHECKLIST FOR TRAVELING WITH A LAPTOP

- Update the antivirus and spyware protection software to the latest virus definitions because one cannot be sure that a network used on the road is fully protected.
- Use a program, such as Norton Ghost, that can make a drive image, which creates an image of the laptop's hard drive, so that if the hard drive crashes, it can be recovered from the image.
- Check the batteries and if time permits, cycle them all the way down and back to full charge again. If possible, take an extra battery that is charged to extend your PC time if you are isolated without power. Consider alternative power sources, such as solar panel chargers, disposable battery replacements and power cells, and a 12-volt adapter for converting power from a car battery to use your laptop.
- Preparations for traveling with a laptop include placing the computer in a hard-shell padded case. It also helps to have an assortment of plugs and adapters and an extra network cable, just in case. Don't forget a power/recharge cable.
- Put everything in plastic baggies, even when the equipment is in its case. If you can find a large enough baggie for your laptop, you can protect it from moisture should your case be exposed to the elements and leak. Temperature changes can cause condensation, so if you do pack your equipment in baggies, throw a couple of silica gel desiccator packs into the baggie, too.
- If you know you will be in an area operating on generator power, take a surge protector to prevent power spikes from damaging your devices.
- At all costs, avoid having your laptop or computer device go through a baggage check—make sure it can be stowed as a carry-on. Try to keep it away from metal detectors because they might erase magnetic media.
- Take a cable lock so that you can secure your laptop somewhat. Although it won't prevent a thief who really wants it, it may deter someone walking by and snatching it while you have your back turned.

longer battery life, a slightly smaller form, and the pen-based input.

When selecting a laptop or tablet PC to take to the field, one will be deluged with hundreds of choices. In selecting a device, it is important to consider the conditions under which the device will be used. There are many "hardened" devices, specifically designed to military standards for shock and vibration resistance, water resistance, and dust impingement. These hardened PCs can be twice the price of the regular off-the-shelf laptop. If a hardened PC is affordable, one can rest assured that it will more than likely survive being taken into the field and be able to keep data safe. An alternative, however, is to purchase an off-the-shelf laptop from a local computer/electronics store and an insurance policy for it. Oftentimes, a $50-per-year policy with a deductible of only a few hundred dollars is available. This would easily cover a catastrophic loss of the device (e.g., major drop, crush, or immersion), but it probably would not cover minor damage such as the disk drive door breaking off. When buying a hardened PC, one should ask the vendor specific questions about drop and immersion tests and whether the device meets Mil standards (Box 20-2).

If at all possible, test a device in various types of weather, from direct sun to night time. Make sure the screen is readable in direct sunlight, can be dimmed for use during night operations, and is ergonomic when held and does not cause undue strain due to weight or bulkiness. Try the doors, accessory ports, and plugs to make sure that by simply plugging a peripheral into the PC, it is not rendered immobile or unwieldy or that its water resistance or another hardened standard is not rendered ineffective.

The Personal Digital Assistant

Another handheld device that is usually smaller than the tablet PC is the palm-sized personal digital assistant (PDA). The PDA has become the peripheral brain for many in the healthcare setting. Rather than wear or carry a laboratory coat full of plastic cards with scores and scales, quick guide books, and other reference texts, a healthcare provider can store all of this information in a PDA. The information can be indexed and referenced quickly. PDAs come in two types: the Palm Operating System and the Microsoft Pocket PC Operating System. Most of the major vendors are authoring software for both platforms, but the Palm platform has been around longer and has more shareware and freeware medical titles. A PDA can be an invaluable resource for the disaster responder. Often in the field, the disaster responder does not have the luxury of ducking into the

BOX 20-2 MIL-STD 810

MIL-STD is a series of specifications set by the U.S. Department of Defense. When purchasing a hardened device for field use, look for vendor affirmatiom that their device meets military standards to ensure that it will survive use in a post-disaster field environment.

emergency department library to look up something in the *Physicians Desk Reference* or another medical text. With a PDA, however, one can "take" those texts to the field (Box 20-3). In many cases, searches can be done with a keyword to rapidly find the needed information.

The address book, calendar, contacts, tasks, and notes are probably the more commonly used built-in applications on a PDA. Other uses of the PDA for disaster response include keeping track of contact information for other disaster responders and agencies. There are also a number of programs that allow for rapid form filling and database applications for recording data and creating quick ad-hoc reports. Some PDAs have built-in cameras, allowing one to rapidly document a disaster scene for later use. With accessories such as an external keyboard, one can even type full documents on the PDA and can print the documents with an infrared-capable printer.

Although PDAs may seem to be stand-alone devices, they require periodic visits to the laptop or desktop for synchronization. During this synchronization process, vendors provide updates to software over the Internet; calendars, address books, tasks, and notes are synchronized with desktop software; and new software can be installed from the desktop to the PDA. If you are recording data on forms on the PDA, this synchronization may also be required to pass the data from the forms tool on the PDA to an application running on the desktop as a full-featured database.

As with the laptop, there are a number of accessories that are useful to have when traveling. An attachable keyboard is helpful to type reports on the PDA for printing later. The PDA should have a hard-shell case, and it is advisable to pack the PDA in a plastic baggie for protection against the elements. With the PDA, hundreds of free medical texts and references available on the Internet can be accessed and would be quite useful if a disaster responder becomes isolated from reference resources. These can be found by searching the Internet for texts and software related to healthcare and disaster and response; some will be free, some will be for sale. A solar battery charger is ideal for a PDA because its batteries do not require much energy to charge. Lastly, make sure that data on the PDA are uploaded to a desktop or laptop computer, and try to store critical files and infor-

mation on the removable memory media. In the event that power is unavailable and the PDA loses its charge, all the data may be lost without that backup.[2]

Like the laptop or tablet PCA, a PDA comes with many choices. For those not familiar with a PDA, it is advisable to borrow one for a day, if possible, to get a feel for the work flow and how it would be used during a typical day. Pay attention to whether the device can fit into your pocket or whether you will have to carry it around in a case that you might put down and forget or not have on hand when you need it. The ideal device is small and unobtrusive; however, the device should have enough computing power, storage, and functionality to meet the user's needs. One should also consider purchasing a hardened PDA. Although not expensive in comparison with a hardened laptop, a PDA that has been designed to take into the elements will still be twice the price of an off-the-shelf model. The small size and highly portable nature of the PDA may make it a better investment because the user may be more likely to take it into the field than a laptop.

Local Area Network/Wide Area Network/Wireless Network

As emergency managers are getting more sophisticated in their use of information technology, it is not uncommon to see disaster responders establish a local area network (LAN) where their incident command is set up (e.g., in the Emergency Operations Center or in the disaster field office). This network links a group of computers together and allows instant messaging between computers; the sharing of files and documents between computers; and, better yet, the centralization of file storage to one large networked hard drive that each workstation has rights to access. Thus, a backup can be taken of just that centralized hard drive periodically rather than each individual workstation. In many cases, a wide area network can be established, which is the linking of more than one LAN. For example, the disaster field office may be linked over a public network through a virtual private network (VPN) to the main office or headquarters. This VPN connection provides a secure tunnel through the Internet from point to point so that sites in between cannot access passing traffic. This creates a wide area network that is not limited by geography or distance, just connectivity.

Wireless networks are fairly new and take advantage of a network access point, which is a transceiver that communicates with a wireless transceiver card on the workstation or laptop. Essentially, this topography creates a wireless network similar to a wired one, but with the convenience of rapid setup without the need to string network cable all over the site. Wireless networks could even be deployed in a tent city, linking treatment areas in the tents to a command tent. Unfortunately, wireless networks, like voice radio frequencies, can be fairly easily received and decrypted by an eavesdropper, thus making them fairly insecure. Sophisticated encryption methods must be put into place to protect sensitive operational security and patient information that may be transferred across a wireless network.

BOX 20-3 USEFUL PDA PROGRAMS FOR DISASTER RESPONDERS

- Epocrates (www.epocrates.com): Enhanced drug and formulary reference with integrated ID treatment guides and tools.
- WISER (http://wiser.nlm.nih.gov/): WISER provides a wide range of information on hazardous substances, including substance identification support, physical characteristics, human health information, and containment and suppression advice.
- Skyscape Books (http://www.skyscape.com): This is a portfolio of medical references for use on handheld devices.
- PEPID (http://www.pepid.com/): PEPID is a physician, critical care, and nursing reference suite.
- Sites that have PDA medical software:
  - http://www.medspda.com
  - http://www.collectivemed.com
  - http://www.medicalsoftwareforpdas.com

Communications Devices

Geographical Positioning System

The Geographical Positioning System (GPS) began as a military system in 1985 and is based on a 24-satellite configuration of transmitters. By measuring the distance to four satellites from the user location, it is possible to establish three coordinates of the user location (latitude, longitude, and altitude). Although originally developed for the Department of Defense, the not-quite-complete system was offered to the civilian community in 1983 by President Reagan after Korean Airlines flight 007 was shot down when it accidentally strayed into Soviet Union airspace. The satellite configuration was complete in the early 1990s, and the Gulf War prompted the sale of thousands of commercial GPS receivers; at that time the military had not manufactured many GPS receivers. Since then, GPS has found its way into the travel, surveying, mapping, and delivery industries. In addition, many casual users take a GPS when they are recreating in remote areas or to locate their favorite fishing spot. For the disaster responder, a GPS unit can be helpful in giving an exact location of a shelter or the location of a landing zone for helicopter evacuation and can assist in the location and mapping of resources to be used to respond to the disaster. There are a number of accessories that will convert a PC or PDA into a sophisticated GPS mapping unit.[3]

Cellular Phones

A cellular phone is probably the most common tool that people use to communicate. Many disaster response agencies consider the cellular phone to be their primary communications tool and issue them to their disaster responders. Consequently, cellular sites after a disaster may experience a high demand as the civilian population makes calls to friends and family to check on their welfare, as responders arrive and begin to arrange resources, as the media arrive and make arrangements to cover the story, and as people shift to cellular as their primary phone if their land line phone is inoperable because of a power outage or other disruption. It is reasonable to assume that a cellular phone may have difficulty in making a connection during a postdisaster response due to the cellular site being overwhelmed. Normally, cellular providers scale their cellular sites to handle only 20% to 30% of their customer base at a time. This is fine for normal traffic, but when a disaster strikes and customers all need to make a contact in a compressed time frame or when outside people come into the area with their cellular phones, the cellular sites may be congested into uselessness. Fortunately, a few initiatives are in place that might reduce this congestion on the cellular systems, especially for disaster responders. Cellular phone providers can deploy a trailer with a cellular antenna, repeater, and generator power, as well as a cell site on wheels (COW) that can be strategically placed in the disaster area and connected to the public telephone network to increase the availability of cellular connections. Also, a few cellular providers have enabled a capability in their systems in which an emergency worker can receive priority on the cellular phone system and get a connection sooner. Unfortunately, there is no legal requirement for them to do so, and as a result of the expense of purchasing additional hardware to make this happen, only a few providers have adopted this technology. Most have not; therefore, this is not a reliable option. After the 2003 summer blackout, only one cellular phone provider in New York City provided priority access.[4]

Satellite Phone Systems

There are a number of satellite phone system providers that use a number of different technologies. IMARSAT is probably the oldest vendor of satellite phone service; it started its service in the early 1990s. The early phone systems consisted of a fold-out, umbrella-like antenna and a briefcase-sized box with a handset. They were portable, although bulky, and the transmission of data over the phone system, if possible, was done at very slow speeds of 300-4800 bits per second (compared with 700-1500 Kbits per second on a broadband cable modem). Satellite phone costs originally were as high as $3 a minute, but most of the current vendors charge about $1 per minute. Phone size also has shrunk to more the size of a laptop. The flip-up lid of the phone, similar to opening the screen of a laptop, acts as the antenna and should be pointed at an angle toward one of the satellites.

Because many of these phone systems use a geostationary orbiting satellite constellation, one must be geographically aware and point the antenna in the correct direction and at the correct inclination to get a good signal on the satellite. There are automatic antenna systems on a number of vendors' satellite phones, which can be mounted to a vehicle so that the phone can maintain a line of sight link to the satellite and be used during travel to the disaster site. Dense leaves or vegetation as well as very dense rain can reduce the signal strength. Some newer phone systems, such as Iridium and Globalstar, have a handset that is not much bigger than a cordless phone for home use. These systems use a constellation of low earth-orbiting satellites and incorporate the group special mobile (GSM) protocol for cellular phone technology, allowing the handset to connect to terrestrial GSM cellular networks while in signal range to a cellular site and then automatically switch to an orbiting satellite when out of the terrestrial GSM range. Unfortunately, satellite phone systems are very expensive to bring into service and maintain. A number of vendors have been close to bankruptcy and been saved by investors.[5]

Mobile Communications Vehicles

Many response agencies have built and deployed vehicles that are outfitted with communications and computer equipment that is capable of performing a variety of functions. These vehicles usually are equipped with their own generators for power and contain a number of different radio systems that can be programmed to communicate on many different radiofrequencies. A radio operator in the vehicle can pass information between disparate radio systems and agencies and may be able to help with some of the lack of interoperability issues. These vehicles also have the ability to patch into a telephone network and the Internet. Depending on their sophistication, they may have satellite phone systems, high frequency radio, and facsimile capability computers with scanners and printers. Specially trained teams of radio operators, both amateur and public safety dispatchers, and information technology personnel usually staff one of these vehicles. Oftentimes, the incident command staff makes use of these vehicles as part of their command post, or the vehicle can support a disaster response team or disaster field office until more permanent communications can be set up. In events such as mass gatherings or disasters of limited duration, a communication vehicle such as this can be used to provide rapidly deployed communications support in a small footprint and then be completely disassembled at the end of the event.

Radio Systems

Whole books have been written on radio communications, even specifically on disaster communications. Professional communications specialists and many amateur radio operators have spent hundreds of hours training themselves on these systems, so this chapter only gives a mile-high view of the communications systems and frequencies that may be used during a disaster response. It is a good idea for the disaster responder to be aware of what systems are in use, when they should and should not be used, and how to best take advantage of these tools.

Radiofrequency (RF) is the part of the electromagnetic spectrum in which electromagnetic waves can be generated and fed through an antenna. There are a number of different modes of the RF spectrum that are most often used for voice and data transmission during a disaster response (Table 20-1). High frequency (HF) is the frequency range from 3-30 MHz and is classically termed "shortwave." HF radio waves are often reflected off the ionosphere, thus frequencies in this range are often used for medium- to long-range terrestrial communications. Sunspot and other solar activity, polar aurora, sunlight/darkness at the transmitting and receiving station, and even the choice of frequency within the spectrum can diminish the relative difference between the signal strength over the background noise (signal-to-noise ratio) and make communication on HF radio unusable at times. In other words, if interference increases the static (noise), a transmitter must be more and more powerful to have the transmitted signal hearable above that noise. HF radio is used in some widely dispersed populations for domestic broadcasting. HF radio is often used for HF networks of radio operators who can, in short term, pass information from one radio station to another, essentially allowing, by a number of "hops," worldwide communications. Amateur radio operators oftentimes provide the first information to the outside world when a disaster site is cut off after a hurricane or a major geological event.

For more local communications, very high frequency (VHF) may be used and ranges from 30-300 MHz. FM radio (88-108 MHz) and various television signals are included in this range. VHF is not usually reflected off the ionosphere so it is limited to local communications. VHF is not as affected as lower frequencies by atmos-

TABLE 20-1 TYPICAL RADIOFREQUENCIES USED IN DISASTER RESPONSE

BAND	FREQUENCY	DESCRIPTION	USES/LIMITATIONS
HF	3-30 MHz	High frequency	Good for long distance because the radio waves bounce off the ionosphere back to earth. Subject to environmental noise and interference.
VHF	30-300 MHz	Very high frequency	Line of sight, less affected by environmental noise. More easily blocked than HF by land features.
UHF	300-3000 MHz	Ultra high frequency	Line of sight, better penetration of land and manmade features. Smaller wave size allows for smaller antennas.
SHF	3-30 GHz	Super high frequency (microwaves)	Passes more easily through the atmosphere and terrestrial features than VHF and UHF. More radio spectrum available in this band.

pheric noise and interference from electromagnetic sources; it does, however, penetrate buildings and other substantial objects more than higher frequencies. Ultra high frequency (UHF) includes frequencies from 300 MHz to 3 GHz. UHF also includes some frequencies dedicated for television signals (in the United States, above channel 13). UHF frequencies penetrate some densely built buildings a little better than VHF frequencies do. UHF wavelengths are very small, allowing for more compact antennas, which some people feel are more convenient and more attractive than the longer VHF antennas. In more sophisticated communications systems, there may occasionally be a super high frequency (SHF) signal, which includes microwaves transmitted from one antenna in line of sight to another. These SHF microwave signals can carry voice and data. Satellite radio bands are contained within this range of frequencies.

With a two-way radio, there are two types of uses of the frequencies. Simplex use of a frequency means that the same frequency is being used to transmit and receive; while one person is talking, nobody else can talk. Duplex use of the frequencies allows duplex conversations, like on a telephone. Additionally, duplex frequency use can allow for a repeater to be placed centrally in the disaster area. The repeater receives on one frequency and rebroadcasts out at higher power on the other frequency. The repeater is usually put in a high location or has a high antenna. Repeater antennas have a high gain, meaning they can pull in weak signals and strong transmitters that can transmit signals farther. A repeater allows the transmission of handheld radios to be extended from just a few miles to tens of miles. Frequencies that do not penetrate buildings well, such as UHFs, have better transmission.[6]

Specialized Informatics Systems and Decision Support Tools

In recent years, the need for specialized information systems composed of databases, surveillance tools, personnel and patient tracking, and evidence-based medicine to support disaster response and management have been recognized. Health departments, which in many cases did not operate 24-hours a day, seven days a week and in some situations did not even have fax capability 10 years ago, now are developing and putting into place sophisticated systems to monitor for bioterrorism, emerging diseases, and ecological impact on a population.

The television cable network CNN is often at the disaster scene rapidly passing on information. This was the case Sept. 11, 2001, when millions of people witnessed the second plane hitting the World Trade Center as broadcasters were on the air covering the event in minutes. Field personnel can send hundreds of e-mails a day from the disaster site back to their agency. Resources come into play faster as response plans gear up and agencies and their personnel begin reporting back their status. There are many ways to communicate, and the amount of information available to decision makers has increased and is dispersed more rapidly. Information can come into the local response center and at agency headquarters oftentimes directly from the source. Each piece of information must be interpreted and requires a familiarity with the source. Assessments, requirements, and needs from the field may come in from many different sources, each with possibly contradictory information. Oftentimes, this can only be correctly interpreted by the local incident commander. In a wide-area disaster, this may be very difficult to consolidate and evaluate at a higher level.

The analysis of the information coming in from field responders is as important as the information flow itself. Consolidation in a meaningful manner and then appropriate communication to the headquarters should be done by someone knowledgeable enough at the local level to pass only that consolidated information gathered by their support personnel. Many examples exist of these types of decision support systems. The CDC makes its decisions based on information consolidated from state health departments. State health departments make their reports to the CDC based on information passed on by local health departments, who, in turn, received their information from the emergency department physician who, for example, may have noticed six patients with the same abnormal symptoms in the last hour. If that emergency physician were to call the CDC directly, the information would be documented but may not account for much until the physician had passed the information through the correct channel for consolidation and communication to a higher level.[7]

Humanitarian Information Systems

Humanitarian information systems (HIS) are specialized systems linking many sources of information and consolidating and reporting them. HIS consists of an early warning and reporting system, which includes the monitoring of specific trends of values, such as rainfall amounts, vegetation mapping, crop production, and market prices, and measures of human factors, such as nutritional status, unemployment, and poverty level. In a smaller-scale disaster, this could include a severity score tabulated from a door-by-door outreach effort to rate the occupants of a dwelling on a number of health, psychosocial, and life safety scores and then map those using a GPS location and a GIS to plot the overall postdisaster health and safety of the community. Thus, a needs assessment is conducted to estimate the needs of the affected population. An HIS should track the resources on hand and the delivery of those resources and then gauge whether the resources are meeting their goals and being delivered to the victims in an efficient manner.[8]

Surveillance and Bioterrorism Detection Systems

Whereas an HIS is a mix of various pieces of software integrated into a single system, bioterrorism detection systems are being developed with federal funds and by private corporations that include continuous surveillance of hospital data from a number of sources. This allows for normalizing and analysis of that data for statistically significant patterns and less specific indicators and rapidly alerting health officials of a developing trend. In the recent past, public health surveillance did not occur in real time, but that has changed and data must begin to be collected often before cases are confirmed and cultures are reported positive. Often there is a narrow window of opportunity after an exposure in which treatment is most effective, such as for anthrax, and rapid identification of similar symptoms from multiple sources can be facilitated if a surveillance system is in place, where real-time reporting can take place. As technology improves, environmental biosensors can be linked to the system to provide even earlier detection before widespread infection and symptoms occur. As most hospital information systems register every patient, de-identification can be done on patient data and the reason for visits can be easily transferred to a local database and even to a national database such as the National Electronic Disease Surveillance System advocated by the CDC. It is more likely that the initial detection of a covert biological or chemical attack will occur at a local level. More and more local and state health agencies are developing ways to detect unusual patterns of disease and injury. Early response to such patterns is essential for ensuring a prompt response to a biological or chemical attack. Unfortunately, many of these projects are at a regional or state level. Local and even some state health agencies budgets are still meager, and the cost of research and development of these systems is still out of reach for many smaller municipalities. If a system is developed, it usually lacks integration with other information systems and often relies on a person to do the daily initial data load or complex schemes of transmitting the data between systems. The Department of Defense system, ESSENCE, which downloads outpatient data from almost 300 Army, Navy, Air Force, and Coast Guard installations around the world each day currently receives the data in one to three days of patient visits, longer than ideal for an optimal reaction to a potential outbreak. Systems that rely on a person interpreting patient visits for key indicators and inputting them into a central database are prone to variations and interpretation of how the data should be tabulated and entered, creating room for error and inconsistency. Furthermore, it has been demonstrated that early detection of just hours can make an enormous difference in a covert attack. Unfortunately, prototype automated surveillance systems have never been able to prove that they can detect a pathogen that quickly and may render a false sense of security. There are very few vendors of bioterrorism surveillance software. Currently the most promising endeavors are those funded by grants from the Department of Defense, CDC, and other federal agencies.[3]

SUMMARY

Disaster informatics and telecommunications have become indispensable tools for disaster managers and responders. As pervasive as these tools are in our daily lives, they are finding their way more and more into the field. E-mail, instant messaging, LANs and intranets, cellular phones, two-way radios, teleconferencing, and many other sophisticated tools are becoming common in handheld devices and in the pockets of disaster responders. Information is a commodity, and the ability to analyze and distribute it to aid in the reduction of human suffering is probably the best money spent.

Device selection will probably be the disaster responder's most difficult task because there are thousands of brands on the market for desktops, laptops, tablet PCs, and PDAs. Vendors may be of help in selecting a product that meets the user's needs, but many vendors are not familiar with the disaster responder's role and may not understand what "punishment" the device may endure. Generally, vendors who sell hardware that is being used in the public safety and field service fields will have a better idea of the harsh environments in which the equipment will have to operate. These vendors are a good first choice to talk with about the different devices.

Protecting the device and data is the next important task for the technologically armed disaster responder. Making sure that the device is stored in a padded, hard shell case for shipping and travel and ensuring that there are redundant backups of the data at multiple points in the preparation, deployment, and demobilization phases are important. This includes taking backup copies of software on a CD in the event that the hardware is damaged in the field.

GPS receivers, cellular phones, radio systems, and the Internet are all tools that a disaster responder may use during a response to help establish and maintain communications with the home agency and other responders. These tools will be a lifeline for ongoing support and the reporting of events. Again, the user will be faced with trying to determine the best radiofrequencies to use for any given circumstance. The disaster responder will need to locate the best vendor for cellular service near the disaster area—one that's large enough or has a large enough customer base that it is in the vendor's best financial interest to supplement local or damaged cellular stations to ensure better usability of the system after the event. Having multiple options for Internet access, such as dial-up, wireless, and fixed LAN ability, will ensure the user flexibility in plugging into whatever is available after a disaster.

As the disaster responder becomes more reliant on electronic equipment for postdisaster duties, he or she will need to consider alternative power sources and methods of recharging batteries, such as solar chargers, hand generators, and disposable power packs. He or she will need to consider taking any number of wall chargers, cords, dongles, adapters, and plugs to the disaster site. The electronic and communications demands for rapid information and assessment in the response and recovery efforts of a disaster mission will prompt the disaster responder to become more computer savvy, more electronically aware, and more technically knowledgeable, and as a result, the disaster responder will be more productive. Reports and assessments must be rapidly tabulated and disseminated through the chain of command. Assessment efforts may rely on computerized surveillance techniques, information gathering and database development for resource tracking, and statistical analysis—all with the ability to rapidly communicate this information to various players and agencies at the disaster site in an organized and succinct manner. As pervasive as each of these technologies is getting in our daily lives, it is obvious that they are becoming equally so in our role in disaster response.

REFERENCES

1. Gantz J. 40 years of IT—An Executive White Paper from IDC. International Data Corp; 2004. Availlable at: http://edn.idc.com/prodserv/downloads/40_years_of_IT.pdf.
2. Bucklen KR. Earthquake in Iran: using the pocket PC for disaster medical relief. *Pocket PC*. June/July 2004;69-72.
3. Zubieta JC, Skinner R, Dean AG. Initiating informatics and GIS support for a field investigation of bioterrorism: the New Jersey anthrax experience. *Int J Health Geogr*. November 2003;2(1):8.
4. Schumer C. Schumer reveals: When cell phones failed during blackout, only one NY cell phone company had emergency plan in place [press release]. Available at: http://schumer.senate.gov/Schumer Website/ pressroom/press_releases/PR01953.html.
5. Requirements on Telecommunications for Disaster Relief from the International Federation of the Red Cross and Red Crescent Societies. Presented at: ITU-T Workshop on Telecommunications for Disaster Relief; 2003; Geneva.
6. Coile RC. The role of amateur radio in providing electronic communications for disaster management. *Disaster Prev Manage*. 1997;6(3):176-85.
7. Henry W, Fisher I. The role of information technologies in emergency mitigation, planning, response and recovery. *Disaster Prev Manage*. 1998;7(1):28-37.
8. Maxwell D, Watkins B. Humanitarian information systems and emergencies in the Greater Horn of Africa: logical components and logical linkages. *Disasters*. March 2003;27(1):72-90.
9. Farrel B. The National Communications System. Available at: http://www.naseo.org/committees/energysecurity/energy assurance/farrell.pdf.
10. Fazio S. The need for bandwith management and QoS control when using public or shared networks for disaster relief work. Presented at: ITU-T Workshop on Telecommunications for Disaster Relief; 2003; Geneva.
11. Garshneck V. Telemedicine Applied to Disaster Medicine and Humanitarian Response: History and Future. Presented at: 32nd Hawaii International Conference on System Science; 1999; Hawaii.

Available at: http://esd12.computer.org/comp/proceedings/hicss/1999/0001/04/00014029.PDF.

12. Teich JM, Wagner MM, Mackenzie CF, Schafer KO. The informatics response in disaster, terrorism and war. *J Am Med Inform Assoc.* March-April 2002;9(2):97-104.

13. Brennan PF, Yasnoff WA. Medical informatics and preparedness. *J Am Med Inform Assoc.* March-April 2002;9(2):202-3.

14. Sessa AB. Humanitarian Telecommunications. Presented at: ITU-T Workshop on Telecommunications for Disaster Relief; 2003; Geneva.

15. Garshnek V, Burkle FM Jr. Applications of telemedicine and telecommunications to disaster medicine: historical and future perspectives. *J Am Med Inform Assoc.* January-February 1999;6(1):26-37.

16. Zimmerman H. Communications for Decision-making in Disaster Management. Presented at: ITU-T Workshop on Telecommunications for Disaster Relief; 2003; Geneva.

chapter 21

Disaster Mitigation

Robert M. Gougelet

The definition of *mitigation* includes a wide variety of measures taken before an event occurs that will prevent illness, injury, and death and limit the loss of property. Mitigation planning commonly includes the following areas:

- The ability to maintain function
- Building design
- Locating buildings outside of hazard zones (e.g., flood plains)
- Essential building utilities
- Protection of building contents
- Insurance
- Public education
- Surveillance
- Warning
- Evacuation

It is of critical importance that emergency planners incorporate the basic elements of mitigation and have the authority and resources to incorporate these changes into their organization/facility/community. Emergency planners should have a basic idea of the concepts of mitigation through their use in natural disasters over the years. The recent federally mandated transition to the all-hazards approach in disaster emergency response has also given a new perspective on mitigation. Although it is not necessary to redefine mitigation, it is essential to understand how the scope and complexity of mitigation and risk reduction strategies have evolved as the United States adapts to new threats. For example, what measures can be taken in advance to protect the population and infrastructure from an earthquake, flood, ice storm, or terrorist attack? As with each mass casualty event, the answers to this question are location-specific and heavily dependent on the circumstances surrounding the event. However, a common understanding of the goals and concepts of mitigation along with knowledge of its policy history and current practices will help a community develop mitigation plans that are both locally effective and economically sustainable. This chapter illustrates how mitigation strategies have evolved, outlines key historical elements of U.S. mitigation policy, highlights critical current mitigation practices, and describes common pitfalls that can hamper mitigation efforts. The realm of mitigation planning is far reaching and complex, and, therefore, the emphasis of this chapter is on the continuity of medical care during a mass casualty event within a community.

GOALS AND CONCEPTS OF MITIGATION

In the simplest of terms, mitigation means to lessen the possibility that a mass casualty event can cause harm to people or property. However, this simple definition covers a broad range of possible activities. For example, an effort to ensure that essential utilities, such as electricity and phone service, continue to be available throughout a natural disaster is very different from efforts to minimize the economic damage of postdisaster recovery from a major flood or attempts to educate the public on how to reduce their risk of exposure during a dirty-bomb incident.

Mitigation strategies can range from focusing exclusively on "hardening" to focusing more on resiliency. Hardening of targets is best described as measures that are taken to physically protect a facility, such as bolting down equipment, securing power and communications lines, installing backup generators, placing blast walls, or physically locking down and securing a facility. Mitigation through hardening has only limited use in systems or facilities such as hospitals where open access to the surrounding community is the hallmark of their operations. In these circumstances, a resilient system capable of flexing to accommodate damage and the ability to maintain or even expand current operations will make that system ultimately more secure. Mitigation through resiliency also has limitations. In many cases, hardening structures is most appropriate, particularly when many citizens may be quickly affected without prior notice or warning. This may include hardening structures in earthquake zones, physically protecting and monitoring the food chain and drinking water systems, and physically securing and protecting nuclear power plants. In these cases, resiliency may come too late to prevent illness and death in large numbers of patients, and planners should target hardening to whatever degree is practically and financially feasible. The threats of nuclear, radiological, chemical, and biological attacks present new challenges for emergency planners. The potentially covert nature of the attack, the wide variety of possible agents (including contagious agents), and soft civilian targets make planning efforts exponentially more difficult than in the past. This complexity has also eroded the distinction between mitigation and response activities. Although it is never possible to mitigate or to plan responses for all contingencies, we do know, however, that there is a basic common response framework. This framework includes coordination, communication to enable inter-agency information sharing,[1] and flexibility to rapidly adapt emergency plans to different sivations.

RECENT HISTORICAL PERSPECTIVE

Traditionally, mitigation in the United States has focused on natural disasters; however, early mitigation planning against manmade disasters included civilian fallout shelters and the evacuation of target cities if a nuclear attack was eminent. The Federal Emergency Management Agency (FEMA) states[2]:

> Mitigation is the cornerstone of emergency management. It's the ongoing effort to lessen the impact disasters have on people's lives and property through damage prevention and flood insurance. Through measures such as; zoning restrictions to prevent building in hazard zones (e.g. flood plains, earthquake fault lines), engineering buildings and infrastructures to withstand earthquakes; and creating and enforcing effective building codes to protect property from floods, hurricanes and other natural hazards, the impact on lives and communities is lessened.

Mitigation begins with local communities assessing their risks from recurring problems and making a plan for creating solutions to these problems and reducing the vulnerability of their citizens and property to risk.[3]

However, since the mid-1990s, mitigation planning has become increasingly more complex. Terrorist attacks, industrial accidents, and new or reemerging infectious diseases are just a few of the threats that have started to consume more planning time and resources. The growing scope of threats that must be addressed in mitigation strategies challenges all aspects of planning and response at all levels of government.[4-6] The importance of sharing intelligence information at the earliest possible stage of a terrorist attack, especially a bioterrorism event, is now recognized in national policy as a critical mitigation asset. Theoretically, if there were the slightest indication of a contagious biological attack occurring within the United States, then early recognition triggered by intelligence alerts followed by appropriate local responses could allow for isolation, treatment, and containment of a potentially widespread event. This intelligence sharing must become a large part of mitigation efforts aimed at limiting the effectiveness of manmade disasters. A similar analogy can be made with the early warning given to the medical community when a surveillance system picks up an unusual cluster of illnesses, long before the initial diagnosis may be made at a physician's office or healthcare facility. The new National Incident Management System (NIMS) states that intelligence must be shared within the incident management structure and states that a sixth functional area, or

Incident Command System Section, covering intelligence functions may be established during the time of an emergency. The elevated status of intelligence within NIMS establishes the importance of early and effective intelligence sharing. The challenge is to establish these sharing relationships before the disaster by incorporating them into an ongoing hazard monitoring process and by integrating them into drills, exercises, and day-to-day activities to ensure that this critical resource is operational when needed to mitigate the consequences of a disaster.[7]

The Disaster Mitigation Act of 2000 (DMA-2000) elevated the importance of mitigation planning within communities by authorizing the funding of certain mitigation programs and by involving the Office of the President. Under DMA-2000, the president may authorize funds to communities or states that have identified natural disasters within their borders and have demonstrated public-private natural disaster mitigation partnerships. DMA-2000 provides economic incentives through promoting awareness and education to prioritize the following objectives for federal assistance to states, local communities, and Indian tribes:

- Forming effective community-based partnerships for hazard mitigation purposes
- Implementing effective hazard mitigation measures that reduce the potential damage from natural disasters
- Ensuring continued functionality of critical services
- Leveraging additional nonfederal resources in meeting natural disaster resistance goals
- Making commitments to long-term hazard mitigation efforts to be applied to new and existing structures

This important legislation sought to identify and assess the risks to states and local governments (including Indian tribes) from natural disasters. The funding would be used to implement adequate measures to reduce losses from natural disasters and to ensure that the critical services and facilities of communities would continue to function after a natural disaster.[8]

Further evidence of the expanding complexity of mitigation efforts can be found in the Terrorism Insurance Risk Act of 2002. This act fills a gap within the insurance industry, which typically does not provide insurance coverage for large-scale terrorist events. The federal government, in the wake of the Sept. 11, 2001, attacks, promptly passed this act, addressing concerns about the potential widespread impact on the economy. The act provides a transparent shared public-private program that compensates insured losses as a result of acts of terrorism. The purpose is to "protect consumers by addressing market disruptions and ensure the continued widespread availability and affordability of property and casualty insurance for terrorism risk; and to allow for a transitional period for the private markets to stabilize, resume pricing of such insurance, and build capacity to absorb any future losses, while preserving State insurance regulation and consumer protections."[9,10] Effective mitigation planning now is expected to include many different aspects of private industry. Private industry is a critical partner; its involvement may range from being a potential risk to the community, such as a chemical plant, to providing assistance in responding to an event. This is especially true in the area of healthcare; most healthcare in the United States is provided by the private sector. It is important to note that the National Fire Protection Association (NFPA) recently released NFPA 1600, *Standard on Disaster/Emergency Management and Business Continuity Programs,* 2004 edition. This standard establishes a common set of criteria for disaster management, emergency management, and business continuity. Planners may use these criteria to assess or develop programs or to respond to and recover from a disaster.[11]

Although mitigation planning has become an essential feature of nearly every industry and institution in the wake of Sept. 11, 2001, healthcare settings are disproportionately affected by new challenges and complexities in mitigation. The severe acute respiratory syndrome (SARS) outbreak shook the foundation of mitigation and prevention in healthcare when healthcare workers and first responders in China and Canada died in 2003 after caring for patients with the SARS virus. Access to several Toronto area hospitals was significantly limited for several months because of illness, quarantine staff, and concerns about contamination. The economic costs to the city of Toronto were in the billions of dollars. Hospitals and their communities were thrown into a complex mitigation and prevention crisis.

The Association of State and Health Officials (ASTHO) has come out with specific guidelines and checklists to help prepare states and communities prepare for a possible outbreak.[12] Pan-influenza planning closely parallels SARS planning, with considerable effort toward preventive vaccination of the population and emphasis on protecting healthcare workers.[13] Effective strategies were learned during the Toronto SARS outbreak, although it was definitely a "learn-as-you-go-along" situation. The most effective mitigation strategies to prepare for the consequences of an outbreak would be to plan for the home quarantine of patients, establish public information strategies to reduce public concern, to close affected facilities until the knowledge base permitted their safe reopening, plan for a coordinated information and command and control center, and have preestablished protocols and procedures in place to protect the health of healthcare workers and first responders.[14]

Vaccination is an essential component of hospital and community mitigation planning. During the fall of 2002, the U.S. government requested that all states prepare for a smallpox attack. The preparations called for each state to present a plan within 10 days to vaccinate all persons within the state, starting with healthcare workers.[15] Each facility and community needs to look at the risk of a disease, the effect of vaccination on healthcare workers, and the ability to maintain continuity of care. If properly informed, healthcare workers could respond and treat patients without risk to themselves or their families. The availability of a vaccination and the ability to mass vaccinate the majority of the population should be considered in all community response plans. The plans for both SARS and pan-influenza now need to address the availability and possible stockpiling of antiviral agents as well as procedures for mass vaccination of the population, if a vaccine were to become available.

We have learned much from the many earthquakes, tornadoes, hurricanes, fires, and floods that the United States has experienced, but it is extremely difficult to plan for terrorist and natural events that can quickly overwhelm communities, states, or even the whole nation. These historical events, policy developments, and shifts in public attention have created a very complex planning and operating environment. The next section of this chapter addresses some of the key current practices that mitigation strategists should consider.

CURRENT PRACTICE

Current mitigation strategies are as varied as the circumstances in which they are formed. This section illustrates the impact of mitigation through a comparison of responses to two earthquakes that were broadly separated in geography and community preparedness. These examples are followed by a discussion of critical elements of mitigation and risk reduction practice in three broad categories: coordination with other organizations and jurisdictions, hospital concerns, and mitigation strategies based in community health promotion and surveillance.

The first step for protecting communities and their critical facilities against earthquakes is a comprehensive risk assessment based on current seismic hazard mapping. This determination of location should also include the assessment of underlying soil conditions, the potential for landslide, and other potential hazards.[15] Communities located on seismic fault lines must also develop and enforce strict building codes.

After the Bam, Iran, earthquake, a large section of the city, at first glance, looked like a burned forest with only the bare trees left standing. It soon became clear that these were steel vertical beams standing upright in mounds of concrete rubble. In comparison, after the Northridge, Calif., earthquake many of the buildings were structurally compromised but did not collapse on their occupants. Undoubtedly, this was the result of the strict building codes and enforcement throughout the state of California. To the victims of the Bam earthquake, the most important lifesaving measures may have been the development and enforcement of strict building codes.[16] Building codes are minimum standards that protect people from injury and loss of life from structural collapse. They do not ensure that normal community functioning might continue after a significant event.[17]

Structural protection of facilities requires the active role of qualified and experienced structural engineers during planning, construction, remodeling, and retrofitting. The immediate response of a structural engineer after a disaster is to assess building damage and to assist in determining the need for evacuation and the measures needed to ensure continuity of function. Extensive analysis of seismic data taken during an earthquake that are compared with subsequent building damage has given structural engineers valuable information on structural failures of buildings. This information allows communities to rebuild with better and stronger facilities.[18]

The following measures to protect the structural integrity of a facility should be in place before an incident[19]:

- A contract with a structural engineering firm to participate in planning, construction, retrofitting, and remodeling
- A contractual agreement guaranteeing the response, after an event, of a structural engineer (with appropriate redundancy) to ensure structural stability, to assess the need for evacuation, and to take additional measures to ensure the continuity of essential functions
- Inventory and classify all buildings
- Conduct a vulnerability assessment
- Ensure code compliance
- Determine public safety risks
- Determine structural reinforcement needs, and prioritize them
- Prepare lists of vulnerable structures for use in evacuation and damage assessment

Extensive resources and technical assistance for structural earthquake protection are available on the Internet. FEMA's Web site itemizes these resources into three major categories: earthquake engineering research centers and National Earthquake Hazards Reduction Program-funded centers, earthquake engineering and architectural organizations, and codes and standards organizations.[20] FEMA has released the *Risk Management Series* publications, which provide very specific guidance to architects and engineers about protecting buildings against terrorist attacks.[21] The Institute for Business and Home Safety is also an excellent source of incident-specific information for both businesses and homes.[22]

The protection of facilities from earthquake damage also involves protecting the facility's nonstructural elements. These nonstructural elements do not comprise the fundamental structure of the building (Box 21-1).

Primary damage to nonstructural elements may be the result of overturning, swaying, sliding, falling, deforming, and internal vibration of sensitive instruments. Relatively simple measures, which do not require a structural engineer, may be taken to prevent damage to or from nonstructural elements. These measures may include fastening loose items and structures, anchoring top-heavy

items, tethering large equipment, or using spring mounts. Other elements, such as stabilizing a generator from vibration damage by placing it on spring mounts or from sliding damage by having slack in attached fuel and power lines, may require the assistance of an engineer. Hospitals and other medical care facilities are especially vulnerable to damage from nonstructural elements. Consider the placement of routine medical care items such as intravenous poles, monitors/defibrillators, and pharmaceutical agents and medical supplies on shelves. Loss of emergency power to key services, such as computed tomography scanners, laboratory equipment, and dialysis units, may also significantly affect the continuity of medical care (E. Aur der Heide, personal communication, February 2005).[23] Loss of generator power may be due to failure of crossover switches, loss of cooling, or loss of connection of power and fuels lines. A process for the continual review of the power needs of new and critical equipment should be a part of a hospital's emergency planning process.

Cooperating with the federal government and understanding the resources, structure, and timeframe in which the federal resources are available are critical to appropriate mitigation planning.[24] NIMS and the National Response Plan are described elsewhere in this book. Each document describes in detail the organizational structure and response authority of the federal government in the time of a disaster.[25,26] Healthcare organizations, communities, and states are mandated to ensure that their strategies for mitigation, response, and recovery are developed in coordination with these national models. Presidential Decision Directive Homeland Security Presidential Directive (HSPD) #5 mandates that by fiscal year 2005, "the Secretary shall develop standards and guidelines for determining whether a State or Local entity has adopted the NIMS,"[27] and all mitigation and risk reductions strategies should be designed accordingly.

In addition to efforts to coordinate with federal plans, mitigation strategists must also build functional partnerships within communities and across jurisdictional lines. This point has been emphasized in several recently published planning guides.[17,28-30] These guides help hospitals and their communities plan for mass casualty events by incorporating key features of planning, risk assessment, exercises, communications, and command and control issues into functional and operational programs.

Hospitals also present special challenges. Presidential Decision Directive HSPD #8 specifies that hospitals qualify as first responders.[31] As such, they have important mitigation activities to consider. What does mitigation mean for a hospital? In the current threat environment, it means minimizing the impact of an event on the institution and ensuring continuity of care.

Accessibility to the public 24-hours a day, seven days a week has been a hallmark of hospital emergency care. However, one of the most important mitigation strategies a hospital can adopt is the ability to limit and control access to patients and families during the time of a mass casualty or a hazardous materials event. Additionally, facilities must have plans and the ability to decontaminate patients, protect essential staff and their families, handle a surge of patients with complimentary plans for

BOX 21-1   NONSTRUCTURAL ELEMENTS

Cabinets
Compressed gas tanks
Fuel tanks
Generators
Equipment and supplies
Signs and pictures
Electrical lines
Communication and information technology lines
Bookshelves
Windows
Electrical fixtures
Storage containers
Hazardous materials
Lockers
Building parapets and facings
Computer hard drives

the forward movement of patients to surrounding areas, set up alternative treatment facilities within the community, to train staff in early recognition and treatment of illness or injury related to weapons of mass destruction, and ensure continuity of care and financial stability during and after an event.

Although hospitals will always form the cornerstone for medical treatment of patients during mass casualty events, best practices for hospitals must now also incorporate healthcare resources within the community.[32] Hospitals will have to work with other first responders within the community to conduct drills and exercises that realistically test the whole hospital's ability to respond to a mass casualty event.[33] Hospitals also will have to ensure that staff members have the proper training to complete hazard vulnerability assessments[34] and to set up and staff outpatient treatment facilities to ensure continuity of care.[35,36] Even with very careful planning, most communities will be overwhelmed for the first minutes to hours or possibly days after a massive event, until an effective and prolonged response can occur. Communities must also look at the continuity of medical care as a communitywide issue and not just emphasize the hospital or emergency medical services aspects of medical care. The loss of community-based clinics, private medical offices, nursing homes, dialysis units, pharmacies, and visiting nurse services can significantly increase the number of patients seeking care at hospitals during a mass casualty event. Risk communication and education, specifically aimed at protecting the affected population, can help prevent surges of medical patients.[1]

Hospitals now have enormous community responsibilities in terms of preparing for and mitigating mass casualty events. Hospitals in hurricane, flood, earthquake, and tornado zones have prepared for many years against these threats. However, a pattern of repeated systems failures within hospitals continues and includes communications and power loss, with additional physical damage to the facility.[37] To prevent such failures, hospitals need to recognize that mitigation and risk reduction planning must approach the level of detail and logistical support that parallels military planning.

Surveillance is another key mitigation strategy for health emergencies. Early recognition of sentinel cases in biological events can significantly affect the outcome, particularly in contagious events. States are funded and required to participate in the surveillance programs mandated in CDC and Health Resources and Services Administration guidelines.[38,39] The earlier an event is recognized, especially if it involves a contagious disease, the earlier treatment can begin and preventive measures can be taken to prevent the spread of illness to healthcare workers and responders, as well as the rest of the community. Public health departments are critical to establishing relationships between local providers and their communities. Local, state, and federal public health agencies must ensure that effective surveillance at the community level occurs. These agencies can also assist in awareness-level and personal protection training for hospital staff, emergency medical service employees, and law enforcement first responders.

PITFALLS

Motivating healthcare facilities to take part in mitigation is one of the largest challenges in disaster medicine. It is always best to take measures beforehand to minimize property damage and prevent injury and death. In the case of hospitals, some preliminary research indicates that four factors affect an institution's motivation to mitigate: influence of legislation and regulation, economic considerations, the role of "champions" within the institution, and the impact of disasters and imminent threats on agenda-setting and policy making. It was discovered during this research that "mitigation measures were found to be most common when proactive mitigation measures were mandated by regulatory agencies and legislation."[40] Tax incentives, government assistance grants, and building code and insurance requirements may also serve to motivate administrators and decision makers to put the necessary time and effort into mitigation planning.[17]

CONCLUSION

Extensive mitigation activities are a necessary prerequisite for the response and recovery activities that must follow a large-scale mass casualty event. We have never seen the number of casualties in the United States we are preparing for today. We do have the threat of an enemy who will strike within the United States with the purpose of inflicting mass numbers of casualties on the civilian population. We must maintain the perspective that even the smallest chance of such an incredibly devastating event, whether manmade or natural, warrants our full attention. If there is no other motivating factor, the possibly such an event must suffice.

REFERENCES

1. Aur der Heide E. Principles of hospital disaster planning. In Hogan DE, Burstein JL, eds. *Disaster Medicine*. Philadelphia: Lippincott, Williams & Wilkins; 2002.
2. Federal Emergency Management Agency. Mitigation Division. Available at: http://www.fema.gov/fima/.
3. State of Vermont Emergency Management Agency. Mitigation. Available at: http://www.dps.state.vt.us/vem/mitigation.htm.
4. Centers for Disease Control and Prevention. Smallpox Response Plan and Guidelines (Version 3.0). Available at: http://www.bt.cdc.gov/agent/smallpox/response-plan/index.asp.
5. Centers for Disease Control and Prevention. Severe acute respiratory syndrome (SARS). Available at: http://www.cdc.gov/ncidod/sars/.
6. Centers for Disease Control and Prevention. Biological and chemical terrorism: strategic plan for preparedness and response. Recommendations of the CDC Strategic Planning Workgroup. *Morb Mortal Wkly Rep*. April 2000;49:RR-4.
7. Federal Emergency Management Agency. NIMS compliance. Available at: http://www.fema.gov/nims/nims_compliance.shtm#nimsdocument.
8. Federal Emergency Management Agency. The Disaster Mitigation Act of 2000. Available at: http://www.fema.gov/fima/dma2k.shtm.
9. U.S. Department of the Treasury. H.R. 3210. Terrorism Risk Insurance Act of 2002. Available at: http://www.treasury.gov/offices/domestic-finance/financial-institution/terrorism-insurance/pdf/hr3210.pdf.
10. Manns J. Insuring against terror? *Yale Law Journal*. June 2003;112(8):2509-51.

11. National Fire Protection Association. NFPA Standard on Disaster/Emergency Management and Business Continuity Programs. 2004 ed. Available at: http://www.nfpa.org/PDF/nfpa1600.pdf?src=nfpa.

12. Association of State and Territorial Health Officials and National Association of County and City Health Officials. State and Local Health Official Epidemic SARS Checklist. Available at: http://www.astho.org/pubs/SARSChecklist.pdf.

13. Association of State and Territorial Health Officials. Preparedness Planning for State Health Officials. Available at: http://www.astho.org/pubs/Pandemic%20Influenza.pdf.

14. Gopalakrishna G, Choo P, Leo YS, et al. SARS transmission and hospital containment. *Emerg Infect Dis*. March 2004;10(3):395-400.

15. Federal Management Emergency Agency. Mitigation ideas: possible mitigation measures by hazard type, a mitigation planning tool for communities. Available at: www.fema.gov.

16. Personal observations during deployment: DMAT NM#-1 Northridge Earthquake 1994, IMSURT-East Bam, Iran 2004.

17. Auf der Heide E. Community medical disaster planning and evaluation guide: an interrogatory format. *Am Coll Emerg Physicians*. 1995.

18. Hays W. Data acquisition for earthquake hazard mitigation—abstract. Presented at: International Workshop on Earthquake Injury Epidemiology for Mitigation and Response; July 10-12, 1989; John Hopkins University, Baltimore.

19. State of California, Governor's Office of Emergency Services. Hospital and Earthquake Preparedness Guidelines. Available at: http://www.oes.ca.gov/Operational/OESHome.nsf/978596171691962788256b350061870e/C38723C529A5CA5188256BBF005E375F?OpenDocument.

20. Federal Emergency Management Agency, National Earthquake Hazards Reduction Program. Publications and resources. Available at: http://www.fema.gov/hazards/earthquakes/nehrp/eq_links.shtm.

21. Federal Emergency Management Agency, Mitigation Division. Risk Management Series publications. Available at: http://www.fema.gov/fima/rmsp.shtm.

22. Institute for Business and Home Safety. Available at: http://www.ibhs.org/.

23. Technical Guidelines for Earthquake Protection of Nonstructural Items in Communication Facilities. Bay Area Regional Earthquake Preparedness Project (BAREPP).

24. Federal Emergency Management Agency, Response and Recovery. A guide to the disaster declaration process and federal disaster assistance. Available at: http://www.fema.gov/rrr/dec_guid.shtm.

25. U.S. Department of Homeland Security. National Incident Management System. Available at: http://www.dhs.gov/interweb/assetlibrary/NIMS-90-web.pdf.

26. U.S. Department of Homeland Security. National Response Plan. Available at: http://www.dhs.gov/dhspublic/interapp/editorial/editorial_0566.xml.

27. U.S. Department of Homeland Security. Homeland Security Presidential Directive/HSPD-5: Management of Domestic Incidents. Available at: http://www.dhs.gov/dhspublic/display?content=4331.

28. Gougelet R, Atther Mughal M. It takes a community: the Army's integrated bioterrorism response model. *Frontline First Responder*. September 2003. Available at: http://www.emsmagazine.com/ffr/ffrsep0003.html.

29. Rosen J, Gougelet R, Mughal M, Hutchinson R. Medical Disaster Conference. Coordination draft: conference report. June 13-15, 2001; Dartmouth College, Hanover, NH. Available at: http://www.dartmouth.edu/~engs05/readings/md/summary/DartMedDisRepv1.2.pdf.

30. Improving Local and State Agency Response to Terrorist Incidents Involving Biological Weapons. Available at: http://www.edgewood.army.mil/downloads/bwirp/bwirp_planning_guide.pdf.

31. The White House. 2003 Homeland Security Presidential Directive/HSPD-8: National Preparedness. Available at: http://www.whitehouse.gov/news/releases/2003/12/20031217-6.html.

32. Joint Commission on Accreditation of Healthcare Organizations. Health Care at the Crossroads: Strategies for Creating and Sustaining Community-wide Emergency Preparedness Systems. Available at: http://www.jcaho.org/about+us/public+policy+initiatives/emergency_preparedness.pdf.

33. Joint Commission on Accreditation of Healthcare Organizations. Revised Environment of Care Standards for the comprehensive accreditation manual of hospitals. *Joint Commission Perspectives*. December 2001;21(12). Available at: http://www.jcrinc.com/subscribers/perspectives.asp?durki=1018.

34. Joint Commission on Accreditation of Healthcare Organizations. Analyzing your vulnerability to hazards. *Joint Commission Perspectives*. December 2001;21(12). Available at: http://www.jcrinc.com/subscribers/perspectives.asp?durki=1007.

35. Acute Care Center: A Mass Casualty Care Strategy for Biological Terrorism Incidents. Available at: http://www.edgewood.army.mil/downloads/bwirp/acc_blue_book.pdf.

36. Neighborhood Emergency Help Center Pamphlet: A Mass Casualty Care Strategy for Biological Terrorism Incidents. Available at: http://www.edgewood.army.mil/downloads/bwirp/nehc_green_book.pdf.

37. Milsten A. Hospital responses to acute-onset disasters: a review. *Prehospital Disaster Med*. January 2000;15(1):32-45.

38. U.S. Department of Health and Human Services, Health Resources and Services Administration. National Bioterrorism Hospital Preparedness Program. Available at: http://www.hrsa.gov/bioterrorism/.

39. Centers for Disease Control and Prevention. Continuation Guidance for Cooperative Agreement on Public Health Preparedness and Response for Bioterrorism—Budget Year Five. Available at: http://www.bt.cdc.gov/planning/continuationguidance/index.asp.

40. RP Connell. *Disaster Mitigation in Hospitals: Factors Influencing Decision-making on Hazard Loss Reduction* [thesis]. University of Delaware; 2003. Available at: http://www.udel.edu/DRC/thesis/connell_thesis.DOC.

SUGGESTED READING

1. Guidelines for Vulnerability Reduction in the Design of New Health Care Facilities. Available at: www.paho.org/english/dd/ped/vulnerabilidad.htm.

2. Principles of Disaster Mitigation in Health Facilities. Available at: http://www.paho.org/English/PED/fundaeng.htm.

3. Protecting New Health Care Facilities from Disasters. Available at: http://www.paho.org/english/dd/ped/proteccion.htm.

chapter 22

Vaccines

Kent J. Stock

HISTORICAL BACKGROUND

The Biological and Toxin Weapons Convention was established in 1972. Members of the convention produced a treaty that prohibited the development, production, stockpiling, and acquisition of biologic weapons. This was the first comprehensive, international effort to ban biologic and chemical weapons since the Geneva Protocol in 1925, and it was the first international treaty to ban an entire class of weapons. The treaty was opened for signature on April 10, 1972, and entered into force on March 26, 1975. The treaty has been signed by 144 nations, including the United States and the Soviet Union.

On Oct. 4, 2001, a case of inhalational anthrax was reported in Florida.[1] Epidemiologists at the Centers for Disease Control and Prevention (CDC) later identified and confirmed 22 cases—11 cases of inhalational anthrax and 11 cases of cutaneous anthrax.[2] The dissemination of these anthrax spores via letters through the U.S. mail appeared to be an intentional act of bioterrorism. In the aftermath of the Al-Qaida attacks on the World Trade Center and Pentagon buildings, this pernicious act illustrated our country's vulnerability to terrorist attacks, particularly those involving the use of biologic weapons. In response to the terrorist attacks the United States, the federal government passed the USA Patriot Act in October 2001 and the Public Health Security and Bioterrorism Preparedness and Response Act in June 2002. These acts created the Department of Homeland Security and empowered the Department of Health and Human Services (DHHS) to begin efforts to protect the civilian population against future attacks with biologic weapons by enhancing surveillance and promoting preparedness.

DHHS, in conjunction with the CDC and National Institutes of Health, convened members of the research community to discuss the development of a research agenda and strategic plan for biodefense research. These efforts to counter bioterrorism focused on a group of microbes that included *Yersinia pestis, Francisella tularemia, Bacillus anthracis,* variola major virus, *Clostridium botulinum,* and the hemorrhagic fever viruses.[3] Variola major virus (smallpox) was particularly feared because of its high mortality rate, the absence of specific therapy, and the highly susceptible general population.[4] The CDC published its *Interim*

Smallpox Response Plan and Guidelines in November 2001.[5] These guidelines were later updated in 2002.[6] This was the first time a U.S. government agency sponsored and implemented a large-scale civilian vaccination strategy in anticipation of a potential threat with a biologic weapon.

The initial debate focused on whether the entire population should be vaccinated to eliminate the threat of a future attack or whether to institute a targeted vaccination program only after an attack occurs or if the likelihood of an attack is deemed high by government officials. CDC officials decided to support a "ring vaccination" approach after a case of smallpox was identified.[5] The vaccination approach focuses on a surveillance and containment strategy. It involves the identification of smallpox cases, isolating those individuals, and vaccinating contacts and household contacts of those contacts.[5] The plan did not recommend mass vaccination in response to a documented case. Additional measures were instituted to voluntarily vaccinate first responders and healthcare and emergency personnel who would be responsible for caring for smallpox victims. Unfortunately the response on behalf of healthcare and emergency personnel was subdued due to concerns regarding vaccine safety and the low likelihood of a smallpox threat.

Large-scale vaccination programs in noncivilian populations have been conducted in the past. In 1998, the U.S. Department of Defense recommended vaccinating military recruits against anthrax. Opposition by some recruits was voiced because of a fear of unwanted side effects. Recent efforts to vaccinate military personnel in Iraq against anthrax have been conducted with substantial compliance and success.[7] Implementation strategies for mass vaccination programs against anthrax in the military are continuing to be studied closely so that the lessons learned can be applied to civilian vaccination programs.

IMMUNITY

Immunization is the method of artificially inducing immunity to prevent the development of disease. The artificial induction of immunity was first demonstrated by Edward Jenner in 1796.[8] He observed that milkmaids who had contracted cowpox were immune to smallpox. He developed the practice of vaccination, inoculating fluid from cowpox lesions into the skin of susceptible individuals. Inoculated individuals typically developed mild illness; however, some did develop disseminated infection with secondary complications.

Immunization can be induced via active or passive methods. Active immunization typically involves the administration of a vaccine to induce the host to produce an immune response against a particular microorganism. Passive immunization refers to the practice of providing temporary protection by passively transferring exogenously produced antibody, such as immune globulin, to a susceptible host. Immunizing agents include vaccines, toxoids, antitoxins, and antibody-containing solutions. Immunizing agents are derived from either animal or human sources.

The initial response of the immune system to the introduction of an antigen occurs after the primary exposure. After a period, one witnesses the development of humoral- and cell-mediated immunity. Circulating antibodies do not typically develop for 7 to 10 days. If an antigen is presented for a second time, an exaggerated humoral- or cell-mediated response occurs, called an "amnestic response." These amnestic responses usually result in antibody formation within 4 to 5 days.

There are multiple determinants of immunogenicity. Immunogenicity is determined by the physiological state (e.g., nutrition, immune status, age) and the genetic characteristics (e.g., major histocompatibility complex polymorphism) of the host, the manner in which the immunizing agent is presented (e.g., route, timing of doses, use of adjuvants), and the composition and degree of purity of the antigen.

VACCINES

The ideal vaccine should possess the following characteristics[9]:

- The agent should be easy to produce in well-standardized preparations that are readily quantifiable and stable in immunobiological potency.
- It should be easy to administer.
- It should not produce disease in the recipient or susceptible contacts.
- It should induce long-lasting (ideally permanent) immunity that is measurable by available and inexpensive techniques.
- It should be free of contaminating and potentially toxic substances.
- Adverse reactions should be minimal and minor in consequences.

Current vaccines do not typically meet all of these criteria. Most possess limited efficacy or have unwanted side effects.

Vaccines typically consist of live-attenuated or killed-inactivated microbiological agents. Many viral vaccines contain live-attenuated virus (e.g., measles, mumps, rubella, oral polio). The vaccines for some viruses and most bacteria are killed-inactivated, subunit preparations

or are conjugated to immunobiologically active proteins (e.g., tetanus toxoids). Live-attenuated vaccines tend to elicit a broader immunological response on behalf of the recipient. Live-attenuated vaccines also tend to elicit a more durable immunological response. Killed-inactivated vaccines, which typically have a lesser antigenic mass, require booster vaccinations.

Currently licensed vaccines are both effective and safe; however, adverse events are associated with vaccine administration. Adverse events can be both trivial and life-threatening. Examples include injection site reactions, fever, irritability, and hypersensitivity reactions. Administration of live viruses can sometimes lead to disseminated infection and therefore is contraindicated in certain populations (e.g., immunocompromised). The National Childhood Vaccine Injury Act was passed by Congress in 1986. This act required the reporting of certain vaccine adverse events to the secretary of the DHHS. It also led to the creation of the Vaccine Adverse Events Reporting System.[10] The system's primary function is to investigate and study new vaccine adverse events or changes in the frequency of known vaccine adverse events. The reporting system has helped identify rare adverse events, including intussusceptions associated with rotavirus vaccine,[11,12] myopericarditis and ischemic cardiac events among smallpox vaccine recipients,[13] and viscerotropic and neurotropic disease after yellow fever virus administration.[14]

The development of vaccines and the implementation of vaccination strategies have had a profound impact on childhood morbidity and mortality.[15] From 1951 to 1954, approximately 16,000 cases of polio occurred each year in the United States, four years before vaccine licensure.[16] The impact on the health of schoolchildren was tremendous. In response to the health hazards posed by polio, the United States began a field trial in 1954, in which thousands of susceptible schoolchildren were administered an unlicensed, live polio vaccine developed by Dr. Jonas Salk. *Life* magazine referred to the study as "the biggest experiment in U.S. medical history." Twenty-five years after this historic experiment, the last recorded case of wild-type poliovirus in the United States occurred.[17] In 1988, the World Health Organization launched the global polio eradication effort. Polio is now eradicated from the Western hemisphere, and in 2003 there were only 677 cases recorded worldwide in six different countries.

BIOLOGIC AGENTS

The CDC has designated three categories of biologic agents according to their potential as weapons of terrorism.[18] Category A agents were given the highest priority because they are easily disseminated or transmitted, associated with high mortality rates, can cause panic and social disruption, and require special action for public preparedness. Category B agents are moderately easy to disseminate, cause moderate morbidity and low mortality, and require enhanced diagnostic capacity and disease surveillance. Category C agents include emerging pathogens that have the potential for becoming biologic weapons in the future. Immunizing agents are available against several bioterrorist agents.

Category A

Anthrax (B. Anthracis)

BioPort Corp. in Lansing, Mich., manufactures the only human vaccine for the prevention of anthrax in the United States. Licensed in 1970, the vaccine was formerly known as Anthrax Vaccine Adsorbed (AVA). Its current name is BioThrax. The vaccine is prepared from a cell-free culture filtrate of a nonencapsulated, attenuated strain of B. anthracis.[19] The antigen primarily responsible for inducing protective immunity is the protective antigen.[20] The immunization schedule involves six immunizations. The vaccine is administered subcutaneously in a 0.5-mL dose at 0, 2, and 4 weeks and 6, 12, and 18 months.[21] Annual boosters are recommended thereafter. The available vaccine is recommended for select laboratory workers and military personnel.[22] The vaccine is effective for the prevention of cutaneous disease in adults. Studies in nonhuman primates suggest protection from inhalational disease as well.[23] Adverse events include injection site reactions, fever, chills, myalgia, and hypersensitivity reactions. The vaccine is not licensed for use in children or pregnant women. The vaccine is not currently licensed for postexposure prophylaxis; however, vaccination with antibiotic administration would be recommended in the event of a biologic attack.[4]

Botulism (C. botulinum)

Therapy for botulism includes passive immunization with antitoxin. Human-derived botulinum antitoxin (formerly known as Botulism Immune Globulin Intravenous [BIG-IV]) is only indicated for use in cases of infant botulism.[24] Efficacy was demonstrated in a randomized trial.[25] In the United States, the California Department of Health can be contacted for procurement of BIG-IV. Trivalent equine botulinum antitoxin (types A, B, and E) and bivalent antitoxin (types A and B) are available for the treatment of foodborne or wound botulism. Equine antitoxin can be obtained from the CDC through state health departments. Intravenous administration of equine antitoxin neutralizes toxin molecules that have not yet bound to nerve endings. One vial (10 mL) of trivalent antitoxin (7500 IU of type A, 5500 IU of type B, and 8500 IU of type E) is administered per patient.[26] No additional doses are recommended. The half-life is estimated to be 5 to 8 days.[27] A hypersensitivity reaction has been reported in 9% of individuals.[27,28] A retrospective study demonstrated that the early administration of antitoxin (within 24 hours of onset of symptoms) was associated with an overall mortality rate of 10%, compared with 15% in patients in whom antitoxin was administered after 24 hours of symptoms and 46% in patients who did not receive antitoxin at all.[29] Equine antitoxin is not currently recommended for use in cases of infant botulism. This is largely due to the concern for hypersensitivity reactions. There are no licensed botulism toxoid vaccines currently available.

Smallpox (Variola Major)

Vaccination against smallpox was first performed by Edward Jenner in 1796.[8] The currently available smallpox vaccine was first licensed in 1903.[30] The last case of smallpox in the United States occurred in 1949. Routine vaccination against smallpox was discontinued in the United States in 1972. Eradication of smallpox was officially declared in 1980 by the World Health Organization. Wyeth Laboratories, Inc., the only licensed producer of smallpox vaccine in the United States, discontinued distribution to the civilian population in May 1983.[31] By 1984, only the CDC in Atlanta, Ga., and the Research Institute of Viral Preparations in Moscow, Russia, possessed variola virus isolates. Because of the threat of bioterrorism, the United States produced 15 million doses of smallpox vaccine derived from the New York Board of Health vaccinia strain.[32] An additional 280 million doses of vaccine were to be available by late 2002. Sanofi-aventis has also identified 70 to 90 million doses of vaccinia vaccine from storage that will be added to the nation's stockpile.[32]

The only licensed smallpox vaccine in the United States is a lyophilized, live preparation of vaccinia virus.[24] The vaccine preparation contains vaccinia virus, distinct from the variola virus, which causes smallpox and cowpox virus that was initially used by Jenner. The vaccine is highly effective in preventing smallpox. Protection typically wanes 5 to 10 years after a single dose.[24] The federal government has recently contracted for the production and purchase of a new vaccine preparation. It is derived from tissue cell culture and may become available for use in the next 1 to 2 years. Modified vaccinia virus Ankara (MVA) may be suitable as a new smallpox vaccine.[33] It is an attenuated strain and may be safer than unattenuated products. Smallpox vaccine is currently approved by the U.S. Food and Drug Administration for use in persons in special risk categories, including laboratory workers. The CDC recommended and implemented a voluntary vaccination plan for public safety and public health personnel because of the threat of bioterrorism.

The vaccine is administered with the use of a bifurcated needle. A droplet of vaccine is held by capillarity action between the two tines. The needle is introduced into the epidermis. Fifteen perpendicular strokes are rapidly made in a 5-mm area. The site should be covered with a loose, nonocclusive dressing. One should avoid touching the area to avoid transferring the virus to other body sites. An evolution of skin lesions will occur at the site of inoculation 3 to 21 days after inoculation.[24] The lesion will eventually scab and leave a scar.

Smallpox vaccine is considered safe, but adverse events are described. Approximately 70% of children experience fever.[24] Injection site pain and myalgia are other minor side effects. Complications include postvaccinial encephalitis (12.3/1 million primary vaccinations), progressive vaccinia (1.5/1 million primary vaccinations), eczema vaccinatum (38.5/1 million primary vaccinations), generalized vaccinia (241.5/1 million primary vaccinations), inadvertent inoculation (529.2/1 million primary vaccinations), rashes (1/3700 vaccinated; erythema multiforme is the most common), Stevens-Johnson syndrome (rare), and myopericarditis (<1/12,000 vaccinated persons).[13,34,35] Death occurs as a result of life-threatening reaction to the vaccine in about 1 per 1 million primary vaccinations.[34] Smallpox vaccine should not be administered to individuals with atopic dermatitis or eczema; acute, active, or exfoliative skin conditions; altered immune states; pregnant or breast-feeding women; children younger than 1 year; or individuals with allergy to any vaccine component.[36]

The smallpox vaccine can be used for postexposure prophylaxis. If administered within 96 hours of exposure, it can prevent or significantly decrease the severity of disease experienced by victims.[37,38]

Plague (Y. pestis)

The commercially available plague vaccine was first licensed in 1911.[30] It was a formaldehyde-killed, whole bacilli vaccine. It was administered at 0 and 4 weeks and 6 months as a primary series. Boosters were administered in 6-month intervals for 3 doses, then every 1 to 2 years thereafter. The vaccine did not prevent the development of pneumonic plague, but it did have some protective effect against bubonic disease.[39,40] Adverse effects included local reactions and headache. Hypersensitivity and severe systemic reactions were rare.[41] The vaccine was administered to high-risk individuals, including military personnel working in endemic areas, laboratory workers working directly with Y. pestis, or researchers working with animals in plague enzootic areas. The manufacturer discontinued production of the vaccine in 1999, and it is no longer commercially available. Research is being conducted to produce a vaccine that is protective against pneumonic plague.[42]

Tularemia (F. tularemia)

The first tularemia vaccine was developed in the Soviet Union in the 1930s. It was a live-attenuated vaccine and was administered to millions of individuals who resided in tularemia-endemic regions.[43] An investigational live-attenuated vaccine derived from the avirulent live vaccine has been administered in the United States. The vaccine was reserved for laboratory workers who work routinely with F. tularemia.[44] This product is currently under review by the Food and Drug Administration and is not currently commercially available. In one retrospective study, the live vaccine offered some protection against acute inhalational tularemia among laboratory workers.[45] The live vaccine did not protect against ulceroglandular disease, but individuals who received the vaccine had milder symptoms. Vaccination is not currently recommended for postexposure prophylaxis due to its limited efficacy.

Hemorrhagic Fever Viruses

This category refers to four distinct families of viruses. Filoviridae includes the Ebola and Marburg viruses. Arenaviridae includes the Lassa virus and New World Arenaviridae. Bunyaviridae includes Nairovirus, Phlebovirus, and Hantavirus. Flaviviridae includes dengue, yellow fever, Omsk hemorrhagic fever, and Kyasanur Forest disease. All of these viruses are associated with clinical disease that produces fevers and a bleeding diathesis in humans. There are no licensed vaccines for any of the hemorrhagic fever viruses, except for yellow fever.

The yellow fever vaccine was initially licensed in 1953.[30] It is a live-attenuated vaccine that is highly effective in travelers to endemic areas.[46] It is not recommended for postexposure prophylaxis because of the virus' short incubation period.

Research is being conducted on the development of vaccines for several hemorrhagic fever viruses, including Ebola virus.[47] Research efforts are limited by the need for BSL-4 laboratory space. BSL-4 laboratory space is designed for maximum containment. This lab is used to provide scientists with a safe environment to study deadly pathogens for which there are no available treatments or vaccines.

Category B

Q Fever (Coxiella burnetii)

No human vaccine is currently available in the United States.

Brucellosis (Brucella Species)

No human vaccine is currently available in the United States.

Glanders (Burkholderia mallei)

No human vaccine is currently available in the United States.

Melioidosis (Burkholderia pseudomallei)

No human vaccine is currently available in the United States.

Encephalitis (Alphaviruses)

Examples include eastern equine and western equine encephalomyelitis and Venezuelan equine viruses. No human vaccine is currently available in the United States.

Typhus Fever (Rickettsia prowazekii)

No human vaccine is currently available in the United States.

Toxins (e.g., ricin, staphylococcal enterotoxin B)

No human vaccine is currently available in the United States.

Psittacosis (Chlamydia psittaci)

No human vaccine is currently available in the United States.

Food Safety Threats (e.g., *Salmonella* Species, *Escherichia coli* 0157:H7)

Two typhoid vaccines are currently licensed for use in the United States. The first oral vaccine was licensed for use in 1990.[30] The oral Ty21a vaccine is indicated for children age 6 and older and for adults.[24] Individuals ingest one enteric-coated capsule every 2 days for a total of 4 doses. Each capsule should be taken with cool liquid, 1 hour before a meal and must be kept refrigerated. The manufacturer recommends a new complete series every 5 years.[24] The oral vaccine is associated with minimal unwanted side effects. Reported side effects include abdominal discomfort, nausea, vomiting, fever, headache, and rash.[24] The first parenteral vaccine was licensed for use in 1917.[24] The Vi capsular polysaccharide vaccine is indicated for individuals age 2 and older.[24] The vaccine is administered intramuscularly, one 25-ug (0.5-mL) dose. Booster doses are recommended by the manufacturer every 2 years.[24] Adverse effects associated with the parenteral vaccine include fever (0%-1%), headache (1.5%-3%), and injection site reactions (7%).[24] The demonstrated efficacy of both vaccines ranges from 50% to 80% after a primary series.[30] Immunization is currently recommended for travelers to endemic areas, people with an exposure to a documented *Salmonella typhi* carrier, and laboratory workers with frequent contact with *S. typhi*.[30] General contraindications include children younger than 2, pregnant women, and people with a history of a hypersensitivity reaction to the vaccine. The oral Ty21a vaccine should not be administered to individuals actively taking antibiotics, especially sulfonamides or mefloquine.[30] One should allow the individual to stop taking these medications for at least 24 hours before administering the vaccine. The oral vaccine should not be administered to immunocompromised individuals.[30]

No human vaccine is currently available in the United States for the prevention of illness caused by *E. coli* 0157:H7.

Water Safety Threats (e.g., *Vibrio cholerae*, *Cryptosporidium parvum*)

No human vaccine is currently available in the United States for the prevention of illness caused by *V. cholerae* or *C. parvum*. Two oral cholera vaccines are available elsewhere (WC/rBS and CDV 103 Hgr).[24] Neither vaccine can be administered to children younger than 2.[24] They are not effective against *V. cholerae* 0139 Bengal.[24] The World Health Organization no longer recommends immunization for individuals traveling to or from cholera-infected regions. Cholera vaccine is not required for entry into any country at this time.

Category C

Emerging Threat Agents (e.g., Nipah virus, Hantavirus)

No human vaccine is currently available in the United States for Nipah virus or Hantavirus.

Miscellaneous Agents

Influenza

The currently available inactivated influenza virus vaccine was first licensed in 1945.[30] The vaccine is produced in embryonated hen eggs. It is composed of inactivated whole virus, split product, or neuraminidase/hemagglutinin subunit vaccines.[24] These vaccines are multivalent and typically contain three virus strains.[24] The vaccines are developed annually to match the predicted strains of influenza that are expected to predominate in the coming season. The opportune time to vaccinate people in the United States is October through November. Peak influenza season typically occurs December through March. The vaccine typically offers protection for 4 to 6 months.[48] Vaccine efficacy is estimated at 30% to 80%.[48] The efficacy is influenced by the population, end points measured, and match between vaccine and circulating virus. Febrile reactions are rare in children younger than age 13.[24] Fever tends to occur within 6 to 24 hours of administration of vaccine in children younger than 24 months.[24] Local reactions occur in 10% of individuals 13 years or older.[24] A slight increase in Guillain-Barré syndrome was seen in vaccine recipients.[24] This resulted in an excess rate of approximately 1 per 1 million people immunized.[24] People with a history of Guillain-Barré syndrome or anaphylaxis to egg protein, chickens, or other vaccine components should not receive the inactivated vaccine.[24] The 2004 Advisory Committee on Immunization Practices recommends the following primary groups for vaccination[49]:

- All children 6 to 23 months old
- Persons older than 65
- Pregnant women
- Persons with chronic medical conditions who are at increased risk for influenza-related complications
- Healthcare workers
- Residents of nursing homes and other chronic care facilities
- Household contacts of persons who live, care for, or have frequent contact with persons at high risk and who can transmit influenza to those persons at high risk

Intranasal vaccines also have been developed. Inactivated intranasal vaccines have been shown to be more immunogenic than the injected vaccine.[50] Nasally administered live-virus vaccines also have been developed. These vaccines are made with cold-attenuated influenza viruses. The advantage of these vaccines is that they are relatively easy to administer and induce mucosal immunity.[48] Vaccine recipients reported rhinorrhea (44%) and pharyngitis (26.6%).[51] Efficacy reached 93% in a study involving healthy children.[52] These unwanted side effects typically occurred within 7 days of administration of the vaccine. Intranasally administered live-virus vaccine should be encouraged for healthy persons ages 5 to 49 years.[49] Pregnant women, healthcare workers caring for severely immunocompromised patients in special care units, and persons caring for children younger than 6 months should not receive the live virus vaccine.[49]

FUTURE EFFORTS

Vaccine research continues to advance. Investigators from both private and public institutions are vigorously pursuing more effective and safer vaccine products. Research interests include developing new vaccine delivery systems (e.g., DNA vaccines, novel routes of administration, the creation of combination products, and eliminating unwanted side effects).

Because of the perceived increase in the threat of bioterrorism, several government agencies have been charged with directing their resources and efforts to develop vaccines that will protect the general population from certain biologic agents. The National Institutes of Health and its subordinate, the National Institute of Allergy and Infectious Diseases, are developing medical countermeasures in the form of therapies, vaccines, and diagnostic tools to protect the country from deliberate attacks with biologic agents.[53] Specific research agendas for agents of bioterrorism are outlined in detail by several government agencies.[54,55] Approximately $652 million of the 2005 National Institutes of Health biodefense research budget will be dedicated to vaccine research.[56]

QUARANTINE AND ISOLATION

Webster's New World Dictionary[57] defines *quarantine* as "the period, originally forty days, during which an arriving vessel suspected of carrying contagious disease is detained in port in strict isolation." The word was derived from the Italian *quarantine,* which meant "space of forty days."[57] *Quaranta* was imposed on Italian merchants arriving home to port during the 1300s at the height of the Black Plague outbreaks in Europe. Modern users have applied the term to several scenarios during the era of bioterrorism to refer to travel limitations, restrictions on public gatherings, and isolation of sick individuals to protect others. This has led to much confusion and miscommunication. Recent efforts by several authors have meant to clarify this situation by providing a contemporary definition. They interpret quarantine as referring to the "compulsory physical separation, including restriction of movement, of populations or groups of healthy people who have been potentially exposed to a contagious disease, or to efforts to segregate these persons within specific geographic areas."[58] Human quarantine is justified under the terms of the public health contract.[58] Adverse consequences that have occurred historically with quarantine actions have included the increased risk of transmission among the quarantined population, precipitation of violent acts, and the potential for ethnic bias influencing decision making.[55,60,61]

Isolation refers to "the separation and confinement of individuals known or suspected to be infected with a contagious disease to prevent them from transmitting disease to others."[58] The terms should not be used interchangeably.

REFERENCES

1. Centers for Disease Control and Prevention. Ongoing investigation of anthrax—Florida. October 2001. *Morb Mortal Wkly Rep.* 2001;50:877.
2. Centers for Disease Control and Prevention. Update: investigation of bioterrorism-related anthrax—Connecticut, 2001. *Morb Mortal Wkly Rep.* 2001;50(48):1077-9.
3. Lane HC, La Montagne J, Fauci AS. Bioterrorism: a clear and present danger [erratum in: *Nat Med.* 2002;8:87]. *Nat Med.* 2001;7:1271-3.
4. Henderson DA, Inglesby TV, Bartlett JG, et al. Smallpox as a biologic weapon: medical and public health management. *JAMA.* 1999;281:2127-37.
5. Centers for Disease Control and Prevention. *Interim Smallpox Response Plan and Guidelines: Draft 2.0.* Atlanta: Centers for Disease Control and Prevention; November 21, 2001.
6. Centers for Disease Control and Prevention. *Interim Smallpox Response Plan and Guidelines: Version 3.0.* Atlanta: Centers for Disease Control and Prevention; November 26, 2002. Available at: http://www.bt.cdc.gov/agent/smallpox/response-plan/index.asp.
7. Folio LR, Lahti RL, Cockrum DS, et al. Initial experience with mass immunization as a bioterrorism countermeasure. *J Am Osteopath Assoc.* 2004;104(6):240-3.
8. Hopkins DR. *Princes and Peasants.* Chicago: University of Chicago Press; 1983.
9. Dennehy PH, Peter G. Active immunizing agents. In: Feigin RD, Cherry JD, Demmler GJ, et al, eds. *Textbook of Pediatric Infectious Diseases.* Vol. 2. 2004.
10. National Childhood Vaccine Injury Act of 1986, at Section 2125 of the Public Health Service Act as codified at 42 USC Section 300aa-26.
11. Centers for Disease Control and Prevention. Intussusception among recipients of rotavirus vaccine: United States, 1998-1999. *Morb Mortal Wkly Rep.* 1999;48:577-81.
12. Zanardi LR, Haber P, Mootrey GT, et al. Intussusception among recipients of rotavirus vaccine: reports to the Vaccine Adverse Event Reporting System. *Pediatrics.* 2001;107:E97.
13. Centers for Disease Control and Prevention. Cardiac adverse events following smallpox vaccination: United States, 2003. *Morb Mortal Wkly Rep.* 2003;52:248-50.
14. Centers for Disease Control and Prevention. Adverse events associated with 17D-derived yellow fever vaccination: United States, 2001-2002. *Morb Mortal Wkly Rep.* 2002;51:989-93.
15. Centers for Disease Control and Prevention. Impact of vaccines universally recommended for children—United States, 1990-1998. *Morb Mortal Wkly Rep.* 1999;48:243-8.
16. Pickering LK, Baker CJ, Overturf GD, et al. Active and passive immunization. In: *Red Book: 2003 Report of the Committee on Infectious Diseases.* 26th ed. Elk Grove Village, IL: American Academy of Pediatrics; 2003:2.
17. Strebel PM, Sutter RW, Cochi SL, et al. Epidemiology of poliomyelitis in the United States one decade after the last reported case of indigenous wild virus-associated disease. *Clin Infect Dis.* 1992;14:568-79.
18. Centers for Disease Control and Prevention. Biologic and chemical terrorism: strategic plan for preparedness and response. Recommendations of the CDC Strategic Planning Workgroup. *MMWR Recomm Rep.* 2000;49(RR-4):1-14.
19. Michigan Department of Public Health. *Anthrax Vaccine Adsorbed.* Lansing: Michigan Department of Public Health; 1978.
20. Brachman PS, Friedlander A. Anthrax. In: Plotkin SA, Orenstein WA, eds. *Vaccines.* 3rd ed. Philadelphia: WB Saunders; 1999:629-37.
21. Franz DR, Jahrling PB, Friedlander AM, et al. Clinical recognition and management of patients exposed to biologic warfare agents. *JAMA.* 1997;278:399-411.
22. Centers for Disease Control and Prevention. Notice to readers: use of anthrax vaccine in response to terrorism: supplemental recommendations of the Advisory Committee on Immunization Practices. *Morb Mortal Wkly Rep.* 2002;51:1024-6.
23. Ivins BE, Fellows P, Mitt ML, et al. Efficacy of standard human anthrax vaccine against *Bacillus anthracis* aerosol spore challenge in rhesus monkeys. *Salisbury Med Bull.* 1996;87:125-6.
24. Pickering LK, Baker CJ, Overturf GD, et al. Summaries of infectious diseases. In: *Red Book Report of the Committee on Infectious Diseases.* 26th ed. Elk Grove Village, IL: American Academy of Pediatrics; 2003:245, 386-91, 557, 688.

25. Arnon SS. Clinical trial of human botulism immune globulin. In: Das Gupta, BR, ed. *Botulinum and Tetanus Neurotoxins: Neurotransmission and Biomedical Aspects*. New York: Plenum Press; 1993:477-82.

26. Shapiro RL, Hatheway C, Swerdlow DL. Botulism in the United States: a clinical and epidemiologic review. *Ann Int Med*. 1998;129:221-8.

27. Hatheway CL, Snyder JD, Seals JE, et al. Antitoxin levels in botulism patients treated with trivalent equine botulism antitoxin to toxin types A, B, and E. *J Infect Dis*. 1984;150:407-12.

28. Black RE, Gunn RA. Hypersensitivity reactions associated with botulinal antitoxin. *Am J Med*. 1980;69:567-70.

29. Tacket CO, Shandera WX, Mann JM, et al. Equine antitoxin use and other factors that predict outcome in type A foodborne botulism. *Am J Med*. 1984;76:794-8.

30. Orenstein WA, Wharton M, Bart KJ, et al. Immunization. In: Mandell GL, Bennett JE, Dolin R, eds. *Principles and Practice of Infectious Diseases*. 5th ed. 2000:3211.

31. Centers for Disease Control and Prevention. Recommendation of the Immunization Practices Advisory Committee (ACIP): vaccinia (smallpox) vaccine. *Morb Mortal Wkly Rep*. 1991;40:1-10.

32. Breman JG, Henderson DA. Diagnosis and management of smallpox. *New Engl J Med*. 2002;346:1300-8.

33. Lane JL, Ruben FL, Neff JM, et al. Complications of smallpox vaccination, 1968: national surveillance in the United States. *N Engl J Med*. 1969;281:1201-8.

34. Centers for Disease Control and Prevention. Executive summary: smallpox response plan. Available at: http://www.bt.cdc.gov/agent/smallpox/response-plan/files/exec-sections-i-vi.pdf.

35. Centers for Disease Control and Prevention. Adverse reactions following smallpox vaccination. Available at: http://www.bt.cdc.gov/agent/smallpox/vaccination/reactions-vacc-clinic.asp.

36. Dixon CW. *Smallpox*. London: J&A Churchill; 1962:1460.

37. Dixon CW. Tripolitania, 1946: an epidemiological and clinical study of 500 cases, including trials of penicillin treatment. *J Hyg*. 1948;46:351-77.

38. Earl PL, Americo JL, Wyatt ES, et al. Immunogenicity of a highly attenuated MVA smallpox vaccine and protection against monkeypox. *Nature* 2004;428:182-5.

39. Speck RS, Wolochow H. Studies on the experimental epidemiology of respiratory infections: experimental pneumonic plague in Macacus rhesus. *J Infect Dis*. 1957;100:58-69.

40. Centers for Disease Control and Prevention. Prevention of plague: recommendations of the Advisory Committee on Immunization Practice (ACIP). *Morb Mortal Wkly Rep*. 1996;45(RR-14):1-15.

41. Orenstein WA, Wharton M, Bart KJ, et al. Immunization. In: Mandell GL, Bennett JE, Dolin R, eds. *Principles and Practice of Infectious Diseases*. 5th ed. 2000:3218.

42. Titball RW, Eley S, Williamson ED, et al. Plague. In: Plotkin S, Mortimer EA, eds. *Vaccines*. Philadelphia: WB Saunders; 1999:734-42.

43. Sjostedt A, Tarnvik A, Sandstrom G. *Francisella tularensis:* host-parasite interaction. *FEMS Immunol Med Microbiol*. 1996;13:181-4.

44. French GR, Plotkin SA. Miscellaneous limited-use vaccines. In: Plotkin S, Mortimer EA, eds. *Vaccines*. Philadelphia: WB Saunders; 1999:728-33.

45. Burke DS. Immunization against tularemia: analysis of the effectiveness of live *Francisella tularensis* vaccine in prevention of laboratory-acquired tularemia. *J Infect Dis*. 1977;135:55-60.

46. Monath TP. Yellow fever: an update. *Lancet Infect Dis*. 2001; 1:11-20.

47. Sullivan NJ, Sanchez A, Rollin PE, et al. Development of a preventative vaccine for Ebola virus infection in primates. *Nature*. 2000;408:605-9.

48. Cifu A, Levinson W. Influenza. *JAMA*. 2000;284:2847-9.

49. Centers for Disease Control and Prevention. Influenza. Available at: http://www.cdc.gov/flu.

50. Muszkat M, Yehuda AB, et al. Local and systemic immune response in community-dwelling elderly after intranasal or intramuscular immunization with inactivated influenza vaccine. *J Med Virol*. 2000;61:100-6.

51. Nichol KL, Mendelman PM, et al. Effectiveness of live, attenuated intranasal influenza vaccine in healthy, working adults: a randomized, controlled trial. *JAMA*. 1999;282:137-44.

52. Belshe RB, Mendelman PM, et al. The efficacy of live, attenuated, cold-adapted, trivalent, intranasal influenza virus vaccine in children. *New Engl J Med*. 1998;338:1405-12.

53. Fauci AS. Biodefence on the research agenda. *Nature*. 2003;421:787.

54. National Institute of Allergy and Infectious Diseases. NIAID biodefense research. Available at: http://www2.niaid.nih.gov/biodefense/.

55. Eidson W. Confusion, controversy, and quarantine: the Muncie smallpox epidemic of 1893. *Indiana Mag Hist*. 1990;LXXXVI:374-98.

56. Hirschberg R, La Montagne J, Fauci AS. Biomedical research—an integral component of national security. *New Engl J Med*. 2004;350:2119-21.

57. *Webster's New World Dictionary*. 2nd College ed. New York: Simon and Schuster; 1982:1162.

58. Henderson DA, Inglesby TV, O'Toole T. *Bioterrorism: Guidelines for Medical and Public Health Management*. Chicago: AMA Press; 2002:222.

59. Merritt D. The constitutional balance between health and liberty. *Hastings Cent Rep*. December 1986:2-10.

60. Markel H. "Knocking out the cholera": cholera, class and quarantines in New York City. 1892. *Bull Hist Med*. 1995;69:420-57.

61. Center for Law and the Public's Health at Georgetown and Johns Hopkins Universities. Public Health and the Protection of Individual Rights. Jew Ho v Williamson, 103 F. 10 (1900). Available at: http://www.publichealthlaw.net/Reader/dl.php?doc_id=7103010.

Occupational Medicine: An Asset in Time of Crisis

Tee L. Guidotti

Corporations and other large institutions have become deeply concerned with continuity of operations and the security of their personnel. The new urgency placed on these functions since Sept. 11, 2001, has drawn attention to a substantial resource already in place in such organizations—their occupational health services. The imperatives of corporate security and homeland defense have, in turn, invigorated and expanded the mission of occupational medicine, one of the oldest recognized medical specialties.[1]

Occupational health services are most familiar in the manufacturing sector and in the setting of a plant's medical clinic. Typically, such services include at least one occupational health nurse (also a professional specialization); an occupational physician (typically on contract); and support staff, all of whom report on a regular basis to a plant manager and are responsible professionally to a corporate medical director, who himself or herself serves as a traveling troubleshooter, in-house resource on health issues, and auditor for health affairs. This physician-led, health-centered team typically is engaged in regular interaction and troubleshooting in collaboration with an industrial hygienist and safety officer, who are usually oriented more toward process and plant operations, documenting regulatory compliance, and identifying and measuring health hazards. These hazard-oriented professionals usually report to a different manager or directly to the plant manager. This basic pattern was once the norm in industry, but the dramatic reorganization in industry, management focus on core business, and the rise of the service sector have forged a new pattern, in which services are outsourced to contractors and consultants.[2]

However, whichever pattern is followed in a particular enterprise, the following essentials are in place in most large operations: a means of monitoring the health of workers, a system for documenting their health, a system for documenting and evaluating hazards, a mechanism for responding to emergencies, and a panel of health consultants.[3]

This is exactly the type of infrastructure that large organizations need so that they can respond to disasters and protect the security and continuity of operations.[4]

Thus, large organizations already have in place a structure on which to build to protect their operations and personnel. Involvement of the occupational health service in emergency management, which was common in the past, is a natural extension into disaster medicine, involving training and preparation for consequence management and mitigation activities,[5] preparedness for a response indigenous to the physical plant, and planning for the management of risks inherent to the operation.[2,6] The occupational health service also has an important place at the table as an active member of the healthcare team, interacting with local prehospital care providers and hospitals on the Local Emergency Preparedness Committee (LEPC).

Box 23-1 presents the usual functions of a corporate medical department, provided or supervised by occupational physicians.[2] These functions have traditionally been clustered in a few broad missions: to protect health, to support productivity, to reduce loss and liability, to manage health affairs, and to ensure compliance with regulations and best practice for the industry. These functions have traditionally been viewed as support functions, not part of the business operations of the organization. Indeed, this is why these functions were subject to outsourcing throughout the private and government sectors during the 1980s and 1990s.

A new realization of the criticality of these functions is spreading in the corporate sector, stirred by the awareness of the profound threat of major industrial incidents and potential terrorist attacks to the continuity of operations and the survival of key personnel.[4,7] The role of the occupational physician is increasingly recognized for its potential to contribute to the survival of the enterprise, not just its efficient operation.[3] For example, Dow received an award from the state of Michigan Public Health Department for assistance to the state, particularly with respect to its efforts in disaster planning.

The usefulness of a trained, well-informed, prequalified medical resource for dealing with incidents on-site is obvious. These incidents may include, but are certainly not limited to, sending infectious material through the mail to company personnel and using company equipment, such as airplanes or, potentially, chemical plants or storage facilities, as instruments of assault. The occupational physician, who is trained in hazard assessment, also may assume the responsibility of determining when a site is safe to re-enter or when a facility can be reopened. He or she also would be responsible for managing the psychological consequences of an assault.

Less obvious, but equally valuable, is the role that such physicians may play in managing the consequences of widespread disruption to business operations due to major threats and in protecting the business, the product, and the brand against catastrophe in cases in which a company's products, facilities, or operations are used to deliver a threat or become targets for terrorist activity. In time of crisis, the occupational physician may help get the community back on its feet by helping to keep an employer open or critical infrastructure functioning.[8]

Similarly, the occupational physician has been called on to manage the corporate response to serious health-related issues, such as traveling to areas in which severe acute respiratory syndrome (SARS) and other emerging infections are a risk; rapidly investigating suspicious outbreaks of disease or exposure to potential hazards; and determining when re-entry and reoccupancy is possible in contaminated facilities, such as post office facilities contaminated with anthrax.[4] Several companies, including Cathay Pacific, participated in an informal monitoring network during the SARS epidemic to share observed trends and experience when the information they needed was not forthcoming from conventional sources. Procter and Gamble, alerted to the emerging problem by its own corporate medical leader for China, instituted SARS precautions a month before any official warnings were advised.

These functions build on the traditional involvement of physicians in disaster planning, as well as health protection for employees.[2,6] Disaster planning has traditionally been one of the core functions of the medical department and occupational physicians in corporate settings. The physician has usually assumed responsibility within the organization for planning the medical response to emergencies, identifying facilities and resources for dealing with serious injuries and mass casualties, and providing health protection for key personnel, if required. Although outsourcing has reduced the direct involvement of occupational physicians in planning emergency management in many organizations, particularly in the service sector, this function has not been completely replaced by external consultants because it requires a practitioner with intimate knowledge of the operations, hazards, workforce, and policies of the organization.

The occupational physician can add value to the management of catastrophic consequences in many other ways. These include the following:

- Survival of key personnel in a catastrophic event
- Continuity of business after a catastrophic event
- Instant connectivity to resources for assistance in a health-related emergency
- Surveillance of the workforce and the early detection of an outbreak
- Integration of emergency response with public health agencies
- Surge capacity in the event of a local event that requires mobilization of all available medical resources
- Vaccination programs and other protective measures
- Establishing on-site consequence management and mitigation programs
- Developing decontamination plans
- Providing specialized, sector-specific expertise to emergency managers
- Advising on effective personal protective equipment (PPE)
- Liasing with the LEPC, prehospital care, and hospitals
- Continuing education and training on-site and in the community of the indigenous risks inherent to the operation
- Accessing material safety data sheet information
- Leading any after-action discussion to bring about process and system improvement

Performing these duties effectively requires committed time for preparedness activities and an occupational health service that is structured and whose providers are trained to play such a role in time of crisis. However, it is costly and inefficient for even large corporations to dedicate a full staff and support structure for the management of an event that may or may not materialize. This is why adaptation of the existing occupational health service makes sense for many employers, especially those in critical or hazardous industries.

Incorporating emergency management into the mission of the occupational health service builds allows for an emergency response system that a business would not otherwise have. The same resources used for tracking employees' health can be used for surveillance to detect potential disease outbreaks due to bioterrorism. The technology of hazard identification and measurement can be applied to detect chemical or radiation threats. The medical staff on duty primarily to monitor health and to provide timely clinical care can provide surge capacity in time of crisis. Health protection for senior executives, and the personal knowledge that this entails, can keep key personnel on the job and safe, especially when they are moved to new locations or are operating under conditions of stress and potential risk. The skills that are normally applied to ensuring a safe workplace can be used to determine when it is acceptable to return to work or to venture into a facility that has been contaminated or damaged. Planning for foreseeable industrial disasters can inform and refine the response to unforeseen threats, given that sophisticated disaster planning is a matter of identifying resources and contingencies, not deriving detailed plans for single-threat incidents.

Perhaps most attractive to cost-conscious managers is that investment in expanding the emergency management capacity within an occupational health service is not "lost" if an event never occurs. The same capacity supports and enhances the traditional occupational health services that industry and government employees require and may lead to cost savings, increased productivity, and reduced liability in their own right.

Occupational physicians, who are conscious of their responsibility and aware of their own position on the firing line along with the employees and executives they protect, have been preparing themselves for an expanded role in emergency management. The principal specialty organization, the American College of Occupational and Environmental Medicine (ACOEM), has for some time offered training in the characteristics of weapons of mass destruction (well before Sept. 11, 2001, and the anthrax assaults), emerging infections (particularly using the model of SARS), and "tabletop" exercises to train participants in emergency management and consequence management for disasters and mass casualties. Immediately after the Sept. 11, 2001, tragedy, an ACOEM task force produced a guide to the management of mental health issues among survivors of mass assaults, disseminated it to all members, and posted it on the ACOEM Web site—all within four days. This achievement was unique and widely admired among medical specialty organizations.

In 2003, leaders within ACEOEM developed the Occupational Health Coordinating Group (OH-CG) as a resource for coordinating responses, accessing management resources, and sharing information in times of crisis. It includes physicians, occupational health nurses, industrial hygienists, and other occupational health professionals. The OH-CG is a working council, sponsored by the Department of Health and Human Services, within what will eventually become a health-sector ISAC (Informational Sharing and Coordination) organization. This is a highly unusual and encouraging development in many respects. ISACs have official status with the Department of Homeland Security and are intended to coordinate the planning response of critical sectors of the American economy and society. They have been formed, for example, in industry sectors such as critical utilities and transportation. The OH-CG was the first health-sector ISAC to be created and is now the Occupational Health Subcommittee of the Healthcare Sector Coordinating Council, the ISAC for healthcare. This is a remarkable achievement for a relatively small medical specialty. Because occupational health is cross-cutting across industries, the OH-CG is expected to serve as a resource for other critical sectors rather than to focus primarily on the health sector per se and in so doing uniquely relate to other ISACs as much as the one of which it is a part. Its mission is to provide occupational health professionals with what they need and when they need it in a time of crisis through channels that do not depend on any one mode of communication.

How might an organization prepare its occupational health department to respond on this scale in a crisis? Partly, the answer is to build an effective and efficient team. Teamwork comes from training and planning but also from regular personal contact and cooperation. A team that functions well in the complex duties of an occupational health service and that already knows the operations, workforce, and facilities is more likely to function well in an emergency than would an outside provider, who may not be around during a crisis.

Another part of the answer is to build redundant information and communication systems that can quickly retrieve critical information on hazards, disease or injury patterns, and individual health records in an adverse environment. Occupational health systems may require upgrading to do this effectively, but the technology is readily available. Partnerships within the LEPC, local industry, and other like facilities not only reduce the initial and ongoing costs but also enable more efficient planning, training, and response.

Acquiring the necessary expertise is obvious. The occupational health staff may require special training to take on the additional functions, but this is not much of a stretch from current duties. County emergency managers are eager to share training opportunities through grants and other programs within the public domain. On-site training and response in coordination with local prehospital care using strategies of consequence management and mitigation, education, decontamination, and PPE will support Occupational Safety and Health Administration efforts to protect workers and may reduce liability exposure for the organization's insurers. The expense for preparedness may be justified by potential reductions in insurance premiums, as well as reduction of loss in the event of an emergency.

Establishing networks and agreements for mutual assistance may be critical. Here, the occupational health staff can coordinate arrangements with local hospitals, specialist practitioners, public health agencies, and first responders in advance and maintain personal relationships required for smooth operation in the event of a crisis. The first step is to forge an active participant's role in the LEPC. Some counties have a more active, dynamic, and responsive LEPC than others do. An occupational health service for a large organization has the opportunity to lead and become the backbone of emergency management in the community.

Facilities planning may be required, taking into account the characteristics of the site for evacuation, securing the premises but preserving access for ambulances and first responders, and defining areas of the plant for operational response (e.g., for staging rescue operations, triage, stabilizing casualties, decontamination, and "incident command"[9] activities). Even locations without special hazards may benefit from such contingency planning in the event of an external threat. For example, the first anthrax assault was in the office of a newspaper, not normally a high-risk location.

Under various contingencies, surge capacity may be projected, as well as whether to call in help for managing mass casualties on-site (especially if local hospitals are not functioning or cannot be reached), to assist other units in a mutual assistance pact, or to perform services such as mass immunizations. On-site decontamination may have to be continued at the hospital or a second location away from the industrial incident. Surge capacity operations may be created away from the hospital under the direction of the LEPC, county emergency manager, or hospital. This may include separate healthcare mutual aid agreements specific for the incident and secondary triage and treatment provided by trained physicians and other healthcare providers through the use of vendor agreements or prepositioned equipment and supplies. This strategy will enable the hospital and community healthcare delivery system to operate at near-standard operations during an industrial incident. Any facility that has potable water, electricity, and shelter may participate. Pre-existing arrangements for accessing these sites should be spelled out under mutual aid agreements, vendor contracts, memoranda of understanding, or special circumstances agreements negotiated in advance between the county emergency management office, the hospital, or the local employer. Documentation of expenditures is a critical function, just as it is in the incident command structure,[9] to reimburse all nonvolunteers and contracts executed in the response.

Certain routine functions can be anticipated and planned. For example, if anthrax or some other threat is determined to be a possibility for a business, procedures can be put in place in advance to protect employees, limit disruption, and rapidly evaluate evolving situations. This was done in a timely manner by DST Output, the nation's largest direct mail operation, on the advice of its medical director. Planning is particularly important to deter inevitable hoaxes and to prevent disruptions to business from ill-defined or unknown hazards. For example, the common scenario of an unknown "white powder" appearing on a loading dock or in an office can shut down operations for a day or more until a toxic substance is ruled out. Having the capacity on hand to show that it is harmless saves time and anxiety.

Confronted with a true emergency, most people behave in an adaptive, rational manner that helps them to get through the crisis and to mitigate personal damage or injury. Some are capable of helping others in an emergency.[10] This response appears to be shaped, at least in part, by whether the emergency arises from a natural disaster or a "technological" event (an incident arising from human agency).[6] The perception of an intentional assault may also shape the psychological response for some people. Some people in situations of perceived catastrophic risk behave irrationally, however, and demonstrate psychogenic symptoms and maladaptive behavior.[11-22] Dealing with anxiety-promoting perceptions and psychogenic symptoms among employees that arise from rumors or incidental illness occurring at the worksite requires skill in rapid assessment and in risk communication but can save an enterprise from devastating loss of confidence and potential loss from employees who may refuse to come to work. Distinguishing between human drama and a true emergency arising from a nonobvious cause is also a challenge that requires specialized expertise that is within the scope of the occupational physician.

An enterprise may be in a position to control its liability and potential loss from claims after a disaster by developing a flexible, effective emergency management capability within its occupational health services before a disaster event. In addition to reducing actual loss through planning and effective consequence management, which is most important, such an enterprise would also be able to show after the fact that it had done its due diligence in anticipating and preparing for plausible threats. This could reduce its exposure to punitive awards or claims based on negligence or omission. Legal opinions on this may vary, but it seems reasonable that a company that appears to be prepared is less likely to be accused after the fact of ignoring a foreseeable threat.

In the classic business model followed during times of business as usual, the priorities of corporate management in descending order are shareholder value and profitability, continuity of production and operations, and loss control and risk management. For government agencies, there is a similar set of priorities, with the mission of the agency coming first. However, in times of crisis, survival of the enterprise and protection of people take precedence. In the past, occupational medicine and occupational health services have always been perceived as support functions, facilitating management priorities, but not core business priorities. In the new era of threats to survival and business continuity, occupational health services and the physicians in them may play a role in the survival of the enterprise and its people. A wise organization, faced with an extraordinary threat, may look within to build its salvation on a functioning system that already serves its interests.

REFERENCES

1. Emmett EA. What is the strategic value of occupational and environmental medicine? Observations from the United States and Australia. *J Occup Environ Med.* November 1996;38(11):1124-34.
2. Guidotti TL, Cowell JWF, Jamieson GG. *Occupational Health Services: A Practical Approach.* Chicago: American Medical Association; 1989:369.
3. McLellan RK, Deitchman SD. Role of the occupational and environmental medicine physician. In: Upfal MJ, Krieger GR, Phillips SD, Guidotti TL, Weissman D, eds. Terrorism: biological, chemical, and nuclear. *Clin Occup Environ Med.* 2003;2(2):181-90.
4. Hudson TW, Roberts M. Corporate response to terrorism. In: Upfal MJ, Krieger GR, Phillips SD, Guidotti TL, Weissman D, eds. Terrorism: biological, chemical, and nuclear. *Clin Occup Environ Med.* 2003;2(2):389-404.
5. Haddow GD, Bullock JA. *Introduction to Emergency Management.* Boston: Butterworth Heinemann; 2003:37-47.
6. Guidotti TL. Managing incidents involving hazardous substances. *Am J Prev Med.* 1986;2:14-154.
7. Guidotti TL, Hoffman H. Terrorism and the civilian response. In: Upfal MJ, Krieger GR, Phillips SD, Guidotti TL, Weissman D, eds. Terrorism: biological, chemical, and nuclear. *Clin Occup Environ Med.* 2003;2(2):169-80.
8. Landesman LY. *Public Health Management of Disasters: The Practice Guide.* Washington DC: American Public Health Association; 2001:145.
9. Hogan A. Municipal and emergency health care planning in disasters. In: Hogan DE, Burstein JL. *Disaster Medicine.* Philadelphia: Lippincott Williams & Wilkins; 2002:108-9.
10. Auf der Heide E. Common misconceptions about disasters: panic, the "disaster syndrome", and looting. In: O'Leary M. *The First 72 Hours: A Community Approach to Disaster Preparedness.* Lincoln, NE: Universe Publishing, 2004:340-79.
11. Guidotti TL, Alexander RW, Fedoruk MJ. Epidemiologic features that may distinguish between building-associated illness outbreaks due to chemical exposure or psychogenic origin. *J Occup Med.* 1987;29:148-50.
12. Amin Y, Hamdi E, Eapen V. Mass hysteria in an Arab culture. *Int J Soc Psychiatry.* 1997;43(4):303-6.
13. Bartholomew RE, Wessely S. Protean nature of mass sociogenic illness: from possessed nuns to chemical and biological terrorism fears. *Br J Psychiatry.* 2002;180:300-6.
14. Boxer PA. Occupational mass psychogenic illness. History, prevention and management. *J Occup Med.* 1985;27(12):867-72.
15. Cardena E, Spiegel D. Dissociative reactions to the San Francisco Bay area earthquake of 1989. *Am J Pyschiatry.* 1993;150(3):474-8.
16. Colligan MJ, Urtes MA, Wisseman C, Rosensteel RE, Anania TL, Hornet RW. An investigation of apparent mass psychogenic illness in an electronics plant. *J Behav Med.* 1979;2(3):297-309.
17. House RA, Holness DL. Investigation of factors affecting mass psychogenic illness in employees in a fish-packing plant. *Am J Ind Med.* 1997;32(1):90-6.
18. Leach J. Why people "freeze" in an emergency: temporal and cognitive constraints on survival responses. *Aviat Space Environ Med.* 2004;75(6):539-42.
19. Magnavita N. Industrial mass psychogenic illness: the unfashionable diagnosis. *Br J Med Psychol.* 2000;73(pt 3):371-5.
20. Norwood AE, Ursano RJ, Fullerton CS. Disaster psychiatry: principles and practice. *Psychiatr Q.* 2000;71(13):207-26.
21. Ryan CM, Morrow LA. Dysfunctional buildings or dysfunctional people: an examination of the sick building syndrome and allied disorders. *J Consult Clin Psychol.* 1992;60(2):220-4.
22. Streuwing JP, Gray GC. An epidemic of respiratory complaints exacerbated by mass psychogenic illness in a military recruit population. *Am J Epidemiol.* 1990;132(6):1120-9.

chapter 24

Worker Health and Safety in Disaster Response

Clifford S. Mitchell, Brian J. Maguire, and Tee L. Guidotti

This chapter addresses worker safety in disaster response, including evaluation and management of workers involved in a disaster, medical surveillance, legal and regulatory requirements related to worker exposures, and specific issues for particular worker populations. Protection of worker safety and health during and after a disaster requires careful planning, training, and integration of occupational medicine, nursing, industrial hygiene, safety, and environmental functions. Recent disasters, including the terrorist attacks of Sept. 11, 2001, and the use of anthrax in the postal system, have demonstrated the importance of integrating emergency preparedness with other aspects of occupational and safety and health.[1]

PRE-EVENT PLANNING

The previous chapter discussed pre-event planning for a disaster, including the need for mutual assistance networks, facility planning and surge capacity, and consideration of potential threat agents. In addition, it is important to consider workforce preparation and training, not only for first and secondary responders, but for others who might potentially be involved in disaster response, including skilled support personnel and other categories of workers.[2] All workers should receive pre-event training and "real-life" drills in certain basic aspects of disaster response, including:

- Egress and evacuation
- Use of personal protective equipment (PPE)
- Recognition of threats/hazards
- Activation of the emergency response system
- Incident command
- Their own specific functional role in an emergency

In addition, certain workers may need additional training, depending on their jobs. Some of these requirements are described in the U.S. Occupational Safety and Health Administration (OSHA) standard for hazardous waste operations and emergency response (HAZWOPER).[3] The HAZWOPER standard describes worker safety requirements for hazardous waste or emergency response sites that could involve chemical, biological, nuclear, radiological, or other hazards. OSHA distinguishes between training requirements for workers who need basic awareness training, those at the "operations level," workers known as hazardous materials technicians (workers involved in stopping the release of hazards), workers with specific knowledge of the hazards involved, and the on-scene incident commanders.

Another aspect of pre-event planning involves PPE. Selection of PPE involves collaboration between industrial hygiene, safety, occupational medicine and nursing, and those involved in evaluating the potential risks and agents involved. The National Institute for Occupational Safety and Health (NIOSH) recently issued standards for respiratory protection against chemical, biological, radiological, and nuclear (CBRN) hazards.[4]

MANAGEMENT OF WORKERS INVOLVED IN DISASTER RESPONSE

During the disaster response, workers should receive limited briefings and training, sufficient to ensure that they are aware of the specific hazards they face on the site, that they are able to use their PPE appropriately, and that they understand the specific command structure and communications systems in place at the site. This applies to workers at the site of a large-scale disaster after the initial response. Hospital workers at receiving hospitals ("first receivers") should also receive training, with the level of training depending on how likely the personnel are to have direct contact with contaminated patients.[5] Training for first receivers should ideally take place well before an incident occurs because such training may not be practical during the emergency phase.[6,7]

The medical management of acutely exposed individuals is discussed elsewhere in this text. There are, however, specific considerations for the management of workers who may be involved in disaster response, particularly if they have been potentially exposed to hazardous agents. These include use of biological monitoring for acute exposures, surveillance for illness and injury after exposures, mental health considerations, and reporting requirements for specific exposures.

In many cases, workers who are designated first or secondary responders will already be enrolled in medical surveillance programs and will have received baseline or pre-event medical evaluations as required under the HAZWOPER standard.[8] Although the standard does not specify the tests that must be performed, it does require "... [a] medical and work history (or updated history if one is in the employee's file) with special emphasis on symptoms related to the handling of hazardous substances and health hazards, and to fitness for duty including the ability to wear any required PPE under conditions (i.e., temperature extremes) that may be expected at the work site...."[9] Typically, such workers also receive a clinical examination that includes laboratory tests (particularly baseline liver and renal function tests and hematological parameters), pulmonary function tests, chest roentgenograms, electrocardiograms, and other tests as indicated clinically. The selection of particular tests is based on the likelihood of exposure to and toxicological properties of possible agents and medical judgment about the utility of the tests as screening tests for disease or injury.

Workers involved in disasters where exposures to hazardous substances may occur should be evaluated as soon as possible after the incident. This evaluation has the following purposes:

- Obtain as complete a picture as possible of the exposure
- Estimate the potential for an internal dose
- Determine which, if any, biological measures of exposure may be appropriate
- Treat for acute exposures as needed
- Determine the need for follow-up, including surveillance

Estimating exposure and internal dose initially requires information about the hazards at the site, the activities and duration of exposure, type of PPE worn, and other relevant factors. For the medical provider, it is often helpful to create a questionnaire, in consultation with a knowledgeable industrial hygienist, that can be given to all of the potentially affected workers. Questionnaires help to standardize information and make it easier to see large numbers of patients efficiently. Questionnaires can include not only information about the current exposure, but also about past occupational and environmental exposures and pertinent medical history. There are several good references available for a standardized occupational/environmental history form.[10]

Medical surveillance requirements will depend on the agent(s) involved and the exposed population. Some substances, such as lead or asbestos, may have specific regulatory requirements for postexposure surveillance related to occupational exposure, but in many cases, it will be up to the healthcare provider to determine surveillance recommendations on a case-by-case basis.

Healthcare personnel should coordinate closely with industrial hygiene, safety, and environmental personnel to understand as completely as possible the nature and extent of exposure. The selection of appropriate biologic exposure indicators may be aided by intra- and post-event environmental sampling. If the exposures occurred at an industrial location, additional information may be available through the company's environmental health and safety office or through the company's public reports submitted in compliance with the Emergency Planning and Community Right-to-Know Act.[11] Material data safety sheets are available online, as are databases such as the National Library of Medicine's toxicology databases. These are useful aids in choosing appropriate surveillance tests.[12] For radiological emergencies, useful resources include the Radiation Emergency Assistance Center/Training Site (REAC/TS) at the Oak Ridge Institute for Science and Education (available at: http://www.orau.gov/reacts/). Resources for chemical exposures include local poison control centers, industry emergency response centers (many of which have 24-hour hot lines or online response), and federal agencies such as the Environmental Protection Agency. The Centers for Disease Control and Prevention maintains a registry of emergency preparedness training opportunities for clinicians, as well as information about biological hazards.[13] Follow-up studies of clean-up workers at the World Trade Center demonstrate the importance of looking systematically for symptoms and biological indicators of exposure.[14]

Mental health issues are a critical component of worker safety and health management in disasters. Numerous studies have addressed the mental health consequences of disasters, and mental health professionals should participate in both pre-event planning and postevent management of workers involved in disaster response. There is still a need for considerable research related to the effectiveness of various mental health interventions used in disaster management.[15] After the disaster, both emergency responders and those who worked at the location may require considerable preparation before resuming their work.[16]

Both occupational disease reporting and workers' compensation, although rarely immediate concerns in the postevent period, are considerations for workers who have been involved in disaster response. OSHA regulations require that employers report occupational illness and injury. Workers in a disaster may still ultimately be covered by OSHA regulations if the workers are responding as a part of their job.[17] Similarly, many states have surveillance reporting requirements for occupational diseases, and in some cases, these could also apply to disaster response workers. Finally, workers who become injured or ill in the process of responding to a disaster may be entitled to workers' compensation.

OCCUPATIONS INVOLVED IN DISASTER RESPONSE

This section considers occupational groups that will typically be involved in disaster response. The experience of Sept. 11, 2001 showed that many individuals and volunteers may also be involved in disaster response, and their health needs should also be considered in the medical response; however, the groups discussed in this section are, in many cases, expected to put themselves in situations in which they are likely to be exposed to potentially life-threatening hazards.

First Responders

First responders are primarily emergency and security personnel; the term "first receivers" has been used to describe those who are first to receive the victims in the emergency room. The overriding priority of first responders is to protect the victims and to secure the location. They rescue or otherwise protect others who are not able to save themselves. If the personal risk is acceptable, their secondary objective is to protect property from destruction or damage. To achieve these priorities, first responders allow themselves to be exposed to hazards that are unusual for anyone else in the community and that would not be tolerated in other occupations.

The occupations normally considered among first responders include the following:

- Police
- Firefighters (often cross-trained as emergency medical services [EMS] and hazardous materials [HazMat] personnel)
- EMS personnel

Two other categories of workers who are often deployed early in disaster response have been termed "second responders" and "skilled support personnel." Secondary responders include a broad range of workers, including certain emergency public health and medical personnel, HazMat personnel, crime scene technicians, urban search and rescue personnel, mortuary personnel, radiation safety experts, structural engineers, and others who may be involved in all aspects of the disaster response. Skilled support personnel are defined in the HAZWOPER standard as workers who are operators of certain heavy equipment, such as hoisting equipment and cranes and earth moving or digging equipment, and who may also be exposed to hazards on-site.

First responders are generally the second to arrive on the scene after concerned nearby passersby and neighbors who rush to provide immediate assistance. In so doing, they are often exposed to hazards that would be intolerable in normal work. In a terrorist event, they would also be intentional targets.

The occupational risks of first responders include the same hazards that threaten the victims. Because first responders often arrive before the site has been secured, decontaminated, or thoroughly searched, they may face threatening situations on arrival. For example, the first arrivals at the site of a terrorist bombing must face the real possibility of a second explosive device intended for them. Even after the site is secured, first responders are confronted with events and circumstances outside the usual experience of humans in their daily lives.

Although each of the occupations that constitute first responders has its own set of hazards, risks, and traditions, first responders share several features in common, including:

- An awareness of personal danger, often accompanied by coping mechanisms that may include denial
- Long periods of relative quiet or routine interrupted abruptly by periods of intense activity, often accompanied by psychological stress
- Rigid codes of behavior and high expectations for performance, often accompanied by complicated job responsibilities and guidelines and high penalties for failure
- A strong ethic of teamwork and camaraderie, always with a strong sense of mutual reliance and social penalties for letting down one's co-workers
- A rigid hierarchy or "chain of command," which is necessary to reduce uncertainty and to make sure that procedures are followed correctly

Firefighters

Occupational hazards experienced by firefighters may be categorized as physical (mostly unsafe conditions, thermal stress, and ergonomic stress), chemical, and psychological.[18,19] The level of exposure to these hazards that a firefighter may experience in a given fire depends on what is burning, the combustion characteristics of the fire, the structure on fire, the presence of nonfuel chemicals, the measures taken to control the fire, the presence of victims requiring rescue, and the position or line of duty held by the firefighter while battling the fire. The hazards and levels of exposure experienced by the first firefighter to enter a burning building and engage in fire suppression, called "knockdown," are different from those of the firefighters who enter later to search for smoldering fuel that could flare up later, a process called "overhaul." In general, the former is exposed to a greater risk of trauma, and the latter is exposed to more hazardous chemicals by inhalation.

There are many physical dangers in firefighting that can lead to serious physical injury.[20] Injuries can be minimized by intensive training, job experience, strict preplacement screening, competency, and physical fitness. However, the nature of the job is such that firefighters may be placed in dangerous situations by miscalculation or circumstance or during rescues. The structure that a firefighter enters is not only on fire but often weakened structurally. Walls, ceilings, and floors may collapse abruptly and trap firefighters or cause them to fall. Exposed wires may present a risk of electrocution.

Injuries associated with firefighting are therefore predictable: burns, falls, and being struck by falling objects. Mortality from these causes is markedly increased among firefighters compared with other workers. Jobs in firefighting with a high risk of burns, especially, include those involving early entry and close-in firefighting, such as holding the nozzle. Burns are also more commonly associated with basement fires, recent injury before the incident, and training outside the fire department of present employment. Falls tend to be associated with self-contained breathing apparatus (SCBA) use, ladder work, and assignment to truck companies.

The energy requirements for firefighting are complicated by the severe conditions encountered in many inside fires. The metabolic demands of coping with retained body heat, heat from the fire, and fluid loss through sweating add to the demands of physical exertion. Firefighters adjust their levels of exertion in a characteristic pattern during simulated fire conditions, as reflected by heart rate. Initially, their heart rate increases rapidly to 70% to 80% of maximal within the first minute. As firefighting progresses, firefighters maintain their heart rates at 85% to 100% of maximal.[21]

Firefighters exert themselves to maximal levels while battling fires. Climbing an aerial ladder, dragging hoses, carrying the traveling ladder, rescuing victims, and raising the ladder are among the most strenuous tasks, in declining order of energy demand. The most demanding activity is building search and victim rescue by the "lead hand" (first firefighter to enter the building), resulting in the highest average heart rate and highest rise in rectal temperature. Serving as "secondary help" (entering the building at a later time to fight the fire or to conduct additional searches and rescues) is the next most demanding activity, followed by exterior firefighting and serving as crew captain (directing the firefighting, usually at some distance from the fire). Other demanding tasks, in decreasing order of energy costs, are climbing ladders, dragging hoses, carrying a traveling ladder, and raising a ladder.

During firefighting, core body temperature and heart rate follow a cycle over a period of minutes: they both increase slightly in response to work in preparation for entry, then they both increase more as a result of environmental heat exposure, and they subsequently increase more steeply as a result of high workloads under conditions of heat stress. After 20 to 25 minutes, the usual length of time allowed for interior work by the SCBA used by firefighters, the physiological stress remains within limits tolerable to a healthy individual. However, in extended firefighting that involves multiple re-entries, there is insufficient time between SCBA air bottle changes to cool off, leading to a cumulative rise in core temperature and an increasing risk of heat stress.

Obviously, burns and other thermal injuries are leading causes of injury to firefighters, although standard "turnout" gear is very effective in minimizing the risk of burns. "Flashovers" are explosive eruptions of flame in a confined space that occur as a result of the sudden ignition of flammable gas products driven out of burning or hot materials and combined with superheated air. Fire situations that lead to "flashovers" may engulf the firefighter or cut off escape routes. Hot air by itself is not usually a great hazard to the firefighter. Dry air does not have much capacity to retain heat. Steam or hot wet air can cause serious burns because much more heat energy can be stored in water vapor than in dry air. Fortunately, steam burns are not common. Radiant heat is often intense in a fire situation. Burns may occur from radiant heat alone. Firefighters may also show skin changes characteristic of prolonged exposure to heat.

Under fire conditions, these physical demands are complicated by the metabolic demands of coping with heat and loss of fluids. The combined effect of internally generated heat during work and of external heat from the fire may result in markedly increased body temperatures that climb to unusually high levels in an intense firefighting situation. Half-hour interval breaks to change the SCBA are not enough to arrest this climb in temperature, which can reach dangerous levels in prolonged firefighting. Although essential, personal protection imposes a considerable additional energy burden on the firefighter, particularly the SCBA.

Heat stress during firefighting may come from hot air, radiant heat, contact with hot surfaces, or endogenous heat that is produced by the body during exercise but which cannot be cooled during the fire. Heat stress is compounded by the insulating properties of the protective clothing and by physical exertion, which result in heat production within the body. Heat may result in heat stress, with the risk of dehydration, heat stroke, and cardiovascular collapse.

Unusual exposures, such as intense exposure to the fumes of burning plastics, can cause severe lung toxicity, reactive airways disease (where none existed before), and even permanent disability. Ordinary firefighting may be associated with short-term changes similar to asthma, which resolve over days. This does not appear to result in an increased lifetime risk of dying from chronic lung disease. However, this generalization may not apply in individual cases in which there has been an unusually intense exposure.

More than 50% of fire-related fatalities are the result of exposure to smoke, rather than burns. One of the major contributing factors to mortality and morbidity in fires is hypoxia because of oxygen depletion in the affected atmosphere, leading to loss of physical performance, confusion, and inability to escape. The constituents of smoke, singly and in combination, are also toxic. The toxicity of smoke depends primarily on the fuel, the heat of the fire, and whether or how much oxygen is available for combustion. Only carbon monoxide and hydrogen cyanide are commonly produced in lethal concentrations in building fires.

Firefighters tend to judge the level of hazard they face by the intensity of smoke, and they decide whether to use an SCBA solely on the basis of what they see. This may be very misleading after the flames are extinguished. The SCBA is an effective personal protection device that prevents exposure to the products of combustion when used properly. Fire services routinely require the use of SCBA during overhaul, but individual firefighters may ignore the requirement and wear it only during knockdown.

There is no apparent correlation between the intensity of smoke and the amount of carbon monoxide or cyanide in the air. Firefighters may also be exposed to nitrogen dioxide, sulphur dioxide, hydrogen chloride, aldehydes, and organic compounds such as benzene, depending on the material involved in the fire.

Certain situations present more airborne hazards than others. Firefighters should particularly avoid smoking during the clean-up, or "overhaul," phase, when burning material is smoldering and therefore burning incompletely because carbon monoxide is likely to be in the atmosphere. Synthetic materials are most dangerous during smoldering conditions, not in conditions of high heat. Concrete retains heat very efficiently and may also act as a "sponge" for trapped gases that are then released from the porous material, releasing hydrogen chloride or other toxic fumes long after a fire has been extinguished. Polymeric plastic materials in building construction and furnishings pose particular hazards because they combust into toxic products. Acrolein, formaldehyde, and volatile fatty acids are common in smoldering fires of several polymers, including polyethylene and natural cellulose. Cyanide levels increase with temperature when polyurethane or polyacrylonitriles are burned; acrylonitrile, acetonitrile pyridine, and benzonitrile occur in quantity in temperatures greater than 800°C but less than 1000°C. Polyvinyl chloride has been proposed as a desirable polymer for furnishings because of its self-extinguishing characteristics due to the high chlorine content. Unfortunately, the material produces large quantities of hydrochloric acid when fires are prolonged.[22]

The introduction of SCBA and other protective equipment within the last 20 years has created a much safer working environment for the firefighter. However, the added weight of the equipment increases the physical exertion required and may throw the firefighter off balance in some situations. The firefighter's typical "turnout" gear may weigh about 51 lb and imposes a high energy cost. The protective clothing also becomes much heavier when it gets wet. A 20% decrement has been found in work performance imposed by those carrying an SCBA, which is a substantial restraint under extreme and dangerous conditions.

Police

In a disaster, police will have several functions: (1) establishing and maintaining order at the scene; (2) protecting the safety of the population at risk in the vicinity of the disaster; (3) protecting the safety of other responders; (4) maintaining the integrity of the scene if a criminal investigation is involved; and (5) in many cases, assisting with rescue operations. In a disaster, one of the most important functions of the police is to maintain the security of the disaster scene from well-meaning volunteers who may inadvertently put themselves and others at risk. Although they are commonly the first or second to arrive on-scene, police officers may not necessarily have access to the same level of PPE as other first responders, and the nature of their work can make it more difficult to consistently use PPE. The nature of the police force is such that in some cases it may be challenging to ensure that all potentially exposed police officers participate in postevent medical management and follow-up.

EMS Personnel

EMS personnel include paramedics, emergency medical technicians (EMTs), and other prehospital care providers. These personnel treat approximately 22 million patients a year in the United States.[23] In addition, they are first responders to natural and manmade disasters and are a crucial component of the nation's disaster response system. Although prehospital care personnel have been operating in the United States for more than a century, it is only recently that the full range of risks associated with this work has been investigated. Recent research has shown that the occupational fatality rate for this group is more than twice the national average[24] and that the rate of nonfatal occupational injuries and illnesses may be more than five times the national average[25,26]; the rate of nonfatal injuries and illnesses among EMS workers exceeds the rates for police and fire personnel.[27] Because these risks are only now being recognized, EMS personnel and managers as well as town council members and mayors, are largely unaware of the extent of the dangers associated with the work.

Historically, the role of EMS was to provide on-scene treatment and then rapid transportation to a hospital.[28] This role has been evolving in recent years as EMS agencies have become more involved not only in disaster preparation and response but also in community health. One agency, for example, instituted a program that reduced the county pediatric drowning rate by 50%.[29] EMS agencies nationwide are becoming more involved in a variety of community health initiatives.[30,31]

The organization of EMS services varies widely by jurisdiction. In larger cities, fire departments typically provide first responder services for critical calls; fire department personnel may have training that ranges between a few hours of basic instruction up to full paramedic training. In some jurisdictions, EMS agencies are private companies contracted by the municipality; in others, the fire department is responsible for EMS and provides either fire personnel on ambulances or hires civilian workers for the ambulances. In other jurisdictions, a municipally owned and operated "third service" is responsible for providing EMS. Finally, hospitals or even police departments may operate a local EMS agency.

There are an estimated 900,000 EMS workers in the United States; approximately 175,000 are full-time workers and 154,000 are paramedics.[23] Volunteers provide much of the nation's EMS.[32] There are more than 40 different levels of prehospital providers in the United States.[32] However, most EMS workers can be divided into two primary job classifications: basic life support personnel, such as EMTs, and advanced life support personnel, such as paramedics. Training requirements for these personnel vary by state, but in general, EMTs have approximately 300 hours of training and paramedics have about 1200 hours more than the EMT level. Protocols also vary by state and local jurisdiction.

On a day-to-day basis, the risks faced by EMS workers include musculoskeletal injuries from carrying patients, assaults, needlesticks, and transportation-related injuries (e.g., from ambulance collisions, helicopter crashes, and by being struck by moving vehicles on the scene of a call). The EMS worker may have to carry a heavy patient down (or up) multiple flights of stairs or over slippery surfaces. EMS workers respond to calls in areas that have high crime rates and enter homes where the occupants are under a great deal of stress. The risk of needlestick injury may be increased when patients require immediate treatment in areas with poor lighting or in the back of a moving ambulance. Transportation incidents have been shown to cause the largest proportion of fatal injuries; they also account for many of the most serious nonfatal injuries.

Psychological stress may be a significant risk factor for EMS personnel, but the short- and long-term effects are not yet well understood. It also is not known how EMS work may affect chronic conditions. Because EMS workers tend to be young and because these workers have a high turnover rate, there are no data on how EMS work may affect workers' risk of cardiovascular disease, cancer, or other conditions. In addition, little is known about the general health of the EMS workforce. Whereas police and firefighting agencies typically have strenuous physical standards and requirements, EMS agencies may have few, if any, such policies.

The availability of PPE is believed to vary widely by agency and jurisdiction. Although all EMS workers likely have ready access to surgical gloves and masks, anecdotal information suggests that many workers do not have access to helmets, rescue gloves, turnout gear, or heavy boots. This paucity of resources may exacerbate the risks faced by EMS workers during disasters.

Other factors that may contribute to increased occupational health risks among EMS workers during disasters include lack of disaster-related training, lack of disaster preparation among EMS supervisors, poor coordination and communication with other public safety personnel, and inadequate equipment. Although little is known about the specific occupational health effects of disaster responses and operations on EMS workers, it is reasonable to presume that a person in an occupation that is becoming more widely recognized as having among the highest rates of nonfatal injuries and illnesses on a day-to-day basis would be at even greater risk of injury during a disaster event.

Secondary Responders and Skilled Support Personnel

Although there are few studies of the exposures or health consequences experienced by secondary responders and skilled support personnel in a disaster, experience suggests they may be at risk for significant exposures, particularly because in some cases these workers receive less training and have less access to PPE than first responders.[1] It is critical that these workers receive adequate training and "real-life" drills before a disaster and that they participate in postevent medical evaluations and surveillance activities.

RECOMMENDATIONS

If one is to reduce the severity of illness and injury experienced by workers in disasters, one must consider every aspect of the disaster, including the inciting agent(s), the worker, and the physical and social environments in which the disaster occurs. In addition, there are steps that can be taken at every stage of the disaster—before, during, and after the event—to decrease injury and illness severity. Healthcare workers, in particular, need to be involved in every aspect of planning the response, offering guidance in training, providing input on selection of appropriate PPE, coordinating triage and transport of injured patients, and ensuring that the facilities

exist to respond in a timely fashion when a disaster occurs. It is particularly important to conduct medical surveillance to detect subtle population-based changes due to exposures that might not be detected in individual workers. Risk communication must be an integral part of any response plan.

REFERENCES

1. Lippy B. Protecting the health and safety of rescue and recovery workers. In: Levy BS, Sidel VW, eds. *Terrorism and Public Health: A Balanced Approach to Strengthening Systems and Protecting People*. New York: Oxford University Press; 2003:80-100.
2. Mitchell CS, Doyle ML, Moran JB, et al. Worker training for new threats: a proposed framework. *Am J Industr Med*. November 2004;46(5):423-31.
3. US Department of Labor, Occupational Health and Safety Administration. Hazardous waste operations and emergency response (29 CFR 1910.120 and 29 CFR 1926.65). 29 CFR 1910.120 available at: http://www.osha.gov/pls/oshaweb/owadisp.show_document?p_table=STANDARDS&p_id=9765. 29 CFR 1926.65 available at: http://www.osha.gov/pls/oshaweb/owadisp.show_document?p_table=STANDARDS&p_id=10651.
4. National Institute for Occupational Safety and Health. CBRN respirator standards development. Available at: http://www.cdc.gov/niosh/npptl/standardsdev/cbrn/.
5. US Department of Labor, Occupational Safety and Health Administration. *OSHA Best Practices for Hospital-Based First Receivers of Victims from Mass Casualty Incidents Involving the Release of Hazardous Substances*. January 2005. Available at http://www.osha.gov/dts/osta/bestpractices/firstreceivers_hospital.html.
6. Auf Der Heide E. Principles of hospital disaster planning. In: Hogan D, Burstein JL, Eds. *Disaster Medicine*. Philadelphia: Lippincott Williams & Wilkins; 2002:57-89.
7. Vogt BM, Sorensen JH. *How Clean Is Safe? Improving the Effectiveness of Decontamination of Structures and People Following Chemical and Biological Incidents*. Oak Ridge, TN: Oak Ridge National Laboratory; 2002.
8. US Department of Labor, Occupational Health and Safety Administration. Hazardous waste operations and emergency response (29 CFR 1910.120[f]). Available at: http://www.osha.gov/pls/oshaweb/owadisp.show_document?p_table=STANDARDS&p_id=9765.
9. US Department of Labor, Occupational Health and Safety Administration. Hazardous waste operations and emergency response (29 CFR 1910.120[f][4][i]). Available at: http://www.osha.gov/pls/oshaweb/owadisp.show_document?p_table=STANDARDS&p_id=9765.
10. US Department of Health and Human Services, Agency for Toxic Substances and Disease Registry. Case Studies in Environmental Medicine: Taking an Exposure History. Available at: http://www.atsdr.cdc.gov/HEC/CSEM/exphistory/pdffiles/exposure_history.pdf.
11. Environmental Protection Agency. RCRA, Superfund & EPCRA Hotline Training Manual (40 CFR 350-372). Available at: http://www.epa.gov/ceppo/pubs/hotline/intepcra.pdf.
12. National Library of Medicine Specialized Information Services. Toxicology and environmental health. Available at: http://sis.nlm.nih.gov/Tox/ToxMain.html.
13. Centers for Disease Control and Prevention. Emergency preparedness and response: agents diseases, and other threats. Available at: http://www.bt.cdc.gov/index.asp.
14. Landrigan PJ, Lioy PJ, Thurston G, et al. Health and environmental consequences of the world trade center disaster. *Environ Health Perspect*. May 2004;112(6):731-9.
15. Wells JD, Egerton WE, Cummings LA, et al. The U.S. Army Center for Health Promotion and Preventive Medicine response to the Pentagon attack: a multipronged prevention-based approach. *Mil Med*. September 2002;167(suppl 9):64-7.
16. US General Accounting Office. *U.S. Postal Service: Clear Communication with Employees Needed before Reopening the Brentwood Facility*. Statement of Bernard L. Ungar and Keith

Rhodes before the Committee on Government Reform, US House of Representatives. GAO-04-205T; October 23, 2003; Washington, DC.

17. US Department of Labor, Occupational Safety and Health Administration. Recording and reporting occupational injuries and illness (29 CFR 1904). Available at: http://www.osha.gov/pls/oshaweb/owastand.display_standard_group?p_toc_level=1&p_part_number=1904.

18. Agnew J, McDiarmid MA, Lees PS, Duffy R. Reproductive hazards of fire fighting. I. Non-chemical hazards. *Am J Ind Med*. 1991;19(4): 433-45.

19. McDiarmid MA, Lees PS, Agnew J, Midzenski M, Duffy R. Reproductive hazards of fire fighting. II. Chemical hazards. *Am J Ind Med*. 1991;19(4):447-72.

20. Hodous TK, Pizatella TJ, Braddee R, Castillo DN. Fire fighter fatalities 1998-2001: overview with an emphasis on structure-related traumatic fatalities. *Inj Prev*. August 2004;10(4):222-6.

21. Eglin CM, Coles S, Tipton MJ. Physiological responses of fire-fighter instructors during training exercises. *Ergonomics*. April 2004;47(5):483-94.

22. Brandt-Rauf PW, Fallon LF Jr, Tarantini T, Idema C, Andrews L. Health hazards of fire fighters: exposure assessment. *Br J Ind Med*. September 1988;45(9):606-12.

23. Maguire BJ, Walz BJ. Current emergency medical services workforce issues in the United States. *J Emerg Manage*. 2004;2(2):17-26.

24. Maguire BJ, Hunting KL, Smith GS, Levick NR. Occupational fatalities in EMS: a hidden crisis. *Ann Emerg Med*. 2002;40(6):625-32.

25. Gershon RRM, Vlahov D, Kelen G, Conrad B, Murphy L. Review of accidents/injuries among emergency medical services workers in Baltimore, Maryland. *Prehospital Disaster Med*. 1995;10(1):14-18.

26. Schwartz RJ, Benson L, Jacobs LM. The prevalence of occupational injuries in EMTs in New England. *Prehospital Disaster Med*. 1993;8(1):45-50.

27. Maguire BJ, Hunting KL, Guidotti TL, Smith GS. Epidemiology of occupational injuries and illnesses among emergency medical services personnel. Abstract available at: http://apha.confex.com/apha/132am/techprogram/paper_92287.htm.

28. Walz BJ, ed. *Introduction to EMS Systems*. Albany: Delmar Publishing, 2001.

29. Harrawood D, Gunderson MR, Fravel S, Cartwright K, Ryan JL. Drowning prevention. A case study in EMS epidemiology. *J Emerg Med Serv*. 1994;19(6):34-8, 40-1.

30. Kinnane JM, Garrison HG, Coben JH, et al. Injury prevention: is there a role for out-of-hospital emergency medical services? *Acad Emerg Med*. 1997;4(4):306-12.

31. Yancey AH 2nd, Martinez R, Kellermann AL. Injury prevention and emergency medical services: the "Accidents Aren't" program. *Prehosp Emerg Care*. 2002;6(2): 204-9.

32. US Department of Transportation, National Highway Traffic Safety Administration. Human Resources. In: *EMS Agenda for the Future*. DOT HS 808 441, NTS-42. August 1996. Available at: http://www.nhtsa.dot.gov/people/injury/ems/agenda/emsman.html#HUMAN.

chapter 25

Disaster Preparedness*

Mark E. Keim and Paul Giannone

To start early is easy going, to start late is breakneck.
                                                    Maori proverb

EVOLVING DEFINITIONS

To communicate effectively about disasters as an empirical endeavor, clear definitions of the specific terms must be used. Unfortunately, "no definition of disaster is accepted universally"[1]; therefore, this chapter begins with a definition of terminology that will serve as a foundation for further discussion of preparedness. For the sake of clarity and external validity, this chapter adheres to widely held definitions but also remains selective of some definitions that are particularly meaningful within the context of disaster preparedness.

The definition of *disaster* now adopted by the United Nations[2] and the World Health Organization[3] describes disasters as: "A serious disruption of the functioning of a community or a society causing widespread human, material, economic or environmental losses which exceed the ability of the affected community or society to cope using its own resources." An event that does not exceed a society's capacities to cope is classified as an *emergency*: ". . . a sudden and usually unforeseen event that calls for immediate measures to minimize its adverse consequences."[3] During disasters, in contrast to everyday emergencies, organizations have to do the following[4]:

- Quickly relate to more and unfamiliar groups
- Adjust to losing part of their autonomy and freedom of action
- Apply different standards
- Operate within closer-than-usual public health and private-sector interfaces

Emergencies and disasters also tend to be conceptually differentiated from catastrophes.

In a catastrophe, as opposed to a disaster, the following take place[4]:

- Most or all of the community built structure is heavily affected.
- Local officials are unable to undertake their usual work roles, and this often extends into the recovery period.
- Most, if not all, of the everyday community functions are sharply and simultaneously interrupted.
- Finally, help from nearby communities cannot be provided.

Communities and nations must therefore evaluate their own unique vulnerabilities and plan accordingly for this entire range of potential events.

Emergencies and disasters are thus part of a relative continuum of events that occurs when a population is both exposed to a "threatening event or potentially damaging phenomenon," referred to as a *hazard*.[3] When a vulnerable population becomes exposed to any particular hazard, there are "lives lost, persons injured, property damaged and economic activity . . . disrupted."[3] These events are defined as *risks*. Risk is the product of hazard and vulnerability. Thus, the disaster is defined by the vulnerability of the population to a hazard event and not by the mere fact of its occurrence.[5] The functional impact is determined by the resources of the community and the community's ability to use its resourcese[6] (referred to as *capacities* or *coping mechanisms*). Many factors increase a person's vulnerability to health emergencies and disasters.[7] Poverty is the single most important risk factor for vulnerability: "The poorest people in the poorest countries are the most vulnerable—and it is vulnerability that kills."[8]

Vulnerability to emergencies and disasters has two sides—the degree of exposure to dangerous hazards (susceptibility) and the capacity to cope with or recover from their consequences (resilience). Vulnerability reduction programs reduce susceptibility and increase resilience. Susceptibility to disasters is decreased by prevention and mitigation of emergencies.[9] Resilience has two components: (1) that provided by nature and (2) that provided through the actions of humans. One example of resilience provided by nature is the manner in which porous soil may allow for more rapid drainage of floodwater as opposed to more occlusive soil types. One example of human actions that affect resilience may be the social order of society and how this organizational

---

*The material in this chapter reflects solely the views of the authors. It does not necessarily reflect the policies or recommendations of the Centers for Disease Control and Prevention or the U.S. Department of Health and Human Services.

structure may facilitate (or hinder) response and recovery. Resilience is composed of (1) the absorbing capacity, (2) the buffering capacity, and (3) the response to the event and recovery from the damage sustained.[1]

As preparedness increases, the ability of the society to absorb the event and thus lessen adverse outcomes is augmented as a dependent variable of preparedness.[1] By increasing preparedness, we increase resilience, decrease vulnerability, and thus lessen the risk of disasters. In addition, effective risk-reduction activities strengthen the buffering capacity of a population to respond to everyday emergencies found in all societies, thus minimizing the change in an essential function for a given change in available resources.[1]

Both predisaster and postdisaster public health responses to disasters may also be considered within a context of preventive medicine.[10] Primary and secondary prevention represent activities taken before a disaster.[11] Primary prevention is done to prevent adverse events from ever occurring. For example, floodplain management in an area of frequent flooding may actually prevent future inundation disasters altogether. In secondary prevention, measures are taken in advance that will decrease or eliminate the impact of risks.[7] It involves mitigation, "structural and non-structural measures undertaken to *limit the adverse impact* of natural hazards, environmental degradation and technological hazards," as well as preparedness, "activities and measures taken in advance to *ensure effective response to the impact* of hazards..."[2] Finally, tertiary prevention activities occur after the disaster response and recovery, when actions are undertaken to minimize loss of life and damage and to hasten the return to predisaster normal functioning.

Recently, the overall approach to emergencies and disasters among nations has shifted from ad hoc postdisaster activities to a more systematic and comprehensive process of risk management that also emphasizes the importance of predisaster activities, including prevention, mitigation, and preparedness.[7] Disaster risk management, including risk-reduction strategies, is part of a more comprehensive system of actions that include prevention, mitigation, response, and recovery from the tragic event, whether that event is an emergency or a disaster.

HISTORICAL PERSPECTIVE

The events of the past three decades have given birth to an understanding of the importance of disaster preparedness. The Guatemala earthquake of 1976 killed 23,000 people and led to the publication of multiple articles analyzing aspects of the international response.[4,9] Postdisaster analyses of this and other subsequent large-scale disaster events revealed a strong case for multihazard disaster preparedness. During the 1980s, new concepts that were based on the notions of hazards and vulnerabilities evolved. These concepts were further validated during the African famine and the 1985 Mexico City earthquake. Governments of industrialized nations began to abandon their disaster relief approaches to

better reflect the new importance of preparedness. This growing awareness was bolstered by a growing body of disaster research; an increasing professionalism in the field that grew to include academic coursework; the development of manuals and standardized tools; a growing "response fatigue" among donor nations and organizations; and an economic appreciation of the cost-effectiveness of prevention and preparedness as weighed against extremely expensive response efforts. The growing burden of disasters on global health was becoming all too clear. During a 20-year period, natural disasters alone killed 3 million people worldwide, affected 800 million lives, and resulted in property damage exceeding $23 billion.[9,12] In response to this growing threat, the United Nations (UN) General Assembly declared the 1990s to be the International Decade of Natural Disaster Reduction (IDNDR) and called for a global effort to reduce the suffering and losses.

In May 1994, one major achievement of the IDNDR was the hosting of the World Conference on Natural Disaster Reduction, which resulted in the *Yokohama Strategy and Plan of Action for a Safer World: Guidelines for Natural Disaster Prevention, Preparedness and Mitigation.*[13] One of the strategies within the Yokohama Plan of Action stated that "[the world] will develop and strengthen national capacities and capabilities and, where appropriate, national legislation for natural and other disaster prevention, mitigation and preparedness, including the mobilization of non-governmental organizations and participation of local communities."

The Johannesburg World Summit on Sustainable Development plan of implementation further stated: "An integrated, multi-hazard, inclusive approach to address vulnerability, risk assessment and disaster management, including prevention, mitigation, preparedness, response and recovery, is an essential element of a safer world in the twenty-first century."[14]

A more recent UN General Assembly resolution on natural disasters and vulnerability takes into account the outcomes of the WSSD and the role of the International Strategy for Disaster Reduction. It coordinated a review of the *Yokohama Strategy and Plan of Action* as a major goal of the Second World Conference on Disaster Reduction held in Kobe during January 2005.[15]

CURRENT PRACTICE

The Approach to Disaster Preparedness

"Emergency preparedness is a program of long term development activities whose goals are to strengthen the overall capacity and capability of a country to manage all types of emergencies and bring about an orderly transition from relief through recovery and back to sustained development."[9]

To be most effective, a disaster preparedness program must be one component of an overall vulnerability reduction strategy and should not be implemented as an isolated project. As stated earlier, vulnerability reduction must also include activities for reducing susceptibility by way of prevention and mitigation.

Disaster preparedness should be guided by a range of principles to adequately protect communities, property, and the environment. To be most effective, the approach must be:

- Comprehensive[16]
- All-hazard[16]
- Multisectoral and intersectoral[16]
- Community based[16]
- User friendly
- Culturally sensitive and specific

A comprehensive approach entails developing and implementing strategies for different phases of the emergency management cycle (i.e., prevention/mitigation, preparedness, response, and recovery) in the context of sustainable development. These phases often overlap each other both in time and scope. The management of emergencies is a process that should be part of the normal development plan of every country.

A widely used international concept is that of sustainable development. Sustainable development is "development which meets the needs of the present without compromising the ability of future generations to meet their own needs."[16a] This concept has been around for a number of decades, starting with the Declaration of the United Nations Conference on the Human Environment at Stockholm from June 5-16, 1972. Principle 1 of this declaration stated: "Man has the fundamental right to freedom, equality and adequate conditions of life, in an environment of a quality that permits a life of dignity and well-being, and he bears a solemn responsibility to protect and improve the environment for present *and future generations.*"[16a]

The 2002 World Summit on Sustainable Development plan of implementation reaffirmed sustainable development as a central element of the international agenda.

The all-hazards approach[17] concerns developing and implementing emergency management strategies for the full range of likely emergencies or disasters, including both natural and technological, which also includes conflict-related hazards of terrorism and warfare.

The multisectoral and intersectoral approach means that all organizations, including government, private and community organizations, and traditional and informal leadership, should be involved in disaster preparedness. If this approach is not used, emergency management is likely to be fragmented and inefficient.[3] The multisectoral and intersectoral approach will also help to link emergency management to sustainable development through the institutionalization of risk reduction and the use of its principles in long-term development projects.

The concept of preparedness at the community level is based on the premise that the members, resources, organizations, and administrative structures of a community should all form the foundation of any emergency preparedness program. As the saying goes, "All disasters are local," meaning all initial disaster responses start at the local level. External assistance in emergency management may be expected, but it should not be relied on as the sole means of risk reduction.

These combined approaches will also help link risk reduction to sustainable development through the institutionalization of emergency management and the use of its principles in development projects. The resulting program becomes the responsibility of all and is undertaken at all administrative levels of both government and nongovernment organizations. The program concentrates not only on disasters but also on sustainable development of the society as a whole. These elements should be created at community, provincial, and national levels. An inherent capacity for risk reduction at each of these levels is a precondition for effective response and recovery when an emergency or disaster strikes. Without these capacities, any link from recovery to development will not be sustainable.

Health Objectives of Disaster Preparedness

Objectives of preparedness for health emergencies have been offered as follows:

- Prevent morbidity and mortality[11]
- Provide care for casualties[11]
- Manage adverse climatic and environmental conditions[11]
- Ensure restoration of normal health[11]
- Re-establish health services[11]
- Protect staff
- Protect public health and medical assets

The actions required to meet these needs can be grouped into the following four categories[11]:

1. Preventive measures (e.g., building codes, floodplain management)
2. Protective measures (e.g., early warning, community education)
3. Lifesaving measures (e.g., rescue and relief)
4. Rehabilitation (e.g., resettlement, rebuilding)

Elements of Disaster Preparedness

Although the terms *preparedness* and *planning* are sometimes used interchangeably or redundantly, planning constitutes only one component of a comprehensive program of disaster preparedness. The elements of emergency preparedness typically include vulnerability assessment, emergency planning, training and education, warning systems, specialized communication systems, information databases and management systems, resource management systems, resource stocks, emergency exercises,[3] population protection systems,[18] and incident management systems.[19]

Processes of a Disaster Preparedness Program

Comprehensive disaster preparedness programs have been described to include the following processes[3,9]:

- Policy development
- Vulnerability assessment
- Disaster planning

- Training and education
- Monitoring and evaluation

Policy Development

Policy development includes legislation that is normally developed by a national government and mainly relates to responsibility for emergency preparedness and special emergency powers. There is also a need for central government, provincial and community organizations, and non-government organizations to develop appropriate policies.

Policy is required to ensure that common goals are pursued within and across organizations and activities, to streamline rapid decision-making, to ensure that actions are legal, to protect people from liability, and to ensure that common practices are followed. Without agreed policies, there will be poor coordination, a lack of a unified direction, and poor results. Policy can take the form of legislation, decisions by executive government, interorganizational agreements, or organizational directions.

Vulnerability Assessment

The vulnerability assessment identifies and prioritizes potential hazards that may affect a community and suggests where damage may occur and which aspects of the community should be modified to lessen vulnerability. The assessment will also identify local capacities or coping mechanisms. It also provides a baseline for recovery strategies, in that it will describe the "normal" state of a community. There are a number of possible ways of assessing vulnerability. The process for vulnerability assessment described here is a series of steps, each of which contains a number of techniques. For example, hazard identification, community and environmental analysis, and hazard description are some of the steps. In turn, there are a number of techniques for identifying hazards, for describing the people, property, and environment that the hazards may affect, and for describing hazards and recommendations for risk reduction. Keim and Rhyne[20] have quantified the preparedness quotient, P_Q, as an objective measure of disaster resilience. This metric of health-sector preparedness has also been factored into a broader assessment of vulnerability that also includes an engineering-based measurement of mitigation.

Disaster Planning

A disaster plan is an agreed set of arrangements for preparing for, responding to, and recovering from emergencies and involves the description of responsibilities, management structures, strategies, and resource and information management. Disaster planning is about protecting life, property, and the environment.

"Planning is more important than the plan."
Mark Keim, MD

The written plan itself is only one outcome of the planning process. The planning process should produce the following:

- An understanding of organizational responsibilities in response and recovery

- Stronger emergency management networks
- Improved community participation and awareness
- Effective response and recovery strategies and systems
- A simple and flexible written plan

A FUNCTIONAL APPROACH TO DISASTER PLANNING

Although the hazards that cause disasters vary greatly, the potential public health consequences and subsequent needs of the population do not.[17] For example, warfare, chemical releases, floods, hurricanes, and earthquakes all force people from their homes. Based on this knowledge, a jurisdiction can develop a plan around the function of finding shelter for the displaced with minor adjustments for the rapidity, scale, duration, location, and intensity of different hazards.

Regardless of the hazard, disasters result in 15 public health consequences and create 32 categories of public health needs. And not all public health consequences are completed by public health staff. For example, public works and other government agencies are also involved in the provision of safe water, sanitation, and shelter. Table 25-1 provides a listing of the public health consequences and population needs caused by all natural and technological disasters, regardless of the precipitating hazard.

A critical aspect of planning for the response to emergency situations is to identify all of these common functions, assign responsibility for accomplishing each function, and ensure that tasked organizations have prepared standard operating procedures that detail how they will carry out critical objectives associated with the larger functions.

Keim and Giannone[21] invented the Automated Disaster and Emergency Planning Tool (ADEPT), which represents software-based technology for assisting public health officials with an easily accessible and evidence-based method for writing, exercising, and improving public health emergency operations and planning. ADEPT identifies all of the functions of public health emergency response according to each major hazard. The tool then guides the user in assigning tasks and performance indicators for each of these functions. It integrates widely held national and international standards for public health, emergency management, humanitarian assistance, continuous quality improvement, and incident management.[22-32]

COMPONENTS OF A DISASTER PLAN

Most disaster plans that use a functional approach consist of the following four basic components:

- A "basic plan" containing a statement of policy, assignment of responsibility, and concept of operations
- A "functional annex" or set of contingencies that organize tasks around the completion of objectives related to each critical function
- "Hazard-specific appendices" or reference tables that

TABLE 25-1 PUBLIC HEALTH CONSEQUENCES AND FUNCTIONS ASSOCIATED WITH ALL DISASTERS

PUBLIC HEALTH CONSEQUENCES	PUBLIC HEALTH FUNCTIONS
Common to all consequences	Resource management
	Mental health services
	Reproductive health services
	Social services
	Occupational health and safety
	Business continuity
Deaths	Mortuary care
	Social services
	Mental health services
Illness and injuries	Health services
	Injury prevention and control
	Epidemiology
	Disease prevention and control
Loss of clean water	Access to safe water
Loss of shelter	Shelter and settlement
	Social services
	Security
Loss of personal and household goods	Personal and household goods
Loss of sanitation and routine hygiene	Sanitation, excreta disposal, and hygiene promotion
Disruption of solid waste management	Solid waste management
Public concern for safety	Risk communication
	Public information
	Security
Increased pests and vectors	Pest and vector control
Loss or damage of healthcare system	Health system and infrastructure support
Worsening of chronic illnesses	Health services
Food scarcity	Food safety, security, and nutrition
Standing surface water	Public works and engineering
Toxic exposures	Risk assessment
	Population protection
	Health services
	Hazardous materials emergency response
	Occupational health and safety

provide additional detailed information applicable to the performance of a particular function in the face of a particular hazard
• Standard operating procedures and/or checklists that detail how responders will carry out the tasks related to each function

Training and Education

Training and education involve training public health personnel and community responders in emergency management skills and knowledge and informing the community of the actions that may be required during emergencies and how the community can participate in emergency management.

The following are objectives of training and education in emergency management:

• The community is empowered to participate in the development of emergency preparedness strategies.
• The community knows the appropriate actions for different types of emergencies and the organizations it can turn to for assistance.
• Emergency management personnel are able to carry out the tasks allotted to them.

There are a number of possible training and education strategies that are suitable for different audiences and purposes. Strategy selection should be based on need, audience, purpose, available time, and available money and other resources.

Training and education strategies may include the following:

• Workshops, seminars, formal education programs, or conferences[16]
• Self-directed learning[16]
• Individual tuition[16]
• Exercises[16]
• Pamphlets, videos, media advertisements, newsletters, or journals[16]
• Informal or formal presentations[16]
• Training of the public, from schoolchildren to professionals[16]
• Public displays or public meetings[16]
• Mentorship and temporary duty assignments

Monitoring and Evaluation

Monitoring and evaluation involve determining how well an emergency preparedness program is being developed and implemented and what needs to be done to improve it. These can be applied to all processes of a disaster preparedness program.

The following four methods for monitoring and evaluating preparedness are described here:

- Project management
- Operational debriefing
- Exercises
- Systems analysis

Project management is a means of monitoring and evaluating during the implementation phase of a project and includes:

- Measuring the progress toward project objectives
- Analysis to determine the cause of deviations in the project
- Determining corrective actions

Operational debriefing uses the process of an after-action study or a discussion of lessons learned after significant or strategically important operations. These evaluation tools are generally conducted immediately after a disaster event, may not be based on statistical analysis, and are more descriptive in nature. In its simplest form, it may be a forum for discussion of what went right and what could have been done better to improve services.

Exercises are a common way of monitoring and evaluating parts of emergency preparedness programs. Exercises can be used to test aspects of emergency plans, emergency procedures, training, feasibility of coordination, communications, etc. The purpose of an exercise, and the aspect of emergency preparedness to be tested, must be carefully decided and fairly specific. An exercise should not be conducted with the purpose of testing an entire emergency plan or all aspects of training.

Some typical types of exercise include:

- **Operational exercises:** where personnel and resources are actually deployed in a simulation of an emergency
- **Tabletop exercises:** where personnel are presented with an unfolding scenario, asked what actions would be required, and how the actions would be implemented
- **Syndicate exercises:** where personnel are divided into syndicates to discuss and consider a given scenario, and the syndicate planning and response decisions are then discussed in an open forum

System analysis is used to study the various components of a preparedness program, searching for the existence of elements of the program that are assumed to be important by using objectives, checklists, and key questions for each element.[33] The national emergency profile and health policy are dealt with in general terms, whereas the element concerning technical and administrative organization is analyzed in greater detail.

Managing the Process of Disaster Preparedness

Whether developing and implementing an entire emergency preparedness program or conducting a vulnerability assessment or emergency planning project, project management methods will be required.

There are three major phases of project management: project definition, project planning, and project implementation.[23] *Project definition* concerns the aims and objectives of a project, as well as its scope and authority. *Project planning* is the process of sequencing tasks to achieve the project objectives and to ensure timely project completion and efficient use of resources. It involves determining tasks, assigning responsibilities, developing a timetable, and determining resource allocation and timing. *Project implementation* consists of project performance, monitoring and evaluation, and taking corrective action.

In the late 1980s and early 1990s a reformation of management theory and structure occurred in American business. Continuous quality improvement (CQI) arose out of the careful and disciplined study of traditional management approaches by a group of separate but similar thinkers.[23] Certain key features are inherent to any CQI approach, regardless of its specific application. These features include the following:

1. Customer focus (or, in the case of disaster management, victim focus)
2. Statistical application of knowledge of variation
3. Focus on process
4. Design and redesign
5. A redefinition of leadership

A rich literature has since developed regarding the implementation of CQI in a wide range of settings in both the manufacturing and service industries, including healthcare.[23] "CQI applications have been particularly relevant to the emergency department, given the process-based focus of quality improvement and the fact that the emergency department is a process rich environment."[23] The same could also be said for all phases of disaster management, which are also process-rich.

CQI as Applied to Disaster Preparedness

To a large extent, disaster planners previously considered the end results of their work to be largely immeasurable. The victim's journey from impact to recovery, although subject to numerous measurements, had been considered to be largely an immeasurable process, particularly with regard to customer satisfaction, cost, outcome, and measurement.[34] This is an odd paradox in a field whose very essence concerns the nature of being able to measure quantifiable differences in public health as the course of the disaster event progresses or improves. Nonetheless, a body of literature is now developing that supports the application of measures of effectiveness for evaluation and monitoring of humanitarian assistance efforts.[35]

Although certain protocols have always existed within the fields of emergency and disaster medicine, there nonetheless has been a substantial degree of freedom on the part of the individual practitioner to diagnose and treat patients according to the preferences of the individual practitioner. The movement toward more clearly defined clinical pathways in medicine and other specialties represents part of the success of CQI principles. There are many examples of successful control of special cause variation through accepted treatment protocols, including the use of the principles outlined in the Advanced Trauma Life Support Course,[36] the Advanced Cardiac Life Support Course,[37] the Advanced Pediatric Life Support Course,[38] and, more specifically related to disaster management, the Sphere Project.[24]

CUSTOMER FOCUS

In simplest terms, a customer is any person who is affected by a process or product. In terms of disaster preparedness and response, this definition includes "external customers," such as communities and their societies, and "internal customers," such as multisectoral first responders and relief workers and their respective agencies.

STATISTICAL APPLICATION OF KNOWLEDGE OF VARIATION

Understanding the implications of variation in process is a critical skill for the disaster manager. Common cause variation refers to naturally occurring, statistically predictable variations that are inherent in all processes. By applying statistical principles, one can determine the variations that are common causes in nature, which helps guide appropriate interventions to improve the system. Because of the lack of understanding of the basic principles of common cause variation, one of the most common problems is tampering with the system as a result of overinterpretation of data.[23] Special cause variation is a natural variation caused by events or circumstances that are nontypical and therefore not inherent in the process. Such special causes are often operator-dependent (caused by variation in individuals providing service within the system). This is particularly true in cases in which different operators provide the service through a process that is inherently different from that of other providers. At its essence, CQI in many respects is the simple application of the scientific method to cross-functional processes that results in a deeper and more fundamental understanding of disaster response and recovery.

FOCUS ON PROCESS

Any project or program, including disaster preparedness, has a series of inputs and processes that produce outputs, which result in outcomes. The inputs of disaster preparedness include people's time and energy, people's perceptions of vulnerability and emergency requirements, money and resources, and commitment and perseverance. The processes, in this instance, are those of disaster preparedness. The outputs include information on hazards and vulnerability; training; resource acquisition; organizations that are aware of their responsibilities in preparing for, responding to, and recovering from emergencies; commitment to an emergency plan; and enhanced emergency preparedness. The outcomes of appropriate and effective disaster preparedness are improved protection of life, property, and the environment and the ability to sustain development.[3]

Virtually all interactions in disaster preparedness and response require interdependent, cross-functional processes for their successful conclusion. It is precisely because the disaster event is a process-rich environment that the precepts of CQI hold so much promise for improvement of disaster medicine. As Deming first noted, 85% of bad outcomes arise from the process itself, whereas only 15% arise from faulty performance by the individual provider.[23] Given this fact, CQI attempts to improve processes and systems rather than focus on individual performance.

EMPHASIS ON DESIGN AND REDESIGN

Another of the key concepts in CQI is the emphasis on design and redesign. As Donald Berwick[39] noted, "Every process provides information by which that process can be improved." This focus on process improvement is a dramatic change from the prior emphasis on outlier activity. In traditional after-action studies or reports, quality improvement is attempted by routing out "bad apples" and adverse events in disaster drills and exercises or anecdotally identifying "lessons learned" from one disaster response rather than by improving entire processes and systems. However, quality is more than the absence of adverse events; elimination of outliers in a system may have minimal impact on mean performance. Quality exists to the extent that value is added in the course of the process itself. This goal of CQI is best achieved when the focus is on analyzing the system in such a way that the entire performance curve can be shifted to the right, so that "average performance" improves rather than placing emphasis primarily on the outliers with bad outcome.

A REDEFINITION OF LEADERSHIP AND EMPOWERMENT

The founders of CQI proved that the "traditional" management approach had certain subtle, inherent, unavoidable, and predictable consequences.[23] The role of the traditional manager was to observe the system and provide feedback to the staff in the form of exhortation, reward, and control. CQI recognizes that the continuous redesign of the system must of necessity include the input of those responsible for providing service to the patient or customer. One consequence of traditional management systems is the development of what Paul Batalden[40] referred to as "functional silos," (otherwise known as "stove-piping"), referring to the situation when units or subunits in the system operate separately without coordination. In effect, this creates artificial functional vertical silos in disaster management processes that are fundamentally horizontal in nature. As these vertical silos occur, the processes of necessity become unlinked (this is usually readily apparent to the disaster victim or the field responder). For this reason, communities, planners, and responders should make an effective transition to collaborative management philosophy in which governance is shared, workers are empowered, and quality is a function of community outcomes and satisfaction. Like the humanitarian charter of the Sphere Project,[24] the Deming method of CQI is rooted in the principles of human dignity and potential.[23] This redefinition of leadership and empowerment of the community also provide for the element of stakeholdership, which has also been described as an essential guiding principle necessary for effective disaster preparedness.[16]

PITFALLS

Pitfalls of Disaster Management in General

In one study of past disaster management problems and their causes, the following problems were categorized[10]:

- Inadequate appraisal of damages
- Inadequate problem ranking
- Inadequate identification, location, transportation, and utilization of resources

Among 22 U.S. disasters in this study, 93 examples of inappropriate management activities were identified. Most disaster mismanagement problems occurred because managers did not know what all of the relief activities were or how they should be accomplished.[10] Difficulties in disaster management also frequently involve breakdowns in communication and coordination.[41] The people of the Caribbean have a saying regarding the frequently recurring themes of disaster mismanagement that occur, "Horses never step in the same hole in the road more than once ... Only people do." Many of the mistakes that we make in disaster response could easily be prevented through adequate preparedness and learning from past mistakes.

Preparedness as a Short-Term Activity

"In disaster-prone countries, constant preparedness is essential."[5] To be most effective, a disaster preparedness program should be one component of an overall vulnerability reduction strategy and should not be implemented as an isolated project.[9]

Lack of Valid Assumptions and Knowledge Regarding the Disaster Phenomenon

"Proper planning and execution of disaster medical aid programs require knowledge of the types of disasters that might occur, the morbidity and mortality that might result and the consequent medical care needs."[12] Health decisions made during emergencies are often based on insufficient or unnecessary health aid, waste of health resources, or counter-effective measures.[42] In addition, the very nature of disasters adds difficulty to empirical or prospective study. These high-profile events also tend to gain a high degree of public and personal attention. The literature is therefore replete with inaccurate anecdotal case reporting, even though studies of disasters have identified variables that contribute to the potential for injury.[41]

Over-Reliance on External Assistance, Mobile Field Hospitals, and Specialized Surgical Teams

It has been the personal experience of the primary author as both a disaster victim[43] and as a disaster responder that "families, friends and neighbors search, evacuate and extricate their own in the aftermath of a disaster"[44] and that by the time external relief teams are functional on-site, a very large majority of the total dead have already died,[11,45-47] or in the case of chemical contamination, victims often arrive at the hospital before undergoing any prehospital decontamination.[48] External emergency relief is, therefore, largely expensive, wasteful, and not particularly effective.[11] These types of medical relief operations have been referred to as the "second disaster."[49]

In addition, response measures do not always lead to the most effective means of recovery. Disasters, such as hurricane Mitch in Central America, may additionally negate the accomplishments of a generation in human, institutional, and economic development and increase the already high dependence on external assistance and financing.[50] This does not imply that disaster relief should be abandoned, but rather that a more comprehensive and cost-effective approach to disaster risk reduction and management is needed.

Misuse of Disaster Exercises

Experience is the key to a successful disaster response. Unfortunately, disaster drills occur infrequently, may not test the plan and the participants effectively, and may create a sense of misplaced security.[41] In addition, an exercise should not be conducted with the purpose of testing an entire emergency plan or all aspects of training.[3]

Problems in Disaster Planning

Standard disaster plans, when completed, are rarely used in operations because of the following:

- They are cumbersome. Disaster plans tend to be extremely thick, nonuser-friendly documents that fulfill legal regulations but do not address operational problems.
- Staff is often not trained on or even aware of a developed disaster plan.
- Health disaster plans are not integrated into the overall planning process. They do not easily fit into the national plans or work on the assumption that other external players or agencies will coordinate or support public health response activities when required.
- Disaster planning that integrates government regulations/requirements and best practices creates plans that are difficult to operationalize.
- There is a tendency to have a single disaster plan and to send the same disaster response regardless of the particular circumstances.[3]

In addition, there are many challenges facing public health planners as they strive to perform these tasks in an efficacious and cost-efficient manner, including the following:

- Many public health officials throughout the world have limited knowledge, experience, and time for developing, evaluating, or improving the quality of emergency operations plans.
- Plans must address a broad range of hazards and contingencies and tend to be a voluminous document that must also be user-friendly and easily accessible during the postdisaster phase.
- Public health response activities must be well-integrated with other government and nongovernment agencies and institutions and be based on scientific evidence.
- Existing models and guidance for emergency operation planning focus on plan content (or tasks) rather than the process (or management system) and lack clear indicators of performance and outcome or measures of effectiveness.

Overemphasis on Mass Casualty Care in Health-Sector Disaster Plans

In the past, health-sector disaster planning tended to focus inordinately on mass casualty care, including surgical and critical care,[20] even though these interventions have tended to play a small role in public health.[44]

Poor Planning for Management of Human Resources

Rescue personnel are generally reluctant to ask for rest, food, and water breaks while victims are in need.[41] This results in high levels of fatigue, thus hindering effective operations, worker safety, and even patient care. Many plans and preparedness programs do not take into consideration the need for employee rest periods, occupational health measures, and critical incident stress management for disaster responders. Personnel problems associated with the inevitable onslaught of well-meaning volunteers can also occur.[41,51]

FUTURE OF DISASTER PREPAREDNESS

The future of disaster preparedness will depend on the maturity of disaster medicine and disaster management as an empirical science. As is the case with the practice of medicine, one universally applicable procedure or template is not applicable to all instances. The "cure" must be based on an accurate diagnosis and appreciation of the unique needs and resources of the population involved. However, there is now a large and ever-growing body of evidence with which to guide well-informed decision-making. Best practices, such as the Sphere Project minimum standards,[24] that are well implemented at the community level and that integrate all sectors may become more commonplace. Qualitative assessment and management methodologies, such as the preparedness

quotient, vulnerability indices, and CQI[23] programs, may provide models for further objectification of disaster preparedness. Computer-driven disaster planning and management tools, such as the Centers for Disease Control and Prevention ADEPT disaster planning software[21] and the Pan American Health Organization SUMA Humanitarian Supply Management System,[52] may further facilitate timely and rapid evidence-based decision-making among a wider audience. A more holistic approach to disaster preparedness within the context of a comprehensive strategy of disaster risk reduction may promote sustainable development on a global scale. This will all depend on the commitment of those now called to the task. Future generations may either admire our thoughtful investment or curse our selfish shortsightedness. The dividends of preparedness, though seldom realized today, often become tragically obvious tomorrow.

REFERENCES

1. Task Force on Quality Control of Disaster Management, World Association for Disaster and Emergency Medicine, Nordic Society for Disaster Medicine. Health disaster management: guidelines for evaluation and research in the Utstein Style. Volume I. Conceptual framework of disasters. *Prehospital Disaster Med.* 2003;17(suppl 3):1-177.
2. United Nations, International Strategy for Disaster Reduction. Terminology: basic terms of disaster risk reduction. Available at: http://www.unisdr.org/eng/library/lib-terminology-eng-p.htm.
3. Koob P. World Health Organization. *Health Sector Emergency Preparedness Guide.* Geneva: The World Health Organization; 1998.
4. Quarantelli EL. *Emergencies, Disasters and Catastrophes Are Different Phenomena.* [Preliminary paper.] Newark, DE: Disaster Research Center; 2000. Available at: http://www.udel.edu/DRC/Preliminary_Papers/pp304.pdf.
5. de Ville de Goyet C, Lechat M. Health aspects in natural disasters. *Trop Doct.* 1976;6:152-7.
6. Koenig K, Dinerman N, Kuehl A. Disaster nomenclature—a functional approach: the PICE system. *Acad Emerg Med.* 1996;3(7):723-7.
7. Clack Z, Keim M, Macintyre A, et al. Emergency health and risk management in sub-Saharan Africa: a lesson from the embassy bombings in Tanzania and Kenya. *Prehospital Disaster Med.* 2002;17(2):59-66.
8. Nelson D. Mitigating disasters: power to the community. *Int Nurs Rev.* 1990;37(6):371.
9. de Boer J, Dubouloz M, ed. *Handbook of Disaster Medicine.* The Netherlands: International Society of Disaster Medicine; 2000.
10. Sidel V, Onel E, Geiger H, et al. Public health responses to natural and human-made disasters. In: Last JM, Wallace RB, eds. *Maxcy-Rosenthal-Last Public Health and Preventive Medicine.* 13th ed. Norwalk, CT: Appleton and Lange; 1992:1173-86.
11. Lechat M. *Disaster as a Public Health Problem.* Brussels: Catholic University of Luvain; 1985.
12. Noji E. Natural disaster management. In: Auerbach P, ed. *Wilderness Medicine.* 4th ed. St. Louis: Mosby; 2001:644-63.
13. *Yokohama Strategy and Plan of Action for a Safer World: Guidelines for Natural Disaster Prevention, Preparedness and Mitigation.* Available at: http://www.unisdr.org/eng/about_isdr/bd-yokohama-strat-eng.htm.
14. Proceedings of the World Summit on Sustainable Development Plan of Implementation, Johannesburg, South Africa. Available at: http://www.un.org/esa/sustdev/documents/WSSD_POL-PD/English/POIToc.htm.
15. Second World Conference on Disaster Reduction to be held in Kobe during January 2005. Available at: http://www.unisdr.org/eng/wcdr/wcdr-index.htm.
16. Emergency Management Australia. *Australian Counter Disaster Handbook. Counter-Disaster Concepts and Principles.* Vol 1. 2nd ed. Canberra: Emergency Management Australia; 1993.

16a. United Nations. Declaration of the United Nations Conference on the Human Environment at Stockholm, June 5-16, 1972. Available at: http://www.unep.org/Documents.multilingual/Default.asp?DocumentID=97&ArticleD=.

17. Federal Emergency Management Agency. *State and Local Guide 101: Guide for All Hazard Emergency Operations Planning, SLG101*. Washington, DC: Federal Emergency Management Agency; 1996.

18. National Institute for Chemical Studies. *Sheltering in Place as a Public Protective Action*. Charleston, WV: Environmental Protection Agency; 2001.

19. The White House. Homeland Security Presidential Directive/HSPD-5. Management of Domestic Incidents. Available at: http://www.whitehouse.gov/news/releases/2003/02/20030228-9.html.

20. Keim M, Rhyne G. The Pacific Emergency Health Initiative: a pilot study of emergency preparedness in Oceania. *Australian J Emerg Med*. June 2001;(13):157-64.

21. Keim M, Giannone P. The PEHI process: an integrated approach to public health emergency operations planning and quality management. Lecture presented at: Sixth National Environmental Public Health Conference:
Preparing for the Environmental Public Health Challenges of the 21st Century; Feb. 16, 2004; Atlanta.

22. Auf der Heide E. *Community Medical Disaster Planning and Evaluation Guide*. Dallas: American College of Emergency Physicians; 1995.

23. Mayer T, Salluzo R. Theory of continuous quality improvement. In: Salluzo R, Mayer T, Strauss R, et al, eds. *Emergency Department Management*. St. Louis: Mosby; 1997:461-79.

24. The Sphere Project. *Humanitarian Charter and Minimum Standards in Disaster Response*. Oxford, UK: The Sphere Project; 2004.

25. World Health Organization. *Handbook for Emergency Field Operations*. Available at: http://www.who.int/disasters/repo/7660.doc.

26. United Nations, Protein-Calorie Advisory Group. *A Guide to Food and Health Relief Operations for Disasters*. New York: United Nations; 1977.

27. Davis J, Lambert R. *Engineering in Emergencies: A Practical Guide for Relief Workers*. London: Intermediate Technology Publications; 1995.

28. *Community Emergency Preparedness: A Manual for Managers and Policy-Makers*. Geneva: World Health Organization; 1999.

29. *Handbook for Emergencies*. 2nd ed. Geneva: United Nations High Commissioner for Refugees; June 2000.

30. *Water Manual for Refugee Situations*. Geneva: United Nations High Commissioner for Refugees; November 1992.

31. Eade D, Williams S, eds. Emergencies and development. In: *The Oxfam Handbook of Development and Relief*. Vol 2. Oxford: Oxfam Publishing; 1995.

32. Sandler R, Jones T, eds. *Medical Care of Refugees*. Oxford: Oxford University Press; 1987.

33. *Guidelines for Assessing Disaster Preparedness in the Health Sector*. Washington, DC: Pan American Health Organization; 1995.

34. Burkle FM. Complex humanitarian emergencies: III. Measures of effectiveness. *Prehospital Disaster Med*. 1995;10(1):48-56.

35. Burkle F. Measures of effectiveness in large-scale bio-terrorism events. *Prehospital Disaster Med*. 2003;18(3):258-62.

36. Committee on Trauma, American College of Surgeons. *Advanced Trauma Life Support Course*. Chicago: American College of Surgeons; 1994.

37. American Heart Association. *Advanced Cardiac Life Support Course*. Dallas: American Heart Association; 1995.

38. American Academy of Pediatrics/American College of Emergency Physicians. *Advanced Pediatric Life Support*. Dallas: American College of Emergency Physicians; 1995.

39. Berwick DM. Continuous improvement as an ideal in healthcare. *New Engl J Med*. 1989;320(1):53-6.

40. Batalden PB, Buchanan ED. Industrial models of quality improvement. In: Goldenfield N, Nas DB, eds. *Providing Quality Care: The Challenge to Clinicians*. Philadelphia: American College of Physicians; 1989.

41. Waeckerle J. Disaster planning and response. *New Engl J Med*. 1991;324(12):815-21.

42. Seaman J. Disaster epidemiology: or why most international disaster relief is ineffective. *Injury*. 1990;21:5.

43. Duclos P, Ing R. Injuries and risk factors for injuries from the 29 May 1982 tornado, Marion, Illinois. *Int Epi Assoc*. 1989;18(1):213-19.

44. Sapir D, Lechat M. Reducing the impact of natural disasters: why aren't we better prepared? *Health Policy Planning*. 1986;1:118.

45. de Bruycker M, Greco D, Lechat MF. The 1980 earthquake in southern Italy: rescue of trapped victims and mortality. *Bull WHO*. 1983;51:1021.

46. Pan American Health Organization. *WHO/PAHO Guidelines for the Use of Foreign Field Hospitals in the Aftermath of Sudden-Impact Disasters*. Available at: http://www.paho.org/english/dd/ped/FieldHospitalsFolleto.pdf.

47. Pluut I. Field hospitals in Bam, Iran. Available at: http://www.disaster-info.net/downloadzone/bam.htm.

48. Levitin H, Siegelson H. Hazardous materials. Disaster planning and response. *Disaster Med*. 1996;14(2):327-48.

49. Lechat MF. Updates in epidemiology of health effects of disasters. *Epidemiol Rev*. 1990;12:192.

50. Anonymous. Impact of hurricane Mitch on Central America. *Epidemiol Bull*. December 1998;19(4):1-13.

51. Quarantelli EL. *Delivery of Emergency Medical Services in Disasters: Assumptions and Realities*. New York: Irvington; 1985.

52. SUMA Humanitarian Supply Management System. Available at: http://www.disaster-info.net/SUMA/.

chapter 26

Policy Issues in Disaster Preparedness and Response

Eric S. Weinstein

At the intersection of public perception, science, the duty of government to act, and the rights of the individual sits public health policy. Guiding the paths of healthcare providers, bureaucrats, and patients is an ongoing collaboration to do the most good for the most people. Citations from the *Bible* and other ancient texts demonstrate meritorious efforts to reduce the spread of disease. Scholars are quick to point out the lack of appreciation of factual scientific knowledge through centuries of political maneuvering to regulate immigration, forcefully separate innocents to protect the fearful, and hide the unfortunately afflicted from view. This chapter discusses recent examples of public health policy in the light of individuals' rights and the science of public health threats.

THE ETHICAL VIEW FOR THE SCIENTIST

In our free, democratic society, policy makers tasked with the authority to protect the public's health must also consider the individual's civil and political rights of liberty, privacy, association, assembly, and expression.[1] No one argues against the need to contain the spread of an illness or reduce the threat to life and property damage by terrorism or a natural or industrial disaster. Gostin[1] writes that it is not improper to restrain the enjoyment of liberty, privacy, or property per se, but it is improper to do so unnecessarily, arbitrarily, inequitably, or brutally. This can take place when government acts against a threat that is not valid or not based on objective, reliable scientific knowledge. Protecting public health is difficult to do when an uncertain, evolving illness begins to affect individuals and there is limited technology and limited acquisition of dynamic relevant information. Many illnesses appear the same early in the course of the illness, and it is not until later that the diagnosis can be affirmed. Consider such an illness affecting dozens, hundreds, or thousands of people spread over continents, with fear mounting and governments pressed into acting immediately. It would be the government's burden to defend and rigorously evaluate the effectiveness of a public health measure adopted to contain and treat this mystery illness in real time. Certainly,

a known illness for which research has identified the agent, vectors, susceptible hosts with evidence-based diagnostics, treatment, and cost to society can be addressed by an effective public health policy. The challenge to a public health agency is to reach this familiarity with a new syndrome or toxidrome in short order.[1]

The balance between the establishment and maintenance of health and the prevention or reduction of transmission of illness with subsequent inhibition or reduction of the individual's rights should follow the doctrine of least-restrictive alternative to reduce the risk or ameliorate the harm. Legal scholars can assume this role alongside public health authorities who are not versed in the ramifications of invasiveness, the intrusion of an intervention on the individual's rights, or the scope and selection of individuals to receive an intervention. The duration of the intervention should be proportionate to the desired effect, with ongoing review to reduce untoward effects that would limit an individual's rights.[1]

A fair public health policy benefits those in need and burdens those who endanger the public's health. These policies should not discriminate against sex, ethnicity, or other demographic factors unless scientifically proven to be accurate and if applied evenly will achieve the intended outcome. A means to address perceived inequalities or lack of sensitivity to individual rights is due process. This check-and-balance opportunity of an individual to seek the decision of others assembled to independently determine the merits of a public health intervention in a timely manner may reduce any further effects of a misapplied policy or ineffective course of action. This unbiased informed decision can fashion redress to rectify any misapplication or unintended consequences of policies. This form of process improvement will achieve more appropriate future policy and build trust in government that permits justice to be served.[2] Unfortunately, time is of the essence when a public health agency is pressured to act against an unknown illness. Review during the course of the dynamics of the response to the threat can and should occur simultaneously to scale back any restrictions on individual rights as the science of the event is established.[3] The uninformed public must trust government to achieve compliance with public health policy as the event unfolds before a wary media. Careful discussions in an open forum will not only make it easier for the policy to be accepted and thus achieve the intended end, but also will help attract unknown individuals or groups to further the policy through their involvement in the process. The common good for the public as a whole can be met by the involvement of the community of individuals. Transparency flushes facts, quells rumors, and dispels myths. Protection of an individual's rights can be ensured if the creation of public health policy adheres to necessity of action through proportional, nondiscriminatory, and fair means.[4]

EVACUATION ORDERS: "YOU MAY WANT TO HEED THIS ADVICE FOR YOUR OWN GOOD"

As fate yields opportunity, the writing of this chapter began with the author under the voluntary evacuation issued for coastal South Carolina in response to the then-impending threat of Hurricane Charley (Aug. 13, 2004).[5] New evacuation measures had been put into place after the infamous 1998 mandatory evacuation of the Charleston, S.C. area in advance of Hurricane Floyd. That evacuation distressed families in that some sat in traffic for 18 hours along a more-than-150-mile stretch along I-26 up to Columbia. At the time of Hurricane Floyd, roughly 1/7th of the S.C. population participated in the evacuation of the entire coastline, with Hurricane Hugo still fresh on most residents' minds.[6] The public outcry after the flawed Hurricane Floyd evacuation enabled the retrospective science of disaster medicine to produce significant changes to the entire data-gathering process that a S.C. governor uses to declare a mandatory evacuation under state law.[7] Exercises have proven that lane reversals, new highway construction, and strategic placement of hundreds of S.C. law enforcement officers and Department of Transportation workers in concert with computer-aided scenarios have been successful to reduce the time of evacuation to up to 10 hours, despite a surge of migration from at-risk coastal S.C. areas.[8] Shortly after the Hurricane Floyd evacuation, honest assessments took place, with a subsequent increased fund of concrete data used to make the executive decision to issue a mandatory evacuation order. An evacuation order can cost a state millions of dollars, disrupt local economies dependent on tourism, and further decrease an already waning public trust. In an effort to make an evacuation easier, the 2003-2004 S.C. General Assembly voted to amend a 1976 law to allow the governor to order that traffic lanes be reversed so that all lanes in an evacuation area flow in one direction away from the evacuation area.[9]

AN OUTBREAK AND THE EMERGENCY MEDICAL TREATMENT AND LABOR ACT: PATIENT CARE ENSURED

The key to any containment strategy is for the local government executive to issue an emergency order or proclamation establishing a new set of operating proce-

dures for public health authorities, the healthcare delivery system, and other government agencies.[10] If an outbreak is local, the county executive or county council would issue the order or proclamation through a well-defined process. If an outbreak is across counties, the governor would issue the order or proclamation. The Emergency Medical Treatment and Labor Act (EMTALA) of 1986 permits regionalization of prehospital care to afford the best possible medical care for victims of trauma; those suffering from an acute cerebrovascular accident (CVA); and patients requiring special services such as pediatrics, obstetrics, and, increasingly, psychiatry. Under an executive order to mitigate the threat of a public health emergency (PHE), patients who meet predetermined criteria developed in a collaborative effort using the most accurate; timely; and, if possible, evidence-based determinations can be directed to an established healthcare facility (HCF) or a newly created facility staffed with the necessary personnel, equipment, and supplies to meet the need.[11] This plan can be accomplished ahead of time in anticipation of an outbreak of known pathogens or in the early phases of a new illness pattern detected through the triggers of syndromic surveillance.

Patients who enter the healthcare system after a telephone call to 911 (or other phone number) for emergency medical transport may be evaluated by an emergency medical technician (EMT) when the ambulance arrives. Currently, certain systems will permit an EMT-paramedic (EMT-P) evaluation for appropriateness of transport via emergency medical services (EMS). This is based on strict criteria developed by off-line medical direction; approved by county officials with appropriate documentation; and, more importantly, communication between the EMT crew, on-line medical control, and subsequent review of each call.[12] In a PHE, the most practical extension of this on-scene or field triage process is for an EMS crew, with an EMT-P, registered nurse (RN), or midlevel provider (physician assistant or nurse practitioner), to perform an evaluation of the patient for preset criteria. These criteria can be determined de novo as the PHE is evolving by the assembled collaborative team process or from prior known, reviewed, and learned outbreak responses. This process must include appropriate education about the outbreak; issuance of equipment, supplies, and personal protective equipment (PPE) to the EMS responders; and a screening process to exclude responders who may be more susceptible or less-than-adequate, placing them more at risk.[13] The patient will enter the PHE evaluation and treatment process, and anyone else at the EMS evaluation site must be considered a contact person and enter the PHE evaluation process. The evaluation site must be assessed for epidemiological concerns and adjudicated accordingly.[13]

The dispatch of this PHE field evaluation team (FET) can be accomplished through use of priority medical dispatch or a similar 911 operating system. In a PHE, a person who calls the 911 system (or another telephone number for ambulance service for those regions not yet using 911) will undergo caller interrogation specific for the symptoms and any other information that can be learned. The caller will then be given instructions on first aid for laypersons or the establishment of containment strategies pending arrival of the FET. Priority medical dispatch or a similar system can then send the FET to the scene to perform the evaluation, separate from the usual standard EMS.

If this evaluation determines that the patient is a potential victim of a PHE, the EMS crew can transport the patient to a HCF established to evaluate and treat the presenting symptom complex. If the patient is in distress, he or she will be attended to as per standard operating procedures and then transported to the HCF.[11] The EMS crew will be told what containment strategies and procedures an HCF has undertaken for the patient. During the executive declared PHE, the destination HCF may not be a standard HCF, such as the closest hospital, but it may be a "fever hospital" or an HCF specifically created for the PHE.[13] This location will have healthcare workers (HCWs) who are trained, equipped, supplied, and donned in appropriate PPE. It may be on the grounds of the closest hospital, public health clinic, or in another building with appropriate air exchanges, water, heating and air, food preparation, restrooms, showers, etc. in the community to contain the PHE while allowing other hospitals and HCFs to attend to their usual patient loads without an influx of patients with special needs that may be incapacitating due to the surge in volume or contamination.[11] In a short period, such an unconventional HCF can be fully operational with prepositioned stores or vendor agreements.

Guidelines can be created, extensively reviewed from the go-forward, and adapted as the outbreak proceeds. If a patient is determined to meet predetermined criteria, then the process will continue with the patient discharged home with close monitoring, to another HCF for long-term care, or to another HCF for containment.[3] If the patient does not meet the criteria, then the patient can receive appropriate diagnosis and care at that location and then be transported to an acute-care HCF (hospital, clinic, or physician office) for further evaluation, care, and discharge.[14] The vehicle used to transport the patient and the accompanying personnel will have to undergo containment strategies from the initial PHE HCF to the next location.

EMTALA requires that the dedicated emergency department (ED) of an HCF perform a medical screening examination (MSE) for patients who present asking for a medical evaluation or when the MSE is requested by another person.[15] Patients who self-refer to the ED during an executive declared PHE could receive an MSE by the hospital designated RN or midlevel provider donned in appropriate PPE. This HCW can be screened to ensure that he or she is fit for the assignment, vaccinated accordingly, and in-serviced to the threat at hand.[3] The patient may receive an MSE, accepted by the physician at the PHE HCF, and sent with the appropriate EMTALA transfer documentation. If the patient requires stabilization before transfer to the PHE HCF or requires admission to the HCF for acute- and/or long-term care, this could commence accordingly, with containment strategies observed.

At the HCFs, containment strategies should include training of all employees to the specific presenting symptoms and signs of the PHE, use of PPE for those who routinely meet and greet people at their work stations, and limitations on entrance locations to the public.[3] HCF-designated HCWs positioned to act as screeners can direct people entering the HCF to a receiving area for a more rigorous evaluation, separate from the ED, if they are coming to the HCF as a visitor or to conduct other business. More importantly, if a patient seeking medical attention enters the HCF though a nontypical entrance, containment strategies can commence accordingly. Signage specific for the PHE can direct patients presenting to the HCF for evaluation to containment areas designed for this initial evaluation.

It is plausible for specially trained HCWs, in tandem with personnel from law enforcement, public safety, department of transportation, or another like agency, to assist in the sorting of patients that self-refer to the HCF at locations removed from the entrance of the HCF. To reduce drunk driving for the public good, law enforcement personnel currently set up road blocks, at which they check driver's licenses, registration, and insurance cards and screen for impaired drivers or passengers or vehicles suspected of being involved in illegal activities.[16] An executive PHE can extend certain powers to law enforcement to assist the public health effort to contain the illness.[17] Queues of traffic at locations safely established in route to a hospital can act as a checkpoint for screening, as previously noted, with direction of patients to the PHE HCF or their usual HCF containment area for an MSE. The vehicle and person(s) in the vehicle will enter the epidemiology evaluation and containment process. If the PHE HCW screening determines that a person fits the PHE symptom complex, the PHE FET can be deployed to conduct further evaluation and transport. The vehicle that carried the patient(s) will then have to be isolated, evaluated for contamination, and decontaminated accordingly.

SMALLPOX VACCINATIONS: THINK BEFORE YOU ACT

The Centers for Disease Control and Prevention (CDC) Advisory Committee on Immunization Practices (ACIP) revised its 1991 recommendations in June 2001 to include the use of vaccinia vaccine if the smallpox (variola) virus was used as an agent of biological terrorism or if a smallpox outbreak were to occur for another unforeseen reason. This plan included pre-exposure vaccination for first responders or treatment teams dispatched to attend to those exposed.[18] Modlin[19] was chair of the ACIP when the 2001 recommendations were released, and he later wrote a cautious editorial in March 2002 asking that policy makers weigh the best available analysis of vaccine-related morbidity and costs against the best available assessment of risk for smallpox release. Fauci[20] followed with similar caution, with a reminder of why the smallpox vaccination program was discontinued in the face of known risks, known transmissions, and known cases worldwide—there were several vaccine-related deaths each year as the risk of contracting the disease continued to decline. He concurred with the "ring-vaccination" strategy, which worked during past decades and involves isolating those suspected or confirmed of being infected with the virus and then tracing contacts and their contacts for vaccination. This minimized the risk of adverse vaccine events (AVEs) and effectively used limited vaccines and other resources, including manpower to adjudicate the plan.[20]

A widespread vaccination program is estimated to produce 4600 serious AVEs and 285 deaths.[21] These numbers are unacceptable to many who are facing no known risk and no substantial proof of smallpox outside of known repositories.[22,23] Meltzer,[24] through the CDC, in December 2001 showed that the number of susceptible persons and the assumed rate of transmission are the most important variables influencing the total number of smallpox cases to be expected from an intentional release of smallpox into a community. Data analysis of known outbreaks showed that one infected person would subsequently infect fewer than three persons; these data are important when deciding strategies of containment. The data showed that the ring-vaccination surveillance-containment strategy would yield the fastest time to contain an outbreak with the least number of deaths, but they did not discuss AVEs, the effect of smallpox morbidity, or the costs to adjudicate the strategy.[24]

Non-peer review medical journals began detailing reservations about the National Smallpox Vaccination Program (NSVP) within weeks of its announcement. In preparation for the program's Jan. 24, 2003, commencement, hospitals openly questioned the financial burden of prescreening examinations, administering the vaccines, monitoring employees for AVEs, and providing treatment if necessary to the intended 500,000 first responder HCWs. They were also concerned that the risks of such a large-scale program for an unsubstantiated rumor based on loose "what-ifs" could reduce an already short staff because vaccinated workers may have to miss work. Hospitals also noted the risk of their HCWs transmitting vaccinia to patients in their facilities as well as HCW family members. Public health policy in this instance did not address the legal ramifications of compensation to inoculated HCWs who suffered an AVE, temporary or permanent. Who should pay the HCW if he or she cannot work? Would subsequent medical costs be paid through workers' compensation or an HCW's own medical insurance?[25] These questions still have not been answered.

The Homeland Security Act of 2002 extended liability protection to the manufacturers of the vaccine, hospitals administering the vaccine, and individuals receiving the vaccine, presumably if they transmit vaccinia to another person. Hospital attorneys debated what locations were protected because it appeared that hospitals themselves were protected only if their vaccination clinic was on-site but not if they chose an off-site HCF such as a clinic.

Reports of HCW AVEs were accumulating with the commencement of the NSVP, slowing the program to a trickle. If 30% of HCWs in some facilities would have had to miss some work, the staffing nightmare could have been dangerous. In April 2003, the CDC ACIP released a supplement, *Recommendations for Using Smallpox Vaccine in a Pre-Event Vaccination Program*, to its 2001 smallpox vaccine recommendation, moving the focus from each hospital establishing and maintaining at least one response team to only the state having a team. The acquired knowledge of AVEs supported vaccinating healthy, screened HCWs who had been previously vaccinated to staff HCF treatment teams. Dressings to cover the vaccination site, changed by a specific team, were stressed, as was vigorous handwashing techniques. The pre-NSVP concern about administrative leave was not required unless specific minor AVEs developed. The CDC released preliminary reports[26] of 10 cases of myopericarditis among approximately 240,000 healthy personnel who received the vaccine for the first time and none among 110,000 who received another vaccine as a booster. The report noted two civilian volunteers with AVEs (one with myocarditis and one with pericarditis), a rate greater than what was previously noted in unvaccinated healthy military personnel from 1998 to 2000. More disturbing were the reports of five civilian volunteers who contracted myocardial ischemia–related AVEs, three with infarction and two with angina. Screening noted that four of these five had known cardiovascular risk factors, and the other had known cardiovascular disease.[26] Based on these findings, the CDC ACIP released another supplement, this time excluding persons with cardiac disease or risk factors from the NSVP.[27]

Sepkowitz[28] answered the question: How contagious is vaccinia? The research showed a risk of secondary transmission of vaccinia, with an 11% fatality rate, with nosocomial transmission apparently occurring through minor contact with a source case. Incidental transmission in the home was noted to occur more often with sustained, intimate exposure that is believed to be related to differences in immunological competency and dermatological differences. With the recommendation to not grant administrative leave for newly vaccinated HCWs, hospitals would have to weigh the risk of a self-inflicted epidemic for an unrealized, unsubstantiated risk.[28] Data gathered from January to July 4, 2003, did not corroborate the conclusions of Sepkowitz's study; there were no transmissions of vaccinia from 37,875 vaccinated volunteer civilians to other persons.[29] These uncertainties of benefit versus the reduced risk combined with the end of the conventional war in Iraq without finding any evidence of weapons of mass destruction and a contentious medicolegal climate in the United States contributed to a less-than-enthusiastic response to the NSVP.

More than a year after the commencement of the NSVP, policy makers showed HCW who volunteered to be vaccinated that they were listening to their concerns by passing the Smallpox Emergency Personnel Protection Act of 2003 (Dec. 13, 2003).[30] Funded at $42 million, the program provides financial and medical benefits to eligible members of a smallpox emergency response plan approved by the U.S. Department of Health and Human Services (HHS) who sustain certain medical injuries caused by a smallpox vaccine. In addition, unvaccinated individuals injured after coming into contact with vaccinated members of an emergency response plan—or with a person with whom the vaccinated person had contact—may be eligible for program benefits. The program also provides benefits to survivors of eligible individuals whose death resulted from a covered injury. HHS recognized the disconnect from the NSVP felt by HCWs when it began implementation of the compensation program by publishing a Smallpox Vaccine Injury Compensation Table in the Aug. 27, 2003 edition of the *Federal Register*.[31] The table became effective upon publication. Moving this from HHS to federal law only contributed to the loss of public faith in the program.

Bozzette and others[32] posted *A Model for Smallpox-Vaccination Policy* on the *New England Journal of Medicine's* Web site on Dec. 19, 2002. This stochastic model of outcomes considered a range of threats, including a hoax, and predicted the number of deaths, but not morbidity nor the extent of AVEs, after the use of various measures to contain the spread of smallpox. The study brought policy implications to the forefront, specifically the benefit of isolation while highlighting the lack of case law with concerns of denial of civil liberties.[32] Federal law gives the U.S. Public Health Service the power to detain individuals, for such time and such manner as may be reasonably necessary, believed to be infected with a communicable disease in the communicable stage to prevent transmission of the disease.[33] Containment strategies have been successful for centuries to combat the spread of smallpox. Smallpox is spread via large droplet respiratory transmission from face-to-face contact. In 1988 the World Health Organization determined that air samples taken in the vicinity of smallpox patients were rarely positive. This, coupled with the observation that most patients with uncomplicated disease are not capable of generating a strong enough cough to propel aerosols long distance, builds the clinical case for smallpox containment strategies.[34] Containment vaccination can be directed at the persons at the highest risk for disease—those who had face-to-face contact within 2 meters.[35]

CONTAINMENT STRATEGIES: LIMIT CONTACT, LIMIT THE SPREAD

Barbera and colleagues[36] published a primer on the containment strategies of quarantine (potentially exposed to an infectious agent) and isolation (suspected infection determined by the manifestation of the agent's symptoms/signs/laboratory confirmation). The term *large-scale quarantine* was defined to assist public health policy planners to distinguish a few patients potentially exposed from the numbers that policy planners envision in bioterrorist scenarios or a pandemic.[36] This clinical strategy is no different than the commonplace school or work excuse that physicians provide ED patients, but on a grand scale to limit the spread of an infectious agent from others. A physician writes an excuse, and the school or employer recognizes that the physician wants to protect the other students or employees from "catching" the illness. The student or employee suffers no consequence or injury from not attending school or showing up for work. Individual citizens appreciate the need for government to prevent significant risk to the health of themselves and others. The public health con-

tract between the individual and the government cedes certain rights and liberties to achieve a healthier and safer society. A federal statute applies to interstate commerce or travel between states or countries, whereas a state statute applies to most all other instances that would require compulsory separation of individuals. The framework for public health powers (necessity, effective means, proportionality, and fairness) must be applied to the draconian police powers of quarantine and isolation through the following questions[1]:

1. Does the science of the known infectious disease process support the separation of those infected or those possibly infected from those not infected?
2. Can those separated be placed into quarters that will not further the infectious process, respect their dignity, and provide reasonable levels of comfort?
3. Does the risk of separation of individuals from their families, livelihood, and communities outweigh the risk of not separating them and thus furthering the disease among their families, workplace, or communities?[36]

SCIENCE CALMS FEARS

Smallpox is not transmitted during the prodromal phase of high fever that precedes the rash. If an individual is exposed to smallpox, he or she can be quarantined to his or her home and can maintain most levels of normal activity until the start of a fever. Then, these individuals can be isolated until it is clear that the fever is not from smallpox. A close contact of a documented smallpox patient should receive the smallpox vaccine if there are no contraindications. If the exposed person is unwilling to accept the risk of the smallpox vaccine or is found to have contraindications, then a full 18-day quarantine is warranted to observe for the tell-tale sign of fevers. The contact is then isolated to reduce the transmission of smallpox to others, with the possibility of vaccination increased since the prodromal now has smallpox or, if the vaccine is contraindicated, other therapies can be administered. This would be the least-restrictive alternative to permit observation without complete disruption of the individual's life and those that depend on him or her.[37]

SEVERE ACUTE RESPIRATORY SYNDROME: REAL-TIME SCIENCE INTERSECTS WITH DIFFERENT GOVERNMENTS

Canada

Dwosh and colleagues[3] showed clear evidence of swift strategy to contain the severe acute respiratory syndrome (SARS) virus at the Richmond Hill Hospital (Toronto, Canada) in March 2003. Patients and hospital staff who had come into close, unprotected contact with two index SARS patients were identified and told to stay home and monitor themselves for a list of symptoms and signs with calls twice a day from public health officials. Fifteen people who began to exhibit the first signs of the illness, specifically a fever, were then isolated. Thereafter, no further cases of SARS were identified.[3]

China

In May 2003, 1 month after the SARS outbreak had peaked, people in the Haidian District of Beijing who had close contact with a suspected SARS patient for more than 30 minutes' duration were quarantined. At first, quarantine lasted for 14 days and was later reduced to 10 days and then 3 days as the results of quarantine strategy were reviewed. A least-restrictive alternative for travelers entering the area was personal surveillance with close medical supervision to permit prompt recognition of infection or illness without restriction of movement. Only persons who had a history of contact with a SARS patient developed SARS during quarantine. In contrast, none of the people who did not come into contact with a SARS patient developed SARS. There were no cases of secondary transmission of SARS to relatives or other contacts during quarantine. Exposed persons were sent home and told to monitor their temperature and to have all members of the household observe strict handwashing precautions and to use respiratory masks. Review of the data showed that if public health authorities had focused only on persons who had contact with an actively ill SARS patient, the number of quarantined persons would have declined by 66%. Persons exposed to a SARS patient in the incubation phase had little to no risk of contracting SARS. It was determined that a person exposed to a SARS patient could monitor his or her temperature alone while on personal surveillance with public health monitoring. If the person developed a fever, then he or she would be removed from the home and isolated. Such modifications would have returned persons to their routines more promptly and reduced the overall resources spent to observe patients in their homes. As the illness is identified as a separate entity through surveillance, data can be collected in real time to permit these changes on a more dynamic basis.[38]

Taiwan

Taiwan public health authorities used different containment strategies; close contacts were quarantined for 14 days from February 2003 until June 10 and then aligned with the World Health Organization 10 days later. Hospital staff and patients in close contacts with SARS patients were quarantined in HCFs; all others were quarantined at home, except for homeless persons, who were asked to go voluntarily to government quarantine centers. This tiered system was extended to travelers to Taiwan from April 28 to July 4. Travelers were quarantined for 10 days in an airport transit hotel, at home, or at a quarantine site designated and paid for by their employer if under business (otherwise by the government). If one of these sites was not available, then the traveler was quarantined at a government center. On June 9, because of pressure from Taiwan business leaders, restrictions were eased for employees of Taiwanese companies based in mainland China who were returning to Taiwan for business. These travelers were allowed to return to work if they wore surgical masks.[39]

Persons under quarantine were required to stay where they were quarantined, to wear masks, and observe other precautions, with frequent readings of their temperature. The differences in Level A quarantine (14 days, close contact) and Level B quarantine (traveler, 10 days) were restrictive and not based on science because a traveler could have just as easily come into close contact with a SARS patient and develop a fever as could an HCW or family member of a SARS patient. Yet the Level A person was not permitted to leave the site unless deemed necessary by public health authorities, with all meals delivered. Level B persons were free to go to an open area to exercise and purchase meals. To clearly show the difference in approach, Taiwanese officials used video monitoring of some persons who were contacts of a SARS patient and were found to have violated their quarantine at home. Due to this commonplace occurrence at the end of the outbreak, most at-home quarantine persons were under video monitoring. Persons who completed their quarantine received a payment of the equivalent of U.S. $147.00 and other social services from local authorities.[39]

Of the 131,132 persons quarantined, 286 (0.2%) were fined for violations of their quarantine. Of the 50,319 persons in Level A quarantine, 4063 (8%) were placed under video monitoring, and 112 developed SARS. Of the 80,813 persons under Level B quarantine, 21 (0.03%) developed SARS. Those with the highest risk of contracting SARS were exposed HCWs (0.34%), family members of SARS patients (0.33%), and those who were on the same airplane flight who sat within three rows of a SARS patient (0.36%). The lowest percentage of patients were those simply traveling from a SARS-affected area.[39]

Hong Kong

On March 1, 2003, the spread of SARS in the Hong Kong Special Administrative Region was traced to Prince of Wales Hospital HCWs and their contacts. After slow implementation of internal containment strategies—specifically, isolation—the outbreak was slowed. The second wave of SARS was traced to a patient who used a toilet in a housing project, which lead to that entire area being quarantined. This was worsened when persons from the affected housing project went to a nearby housing project, not observing quarantine or partially adhering to guidelines. The third wave inundated hospitals as the entire region was in the midst of the outbreak. By April 10, "home quarantine" was implemented for household contacts of confirmed SARS patients. The time lag to identify SARS patients led to a peak on April 17. It was not until April 25 that "home confinement policy" was extended to households with contacts of suspected SARS patients.[40]

LEGISLATING PUBLIC HEALTH

The Model State Emergency Health Powers Act was enacted Dec. 21, 2001, to provide a framework for governors, legislatures, and public health officials to review their statutes and regulations to adhere to the following principles: preparedness, surveillance, management of property, protection of persons, and communication.[41] Gostin noted that the body of public health statutes is layered on old statutes implemented in response to a public health threat decades ago and that a review for current evidence-based medicine or a review grounded in sound science are unlikely. As medical theory has expanded with technology,[1] legal appreciation of an individual's rights have also been defined without benefit of public health law keeping pace. Old legal remedies may not apply to current public health dilemmas; insufficient authority may limit effective action; and coordination between local, state, and federal authorities may be hindered by conflicting statutes that have been rendered moot through technology.[41] Coercive powers may be the only means to ensure the safety and health of the public and must not be taken lightly. Public health law gives government the authority to limit personal interests to safeguard the public health through powers bounded by necessity, effective means, proportionality, and fairness; in return individuals forgo autonomy, liberty, or property. The model act itself is divided into the pre-emergency environment for predeclaration powers and the powers that become the governor's to use after declaration of an emergency. The declaration of a public health emergency must meet the following criteria: (1) an occurrence or imminent threat of an illness or public health condition that (2) is caused by bioterrorism or a new or re-emerging infectious agent or biological toxin previously controlled that also (3) poses a high probability of a large number of deaths, serious or long-term disabilities, or widespread exposure to an infectious or toxic agent that poses a significant risk of substantial future harm to a large number of persons.[41]

The model act filters redundant statutes, removes statutes that have become irrelevant, and enhances traditional public health powers with an extensive set of conditions, principles, and requirements governing the use of personal control measures. Specific advancements include the use of home confinement or other creative less-restrictive alternatives for containment rather than compulsory isolation or quarantine and permits persons so contained to be afforded due process, appropriate medical care, activities, hygiene, and food.[41] Transparency of communication with the public to explain protective measures and access to mental health will reduce public misperceptions. Immunity is afforded to persons exercising authority under the specific declarations of the governor. As of July 2004, 20 states had enacted laws along the model act guidelines of the 29 states that have introduced similar legislation.[42]

Civil libertarians point out the evolution of public health powers, with the federal government retaining authority over interstate and foreign commerce, national defense, and the expenditure of money. Even with the creation of the Department of Homeland Security, the CDC still remains the lead advisory consequence agency in a PHE. In the event of a bioterrorist outbreak, the Federal Bureau of Investigations will provide federal crisis management that is coordinated with a state crisis management agency. In most states, the lead state consequence management agency lacks the depth required in current state law for basic public health to function appropriately.

Annas[2] stated that the model act should respond to real problems, but the scenarios that would require use of these powers are not known and are left to the transparency of the process of a state government to recommend to the governor to use in a PHE. These powers are for all biological agents and their toxins, regardless of entry into the public. Annual influenza epidemics, by definition, are a PHE with the full depth of the government prepared to prevent a pandemic. The fear and panic after the anthrax incidents in the fall of 2001 cannot be compared to the reality of a true PHE involving the deployment of community HCWs. There is no empiric evidence that certain containment strategies are unfounded.

THE DIRECTION FROM HERE

Civil libertarians and legal scholars are becoming more familiar with the science of outbreaks and other elements of public health threats. Scientists are becoming more astute in the ethical and legal ramifications of intended therapies and interventions. The synergy and collaboration between these guardians of public interest will increasingly contribute to the government's ability to formulate effective public health policy.

REFERENCES

1. Gostin L. Commentary: When terrorism threatens health: How far are limitations on human rights justified. *J Law Med Ethics.* 2003;31:524-8.
2. Annas G. Bioterrorism, public health, and civil liberties. *New Engl J Med.* 2002;346(17):1337-42.
3. Dwosh H, et al. Identification and containment of an outbreak of SARS in a community hospital. *Canadian Med Assoc J.* 2003; 168(11):1415-20.
4. Gostin L, Bayer R, Fairchild A. Ethical and legal challenges posed by severe acute respiratory syndrome: implications for the control of severe infectious disease threats. *JAMA.* 2003;290(24):3229-37.
5. State of South Carolina, Office of the Governor. Gov. Sanford expands voluntary evacuation to entire SC coast [press release]. Available at: http://www.scgovernor.com/interior. asp?Site ContentId=6&pressid=119&NavId=54&ParentId=0.
6. Dow K, Cutter S. South Carolina's response to hurricane Floyd. Available at: http://www.colorado.edu/hazards/qr/qr128/qr128.html.
7. South Carolina Code of Laws. §25-1-440 (Additional powers and duties of governor during declared emergency). Available at: http://www.scstatehouse.net/code/t25c001.htm.
8. Intelligent Transportation Systems. Summary of Regional Hurricane Traffic Operations Workshops. Available at: http://www.itsdocs. fhwa.dot.gov /jpodocs/repts_te/13788.html.
9. South Carolina Legislature Online. South Carolina General Assembly 115th Session, 2003-2004. Available at: http://www.scstatehouse. net/sess115_2003-2004/prever/246_20030122.htm.
10. Center for Law and the Public's Health at Georgetown and Johns Hopkins Universities. The Model State Emergency Health Powers Act. Article IV. Section 401. Declaration. Available at: http://www. publichealthlaw.net/MSEHPA/MSEHPA2.pdf.
11. Rosenbaum S, Kamoie B. Finding a way through the hospital door: the role of EMTALA in public health emergencies. *J Law Med Ethics.* 2003;31(4):590-601.
12. Frew S, Aranosian R. Medical-legal concerns of EMS. In: Roush W, ed. *Principles of EMS Systems.* 2nd ed. Dallas: The American College of Emergency Physicians; 1994:351.
13. McIntosh B, Hinds P, Giordano L. The role of EMS systems in public health emergencies. *Prehospital Disaster Med.* 1997;12(1):30-5.
14. Centers for Disease Control and Prevention. Use of quarantine to prevent transmission of SARS—Taiwan 2003. *Morb Mortal Wkly*

Rep. 2003;52(29):680-3. Available at: http://www.cdc.gov/mmwr/ preview/ mmwrhtml/mm5229a2.htm.

15. emtala.com. Emergency Medical Treatment and Labor Act, 42 USC §1395dd, Stat a (Medical screening requirement). Available at: http://www.emtala.com/statute.txt.

16. Roadblock Registry. U.S. Supreme Court. Delaware v Prouse, 440 US 648 (1979). Available at: http://www.roadblock.org/federal/ caseUSprouse.htm.

17. Center for Law and the Public's Health at Georgetown and Johns Hopkins Universities. Model State Emergency Health Powers Act. Article IV. Section 404. Enforcement. Available at: http://www. publichealthlaw.net/MSEHPA/MSEHPA2.pdf.

18. Rotz LD, Dotson DA, Damon IK, Becher JA, Advisory Committee on Immunization Practices. Vaccinia (smallpox) vaccine. Recommendations of the Advisory Committee on Immunization Practices (ACIP), 2001. *Morb Mortal Wkly Rep.* 2001;50(RR-10):1-25. Available at: http://www.cdc.gov/mmwr/preview/mmwrhtml/ rr5010a1.htm.

19. Modlin J. A mass smallpox vaccination campaign: reasonable or irresponsible? *Eff Clin Pract.* 2002;5(2):98-9.

20. Fauci A. Smallpox vaccination policy—The need for dialogue. *New Engl J Med.* 2002;346(17):1319-20.

21. Kemper A, Davis M, Freed G. Expected adverse events in a mass smallpox vaccination campaign. *Eff Clin Pract.* 2002;5(2):84-90.

22. Mack T. A different view of smallpox and vaccination. *New Engl J Med.* 2003;348(5):460-3.

23. Schneider C, McDonald M. "The king of terrors" revisited: the smallpox vaccination campaign and its lessons for future biopreparedness. *J Law Med Ethics.* 2003;31(4):580-9.

24. Meltzer MI, Damon I, LeDuc JW, Millar JD. Modeling potential responses to smallpox as a bioterrorist weapon. *Emerg Infect Dis.* 2001;7(6):959-69.

25. Piotrowski J. Smallpox, big worries. Preparing medical-response teams is easier said than done, according to healthcare providers across the nation. *Mod Healthc.* 2003;33(1):6-7, 12-3, 1.

26. Wharton M, Strikas RA, Harpaz R, et al, Advisory Committee on Immunization Practices, Healthcare Infection Control Practices Advisory Committee. Recommendations for using smallpox vaccine in a pre-event vaccination program: supplemental recommendations of the Advisory Committee on Immunization Practices (ACIP) and the Healthcare Infection Control Practices Advisory Committee (HICPAC). *Morb Mortal Wkly Rep.* 2003;52(RR-7):1-16.

27. Supplemental recommendations on adverse events following smallpox vaccination program: recommendations of the Advisory Committee on Immunization Practices. *Morb Mortal Wkly Rep.* 2003;52(13):282-4.

28. Sepkowitz K. How contagious is vaccinia? *New Engl J Med.* 2003;348(5):439-44.

29. Centers for Disease Control and Prevention. Update: adverse events following civilian smallpox vaccination—United States, 2003. *Morb Mortal Wkly Rep.* 2003;52(34):819-20.

30. Health Resources and Services Administration. Smallpox Emergency Personnel Protection Act of 2003. Available at: ftp://ftp.hrsa.gov/smallpoxinjury/pl10820.pdf.

31. Health Resources and Services Administration. Smallpox Vaccine Injury Compensation Program. Available at: http://www.hrsa.gov/ smallpoxinjury/frn082703.htm.

32. Bozzette SA, Boer R, Bhatnagar V, et al. A model for a smallpox-vaccination policy. *New Engl J Med.* 2003;348(5):416-25.

33. 42 USC chapter 6A, subchapter II, part G, §264. Available at: http://www.cdc.gov/ncidod/dq/42USC264.htm.

34. Fenner F, Henderson DA, Arita I, Jezek Z, Ladnyi ID. Smallpox and its eradication. Available at: http://www.who.int/emc/diseases /smallpox/Smallpoxeradication.html.

35. Kaplan E, Craft D, Wein L. Emergency response to a smallpox attack: the case for mass vaccination. *Proc Natl Acad Sci USA.* 2002;99(16):10935-40.

36. Barbera J, Macintyre A, Gostin L, et al. Large-scale quarantine following biological terrorism in the United States. *JAMA.* 2001;286(21): 2711-17.

37. Epstein J, Cummings DAT, Chakravarty S, Singa RM, Burke DS. Toward a containment strategy for smallpox bioterror: an individual-based computational approach. Center on Social and Economic Dynamics. [Working paper 31.] December 2002. Available at: http://www. brookings.edu/dybdocroot/ es/dynamics/papers/bioterrorism.pdf.

38. Centers for Disease Control and Prevention. Efficiency of quarantine during an epidemic of severe acute respiratory syndrome—Beijing, China, 2003. *Morb Mortal Wkly Rep.* 2003;52(43):1037-40.

39. Centers for Disease Control and Prevention. Use of quarantine to prevent transmission of severe acute respiratory syndrome—Taiwan, 2003. *Morb Mortal Wkly Rep.* 2003;52(29):680-3.

40. Chau P, Yip P. Monitoring the severe acute respiratory syndrome epidemic and assessing effectiveness of interventions in Hong Kong Administrative Region. *J Epidemiol Community Health.* 2003; 57(10):766-9.

41. Gostin LO, Sapsin JW, Teret SP, et al. The Model State Emergency Health Powers Act: planning for and response to bioterrorism and naturally occurring infectious diseases. *JAMA.* 2002;288(5):622-8.

42. The Center for Law and the Public's Health at Georgetown and Johns Hopkins Universities. The Turning Point Model State Public Health Act: State Legislative Table. Available at: http://www. publichealthlaw.net/Resources/ResourcesPDFs/MSPHA%20Legis Track. pdf.

chapter 27

Mutual Aid*

James Geiling and Kerry Fosher

Disaster strikes, and first responders gather their resources, move to the scene, and begin to execute a well-rehearsed response. Personnel, supplies, and equipment meet the requirements of the operation, and once completed, they are refitted and resupplied for the next calamity. But what happens when the disaster evolves slowly over time and distance, involving many organizations across jurisdictional boundaries? Or when, given the just-described scenario of a sudden-impact disaster, local resources become rapidly depleted? Victims of disaster require and, whether in the form of a warm bed or a hot meal, these requirements may exceed the local resources.

Just as an individual who is baking a cake may need a cup of sugar from a neighbor, organizations responding to emergencies occasionally need the assistance of others. Mutual aid is one of the earliest and most organic forms of interagency cooperation and coordination in public safety and health services. Without prearranged mutual aid agreements, events that deplete or exhaust community resources jeopardize the health and safety of not only the victims directly affected by the disaster, but also the rescuers and emergency management personnel themselves.

This chapter introduces a brief history of the federal plan to support disaster response as it applies to working with state and local governments. The chapter also covers the basic concepts of developing mutual aid agreements; organizational leads at the local, state, and federal levels for developing plans; and two common pitfalls that undermine mutual aid plans and operations.

THE MUTUAL AID CONCEPT

Response, Recovery, and Regional Capacity Building

The mutual aid concept in its most basic form is simply the sharing of resources among organizations in times of need. Mutual aid can provide an organization with personnel, equipment, supplies, and pharmaceutical agents in an existing or anticipated emergency. Mutual aid agreements serve to regulate the sharing process, with the identification of what resources can be shared and under what circumstances. Agreements also address potential problems, such as the liability of sharing organizations and responders, reciprocity of credentialing and licensure, the ability of the sharing organization to hold back resources to protect itself, and expectations regarding accounting and reimbursement.

Mutual aid agreements tend to be made between like organizations. Hospitals make them with hospitals, law enforcement agencies with other law enforcement agencies, utility companies with utility companies. Even libraries and museums have mutual aid agreements for coping with disasters.[1,2] However, agreements also are made among jurisdictions, such as state-to-state or county-to-county mutual aid, covering a range of public safety, health, and public works organizations.

When most people think of mutual aid, they picture a cluster of fire trucks or ambulances from different jurisdictions at the scene of a disaster. Mutual aid for dealing with an emergency or a disaster is a very common arrangement, but the concept is not limited to response alone. Mutual aid agreements are often written to include recovery operations as well. These arrangements allow sharing of public works and administrative assets that might not be needed until the crisis has passed. In fact, there is nothing to preclude even pre-event mutual aid in the form of cooperative planning and training agreements, although this is currently rare.

Mutual aid for response and recovery has become part of the decision matrix for planners in many areas of the United States.[3] As the technical base for response equipment and training expands, planners must make decisions about where to place specialized resources for the maximum value to the region. These decisions can be made more resilient through the use or development of mutual aid agreements that address how these regional assets can be shared. Resource placement can then be determined based on the best access to potential users who are partners in the mutual aid agreement.

*The opinions and assertions contained herein are those of the authors and are not to be construed as official or necessarily reflecting the views of the Department of Veterans Affairs or the United States Government.

Conceptual Planning Concerns

The use of mutual aid as a planning tool is very valuable for overall capacity building in a state or region. In times of fiscal constraint, many regions are not able to provide exactly equal resources in every area or in each facility. Good agreements allow planners to consider the capacity of the entire mutual aid network when choosing how to allocate resources for overall preparedness. Of course, this type of planning has always taken place on an informal level. Planners tend to know what other organizations in their area have available to share. However, the use of mutual aid agreements can systematize the process and make it more accountable, minimizing the chances of gaps or misunderstandings. As previously mentioned, most mutual aid agreements address issues of finance, liability, licensing, and the need for organizations to withhold aid based on judgments of their own vulnerability. More sophisticated agreements may also contain annexes of protocols to address common operational interests.

Most conceptual planning concerns are ultimately problems of definition, management, or sustainability. When an organization, such as a hospital, realizes it is overwhelmed, it usually requests mutual aid. However, this means that somebody has to decide what "overwhelmed" means and, hopefully, recognize that operations are approaching capacity in time for mutual aid assets to make a difference. Advance work to define what "almost overwhelmed" might look like in various scenarios goes a long way toward smoothing actual operations. Organizations must also work to "type" their resources, categorizing assets they can share or expect to receive based on the type of emergency. Requests made under mutual aid agreements may be easier to fulfill when requestors ask for a capability rather than a specific organization. Again, advance definition of resources can greatly facilitate the delivery of aid.

Plans to manage mutual aid must include how aid is dispatched, received, managed on-scene, and demobilized. Appropriate dispatch depends on the organization being able to make a considered and coherent request for resources. The receiving organizations must also have protocols for receiving the aid and incorporating it into ongoing operations. Finally, the receiving organization must understand how to demobilize human resources and return or dispose of material ones.

For many types of emergencies and for all disasters, sustainability is a critical element of response and recovery success. Mutual aid often can provide the resource "depth" for an organization or jurisdiction to sustain response until state or national assistance is deployed. Problems can arise if resources are requested too quickly and are exhausted or if they are recalled before they can be useful in extending the duration of response. Some mutual aid planners now want their agreements to include discussions of response sustainability and to provide guidelines to help those on-scene make sound judgments about response timeframes.

Under incident management, it becomes the responsibility of the incident command structure to handle whatever assets arrive through mutual aid. However, incident management is only a system for regularizing the activities of the organization in an emergency or disaster. The system depends on good operational guidelines to ensure that the only unpredictable element in the response is the disaster itself.

Groups such as the National Emergency Management Association and the American Hospital Association[4] have developed model agreements for organizations, localities, and states to use when developing their own mutual aid agreements. A well-known example of this standardization trend is the Emergency Management Assistance Compact (EMAC), a template plan for state-to-state mutual aid.[5] EMAC, described in more detail later in this chapter, is a national mutual aid system for states, but allows some tailoring to meet local needs. Currently, only two states, California and Hawaii, have not adopted the EMAC.

Although each agreement must be tailored to meet organizational and regional needs, the opportunity for standardization has benefits beyond saving keystrokes. In some cases, time and resources saved in creating the agreement can be used for training people to implement it, an element of mutual aid that is sometimes neglected due to other training priorities. Standardization can also help ensure that agreements address operational concerns and are consistent with national plans, such as the National Response Plan[6] and the National Incident Management System.[7]

HISTORICAL PERSPECTIVE

Although discussed in detail elsewhere in this textbook, a brief review of the national disaster response history may provide a perspective on how mutual aid agreements and processes at differing government levels have matured over time. Recent disaster response organization in the United States at the federal level dates to the early 1960s when the newly formed Federal Disaster Assistance Administration of the Department of Housing and Urban Development managed several massive disasters. For example, after the Alaska earthquake of 1964 in which needs far exceeded available local resources, many questions arose as to the federal government's capability to appropriately respond. Review of this disaster and others in subsequent years led to the establishment of a process for presidential disaster declarations through passage of the Disaster Relief Act in 1974. This act provided the legal processes under which state governors could formally request federal assistance after disasters for support that exceeded the state's response capabilities.[8] It was, in essence, the first state-federal government, disaster-specific mutual aid agreement.

However, disaster response at the federal level remained fragmented. More than 100 federal agencies could be called on to respond to disasters ranging from natural events to accidents involving the transportation of hazardous materials.[9] In 1979, President Carter issued Executive Order 12127, which merged many disaster-related responsibilities into the Federal Emergency Management Agency (FEMA).[10] By 1989, with the fall of the Berlin Wall and the decline in the global threat of nuclear warfare, FEMA was funded and empowered to focus its efforts on non-nuclear disaster response as well. The current basis for federal disaster response stems from the Robert T. Stafford Disaster Relief and Emergency Assistance Act (most commonly known as the "Stafford Act"). This law gives the federal government operational guidelines and funding to execute disaster response.[11]

CURRENT PRACTICE

This section describes many local, state, and federal assets or policies that can be used when an organization sets out to develop a mutual aid plan. The activity level and effectiveness of organizations and policies vary, and although each possibility described in this section may not have all the answers, each provides a place to start and is part of the overall context of mutual aid.

Local Community Assets

All disasters begin as local events. Community-level first responders typically serve on the front lines for disaster response, often placing their own personal safety in jeopardy in the process. Some disasters, such as biological terrorist events, may develop slowly over time and great distances, yet the first case is often identified by a local healthcare worker or rescuer who notes an unusual incident, such as the physician who diagnosed the incident case of anthrax in 2001.[12]

Disaster or emergency planning in communities has historically been developed by fire departments, in part as a result of their personnel's ongoing training and experience in managing day-to-day emergencies. Town managers or mayors have overall responsibility; however, fire departments have typically served as both planner and operator. Law enforcement agencies also play a major role in developing the overall response plan. Close integration of these two departments remains critical to the successful planning and execution of emergency and disaster response plans, the goal of which is public safety for the community's residents. These departments develop mutual aid relationships with other towns or localities to provide support for events that exceed their departments' capabilities. Other agencies have been less involved in such preparation.

Local Emergency Planning Committees

Although since 1986, communities, by law, have had to develop a Local Emergency Planning Committee (LEPC), the events of Sept. 11, 2001, dramatically increased the emphasis placed on these organizations to expand their disaster planning process. Planning now must occur not only across some jurisdictional boundaries, but it also must entail other entities beyond industry, fire, and law-enforcement personnel. Specifically, the federal government in 1986 mandated the formation of State Emergency Response Commissions (SERCs); these SERCs were tasked to develop emergency planning districts to ". . . facilitate preparation and implementation of emergency plans."[13] Within these districts, the state is to ". . . appoint members of a local emergency planning committee for each emergency planning district. Each committee shall include, at a minimum, representatives from each of the following groups or organizations: elected State and local officials; law enforcement, civil defense, firefighting, first aid, health, local environmental, hospital, and transportation personnel; broadcast and print media; community groups; and owners and operators of facilities subject to the requirements of this subchapter."[13] In areas where an LEPC is active, it can serve as the focal point in the community for information and discussions regarding all aspects of emergency planning as well as health and environmental risks.

US Citizen Corps

The federal government created the USA Freedom Corps after Sept. 11, 2001, in an effort to provide opportunities for citizens to serve their community and foster a culture of service, citizenship, and responsibility. Although federally managed, components of the US Citizens Corps, an arm of USA Freedom Corps, are designed to be staffed by local volunteers and serve in local events. The Community Emergency Response Team (CERT) program helps train individual volunteers to be better prepared to assist their community, serving as support to first responders, directly assisting victims, and organizing volunteers who arrive on-scene. They also can assist in projects designed to enhance public safety.[14]

The other major component of the US Citizen Corps available for assistance at the local level is healthcare personnel who serve as part of the Medical Reserve Corps (MRC). "The MRC program coordinates the skills of practicing and retired physicians, nurses and other health professionals as well as other citizens interested in health issues, who are eager to volunteer to address their community's ongoing public health needs and to help their community during large-scale emergency situations."[15] The Office of the Surgeon General within the U.S. Department of Health and Human Services oversees the program, but its components, tasks, activation, utilization, etc. are governed locally and through state Citizen Corps Councils. Local community leaders develop MRCs and outline their roles and responsibilities in disaster response. MRCs may also play a role in day-to-day public health and safety campaigns or other volunteer efforts. Finally, they may cooperate with the local Metropolitan Medical Response System (MMRS) and assist with local disaster medical assistance teams.

Metropolitan Medical Response System

Many areas around the country now have MMRS projects. This national program started in 1996 under the U.S. Department of Health and Human Services, but it has shifted to the Department of Homeland Security under FEMA's oversight. Each MMRS contract is awarded to a region that agrees to complete a series of steps toward regionalizing its medical response capacity and preparedness. The main thrust of the program is to develop robust regional systems that coordinate existing plans and resources and assist agencies in planning, training, and exercising together. Initially developed to regionalize response around major cities, MMRS projects now exist in broader regions. The most recent MMRS project, started in 2003, covers three northern New England states. (More information is available at: http://www. nnemmrs.org.)

Like the LEPCs, MMRS projects have a mandate to include people from a wide variety of disciplines in a coordinated planning effort. As a result, they make an excellent starting point for finding pre-existing knowledge of resources and cooperative agreements that helps make new mutual aid agreements strong.

Other Government Agencies

A variety of other government organizations may play a prominent role in local disaster response. Search and rescue organizations may come from state Fish and Game agencies, private organizations, Civil Air Patrol, and others, although federal agencies, local military, Veterans Affairs, federal law enforcement agencies, etc. may serve as first responders for some communities and hence need to clearly predetermine their roles, responsibilities, and command relationships during disaster planning.

Voluntary Organizations and Volunteers

The American Red Cross (ARC) plays an active role in the health and safety in most communities, and although it is not a government entity, it has a federal mandate to assist in disasters.[16] It is a lead primary agency for Emergency Support Function #6 (Mass Care) in the National Response Plan. Staffed by both professionals and volunteers, ARC's disaster relief is designed to meet the immediate, disaster-related needs of victims as well as emergency workers. It provides shelter, food, and health and mental health services to address basic human needs during the event and later provides services to help disaster victims and emergency workers return to some form of normalcy. Its special shelters could also be called on to assist in the care and management of hospitalized patients who are discharged because of low acuity or evacuated because of disruption of the hospital facility. The ARC normally provides care to all victims who arrive at one of its shelter for support, but pre-event mutual aid agreements and discussions can help coordinate disaster health services within a given community.[17]

Other relief agencies appear at disasters and play a role in supporting both victims and rescue workers. At the Pentagon disaster on Sept. 11, 2001, the first agency to arrive was the Salvation Army (J. Geiling, personal observation). The Salvation Army is a Christian-based international organization whose mission includes ". . . To provide support, training and resources to respond to the needs of those affected by emergencies without discrimination."[18] Additional religious or other cause-related organizations serve, in part, to assist their community in times of need.

Individual volunteers also tend to flock to disaster scenes, in part to assist with the rescue effort. This "convergent volunteerism" can be defined as ". . . The arrival of unexpected or uninvited personnel wishing to render aid at the scene of a large-scale emergency incident [and

who often] engage in freelancing, [that is,] operating at an emergency incident without knowledge of or direction by the on-scene command authority."[19] These volunteers are not limited to medical personnel, but also can include fire and law enforcement representatives and others. They migrate to the scene, in part as a result of misinformed requests for help often by well-intended media reporters, politicians, or professionals from their specific organizations.

Challenges facing these volunteers and those tasked to oversee the response effort include volunteer safety; interference with the operations; security, especially at a crime scene; and qualifications as responders. These "credentials" may be typical medical skills and licensures of healthcare providers who arrive on-scene, but they apply to others who appear as well. For example, incident managers often need to deal with firefighters who self-dispatch to a scene—they may be helpful with their specific skill sets but are unproven, unknown, and may pose safety hazards on-scene. Hence, some have posed the establishment of a national system of fire service credentialing.[20] Finally, for large-scale disasters, sustained operations will require the expertise of professionals working later shifts in their normal place of employment; organizations' effectiveness will be depleted if their personnel report to the disaster scene as unsolicited volunteers.[19]

Volunteers will likely continue to converge on disasters because of two reasons: (1) volunteers, especially first responders, are genuinely altruistic and want to help, and (2) they often are unsure as to the exact need, so assuming any help is better than none, they migrate to the scene. People who are used to going to disasters will likely continue in their quest to provide aid. However, rapidly obtaining a needs assessment and disseminating such information may prevent unnecessary aid; this communication depends on a functioning, well-tested, interorganizational mutual aid two-way radio system. Key responders to area disasters should proactively determine such roles and responsibilities, especially in scenarios that typically involve multiple organizations or jurisdictions.

Convergence behavior is often not limited to the movement of personnel. Unnecessary donations of equipment, clothing, and medical supplies (including blood products that require significant logistical and administrative support) can also appear at a disaster scene. Managing this collection can, unfortunately, use critical assets needed to manage the disaster itself.[21]

Local Emergency Management Plans and Mutual Aid

A review of the agencies and personnel available as well as thought given to who else may show up at a disaster are important aspects of the planning or mitigation phases of disaster response. Formalizing this information into a plan and developing mutual aid agreements optimize the chances for successful disaster relief operations. Developing a plan at the local level can be a daunting job for the individual(s) tasked (or who volunteer) to complete it. The National Response Plan outlines the basic components for a plan, but often state governments provide their towns with a template. For example, the state of Vermont's "Model Town Emergency Operations Plan" guides communities through purpose statements, hazard vulnerability analysis, operations, support resources, exercise and training, and other components needed to complete a town plan. Details on specific emergency support functions can be found in its 13 annexes.[22]

Other locations, typically large cities, may present more complicated situations—multiple agencies from a variety of jurisdictions and levels of government not only interact for daily operations, but also for emergencies and disasters. The metropolitan Washington, D.C., area has established a 17-member Council of Governments (COG) to help in a coordination effort for the region. Collectively, with input from the state of Maryland, the Commonwealth of Virginia, the federal government, public agencies, the private sector, volunteer organizations, and local schools and universities, the COG has established a Regional Emergency Coordination Plan (RECP) to provide a vehicle for collaboration in planning, communication, information sharing, and coordination activities before, during, or after a regional emergency.[23] The plan describes the purpose and scope, as well as the roles, responsibilities, communication, and coordination relationships among member organizations. In a manner similar to the Vermont plan, the RECP delineates its emergency support functions into 15 areas, or regional emergency support functions (R-ESFs), which "identify organizations with resources and capabilities that align with a particular type of assistance or requirement frequently needed in a large-scale emergency or disaster."[23] The 15 R-ESFs are transportation; communications infrastructure; public works and engineering; firefighting; information and planning; mass care; resource support; health, mental health, and medical services; urban search and rescue; hazardous materials; food; energy; law enforcement; media relations and community outreach; and donations and volunteer management.

These regulatory structures and component organizations all desire to serve the public in time of need. However, the political, economic, and structural viability of each one and its individual members depends to a large extent on prearranged relationships and mutual aid agreements that are designed to provide emergency assistance to each other in the event of an emergency or disaster. The conditions of these arrangements may be to provide reciprocal services or to receive direct financial reimbursement for labor, supplies, or equipment. Ideally the arrangements are codified in writing before an event, although they may be based on unwritten mutual understanding and may even occur after an event has taken place. FEMA's Mutual Aid Agreements for Public Assistance (Recovery Division Policy Number 9523.6) specifies criteria by which FEMA recognizes the eligibility for reimbursement of costs under the Public Assistance Program incurred by such mutual aid agreements.[24]

Well-developed mutual aid arrangements, particularly in major metropolitan areas, such as that previously outlined for the Washington, D.C. area, make reimbursement for services more likely. For example, the Washington, D.C. area COG received recognition and congressional support in December 2004 for its National Capital Region Mutual Aid Act, which it then adopted in April 2005.[25]

First responders outside of regions with developed mutual aid agreements, such as in very remote areas, must also consider how they will share their resources. Often their assets are very limited in scope and are charged to cover large areas. Funding for such enterprise has been limited in the past. However, the federal government's 2003 budget earmarked $140 million to assist rural communities with planning and establishing mutual aid agreements.[26]

Finally, even though well-defined, codified mutual aid agreements serve all parties who participate in disaster response, it is the *process* by which disaster planning and mutual aid arrangements develop that is most crucial to a successful disaster response. It is through the planning process that relationships among emergency response organizations, both inside and outside of the planners' jurisdiction, develop. Exchanging business cards, rehearsing plans through exercise drills, refining communications plans, and other activities during disaster preparedness all foster a sense of trust among the participating organizations, thereby improving overall interorganizational and intraorganizational communications in a disaster.[27]

Hospitals

Hospital disaster preparation and incident planning have had a dramatic surge in importance since Sept. 11, 2001. Legislation delegating hospitals as first responders also makes them eligible for funding to support the planning process, an often-quoted impediment to their preparation.[28] Individual hospital preparation and response to an incident have been reviewed in detail elsewhere.[29] However, outside organizations and agencies continue to expand their expectations for hospitals to be adequately prepared. Unfortunately, though, hospitals often tend to conduct their disaster preparations and training in isolation, which impairs their ability to interact with these groups when disaster strikes.

As previously outlined, LEPC guidelines recommend that local hospitals participate in the community's emergency preparation. In addition to routine agreements on patient receiving and treatment, these preparations now call for expensive and underfunded capabilities such as planning for the reception of contaminated chemical casualties. Hospitals' primary credentialing oversight comes from the Joint Commission on Accreditation of Healthcare Organizations (JCAHO). This body also mandates a variety of emergency preparations that, again, require additional expensive preparations. If hospitals do not receive adequate financial support and therefore are not prepared, victims of mass casualty incidents may end up riding "ambulances to nowhere."[30]

JCAHO, however, continues to refine its requirements. The bulk of JCAHO's requirements for emergency preparedness lie in its Environment of Care (EC) section. Elements of performance for EC 4.10 require hospitals to establish with the community a hazard vulnerability analysis, the hospital's role relative to the community's emergency management plan, and an "all-hazards" command structure that easily melds with the community's command structure. Exercises that test the plan must be conducted twice each year, one of which must include participation in a community-wide exercise (EC 4.20).[31]

Hospitals affected by disasters often become inundated with victims seeking care, who in reality need minimal medical attention. Additionally, individuals who may simply need observation during the latency period of a potential biological hazard may overwhelm a hospital's requirements to treat the more seriously ill or injured. To prevent this increased burden, hospitals should explore mutual aid agreements with special shelters, such as those managed by the ARC or other volunteer organizations, as previously discussed. Additionally, urgent care centers, individual physician or healthcare worker clinics, mental health clinics, surgicenters, nursing homes, etc. may all be additional locations to provide care for low-acuity cases. These facilities and others may also help individuals seeking care who really only need shelter. In combination, hospitals may be able to work with these organizations to accommodate much-needed surge capacity, a topic covered in detail elsewhere in this textbook.

There are other models that communities can use to develop scalable triage, treatment, and dispensing facilities external to normal care centers. One such example, developed by a team of military and civilian specialists, is the *Modular Emergency Medical System*.[32,33] Along with general planning guidance for mass casualty incidents, this series of publications includes detailed plans for two types of centers that can be quickly set up to help relieve the burden on hospitals. The Neighborhood Emergency Help Center concept is designed to manage asymptomatic and noncritical patients, providing limited care and treatment.[34] The Acute Care Center (ACC) concept provides a means of caring for those who need inpatient treatment but do not require advanced life support or intensive care.[35] These models can be tailored to area needs and resources and provide a realistic way for communities to manage mass care incidents. In fact, the ACC concept is recommended in the current Health Resources and Services Administration (HRSA) grant guidance.[36] Finally, the U.S. Department of Health and Human Services is developing a series of Federal Medical Contingency Stations to use to support surge capability needs of local healthcare facilities.[37] Each of these center concepts was designed to encourage communities to make use of existing facilities to house the centers and requires advance effort to develop memoranda of understanding with facility owners and mutual aid agreements to ensure that the center can be set up, staffed, and demobilized without depleting hospital resources.

Volunteers present a significant challenge to those planning for and managing a response. As previously discussed, well-intending volunteers tend to converge at a disaster to provide their assistance. This sense of duty also applies to healthcare providers who arrive at an overwhelmed or damaged hospital to assist in needed patient care activities. During disaster planning, the facility needs to decide whether volunteers will be used or in what roles they will be used; if nurse or physician volunteers will be used; and if so, how will the credentials of volunteers be verified.[38] The American College of Emergency Physicians recommends that all hospitals have a detailed process in place to allow for the emergency privileging of additional physician staff who arrive at a facility to support response efforts to a declared hospital disaster. So-called "disaster credentialing" should ideally be completed before an event and mirror the credentials of the providers at their "home hospitals." In the event of a disaster, immediate credentials can then be granted with proper identification. Hospitals providing these disaster credentials must also be prepared to provide professional liability coverage for physicians who provide care during a disaster in their institution and be prepared to address issues of compensation for injured workers.[39,40] The provision of disaster credentials must follow the medical staff guidelines outlined by JCAHO under Medical Staff (MS) 4.220. The elements of performance for this standard include identifying the individual(s) responsible for granting such privileges, a mechanism to manage those with these credentials, and the development of a priority pathway to verify credentials as soon as practical after an event.[31]

Identification and credentialing are topics that can be included in mutual aid agreements to the benefit of the entire community or state. As responders and volunteers appear on-scene, it is critical that security personnel are able to determine who is allowed to work and in what capacities, often without the benefit of a sophisticated understanding of licensure and credentialing. Coordinated standards for identification can increase the speed and accuracy of this process. Some national initiatives are under way, such as the fire service credentialing proposal previously described. Another initiative is HRSA's funding for the Emergency System for the Advance Registration of Volunteer Health Professionals (ESAR-VHP) program, which is an attempt to provide standardized credentialing and identification protocols. (The basis for the ESAR-VHP initiative is U.S. Public Law 107-188, the Public Health Security and Bioterrorism Preparedness and Response Act of 2002 [section 107, Emergency system for advance registration of health professions volunteers]). (PL 107-188 is available at: http://thomas.loc.gov/.) The 2005 HRSA guidelines require awardees to develop ESAR-VHP activities in their regions. The most recent ESAR-VHP guidelines were released in June 2005. However, healthcare facilities should seek out local initiatives and actively participate to ensure that their needs are addressed and that they are aware of the systems that are developed in their communities.

Like other community-based organizations, hospitals must share resources and plans with other entities in the community. Mutual aid agreements or memoranda of understanding formalize and delineate each other's roles and responsibilities. Agreements need to include not only representatives from public safety and community industry, but also those from other nearby healthcare facilities. Developing a detailed, yet functional, mutual aid agreement between medical facilities can be a challenging task. Much coordination, inspection, discussion, legal review, etc. must occur before most signatories will agree to such arrangements.

Fortunately, several templates exist to aid the process.[41-44] These models include information such as the purpose of the memorandum of understanding, timing and method of communicating requests, documentation standards, guidance on patient transport, hospital supervision, financial and legal liabilities, and notification of next of kin and the patient's physician. It is also important that these topics be discussed not only in general principles of medical operations, but also as they apply to the evacuation of patients and the transfer of personnel, pharmaceuticals, supplies, or equipment.

Command Structure

When disaster strikes a community, local, community-level assets typically respond first. The majority of organizations in the first responder community attempt to establish command and control of the scene using principles of the Incident Command System (ICS). Discussed in detail elsewhere in this textbook, ICS establishes a proven organizational template that can be expanded or contracted in a modular fashion to meet the demands of the event. The emergency medical services (EMS) branch of the operations section is supposed to manage medical support to the operation. Under the National Incident Management System (NIMS), which is discussed in detail elsewhere in this textbook, a medical unit is also established under the logistics section to provide medical support to the emergency responders themselves.[7] If the incident is primarily a mass casualty event involving essentially all medical assets, then the operations section chief, or even the incident commander, may be from the health sector.[45]

This organizational paradigm is often not followed by hospitals in their response to either an internal or external disaster; they tend to rely on their own organizational structure that has evolved to support their day-to-day operations. However, when disaster strikes, hospitals need to move toward an emergency management structure to ensure institutional and personnel safety and security, optimize patient care, and efficiently use scarce resources. As previously mentioned, JCAHO mandates an emergency management system that easily integrates into that of the community.

The Hospital Emergency Incident Command System (HEICS) is fast becoming the standard for healthcare systems' disaster response. The organization of HEICS mirrors that of ICS, with five functional areas: command, operations, planning, logistics, and finance and administration. Job action sheets provide checklist tools for providers in each position to prioritize and categorize their efforts into immediate, intermediate, and extended tasks. HEICS is not a turnkey system; rather it is a process that must be adapted to each event and is supported by specific emergency management policies and procedures.[46] The HEICS structure focuses on management of internal disasters. As previously discussed, coordination with external agencies becomes necessary for the facility to effectively integrate itself into any community disaster response. HEICS can begin to facilitate that process by ensuring that outside groups and leaders that follow ICS principles can (ideally) find their hospital-based counterpart in the ICS structure to better coordinate the disaster response.

State and federal assets that arrive on-scene will similarly fall in line with their own form of an ICS; any interorganizational variations will likely change to adhere to new guidelines published in NIMS.[7] A major event may result in the establishment of multiple incident command posts (ICPs) and agency Emergency Operations Centers (EOCs). To manage the entire event, representative agencies may meet to form a Joint Operations Center (JOC), usually off-site to effectively provide a strategic, unified command (J. Geiling, personal observation).

Healthcare workers often believe that daily emergency care and practice suffice in the translation to disaster preparedness. Although medical and administrative skills normally work in common emergencies, they do not adequately prepare the individual healthcare worker or institution for the chaos of a disaster. For example, disasters often require the completion of tasks that do not normally occur in routine emergencies, such as scene security, search and rescue operations, patient movement and evacuation activities, media operations, and overwhelming requests for information. Failure to understand the organizational milieu of a disaster setting risks putting various types of providers into settings where independently they seek to do good but collectively they endanger themselves, their patients, and the scarce resources on hand.[47] Hence, an understanding of disaster organization becomes imperative for a safe and effective individual and organizational response. This understanding is also essential for the effective requesting and management of mutual aid assets.

State Assets

As previously discussed, most disasters begin as local events and are managed with local, community-level assets. State and federal agencies located in the vicinity may also serve as first responders without full escalation of the response outside of the community. When community resources become overwhelmed or other characteristics of the disaster mandate state or federal involvement (such as in multijurisdictional fire response or events related to terrorism), individual state emergency management organizations respond.

National Guard

Many state assets can be called on to support a state-managed disaster response. Integrating them into the state emergency management plan naturally requires detailed planning. One organization that is often overlooked, in part because of its perceived complexity, is the National Guard. At the disposal of the governor, National Guard units serve the public interest in their state in time of disaster, unless they are called on for federal service. Recently, the National Guard Bureau formed new units, called Civil Support Teams, Weapons of Mass Destruction (CST (WMD)). These teams, under the operational control of the adjutant general and ultimately the governor of each state, are designed to mobilize within 2 hours to augment local and regional terrorism response, principally for events known or suspected to involve weapons of mass destruction, including nuclear, chemical, or biological agents. When deployed to an event, these teams report to the incident commander and provide assessment capabilities, advice, and assistance to the response effort. In essence, they supplement other fire and hazardous materials teams that may be on location, serving as a bridge until other state or federal assets arrive.[48]

State Emergency Response Commission

Each state develops its own disaster organizational system. However, the same legislation that mandated the establishment of LEPCs previously described, also directed the establishment of SERCs.[13] Appointed by each governor, "... SERCs [normally] have been formed from existing organizations such as state environmental, emergency management, transportation, or public health agencies. In others, they are new organizations with representatives from public agencies and departments, along with private groups and associations."[49] SERC duties include the establishment of local emergency planning districts and LEPCs within each district, coordination and supervision of LEPC activities, oversight of proposals for and distribution of training funds, and annually reviewing local emergency plans.

Emergency Management Assistance Compact

Disasters that cross state boundaries may be managed at the state level, without necessarily invoking the need for a federal response, under the auspices of the Emergency Management Assistance Compact (EMAC). Legislated in 1996 as Public Law 104-321, EMAC is a mutual aid agreement and partnership between states that exists because of the common threat from a variety of disasters; it is a legal mechanism and not an organization. Out-of-state aid organized through EMAC helps ease the movement of personnel and equipment across state borders. Requests for EMAC assistance are legally binding contracts, obligating the requesting state to reimburse all out-of-state costs and liability complaints for out-of-state personnel. Finally, EMAC permits states to both ask for assistance and to provide available resources with a minimal amount of "bureaucratic wrangling."[50]

Model Intrastate Mutual Aid Legislation

Produced by the National Emergency Management Association, in concert with the Department of Homeland Security, FEMA, and other emergency responders, the Model Intrastate Mutual Aid Legislation provides a robust template to expand on the mutual aid agreement legislated under EMAC. A multidisciplinary group of subject matter experts gathered in January 2004 to review a variety of mutual aid agreements, from all levels of government, and on thorough review and evaluation of "best practices" developed this template. Covering 11 basic articles, "... The model is meant to be a tool and resource for states and jurisdictions to utilize in developing or refining statewide mutual aid agreements. It is anticipated that states and jurisdictions may wish to modify the model to conform to their own state

laws and authorities, or to address unique needs and circumstances. Further, the proposed articles and provisions in the model are complementary to the recommended minimum elements to be included in mutual aid agreements that are a part of the draft National Incident Management System Plan."[51]

Federal Assets

Once a the disaster response exceeds the capabilities of local, state, or inter-state capabilities or the disaster results from a recognized act of terrorism, federal resources mobilize to assist the community. A large number of diverse organizations with many differing capabilities can be called on to assist; many of these are discussed in detail elsewhere in this textbook. In larger metropolitan areas, but also in local areas adjacent to federal facilities, these assets may appear immediately on-scene, serving in a first responder capacity. However, outside of this example, federal assets mobilize in a specified manner, according to federal policy.

The governing document for the federal response is the National Response Plan (NRP). As previously noted, this plan serves as the basis for tailoring the federal response to the needs of the disaster. Under the guidance of FEMA, now assigned to DHS, lead agencies and supporting agencies for the 15 Emergency Support Functions (ESFs) provide a robust response capability.[6]

The NRP has entirely replaced the Federal Response Plan. "National" is an intended change to the name of the plan, emphasizing the federal government's ability to tailor its response, across the spectrum of government, to assist local officials and agencies.[52]

The Disaster Declaration Process and Federal Disaster Assistance

When disaster strikes, individual communities, states, and other organizations cooperating through mutual aid agreements respond to assist the afflicted area and its victims. As noted, some federal assets may be on hand, and depending on the scenario (for example, a terrorist event), others may preemptively deploy to the scene. Outside of these settings, the federal disaster declaration process to request federal assistance follows the guidelines outlined in the 1988 Robert T. Stafford Disaster Relief and Emergency Assistance Act. This Stafford Act requires that "all requests for declaration by the President that a major disaster exists shall be made by the Governor of the affected State."[53]

The governor's request is processed through the regional FEMA office. The first step is a preliminary damage assessment (PDA) conducted by state and federal officials. This assessment, in concert with the governor's request, must demonstrate a need beyond the capabilities of the local and state governments. The PDA normally precedes the governor's request, though it may follow for obviously catastrophic events. Pending the approval of federal assets, the governor must initiate the state's emergency plan, documenting the resources used for the state's response. Also required is an impact estimate, which is a projection of the financial cost to the public and private sectors. Finally, the governor must provide a needs assessment on the assistance required. Based on this information and with the governor's appeal, the president decides on the validity of the request; declaration of the event as a federal disaster activates a broad scope of federal programs and services to assist in the response, rescue, and recovery operations.[53]

National Mutual Aid and Resource Management Initiative

As higher levels of government respond, the greater the capabilities, but also the complexities of the response. Pre-established mutual aid agreements and packages of response capability may enhance the timeliness of the entire response effort. An effort to streamline the process of developing mutual aid agreements and managing resources, the National Mutual Aid and Resource Management Initiative, is being spearheaded by FEMA in concert with the National Emergency Management Association. Through this initiative, FEMA hopes to provide for an efficient and effective all-hazards disaster response.

Once implemented, the system should enhance readiness and response, at all governmental levels, by allowing emergency management personnel to identify, locate, request, order, and track outside resources quickly. Key concepts of this program include use of preincident mutual aid agreements; protocols for the documentation and inventory of disaster response resources; a national deployable inventory of preidentified, credentialed, categorized, and capability-typed resources; and an automated resource management system to track all disaster resource requests.[54] Finally, to help ease the burden on emergency managers in deciding the resources required for the disaster, this initiative seeks to type, or group, federal, state, and local assets into eight disciplines. These groupings will help ensure that the needed support capability reaches the requestor at the disaster.

OPERATIONAL PITFALLS

This section describes two of the most common pitfalls that can undermine even the best mutual aid plan or response operation.

Two-Hat Syndrome

Although the organizational construct for disaster response introduced here, and detailed elsewhere in this textbook, is designed to ensure a thorough, robust, and responsive disaster response capability, vulnerabilities jeopardize response effectiveness. Many weaknesses have been described and experienced by emergency management personnel. However, no disaster response can be affected without experienced, healthy, and available responders.

As government budgets become strained with daily needs and now the additional demands of homeland security, available personnel assets become less available. To help continue with necessary services, many agencies require individuals to perform a "dual-hat" mission, carrying the burden of two positions. People, who are asked, required, or who volunteer for such duties may jeopardize response efforts in the event of a disaster. This "two-hat syndrome" also often extends beyond the public sector. For example, asking part-time or off-duty persons to assist in relief efforts means they may not be available for other needed services that they normally perform. Agencies that have mutual aid arrangements may, in fact, be sharing personnel. These challenges are magnified during military activation of Guard or Reserve forces—many of these personnel also work in other public sector jobs. Surveys have determined that of all of the public service sectors, fire and rescue operations, private ambulances, and emergency management services suffer the most from this "syndrome."[55] Clearly this issue complicates disaster response and necessitates consideration during predisaster planning and training.

Complicated Wire Diagram—Who's in Charge?

Finally, the detailed emergency response capabilities described in this textbook all may eventually meet "on the battlefield" at the disaster scene. Defined command and control relationships, policy guidelines, regulatory edicts, mutual aid agreements, memoranda of understanding, or simple "gentlemen's agreements" outline the ideal mechanism for all parties to execute a disaster response. However, when disasters occur, the agencies that arrive to assist often come from different locations with differing and, oftentimes, competing ideas on management of the disaster. Mutual aid and working arrangements, even if prearranged rather than being developed on scene, often have not been rehearsed. Consequently, individuals who respond to a disaster need to have both the flexibility and the authority granted by their parent organizations to improvise on-scene. This "planned improvisation" should be both expected and, ideally, rehearsed during disaster planning.[56]

Additionally, the decision makers who arrive on-scene tend to come from lower levels in their organizations' hierarchy. They often fail to understand their organization's participatory role in the overall disaster response, focusing instead on their more familiar intraorganizational policies and procedures. In disaster parlance this is known as the "'Robinson Crusoe Syndrome' (i.e. 'we're the only ones on the island'). This narrow focus on one's organizational goals has been observed not only in disaster response, but in planning as well."[57] This dilemma also highlights the importance of training that focuses on interagency or interorganizational response, which unfortunately does not occur very often.

SUMMARY

Mutual aid arrangements among agencies likely to operate in a disaster clearly enhance the probability of success, giving robust and redundant response capabilities. The key to the success of the effort lies in the people—their availability, physical stamina, understanding of the disaster response milieu, and pre-event training. Only through rehearsal will the nuances of these arrangements and capabilities be delineated and repaired to meet the needs of the victims who depend on the responders and their plan.

REFERENCES

1. Inland Empire Libraries Disaster Response Network. Available at: http://www.ieldrn.org/mutual.htm.
2. Lower Hudson Conference of Historical Agencies and Museums. Available at: http://lowerhudsonconference.org/empart/Planning/Page10564/page105644.html.
3. National Emergency Management Association. If disaster strikes today, are you ready to lead? A governor's primer on all-hazards emergency management. Available at: http://www.nemaweb.org/docs/Gov_Primer.pdf.
4. American Hospital Association. Model Hospital Mutual Aid Memorandum of Understanding. Available at: http://www.aha.org/aha/key_issues/disaster_readiness/resources/content/ModelHospitalMou.doc.
5. Emergency Management Assistance Compact. Available at: http://www.emacweb.org/.
6. U.S. Department of Homeland Security. National Response Plan. Available at: http://www.ccep.ca/responseplan.pdf.
7. U.S. Department of Homeland Security. National Incident Management System. Available at: http://www.fema.gov/nims/.
8. Federal Emergency Management Agency. Robert T. Stafford Disaster Relief and Emergency Assistance Act, as amended by Public Law 106-390, October 30, 2000. Available at: http://www.fema.gov/ library/stafact.shtm.
9. Federal Emergency Management Agency. FEMA history. Available at: http://www.fema.gov/about/history.shtm.
10. Federal Emergency Management Agency. Executive Order 12127: Federal Emergency Management Agency. Available at: http://www.fema.gov/library/eo12127.shtm.
11. Roth PB, Gaffney JK. The federal response plan and disaster medical assistance teams in domestic disasters. *Emerg Med Clin North Am.* 1996;14(2):371-82.
12. Bush LM, Abrams BH, Beal A, Johnson CC. Index case of fatal inhalational anthrax due to bioterrorism in the United States. *New Engl J Med.* 2001;345(22):1607-10.
13. 42 USC chapter 116, subchapter I, section 11001. Available at: http://www4.law.cornell.edu/uscode/42/11001.html.
14. U.S. Citizen Corps. Community Emergency Response Team (CERT). Available at: http://www.citizencorps.gov/programs/.
15. U.S. Citizen Corps. Medical Reserve Corps (MRC) program. Available at: http://www.citizencorps.gov/programs/.
16. American Red Cross. Disaster services. Available at: http://www.redcross.org/services/disaster/0,1082,0_319_,00.html.
17. American Red Cross. Frequently asked questions. What health services does the American Red Cross provide during a disaster? Isn't this the government's responsibility? Available at: http://www.redcross.org/faq/0,1095,0_378_,00.html.
18. Salvation Army. Relief work. Available at: http://www1.salvationarmy.org/ihq/www_sa.nsf/vw-search/E5C6EB09E25BC2A080256D4B004CEF40?opendocument.
19. Cone DC, Weir SD, Bogucki S. Convergent volunteerism. *Ann Emerg Med.* 2003;41(4):457-62.
20. Fire Chief. National credentials? Available at: http://www.firechief.com/preparedness/firefighting_national_credentials/.
21. Auf der Heide E. Convergence behavior in disasters. *Ann Emerg Med.* 2003;41(4):463-6.
22. State of Vermont, Department of Public Safety. Model Town Emergency Operations Plan. Available at: http://170.222.24.9/vem/ MODEL.doc.
23. Metropolitan Washington Council of Governments. Regional Emergency Coordination Plan (RECP). Available at: http://www.mwcog.org/security/security/plan.asp.
24. Federal Emergency Management Agency. Public Assistance: 9523.6 Mutual Aid Agreements for Public Assistance. Available at: http://www.fema.gov/rrr/pa/9523_6.shtm.
25. Metropolitan Washington Council of Governments. Resolution requesting congressional support for national capital region mutual aid. Available at: http://www.mwcog.org/uploads/committee-documents/v15ZXVg20040416070148.pdf.
26. US Department of Homeland Security. Mutual aid agreements: support for first responders outside major metropolitan areas. Available at: http://www.dhs.gov/dhspublic/display?theme=63&content=233&print=true.
27. Auf der Heide E. Inter-agency communications. In: *Disaster Response: Principles of Preparedness and Coordination.* Available at: http://orgmail2.coe-dmha.org/dr/index.htm.
28. White House. Homeland Security Presidential Directive/HSPD-8. Available at: http://www.whitehouse.gov/news/releases/2003/12/print/20031217-6.html.
29. Geiling JA. Hospital preparation and response to an incident. In: Roy M, ed. *Physician's Guide to Terrorist Attack.* Totowa, NJ: Humana Press, Inc; 2004:21-38.
30. Barbera JA, Macintyre AG, DeAtely CA. *Ambulances to Nowhere: America's Critical Shortfall in Medical Preparedness for Catastrophic Terrorism.* Cambridge, MA: John F. Kennedy School of Government, Harvard University; October 2001. BCSIA Discussion Paper 2001-15, ESDP Discussion Paper ESDP-2001-07.
31. Joint Commission on Accreditation of Hospital Organizations. *Comprehensive Accreditation Manual for Hospitals: The Official Handbook (CAMH).* Update 2, May 2005. Oakbrook Terrace, IL: Joint Commission on Accreditation of Hospital Organizations; 2004.
32. U.S. Army Soldier and Biological Chemical Command. Improving local and state agency response to terrorist incidents involving biological weapons. 2003. Available at: http://www.nnemmrs.org/surge.html (Community Planning Guide).
33. U.S. Army Soldier and Biological Chemical Command. *Modular Emergency Medical System: A Mass Casualty Care Strategy for Biological Terrorism Incidents.* 2002. Available at: http://www.nnemmrs.org/surge.html (Modular Emergency Help Center).
34. U.S. Army Soldier and Biological Chemical Command. Neighborhood emergency help center pamphlet: a mass casualty care strategy for biological terrorism incidents. 2001. Available at: http://www.nnemmrs.org/surge.html (Neighborhood Emergency Help Center).
35. U.S. Army Soldier and Biological Chemical Command. Acute Care Center: A mass casualty care strategy for biological terrorism incidents. 2003. Available at: http://www.nnemmrs.org/surge.html (Acute Care Center).
36. Health Resources and Services Administration Special Programs Bureau. National Bioterrorism Hospital Preparedness Program FY 2004 Continuation Guidance. May 2004. HRSA grant materials are available at: http://www.hrsa.gov.
37. U.S. Department of Health and Human Service. Federal Medical Contingency Stations Type III (Basic) demonstration. Presented at: Denver Convention Center; January 6, 2005; Denver.
38. Burrington-Brown J. Practice brief. Disaster planning for a mass-casualty event. *J AHIMA.* 2002;73(10):64A-64C.
39. American College of Emergency Physicians. Hospital disaster planning. *Ann Emerg Med.* 2003;42(4):607-8.
40. 2003 American College of Emergency Physicians' Board of Directors. Hospital Disaster Privileging, Policy No. 400326, Approved February 2003. Available at: http://www.acep.org.
41. American Hospital Association. Model hospital mutual aid memorandum of understanding. Available at: http://www.kyha.com/documents/ModelMOU.pdf.
42. New Hampshire Hospital Association and Vermont Hospital Association. Draft model language for hospital mutual aid agreements. Available at: http://www.mhalink.org/public/Disaster/files/prep-2003-13-2.pdf.
43. New Hampshire Hospital Mutual Aid Network. Memorandum of understanding. Available by permission from Bizzarro K, New Hampshire Hospital Association. Available at: http://www.nhha.org.
44. Vermont Association of Hospitals and Health Systems. Guidelines for inter-hospital mutual aid response: letter agreement. Available at: http://www.vahhs.org/lucie/mutualaid/LetterAgreement.htm.
45. Auf der Heide E. The Incident Command System. In: *Disaster Response: Principles of Preparedness and Coordination.* Available at: http://orgmail2.coe-dmha.org/dr/index.htm.
46. San Mateo County Health Services Agency Emergency Medical Services. HEICS, the Hospital Emergency Incident Command System. Available at: http://www.emsa.cahwnet.gov/dms2/heics3.htm.

47. Bissel RA, Becker BM, Burkle FM. Health care personnel in disaster response: reversible roles or territorial imperatives? *Emerg Med Clin North Am.* 1996;14(2):267-88.

48. 103rd Weapons of Mass Destruction Civil Support Team. General fact sheet. Available at: http://c21.maxwell.af.mil/wmd-cst/cst_factsheet_103rd.pdf.

49. The Right-To-Know-Network. What are LEPCs and SERCs? Available at: http://65.108.196.28/Downloads/LEPC_Bulletin.pdf.

50. Emergency Management Assistance Compact. About EMAC. Available at: http://www.emacweb.org/.

51. National Emergency Management Association. Model Intrastate Mutual Aid Legislation. Available at: http://emacweb.org/docs/Wide%20Release%20Intrastate%20Mutual%20Aid.pdf.

52. U.S. Department of Homeland Security. Initial National Response Plan fact sheet. Available at: http://www.dhs.gov/dhspublic/display?theme=43&content=1936.

53. Federal Emergency Management Agency. A guide to the disaster declaration process and federal disaster assistance. Available at: http://www.fema.gov/rrr/dec_guid.shtm.

54. Federal Emergency Management Agency. National mutual aid and resource management initiative. Available at: http://www.fema.gov/preparedness/mutual_aid.shtm.

55. Denlinger RF, Gonzenbach K. The "two-hat syndrome": determining response capabilities and mutual aid limitations. *Perspectives on Preparedness.* 2002;11:1-11.

56. Auf der Heide E. Principles of hospital disaster planning. In: Hogan DE, Burstein JL, eds. *Disaster Medicine.* Philadelphia: Lippincott Williams & Wilkins; 2002:57-78.

57. Auf der Heide E. Disasters are different. In: *Disaster Response: Principles of Preparedness and Coordination.* Available at: http://orgmail2.coe-dmha.org/dr/index.htm.

chapter 28

Surge Capacity

Julie Ann P. Casani and Albert J. Romanosky

The events of 2001 are often cited as being pivotal for a new definition of preparedness. In actuality, there were multiple factors forcing the healthcare industry to look at surge capacity before the 2001 terrorist attacks on the United States. Beginning more than two decades earlier, crises in emergency department overcrowding provided insight into the necessity for flexing the number of hospital beds, providing rapid discharge of inpatients, delaying scheduled surgeries, diverting ambulances based on triage criteria, and altering practice paradigms to allow "auxiliary" nursing staff to provide necessary emergency care. Since 2001, events such as severe acute respiratory syndrome (SARS) and smallpox preparedness have illustrated the need for surge capacity and the ability of facilities not only to flex upward the number of beds but also to supply specialized or specified treatment (e.g., high-level respiratory isolation). The majority of surge planning has focused on trauma care for victims of multicasualty incidents; terrorist and industrial chemical incidents; and public health emergencies, such as bioterrorism and natural epidemics. There are discrete differences in the type of capacity needed for each type of incident, but there are overarching principles that can benefit surge capacity planning for all-hazards disaster planning.

One of the great challenges has been funding for surge capacity. Health economics in the United States, in an attempt to limit escalating healthcare costs, has resulted in the overall reduction of acute care inpatient beds and has eventually led to a vastly expanded network of industry related to home care and intermediate care facilities. In most acute care hospitals, making the "bottom line" is a challenge in itself, let alone providing services and capacity for an event that may never happen, developing resources that are costly with limited or no pre-event funding, and planning for expenditure of resources that may not be reimbursed. The end result is opposing forces and policies in which preparedness efforts are attempting to increase surge capacity while cost containment measures are shifting care away from acute care centers (ACCs).

Surge capacity has been defined as encompassing "potential patient beds; available space in which patients may be triaged, managed, vaccinated, decontaminated, or simply located; available personnel of all types; necessary medications, supplies and equipment; and even the legal capacity to deliver health care under situations which exceed authorized capacity."[1] Integral to this definition are the multiple elements, not solely facilities or beds. Hick and colleagues[2] go on to define surge capability as the "ability of the health care system to mange patients who require specialized evaluation or interventions." This distinction is important because it focuses on the more specialized resources and nonfixed bed capabilities. Historical events and theoretical models provide estimates of the number of acutely ill people requiring care after disasters. However, the definition of an "acutely ill or injured" patient is case-dependent and does not reflect the *level of care* the victim may require. Trauma-related projections range from 100 to 300 patients/1 million population after mass casualty incidents (MCIs) to 300 to 600 patients/1 million population, according to the National Disaster Medical System (NDMS) plans. There are limited projections for bioterrorism or large-scale communicable disease models. These include the NBC-CREST (Department of Defense) model estimates of 500 patients/1 million population and pandemic influenza planning estimates of 15% to 35% of the population. The pandemic influenza model assumes a gross attack rate of 30% and would result in five times as many influenza-related hospitalizations and deaths as in a regular influenza epidemic with the current levels of vaccination in the population, mostly in persons ages 65 and older.[3] Based on data from the influenza pandemic of 1918 to 1920, projections were made with respect to the current population of Germany (approximately 82 million). An estimated 20 million to 25 million cases of influenza will occur, with 200,000 admissions to hospitals, resulting in a total of 1.6 million days of hospitalization, 120,000 deaths from influenza, and an annual excess mortality of 175,000. This is a ratio of 2500 hospital patients/1 million population. Approximately 1.2 million cases of pneumonia as a secondary infection also should be expected.[4]

Because of the wide spread of estimations, which are dependent on the causative agent, for planning purposes, many use 500 adult and pediatric victims/1 million population above the daily capacity to calculate surge capacity. A regional capacity requirement example is found in Table 28-1; Region A is an intrastate region in which City A is located.[5]

TABLE 28-1 REGIONAL CAPACITY REQUIREMENT

	POPU-LATION	SURGE (BEDS/PATIENTS)	CURRENT DAILY CAPACITY	INCREASE
State A	5,595,211	2798	10,006 (48 facilities)	28%
Region A	2,571,695	1286	6129 (22 facilities)	21%
City A	628,670	314	3827 (12 facilities)	8%

Most projection prototypes assume the current health-care delivery model, which may or may not be attainable or sustainable at high levels of patient load. Regardless of cause, to approach projected levels of surge demands, multidisciplinary, multientity, regional, collaborative planning must be undertaken because no single component can provide all of the necessary resources. The authors of the Agency for Healthcare Research and Quality document, *Regionalization of Bioterrorism Preparedness and Response,*[6] conclude that "regionalization is likely to benefit elements of a bioterrorism response including the provision of surge capacity in essential response services such as triage, the provision of medical care, distribution and dispensing of prophylactic therapies, outbreak investigation, security management, and emergency management.... Coordination of these organizations may benefit from implementation of information management strategies and pre-event agreements that specify response roles, remuneration, and chain of command."

Overall coordination of planning and response is critical for implementation. The introduction of new modalities and paradigms presents a challenge to responders and the public who will instinctively react as they have in the past. If new programs and responses are expected to be implemented, then adequate communication, education, and exercises will reinforce this implementation. Incident management systems and Incident Command Systems must be integrated along with communications systems and protocols.

Multiple models have been postulated for the systematic, graded response necessary to provide a capacity to care for an overwhelming influx of patients.[7,8] These models provide tool kits for evaluating the utilization of current resources and defining supplementary resources to provide the necessary location, staff, and supplies for response. Additionally, the type of incident may require a shift in necessary assets and availability of these assets. For example, the immediate response required in a catastrophic explosion will require a different strategy than the sustained nature of a wide-scale communicable disease event. Few of these models allow for healthcare staff to be among the ill or injured. In the Toronto SARS experience, the incident rates among nurses who worked in emergency departments, intensive care units, and coronary care units ranged from 10.3% to 60.0%.[9] In addition, non-ill providers who fail to report for duty may further affect response. The potential unreliability of

the assessment of available resources may be especially troublesome if the healthcare workforce is particularly vulnerable physically or psychologically, as in the SARS outbreaks of 2003 and the early outbreaks of Ebola hemorrhagic fever. Likewise, few of these models anticipate the loss or compromise of a healthcare facility or access to it if it is located in close proximity to the event.

There are a number of dynamics that must be considered to prepare overall for a surge of acutely ill or injured patients. On a daily basis, the healthcare system attempts to provide the necessary triage, treatment, and health maintenance at a level that is determined as "normal operations." A tentative balance of supply and demand is struck, based on dynamic shifts within a health system that is typically already at capacity. The actions implemented are variably applied and do not address the root causes behind the immediate crisis of overload: the critical nursing shortage, health insurance inequities, national malpractice concerns, and health economic trends. In many cases, the immediate demand is met and the system returns to an ever-increasing new normal of stress.

During the day, week, month, or season, if a peak in the number of patients is observed, then local, facility-specific provisions adapt to this increased demand by implementing "emergency operations." This may result in longer office hours, emergency department diversion, longer wait time for ambulances, early discharge protocols, etc. A 2001 American Hospital Association survey showed that 60% of all and 80% of urban hospitals described their emergency departments as "at" or "near" capacity, as did 90% of all Level 1 trauma centers with more than 300 beds.[10] One in eight hospitals reported emergency department diversion 20% or more of the time. About 20% of the hospitals' capacity can be freed up by discharging existing patients, canceling elective surgery, and calling in off-duty staff. This response is usually (1) area limited, (2) time limited, (3) difficult but manageable, and, (4) occasionally "routine." Repeated or prolonged stress at this level results in either a short-term (weeks) decay or, optimally, long-term solutions, such as increased staff, re-engineered space, etc. Close examination of these solutions provides important insight into potential solutions to a larger-scale, longer-term surge capacity situation. The incremental costs of re-engineering space to provide flexible utilization is much more cost-effective and allowable under most regulatory systems than is a fixed building or permanent assignment of space. The process involved in changing operations, such as surgery scheduling and staff shift flexibility, provides insight into the impact of long-term disaster services. For example, Rambam Medical Center in Haifa, Israel, can increase the number of burn victims it can handle from 15 to 136 by altering staff allocations and re-engineering space.[11]

Larger-scale events, longer-term events, or those requiring specified care will place unique demands on a system, regardless of emergency operations preparedness. It should not be assumed that 100 times as many patients require 100 times the amount of response. At some point, which will vary depending on resources, community, and type of event, a critical threshold will be met in which "emergency operations" no longer suffice. At this point, "disaster operations" are implemented. Efforts such as (1) "aggressive diversion" of patients to triage and decontamination facilities, (2) implementation of treat and release/refer protocols, (3) transfer of nonacute admissions to long-term care facilities, and (4) institution of widespread home care plans may be put into operation (Fig. 28-1). "Aggressive diversion" of patients refers to the direction or redirection of ambulances and patients away from acute care facilities to locations that provide triage, decontamination, and/or treatment. This may be done by transportation away from facilities, public information campaigns instructing people *not* to go to hospitals but rather to seek care at off-site centers, etc. Treat and release protocols and referral protocols may be implemented to allow for expedient care and throughput in alternative facilities or by physician and nurse extenders. Each of these programs requires extensive planning, policy and statutory research, and public dialogue in preparation for implementation.

CURRENT PRACTICE

A matrix of planning capacities is offered (Table 28-2). It is recognized that this is only one approach to maneuvering through the very difficult process of assigning resources and anticipating needs. This matrix is prepopulated and is provided as a starting point for planners. It is fully expected that communities may add or delete components that reflect available resources and cultural acceptance of their uses. A discussion of the components follows.

Arenas of care have been delineated with the assumption that there will be a continuum of care and that patients may not attend every arena. The "prehospital" arena is care delivered between the scene of the incident and definitive care. The care may be provided by tradi-

tional first responder entities (law enforcement, fire/rescue/emergency medical services [EMS], etc.) or via portable emergency triage and decontamination centers for large-scale events. This arena may also include any ad hoc informal community first aid centers. Integration of these may be a challenge, especially in light of limited communications and information systems. However, general public community education and preparation may eliminate a portion of the system's surge demands. It may be assumed that not every person needs to be treated in a formal medical care unit. It may also be assumed that not every patient will be cared for in a prehospital arena and may self-refer directly to "traditional facilities." In fact, the overwhelming majority of ambulatory patients are likely to self-refer to the nearest known traditional facility (hospital) in an acute disaster, such as natural disasters, explosions, etc. In some public health emergencies that develop and progress more slowly, this may or may not be the case. Education efforts and consistent, clear information programs and policies could affect this behavior.

"Traditional facilities" refers to locations where acute and general care is routinely delivered. These include emergency facilities, hospital- and nonhospital-based; private healthcare provider offices; small and large group practices; and community health centers, both private and those operated by public health entities.

During a health emergency, care may be shifted away from traditional facilities, either through naturally occurring forces or through policy and procedure implementation. It is commonly assumed that an expanded capacity within traditional facilities will provide the answer to surge demands. It is postulated here that if that were the case, then surge capacity would not be an issue at all other than building and supplying more traditional facilities. As elaborated earlier, this is antithetical to current market and overall health policy forces and is the very reason surge capacity becomes problematic. Therefore, to supply services during the increased stress of a health emergency, the system will need to look to "nontraditional facilities" in addition to the traditional facilities for resources. For a biological event or communicable disease public health emergency, this may include establishing treatment and triage centers not in hospitals but in other locations, such as long-term care facilities, hotels, and schools, perhaps using the Soldier Biological and Chemical Command (SBCCOM) Modular Emergency Medical System model.[12,13] For a chemical event, this may be establishing locations for decontamination, triage, and treatment away from emergency departments, for example, in an off-site triage, treatment and transportation center (OST³C)[14] if such a center can be established quickly and in close proximity to the event so that it is visible and accessible.

Finally, there can be many patients who are either not treated in an acute care facility of any kind but are referred home and are treated and/or followed-up at home or at a later time as referrals. This "nonfacility" domiciliary environment should not imply noncare. Instead this may require quite complex care and complex case management and will engage the medical and nonmedical communities and family resources.

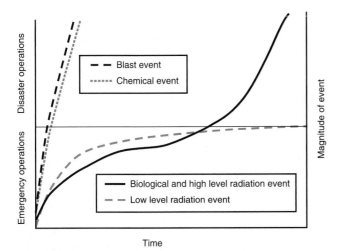

FIGURE 28–1. Response and magnitude of event plotted against time. Depending on the nature of the event, the healthcare system will attempt to respond to the increased demands. As demand for services increases, "normal operations" will be replaced by "emergency operations." As the system is again stressed, the response shifts to "disaster operations."

TABLE 28-2 SURGE PLANNING MATRIX*

COMPONENT	PREHOSPITAL ARENA	TRADITIONAL FACILITIES ARENA	NONTRADITIONAL FACILITIES ARENA	DOMICILIARY CARE ARENA
Facilities	Triage facilities Decontamination facilities Private offices, community health centers, large group practices Transport vehicles (emergency medical service [EMS], private carriers, transportation sector resources)	Emergency departments, urgent care centers Hospitals Public health centers	Off-site treatment centers (acute care facilities) Long-term care facilities (off-site triage, treatment, and transportation center [OST³C])	Homes Dormitories Hotels
Personnel	EMS providers (ALS/BLS) Public health and hospital workers Volunteers Disaster medical assistance teams (DMATs), U.S. Public Health Service (USPHS) Metropolitan Medical Response System (MMRS)	Healthcare providers Volunteers	Healthcare providers Public health Volunteers DMATs, USPHS Nongovernment organizations Medical professions students Strategic National Stockpile	Public health: epidemiological investigation and tracking Home healthcare agencies Community and faith-based groups Nongovernment organizations
Medication and supplies	MMRS DMATs Planned caches Vendors	Strategic National Stockpile Planned caches Vendors	Strategic National Stockpile Planned caches	Strategic National Stockpile Vendors Planned caches Coordination
Policy (including legal and statutory issues)	Triage protocols Mutual aid agreements Credentialing of volunteers	Specialty hospital designation Triage protocols Discharge planning Transfer protocols Credentialing of volunteers	DMATs Vendors Transfer protocols Credentialing of volunteers	

*This matrix is prepopulated with elements to begin planning efforts for surge capacity. Please refer to the chapter text for descriptions and discussion of the elements listed.

Facilities

Prehospital Arena

In areas where private-sector ambulances are not typically used for emergency transport, prior memoranda of understanding (MOUs) may be necessary to ensure availability, credentialing of personnel, emergency reimbursement, dispatch protocols, medical direction, etc. Additional resources from the transportation sector may be engaged, optimally with prior planning. Buses, taxis, and vans, both public and private service, can be used to transport large numbers of patients. Public-sector transportation vehicles are typically rapidly and easily accessible to government authorities. Many government authorities contract with private conveyance systems for more routine transportation needs. There may be opportunity to expand those contractual services to include emergency availability for transport not only of patients but, potentially, personnel. Finally, use of mass transportation vehicles may offer shelter for victims during the initial phases of a disaster.

Traditional Facilities Arena

Much has been done in the United States to prevent damage to critical structures from natural hazards such as earthquakes and floods. Seismic design provides stability of hospitals and allows for maintenance of care in high-risk areas.

Traditional facilities typically provide surge capacity for beds by reallocating designated beds to the event. For example, postanesthesia areas that have cardiac monitoring capabilities may be turned into intensive care units. Hospital-based same-day surgical suites may be used in the treatment of acute injuries because they also house minor surgical supplies. Rooms with additional oxygen outlets that are used on a daily basis as a single-bed room can be used to cohort contagious patients.

As demand increases, patients requiring isolation who are dispersed throughout the hospital can be gathered into specialized multiroom units. Specialized needs for high-level respiratory and isolation units may be "created" by relatively low-cost engineering with the installation of ventilation deflectors that allow for negative air flow to those rooms individually or to a unit. In an incident, air flow and air exchanges can be adapted to provide flexible utilization of nonspecialty bed capacity. The authors of *Regionalization of Bioterrorism Preparedness and Response*,[6] through retrospective analysis, determined that "pre-event hospital designation contributes to lower costs and improved patient outcomes. The evidence from trauma care regionalization suggests that a key component of high-quality, cost-effective care is limiting high-cost specialty care to specifically designated hospitals with increased experience in treating severely injured patients. A bioterrorism response system may benefit from the pre-event designation of hospitals." However, in the SARS events in Toronto, it was found that the transfer of patients to designated facilities may have contributed to further spread of the disease, especially early in the outbreak when control measures were still being clarified and made universal.[15,16] Well documented in the literature and further described by Einav and colleagues[17] in a study of terrorist-related MCI blast incidents, the most urgent and nonurgent victims are taken to the nearest hospital, even if it is not a designated trauma center. The authors suggest a paradigm shift in trauma care in which all hospitals should have some minimal level of capability for trauma care. In fact, the most recent model in Israel designates the nearest hospital as the evacuation hospital to which all trauma victims are taken. Only the most seriously wounded get surgical intervention while other less critical victims are sent to surrounding facilities after stabilization of life-threatening injuries, thereby making the facility serve as a triage center. In a mass-casualty event, referral and transfer to tertiary care facilities for advanced specialty care may be necessary and desired; however, in the disaster operation phase, these specialized services may no longer be available, either because the services have been diverted to general care or the specialty services are overwhelmed. Additionally, until or even after aggressive diversion of patients to triage centers is well established, patients may still self-refer to the hospital of their choosing for a number of reasons, including proximity, insurance coverage, and personal preference. It may be unpredictable as to which facilities will become a focus for care and likely that many, if not all, hospitals will become primary institutions. For this reason, *every* facility must be prepared to care for patients.

In addition to hospitals, other traditional facilities will be used through self-referral or through a planned, graded diversion triage plan. Patients with minor illness and injuries can be triaged to urgent care centers, public health centers, and community health centers. The results of a pre-event inventory of laboratory and radiologic capabilities will determine optimal triage protocols.

In disasters in which access to critical routine healthcare is disrupted, such as for patients undergoing hemodialysis and those with a chronic fragile health status, diversion to traditional facilities may place a surge capacity need in a different manner. Traditional facilities will need to be capable of maintaining critical services while also contributing to the community's surge capacity.

Nontraditional Facilities Arena

The OST³C model uses a rapidly deployable center that would accept patients, either self-referred or transported by ambulance from an explosion or chemical event. It has been suggested that early deployment of local medical centers can alleviate the burden placed on local hospitals.[18] Decontamination facilities may need to be established rapidly to prevent further contamination of the center. Patient care flow in the center directs

patients first to a triage process and then to either a transportation section for transfer to a hospital or to a treatment area for definitive care. The duration of care is anticipated to be relatively brief (24 hours or shorter) and may consist simply of observation for further symptoms. Because most casualties in an acute, rapid-onset event (explosion, structure collapse, or chemical release) will be rapidly transported, the most significant weakness of the OST³C model is the need for rapid deployment and implementation. Therefore, the OST³C facility must be well planned, well integrated, and well rehearsed. This frequently limits its utilization; however, two additional potential roles for such a facility include short-term (12- to 24-hour) observation units and predeployment for large-scale events, such as mass gatherings. Physical requirements include access to controlled vehicular traffic for ambulance use, male and female lockers and shower facilities or an external water supply for outside decontamination, heating and air conditioning, electricity with generator back-up, etc. Potential buildings to be used for an OST³C are gymnasiums, fitness centers, hotels conference centers, and any other building with large space capacity.

The acute care center (ACC) component of the Modular Emergency Medical System (MEMS) provides a care center approach. As described in *Modular Emergency Medical System: Concept of Operations for the Acute Care Center,*[19] the ACC is designed as an organized, equipped, and staffed facility specifically to provide services to those affected by a biological or communicable disease event. It is designed to treat patients who require acute care but not mechanical ventilation for a duration of days to weeks. Patients who require intensive life supportive care would be admitted to a traditional hospital. The ACC would be near a traditional hospital but transparent to the public who should self-refer or be referred to the center's emergency department for initial evaluation and subsequent triage.[19] However, the ACC also could be integrated into diversion protocols to alleviate emergency departments from this triage function and optimize the ACC's utility. The ACC module is a 250-bed pod system (5 × 50-bed nursing units) that is expandable to a maximum of 1000 patients and requires 40,000 to 48,000 square feet. Ideal buildings include armories, schools, hotel conference rooms, and community centers. These buildings offer adaptable space, heating and air conditioning, kitchen facilities, adequate plumbing facilities, and power and water supply. They also may supply necessary Internet access.[19]

Long-term care facilities (nursing homes, assisted living facilities, and rehabilitation centers) may be available either for acute care patients or for patients who were discharged early from traditional acute care facilities to make beds available for disaster victims.

Special medical needs shelters that focus on attending to people requiring specialized services may allow the healthcare community not only to provide acute services to this population but may also allow for continuing care and domiciliary care for subacute and longer terms of treatment. The need for this type of shelter and the specific resources necessary must be planned for after an assessment of the community, optimally before an event.

Domiciliary Care Arena

Patients who are discharged from a hospital, treated and released home from triage centers, or those being observed at home for symptoms will require specific facility resources. Adequate home care accessories (e.g., wheelchairs, crutches, bandages) may need to be made available. Patients being monitored by public health authorities either for epidemiological information or symptoms will require adequate access to telephone monitoring or access to providers visiting at the home. As required, the homes must be able to provide heat or air conditioning, power, water, a food supply, and the basic needs. If homes are not available, alternative domiciliary care can be provided at locations such as hotels and college dormitories.

There are additional considerations for all of the previously cited facilities. Care should be taken not to identify facilities assumed by other response agencies (e.g., American Red Cross, National Guard Armories). In addition, portable structures, either hard shell or tent type, can be used and provide cost-effective, nonconstruction solutions. The length of use may be affected by the choice of shell, weather elements, and actual use. MOUs with facilities, especially if not publicly held, should be instituted to allow for availability and postevent reimbursement and recovery. Alternatively, adequate legal authority of local or state officials to commandeer facilities must be established and used.

Personnel

During the evolution of the event through to disaster operations, the roles of personnel may change and practice paradigms may shift. Table 28-3 illustrates this shift in roles.

Prehospital Arena

For formal incident scene triage, treatment, and transport, traditional fire/rescue/EMS and other first responder agencies will provide the necessary care. Informal triage and transportation will also be performed by bystanders and the casualties themselves. The formal resources can be supplemented with community teams, such as the Community Emergency Response Teams (CERTs). The CERT program is an all-risk, all-hazards training in which citizens may initially take actions on their own, and these actions can make a difference. The CERT program was developed by the Los Angeles Fire Department (LAFD) to engage citizen volunteer efforts to augment the response capacity before and during the department's response. In 1993, the Federal Emergency Management Agency (FEMA) made the concept and program available to communities nationwide. The Emergency Management Institute (EMI), in cooperation with the LAFD, expanded the CERT materials to make them applicable to all hazards. In January 2002, CERT became part of the Citizen Corps, a unifying structure to link a variety of related volunteer activities to expand a community's resources for crime prevention and emergency response. As of December 2004, 50 states, three territories, and six foreign countries were using the CERT training for a total of 1900 CERT teams.[20]

Because of the magnitude of a catastrophic event, such as an explosion, adaptations will be made as MCI operations are instituted. Triage will be abbreviated with use of systems such as the Sacco Triage Method or START (Simple Triage and Rapid Treatment Plan) method, which were both developed for use by rescuers with basic first aid skills to triage patients in 30 to 40 seconds or less. The Sacco Triage Method attempts not only to assign a level of acuity to a patient but also allows available resources to be assigned to the patient. Optimally, treatment will be limited and patients will be transported per MCI protocols.

Central collection points, such as portable triage shelters or the OST³C, can be staffed with personnel other than traditional first responders. Care at these intermediary centers is not expected to be a substitute for that provided in a traditional emergency department; staff should be able to provide, at a minimum, basic life support functions. Individual jurisdictions may decide to staff these centers with personnel who can provide a higher level of care if, for example,

TABLE 28-3   HEALTHCARE PROVIDER ROLES*

PROVIDER	DAILY ROLE	ROLE DURING SURGE
Public health: State and local	Mental health, epidemiological investigations, disease monitoring, alerting, healthcare regulation and oversight, expertise resource, laboratory analysis	*Crisis and resource management and coordination, regulatory relief Neighborhood Emergency Help Centers (NEHCs), ACCs, OST³C*
Hospitals	Diagnosis and treatment of all patients	Diagnosis and treatment of *critically* ill patients
Community health providers: Private practitioners, large group practices, community health centers, surgicenters	Care and treatment of noncritically ill patients (general medical and mental healthcare)	Care and treatment of *less critically* ill patients (minor trauma and surgical patients)
Fire/Rescue/EMS: Public and private	Scene Incident Command System and control Triage, treatment, and transport	Triage, treatment, and transport; *greater role in crisis and resource management and coordination*

*The roles of providers may shift as the event unfolds and evolves. This table reflects (in italics) new or differences in roles that may be required of providers.

screening and dispensing of prophylactic antibiotics or vaccinations are to occur. Several models are offered for establishing a triage and dispensing site, optimizing personnel resources, and projecting the number of persons to be vaccinated or dispensed medicines.[21,22] The Bioterrorism and Epidemic Outbreak Response Model (BERM)[23] provides a computer model for determining the number and types of personnel necessary for such a clinic site and can be used for planners to provide adequate resources. Most dispensing site plans are based on the medical model and, therefore, provide for some degree of triage for ill patients. It is anticipated that these providers will be public health and community volunteers because hospital employees will be occupied in their respective facilities.

Additional resources available for "prehospital" arena care include those involved with volunteer corps, disaster medical assistance teams (DMATs), and the Metropolitan Medical Response System (MMRS). These resources allow for reliance on personnel responding directly to the emergency rather than staff required to report for duty at traditional facilities.

A federal DMAT, which is part of the National Disaster Medical System (NDMS), is a group of medical and support personnel designed to provide emergency medical care during a disaster or other unusual event at a location usually remote from the origin of the team. DMATs deploy to disaster sites with adequate supplies and equipment to support themselves for 72 hours and provide medical care at a fixed or temporary medical site. They may provide primary healthcare and/or augment overloaded local healthcare staff. DMATs are designed to be a response element to supplement local medical care until other federal or contract resources can be mobilized or the situation has resolved. Each DMAT deployable unit consists of approximately 35 individuals; however, teams may consist of more than three times this number to provide some redundancy for each job role. This ensures that an adequate number of personnel are available at the time of deployment. A team is composed of medical professionals and support staff who are organized, trained, and prepared to activate as a unit. Some states and regions are developing intrastate DMATs or Medical Reserve Corps. In a large-scale disaster, a DMAT's ability to provide local personnel surge capacity may be limited because these teams frequently draw on the same pool of professionals already expected to respond during the disaster.

The MMRS, directed by U.S. Department of Homeland Security and FEMA, directly supports enhancement of existing local first responder, medical, public health, and emergency management by increasing systematic, integrated capabilities to manage a weapons of mass destruction MCI until significant external resources arrive and are operational (typically 48 to 72 hours). The program provides training, supplies, medical caches, and coordination within a metropolitan jurisdiction. It does not supply additional personnel but provides an organizational structure and resources for response in a region. There are 125 MMRS operations in the United States.

Traditional Facilities Arena

Care of patients at traditional facilities may require additional resources, the reapportioning of staff to different staffing patterns, etc. Relative to the amount of surge capacity within the hospital, planners could calculate the number of necessary additional staff as follows:

168 hours per week ÷ 40 hours per week workload = 4.2 full-time equivalents (FTEs)

Each staff position requires 4.2 FTEs for 24-hour operations, 7 days a week.

If a 1:4 staff-to-patient ratio is maintained, then:

(No. of surge beds ÷ 4) = No. of staff positions

(No. of staff positions) × (4.2 FTEs) = No. of additional healthcare providers necessary per week

If a 1:6 staff-to-patient ratio is maintained, then:

(No. of surge beds ÷ 6) = No. of positions

(No. of staff positions) × (4.2 FTEs) = No. of additional healthcare providers necessary per week

If a 1:10 staff-to-patient ratio is maintained, then:

(No. of surge beds ÷ 10) = No. of staff positions

(No. of staff positions) × (4.2 FTEs) = No. of additional healthcare providers necessary per week

Table 28-4 presents the calculated staffing needs for the various staffing ratios calculated for the regional surge beds presented in Table 28-1.

An additional staff resource to hospitals is a preestablished system of volunteers. Healthcare provider volunteers who are not full-time employees, who are retired, or who are no longer in clinical practice but maintain a license may be available for emergency staffing. Volunteer management programs must provide for the recruitment, confirmation of credentials, emergency notification/ deployment, and training/orientation of these valuable individuals. Individual healthcare entities

TABLE 28-4 ADDITIONAL STAFF REQUIRED FOR SURGE

	POPULATION	SURGE (BEDS/ PATIENTS)	HEALTHCARE PERSONNEL (1:4)	HEALTHCARE PERSONNEL (1:6)	HEALTHCARE PERSONNEL (1:10)
State A	5,595,211	2798	2938	1958	1175
Region A	2,571,695	1286	1350	900	540
City A	628,670	314	329	220	131

must decide whether to accord any particular healthcare worker emergency privileges to practice in facilities for which it has responsibility. Approaches include accepting the credentials maintained by other accredited healthcare facilities during an emergency into facility emergency preparation plans, relying on government programs that develop volunteer medical corps, and/or establishing mutual aid agreements. The Emergency Systems for Advance Registration of Volunteer Health Care Personnel (ESAR-VHP) is an additional step to provide for coordinated emergency increases in staffing of physicians, nurses, pharmacists, behavioral health professionals, emergency medical technicians, and other appropriate healthcare professionals. The ESAR-VHP system, still in development, would establish a regionally accepted, standardized advanced registration system for healthcare professionals through collaboration of hospitals, licensing boards, professional organizations, etc.

Managing the number of spontaneous volunteers by providing rapid credential verification and logistic requirements increases organizational burdens. Providing adequate coordinated efforts for volunteers and integrating these well-intentioned and needed individuals would yield positive results for all parties.

Nontraditional Facilities Arena

Once the provision of care is shifted or augmented to a nontraditional facility, the targeted reserves of healthcare providers likewise shifts away from those in traditional hospitals. Out-of-hospital primary providers, public health providers, volunteer corps, DMATs, and other federal assets will be relied on to deliver care in these locations. In addition, nongovernment agencies, such as the American Red Cross Disaster Relief Services and Salvation Army, may deliver care. A pre-event inventory of agencies, type of care provided, and number and identity of providers must be conducted to provide a responsible plan without "double counting" assets. For example, the use of National Guard medical personnel may be a pivotal piece of a community's plan. However, many of these personnel are also providers at local hospitals or may become an essential federal asset and may not be accessible for local response.

It is recommended in the ACC model to have the following minimal staffing per 12-hour shift for a 50-bed nursing subunit:

- Physician (1)
- Physician's assistant (PA) or nurse practitioner (NP) (physician extenders) (1)
- Registered nurses (RNs) or a mix of RNs and licensed practical nurses (LPNs) (6)
- Nursing assistants/nursing support technicians (4)
- Medical clerks (unit secretaries) (2)
- Respiratory therapist (RT) (1)
- Case manager (1)
- Social worker (1)
- Housekeeper (1)
- Patient transporter (1)

The minimal number of staff providing direct patient care on the 50-bed nursing subunit per 12-hour shift is 12, which includes the physician, physician extenders, nurses, and nursing assistants.

While the absolute number of providers necessary changes as the event progresses from "emergency operations" to "disaster operations" so, too, do the roles change. As illustrated in Table 28-3, as "disaster operations" and aggressive diversion are implemented, community providers may be tasked with providing care to the less critically ill and injured patients, whereas the hospital providers will be responsible for the more critically ill and injured patients.

Domiciliary Care Arena

Domiciliary care will, of necessity, require case management. This case management may be provided by several resources at various stages of the event and the patient's course. If the patient is hospitalized, the case management through hospitalization and through to discharge may be assumed by the facility. However, if the person is never hospitalized or is discharged from a facility, public health, community practitioners, etc., may be responsible for assuming this role. A pre-event inventory of resources for domiciliary care will reveal what currently exists in a community, what the needs may be, and any gaps that will occur during a disaster, which may be addressed through preparedness activities.

Public health authorities will be engaged in the epidemiological investigation, including case investigation and case contact. They are also likely to be responsible for the monitoring of symptoms and the initiation and maintenance of quarantine in communicable disease outbreaks. In addition, public health agencies typically provide telephone hot lines with information for providers and the general public. In Toronto, 225 residents met the case definition of SARS. Toronto Public Health investigated 2132 potential cases of SARS, identified 23,103 contacts of SARS patients as requiring quarantine, and logged 316,615 calls on its SARS hot line.[24] Temporary suspension of nonessential services may result in additional public health personnel; however, a long-term event will require regular re-evaluation of the need to reinitiate these services.

Providers of domiciliary care may come from professional and nonprofessional resources. Home health agencies and nongovernment agencies, such as the American Red Cross, may be available and have capacities to provide professional level services. Basic services, such as oral hydration, dressing care, and activities of daily living, may be provided by community-based formal and informal networks. Families, churches, and community organizations can be engaged to deliver such services and may be willing to do so, provided they are given the resources, minimal-but-meaningful education, and appropriate protection to do so. Pre-event outreach can organize these groups and allow for adequate support.

Medications and Supplies

Medications and supplies are commonly regarded as a short-term need and vulnerability. In fact, in a long-term event, such as a communicable disease event, supply shortages may become an increasing and broader issue. A disaster may quickly exhaust available supplies, including medications, or may prevent the further replenishment of supplies from outside of the affected area. It is important to conduct a needs assessment and have an ongoing materials management process to assess current and anticipated needs and acquisition and appropriation of supplies on hand. In many U.S. disasters, supply shortages have not occurred, but rather, excessive donations have created a different challenge (see Chapter 35). Unfortunately, the pre-event purchase and stockpile of equipment can be costly and difficult to justify in the current economic environment and as healthcare facilities continue to shift to "just in time" inventories. Graded increases in par levels of supplies, regionally leveraged purchases, and rotation into stock can ease the financial burden of preparedness. Federal response systems anticipate this need and purchase, and strategic forward deployment has been under way at that level. However, depending on the nature of the incident, it is prudent to assume that facilities and agencies should plan on being self-sufficient for the first 48 to 72 hours after an event. This places an additional burden on planning for an event, such as an explosion or chemical event, which will require adequate resources within the first hours or sooner. In this case, outside resources should be used to provide subsequent care and to restock used supplies.

If additional supplies are warehoused at central locations, numerous factors will need to be taken into consideration, including apportionment decisions, speed and mechanism of delivery, and access to delivery location. Limited material supplies may not meet demands, and an apportionment policy should be decided on before an event to allow for dialogue, education, and evidence-based decisions by officials. The speed and mechanism of delivery may vary, depending on the incident. Natural disasters may impede surface transportation of surge supplies. During the Sept. 11, 2001, attack on the Pentagon, emergency response vehicles, police closing of roads, and the ordered evacuation of federal facilities created a transportation gridlock, limiting the delivery of anticipated supplies to some hospitals in the District of Columbia (MedStar Health System, personal communication, January 2004).

Adequate personal protective equipment (PPE) for the anticipated surge capacity staff will be necessary to maintain a healthy staff. Depending on the nature of the event, the type of PPE used will likely be the most protective until the causative agent is defined. Standards for such PPE are well defined by the Occupational Safety and Health Administration. In disasters with noncontaminated physical hazards, such as an earthquake with building collapse, PPE should consist of protection for the extremity, head, ears, and eyes. In the prehospital arena, for suspected chemical, contaminated explosive, or unknown contamination scenes, personnel functioning within a "hot zone" are likely to be in Level A protection. Level A PPE offers the highest level of protection. It encompasses positive pressure breathing apparatus, SCBA, with a fully encapsulating chemical suit. After the removal of victims and subsequent decontamination, graded "step-down" in protection can be made until a level appropriate for definitive protection is attained. For example, initial evaluation of patients with an unknown communicable disease may

first be approached with the provider in full high-efficiency particulate air (HEPA) respiratory and splash precautions. Once the infectious agent is identified and other potential preventative steps are taken (e.g., vaccination), PPE can be shifted to the appropriate mask and Universal Precautions. Amounts of PPE required to sustain a response is dependent on the durability and lifespan of the equipment (single-use versus multi-use), inter-user transfer of equipment (sharing), and the anticipated number of changes per provider. Durable hazardous materials gear may have longevity of several days into an event, may be able to pass from one worker to another, and is not necessarily disposable after each use. N95 respirators used for smallpox respiratory protection may be usable by a single user over a 12-hour shift but would *not* be shared and would be disposed of after the shift. Estimation of PPE requirements can be made by the following formula:

No. of personnel per day × No. of exchanges per day per person = No. of anticipated PPE sets per day

Medical supplies such as antibiotics, chemical antidotes, bandages, and splints can be maintained at traditional facilities and/or cached at central locations. Anticipating the number of needed supplies will depend on the anticipated surge needs and will likely be proportionate to those needs. Adjustments will need to be made with materials managers' assistance to accommodate differences in durable and nondurable goods. Additional resources include prepositioned caches in traditional first responder agencies (police, fire/rescue/EMS) and in agencies such as emergency management agencies and public health agencies. Deployable assets such as the Strategic National Stockpile, the CHEMPAK program, DMATs, and MMRS, have caches of medical materials not only to sustain the function of the teams but for treatment of casualties and patients. There are numerous community resources that should be inventoried and may be available for use. Pharmaceutical vendors, veterinary pharmacies and practices, dentists and dental supply warehouses, etc., may have supplies that are usable and available. Planning for use should include emergency procurement plans, apportionment policies, and MOUs with these entities to expedite postevent recovery.

Delivery of essential supplies such as power, food, and water must be considered for those people who, because of their injuries or illnesses, cannot access these services on their own. Traditional formal disaster relief services, such as the American Red Cross and Salvation Army, and nonformal services, such as community and faith-based groups, should be integrated so that patients in domiciliary care are identified to them and the organizations are part of an individual's case management plan.

Legal and Policy Issues

Policy development and decisions, to the extent possible, are best made or planned for in the pre-event stages when level heads prevail; there is the ability to adequately review current literature and science; and dialogue, debate, and education can be accomplished.

Triage, treatment, and transfer protocols; mutual aid agreements; and credentialing programs will require the input and review by legal counsel. Additional statutory and regulatory changes may need to be sought to provide the bases for emergency powers of officials, medicolegal protection as practice paradigms shift, and compensation and liability for surge personnel.

Aggressive diversion of patients described earlier raises several critical legal concerns and questions. Issues related to malpractice liability, state regulations, and the Federal Emergency Medical Transfer and Labor Act (EMTALA) must be well researched and addressed.

EMTALA provides for, among other items, adequate screening before patient transfer, maintenance of level of care during transfer, and an accepting physician at the receiving facility. Triage away from a facility without well-established protocols that have been reviewed and approved by legal authorities will result in unwelcome anxiety and noncompliance by healthcare providers. During *nationally* declared disasters, EMATLA regulations may be suspended by authorities, but during *local* or *state* disasters, they will be in force.[25]

Even with effective planning and use of resources, an overwhelming event may outstrip resources and result in the re-evaluation and acceptance of a degradation of the standards of care. Serious discussions of this potential must be conducted before an event, not only with policy makers and legal experts but also with the general public.

CONCLUSION

Overall, the goal of surge capacity planning is to provide a series of prepositioned processes to ensure the delivery of appropriate care with appropriate resources in a graded, phased response. A potentially overwhelming response can be planned and provided for with adequate assessment of the population's needs and community resources and the development of plans for matching these needs with resources, augmenting as necessary. Planning may not necessarily include large capital expenditures but will provide stimulus for creative collaborative processes. The integration of disciplines and practices is essential because no single healthcare component can shoulder this alone. Integration of the general public through to multiple government agencies in response to a disaster will ultimately provide for an overall surge capacity.

REFERENCES

1. Joint Commission on Accreditation of Healthcare Organizations. Health Care at the Crossroads: Strategies for Creating and Sustaining Community-wide Emergency Preparedness Strategies. Available at: http://www.jcaho.org/about+us/public+policy+initiatives/emergency_preparedness.pdf.
2. Hick JL, Hanfling D, Burstein J, et al. Health care facility and community strategies for patient care surge capacity. *Ann Emerg Med*. 2004;44(3):253-61.
3. van Genugten MLL, Heijnen MA, Jager JC. Pandemic influenza and healthcare demand in the Netherlands: scenario analysis. *Emerg Infect Dis*. 2003;9(5):531-8. Available at: http://www.cdc.gov/ncidod/EID/vol9no5/02-0321.htm.
4. Fock R, Bergmann H, Bussmann G, et al. Influenza pandemic: preparedness planning in Germany. *Euro Surveill*. 2002;7(1):1-5.
5. Health Resources and Services Administration. National Bioterrorism Hospital Preparedness Program, FY 2004 Continuation Guidance. Available at: ftp://ftp.hrsa.gov/hrsa/04guidancedot/hrsa04biot.pdf.
6. Stanford-UCSF Evidence-based Practice Center. *Regionalization of Bioterrorism Preparedness and Response: Evidence Report/Technology Assessment No. 96*. Rockville, MD: Agency for Healthcare Research and Quality;April 2004. AHRQ publication 04-E016-2.
7. Allswede MP, Watson SJ. *AHRQ Partnership for Quality*. 2002. Available at: http://www.ahrq.gov/news/ulp/surge/allswedetxt.htm.
8. Cantrill SV, Eisert SL, Pons P, et al. Rocky Mountain Regional Care Model for Bioterrorist Events: Locate Alternate Care Sites During an Emergency. Available at: http://www.ahrq.gov/research/altsites/.
9. Varia M, Wilson S, Sarwal S, et al. Investigation of a nosocomial outbreak of severe acute respiratory syndrome (SARS) in Toronto, Canada. *CMAJ*. 2003;169(4):285-92.
10. American Hospital Association. Emergency Department Overload: A Growing Crisis. Available at: http://www.aha.org/aha/press_room-info/content/EdoCrisisSlides.pdf.
11. Posner Z, Admi H, Menashe N. Ten-fold expansion of a burn unit in mass casualty: how to recruit the nursing staff. *Disaster Manag Response*. 2003;1(4):100-4.
12. Expanding Local Healthcare Structure in a Mass Casualty Terrorism Incident, Modular Emergency Medical System. U.S. Army, SBCCOM; June 2002. Available at: http://www.edgewood.army.mil/hld/ip/mems_copper_book_download.htm.
13. Neighborhood Emergency Help Center, A Mass Casualty Care Strategy for Biological Terrorism Incidents. U.S. Army, SBCCOM; May 2001. Available at: http://www.edgewood.army.mil/hld/ip/mems_copper_book_download.htm.
14. An Alternative Health Care Facility: Concept of Operations for the Off-site Triage, Treatment and Transportation Center (OST³C), Health and Safety Functional Workgroup, CWIRP. U.S. Army, SBCCOM; March 2001. Available at: http://www.edgewood.army.mil/hld/ip/mems_copper_book_download.htm.
15. Dwosh HA, Hong HH, Austgarden D, Herman S, Schabas R. Identification and containment of an outbreak of SARS in a community hospital. *CMAJ*. 2003;168(11):1415-20.
16. MacDonald RD, Farr B, Neill M, et al. An emergency medical services transfer authorization center in response to the Toronto severe acute respiratory syndrome outbreak. *Prehosp Emerg Care*. 2004;8(2):223-31.
17. Einav S, Feigenberg Z, Weissman C, et al. Evacuation priorities in mass casualty terror-related events: implications for contingency planning. *Ann Surg*. 2004;239(3):304-10.
18. Peleg K, Reuveni H, Stein M. Earthquake disasters—lessons to be learned. *Isr Med Assoc J*. 2002;4(5):373-4.
19. Modular Emergency Medical System: Concept of Operations for the Acute Care Center (ACC). U.S. Army, SBCCOM; May 2003. Available at: http://www.edgewood.army.mil/hld/ip/mems_copper_book_download.htm.
20. Federal Emergency Management Agency. CERT Overview. Available at: http://training.fema.gov/emiweb/CERT/overview.asp.
21. Centers for Disease Control and Prevention. Download Maxi-Vac Version 1.0 (Draft). Available at: http://www.bt.cdc.gov/agent/smallpox/vaccination/maxi-vac/index.asp.
22. Centers for Disease Control and Prevention. Smallpox Response Plan and Guidelines (Version 3.0). Annex 3: Guidelines for Large Scale Smallpox Vaccination Clinics. Available at: http://www.bt.cdc.gov/agent/smallpox/response-plan/files/annex-3.pdf.
23. Weill/Cornell Bioterrorism and Epidemic Outbreak Response Model (BERM). Available at: http://www.hospitalconnect.com/aha/key_issues/disaster_readiness/resources/vaccination.html.
24. Svoboda T, Henry B, Shulman L, et al. Public health measures to control the spread of the severe acute respiratory syndrome during the outbreak in Toronto. *New Engl J Med*. 2004;350(23):2332-4.
25. Mitchiner JC. EMTALA: What Everyone Needs to Know. Available at: http://www.mpro.org/IT/webex/emtala/emtala_handouts.pdf.

chapter 29

Operations and Logistics

David Jaslow

Effective disaster management relies on the ability of responding organizations or personnel to organize themselves into cohesive work units under a defined leadership structure that can coordinate with each other to meet specific goals and mitigate the disaster. One of the hallmarks of a developed country from the emergency response perspective is its ability to effectively respond to and manage a complex disaster event in an organized fashion.[1,2]

The terms "operations" and "logistics" refer to two of the five management functions that compose the foundation of the Incident Command System (ICS). This terminology is also used to describe the actual components or work units that accomplish specific tasks at a disaster event. Such terminology has now become commonplace, and it is routinely used to describe identical functions at local or regional emergency incidents, not just disasters.

The operations section is responsible for taking a set of incident objectives that the incident commander has developed and designing a strategic plan to mitigate the disaster incident and its consequences. Such a plan necessitates organization, assignment, and supervision of tactical resources, all of which are housed in the operations section. The logistics section is responsible for services and support needs, which are necessary to sustain the tactical objectives of the operations section. In simple terms, the logistics section is the "go to" function for any wish list of equipment, personnel, or services necessary to support disaster response operations. Even though operations and logistics are two completely separate functions and functional entities, the efficiency and effectiveness of an operations sector at a major incident are due in some degree to a well-organized and properly functioning logistics sector, much like the relationship between a race car driver and his or her pit crew.

HISTORICAL PERSPECTIVE

Federal response to disasters in the United States probably goes back to an 1803 act of Congress that made provisions available to New Hampshire after a devastating fire. Obviously, the federal government has grown considerably since then and has increased and codified the

response to disasters. It is important to state that, like most laws in the United States, provisions for disaster response, like the provision after the New Hampshire fire in 1803, are reactive and not proactive. Myriad laws and acts such as the Flood Control Act and the Fire Response Act resulted in a relatively fragmented approach to federal disaster response in which a disaster required response from literally hundreds of agencies until the enactment of the Robert T. Stafford Disaster Relief and Emergency Assistance Act in 1974.[2] To further unify the federal response to disasters, the Federal Emergency Management Agency (FEMA) was established in 1979 under President Carter and was charged with coordinating federal disaster response.

Even though disaster response is often legislated at the federal level, response and coordination of deployed resources historically have fallen on the jurisdiction legally responsible for the location in which the disaster occurs. In other words, like politics, all disasters are "local," or at the very least, start out as "local." In most jurisdictions across the United States, the fire chief (or his designee) of the authority having jurisdiction (known as the AHJ) becomes the de facto incident commander at an event that involves imminent danger to life or property, with the exception of purely law enforcement–related situations (e.g., sniper, hostage situation), regardless of training, experience, abilities, knowledge, or competence in responding to major incidents. It is the incident commander who has overall authority for disaster operations, regardless of the size or scope of the disaster, unless or until he or she transfers command to another individual.

For many decades, the standard practice among incident commanders who determined that they lacked the resources to manage an incident was to summon additional manpower supplies, equipment, and emergency vehicles from neighboring communities as quickly as possible. This concept is known as *mutual aid*. Mutual aid compacts or agreements are drawn formally or informally between individual agencies or political jurisdictions, but there is still no national mutual aid system or standardized guidelines for how to develop such a plan in the United States. In more progressive fire-rescue systems, mutual aid resources are dispatched according to a predefined algorithm or plan, and this concept is known as *automatic aid*. One of the greatest challenges of developing mutual aid systems has been to overcome the "more is better" philosophy in the fire service, which leads to large amounts of resources dispatched to a disaster regardless of whether they are proper, necessary, or even requested. This is a particularly thorny issue in regions of the country covered by mostly volunteer departments.

If regional resources do not satisfy the needs of a disaster response, the traditional next step has been to request aid from the state Emergency Management Agency. Governors can declare a state of emergency, which releases materials and financial resources and activates the National Guard. Only in the last 10 to 15 years have many states developed unique specialty response teams capable of mobilizing for disaster response, such as urban search and rescue (US&R) and hazardous materials/weapons of mass destruction (WMD) task forces, emergency medical service (EMS) strike teams, and similar entities. In 1996, Congress enacted the Emergency Management Assistance Compact, a mutual aid agreement that allows human and material resources to cross state lines and operate in a declared disaster situation when requested through the proper channels and approved by the governor of the affected state.

There was no coordinated federal contribution or response to disaster operations and logistics support until the creation of FEMA in 1979. This agency is charged with responding to, planning for, recovering from, and mitigating against disasters. Despite the creation of this agency, it was not until problematic response to several large-scale disasters, including hurricanes Hugo and Andrew and the Loma Prieta earthquake, that FEMA's role in disaster operations and logistics became better defined and coordinated. James Lee Witt, FEMA director under President Clinton, is largely credited with the transformation of the agency from an organization that predominantly handled the recovery phase of a disaster to one that took on a prominent role in the response phase.

CURRENT PRACTICE

Operations

Most disaster response begins with a call to 911, and police or fire personnel are the first responders to the disaster. Those first on-scene begin the initial response that will most typically include assessing the possibility for immediate mitigation and then summoning more resources and setting up an initial Emergency Operations Center (EOC) or command. Even though they will be few, first responders will bear the responsibility for initially assessing the scope and extent of the disaster until more resources arrive. When more resources arrive, the first priority will be to effect mitigation to save lives immediately in danger, but soon after, priorities will grow to include making an assessment of the potential short- and long-term consequences of the disaster; determining the need for resources beyond the local jurisdiction, including state and federal; and organizing an ICS.

Disaster operations increase in size and complexity depending on the nature of the event; duration of the event; and resources, which are necessary to stabilize the incident. Common tactical resources at a disaster incident include fire suppression, technical rescue, hazardous materials containment, and EMS, to name a few. Exactly what kind and quantity of resources will be necessary to deploy at a disaster event depends on the nature of the event and the tactical objectives set by command personnel.

The ICS, discussed in greater detail elsewhere in this textbook, is the national standard for management of personnel and operations at an emergency incident of any size or complexity. ICS is a flexible management structure, which allows for expansion and contraction of all sectors, including operations, based on the dynamics of the incident. In late 2004, the Department of Homeland Security released the National Incident Management System (NIMS) as a template to complement ICS. NIMS builds on the concept of a unified command structure and provides a framework for interoperability and compatibility among various public and private organizations that respond to large-scale disasters within the United States.

The operations section chief is the individual designated by the incident commander to manage and command the operations section and who is ultimately responsible for developing and implementing strategies and tactics to meet the incident objectives. Tactical decision-making (i.e., how, when, and where to deploy certain resources to mitigate a disaster) is the responsibility of the operations section chief. However, the ability to make these decisions in a competent fashion is predicated on a continual flow of information both from the field and from the command sector. If an incident spans more than one operational period (usually one work cycle), the operations chief may assign a deputy to work the opposite shift to ensure adequate time for nourishment and rest.

There are several very difficult obstacles to overcome when establishing a robust operations section during disaster response. Personnel from different agencies may not be accustomed to working together or may not speak the same response vernacular. Communications systems may be different among responding agencies. Tactical objectives may be accomplished differently by different agencies or resource types. Another often-misunderstood pitfall is the influence of politics and egos that may tend to drive decision-making despite the known dangers, which these behaviors engender.

From a field perspective, there are several goals that the operations chief must accomplish during the initial stages of the response to a disaster. First, he or she must develop an incident action plan (IAP). This plan details the objectives of the mission and how they will be met. An IAP should be written for every operational period during the disaster. Second, the operations chief must decide how much to expand his or her organizational structure. Supervisory personnel should be titled and placed in charge of subsidiaries within the operations section based on who is most qualified to perform the task rather than on a person's rank or predisaster title.

Span of control should not exceed seven personnel in the organizational structure. Third, the operations chief must decide in conjunction with the incident commander and safety officer what degree of risk he or she is willing to assume when sending emergency responders into an unstable environment to perform search, rescue, evacuation, medical care, and mitigation activities related to the disaster event. Fourth, the operations chief must maintain an effective line of communication with the various components within the section as well as with the other ICS sections and the incident commander. Fifth, the operations chief must understand the concept of flexibility when making decisions. Disaster events may appear static to the civilian population, but emergency responders understand that these events are dynamic in nature. Changing environmental conditions, secondary hazards, fatigue, resource availability, and many other factors contribute to ever-changing disaster conditions, and these conditions require adaptability and flexibility in decision-making by those whose job is it to mitigate the incident.

Expansion of the operations section of the ICS is usually a rare event during local emergencies. However, an event that the Department of Homeland Security labels an "incident of national significance" may necessitate creation of divisions, groups, branches, task forces, and strike teams. These entities represent functional and geographical separation of duties. Such was the case at the 2001 World Trade Center disaster. The Fire Department of New York (FDNY) retained command and control of the entire incident and eventually developed a unified command structure according to principles of the ICS. The 16-acre size of the disaster site required a large-scale expansion of the operations section. Divisions were created according to street names that bordered the scene. Groups included functional components such as technical rescue, fire suppression, and EMS. Branches of each group were composed of personnel attached to a specific type of resource, such as the US&R branch. Within the US&R were individual US&R task forces. EMS strike teams from FDNY and surrounding mutual aid organizations were deployed in support of US&R task forces and other specialized resources.

A variety of federal resources are available to assist local incident commanders in handling large-scale disasters and their aftermath. Such resources and directions for their interaction and coordination can be found in the National Response Plan (NRP), which debuted in December 2004. The NRP aligns federal coordination structures, capabilities, and resources into a unified, all-discipline and all-hazards approach to domestic incident management. An outline of the contents of the NRP can be found in Box 29-1.

Two of the most common emergency response resources deployed from the Department of Homeland Security are US&R task forces and disaster medical assistance teams (DMATs). US&R task forces specialize in response to collapse of reinforced concrete buildings, and their primary mission is to rescue persons trapped in confined spaces regardless of the etiology of the event. DMATs are mobile field hospitals staffed with a

multidisciplinary team of healthcare professionals that can provide medical care for prolonged periods when local infrastructure is incapacitated. Additionally, there are specialized DMATs for the care of children, burns, victims of WMD incidents, animals, and deceased persons.[3]

Logistics

Typical logistics functions during a disaster include obtaining, maintaining, and tracking essential personnel, supplies, and equipment; providing communications hardware and installation of communications systems; setting up food services; setting up and maintaining incident facilities such as dining halls, the incident command post, and bed-down areas; obtaining necessary transportation resources for personnel and supplies; and providing medical services to incident personnel. The size, duration, and specific needs of an incident dictate whether a separate logistics functional element must be created within the ICS. Most disasters, by definition, meet the criteria that any incident commander would use to establish a logistics section. Essentially, the logistics section, or function, is to figure out how to get what is needed and get it to where it is needed. An often daunting function, there are many examples from history that show us the difficulty of getting what is needed, but more often than not, it is getting the required resources, including manpower, to the needed place that proves the most challenging.

The logistics section chief manages and commands this section and is ultimately responsible for its performance. If an incident spans more than one operational period (usually one work cycle), the logistics chief may assign a deputy to work the opposite shift to ensure adequate time for nourishment and rest.

The logistics section is typically divided into two branches: service and support. Units located within the service branch provide direct service functions that require human interaction, including communications, medical care, and nourishment. The support branch is composed of functions that typically do not involve human interaction, such as vehicles and transportation, supplies, and facilities.

The medical unit located within the service branch of the logistics section warrants special attention since it is often confused with the delivery of routine EMS at a large-scale incident. Emergency medical functions fall within two distinct categories in the ICS. EMS is typically a branch within the operations section. The responsibility of the EMS branch is to provide emergency medical care and treatment to victims of the disaster. The medical unit is designed only to provide emergency medical evaluation and treatment to disaster responders.

This is an important distinction, both theoretically and functionally. The medical unit is akin to the rehabilitation, or "rehab," sector at a fire scene. The goal of the rehabilitation sector is to monitor firefighters and other emergency response personnel for signs and symptoms of physical and psychological stress induced by the incident. These conditions are usually successfully mitigated with hydration, nutrition, and rest. The rehabilitation sector is a separate function from the treatment sector established by EMS personnel to treat victims of the fire itself. At a disaster scene, the victim treatment area and the responder treatment area should be physically separate, especially since responders do not typically require medical treatment per se and will have difficulty recuperating amidst the chaos of a victim treatment area.

The logistics section chief works closely with the chiefs of planning and finance/administration. He or she monitors the incident action plan because it provides valuable information about what supplies and equipment may be necessary as the disaster event progresses and as incident objectives change. The logistics section chief is also mindful that supplies and equipment may have to be contracted and purchased or bartered. Thus, the logistics section chief must interact frequently with his or her counterpart in finance/administration since lack of funding may have a direct impact on the performance of the logistics section.

Massive relief operations, such as was seen during the response to the Southeast Asia tsunami disaster of 2004, provide insight into why logistics is such an important part of disaster response. Described as a "logistics nightmare" by United Nations personnel, the response to the tsunami disaster of unprecedented proportions was quite complicated, especially considering the difficulties with the development of a unified command structure among representatives of state and nongovernment agencies from different countries. At one point early in the response, flights to an airport in Indonesia had to be suspended because there were too many airplanes already on the ground that were unable to unload their cargo due to lack of space at the airport; this was due to ineffective ground transportation to deliver the goods to the end user. This problem, in turn, was partially a result of a lack of vehicles and partially a result of the inability for the available vehicles to reach certain areas due to wash-out of the roadways.[4] Ironically, the biggest ongoing logistical challenge in the response to the Southeast Asia tsunami was how to distribute the abundance of supplies and funding. Similar problems have occurred in various disaster events in the United States during the past 20 years.

The Operations Support Directorate (OSD) exists within FEMA to provide the agency with logistics, security, health and safety, and other mission support services essential to the accomplishment of the agency's all-hazards management program (Box 29-2). FEMA's Mobile Operations Division includes five regional Mobile Emergency Response Support (MERS) detachments and the Mobile Air Transportable Telecommunications System. MERS provides a large fleet of specialized vehicles and dedicated personnel to deliver food, water, fuel, sophisticated com-

BOX 29-2 RESPONSIBILITIES OF FEMA'S OPERATIONS SUPPORT DIRECTORATE

- Logistical support in the areas of agency-wide logistical systems, disaster support facilities operations for FEMA, and the agency's emergency management partners
- Protection of personnel, facilities, and equipment to ensure a secure environment for FEMA and its emergency management partners
- The agency-wide Occupational Safety and Health Program
- The FEMA mitigation program for employees
- Numerous essential mission support functions, such as printing, graphics, storage, and distribution of FEMA publications, forms, and records; management program; space management; and procurement of operational supplies, equipment, and services

munications capability, and other logistics support wherever needed. These resources support local, state, and federal emergency responders, not disaster victims.

PITFALLS

Management of large-scale disasters is fraught with difficulty despite the fact that most problems are predictable and recur at every major disaster to some degree (Box 29-3). There is no disaster incident in which everything goes according to plan. The ability of the incident commander and the operations and logistics chiefs to be flexible in decision-making, delegate authority when necessary, and adapt to changes in incident conditions and mission priorities is essential.

Most communities have developed fairly comprehensive emergency management plans to address the hazards in their region. However, too often these plans lack a significant public health and medical component or that component is poorly defined in terms of what its relationship is to the overall disaster incident. Drs. Joe

BOX 29-3 PARTIAL LIST OF FACTORS ASSOCIATED WITH INEFFICIENT OR INEFFECTIVE DISASTER OPERATIONS

- Lack of accountability, including inadequate supervision and ambiguous or absent chains of command
- Poor communications due to inefficient uses of available communications, failure of and lack of redundancy in communications systems, and conflicting codes and terminology
- Lack of an orderly, systematic planning process
- No common, flexible predetermined management structure to enable delegation of responsibilities and manage workloads efficiently
- No predefined methods to integrate interagency requirements into the management structure and planning process effectively
- Inability to control access to the disaster site, to manage a large influx of unsolicited disaster volunteers, and to curb "freelancing" among emergency response personnel
- Difficulty in coordinating, tracking, and documenting human and materials resources

Barbera and Anthony MacIntyre, disaster medicine experts from George Washington University, designed a comprehensive model for the management of mass casualty incidents as well as more routine emergency incidents, which have predominantly a health and medical focus. The Medical and Health Incident Management (MaHIM) System describes an "overarching system for organizing and managing the many diverse medical and public health entities involved in mass casualty response." It is based on principles of public health and emergency management and attempts to point out the community approach to problem-solving and emergency response in the setting of a mass casualty incident rather than the individual response of an EMS service, hospital, or public health department.[5] The MaHIM can be found at: www.gwu.edu/~icdrm/publications/index.html.

CONCLUSION

The United States has long set the pace among developed countries in emergency response to catastrophic incidents, perhaps because it has successfully merged many principles of organizational behavior, emergency medicine, and emergency management. Coordination of emergency responders, development of a unified command structure, tracking of resources, and maintenance of functional communications systems remain challenges that will meet us at every disaster event. The NIMS and the NRP represent the federal government's most important contributions to improving disaster response and logistics capabilities in the last decade. Anticipation of pitfalls in disaster response and logistics support and development of adequate contingency planning may be the most important lessons to teach to those who will fill command and leadership positions at a disaster incident.[6] Individuals who wish to learn more about disaster response, the ICS, NIMS, or the NRP can complete self-study courses created by FEMA at http://www.training.fema.gov/emiweb.

REFERENCES

1. Lewis CP, Aghababian RV. Disaster planning, Part I. Overview of hospital and emergency department planning for internal and external disasters. *Emerg Med Clin North Am.* 1996;14(2):439-52.
2. Dara SI, Ashton RW, Farmer JC, Carlton PK Jr. Worldwide disaster medical response: an historical perspective. *Crit Care Med.* 2005;33(1 suppl):S2-6.
3. Roth PB, Gaffney JK. The federal response plan and disaster medical assistance teams in domestic disaster. *Emerg Med Clin North Am.* 1996;14(2):371-82.
4. VanRooyen M. After the tsunami—facing the public health challenges. *New Engl J Med.* 2005;352(5):435-8.
5. Barbera JA, Macintyre AG. Medical and Health Incident Management (MaHIM) System: A comprehensive functional system description for mass casualty medical and health incident management. Institute for Crisis, Disaster, and Risk Management. Washington, DC: The George Washington University; October 2002.
6. Auf der Heide E. Disaster planning, Part II. Disaster problems, issues, and challenges identified in the research literature. *Emerg Med Clin North Am.* 1996;14(2):453-80.

chapter 30

The Incident Command System

Nicholas Sutingco

Many incidents, whether major disasters or minor accidents, often require a coordinated response from a variety of agencies along with an established system of command and control. The Incident Command System (ICS) was created to be used at the scene of emergencies and has become a model tool for command, control, and coordination of an effective emergency response. ICS applies leadership and business principles to emergency response command to improve efficiency and effectiveness. The ICS is designed to organize people and resources and to activate necessary services during an emergency response while providing an easily recognizable and accepted organizational structure that can be used for a variety of incidents. Overall, the ICS provides a means to coordinate the efforts of individual agencies as they work toward protecting life, property, and the environment—all while ensuring the efficient, safe use of resources.

Federal law requires the use of ICS for response to hazardous materials (HazMat) incidents. In fact, many states are adopting ICS as their standard system for responding to all incidents. ICS is also promoted by national organizations, such as the Federal Emergency Management Agency (FEMA) and the National Wildfire Coordinating Group, and has been adopted by the National Fire Academy as its standard for incident response. In addition, the ICS is endorsed by the American Public Works Association and the International Association of Chiefs of Police. It was also included in the National Fire Protection Association's (NFPA) 1995 *Recommended Practice for Disaster Management (NFPA 1600)* and is also a part of the National Interagency Incident Management System (NIIMS).

HISTORICAL PERSPECTIVE

In the fall of 1970, Southern California was devastated by a number of wildland fires that burned more than 6 million acres. After 13 days, 772 structures and 16 lives were reported lost.[1] In a report on the overall emergency response to this disaster, numerous coordination problems were identified. Consequently, Congress funded a consortium of state, county, and city fire departments, led by the U.S. Forest Service, to investigate and

address these problem areas. This consortium was known as the Firefighting Resources of California Organized for Potential Emergencies (FIRESCOPE). The consortium identified several recurring problems involving multiagency responses, including nonstandard terminology, nonintegrated communications, lack of consolidated action plans for designated facilities, and an inability to expand and contract as required by the situation.[1] Efforts by FIRESCOPE to address these problems led to the development of the original ICS model for incident management.

ICS later evolved into a system that is now essentially an "all-hazards" tool appropriate for all types of fire and nonfire emergencies. Much of the success of ICS can be attributed to its flexible yet standardized organizational structure and set of procedures. Not surprisingly, users of the ICS have found it to be useful and widely adaptable in a variety of large-scale emergencies and incidents. Over the years, the original FIRESCOPE ICS has been modified and adapted in numerous ways by many, resulting in a number of variant systems. These variants may indeed be easier to use, but their application in large-scale incidents, such as earthquakes and floods, often falls short when compared with the original FIRESCOPE ICS.

Individual communities often have slightly different approaches toward emergency planning and response. Coordinating various communities during a large-scale incident can be complicated by existing differences. Again, ICS use has evolved by incorporating new emergency management concepts into the municipal Emergency Operations Center (EOC) to allow for an easier application of the original ICS model. As a result, more local governments are using the ICS to organize and manage their emergency responses.[2-6] On a different scale, several hospital models exist. However, an increasingly popular configuration is the Hospital Emergency Incident Command System (HEICS).

In 1987, the Hospital Council of Northern California completed work on an adaptation of the ICS to hospital emergency response functions. In a publication entitled *Earthquake Preparedness Guidelines for Hospitals,* ICS principles were used in a system intended to unify hospitals with other emergency responders.[7] That document in particular served as a cornerstone in the development of the original HEICS, written by Orange County (Calif.) Emergency Medical Services in 1991. Since then, there have been three editions of HEICS; however, all original attributes, steeped in ICS basic principles, remain as before. HEICS is discussed later in the chapter.

CURRENT PRACTICE

No disaster or emergency is ever the same. Likewise, no one emergency management tool is perfect for all types of incidents. With this in mind, it is not surprising that the major desirable factor in an effective emergency management tool is its flexibility—its ability to be modified to meet the needs of different circumstances without losing compatibility with the entities involved. It also must be effective regardless of the size of incident. Some fire departments use the ICS in nearly every response.[5,6] In so doing, these departments become more familiar with its application. Users become more comfortable with the system, and when applying it in its larger scope during a larger incident, a resource-intensive emergency becomes relatively simpler.

The original ICS organization is built around five major components: command, planning, operations, logistics, and finance/administration (Fig. 30-1).[8-10]

These five components are present at every incident—from a routine emergency to a major disaster response. In small-scale incidents, these five major components may be managed by the incident commander (IC) alone. In larger-scale incidents, it may become necessary to set up each component separately, with a leader for each component (a section chief) reporting directly to the IC. All incidents, regardless of size or complexity, will have an IC who is ultimately responsible for the execution of each of these five basic ICS activities. The IC is able to expand or contract the ICS organization as required by the situation.

Command Function

The command function is under the immediate authority of the IC. Responsibilities of the IC include the following[8-10]:

- Establishing command and developing an appropriate organizational structure
- Establishing the incident command post (ICP), where primary command functions are executed
- Developing and implementing the incident action plan (IAP)
- Preserving life and property

- Managing resources, including personnel
- Establishing and supporting effective communications with outside agencies (this includes the EOC, when it is activated)
- Ensuring responder and public safety
- Maintaining accountability for task accomplishment
- Authorizing the release of information to the media
- Keeping track of incident finances

As the incident grows in complexity, the IC may find it necessary to delegate authority for performing some of these activities. When such expansion of the command function organizational structure is required, the IC can establish the following command staff positions (Fig. 30-2)[8-10]:

- The information officer deals with the media, coordinating the release of information, alongside the public affairs office at the EOC.
- The safety officer assesses and monitors safety conditions and develops plans to ensure personnel safety.
- The liaison officer is the on-scene contact person for all additional agencies involved in the incident response.

In addition, each of these positions may have a number of subordinates, depending on the size and complexity of the incident.

By delegating the authority to make decisions regarding problems in these three specific areas of incident management, the IC's effectiveness can be improved.

When deciding to expand or contract the ICS organization, the IC should consider the following three major incident principles[4,5,11]:

- Life safety
- Incident stability
- Property conservation

The first priority is always the safety of the public and all incident responders. Second, the IC must consider the stability of the incident when developing an efficient plan that maximizes the response effort and efficiently uses the resources available. Third, the IC is responsible for minimizing property damage while implementing the IAP.

After careful consideration of these principles and more, the complexity of the incident may cause the IC to activate any one or all additional general staff sections. Again, these include planning, operations, logistics, and finance/administration. Each section chief, in turn, can expand internally as needed. Finally, it should be reiterated that the complexity of the ICS organizational structure is dictated by the complexity of the incident—not the size, which is based on the geographical area or the number of resources involved.

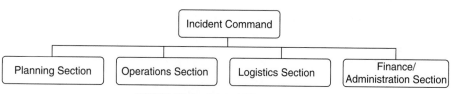

FIGURE 30–1. Original ICS organization.

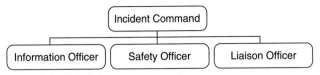

FIGURE 30–2. Command IC staff positions.

Planning Section

In small-scale incidents, the IC often assumes the responsibility of planning. However, when the complexity of the incident is of a larger scale, the planning section is activated by the IC. The planning section serves to continually evaluate the incident situation. Responsibilities of the planning section can be described by a number of functional units (Box 30-1).[8-10]

The situation unit collects incident information, processes it, and disseminates reports to all sections and agencies involved. The resources unit is responsible for accounting for all personnel and equipment, and the documentation unit maintains incident records. The damage assessment unit appraises property damages. A special needs population unit devises plans to protect those with special needs. A technical specialist and/or volunteers unit enables the response to access persons with specialized skills and knowledge related to the incident at hand. Finally, the demobilization unit organizes the de-escalation of all resources when an incident response comes to a close.

It should also be noted that a major responsibility of this particular general staff section is the creation of the IAP. The IAP defines incident response activities and which resources are to be used over a clearly specified period.[1,4,8,10] Overall, the planning section has the critical task of anticipating the problems and needs of other ICS general sections and providing incident status updates to the IC.

Operations Section

The operations section is responsible for implementing the IAP developed by the planning section. The operations section chief has the primary responsibility of coordinating operations section activities in accordance with the IAP. Other responsibilities of the operations section chief include determining required resources and the organizational structure within the section, informing the IC of situation and resource status within the section, and assisting the IC in creating objectives for the incident.[8-10]

The responsibilities of the operations section as a whole take place on the actual scene of the incident. These activities include, but are not limited to, triage, rescue, emergency medical services (EMS), firefighting, and disaster relief services for victims (e.g., shelter).[8-10] These branches, as they are called in ICS, may be broken down further into divisions or groups, as required by the complexity of the incident. The operations section chief decides whether the formation of these branches is necessary. It should also be noted that during an active response, the operations section is the only general staff section that has direct contact with the public. All other activities under the control of the remaining general staff sections are in support of the operations section.

Logistics Section

The logistics section functions to support all incident responders. This section is responsible for organizing the necessary facilities, personnel, and materials, including equipment, as determined by the operations section and requested through the IC. Like the planning section, the logistics section can be described by a number of functional units (Box 30-2).[8-10]

Remembering again that every general staff section can be expanded or contracted as needed, the logistics section can include a communications unit responsible for devising a communications plan and maintaining the lines of communications between ICS general staff sections and outside agencies. An information systems unit establishes and maintains the technology necessary to disseminate situation information to emergency workers. The medical unit in the logistics section provides care for incident responders, *not* civilian victims—civilian victims are cared for by EMS organized by the operations section. A food unit supplies food and water to emergency workers. A supply unit orders personnel and supplies for emergency workers. A donated goods unit manages the inventory of donated goods, which historically can be exceedingly large in disaster responses.[12] Finally, a facilities unit creates and maintains any necessary facilities used by emergency workers.

BOX 30-1 PLANNING SECTION FUNCTIONAL UNITS

Situation unit
Resources unit
Documentation unit
Damage assessment unit
Special needs population unit
Technical specialist and/or volunteers unit
Demobilization unit

BOX 30-2 LOGISTICS SECTION FUNCTIONAL UNITS

Communications unit
Information systems unit
Medical unit
Food unit
Supply unit
Donated goods unit
Facilities unit

Finance/Administration Section

Simply stated, the finance/administration section tracks incident costs. Careful records of all financial operations are necessary to ensure adequate reimbursement of costs. This is especially important when the incident is of such a large scale that a presidential declaration has been made. This general staff section has four key activities, which are assigned to functional units (Box 30-3).[8-10]

The time unit records all personnel time during a response. A procurement unit handles all contractual paperwork (e.g., for equipment). A compensation or claims unit handles injury and damage claims. A cost unit makes cost-saving recommendations. Of note, these activities usually occur within the EOC, which is discussed later in the chapter.

CONCEPT AND PRINCIPLES OF THE ICS

ICS concepts and principles have been time-tested and proven in all levels of governmental agencies and industry. To ensure that all persons who may become involved in an incident are familiar with ICS principles, ICS training is available.[8-10] There are a number of core principles included in the ICS structure (Box 30-4).[4]

Common Terminology

Whenever an incident response involves more than one agency, common terminology within the emergency management system becomes a critical feature. Clearly, confusion and inefficiency can result when agencies have slightly different terms for major functions, facilities, personnel, equipment, and/or units. In ICS, terminology for all of these components has been predesignated and standardized.[4,8,10]

Infrequently, multiple incidents occur at the same time within a common jurisdiction. In such cases, the IC will assign his or her incident a unique name.[5] This is particularly useful when a radio frequency must be shared for multiple incidents. In addition, inherent to this concept of common terminology is the guideline that plain English should be used in radio transmissions (i.e., without "ten" codes or agency-specific codes).

Modular Organization

The principle of modular organization is exemplified in Fig. 30-1. It develops as the first-arriving officer (who becomes the IC) assesses the complexity of the incident

BOX 30-3	FINANCE/ADMINISTRATION SECTION FUNCTIONAL UNITS

Time unit
Procurement unit
Compensation or claims unit
Cost unit

BOX 30-4	CORE ICS PRINCIPLES

Common terminology
Modular organization
Integrated communications
Unity of command
Unified command structure
Consolidated IAP
Manageable span of control
Designated incident facilities
Resources management

and activates other functional areas as needed. For example, in ICS this means activating the planning section to assist in the creation of the IAP for a larger-scale incident.

Integrated Communications

Integrated communications refers to a system that establishes a single communications plan with a set of standard protocols that uses common terminology.[4,8,10] The complexity of coordinating a hospital's emergency response with the surrounding community illustrates the importance of a universally accepted communications system.

With regard to hospital and emergency department (ED) preparedness, internal and external communications are vital. Phone numbers for the Centers for Disease Control and Prevention, the Federal Bureau of Investigations, and the local public health department should be kept in the ED and laboratory.[13] Unimpeded contact with agencies is important when reporting a possible bioterrorism attack, activating epidemiological surveillance, or requesting antibiotics or other supplies. Moreover, communications are needed to access assets such as Metropolitan Medical Response Teams, disaster medical assistance teams, and the National Guard Weapons of Mass Destruction-Civil Support Teams.[14]

Unity of Command

When attempting to establish a common set of incident strategies and tasks, it helps when multiple agencies and all personnel involved report to one designated person—the IC. This concept of unified command does *not* mean that any single agency gives up specific authority or accountability. All involved agencies contribute to the command process under the concept of unified command. Consequently, this allows the incident to function under a single IAP.[4,8,10]

In addition, it is recommended that agency leaders regularly communicate before the onset of any large-scale emergency in an effort to get to know one another. Not surprisingly, such personal familiarity fosters cooperation among agencies that work together during any emergency response.

Consolidated Incident Action Plan

A complex incident response benefits from a consolidated IAP. By detailing operational objectives and support activities, order can be established amidst the chaos that often surrounds complex incident responses.[4] The IC decides whether a written IAP is necessary. At the minimum, ICS requires a written IAP whenever several agencies pool resources or multiple jurisdictions are involved. When written, an IAP may include a number of forms as attachments (e.g., traffic plan, safety plan, communications plan). Overall, a written plan is preferred over an oral plan because it protects against liability suits and provides necessary documentation when applying for state and federal assistance.[8,10]

IAPs should be devised around a timeframe called an *operational period.* By using such operational periods, measurable goals are more easily achieved as response initiatives are focused for a shorter period, rather than over an undetermined length of time. Operational periods can be of various lengths but are usually no longer than 12 hours.[8,10] The IC determines the length of the operational period after careful consideration of the incident complexity and size.

Manageable Span of Control

In ICS, manageable span of control is a concept that serves to control the number of resources that operate under an organizational structure to ensure efficiency. In particular, it demands that the number of individuals under one supervisor optimizes the effectiveness of the organization. Often the span of control of a supervisor averages five resources or individuals.[4,8,10]

Designated Incident Facilities

At the minimum, there should be a designated facility where the IC, the command staff, and the general staff can collectively manage incident operations—the EOC.[8,10] Staging areas are also required to prepare and organize all necessary resources before their deployment. Other facilities may be deemed necessary and can be assigned in a large variety of geographical locations.

The Emergency Operations Center

The EOC is where critical members of the ICS structure gather to collectively manage overall incident operations. Most jurisdictions maintain an EOC as part of their emergency preparedness program. During larger-scale incidents, the EOC may take on additional functions and will often extend its reach in several ways.[5] For example, a forward command center may be established near the disaster area. In addition, a logistics center and/or EMS area can be established. However, with today's technology, the EOC itself can be located nearly anywhere.

Comprehensive Resources Management

The principle of comprehensive resources management serves to maximize resource use by consolidating control of resources. In doing this, there is more accountability, and freelancing is reduced.[4,8,10] It is important to remember that personnel is a critical resource, and just like all resources, it can be assigned a status condition. For instance, "assigned" resources are active in an incident response, "available" resources are in the staging area awaiting assignment, and "out-of-service" resources are unavailable for assignment.

HOSPITAL EMERGENCY INCIDENT COMMAND SYSTEM

The HEICS is an emergency management system for hospitals and is made up of positions on an organizational chart (Fig. 30-3). Each position represented in Fig. 30-3 has a specific mission, and each position has an individual checklist designed to direct the assigned individual in emergency response tasks. These checklists are called *job action sheets.* In addition, the HEICS design includes standardized forms to simplify and enhance the overall system. Every job action sheet begins with the job title, the supervising officer, where the location of the section operations center is, and a mission statement to define the position responsibility.[7]

HEICS core attributes, some of which are based on basic ICS principles, include the following:

- HEICS provides a manageable scope of supervision for all personnel, similar to the ICS principle of manageable span of control.
- HEICS is a flexible system by virtue of its "modular organization"—another core ICS principle. It can be expanded or scaled back to meet the demands of a variety of crises, regardless of complexity.
- Job action sheets are position descriptions that have a prioritized list of emergency response tasks. They also serve to remind personnel of the standard established lines of reporting.[7]
- The job action sheets and the associated forms promote documentation of details and the overall response to the crisis. Such comprehensive documentation proves essential when trying to recuperate expenses and reduce liability.[7]

The HEICS organizational chart (see Fig. 30-3) imposes structure and understandable lines of authority within the hospital system. Just as in the original ICS, HEICS incorporates four sections of command under the overall leadership of an emergency incident commander. Each of the four sections—planning, operations, logistics, and finance—has a chief, appointed by the emergency incident commander, who is responsible for his or her section and the resources directly involved.*

SUMMARY

The ICS is capable of handling both small, routine operations and very large incidents that cover many square miles or involve multiple communities or states. Although many incidents will not require the activation of any of the four general staff sections, others will require some or all of the sections to be established.

---

*For more information about HEICS, contact the California Emergency Medical Services Authority at (916) 322-4336, or visit its Web site at http://www.emsa.cahwnet.gov/.

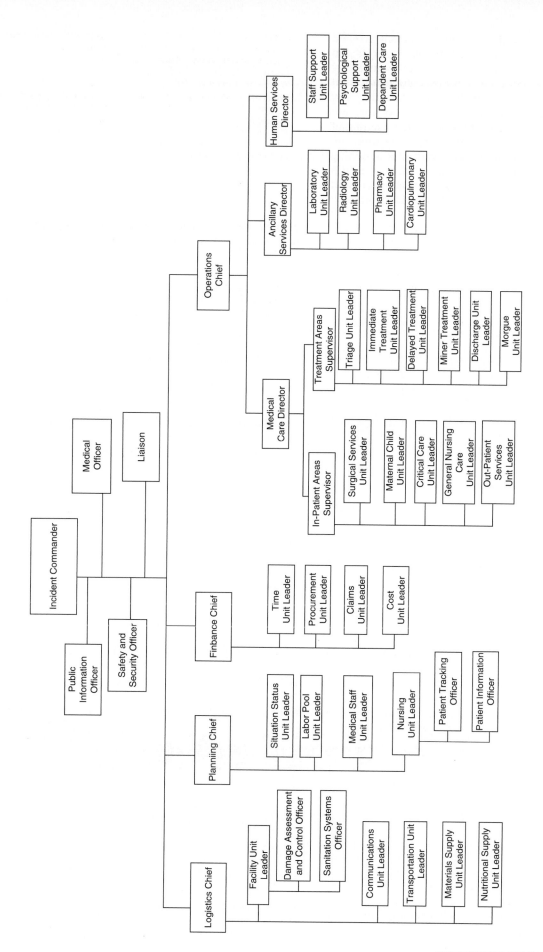

FIGURE 30–3. The Hospital Emergency Incident Command System organizational chart. (Reproduced with permission from State of California Emergency Medical Services Authority.)

ICS is a simple yet detailed system. It is easily grasped but takes practice and familiarity to use it to its full potential. In an effort to promote and continually enhance the principles of ICS, training is offered through the FEMA, the Emergency Management Institute, and other like agencies. Through such courses or through independent study, one can achieve an understanding of the details of ICS and HEICS, which are far beyond the scope of this chapter. (For example, current ICS training and even hospital-based disaster plans such as HEICS now include standardized forms that simplify and enhance the implementation of these flexible systems.)

REFERENCES

1. FEMA (Federal Emergency Management Agency) [1987]. *Exemplary Practices in Emergency Management: The California FIRESCOPE Program.* Emmitsburg, MD: FEMA, National Emergency Training Center, Emergency Management Institute.
2. Auf der Heide E. *Community Medical Disaster Planning and Evaluation Guide.* Dallas: American College of Emergency Physicians; 1995.
3. Auf der Heide E. Disaster planning, part II: disaster problems, issues, and challenges identified in the research literature. *Emerg Med Clin North Am.* 1996;14:453-80.
4. Auf der Heide E. *Disaster Response: Principles of Preparation and Coordination.* St. Louis: Mosby; 1989. Available at: http://orgmail2.coe-dmha.org/dr/flash.htm.
5. Burstein J, Hogan D. *Disaster Medicine.* Lippincott Williams and Wilkins; Philadelphia; 2002.
6. Christen HT, Maniscalco PM. *The EMS Incident Management System: EMS Operations for Mass Casualty and High Impact Incidents.* Jersey City, NJ: Prentice Hall; 1998:1-15.
7. State of California Emergency Medical Services Authority. Hospital Emergency Incident Command System. Sacramento, CA: Emergency Medical Services Authority. Available at: http://www.emsa.cahwnet.gov/dms2/heics_main.asp.
8. Wildland Fire Net. Incident Command System training curriculum. Available at: http://www.firescope.org.
9. U.S. Coast Guard. Incident Command System field operations guide. Available at: http://www.uscg.mil/hq/g-m/nmc/response/.
10. FIRESCOPE. Available at: http://www.firescope.org/.
11. Waeckerle JF. Disaster planning and response. *N Engl J Med.* 1991;324:815.
12. Hogan DE, Waeckerle JF, Dire DJ, et al. Emergency department impact of the Oklahoma City terrorist bombing. *Ann Emerg Med.* 1999;34:160-7.
13. Kortepeter M. *USAMRIID's Medical Management of Biological Casualties Handbook.* ed 4. Washington, DC: U.S. Army; 2001: k14-k27.
14. Garshnek V, Burkle FM Jr. Telecommunications systems in support of disaster medicine: applications of basic information pathways. *Ann Emerg Med.* 1999;34:213-18.

chapter 31

Scene Safety in Disaster Response

Robert L. Freitas

Emergency medical services (EMS) personnel receive training in scene operations and safety during the didactic portion of their training. The training covers the events and concerns in normal EMS response, such as motor vehicle accidents, acts of violence, and electrical hazards, to name a few. Despite this training, prehospital personnel are still injured or killed in the line of duty every year. A study in the *Annals of Emergency Medicine*[1] places the fatality rate of EMS workers at 12.7 fatalities per 100,000 workers compared with 5.0 fatalities per 100,000 workers for the general population. Because of poor data collection, less is known about EMS injury rates compared with those of other public safety personnel, although a study[2] by the Rand Corporation that examining injury rates for all public safety personnel does address the subject. In-hospital medical personnel are less likely to receive any training regarding scene safety for emergency medical response, although the emphasis on hazardous materials training for hospital personnel in recent years does provide some exposure to the concept.

Responding to a disaster presents a unique set of circumstances usually not found in the normal EMS response. Depending on the type of disaster, this could include secondary collapse of structures, operating in unfamiliar surroundings, exposure to smoke and dust, fatigue and dehydration, lack or disregard of safety equipment, and a host of other hazards. Ten emergency medical technicians (EMTs) and paramedics were killed at the 2001 World Trade Center (WTC) disaster, and at least 116 were injured.[3] Both volunteer in-hospital personnel who respond to a disaster because of its proximity to a work site and EMS personnel called to respond to a disaster must be cognizant of the hazards and risks associated with such a response and be prepared to take measures to mitigate those risks. Responders who get injured or incapacitated add to the burden of other public safety personnel who must treat them as well as those injured in the original incident. Medical responders who get injured reduce available resources to the original victims.

HISTORICAL PERSPECTIVE

Healthcare personnel, both prehospital and hospital-based, have routinely responded to disasters with little regard for their own safety. The body of literature on disaster medicine and management both in the United States and internationally is considerable, but little of this literature deals with the safety of emergency medical responders. Formal prehospital care has been evolving for four decades, with better training programs, teaching methods, and protocols; however, safety training and equipment for medical responders have lagged behind.

The formal Incident Command System (ICS), even though in use since the 1970s for some fire services, has only recently become a true component of healthcare operations. EMS agencies have been slowly adopting the ICS during the last 10 years, and the hospital community is now implementing formal training, as mandated by the Joint Commission on Accreditation on Healthcare Organizations.[4] Within the ICS and reporting directly to the incident commander is the incident safety officer (ISO), who has final authority over all operations in regard to responder safety. However, historically this organizational structure has not always been effective, especially when it comes to disasters. In large disasters, one safety officer often has not had enough resources to control the large number of responders, including volunteers, who arrive wholly unprepared for the tasks ahead. In the WTC terrorist attack of 2001, it was observed that "physicians dressed only in scrubs, clogs and surgical masks attempted to negotiate the jagged metal debris to carry out their well-meaning medical interventions."[5] In some situations, firefighters gave up their own personal protective equipment (PPE) to protect the volunteers.[6]

Many hospitals have had "crash boxes" of essential medical and surgical equipment for out-of-hospital response for years, but rarely has the equipment included safety gear. Clinical personnel from hospitals have routinely responded to disasters (and still do) with little or no safety training and even less PPE appropriate for the type of incident. In the 1995 bombing of the Murrah Federal Building in Oklahoma City, a volunteer nurse dressed only in jeans and a sweatshirt suffered a fatal head injury from falling debris.[6] With the vast volume of literature that has come out after the WTC attacks, a true understanding of the problem of keeping responders safe has now come to light.

CURRENT PRACTICE

The current practice of scene safety for disaster response is still evolving, largely in response to review of the WTC disaster in 2001. The Rand Corporation, in concert with the National Institute for Occupational Safety and Health (NIOSH), has published a series of reports that attempts to broaden the knowledge base of this problem. Based on earlier research examining response to disasters, Rand and NIOSH undertook more research into the problem, publishing *Emergency Responder Injuries and Fatalities,*[2] which brings forth the discussion on understanding the types and causes of injuries to public safety personnel while also citing the current lack of adequate tracking methods for including EMS personnel in the data and offering suggestions on how to capture better data on EMS injuries and fatalities. Three other volumes look at the problems faced with protecting public safety personnel when they respond to disasters and offer solutions to better protect those personnel.[7-9]

Still, more effort needs to be expended in understanding how disaster response is different than situations normally encountered by both EMS and hospital personnel. Auf der Heide[10] argues that the difference between the normal mission of emergency response and disaster response is not just one of magnitude managed by bringing into play larger numbers of people and equipment, but rather it is the interplay of a variety of factors. In normal response situations, responders might be exposed to a minimal number of hazards or risks, and usually for a very short period. In contrast, in disaster operations, responders may be exposed to multiple hazards and risks for prolonged periods and often without adequate rest (Box 31-1).

Large Geographical Scale and Unfamiliar Surroundings

In most emergency medical responses, activities are confined to a small area. Responders can readily identify hazards, see who else is responding, quickly estimate the extent of the emergency, and get a sense of how many victims there are. In disasters, especially natural disasters, the geographical scale of the disaster may be overwhelming. The destruction from hurricane Andrew in Florida and Louisiana in 1992 covered more than 1000 square miles.[9] In late 2004, a tsunami in southeast Asia spanned a vast area over three continents. Because of the possible large geographical scale and the loss of familiar surroundings that can occur during a disaster response, it may be difficult to request assistance if responders are not certain of their surroundings. They may be unable to see hazards that could affect them but are not in their immediate field of vision. The large geographical scale may also mean that responders are on-scene for many hours, days, or even weeks to ameliorate the effects.

It is reported that after the 2001 terrorist attacks in the United States at least "six federal and municipal fire and EMS departments, three private ambulance services and a number of volunteer fire departments and ambulance squads responded to the Pentagon" and that an ambulance as far away as Texas responded to the WTC disaster.[3,6] Even though these efforts can be commended, responders unfamiliar with the local surroundings can present safety problems. Finding the way to a staging area or to the scene of a disaster will take more effort for personnel responding from long distances than it will for local units. Responders unfamiliar with the area can inadvertently end up in locations that might contain hazardous materials, as happened during the hurricane Andrew response.[9] Even local responders can have difficulty navigating unfamiliar surroundings if local landmarks and signs have been destroyed, which also occurred during the hurricane Andrew response.[9] Complicate this with the fact that during the initial stages of a disaster, the public may be evacuating the area, causing highway congestion that can contribute to motor vehicle accidents.[11] Responders unfamiliar with the area may not be aware of alternative routes to arrive at their assigned destination if roads are blocked or cannot be navigated due to damage or debris. Hospital personnel who respond to disaster sites are generally not familiar with operating in situations with little light, limited resources, and multiple hazards. Escape routes and safe areas may be difficult to find for those not accustomed to operating in a particular area. Electrical hazards, a problem even when responders are familiar with the area, become more of a problem in unfamiliar surroundings when responders who are trying to orient themselves might not be as vigilant as they normally would be and could walk or drive into hazards, such as live electrical wires. It is essential for responders to ensure that they know where they are going, how to find alternative routes if original routes are blocked, and how to contact coordinating agencies if they become lost. Global positioning systems, although not widely used in medical response, offer hope in allowing response units to navigate unfamiliar territory. It may be difficult to obtain maps in the early phases of a disaster, but having a map of the area is advisable, even if it is hand drawn.

Falling or Flying Debris

Debris from buildings, either damaged during the initial disaster impact or debris that is dislodged due to rescue operations, can be a problem. Medical personnel

---

BOX 31-1 RISKS AND HAZARDS ASSOCIATED WITH DISASTER RESPONSE

- Large geographical scale
- Unfamiliar environments and surroundings
- Falling debris
- Secondary collapse of damaged buildings
- Exposure to hazardous materials
- Excessive noise from machinery and equipment
- Adverse weather
- Inadequate PPE
- Debris fields, causing fall or trip hazards
- Convergent volunteers
- Secondary explosive devices planted by terrorists
- Prolonged duration, causing excessive fatigue, lack of sleep, and inadequate food and hydration

on-scene who are focused on treating patients may not be aware of hazards overhead, and noise from equipment operating at the site can mask the sound of the debris as it falls. Appropriate head and eye protection is critical for all personnel at the scene. The typical eye protection provided to healthcare workers for body fluid splashes offers little protection in a high dust or smoke environment, as was found during the WTC disaster; more than 1000 eye injuries were reported during the first 10 weeks of the WTC operations.[7]

Secondary Collapse of Damaged Buildings

Buildings that survive the initial shock in earthquakes can collapse due to aftershocks or from rescue efforts. WTC Building 7 did not collapse until after 5 PM on Sept. 11, almost 8 hours after the first plane struck one of the other buildings.[6] Responders who plan to set up triage or treatment stations in buildings should first ensure that the buildings have been deemed safe by building engineers or ISOs and are at a safe enough distance from other damaged buildings in the event of collapse. Escape routes and safe zones should be determined while operating within the vicinity of damaged buildings.

Exposure to Hazardous Materials

There is always a risk of unintentional hazardous materials exposure at every disaster site. Intentional hazardous substance exposure through terrorism is covered in other chapters of this text, but hazardous materials are ubiquitous and can be found in hospitals, laboratories, railways, universities, and transportation centers, to name a few. During earthquakes, underground pipelines or above-ground storage tanks may be damaged, leaking hazardous materials into the environment.[11] Buildings damaged during explosions or earthquakes may have leaking fuel tanks, or chemicals used in manufacturing processes may be leaking or mixing together to form new, more toxic compounds.

Exposure to smoke, dust, and other airborne contaminants represents a major problem in disasters where there are large fires or when buildings collapse. NIOSH continues to study the effects of smoke and dust on rescue workers from the WTC attacks. It found that 60% of a subset (1138) of study participants who were evaluated from July 16 and Dec. 31, 2002, suffered from new-onset lower respiratory symptoms and 74% reported new-onset upper respiratory symptoms.[12] Proper PPE must be available and its use mandated on-scene by the ISO, and all disaster responders should have at least hazardous materials awareness training before venturing into disaster scenes. When in doubt about a situation, wait for special operations teams who have testing devices that can determine whether the scene is safe for operations.

Excessive Noise from Machinery and Equipment

Depending on the nature of the disaster, heavy equipment may need to be brought in to facilitate the response. This equipment may create excessive noise either through the exhaust or from moving debris. This makes communication with other medical team members difficult and may make it difficult to hear warning signals indicating aftershocks, secondary explosions, etc. Although wearing hearing protection is advisable, it creates limitations similar to the original source of the noise. It is also usually designed for blocking high-frequency noises and not the low-frequency noises associated with heavy equipment.[7] Additionally, it is difficult to hear radios and other communications devices while wearing the protectors.

Adverse Weather

Because healthcare workers generally dress for their immediate shift, they may be unprepared to deal with the prolonged nature of disasters. EMS workers accustomed to short-sleeve uniform shirts for daytime wear in the summer might find themselves getting chilled by evening, and hospital personnel who respond in hospital garb might be unprepared for sudden rainstorms. Responders to the Oklahoma City bombing had to deal with temperatures that fluctuated from 80' to 40'F, strong winds, rain, and lightning.[13] Healthcare workers both in and out of the hospital who might be called on to respond to disasters should have clothing appropriate for a wide range of weather conditions, including cold weather gear and rain gear.

Inadequate Personal Protective Equipment

EMS and hospital workers are commonly not well prepared and inadequately trained for disaster response when it comes to PPE. Administrators' budgets are often thought to be too lean to spend money on something that happens infrequently and requires a large outlay of funds and training time.[8] It is also suggested that because there is no central federal authority responsible for monitoring PPE for medical response personnel, unlike firefighters and the National Fire Protection Agency (NFPA), funding from government sources for PPE is reduced.[8] Even NFPA's *Standard on Protective Clothing for Emergency Medical Operations*[14] only deals with exposures from body fluids and not the types of hazards likely encountered in disaster operations. Experiences from recent disasters indicate that even with good PPE, the multihazard nature of disasters makes it difficult to have the right equipment all of the time.[7] In a disaster environment, PPE must not only protect the wearer from bloodborne pathogens but also offer protection from other disaster-specific hazards. In addition, due to the extended nature of disaster response, agencies must be able to replenish PPE as it wears out, becomes wet, or breaks down from exposure to chemicals. The multiagency response aspect of disasters can also make the sharing of equipment difficult. With multiple standards for PPE across public safety entities, the chance of cross-agency compatibility of PPE is small. PPE that might be adequate for firefighting is generally not acceptable for the treatment phase of patient care, although it might be appropriate for the patient access phase. Having access to bunker gear is not the answer either, as experiences have indicated that too often bunker gear is too heavy and cumbersome for the prolonged response required to deal with disasters.

Eyewear designed to prevent exposure to body fluids is not adequate for removing patients from rubble piles in high dust environments. Face shields or glasses designed to offer splash protection may not be appropriate in situations in which dust or smoke can penetrate the sides of the glasses/shields. Safety goggles of the kind used in construction may be more appropriate, although they may be uncomfortable for prolonged periods, may fog, and can hinder peripheral vision.[7] Resources should be available for rinsing off glasses because dust and dirt particles can lead to scratched lenses, hindering visibility. Many medical responders are not issued hand protection that complies with Occupational Safety and Health Administration standards for protection from "absorption of harmful substances; severe cuts or lacerations; severe abrasions; punctures, chemical burns; and harmful temperature extremes."[15] Gloves designed to protect against bloodborne pathogens, even though appropriate for general patient care, should be worn underneath a more durable glove when operating in the multihazard environment often encountered in disaster situations; leather is not advised because it absorbs water and cannot be decontaminated. A glove that resists wear, cuts, and punctures but is pliable enough to provide treatment is necessary.

Relying on other agencies or resources to provide adequate equipment is not advised. The different agencies responding to disasters use a variety of brands and models of equipment, making compatibility with respirators, face masks, and cartridge filters not guaranteed. Responders should not use equipment offered by others without at least some training in its use (Box 31-2).

Debris Fields, Causing Fall or Trip Hazards

Most disasters, with the exception of chemical and biological exposures, will cause debris, often over large areas. Hurricanes may leave huge debris fields. Hurricane Andrew destroyed or damaged more than 130,000 homes, including 90% of all the mobile homes in Miami-Dade County.[16] This caused a huge debris field that had to be carefully negotiated by rescue workers. In the aftermath of the Murrah Building bombing, debris was piled 35 feet deep.[9] Debris may consist of wiring, pipes, pieces of concrete, and other building materials; is sharp; and may wear down protective clothing. The southeast Asia tsunami left debris fields kilometers deep along the coastline of the vast area it affected. Debris may need to be cleared to gain access to patients or set up treatment areas. Wind may cause debris to be blown about long after the initial disaster. Being on the lookout for responding apparatus or overhead hazards may cause responders to not look where they are going, resulting in injuries from trips and falls. It is imperative for responders to have a good light at all times, even if the initial response is during the day. Trying to navigate through debris after dark is a perilous operation, even with a light. Furthermore, it may be necessary to enter buildings that have lost power during the day. The penlights used in hospitals are not adequate for this purpose. Lights with disposable batteries or those that can be recharged if the responder has the charging device on hand are recommended. Units without rechargers will only be useful as long as they can be charged. The prolonged nature of disasters may preclude the responder from having the ability to retrieve the charging device.

Convergent Volunteers

Part of the healthcare ethos is the spirit of volunteerism. This is especially true in disasters. Responders want to help those in need, whether this is done in an organized fashion through disaster medical assistance teams (DMATs) or Salvation Army or Red Cross volunteers or through individuals who respond to the scene, often without any training or equipment. Responding agencies may have different protocols, equipment, and staffing configurations. Most of the official volunteer agencies at a disaster scene will be there due to a request for a response. Even though they may present logistical challenges, most usually do not present safety challenges. Failure to communicate between those on official response to the scene and those freelancing causes a breakdown in the ICS and may cause resources to be used in a haphazard manner, potentially endangering responders. Freelancers generally will not have radio communications with command centers or other responders, causing inadequate resource utilization. The response to an airliner crash in 1988 at the Dallas-Fort Worth airport demonstrated this point. Freelancing response units unfamiliar with the airport disaster plan set up a triage site outside the airport, causing responders to continue to look for patients and victims at the crash site who had already been evacuated.[6] Accountability for the safety of all on-scene also suffers when ISOs are unaware of all personnel operating on the scene. Accounting for all responders on-scene is also important in the event of postincident monitoring for hazardous exposures, as in the WTC disaster. There is evidence to

---

BOX 31-2 LEVEL D PPE FOR DISASTER RESPONSE UNDER HAZARDOUS CONDITIONS*

- Long-sleeve shirts
- Protective head gear to protect against falling debris or walking into objects
- Waterproof boots when there is the potential of rolling or falling objects or objects piercing the sole (steel toe boots may cause blistering after prolonged wear)
- Gloves that protect responders' hands from absorption of harmful substances, cuts, lacerations and punctures, and burns
- Eyewear with detachable side protection when there is exposure to dust or other harmful particles
- Battery-operated or rechargeable hand light if the charging unit is with the responder
- Foul weather gear
- Cold weather gear

* Not indicated for response to chemical, nuclear, biological, or radioactive incidents

suggest that most of the convergent volunteer organizations that respond as freelancers come without proper equipment, either pulling equipment out of the hospital that might be needed there or using equipment from other responders on-scene, neither of which is an optimal situation.[6] Volunteers cannot always be counted on for completing tasks, especially if they have not received proper training on how to do the task and are unfamiliar with terminology used by other responders.[10] Directions to volunteers should always be clear and easy to understand. In addition, the person issuing the directions should be certain the volunteer understands the task. For in-hospital personnel interested in responding to disasters outside the hospital, joining a professional group within a disaster section or other volunteer disaster medical organizations, such as the National Disaster Medical Service, is beneficial.[17] These organizations provide training and decrease the chance that volunteer responders will arrive unprepared, creating liability for others. Because volunteers at disasters are a fact of life, coordinating agencies should develop clear strategies for dealing with them and for integrating them into the response, delegating an individual in advance to have responsibility for managing the volunteers.[10]

Secondary Explosive Devices Planted by Terrorists

Every disaster or incident as a result of terrorism has the risk of secondary devices that can cause injury to medical personnel already on-scene. Two Atlanta area bombings in 1997, though not classified as disasters, are noteworthy for having secondary explosive devices: one at a family planning center where the secondary device exploded 1 hour after the first device exploded, injuring four public safety personnel from shrapnel and blast effects, and another at a lounge where the secondary device failed to explode (if it had, it would have injured responders in the vicinity).[18] In the WTC attacks, the second plane struck the south tower approximately 15 minutes after the north tower had been struck by the first plane; many responders were already on-scene by the time second plane struck.[7] Responders must always exercise caution for secondary devices in terrorism attacks, being on the lookout for strange packages or people in the disaster area who clearly have no readily identifiable purpose there. A plan for retreat or an understanding where safe zones are is essential during operations.

Prolonged Duration, Causing Excessive Fatigue, Lack of Sleep, and Inadequate Food and Hydration

Because of the long-term nature of disaster response, it is easy to get fatigued, not get adequate sleep, and not take the time to eat or drink appropriate amounts of fluids. Responders at Oklahoma City reported working shifts longer than 24 hours, with a deleterious effect on their scene awareness and judgment.[19] The Rand research indicates that responders have a tendency to do what their leaders do, and if the leaders do not take adequate

time for rest and rehabilitation, neither will their subordinates.[9] Disasters commonly require calling in off-duty personnel to take over operations when initial responders become fatigued.[10] It is recommended that all responders, including senior personnel, work no more than one 12-hour shift daily.[19] This may need to be adjusted down, depending on the working conditions. Having adequate food and drink nearby that are consistent with one's personal dietary habits is also important.

SCENE SAFETY AT THE DISASTER SITE

According to Garrison, "Avoiding danger is counterintuitive to rescuers."[20] Eliminating all hazards and risks associated with disaster medical response is impossible, and most EMS personnel know the job is dangerous at times. As can be seen in Table 31-1, disasters are complex situations, and every one is different. Therefore, the challenge in disaster response is to manage the risks by having an appropriate mechanism for understanding the dynamic nature of disaster operations. Managing risks is best done by using the safety management cycle (Fig. 31-1). It involves three functions that must be performed continuously throughout the incident: (1) gather information about the current situation, (2) analyze the available options and come up with decisions, and (3) implement decisions.[9] Gathering information at disaster sites is a challenge. The sharing of information across agencies is key to protecting those on-scene. The number of organizations responding to disasters, especially those caused by terrorism, is enormous, with one report citing 159 public-sector agencies responding to the Sept. 11, 2001, WTC disaster and another 290 organizations involved in the response.[21] Many of the different agencies involved in a typical response focus solely on their own organizational tasks and do not see how their activities fit into the big pictures. Auf der

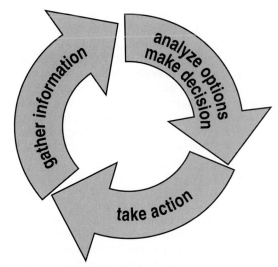

FIGURE 31–1. Safety management cycle. (Redrawn from Jackson B, Baker J, Ridgely M, et al. *Protecting Emergency Responders, Volume 3: Safety Management in Disaster and Terrorism Response.* Santa Monica, CA: The Rand Corporation, Science and Technology Policy Institute [for the National Institute for Occupational Safety and Health]; 2004.)

Heide[10] describes this as the "Robinson Crusoe syndrome," causing responders to believe "we're the only ones on the island." Many of these agencies may possess needed information on the hazards already encountered and hazards already mitigated, may have special expertise in disaster activities or risk assessment, and may possess information on the locations of victims, or resources needed by other groups, etc. Use of the ICS, covered in Chapter 30, is essential. It is this author's belief that in disaster activities, there is no single activity that can have a greater impact on scene safety than a properly functioning ICS, in which all agencies share information. Of equal importance, the incident commander must share all the appropriate information with those on-scene.

Because of the large geographical scale of many disasters, the ISO may not have an accurate picture of all the hazards present, especially if there is limited communication between all of the responding agencies, a common problem in most disaster situations. Medical organizations that routinely respond to disasters are encouraged to have their own safety officers or have one of their members appointed as an assistant ISO, with communications channels to the ISO. Using the NFPA's *Standard for Fire Department Safety Officer*[22] as a guideline, the role of the safety officer is to determine when activities are unsafe or involve significant hazards and then exercise the authority to immediately "alter, suspend, or terminate those activities." When the ISO determines that hazards or activities do not represent an immediate danger, the ISO "takes appropriate action through the incident commander to mitigate or eliminate the hazards."

Once the information has been gathered, the next step is to look at the options available and make a decision, taking into account as many variables as are known. For example, in the initial response of medical personnel to the scene of a disaster, patients requiring rescue may be present. Many victims may also present either self-rescued or rescued by other victims, requiring treatment. Taking the time to analyze the options may make responders realize that there are trained search and rescue personnel nearby and the available resources may be better used in setting up a treatment site first and leaving the rescue to personnel appropriately trained and equipped for the task. Once the decision is made, the next task is to follow through on the decision by taking action. The decision for any action related to safety must be communicated to all those within the immediate span of control and also up the chain of command to the incident commander. It is of great importance to know who is on-scene and how to communicate to them. As happens in many disasters, off-duty personnel will respond from home and therefore may not have adequate communications equipment (e.g., portable radios, pagers). Knowing where they are at a given moment may be a difficult task. If electronic communications are not possible, the use of runners is always an option and is often a good use of volunteers if communications to them are clear and concise.

Crew Resource Management for Safety

If a decision is made regarding safety, there must be an understanding in advance that good safety practices are not optional and that the action to be taken is mandatory for all within the scope of the organization. The ISO might ultimately make a safety decision, but reasonable input and discussion should take place with those involved on-scene. Crew resource management (CRM) for safety practices has been in existence for approximately 25 years. Originally called *cockpit resource management,* it came out of an examination by NASA of air crashes and the role that human error played in them. It has since been adopted for use in medicine, both in the training of emergency department, labor and delivery, and operating room staffs and air-medical operations.[23] The primary tenets of the training are to discuss how errors are caused and how operating in high-stress environments with high workloads, fatigue, and dealing with emergency situations contributes to errors. The principles of the training include seeking information by asking questions, advocating positions, communicating actions, and discussing and resolving conflicts. CRM is not something taught en route to or on-scene at a disaster; it is put into place during the preplanning and preparations phases of the disaster and may present a challenge to the medical community if not discussed in advance. For example, the medical director of an EMS agency must understand that a decision regarding safety applies to him or her as well, even if the decision is made by a safety officer who is a basic EMT. Obviously, safety concerns or mandates must be reasonable for the current conditions; mandating the wearing of safety helmets in a treatment center remote from where there is little risk of falling debris would not make much sense. The same mandate in an active incident area, where there is a chance of falling debris and therefore not allowing clinicians without adequate head protection to enter, would clearly be within the bounds of the safety officer. CRM also teaches that the same medical director just described should feel comfortable telling the ISO that he or she has noticed a crack in the building foundation and inquiring without risk of being ostracized whether it is safe for the treatment team to be there. As has been stressed here, disaster operations are not a static event; the hazards present 8 hours ago may have been dealt with or were determined to be unfounded, but those responsible for safety must constantly reassess the situation and gather new information, analyze the current options, and make new decisions, all of which may result in taking new actions. This safety management cycle must be repeated throughout the event until the incident is considered closed. Good preplanning and preparations before the actual response, with training that includes scene safety procedures, will reduce injuries.

Response to Disasters

Initial notification of a disaster may come in many ways—some informal, others formal. Hospitals may become aware of a disaster when the first patients arrive at the ED door. Public safety agencies may find out through a flood of phone calls to the public safety answering point (PSAP) or if the disaster directly affects the building they are located, such as if the dispatch building trembles from an earthquake. For many, the initial notification may be through media outlets; others will be directed to the scene via official dispatch. Once the decision is made that a response to the disaster is indicated, based on an official request of some sort for assistance, the first thoughts of the medical responder should be personal safety, and this should generate some questions:

- *What PPE will I likely need, and if I don't have it, where will I get it?* Expecting others to provide adequate PPE once you arrive on-scene, unless this has been prearranged, is a dangerous thought. The PPE that awaits you may be equipment you are unfamiliar with or the wrong size. At a minimum, responders should be equipped with appropriate Level D gear, including a safety helmet, adequate footwear, easily visible identification (e.g., reflective vests with skill level clearly stated on it), safety gloves, eye protection, a hand light, and equipment for bodily substance isolation precautions.
- *What hazards are likely to be present based on the location?* If responding to an industrial site, the presence of hazardous materials must always be suspected and different PPE or a different approach to the scene might be needed. If responding to an explosion, the concern over terrorism or secondary explosions must always be considered. Responses near water might require the use of personal flotation devices for responders. Practice an all-hazards approach with the expectation that there will be hazards on-scene, and be prepared to mitigate them.
- *Where am I going, and how do I get there?* If the incident is very large, such as Hurricane Andrew was, responders may be called in from great distances. On occasion, specialized resources (e.g., a surgical team) may get an escort directly to the scene. Badly needed specialized resources do not want to spend hours lost looking for an appropriate rendezvous point or the active incident, and the people on-scene may not have the time to wait. Know where you are going; if you do not, request an escort. Have maps, but keep in mind that local landmarks may have been destroyed. Take the time to download directions from an online map service; it is better to take 5 minutes to get detailed directions than to spend 1 hour trying to find the final destination.
- *Who will I report to when I get there?* If the ICS has not been established yet, then it may be more important to understand that as the first arriving unit, you will be expected to size up the scene and report the situation to the communications center instead of providing treatment to the first patients encountered. If the ICS has been set up, it is important to know who you are reporting to, where to find them, and let them know you have arrived. Updates on your situation are recommended every 30 minutes, unless other rules are in effect.

Scene Size-Up

Once the actual response is under way and regardless of whether response time is expected to be 30 minutes or 30 hours, try to get an update, if possible, of the current conditions on-scene. As responders approach the scene, they should begin determining the scope of the situation and continue to do so until preparing to depart the scene after disaster operations are completed. In the initial early minutes of the response, communications center personnel may be too busy receiving calls and dispatching units to be of much help, but even information being relayed to other units may be useful (e.g., traffic congestion or the presence of hazards). Responders must be vigilant for bystanders and victims fleeing the scene or curious onlookers running toward it. Once near the scene, responders must look and listen for other emergency responders because some who are heading to the scene may be unaware of your presence or where they are going. Responders should look for signs of power outages, which could indicate downed power lines, and look for smoke or fumes.[24,26] If being transported to the scene by someone from another agency, the responder should not assume that the person operating the vehicles has more knowledge about scene safety than himself or herself; throughout disaster operations, one must take responsibility for one's own safety.

As the responder gets closer to the scene, the presence of odors may indicate chemicals, fire, or other hazardous materials. One must quickly make an assessment whether hazardous materials are evident and if they pose a direct hazard, either as a by-product or the direct cause of the disaster, so that the responder does not end up as a victim.[26] The U.S. Department of Transportation's *2000 Emergency Response Guidebook*[25] is a very good field resource for responders who believe there is a danger of hazardous materials present.

As discussed, downed power lines are a common and deadly hazard. If the power is out and you observe damaged poles, count the number of wires at the damaged poles and then at the next undamaged pole down the line. If the number of lines atop the damaged pole is the same, there is a good chance the lines are intact.[25] On arrival at the actual disaster scene, even before the vehicle comes to a stop, a decision will need to be made about where to park the vehicle. Vehicles should park upwind and uphill if possible to avoid toxic fumes or smoke. Scanning for the direction that flags or smoke are blowing may be good indicators of wind direction. Typically, emergency vehicles will try to get as close to the area as possible. Events at the WTC indicate that this may not be the wisest approach. One witness reported seeing a row of 15 ambulances, stating, "They were crushed, completely gutted by falling debris."[3] If a vehicle is not likely to be needed for emergency transport of patients and if it does not have needed supplies, PPE, or communications equipment, it should be relocated to another location safely away from the scene. If it does have needed equipment, consider offloading the equipment and having the vehicle relocate to a safe location. Other vehicles may also be vying for the same space you are occupying and may be more urgently needed; an example would be an aerial ladder truck for rescue efforts. If there are burning vehicles, response units should park no closer than 100 feet from any of them to minimize explosion hazards or the risk of being exposed to leaking fuel.[26]

Lookouts, Communications, Escape Routes, Safety Zones

Wildland firefighters and urban search and rescue technicians use an easy-to-remember system that can be adapted for disaster operations, known as LCES (*l*ookouts, *c*ommunications, *e*scape routes, and *s*afety zones).[11,27] Being a lookout is normally the function of the ISO, but due to the scope of a disaster, the ISO may not be in proximity to all operations or not all responders may have communications with the ISO. In the event there are hazards present, it is important to have an individual who has good visual access to the operations and is not involved in patient care as a lookout, or site-specific safety officer. This person should be free to watch over the operation; identify hazards or potential hazards; and if appropriate, mitigate them. He or she must be readily identified, either by his or her location or by wearing a vest identifying him or her as a lookout or safety officer.

Communications should be established on arrival, not only with the incident commander but also with dispatch centers. On arrival, an exact location should be established for responding teams. This may be difficult if street signs have been destroyed, but it is imperative for all assets to have known locations. Using easily identifiable landmarks, such as buildings in the area, can be of assistance. For example, stating "we are on the south side of the lake" is not an exact location, but it can be useful. Global positioning system devices can be of great assistance in establishing location.

Radios may not be functioning, may be overloaded with emergency traffic, or may not have common frequencies, and the use of runners may be necessary. The lookout or communications person should be alert for other forms of communications that may be used at disaster sites. Search and rescue technicians use an emergency alerting system that consists of an air horn or siren to be used in the event of emergencies:

- Three short blasts of one second each is an indication to evacuate.
- One long, 3-second blast means to cease operations or work noiselessly.
- One long blast and one short blast means to resume operations.

Depending on the nature of the disaster, it may be important to determine escape routes in advance of needing them. During rescue operations at the Oklahoma City bombing, there were three bomb scares, causing evacuation of the treatment areas.[13] Personnel or vehicles may become trapped in a location by other responders and may need to relocate. On occasion, the shortest route to safety may not be the most direct, as in the case of a building collapse in which the shortest route to safety may direct one into the collapse zone. Clearly in this event a more circuitous route may be the safest.

The establishment of safe zones may be important in disasters where the risk of ongoing hazards is great. The safe zone is an area determined to be relatively safe from hazards and might be an area removed from collapsed or damaged buildings, an area remote from hot or warm zones in hazardous materials incidents, or an area where additional measures have been taken to increase building structural integrity. If team members are evacuated to the safe zone, a head count should be the first task done when members arrive to ensure that all members are accounted for.

PITFALLS

A lot has been learned about responder safety since Sept. 11, 2001. The Rand/NIOSH collaboration has brought great resources to emergency managers for keeping all responders safer.[2,7-9] Measures are being put into place to keep better data about medical responder injuries at all incidents, but there are still pitfalls in all of this. Disaster medical services are provided by many organizations, with different standards. The federal government should determine a standard of safety for emergency medical response, as has been done with firefighting through the NFPA. Research is essential; journal articles and educational materials help keep the subject in the spotlight. The Rand studies illustrate the problem with designing PPE that allows medical responders to do their jobs safely. Complacency is the major pitfall to all of this, and if it does not turn into action, medical responders will still face injury or death while responding to disasters. Standards, PPE, and training must be implemented while disasters such as the WTC and the southeast Asia tsunami are still fresh in our minds.

REFERENCES

1. Maguire BJ, Hunting KL, Smith GS, et al. Occupational fatalities in emergency medical services: a hidden crisis. *Ann Emerg Med.* 2002;40:625-32.
2. Houser AN, Jackson BA, Bartis JT, Peterson DJ. *Emergency Responder Injuries and Fatalities: An Analysis of Surveillance Data.* Santa Monica, CA: The Rand Corporation; 2004.
3. 9-11 attack on America: united we respond. *EMS Insider.* 2001;28:1-8.
4. Joint Commission on Accreditation of Healthcare Organizations. *Guide to Emergency Management Planning in Health Care.* Oakbrook Terrace, IL: Joint Commission Resources; 2002.
5. Martinez C, Gonzalez D. The World Trade Center attack. Doctors in the fire and police services. *Crit Care.* 2001;5(6):304-6.
6. Green W. Freelance response to the site—medical staff option of choice? American Academy of Medical Administrators. Spring 2003. Available at: http://www.aameda.org/MemberServices/Exec/Articles/spg03/freelance-%20Green.pdf.
7. Jackson B, Peterson DJ, Bartis J, et al. *Protecting Emergency Responders: Lessons Learned from Terrorist Attacks.* Santa Monica, CA: The Rand Corporation; 2002.
8. Latourrette T, Peterson DJ, Bartis J, Jackson BA, Houser A. *Protecting Emergency Responders, Vol 2: Community Views of Safety and Health Risks and Personal Protection Needs.* Santa Monica, CA: The Rand Corporation; 2003.
9. Jackson B, Baker J, Ridgely M, Bartis JT, Linn HI. *Protecting Emergency Responders, Vol 3: Safety Management in Disaster and Terrorism Response.* Santa Monica, CA: The Rand Corporation; 2004
10. Auf der Heide E. Disasters are different. In: Auf der Heide E, ed. *Disaster Response: Principles of Preparation and Coordination.* St Louis: Mosby; 1989.
11. Federal Emergency Management Agency, US&R. Structural collapse technician course—student manual. Available at: http://www.fema.gov/usr/sctc.shtm.

12. Physical health status of World Trade Center rescue and recovery workers and volunteers—New York City, July 2002—August 2004. *Morb Mortal Wkly Rep.* 2004;53(35):807-12.

13. FEMA urban search and rescue (USAR) summaries. In: Smith C, ed. *Alfred P. Murrah Federal Building Bombing April 19, 1995 Final Report.* Stillwater, OK: Fire Protection Publications; 1996.

14. National Fire Protection Association. *NFPA 1999: Standard on Protective Clothing for Emergency Medical Operations.* Quincy, MA: National Fire Protection Association; 2003.

15. US Department of Labor, Occupational Safety and Health Administration. Inspection guidelines for 29 CFR 1910. Subpart 1, the revised Personal Protective Equipment Standards for General Industry. Available at: http://www.osha.gov/pls/oshaweb/owadisp. show_document?p_table=DIRECTIVES&p_id=1790.

16. Florida Division of Emergency Management. Introductory statement to the inaugural meeting of the state Hazard Mitigation Plan Advisory Team. Available at: http://www.floridadisaster.org/brm/ state-mitigation-strategy/shmpat/introductory-statement.htm.

17. US Department of Homeland Security, National Disaster Medical System. DMAT: Questions & answers. Available at: http://www. ndms.dhhs.gov/dmat_faq.html.

18. Eric Rudolph charged in Centennial Park bombing [press release]. Washington, DC: US Department of Justice; October 14, 1998.

19. US Department of Homeland Security, Lessons Learned Information Sharing. Setting and enforcing maximum shift lengths at incident sites. Available at: http://www.llis.gov/member/secure/getfile.cfm/ LL%202D%20setting%20and%20enforcing%2epdf?ID=6656.

20. Garrison H. Keeping rescuers safe. *Ann Emerg Med.* 2002; 40(6)633-5.

21. Lyman F. *Messages in the Dust: What Are the Lessons of the Environmental Health Response to the Terrorist Attacks of September 11?* Washington DC: National Environmental Health Association; 2003.

22. National Fire Protection Association. *NFPA 1521: Standard for Fire Department Safety Officer.* Quincy, MA: National Fire Protection Association; 2002.

23. Agency for Healthcare Research and Quality. Making Health Care Safer: A Critical Analysis of Patient Safety Practices. Evidence Report, Technology Assessment No. 43. Available at: http://www.ahrq.gov/clinic/ptsafety.

24. Borak J, Callan M, Abbott W. Hazardous materials exposure. Englewood Cliffs, NJ: Brady; 1991:8.

25. US Department of Transportation Research and Special Projects Administration. *2000 Emergency Response Guidebook.* Neenah WI: J.J. Keller and Associates; 2000.

26. Limmer D, O'Keefe M. *Emergency Care.* 10th ed. Upper Saddle River, NJ: Brady; 2005:180-4.

27. US Department of Agriculture, Fire and Aviation Management Division. LCES: Lookouts-Communications-Escape Routes-Safety Zones. Available at: http://www.fs.fed.us/fire/safety/lces/lces.html.

chapter 32

Needs Assessment

Shan W. Liu

Development of the field of needs assessment, or rapid surveillance, has been critical to improving the efficiency and effectiveness of public health interventions. Needs assessments have served organizations on all levels—local, state, and federal—as the essential foundation for policy and program development and resource allocation. In fact, needs assessment, along with policy development and assurance, is one of the core functions of public health.[1]

Disaster medicine is no different in terms of the critical role that needs assessment plays in maximizing appropriate response. In sudden-impact disasters, the most effective efforts to minimize mortality are based on very specific, precisely targeted interventions against demonstrated causes of death.[2,3] Too often, relief responses are based on intuition rather than data. Disaster needs assessments can be used to understand the impact of disasters on public health and the infrastructure of the medical system, enabling the relief community to respond much more effectively. The purpose of a needs assessment is to rapidly survey a postdisaster situation, provide data describing the magnitude of the extent of the emergency, and alert the relief community so that appropriate interventions can be mobilized and certain assets brought to the scene. In essence, it attempts to bring order to the chaos that results from a disaster.[2] By necessity, needs assessments must be performed even as emergency services are being provided.[4] These assessments provide a medium for advocacy that ensures that the response to a disaster is not just what pleases donor political constituents, but addresses the real problems of the affected community.[5] It is the goal of this chapter to introduce the main components of and rationale behind disaster rapid needs assessment.

HISTORICAL PERSPECTIVE

Historically, the perception has been that charity manages relief efforts, in which groups or individuals provide supplies and efforts, regardless of the needs of the situation. Consequentially, the health response to emergencies in the past usually was ad hoc, inappropriate, and inefficient.[6]

The introduction of disaster needs assessments may have started with the practical application of epidemiology during the massive international relief operations in response to the Nigerian civil war in the 1960s. Centers for Disease Control and Prevention epidemiologists developed new techniques for the rapid assessment of nutritional states as well as for conducting surveys. However, widespread implementation of such techniques lagged behind in disaster relief efforts. By the 1970s, the need for disaster epidemiology was evident. Directors of major relief efforts doubled as managers and planners and often lacked sufficient public health experience to successfully respond to major catastrophes. Disaster scenes continued to be cluttered by outdated, unlabeled, and inappropriate medications.

The 1980 Mount St. Helens' disaster served as a historical milestone in terms of shaping the way the federal government responds to disasters, particularly regarding coordination between multiple levels of government agencies. Epidemiological research subsequently became central to targeting strategies according to the needs of the disaster, leading to more appropriate responses and resulting in decreased mortality and morbidity from disasters. By the late 1980s and into the 1990s, interest in the public health of disasters accelerated, notably with the emergence of new professional societies and scientific forums.[7]

CURRENT PRACTICE

Although each particular disaster merits a specific needs assessment, the World Health Organization (WHO) has designed rapid health assessment protocols for common emergencies. In general, the major steps of a rapid health assessment include description of purpose, preparedness, planning, conducting the assessment, analysis of data, and presentation of results.[8] The main priorities are to determine the location of the problem, the magnitude of the crisis, and the immediate priorities.[2]

Before addressing the many steps involved in conducting a needs assessment, two major questions to be asked and answered are: Who performs the needs assessment, and who receives the reports? Ideally, such a project would be performed by an agency that will ultimately implement the relief program. A team should consist of interdisciplinary staff trained in collection of accurate and precise data, such as an epidemiologist, statistician, engineer, and health planner. Such a team should also have members from the host country and/or community as well as from local nongovernment groups, as deemed appropriate.[9]

A critical aspect of performing a needs assessment is directing the report to the appropriate audience. The main recipient will, of course, be the agency that sponsors the survey. However, it is imperative to keep in mind that such information should be dispersed as widely as possible. Hence, the audience will undoubtedly include survivors, nongovernment organizations (NGO), United Nations agencies, donor governments, and media representatives. Each group will have varying roles and consequentially differing informational needs.

Purpose

In disasters, the rapid assessment entails collecting subjective and objective data that measure damage and identify the critical needs of the affected community to design appropriate, immediate response priorities. By virtue of being a rapid assessment, it must be performed in a limited amount of time, either during or immediately after the emergency phase. Ongoing assessments will need to be performed during the rehabilitation and recovery phases of the disaster.[2]

The major parts of a needs assessment are as follows[8,9]:

- Confirm emergency
- Describe type, impact, possible evolution of disaster
- Alert international community to gravity of situation
- Measure present and potential health impact
- Assess adequacy of current response capacity and immediate needs
- Recommend immediate response

Being mindful of the main parts of needs assessments will help focus efforts and preparedness.

Preparedness

Though impossible to plan for all potential disasters, it is imperative that health systems have at least basic infrastructures in place to be able to immediately implement an appropriate rapid assessment and response. Disaster preparedness includes the following:

- Training and evaluation
- Monitoring
- Emergency planning
- Vulnerability assessment

Most of the preparation entails anticipation of needs and organizing a response system that can be quickly deployed when emergencies arise. According to WHO rapid health assessment protocols, emergency preparedness ought to include the following questions:

- Does a national health policy exist regarding emergency preparedness, response, and recovery?
- Who is the person within the ministry of health in charge of emergency preparedness?
- What type of coordination exists between the health sector, civil defense, and other key government ministries?

- What type of coordination exists between ministries of health, the United Nations, and NGOs?
- What operational plans exist for disasters?
- Do national and local health plans exist for disaster management?
- Are surveillance measures in place that can detect early signs of disasters?
- Have environmental health services taken preparedness steps?
- Have facilities and areas been identified to serve as shelter sites?
- What training activities exist for disaster preparedness? Who is involved? Have disaster drills been administered?
- What resources exist to facilitate rapid response to disaster (e.g., emergency budget, supplies)?
- Does a system exist for updating information on key human and material resources needed in a disaster?

Even though each disaster situation requires its own rapid needs assessment, the most effective disaster efforts begin with proper preparedness and planning, long before any disaster occurs.[8]

Planning

On hearing reports or even rumors of a disaster, the preparedness checklist should be updated. However, different types of disasters will require varying timeframes for response. Rapid-onset emergencies (e.g., earthquakes) require immediate assessment within hours of the event. On the other hand, assessment in floods and population displacement emergencies can be done within 2 to 4 days.

With disaster emergencies, there are generally four main stages included in the planning of rapid needs assessment:

- *Stage I (day 1):* Generally when the local community responds to the crisis with little to no information. Initial injury and death estimates are necessary within 24 hours, as a preliminary guide to which resources will be needed.
- *Stage II (day 2):* Largely entails focusing the rapid assessment on resources needed in less accessible areas; shortages in primary healthcare resources; and secondary needs, such as shelter, food, and water. It is at this time that needs for additional aid, such as national or international assistance, should be assessed.
- *Stage III (days 3-5):* Securing shelter and restoring primary healthcare become essential. As such, the assessment focuses more on environmental health, food, special protection, and the restoration of primary health facilities for vulnerable groups.
- *Stage IV (after day 5):* By this time, disaster responses should be fully implemented. The assessment at this point should be focused on establishing a surveillance system and analyzing health trends.

Final preparation includes deciding what information to gather, coordinating different organizations, selecting team members and leaders, and delegating administrative assignments. Team members should include those with familiarity of the region and population affected, experience with the type of emergency, epidemiological analytical skills, and the capacity to make decisions with sparse data. Logistics, such as travel clearance, transportation, safety protocols, and developing communications systems, must also be addressed before conducting the assessment.

Conducting the Assessment

The specific information gathered during the immediate emergency phase of the disaster should include the following[2]:

- Establishing the boundaries of the affected area.
- Identifying transportation issues on main routes to affected areas.
- Identifying major threats to survivors (e.g., landslides, damage to chemical plants).
- Determining damage to broadcasting facilities.
- Determining needs for establishing/restoring communications between major responders.
- Assigning surveyors first to areas where there have been no reports received.
- Assessing the status of hospitals—specifically regarding access to affected areas, damage to hospital structures, operational capability, and availability of personnel and essential equipment.
- Beginning to survey isolated and severely affected communities and assess adequacy of treatment of injured people in those areas.
- Prioritizing areas that need organized search and rescue efforts.
- Assessing level of damage to air-traffic centers—runways, fuel storage, etc.
- Reviewing government stockpiles of accessible essential items.
- Assessing integrity of lifeline services in order of priority: communications, water supply, electric power, road networks, and sewage system.

Rapid surveillances must be systematic and neutral.[5] Despite having to conduct an assessment during the chaos of a disaster, it is imperative that data collection and analysis be performed in a standardized fashion. The four main types of information collection methods are: (1) review of existing data, (2) inspection of affected area, (3) key informant interviews, and (4) rapid surveys. When reviewing existing data, government and international and national NGOs may be sources of information regarding the geographical characteristics of the area, the size and prior health status of the community, and the existing health services. They can also serve as resources for an emergency response operation.

Inspection of the area can be accomplished by air and/or on the ground. Aerial assessments are most helpful in determining the extent of the area affected and conditions of the infrastructure and environment. Group assessments will provide a better sense of shelter and food availability, potential hazards, and a gross sense of the size and type of population affected. Whether by air or ground, observations from the initial inspection should be used to create maps that include the area affected and location of pertinent resources, such as health facilities, water sources, shelter, and food distribution sites.[8] Another vital aspect of aerial inspection is to estimate a reliable denominator. Since rates depend on a somewhat accurate estimate of the population at risk, estimates of population counts (i.e., house counts multiplied by average family size) can be used as an initial estimate of the denominator.[6]

Key informant interviews should be conducted from each sector of the affected community and are central to the assessment. These interviews will include community leaders, local government officials, health workers, and personnel from other emergency response groups. The information from these informants should include the following:

- Subject's perception of the event
- Previous condition of the area
- Size of the affected community
- Adequacy of security, prevalence of violence
- Estimated morbidity and mortality rates
- Existing food supplies and needs (e.g., approximately 1900 to 2100 kcal/person/day)
- Supply and quality of water (e.g., generally 15 L clean water/person/day)
- Adequacy of sanitation (e.g., 1 latrine per 20 persons)
- Existing fuel and communications lines
- Existing resources in community

Although key informant interviews can rapidly provide information, surveyors should always keep in mind that such data are likely to be exaggerated.[8,9]

Aside from inspection of the area and key informant interviews, surveys are central to accurate situational assessments. However, although rapid surveys are likely to be less biased, they take more time and resources. Hence, surveys should be conducted when the information cannot be reliably obtained from other sources. Some of the more common methods of rapid surveillance during disasters are the following: sentinel surveillance, sampling methods, and detailed critical sector assessments.

Sentinel Surveillance

This method is largely used when professional staff create a reporting system that detects early signs of particular problems at certain sites. This is particularly useful during the early warning phase.

Surveys by Specialist Teams (Sampling Methods)

Well-designed surveys from reliable samples allow researchers to confidently generalize findings and apply them to a larger population. There are multiple methods for sampling:

- *Simple random sampling:* When every member of the population at risk is equally likely to be selected and such selection has no effect on other selections.
- *Systematic random sampling:* Choosing every 20th subject, for example, on a list. This is potentially inaccurate if the list is nonrandom or incomplete.

- *Stratified random sampling:* Divide the population into strata, randomly select subjects, and then combine them to give an overall sample.
- *Cluster sampling:* Samples are restricted to a limited number of geographical areas, called clusters. For each geographical area selected, randomly sample and then combine to give an overall sample.

Detailed Critical Sector Assessments by Specialists

This is necessary for evaluations of water supply and electric power and can be performed by staff from within or outside of these systems.[2]

Assessing the effect of a disaster on health entails addressing injuries, missing persons, illnesses, and death rates. Rapid assessment of primary injuries should estimate the number of persons injured and the severity, types, and sites of injuries. Primary injuries are those that are the result of the disaster itself, whereas secondary injuries occur during the postimpact phase of a disaster, such as injuries related to the clean-up. Analysis of where survivors seek care for such injuries provides one major data source.

The severity of a disaster is also closely related to the number of persons missing. Though difficult to obtain precise numbers, preliminary data can come from families as well as estimates from search teams, such as the fire department.

Even though communicable diseases are relatively rare in the immediate days after a disaster, surveyors should identify pathogens already present and pose a danger of spreading. Assessors should also design a preliminary plan for the best measures for disease control.

In emergencies, mortality is usually limited to reports of bodies recovered. Data should also include age- and sex-specific death rates, causes, and risk factors.[8] For example, in complex humanitarian situations, crude mortality rates (CMR) can be measured by designating a burial site and using guards to count burials. Death rates should usually be reported as per 10,000 per day. Generally speaking, rates for emergencies such as humanitarian crises are approximately 0.4 to 0.6 deaths per 10,000 per day. A rate greater than 1.0 is considered elevated, and a rate of more than 2.0 is considered critical.[9] Rapid-onset disasters will obviously have more front-end mortality rates.

Besides assessing the effect of a disaster on health, evaluating the potential effect on health services is also important. The top priority is determining the extent of damage to medical services and which medical facilities are still functioning. Surveyors should gather data regarding location and type of facilities, structural integrity postevent, capacity, injuries and deaths of staff, and any gaps in personnel or supplies. If time permits, data should also be collected concerning injuries treated at facilities, the need to evacuate patients for specialized care, and the types of medicines and other supplies most urgently needed.

Beyond health assessment, surveyors must also examine the integrity of the environmental situation postimpact. Analysis of water supply, sanitation, shelter, and transport is essential. Adequate supply of clean water is of paramount importance, so particular attention should be made to estimate the size of communities without water, potentially contaminated sources of water, and the magnitude of damage to water supplies.

Challenges

Most assuredly, those performing rapid assessments face large obstacles. There may be blocked access to restricted areas, physical danger, nonstandardized reporting, and inaccurate baseline information.[4] Data are usually collected rapidly under extremely adverse conditions, and sources of information must be integrated.[7] Given the constraints of time, pressure, and limited initial research resources, it is likely that more accurate data will be collected during later phases, such as rehabilitation and recovery. Hence, needs assessment has to be an ongoing procedure.[10] Consequently, those reviewing the information must understand the data-gathering methodologies, their inherent limitations, and sources of bias.[2]

Analyzing and Presenting Data

Data analysis should be performed with the use of standard techniques to ensure comparability with other situations. Analysis should be as specific as possible to facilitate the design of appropriate interventions. Presentation of data should be done in a standardized manner, with results that clearly indicate the greatest priorities for the response organization. All results should be widely distributed so that information can be verified and/or complemented. In general, the following format can be used as a standard for a presentation[8]:

- Reason for emergency
- Area affected
- Description of community affected, including injuries and deaths
- Impact of disaster (e.g., daily mortality, financial losses projected)
- Existing resources
- Additional requirements—immediate, medium, and long term

Despite the time constraints and difficulty in collecting data under chaotic environments, it is imperative that final analysis and presentation be as clear as possible, given that relief funding and response will directly result from how the data are reported.

PITFALLS

One major challenge of rapid needs assessment is finding a suitable body or organization with sufficient credibility or authority to disseminate the information and to ensure that the humanitarian response reflects the findings of the assessment. If assessments are not properly linked with decision makers, they are reduced to mere hospital records rather than critical information. Such surveys need credibility and coordination with other agencies to avoid duplicated efforts. A major pitfall is that they are often performed too late, and as a result, their findings may be ignored. A second pitfall is that they are often performed by those without appropriate skills.[5] Poor data collection and analysis are possibly worse than no data at all. A third pitfall is when assessment focuses on areas thought to be most affected instead of taking an overview of the entire area. This is problematic in two ways: first, the sites thought to be worst off may not actually be the most affected. Secondly, by focusing on the hardest-hit areas, there will be biased reporting and subsequent miscalculation of mortality. In general, bias can be a serious problem in rapid needs assessments during disasters. Sample sizes are often too small and not random. Furthermore, obtaining information based on hospitals or clinics can be misleading because those who seek care may not be the ones who actually need care the most because many in need cannot or do not visit health facilities.[6]

Standardized disaster surveillance algorithms have great potential to rapidly identify the acute needs of populations in the midst of disasters and to direct resources to areas most in need during the response and recovery phases.[11] Though such assessments are conducted amidst the upheaval of a disaster, it is imperative that experienced surveyors take a rational, systematic approach to their surveillance. It is such information that will ultimately guide intervention immediately and for future disasters, thereby directly contributing to the prevention of morbidity and mortality.

REFERENCES

1. Petersen D, Alexander G. *Needs Assessment in Public Health: A Practical Guide for Students and Professionals.* New York: Kluwer Academic; 2001.
2. Stephenson RS. *Disaster Assessment. Disaster Management Training Programme.* 2nd ed. United Nations Development Programme/Office of the United Nations Disaster Relief Coordinator; 1994.
3. Gregg M. Surveillance and epidemiology. In: *The Public Health Consequences of Disasters 1989.* CDC Monograph. Atlanta: US Department of Health and Human Services; September 1989.
4. Briggs S, ed. *Advanced Disaster Medical Response Manual for Providers.* Boston: Harvard Medical International Trauma and Disaster Institute; 2003.
5. O'Toole M. Medical and public health needs: the role of the rapid assessment. Presented at: Proceedings of the First Harvard Symposium on Complex Humanitarian Disasters; April 10-11, 1995; Boston.
6. Guha-Sapir D. Rapid assessment of health needs in mass emergencies: review of current concepts and methods. *World Health Stat Q.* 1991;44(3):171-81.
7. Noji E, ed. *The Public Health Consequences of Disasters.* New York: Oxford University Press; 1997.
8. World Health Organization. *Rapid Health Assessment Protocols for Emergencies.* Geneva: WHO; 1999.
9. Leaning J, Briggs S, Chen L. *Humanitarian Crises.* Cambridge, MA: Harvard University Press; 1999.
10. Auf der Heide E. *Disaster Response: Principles of Preparation and Coordination.* St. Louis: Mosby; 1989.
11. Lillibridge SR. Disaster assessment: the emergency health evaluation of a population affected by a disaster. *Ann Emerg Med.* November 1993;22:1715-20.

chapter 33

Disaster Communications

Khama D. Ennis-Holcombe

Facilitating efficient and effective communications is integral to the success of disaster management. Preparations for proper communications should begin long before the first "911" telephone call is made by anticipating and exploring potential communications needs. Communications infrastructure must then be established and tested before it is implemented.

The planning necessary for medical facilities to provide adequate communications in the event of a disaster or mass casualty incident is described in this chapter.

HISTORICAL PERSPECTIVE

At one time, the U.S. government's response to disasters involved dozens of federal agencies handling various individual components. Communications planning was rarely addressed explicitly. Instead, often the assumption was that existing communications infrastructure would be sufficient.

In 1979, President Jimmy Carter created the Federal Emergency Management Agency (FEMA) to coordinate domestic disaster response. Although FEMA represented a consolidation of response efforts, communications planning initially was not directly addressed. Furthermore, disaster management remained largely focused on natural catastrophes, such as hurricanes and earthquakes, or unintentional manmade events, including oil spills and radiation leaks.[1]

With the terrorist attacks of Sept. 11, 2001, the United States experienced unprecedented challenges in domestic disaster management, including a substantial strain on its communications systems. Within minutes of the first plane hitting the World Trade Center, the New York City Police Department established command central in a conference room at Bellevue Hospital's emergency department and began coordinating with emergency medical services. As the media and public picked up on events, telephone lines became jammed and connections were unreliable. Additionally, the Emergency Operations Center that had been designed to handle large-scale disasters affecting New York City was evacuated and most of its structures were destroyed; it had been located at 7 World Trade Center.[2] Communications within the emergency department grew difficult as misinformation

regarding the attacks circulated. Police and administrators were able to correspond through direct conversation, radios, and pagers; however, cell phones and land lines remained unreliable.

In the wake of Sept. 11, many changes have taken place in U.S. disaster management. The Department of Homeland Security was established, bringing FEMA under its auspices. With this reorganization, the conception of disasters has been expanded to focus on intentional terrorist acts, and greater attention has been paid to establishing and protecting emergency communications infrastructure.[3]

CURRENT PRACTICE

There are numerous means of communicating during emergencies, including the standard systems at given facilities and backup resources.[4]

The National Incident Management System (NIMS) was approved in March 2004 as a means to coordinate first responder disaster management between federal, state, and local levels.[5,6] One goal of NIMS is to ensure that the systems necessary for disaster management are in place so that time is not lost devising a plan during a time of need. One of the cornerstones of the communications guidelines is that local systems comply with national interoperable communications standards. A system that works perfectly in one area but cannot interact successfully with neighboring areas and additional agencies is likely to be of limited use. Local systems should be able to fit into a larger scheme of communications when needs exceed local capabilities to interface with expanded disaster response.

There are multiple formats for regional emergency response systems. In most situations, a 911 telephone call is routed through a public safety answering point (PSAP), sometimes at the police department, before being referred to the agency or agencies that will provide initial response, including fire, police, and emergency medical services.[7] These systems use technologies for their operations, including a radio and telephone with originator site localization. The location from which a call is being made is immediately available, with the exception of many cellular phone calls. First responders can be notified immediately, and hospitals also can be notified of potential patients.

Hospitals with emergency departments have means by which ambulances can call in entry notifications. Such calls can be placed while ambulances are en route and allow the facility time to prepare for the patient. In most areas, this communication is based on radio transmissions on ultra high frequency (UHF) and very high frequency (VHF) that are broadcast via radio towers located at specific sites throughout a service region. CMED (Coordinated Medical Emergency Direction) is one such system in operation in Massachusetts and Connecticut. UHF and VHF systems both vary widely. For example, a 24-watt transmitter can transmit signals up to a distance of 50 miles; however, this distance can be increased substantially by a relay tower, and most towers in use are much more powerful.

Medical facility plans are initiated from the moment of disaster notification, based on the patients that may present. A designated regional hierarchy for command and a location for command central will enhance communications efficiency for individual medical facilities. In some systems, the role of incident commander (IC) is fulfilled by the highest-ranked person within the first unit to respond. Within an emergency department, the person in charge may be the most senior attending physician present. Communication and coordination with other local medical facilities are priorities for the IC to ensure the best care for patients.

In addition to establishing a hierarchy, it is also essential to clarify the means by which information will be relayed. This includes communications within any given institution and between multiple institutions and agencies. Within a hospital, for example, there are means to alert the chiefs of each department of potential disasters. Overhead announcements are often possible, but text paging is a simpler and arguably better means of communicating this is information. A list of key personnel is distributed to page operators, and in the event of a disaster, a single message can be sent to all parties via a group page. This is an approach that requires advance discussion and preparation but one that can save considerable time and minimize confusion. Text paging may also be an effective means of communication within individual departments.

The IC will assign roles to senior staff present. Areas to be addressed should include the following:

- Media communications
- Interfacility communications
- Intrafacility/interdepartmental communications
- Emergency department medical care
- Transfer of stabilized patients out of the emergency department
- Communications between the emergency department and the hospital command center

One person is often assigned to supervise and coordinate each of these tasks. In many cases, hospitals already have public relations staff members who handle media communications so that the main focus of practitioners can remain on patient care. Additionally, the local IC must be able to maintain two-way communication with the disaster site. Information that should be prioritized in such communications includes emergency department capacity, hospital capacity, and potential hazards.

Interfacility communications may provide relief when a disaster overwhelms a medical facility. E-mail, telephone, and radio communications are excellent means by which hospitals can maintain contact and ensure that patient care is optimally coordinated. For example, if two hospitals are fairly close in location, specific patients may be directed to the site that is best equipped to manage their presenting concerns. In another scenario, if evidence of potential hazards to caretakers becomes apparent at one facility, it is essential that other facilities at risk be notified. This is especially important, given increasing concerns about biological, chemical, and radiological weapons.

A robust intrahospital communications system is beneficial to normal hospital operations in the absence of disaster. These systems may be used to facilitate movement of patients in the hospital and assist in coordinating tasks that could increase overall efficiency of operations.

Whether a disaster is natural or manmade, it may present enormous stress for all response workers involved. Accurate communications regarding the status of events can serve to minimize confusion. Even though effective communication should be a goal in any workplace, it is crucial in disaster management.

All pathways of communication should be designed to function both up and down the chain of command. Nurses, residents, and physicians should be able to discuss trends or concerns regarding patients with their supervisors, who can then relay these details to superiors to avoid loss of valuable information.

Also a link in the loop of communications and information-gathering is the patients themselves. Patient populations, including the methods of communication that they are most likely to use for health systems information, are elements that require consideration in communication plans.[8] During the August 1999 earthquake in Turkey, which left more than 17,000 people dead, one needs assessment team found that 81% of the population relied on word of mouth for communications, and (only) 23% relied on public address systems, 20% on television, and 15% on radio.[9]

PITFALLS AND STRATEGIES

There are many resources available to reinforce health systems communications. The Centers for Disease Control and Prevention has established the Health Alert Networks, which aims to ensure high-speed Internet access for local health officials, increase capacity for secure communications, improve early warning broadcast alert systems, and optimize general organizational capacity of local systems.

To allow for the efficient transmission of airwaves, radio towers require a degree of unobstructed space; this lack of obstruction makes them difficult to protect. Even though this type of infrastructure presents a vulnerability, strategic duplication of radio towers may serve as a buffer in the event of distress.

If a local system is overwhelmed by the scope of a disaster, federal backup is available. FEMA has established Mobile Emergency Response Support (MERS) systems to provide support throughout the United States. In this system, the country is divided into 10 regions. Mobile units are located in each region and can provide assistance in the form of telecommunications with satellite, line of sight microwave, and radio (high frequency [HF], UHF, and VHF) communications as well as generators in the event of power failure. HF radio is used to communicate with federal, state, and local emergency centers via the FEMA National Radio Network and FEMA Regional Radio Network. VHF and UHF can be used for local radio communications.[10]

In addition to these established systems, in California, there is also a reserve radio system, called the Hospital Disaster Support Communications System and RACES (radio amateur civil emergency services), that uses certified volunteer personnel to perform many tasks related to communications.[11] This public service is intended to assist communications among government agencies and healthcare facilities in times of extraordinary need and could potentially be expanded and developed across the country.

Power outages can occur at any time, in any location. They can be due to system overload during times of excessive use, such as the 2003 blackouts in the Northeastern United States, or to interruptions in service caused by intentional destruction. Regardless of the cause, the possibility of power loss must be anticipated by establishing backup generators that will activate immediately on power interruption. Such generators should be maintained and tested on a regular basis. One aspect of disaster management for which electricity is essential is the operation of most communications technologies and medical equipment.

Finally, testing the plan at regular intervals ensures competency among users. It is even desirable to incorporate as much of disaster communications systems as possible into routine daily operations. In Rhode Island, a disaster communications system that links all of the acute-care hospitals in the state is used three times a day, every day, to provide ambulance diversion status.

SUMMARY

The most important principles of communications related to disaster management are preparation, efficiency, and backup plans. Preparation will ensure that disaster management workers know their responsibilities and how to complete them. Efficient communications systems at each facility will optimize the use of technology and help to maintain an effective chain of command. Finally, establishing backup plans will ensure that response workers can carry out their tasks, even in the midst of unpredictable concerns that are so often part of both natural and manmade disasters. In essence, the more focus that is given to communications before a disaster, the better workers will be able to carry out their roles in the event that a disaster occurs.

REFERENCES

1. Federal Emergency Management Agency. Available at: http://www.fema.gov/about/history.shtm.
2. Kendra JM, Wachtendorf T. Elements of resilience after the World Trade Center disaster: reconstituting New York City's Emergency Operations Centre. *Disasters.* 2003;27(1):37-53.
3. American College of Emergency Physicians, Terrorism Response Task Force. *Positioning America's Emergency Health Care System to Respond to Acts of Terrorism.* October 2002. http://www.acep.org/webportal/PracticeResources/IssuesByCategory/MassCasualty/default.htm.
4. Stephenson R, Anderson P. Disasters and the information technology revolution. *Disasters.* 1997;21(4):305-34.
5. Perry RW. Incident management systems in disaster management. *Disaster Prev Manage* 2003;12(5):405-12.
6. US Department of Homeland Security. National Incident Management System. Available at: http://www.dhs.gov/interweb/assetlibrary/NIMS-90-web.pdf.
7. Federal Communications Commission. Communicating during emergencies. Available at: http://www.fcc.gov/cgb/consumerfacts/emergencies.html.
8. Perry RW, Lindell MK. Preparedness for emergency response: guidelines for the emergency planning process. *Disasters.* 2003;27(4):336-50.
9. Daley W, Karpati A, Sheik M. Needs assessment of the displaced population following the August 1999 earthquake in Turkey. *Disasters.* 2001;25(1):67-75.
10. Federal Emergency Management Agency.
11. HDSCS home page. Available at: www.hdscs.org.

chapter 34

Media Relations*

Daniel F. Noltkamper

Emergency management organizations and media representatives have different and, not infrequently, competing roles in a disaster.[1] Emergency management organizations are focused on response, containment, search and rescue, recovery, and rehabilitation, whereas the media concentrates on gathering information and disseminating it to the public. Both have their own objectives, and even though not the same, they can be complementary if coordinated properly.

As recent events have unfortunately demonstrated, a disaster provides all the ingredients of a hit reality television show or movie. It includes drama, challenges, action, heroism, and suffering.[2] These qualities make it of interest to a national and sometimes international audience and may provide the opportunity for certain organizations or individuals to gain status or popularity. Although often an unintended consequence, this can pose a problem when it becomes a primary motivator. At the World Conference on Natural Disaster Reduction and the Roundtable on the Media, Scientific Information, and Disasters, Dr. Olavi Elo, director of the International Decade for Natural Disaster Reduction (IDNDR), stated: "We are not helped by how the priorities are perceived in the eyes of the media: human misery is far more newsworthy than a population made safe and sound."[1] One study estimated that 25% of all news stories involve natural disasters, technological hazards, and civil disturbances.[2]

New technology has allowed easier, and often instantaneous, broadcasting to a larger population, and the proliferation of television channels and Internet reporting has increased the competition for newsworthy items.[3] Journalists and media organizations have a job to perform, employers and advertisers to satisfy, and a public to inform.

Disaster response organizations work to mitigate hazards, protect the public, restore infrastructures, and assist in recovery. Many times this is completed with small, local agencies in the first few days. Although they need to get information to the people at risk, they may be overtaxed with their other duties. In past times, journalists were seen as a drain on resources and obstruction of emergency response. Attitudes about the media have changed, and a role for the media in disaster management has been identified.

The media need to be included in disaster planning. Their participation will improve their understanding of the response plan, how they can assist, and establish points of contact. An early, good relationship will lead to better cooperation when emergencies present. Even though panic is rare in disasters,[4] properly communicated media information will lessen the disruption produced by horrific events and will reduce individual anxiety.

HISTORICAL PERSPECTIVE

Print and Broadcast

The first American newspaper, known as *Publick Occurrences,* was established in 1690 and was quickly suppressed; the first successful newspaper was the *Boston News-Letter,* which started in 1704. One of the greatest natural disasters of the 20th century was the Galveston, Texas, hurricane of 1900. The *Daily News,* a local Galveston paper, ran a one-paragraph article on page 3 the day the hurricane struck, yet the category 4 hurricane left 6000 people dead and destroyed 3600 homes. In 1906 an earthquake struck San Francisco, and secondary fires disabled all three newspapers in the city. The three competitors teamed up to publish the *Call-Chronicle-Examiner* in Oakland and distributed the paper containing the account the next day in San Francisco.[5]

One of radio broadcasting's greatest moments was May 6, 1937, when reporter Herb Morrison recorded a live account of the Hindenburg disaster in Lakehurst, N.J. It was later aired by WLS of Chicago.[6]

Television's first broadcast of a disaster was also a delayed broadcast. On March 10, 1933, an earthquake struck Los Angeles. Pictures of the damage were aired the next day by station W6XAO. The first telecast of an unscheduled event occurred in New York in 1938 when a mobile unit for RCA was in a park in Queens when a fire broke out on Ward's Island.

---

*The views expressed in this article are those of the author and do not necessarily reflect the official policy or position of the Department of the Navy, Department of Defense, or the U.S. government.

Emergency Advisory System

President Harry S. Truman approved the CONELRAD (Control of Electromagnetic Radiation) program in 1951 to deliver emergency broadcasts over television and AM and FM radio stations. It allowed the president to deliver a message via the mass media to the public.[7] In 1963, President Kennedy converted CONELRAD to the Emergency Broadcast System. It became an interagency effort of the Federal Communications Commission (FCC), Federal Emergency Management Agency (FEMA), and National Weather Service (NWS). He permitted it to be used for state and local emergencies.

Although never used for war announcements or a nuclear attack, as originally intended, the Emergency Broadcast System was used just over 20,000 times between 1976 and 1996 to broadcast civil emergencies. Most (85%) of these announcements were weather-related. In 1997, it was renamed the Emergency Alert System (EAS), and in 1998, it included cable television systems with more than 10,000 subscribers. The EAS also includes the U.S. Weather Bureau tone-alert radio system. FEMA provides information for system use by state and local emergency planners.[2,8-10]

CURRENT PRACTICE

Media: Benefit or Hindrance

The media have the potential to be both a hindrance and a benefit in disaster response. Every disaster response or emergency management system must have plans to deal with the media. Although they may often get in the way, the media may also afford a remarkable opportunity for communication. The media is a cost-effective means of transmitting information to the public to save lives, reduce damage to property, and increase public awareness of hazards.[1] Sirens may provide an initial alert, but most individuals then turn to the broadcast media to determine if the threat is real and obtain more information. In disasters in which warnings are possible, if used properly with careful planning, the media can be a factor in preventing injury or death by serving as an initial warning source for the public. During a disaster, agencies involved directly in the response may use media information as a resource. This may be due to overloaded radio communications or because views from a media helicopter are being shown. Many hospitals first learn about disasters from media sources and initiate preparations for receiving casualties based on the broadcasted accounts of the event.[11]

The media can serve many positive functions in disaster response. They can convey instructions to the target population for protection and evacuation, which can reduce the need for further emergency response personnel. Although often counter to their mission, reporters and news anchors may provide reassurance to the masses when specifically requested to do so. Another important consequence of media coverage is that it may stimulate donations from areas not directly affected by the disaster and initiate government financial support.[2] Political and public support may increase due to the coverage and draw attention to future hazards.[3] If the media report on areas unaffected by the disaster, this may result in a reduction of inquiries from concerned persons outside of the immediate area of the disaster. Finally, follow-up stories may facilitate future emergency services funding and assist in the re-election efforts of politicians in the disaster area.[2]

The news media can stimulate public interest in donations and many times initiate their own "drives." Many times, local leaders suggest donations while being interviewed. Even though the intentions are good, there are many instances in which media involvement regarding donations has turned into a problem. Donations require manpower and storage. Many items may rot if adequate storage is unavailable. Manpower is then needed to dispose of goods that can become a public health issue. Trucks delivering the goods increase traffic into the area. Often, undesired items are received and require storage or disposal. On the other hand, as items arrive, the media may report on the large amount of outside support. False perceptions by the public may lead to a halt in donations of still-needed supplies.[12]

Not all consider the media an easy partner in disaster situations. A major concern is increased resource allocation that diverts attention away from command and control, casualty care, search and rescue, and evacuation. Resources affected can include response personnel and public officials (who are requested for interviews and tours), transportation, communication facilities, electrical power and lighting, work spaces, housing, food, and water. The media may pressure officials for numbers pertaining to casualties and damage. If conflicting numbers are presented, it could be portrayed as incompetence on the part of the command and control organization. Officials may also feel pressured by the media to make decisions prematurely.[2]

Exaggeration may be perceived if the media reports on interesting news items only. Examples include showing a damaged section repeatedly but not showing the unaffected area or reporting looting to be widespread, even if it is not. This is especially true if multiple sources report on the same few instances. Panic is often reported by the media even when it has not occurred. These exaggerations lead to increased inquiries by loved ones outside the area, taxing resources already engaged in other aspects of the emergency. Evacuations may be hampered as people watch pictures of long lines at gas stations and crowded highways and decide not to evacuate.[3]

Media helicopters have been known to assist with search and rescue missions, help analyze disasters, and provide current information on the situation for officials. As of October 2001 there were 200 reported helicopters used for media reporting; 125 of these were in major cities.[13] However, with helicopter use to report stories, there have been concerns raised about the crowding of airspaces and possible further damage to degraded structures. The Federal Aviation Administration (FAA) has the ability to create temporary flight restrictions over scenes of accidents, disasters, and special events under Federal Aviation Regulation 14 CFR Section 91.137 allows for safe operating of disaster relief aircraft. To protect fragile structures and people inside who are at risk of injury in the event of collapse, the suggested restricted airspace is 2000 feet above and a radius of 1 nautical mile from the area. In addition to rotorwash and vibration possibly harming buildings, the noise of aircraft could interfere with sensors being used to locate trapped individuals.[14]

Media Formats

Media types can be separated into broadcast and print. Broadcast media includes television and radio. Print involves newspapers and magazines. Internet reporting is a hybrid of both types. There are differences in their needs and roles in disaster reporting. They will all show up at a disaster to fill the public's need for news. It is also their livelihood, and they are professionals at seeking out newsworthy stories.

The 24-hour satellite and cable television news stations have a need to fill their airtime with items that capture and inform viewers. Local news programs compete to fulfill their obligation to nearby residents, and many people stay tuned to the network news afterward. No area is outside of the reach of television reporting when helicopters and satellite-dish trucks are used. Technology has created smaller and cheaper cameras and transmitting equipment. Fewer crew members are required, making the teams more mobile. When local stations are incapacitated, information can be transmitted to stations in unaffected areas. Those stations can, in turn, send reports back into the affected zones.[2,15,16]

Television is visual, and stations desire graphic images to capture viewers. Most disasters provide many images useful for this purpose. Action is constantly occurring and provides a good background for reporters. Television media have a need for short, succinct reports from officials—approximately a 20- to 30-second report that covers the most important facts. They also will need updates approximately 2 hours before their scheduled news programs air. In some instances they may interrupt regular programming to bring breaking news stories to attention. Since television is visual, officials should remain calm in their appearance and manner while giving interviews.

Radio provides the ability to get the word out quickly. Radio media also can interrupt regular programming to bring unfolding stories to the public. Their desire also is usually brief and concise reports from officials.[3] Since audio is their form of media, they may wish for some degree of background noise, but it may interfere with the message being relayed.[16]

Print media does not have the hour-to-hour deadlines seen with broadcast media so they may be interested in more details and background information.[2] Names of officials and technical words should be spelled out to print media. They may run the disaster stories for a longer period and in more detail, which may assist in future funding. They also have less equipment requirements and rely less on power sources at the site. When Guam was struck by super typhoon Pongsona in December 2002, it knocked out power and telephone lines, disabling television and radio media. Using a computer and generator, the *Pacific Daily News* was able to publish the effects of the storm in print and on its Web site, using a server in Virginia. The newspaper was delivered to residents in shelters since most roads were impassable. Loved ones outside of Guam, the U.S. Weather Service, and the FAA were able to obtain information from the Web site.[17] In this instance, the form of media with the least technology requirements was able to get information to the public.

Internet reporting has features of both broadcast and print media. Internet reports can be presented 24 hours a day and combine visual, audio, and printed forms of communication. Internet accessibility affords disaster response officials the opportunity to provide information and updates to the public and media using fewer resources. Preprinted public safety announcements about multiple hazards that could exist in a disaster situation can be placed on an organization's Web site. Electronic mail groups to media contacts can speed information updates.

In all types of media, special consideration should be given to special groups in the affected areas. Language and cultural barriers should be addressed as well as hurdles involving sight- and hearing-impaired individuals.[2]

Whether dealing with broadcast or print media personnel, disaster officials should get contact names, phone numbers, and e-mail addresses to provide updates as they arise. Also, any background materials about the region affected would be helpful. They may also provide reports with unique aspects and human-interest stories that stimulate attention from areas beyond the local region.

National and Local Media Differences

National media organizations are interested in the overall picture. They also may provide stories with unique aspects and human-interest stories. Questions may be asked about prominent figures, historical and important structures, and significant national treasures. Their resources outweigh those of local media agencies, and they may quickly overwhelm and capture official attention initially given to the local groups. Their resources include star correspondents; subject-matter experts; and logistical coordinators for lodging, power, and telephone lines. Many national networks will also cooperate together because they interact frequently.

Reporters from local media organizations are usually the first on the scene. Many live in or near the disaster area and understand the local impact. They may be present during all phases of the disaster (e.g., mitigation, planning, response, and recovery). During the mitigation phase, they may report on local hazards and minimize the risk of disaster. Reporting of hazards and risks may lead to political and financial support for emergency response organizations. They should be involved in the disaster planning phase, where they can come to a better understanding of the emergency response plan and establish points of contact. In the response phase, they can offer initial warnings of impending emergencies, public safety announcements, evacuation instructions, utility limitations, and information on the progress of the response. Their long-range reporting after the disaster can assist in the recovery phase.[2,18,19] In general, the local media are more interested in their community's welfare than are the national media.[11]

Many times, local news agencies are displaced by the attention given to the national media organizations. It should be remembered that the local reporters are a valuable resource. As relationships and friendships are formed, they may demonstrate more favorable reporting of the emergency response. They can assist in coordinating media pools and press releases as well as tours. If involved in the planning phase, they can become an extension of the usually overtasked public information officer (PIO).

Public Information Officer

The PIO reports to the incident commander in the Incident Command System. The PIO is responsible for developing and maintaining a media contact list, scheduling interviews, selecting and preparing appropriate team members for the interviews, escorting media and VIPs through the site, preparing and issuing press releases, and gathering and verifying information. To complete these tasks, the PIO must have a knowledge of local plans, disaster management concepts, capabilities of the response team, and the state and federal response plan.[3]

Specialized training as a PIO can make the incident commander's representative a valuable asset. The PIO must be equipped with resources such as computers and Internet and telephone access. In some instances, a media relations team may be required. The PIOs from all agencies involved in the disaster response may form the team and may appoint a single spokesperson to disseminate coordinated information.[11] An experienced and well-equipped PIO may be able to defuse many difficult situations involving the press. The PIO should remain accessible to the media at all times and should establish contact with counterparts at other response organizations, such as hospitals and government organizations.[19] In many situations, the PIO can suggest interesting stories to the media. This may include stories that educate the public on the role of emergency management planners and disaster responders.

Web sites can assist the PIO in disseminating information. Preprinted public safety advisories and press releases can be posted on the Web site. These may ensure more accurate information is supplied to the press. News agencies can remain updated through the Web site or by e-mail. A 24-hour hot line with prerecorded messages can also be useful. The PIO should also maintain a communications log that documents all interactions with the press. It should include who said what and when it was said to ensure accurate information is provided during the course of the disaster. This may be used in the recovery phase to update contact lists and produce lessons learned. To improve future plans, consider a survey of local and national media organizations who reported on the disaster.[18]

Press Conferences

Information should be provided as quickly as possible so it may be passed to the public. A media center can meet this need. The center should be established in a safe location to protect the media from hazards, including infectious casualties. Access to food, drinks, and restrooms should be provided. In certain locations, such as hospitals, an area where cellular phones may be used without interfering with patient monitoring should be identified. Most media organizations share information in a major disaster and will appreciate a single location to gather the information. This allows quick access to a lot of information and assists reporters in meeting deadlines.[20,21]

Centralize information as much as possible to send out one consistent message. One identified person, who comes across as trustworthy, will build credibility. That person should be knowledgeable about the disaster response process but may invite other experts to assist as needed. The speaker should be from the command post if possible so the news can report the information as originating from an official source. Names and titles of those speaking, as well as background information, can be disseminated in advance. Question cards can be distributed to the press before the conference, and repetitive questions can be answered by the lead spokesperson. During the initial conference, the schedule for future ones may be announced.[21]

If the center becomes too crowded, media pools may be established. One reporter or a small group of reporters attends the conference and shares the information gathered with media members who were not at the conferences. This also works for tours of the damaged areas once safe access is established. This process is well accepted and should involve one representative each from television, radio, and print. A local reporter involved in the planning stages may be ideal in coordinating the pool and tour representatives.

Interview Basics

Questions from the media are fairly predictable and can be prepared for in advance. Appear calm and professional. Avoid anger and frustration. Think about your answers and avoid rushing; the media can edit out pauses. Speak about the response teams involved, the disaster and its effect, and any casualties that are known. Avoid speculation; specific numbers; technical jargon; and phrases such as "off the record," "I think," and "no comment." Inform the press when you don't know the answer to their question and offer to provide it later. Take the offensive, and offer all available information initially. A leading statement, such as "The most important information is...," will satisfy many reporters' needs, especially those in broadcast media.[3,22] The interview is also a chance to verify information and expose myths. The media will often withhold information that the speaker identifies as being dangerous for public consumption, but care should be taken to emphasize that the information should not be released. Critical messages to convey include the following[23]:

- Personnel in senior leadership know what they are dealing with
- Emergency management knows how to respond to the disaster

- The response plan is . . . .
- The public needs to know . . . . to protect itself
- (If terrorism is involved), steps are being taken to find the guilty parties

Other expected questions will involve who is in charge of the disaster response, whether the situation is under control, how the injured are being cared for, why did this happen and was it preventable, and what else can be expected. Identify locations where other information can be obtained, such as Web sites or hot lines.

Other details may be requested during the interview. Casualty questions may include how many were killed or injured, how many escaped injury, and were any prominent figures involved. Property damage details may focus on important buildings, arts and treasures, prominent owners, measures to protect other properties, and insurance issues. Response questions focus on who discovered the disaster first, who responded and how quickly, whether there were any heroic acts, and where the homeless and displaced are being taken. Questions about cause may involve any previous indications of problems or threats and whether any criminal investigations or lawsuits have been initiated. Other possible questions include whether blasts or explosions were detected, were crimes or violence observed, were there any acts of self-rescue, and the expected extent and duration of the response.[2]

PITFALLS

1. *Not including the media in disaster planning:* Local resources can assist in obtaining public support and funding, educating and informing the public, and assisting with media pools. Also do not ignore the local media organizations when national reporters arrive.
2. *Assuming the media will not appear at the disaster:* They will come, and large disasters may include international representatives.
3. *Sequestering and ignoring the media:* Without information, the media will create stories based on what little facts they have.
4. *Using an untrained, inexperienced PIO:* Emergency management organizations are best represented when a trained, experienced PIO can organize and guide the media.
5. *Hiding the truth:* Using the phrase "no comment" makes the media and public suspicious that there are hidden issues.
6. *Going "off the record":* Odds are that "off-the-record" comments will appear in print or broadcast.
7. *Speculating:* Any assumptions may be incorrect, and when the true information is discovered, it may reflect incompetence.
8. *Failing to check with the potential recipient organizations before issuing appeals for donations or volunteers on their behalf:* Be proactive in announcing when donations or volunteers are not needed.

9. *Failing to provide details on the disaster that will allow the public to determine whether their friends and family are safe:* These details can include maps of the affected area with specific comments on areas not involved. This will reduce the number of inquiries to officials involved in the disaster response.

REFERENCES

1. The Role of Media in Disaster Mitigation: Roundtable on the Media, Scientific Information, and Disasters. Available at: http://www.annenberg.northwestern.edu/pubs/disas/disas32.htm.
2. Auf der Heide E. The Media: Friend or Foe. In: Auf der Heide E, ed. *Disaster Response: Principles of Preparation and Coordination.* St Louis: Mosby; 1989. Available at: http://orgmail2.coe-dmha.org/dr/flash.htm.
3. Burkholder-Allen K. Media Relations and the Role of the Public Information Officer: What Every DMAT Member Should Know. Available at: http://www.mediccom.org/public/tadmat/training/NDMS/MediaRelationsArticle.pdf.
4. Auf der Heide E. Common Misperceptions about Disasters: Panic, the "Disaster Syndrome," and Looting. In: O'Leary M, ed. *The First 72 Hours: A Community Approach to Disaster Preparedness.* Lincoln, NE: iUniverse Publishing; 2004:342-7.
5. Earthquake and Fire: San Francisco in Ruins. Web reprint from: The Virtual Museum of the City of San Francisco. Available at: http://www.sfmuseum.org/1906/callchronex.html.
6. Widner J. Hindenburg Disaster, Herb Morrison Reporting. 2003. Available at: http://www.otr.com/hindenburg.html.
7. Wikipedia, the Free Encyclopedia. CONELRAD. Available at: http://en.wikipedia.org/wiki/CONELRAD.
8. Wikipedia, the Free Encyclopedia. Emergency Broadcast System. Available at: http://en.wikipedia.org/wiki/Emergency_Broadcast_System.
9. Wikipedia, the Free Encyclopedia. Emergency Alert System. Available at: http://en.wikipedia.org/wiki/Emergency_Alert_System.
10. Federal Communications Commission. Fact sheet: the Emergency Alert System (EAS). Available at: http://www.fcc.gov/eb/easfact.html.
11. Auf der Heide E. Principles of hospital disaster planning. In: Hogan DE, Burstein JL, eds. *Disaster Medicine.* Philadelphia: Lippincott Williams & Wilkins; 2002:74-5.
12. National Voluntary Organizations Active in Disaster. Donated Goods in Disaster Response. Available at: http://www.nvoad.org/history5.php.
13. Association of Electronic Journalists. Testimony of Barbara Cochran: U.S. House of Representatives Committee on Transportation and Infrastructure Committee on Aviation. Available at: http://www.rtnda.org/foi/chopperban.html.
14. FAA Office of Communications, Navigation, and Surveillance. Temporary flight restrictions. In: AC No. 00-59: Integrating Helicopter and Tiltrotor Assets in Disaster Relief Planning. Available at: http://www.faa.gov/and/AC0059/ACNo0059.htm#TemporaryFlight.
15. Staten C. Emergency Services Guideline for Media Affairs. Available at: http://www.emergency.com/emsmedia.htm.
16. International Federation of Red Cross and Red Crescent Societies. Communications Guide: The News Media. Available at: http://www.ifrc.org/publicat/commsguide/html/Archive/Chapter3.PDF#xml=http://www.ifrc.org/.
17. Federal Emergency Management Agency. When the Media is a Disaster Victim. How One Small Paper Kept the World Informed. Available at: http://www.fema.gov/nwz03/nwz03_media.shtm.
18. Telg R. Getting the News Out in Times of Disaster. Available at: http://edis.ifas.ufl.edu/WC034.
19. Telg R. Firefighter Public Information Officers' Communication Effectiveness with the Media During the 1998 Florida Wildfires. Presented at: Southern Association of Agricultural Scientists, Agricultural Communications Section; January 2000; Lexington, KY. Available at: http://agnews.tamu.edu/saas/paperrt.htm.

20. St. Luke's, News and Media Center. Disaster/Crisis Guidelines. Available at: http://www.callstlukes.org/news/disaster/guidelines.html.

21. Pan American Health Organization. Media Relations in Emergencies. Available at: http://www.paho.org/English/PED/medios.htm.

22. Center for Disease Control and Prevention. Media Relations Division: Crisis Plan (Draft). Available at: http://www.nphic.org/revised.doc.

23. Medical News Report. Special Report: Federal Anti-terrorism Disaster Drill Has Important Lessons for PR. Available at: http://www.medicalnewsreport.com/med0007.htm.

chapter 35

Managing Volunteers and Donations

Andrew M. Milsten

Offering help to people in need is a basic human instinct. During the war in Yugoslavia (1999), thousands of people were able to survive because of donations from foreign governments and private individuals and organizations.[1] Donations and volunteerism can be a help or hindrance, though, depending on whether the right amount of goods, people, and materials are sent to the disaster region. There is a common misperception that when a disaster occurs, people should send everything they have as rapidly as possible. Misperceptions such as this can result in large amounts of wasted human and nonhuman resources.

There are two types of donations: in-cash and in-kind. Cash donations are often ideal because of flexibility and ease of coordination and because cash allows materials to be purchased through normal channels while supporting the local economy. The Internet has recently become an efficient method for obtaining cash donations. After the southeast Asia tsunami in 2004, large amounts of money were donated rapidly through the Internet, with sites such as Amazon.com collecting upwards of $3 million within days of the event.[2] The downside to cash donations is that they are susceptible to misuse.[1] Donations in-kind are less standardized and, although immensely helpful, can cause problems unknown to the donor.[1] This chapter specifically examines disaster volunteerism and in-kind drug and blood donations.

INTRODUCTION TO DONATIONS

Drug Donations

During times of crisis many different entities provide drug donations, including private individuals and companies, nongovernment organizations (NGOs), international agencies such as the United Nations (UN), and foreign governments.[3] The literature on this subject, which focuses on disasters as well as complex humanitarian emergencies such as refugee situations, indicates that many disaster-stricken regions become dependent on foreign medical aid (for both acute emergencies and long-term aid).[3,4] Drug donations are a complex issue, however, and although such donations can help disaster-stricken countries retain their treatment quality and

meet healthcare needs, numerous negative outcomes also can occur. For example, the common misperception that it is better to send any drug rather than none at all results in often-inappropriate medical materials arriving in the recipient country.[5] Despite the donors' good intentions, donated drugs are often inappropriate to treat local diseases and are nutritionally inadequate (e.g., commercial soft drinks sent to treat cholera in Zaire in 1994).[6-8] In addition, a practice known as "drug dumping" often results in large quantities of useless drugs arriving in the disaster-struck region.[9,10] *Drug dumping,* a term meaning the donation of defective products, has been studied both in terms of quantity and quality (e.g., amount, appropriateness, usability).[3,11]

HISTORICAL PERSPECTIVE

Drug Donations

Standardization and management of medical donations have been issues for years and were under the domain of the Red Cross Movement until 1957. After World War II, national and international organizations focused on these issues. It was not until after the Persian Gulf War, however, that emergency relief deficiency came under the scrutiny of the UN.[12]

Starting in 1976, reports began appearing about the deleterious effects that large amounts of inappropriate donated drugs can have on a recipient country. In 1996, the UN designated the World Health Organization (WHO) as coordinator of health-related international agency work.[12] WHO took several actions in Bosnia to facilitate this mission, including establishing interagency coordination committees, assessing needs, coordinating drug supplies, disseminating drug lists and guidelines, and promoting the use of essential drug kits.[13] Despite WHO's efforts, drug donations to Bosnia and Herzegovina were criticized for the following[1,3,14-16]:

- Being of low quality and frequently expired
- Adding to postwar chaos
- Being unequally distributed
- Allowing an NGO to deliver materials to an area that had recently received similar materials from a different NGO

- Often being inappropriate
- Allowing the media too big a role in swaying what donors gave and how much

Some authors believed that these criticisms were "elitist" and noted that, for example, drug expiration dates are extremely conservative and that a possible solution to the problem of expired drugs could be to "perhaps double the usual dose."[17] These authors also noted that human suffering would be worsened by not using donated drugs.[17] The use of expired drugs generally has not been acceptable for reasons including problems related to toxic metabolites; unknown efficacy; opening the door to bad donation practices; loss of credibility for the donor; and violating the Basal Convention, which regulates the transnational movement of hazardous waste, including unused drugs, and its disposal and requires the owner, the receiver, and the transporter of any chemical that could be toxic, poisonous, or ecotoxic to get clearance from the relevant authority in charge of the Basal Convention.[1,3,6,18]

Examples of inappropriate donation practices are shown in Table 35-1. During the Sudan war (1985) inappropriate pharmaceutical donations included contact lens solution, appetite stimulants, cholesterol-lowering drugs, and expired antibiotics.[5] In Lithuania (1993), 11 women were temporarily blinded after taking a drug donated by Caritas (closantel—a veterinary anthelmintic) that was mistakenly given to treat endometriosis because of poor labeling.[5,19] In Georgia (former USSR) (1995) 20 tons of expired silver sulfadiazine were received, and Eritrea, Africa, (1994) received seven truckloads of expired aspirin, a shipping container of unsolicited cardiovascular drugs with 2 months to expire, and 30,000 bottles of expired amino acid infusion (that could not be disposed of due to the smell).[5,20] Other examples of completely nonsensical donations—although not drug donations per se—include bikinis sent to Gujarat, India (earthquake), crates of double-D bras sent to Kobi, Japan (earthquake), breast implants sent to a hospital in Malawi, Africa, and ski jackets sent to Sri Lanka.[19,21]

U.S. pharmaceutical companies often are saddled with a negative image for their poor donation practices, which is not entirely unjustified. For example, Eli Lilly donated 6 million poorly labeled cefaclor (Ceclor CD) tablets, even though the tablets were nearing expiration and had not received approval from the Food and Drug Administration for sale in the United States.[19] There are worthwhile long-term sustainable U.S. pharmaceutical programs, however, including Merck's Mectizan Donation Program (providing free drugs [ivermectin] to treat river blindness since 1988); Sanofi Aventis' partnership with WHO and the medical NGO Médecins Sans Frontières to distribute medicines for African sleeping sickness; and Roche's policy to make HIV protease inhibitors (nelfinavir and saquinavir) available to developing countries at much reduced costs.[19,22]

In 1999, WHO identified six specific problems associated with drug donations, which led to the development of "good practice" guidelines.[15,23,24] WHO identified the following problems[5,23,25]:

1. Donation of drugs irrelevant to the recipient country's situation
2. Unsorted and poorly labeled drugs
3. Low-quality drugs (e.g., expired, returns)
4. Ignorance of local administrative procedures
5. High custom charges to the recipient (due to high declared drug value)
6. Donation of incorrect quantities (too much of some drugs and too little of others).

TABLE 35-1 EXAMPLES OF DRUG DUMPING

YEAR	LOCATION	AMOUNT DONATED (METRIC TONS*)	INAPPROPRIATE AMOUNT	NOTES
1976[9]	Guatemala earthquake	100 (7000 cartons)	90% unsorted	1120 hours of sorting time
1984-1985[36]	Ethiopia famine	Not listed	Not listed	US $500,000 worth of inappropriate drugs were destroyed
1985[42]	Mexico earthquake	1088 Drugs: 31% Food: 14% Supplies, clothes, and blankets: 24%		Heavy machinery 6%-14% (most needed)
1985-1987[11]	Sudan famine	Not listed	8 million chloroquine and 500,000 piperazine were expired	380,000 Citramon tablets were banned Vitamins and baby food were not registered.
1989[5,27]	Armenia earthquake	5000 Drugs: 65% IV: 20% Consumables: 15%	70% Expired: 8% Frozen: 4% Unsorted: 18% Useless: 11% Unidentifiable: 12%	Poorly labeled antibiotics (238 names in 21 languages) Sorting time was 6 months with 50 people
1992-1996[3]	Bosnia and Herzegovina	27,800-34,800	50%-60%	
1994-1997[23]	Armenia, Haiti, and United Republic of Tanzania	16,500 shipments (no weight listed)	10%-42%	6% expired
2000[19]	Venezuela floods	Not listed	70%	$16,000 spent to sort drugs

*1 metric ton = 2204.6 pounds; 1 ton is approximately 40 cubic feet.

Many authors agree with WHO's assessment and add other factors to consider.[15] For instance, Berckmans[3] noted three categories of donations that were sent to Bosnia and Herzegovina: those that conformed to WHO's interagency guidelines for drug donations, miscellaneous medicines (e.g., unsorted, free samples), and large quantities of donated drugs that were useless or unusable (e.g., 1961 plaster tape, WWII supplies). During the 1985 war in Sudan, the country received drugs that were in small packets and partly used (open blister packets).[4] Another problem with donations to Sudan was that local doctors often were unfamiliar with newly introduced drugs. Further, once the stock of new drugs ran out, patients wished to continue the often more expensive drug, which led to treatment interruptions.[4] In Croatia (1990-1994), it was found that drug donations led to "changes in therapeutic principles" as well as changes in prescribing patterns and organized drug acquisition at University Hospital Center of Rijeka (e.g., decreased use of cotimoxazole, ampicillin, and cephalexin and increased use of amoxicillin plus clavulanic acid, gentamycin, and cefuroxime).[10] Médecins Sans Frontières also notes that the practice and culture of corporate drug donations do not encourage local production of generic drugs and may hinder the recipient countries' attempts at a sustainable cost-recovery program.[19] Finally, Hogerzeil points out that donation of excessive quantities leads to stockpiling, pilfering, and black market sales.[5,26]

There are many reasons to donate medical materials to a disaster-stricken region, and most donations are sent with good intentions.[6,13] However, there are several non-altruistic reasons for donating drugs, such as avoiding drug destruction costs, publicity, disposing of surplus or wasted medicines, political pressure to take action (drug donations "film well"), tax benefits for donor companies and private voluntary organizations, and stimulating the market for certain products (brand recognition in a potential new market).[3,6,15,9,25] Whether these motivations are viewed as morally corrupt and self-serving or well intentioned but gone awry depends on perspective and constitutes a debate beyond the scope of this chapter.

Whatever the reasons behind a donation, there are definite consequences to drug dumping, and the resource-strapped recipient country usually suffers them. It is difficult to store, sort, organize, and handle large quantities of donated medical supplies. Researchers studying the situation in Bosnia and Herzegovina had difficulty in locating unused medical supplies because the warehouses were subject to restricted access and their whereabouts were often unknown.[3] There can also be high destruction costs associated with donating unusable drugs: 1 ton of drugs in Bosnia and Herzegovina cost US $2000 to destroy, costing the recipient country $34 million and requiring the construction of incinerator plants—a situation that occurred in Macedonia and Armenia as well.[3,6,24,27] In cases in which the drugs are inappropriate to the situation but not unusable, the drugs could be shipped to another country rather than be destroyed; however, shipment can cost $2 to $4 million per 1000 metric ton.[24] Other less-tangible destruction costs include health and environmental hazards,

storage, handling, and transportation, which are often greater than the donated drugs.[3,5] In the wake of the southeast Asia tsunami disaster of 2004, there were concerns about empty water bottles littering the environment as well as no-longer-needed medicines (morphine) being loose and uncontrolled in Sri Lanka.[21] WHO has developed guidelines for the safe disposal of drugs, including the use of sanitary landfills, encapsulation, inertization, discharge to a sewer, high-temperature (1200°C) incinerators, and chemical waste treatment centers.[6,13,24,27]

The Armenian earthquake situation vividly demonstrates the local costs associated with poor donation practices. In December 1988, Armenia, Turkey, was rocked by an earthquake (6.9 on the Richter scale) in an area populated by 700,000 people. Deaths were estimated between 24,000 and 60,000 people. Three days after the earthquake, international relief from 74 countries arrived, including 5000 tons of medical materials (valued at US $55 million), money, and human resources.[27] Local resources in the ill-prepared region were depleted, and disorganization reigned. The Armenian airport handled 150 landings a day, where unaccompanied shipments were dropped onto the airstrip and left behind. Armenian personnel were quickly overwhelmed attempting to locate specific supplies amidst the sea of donations and to deliver medical materials to the field. It took 1 month to set up an efficient donation management strategy.[27] Pharmacists spent two-thirds of their time searching for appropriate drugs, and it took 50 people 6 months to sort the donations (mostly nonmedical personnel using pharmaceutical textbooks and cross-indexes to decipher the donated drugs).[5,27] There were also problems handling large heavy packages, finding adequate storage space (32 new storage buildings were constructed that held 70% of donations while the rest were shipped to Moscow), and disposing of drugs destroyed by cold temperatures (4%).[27]

CURRENT PRACTICE

Drug Donations

Suggested solutions to problems associated with drug donations are based primarily on basic disaster planning techniques, such as preparing for anticipated needs, recognizing that each disaster is different and that priorities change, and performing realistic needs analyses.[28,29] Many have advocated for better communication of needs and the exchange of more reliable information between recipient countries and donors.[5,6,13] Mitigation planning should be done by recipient countries to help strengthen legislative policies toward donors, centralize drug donations and emergency aid (using principles of good pharmacy practice), put registration and quality assurance procedures into place, and develop a national essential drugs list.[3,5,23]

Pan American Health Organization (PAHO)/WHO's Supply Management System (SUMA, 1992) is a good example of an information management tool that could help disaster-stricken countries deal with donations more effectively. To help disaster managers sort through large amounts of donations, SUMA uses simple tracking software. SUMA works by prioritizing and collecting data at donation entry points (airport, seaport, or border) and categorizing these items. Other SUMA team members gather data at warehouses and distribution centers and then electronically send this information to the central area. From this area, customized reports detailing donation activity and status can be generated.[30]

WHO has taken the lead on setting standards for good donation practices with guidelines promulgated in 1999.[24] WHO started work on these guidelines in 1990 and finished them through an international consultative process involving more than 100 agencies.[5] WHO's guidelines provide core donation principles and contain four categories (Box 35-1 and Table 35-2).[5,14,23,31-33] WHO also maintains a list of essential drugs (the Model List, revised in 2003) and encourages each country to produce its own national drug list (focusing on safety, appropriateness, efficacy, and cost-effectiveness).[6,34]

Although WHO's guidelines have not been followed on a consistent basis, such as in Albania, Rwanda, and Somalia, their acceptance appears to be growing and has led to a large change in donation practices.[20,24,31] As Autier[18] points out, however, the development of guidelines only will not be sufficient for effective coordination. For example, guidelines alone cannot resolve the problems associated with massive quantities of unsolicited donations, weak monitoring systems, high costs of dealing with useless drugs, training gaps, poor coordination, unclear responsibilities, local and traditional values not being respected, dependency on donated goods, and involvement of military personnel unfamiliar with humanitarian work (during the Kosovo crisis in 1999, NATO military staff were unaware of standard humanitarian distribution procedures).[35] Ideally, donation management and coordination would be carried out by small teams of experts who are familiar with disasters and able to continually adjust donation demands for community health needs. Organizations with minimal bureaucracy are best suited for this task, especially if they are willing to apply some donated monies earmarked for material purchases (such as drugs) to setting up a coordination system.[18]

WHO also developed the emergency health kit, a standardized kit containing sufficient drugs and medical supplies for 10,000 people and designed for immediate release to a refugee situation.[5,36,37] UNICEF and the International Dispensaries Association stock emergency health kits as well.[4] The emergency health kits were put together as a short-term use (3 months) commodity that could be used while more specific needs

TABLE 35-2 WHO DRUG DONATION GUIDELINES (1999)

Selection of drugs	• All drug donations should be based on an expressed need and be relevant to the disease pattern in the recipient country. Drugs should not be sent without prior consent by the recipient.
	• All donated drugs or their generic equivalents should be approved for use in the recipient country and appear on the national list of essential drugs, or, if a national list is not available, on the WHO Model List of Essential Drugs, unless specifically requested otherwise by the recipient.
	• The presentation, strength, and formulation of donated drugs should, as much as possible, be similar to those of drugs commonly used in the recipient country.
Quality assurance and shelf life	• All donated drugs should be obtained from a reliable source and comply with quality standards in both donor and recipient country. The WHO Certification Scheme on the Quality of Pharmaceutical Products Moving in International Commerce 7 should be used.
	• No drugs should be donated that have been issued to patients and then returned to a pharmacy or elsewhere, or were given to health professionals as free samples.
	• After arrival in the recipient country all donated drugs should have a remaining shelf-life of at least one year.
Presentation, packing, labeling	• All drugs should be labeled in a language that is easily understood by health professionals in the recipient country; the label on each individual container should at least contain the International Nonproprietary Name (INN) or generic name, batch number, dosage form, strength, name of manufacturer, quantity in the container, storage conditions, and expiry date.
	• As much as possible, donated drugs should be presented in larger quantity units and hospital packs.
	• All drug donations should be packed in accordance with international shipping regulations, and be accompanied by a detailed packing list which specifies the contents of each numbered carton by INN, dosage form, quantity, batch number, expiry date, volume, weight and any special storage conditions. The weight per carton should not exceed 50 kilograms. Drugs should not be mixed with other supplies in the same carton.
Information and management	• Recipients should be informed of all drug donations that are being considered, prepared or actually under way.
	• In the recipient country the declared value of a drug donation should be based upon the wholesale price of its generic equivalent in the recipient country, or, if such information is not available, on the wholesale world-market price for its generic equivalent.
	• Costs of international and local transport, warehousing, port clearance, and appropriate storage and handling should be paid by the donor agency, unless specifically agreed otherwise with the recipient in advance.

From World Health Organization. Guidelines for Drug Donations–Revised 1999 (Second edition). Available at: http://www.who.int/medicines/library/par/who-edm-par-1999-4/who-edm-par-99-4.shtml.

assessments were accomplished and purchases were organized within the country.[36] The kits are prepackaged (easing logistics), include suggested treatment schedules, and contain equipment and two drug lists (the "A" list has 25 drugs for use by minimally trained health workers, and the "B" list has 31 drugs for physician prescribing). The emergency health kit evolved after 1990 (updated in 1998), and it was requisitioned and used more than once within the same disaster, which prompted fears of dependency on international suppliers. To combat dependency on the kit, WHO promotes the development of country-specific emergency drug lists and supplies based on local disease patterns. Emergency health kits were designed for use during the emergency phase of drought, famine, or war. The kits were not recommended in acute-onset disasters, such as hurricanes or earthquakes (where there is assistance within 24 to 48 hours of the disaster and health needs widely vary); in situations in which the cost of transportation is more than the kit itself; and in countries that have a national emergency formulary. Even though the kit has proved useful, it is the drugs that it contains that make it valuable.[36]

There have been other ideas and regulations put forth to help encourage good donation practices and eliminate the undesirable practice of drug dumping. The ideas are wide ranging but focus primarily on providing quality assurance monitoring and holding donors accused of dumping accountable for their actions.[38] Snell[6] notes that donors and "relief agencies need to educate the public about donations and maintain a commitment to high standards of excellence through consultation with media, and policy makers." Hillstrom[25] suggests allowing a donation to be used only for care of the ill, needy, or infants, and not to be transferred in exchange for money. Furthermore, donations should comply with WHO's guidelines, include proper documentation, and be valued at reasonable market rates to prevent donations being made solely for tax deductions.[25,39] Thomas[19] recommends that any British pharmaceutical company taking a deduction in its tax bill for donations should list the donation in its annual accounts (published publicly). Thomas[19] also suggests a change in the laws that would give the tax credit to the recipient country and not allow any donations that fall outside of WHO guidelines to qualify the donor for benefits. In 2002, Britain announced a series of measures that would ease access to essential medicines for many poor people living in developing countries. These measures include funding research into new treatments for the three "target" diseases identified by the UN (malaria, tuberculosis, and AIDS) as well as legislation encouraging donations of medicines by UK-based pharmaceutical companies.[19] WHO recommends that donors pay attention to logistical issues, such as proper documentation, looking into applicable local laws, considering warehouse costs and weather, and obtaining better information from the recipient.[1] Other WHO suggestions include allocating resources at the beginning of an emergency situation for coordinating donations, creating collection centers, setting donation and national drug policies, and educating the public.[1,39]

Blood Donations

Blood donations are "part of the altruistic response of the general public."[40] After a disaster, people donate blood because of an awareness of the need for blood in the community, sense of social obligation or duty, personal social pressure, need to replace blood used by a friend or relative, and to increase self-esteem.[41] These reasons seem to outweigh the reasons people do not donate, such as fear, inconvenience, perceived medical disqualification, being too busy, not being asked, and apathy.[41]

Staggering amounts of blood are donated after a disaster.[42] Within 5 days after the 1989 San Francisco earthquakes, donations were up 200% from baseline (in affected and unaffected cities).[40] After the terrorist acts on Sept. 11, 2001, blood donations increased 1.3- to 2.5-fold. Mass appeal and blood drives led to the collection of 572,000 units, with enough blood collected by the second day to serve the situational needs. The overwhelming response included 12,000 phone calls (to blood banks) and 5000 units donated in 24 hours, 1800 units of blood escorted by police into the area, and the public lining up for hours and organizing themselves by blood type.[43] Although flights were grounded, the American Red Cross activated its aviation incident response team and mobilized 50,000 units of blood from around the country to be shipped by military transport.[41,43]

Further reports from American Blood Centers (75 centers collecting half of the volunteer blood supply in the United States) noted that 259,000 people donated during the four days after the attacks (three times the normal level).[44] Also, the Red Cross reported 615,995 donations at 36 sites (two times the normal level).[44] So much blood was donated outside of hospitals that 208,000 units of blood were discarded in the weeks after Sept. 11 (five times the normal level), and in the end, only 206 units of blood were used for individuals injured in the attacks.[45]

INTRODUCTION TO VOLUNTEERISM

Disaster Volunteerism

Volunteer numbers also surge after disasters. With proper management and direction, volunteers can accomplish a lot. Otherwise, they may hinder the response and become a logistical problem.[28] Some authors believe that "what the public does (individually and collectively), will make the biggest difference in the outcome of a disaster" and that volunteers can be integrated into the disaster response.[46,47] Others note, however, that "freelancing" medical personnel and "convergent volunteerism" are system problems and disruptive to disaster management.[46,48] *Convergent volunteerism* has been defined as the unexpected or uninvited arrival of personnel wishing to render aid at the scene, who then engage in freelancing (operating at an emergency incident scene without knowledge of the command authority).[48] Most volunteer convergence occurs for two reasons: first, officials overestimate the damage and issue requests from the scene to "send everything you've got," and second, the immediate shortfall of official responders is filled by bystanders.

Certainly, most disasters can benefit from volunteers. Civilian volunteer organizations such as the Red Cross, Voluntary Organizations Active in Disasters (VOAD), and NYC Mayor's Voluntary Action Center allow people to get involved and be helpful where needed.[49] New York City has civilian volunteer managers who are experts in this field but were underused during the initial phases of the Sept. 11, 2001, terrorist attacks.[49] Aside from large civilian volunteer organizations, most volunteers in disasters take part because of timing, the situation, and a desire to help others. Spontaneous volunteers are particularly important for early search and rescue efforts. During the Nimitz Freeway collapse in the 1989 Loma Prieta, Calif., earthquake, 50 people were rescued—49 by bystanders. The volunteers fashioned backboards out of road signs, then waited hours for emergency medical services (EMS) to arrive.[47] Bystanders commonly conduct immediate uncoordinated search and rescue efforts (mostly during large, multisite disasters when EMS is disrupted) and will leave once they feel that EMS on-scene is adequate.[46,47,50,51] Since bystanders and victims accomplish the most immediate search and rescue efforts, it seems wise to plan around this instead of completely discouraging it. Emergency responders can be trained to direct and coordinate these efforts, especially since it is the spontaneous volunteers who often know who is missing and where they were last seen. During the 1998 Swissair crash, local firefighters and fishermen were organized into search and rescue boat groups ("recovery volunteers"), while other local residents ("instrumental volunteers") performed supportive roles. Unfortunately, and not for lack of effort or organization, they found no survivors, but only wreckage and human remains. In addition, these volunteers were given inadequate support after the disaster (46% to 71% of volunteers suffered from posttraumatic stress disorder).[52]

Nevertheless, volunteers can become a liability at disasters when they hinder logistics, cross roles, compromise safety and control, and do not follow proper incident command structure or medical oversight.[53] There are anecdotal stories from the Sept. 11, 2001, terrorist attacks of surgical medical students wearing scrubs and carrying sterile thoracotomy kits around the World Trace Center collapse zone. Clearly, though well intentioned, these types of efforts are ill conceived and have substantial risks with minimal benefits.[48] For example, a nurse who attempted to offer assistance without proper on-scene protective gear after the bombing of the Murrah Federal Building in Oklahoma City was killed by falling debris.[54]

HISTORICAL PERSPECTIVE

Volunteerism

Volunteers have been referred to as the "silver lining" in the cloud of disaster and have been seen as heroes with a badge of honor. Feelings of patriotism, courageousness, spirituality, sense of duty, and even guilt compel people to volunteer.[49,55,56] Volunteerism benefits the community as well as the individual donating his or her efforts by allowing the individual to do something "constructive and communal for his or her own mental health, as an outlet for

rage, and to overcome the sense of powerlessness."[49] Generally, volunteers tend to be people who believe in the good intentions and honesty of others and are agreeable, altruistic, and sympathetic.[57] Furthermore, in a study conducted by Elshaug,[57] volunteers were easy going, active, energetic, and able to concentrate on the task at hand.

Understanding the public's disaster response is important for realistic disaster planning.[46,47] Studies of public behavior during disasters have shown that panic is extremely rare in these situations. Certain situations, though, such as being trapped in a burning building, can lead to panic (Coconut Grove nightclub fire of 1942), but again, this is rare. Extensive studies of more than 900 building fires (including the World Trade Center attacks in 1993 and 2001 and the Beverly Hill Supper Club Fire) failed to find any panic.[58,59]

The role that volunteers play during a disaster is another issue. The literature deals primarily with convergent volunteerism by medical, fire, law enforcement, and civilian personnel.[48] Bissell[51] put forth some general rules for individual roles in disaster situations, including that physician intervention should be at the triage area (except in entrapment situations), that only specially trained physicians and nurses should work in the field environment, and that a physician's primary role is at the hospital. Most physicians are not trained to work in austere environments, such as a California bus accident where on-scene volunteer physicians and nurses contributed to a chaotic scene by "performing poorly" (such as not knowing basic cardiopulmonary resuscitation).[48,60] Physician roles can become even more confused when individuals with various academic training levels are on-scene (medical student, resident, attending), and most of the rescue personnel do not understand the differences between them or are not able verify credentials. Medical personnel perform best when they do tasks similar to their day-to-day activities.[28,54,61]

Convergent volunteers often tend to be viewed as an unwanted nuisance by disaster planners, whose conception of a disaster response often focuses exclusively on the activities of authorized agencies.[47] Some, for example, have complained that convergent volunteers create problems with protocol adherence, crowd control, security, safety, patient tracking, and liability and accountability and that they have to be given food, shelter, and sanitary facilities.[48,62] However, field disaster research studies have shown that most initial search and rescue, casualty care, and transportation efforts in disasters is not carried out by police, fire, and EMS personnel according to a disaster plan; rather, these tasks are performed, on an ad hoc basis, by untrained citizens (family members, co-workers, neighbors, and persons who just happen to be in the area).[47,63]

This often occurs because early in the disaster response there are not enough authorized and trained people available to do the job, when and where it needs to be done. In such a case, bystanders, the victims themselves, and other persons fill in the gap. Sometimes, some simple measures by the first arriving police, fire, or EMS units can help to guide and channel the efforts of bystander volunteers and make their efforts more effective. For example, after a tornado struck Waco, Texas, in 1953, initial search and rescue efforts were uncoordinated and inefficient. However, military workers subsequently brought organization to the rescue efforts by incorporating civilian volunteers into their teams. Most of the teams were composed of 15 men under a leader and an assistant leader, along with another person carrying a walkie-talkie to keep in contact with headquarters and other nearby teams. Signs were put up showing each team's area of operation.[64] Disaster plans should include provisions indicating who is responsible for coordinating spontaneous volunteers working at the scene. Disaster training and drills should also address this responsibility.

Volunteer convergence at hospitals can lead to problems with safety and quality care.[65] Hospitals have to comply with Joint Commission of Accreditation of Healthcare Organization (JCAHO) standards for emergency credentialing of physicians and nurses. Acceptable sources of identification include a current picture hospital identification card, a current license to practice with proof of membership to a disaster medical team, or verification of the volunteer's identity by a current member of the hospital staff.[65] A volunteer's licensure and competency should be verified through a set process as well as shadowing a staff physician.[65]

CURRENT PRACTICE

Volunteerism

The effectiveness of physician volunteers may be enhanced to the extent that they are integrated into a planned response (e.g., one coordinated by the local medical society, Metropolitan Medical Response System, or Medical Reserve Corps). Knowledge of the Incident Command System is also a useful asset.[28] This type of integration worked in the wake of the 1995 Murrah building bombing, the 1985 Mexico earthquake, the 1953 Waco tornado, and the 1994 Northridge, Calif., earthquake (where volunteering nurses were integrated into the Visiting Nurse Association through the local EMS agency).[42,47,62,66] Physicians who become involved with patient care outside of the hospital should try not to deter EMS personnel from following their protocols unless there is a compelling reason to do so and after consulting with their base station physician, if that is possible.[48] Medical personnel should ignore overly hyped media reports and understand credible calls for help and the normal channels they go through.[46] On the other side, the government officials or news media that are calling for volunteers or donations should check with the intended recipients to see what kind of help is really needed. Furthermore, government officials should inform the news media proactively when volunteers or donations are not needed.[47]

Various guides, such as those produced by the states of California and Florida, discuss ways of handling volunteer convergence among the public.[67,68] Some authors report that the public is "treated as an unwanted nuisance by professionals" and the yellow tape perimeter acts as physical and psychological barrier.[47] Instead of pushing the public into a secondary role, Glass[47] suggests

getting the public involved through announcements, forming partnerships, and mobilizing local organizations. Since it is a virtual certainty that untrained members of the public will become involved in casualty care in widespread disasters, it is important to provide them with information on how they can protect themselves and help others. This can be done before an event and can be supplemented with real-time information during a disaster. Examples include how to shelter-in-place; how to decontaminate exposed persons; how to shut off gas and electricity; where to obtain antidotes, potassium iodide, or prophylactic antibiotics; and what hospitals and medical facilities are open, the least crowded, and where they are located.

Furthermore, disaster personnel should enlist the media as an ally, as was done during hurricane Andrew and a Homestead, Fla., area AM radio announcer who was credited with saving many lives by instructing people to get into their bathtubs and cover themselves with mattresses.[47] Also, it is important to educate volunteers, perform community-wide rapid needs assessment, set up statewide medical mutual aid radio systems, and announce what type of donations and volunteers are needed.[46] JCAHO recommends promoting community emergency preparedness plans. This comprises enlisting the community in local response preparations, encouraging an emergency preparedness focus, developing emergency planning and preparedness templates, preserving local healthcare, and establishing leadership and sustainment guidelines.[69]

REFERENCES

1. World Health Organization. EDM 18 Private Donations: An Ounce of Prevention is Worth a Pound of Cure. Available at: http://www.who.int/medicines/library/monitor/edm18b.html.
2. Markon J, Smith L. Internet sparks outpouring of instant donations. *Washington Post*. 2004:A1,A23.
3. Berckmans P, et al. Inappropriate drug-donation practices in Bosnia and Herzegovina, 1992 to 1996. *N Engl J Med*. 1997;337(25):1842-5.
4. Khare AK. Drug donations to developing countries. *World Hosp Health Serv*. 2001;37(1):18-19, 33-4.
5. Hogerzeil HV, Couper MR, Gray R. Guidelines for drug donations. *BMJ*. 1997;314(7082):737-40.
6. Snell B. Inappropriate drug donations: the need for reforms. *Lancet*. 2001;358(9281):578-80.
7. Smego RA Jr, Gebrian B. Donation of medicines to developing countries. *Clin Infect Dis*. 1994;18(5):847-8.
8. World Health Organization. Getting the best from drug donations. Available at: http://www.who.int/medicines/library/monitor/edm_en21.pdf.
9. Lacy E. Pharmaceuticals in disasters. In: Hogan DE, Burstein JL, eds. *Disaster Medicine*. Lippincott Williams & Wilkins: Philadelphia; 2002:34-40.
10. Vlahovic Palcevski V, Vitezic D, Palcevski G. Antibiotics utilization during the war period: influence of drug donations. *Eur J Epidemiol*. 1997;13(8):859-62.
11. Ali HM, Homeida MM, Abdeen MA. "Drug dumping" in donations to Sudan. *Lancet*. 1988;1(8584):538-9.
12. Gray R. Standardization of health relief items needed in the early phase of emergencies. *World Health Stat Q*. 1996;49(3-4):218-20.
13. Forte GB, Alderslade R. Inappropriate drug-donation practices in Bosnia and Herzegovina. *N Engl J Med*. 1998;338(20):1473-4.
14. Bonn D. Call made for application of drug-donation guidelines. *Lancet*. 1999;353(9170):2131.
15. Saunders P. Donations of useless medicines to Kosovo contributes to chaos. *BMJ*. 1999;319(7201):11.

16. Kent D, Glatzer M. Inappropriate drug-donation practices in Bosnia and Herzegovina. *N Engl J Med.* 1998;338(20):1472-4.

17. Hoehn JB. Inappropriate drug-donation practices in Bosnia and Herzegovina. *N Engl J Med.* 1998;338(20):1472-4.

18. Autier P. Inappropriate drug-donation practices in Bosnia and Herzegovina. *N Engl J Med.* 1998;338(20):1472-4.

19. Thomas M. Drug Donations: Corporate Charity or Taxpayer Subsidy [press release]? Available at: http://www.waronwant.org/textonly/0143/www.waronwant.org/?lid=141.

20. Schouten E. Drug donations must be strictly regulated. Georgia has tight guidelines. *BMJ.* 1995;311(7006):684.

21. Barta P, Bellman E. Sri Lanka is grateful, but what to do with ski parkas? Well-meaning donors send heaps of useless stuff; pajama tops, no bottoms. *Wall Street Journal.* 2005:A1.

22. Roche. *Roche Drug Donations Policy.* Available at: http://www.roche.com/pages/downloads/sustain/pdf/drug_don_pol.pdf.

23. Reich MR, et al. Pharmaceutical donations by the USA: an assessment of relevance and time-to-expiry. *Bull World Health Org.* 1999;77(8):675-80.

24. World Health Organization. WHO calls for good drug donation practice during emergencies as it issues new guidelines. Available at: http://www.who.int/inf-pr-1999/en/pr99-45.html.

25. Hillstrom S. Charitable Donations of Drugs by Corporations. Available at: http://www.drugdonations.org/eng/eng_nieuws7.html.

26. Aplenc R. Inappropriate drug-donation practices in Bosnia and Herzegovina. *N Engl J Med.* 1998;338(20):1472-4.

27. Autier P, et al. Drug supply in the aftermath of the 1988 Armenian earthquake. *Lancet.* 1990;335(8702):1388-90.

28. Waeckerle JF. Disaster planning and response. *N Engl J Med.* 1991;324(12):815-21.

29. Rottman SJ. Priorities in medical responses to disasters. *Prehospital Disaster Med.* 1989;5(1):64-6.

30. Humanitarian Supply Management System. Available at: http://www.disaster-info.net/SUMA/english/Links.htm.

31. Ahmad K. WHO releases stricter guidelines on emergency drug donations. *Lancet.* 1999;354(9182):928.

32. Pan American Health Organization. Drug Donations. Available at: http://www.paho.org/english/PED/te_ddon.htm.

33. World Health Organization. Guidelines for Drug Donations—Revised 1999 (Second edition). Available at: http://www.who.int/medicines/library/par/who-edm-par-1999-4/who-edm-par-99-4.shtml.

34. World Health Organization. The WHO Model List of Essential Medicines. Available at: http://www.who.int/medicines/organization/par/edl/eml.shtml.

35. Borrel A, et al. From policy to practice: challenges in infant feeding in emergencies during the Balkan crisis. *Disasters.* 2001;25(2):149-63.

36. Simmonds S, Mamdani M. Essential drug lists and health relief management. *Trop Doct.* 1988;18(4):155-8.

37. World Health Organization. The New Emergency Health Kit 1998. Available at: http://www.who.int/medicines/library/par/new-emergency-health-kit/nehken.shtml.

38. World Health Organization. WHO Medicines Strategy 2004–2007: Countries at the Core. Available at: http://www.who.int/medicines/strategy/MedicinesStrategy2004_2007.shtml.

39. World Health Organization. Managing Drug Supply. Available at: http://www.who.int/medicines/library/monitor/EDM2526_en.pdf.

40. Busch MP, et al. Safety of blood donations following a natural disaster. *Transfusion.* 1991;31(8):719-23.

41. Glynn SA, et al. Effect of a national disaster on blood supply and safety: the September 11 experience. *JAMA.* 2003;289(17):2246-53.

42. Zeballos JL. Health aspects of the Mexico earthquake—19th September 1985. *Disasters.* 1986;10(2):141-9.

43. Becker C, Galloro V. An overwhelming response. Within hours of the disaster, medical supplies were on their way to N.Y., D.C. *Mod Healthc.* 2001;31(38):18-19.

44. Villarosa L. Out to do good, some first-time blood donors get bad news. *New York Times.* Dec 20, 2001:B6.

45. Meckler L. Five times more blood discarded than is usual. *Standard-Times.* Sept 10, 2002:A7.

46. Auf der Heide E. Convergence behavior in disasters. *Ann Emerg Med.* 2003;41(4):463-6.

47. Glass TA. Understanding public response to disasters. *Public Health Rep.* 2001;116(suppl 2):69-73.

48. Cone DC, Weir SD, Bogucki S. Convergent volunteerism. *Ann Emerg Med.* 2003;41(4):457-62.

49. Ellis SJ. A Volunteerism Perspective on the Days After the 11th of September. Available at: http://www.energizeinc.com/hot/01oct.html.

50. Barbera JA, Lozano M Jr. Urban search and rescue medical teams: FEMA Task Force System. *Prehospital Disaster Med.* 1993;8(4):349-55.

51. Bissell RA, Becker BM, Burkle FM Jr. Health care personnel in disaster response. Reversible roles or territorial imperatives? *Emerg Med Clin North Am.* 1996;14(2):267-88.

52. Mitchell TL, et al. 'We Will Never Forget.': the Swissair flight 111 disaster and its impact on volunteers and communities. *J Health Psychol.* 2004;9(2):245-62.

53. Cook L. The World Trade Center attack. The paramedic response: an insider's view. *Crit Care.* 2001;5(6):301-3.

54. Martinez C, Gonzalez D. The World Trade Center attack. Doctors in the fire and police services. *Crit Care.* 2001;5(6):304-6.

55. Ruderman SR. Convergent volunteerism. *Ann Emerg Med.* 2003;42(6):847.

56. Adelman DS. Reaction to disaster volunteering not what I expected. *Nurse Educ.* 2002;27(1):5.

57. Elshaug C, Metzer J. Personality attributes of volunteers and paid workers engaged in similar occupational tasks. *J Soc Psychol.* 2001;141(6):752-63.

58. Noji EK. The nature of disaster: general characteristics and public health effects. In: Noji EK, ed. *The Public Health Consequences of Disasters.* New York: Oxford University Press; 1997:3-20.

59. Auf der Heide E. Common misconceptions in disasters: panic, the "disaster syndrome," and looting. In: *The First 72 Hours: A Community Approach to Disaster Preparedness.* Lincoln, NE: iUniverse; 2004:340-80.

60. Lewis FR, Trunkey DD, Steele MR. Autopsy of a disaster: the Martinez bus accident. *J Trauma.* 1980;20(10):861-6.

61. Wegner D, James TF. The convergence of volunteers in a consensus crises: the case of the 1985 Mexico City earthquake. In: Dynes RR, Tierney KJ, eds. *Disasters, Collective Behavior, and Social Organization.* Newark: University of Delaware Press; 1994:229-43.

62. Team OCDM. *Final Report: Alfred P. Murrah Federal Building Bombing, April 19, 1995.* Stillwater, OK: Fire Protection Publications; 1996:B-114, C-246.

63. Auf der Heide E. Principles of hospital disaster planning. In: Hogan D, Burnstein JL, eds. *Disaster Medicine.* Philadelphia: Lippincott Williams & Wilkins; 2002:57-89.

64. Moore HE. *Tornados over Texas: A Study of Waco and San Angelo in Disaster.* Austin: University of Texas Press; 1958.

65. Downs K, Jefferies C, Klass M. Credential volunteers during disasters. *Hosp Peer Rev.* 2003;28(8):108-10.

66. Stratton SJ, et al. The 1994 Northridge earthquake disaster response: the local emergency medical services agency experience. *Prehospital Disaster Med.* 1996;11(3):172-9.

67. State of California, Governor's Office of Emergency Services. They Will Come: Post-Disaster Volunteers and Local Governments. Available at: http://www.oes.ca.gov/Operational/OESHome.nsf/PDF/They%20Will%20Come%20Post-Disaster%20Volunteers%20and%20Local%20Government/$file/TheyWillCome.pdf.

68. Volunteer Florida. Unaffiliated Volunteers in Response and Recovery. Available at: http://www.volunteerflorida.org/publications/docs/unaffiliatedvolunteers.pdf.

69. Joint Commission on Accreditation of Healthcare Organizations. Introduction to Health Care at the Crossroads: Strategies for Creating and Sustaining Community-wide Emergency Preparedness Systems. Available at: http://www.jcaho.org/about+us/public+policy+initiatives/emergency_preparedness.pdf.

chapter 36

Personal Protective Equipment

John L. Hick and Craig D. Thorne

Personal protective equipment (PPE) recently has become a rather common acronym in the lexicon of healthcare providers, even though it has been common in the fire services, emergency medical services (EMS), and military for quite some time. Essentially, PPE helps ensure that individuals are safe from physical hazards that they may encounter in their work environment. PPE may be used to protect workers from general environmental threats (e.g., temperature extremes, noise), specific work-related threats (e.g., falling objects, falls from heights), or threats faced in an emergency situation (e.g., hazardous chemical and infectious agents). No equipment is appropriate for all individuals and threats, but it must be selected and properly used according to the setting of use and the level of risk.

The critical problem with most PPE, particularly in regard to chemically protective suits and respirators, is that with higher levels of protection come not only higher prices and required training levels, but also a higher physiological and physical burden to the user. Thus, a structured approach to assessment of risk and selection of proper equipment is important to achieve a reasonable level of protection in relation to the hazard.

This chapter reviews the concepts of PPE, recent lessons learned in regard to PPE, types of respirators, key regulations, and issues in the selection of PPE for emergency medical care and decontamination operations.

HISTORICAL PERSPECTIVE

Until recently, PPE for medical providers received little attention short of the "standard precautions" of gloves, with the addition of simple masks and barrier precautions, when needed. The 2003 severe acute respiratory syndrome (SARS) pandemic, the 1995 Tokyo subway sarin attack, the 1995 Murrah Federal Building bombing in Oklahoma City, and the terrorist attacks of September 2001 are some examples of situations in which the lack of proper PPE resulted in adverse health effects for healthcare providers and thus focused attention on PPE as a critical issue in disaster response.

In March 1995, a crude form of the nerve agent sarin was released in the Tokyo subway system on separate cars bound for a common downtown station. This attack resulted in 12 deaths and more than 4000 persons presenting to the hospital for medical evaluation. None of the casualties was decontaminated before treatment or transport. Retrospectively, 135 prehospital and 100 hospital personnel reported symptoms consistent with nerve agent exposure. Fortunately, none required emergency treatment.[1,2] Eleven physicians caring for the sickest victims (including one in cardiac arrest and one in respiratory arrest) were most affected, and six of them required antidotal therapy. Fortunately, all recovered fully and did not have to cease their patient care efforts due to symptoms.[3] Approximately 80% of victims self-referred to hospitals, which is consistent with U.S. experiences indicating that few victims of chemical contamination events undergo decontamination before arrival at a medical facility.[2,4] This has caused most jurisdictions to reconsider historical plans that contaminated patients would not be in contact with medical care personnel until they were "clean." EMS and hospital personnel need to be prepared for contaminated patients presenting directly to them and to recognize that in certain situations, PPE may be required to safely provide care.

SARS posed unique risks and challenges to healthcare workers. This novel viral agent with incompletely defined transmission characteristics was controlled in 2002 with aggressive quarantine measures and use of PPE. In the first wave of SARS in Toronto, 79.2% of all cases were acquired in a healthcare setting.[5] Aggressive use of PPE, including N95 masks, barrier precautions, and gloves, was generally effective at preventing spread, although during one difficult and prolonged intubation attempt, at least six providers contracted SARS from a patient despite complying with PPE recommendations.[6] This case led to recommendations that higher levels of PPE may be required during procedures that are likely to generate aerosols or provoke coughing, such as intubation, airway suctioning, positive pressure ventilation, and nebulization treatments.[7]

The National Institute for Occupational Safety and Health (NIOSH) and the RAND Corporation produced a comprehensive "lessons learned" report summarizing issues from the 2001 terrorist bombings at the World Trade Center (WTC), anthrax incidents, and the 1995 Oklahoma City Murrah Federal Building bombing. The report, titled "Protecting Emergency Responders: Lessons

Learned from Terrorist Attacks" describes in detail many of the challenges responders faced (Box 36-1).[8]

It is clear from the WTC events that a large number of jurisdictions responding, conflicting messages regarding use of PPE and safety of the environment, and lack of a plan to implement respiratory precautions can complicate a response and potentially place providers at risk. WTC responders continue to suffer respiratory symptoms attributable to exposures at "ground zero."[9]

CURRENT PRACTICE

Hazard Vulnerability Analysis

Selection of appropriate PPE begins with an analysis of the hazards that responders may encounter and an assessment of responders' roles and responsibilities. Hazard vulnerability analyses (HVA) are required for community emergency planning grants and are required of healthcare facilities that are accredited by the Joint Commission on Accreditation of Healthcare Organizations (JCAHO).[10] The HVA uses a numerical ranking of factors for specific threats (e.g., chemical release), including the risk of the event occurring, the current preparedness for the threat, and the risk to life. The numerical score determines the gravity of each threat to the community. Each community's HVA will reflect the unique risks that must be considered by its emergency responders. Choice of PPE may be affected by factors within the HVA such as:

- Population density of the community and surrounding area
- High- or moderate-risk terrorist targets in the community (e.g., government buildings, centers of commerce, or another symbolic site)
- Chemical hazards posed by community industry (e.g., use of cyanide and hydrofluoric acid in the electronics industry)
- Risk of transportation incidents and major transportation routes, particularly highways and railroads
- Proximity of healthcare facilities, schools, or other key locations to these potential targets and industrial and transportation hazards
- Frequency of hazardous materials (HazMat) incidents in the community
- Resources available to respond to HazMat incidents (e.g., rapid access to on-site decontamination may decrease, but not eliminate, contaminated persons leaving the scene)

Defining the Agency/Facility Role

Stakeholders in emergency response, including EMS and healthcare facilities and fire and rescue, emergency management, and law enforcement agencies, must clearly define the responsibilities of each entity and the support and resources that each may need or offer during an emergency, particularly one involving a HazMat release.

EMS roles in a HazMat event vary depending on jurisdictional planning. Fire services personnel may or may

---

BOX 36-1 HISTORICAL HAZARDS FACED BY RESPONDERS TO TERRORISM EVENTS

- Physical hazards including fires, burning jet fuel and explosions, rubble piles with sharp rebar and heated metal, falling debris (which resulted in the death of a nurse in Oklahoma City), hazardous materials, electrical hazards, structures prone to collapse, heat stress, exhaustion, and respiratory irritants
- Heat-related seizures while wearing chemically protective suits
- Eye injuries (usually related to particulate exposure), which accounted for 12% of all WTC disaster response worker injuries
- Potential for secondary hazards, including explosive devices and chemical, biological, and radioactive agents
- PPE shortcomings:
  - Heavy helmets hindered performance
  - Self-contained breathing apparatus (SCBA) was heavy and cumbersome
  - SCBA face pieces fogged (reducing visibility), and the equipment hindered verbal and radio communication
  - SCBA air bottle made it difficult to enter small spaces, and the limited air supply (up to 1 hour) necessitated leaving the operation to exchange the air bottle
  - Air tanks and/or filters were not interchangeable between teams, and teams worked under different standards
  - Powered air-purifying respirator (PAPR) filters became clogged and were uncomfortable for long duration use. Many workers instead opted to use dust masks (which offered little protection and caused nose-bridge chafing) or to wear the masks/hoods around their necks ("neck protectors")
  - Use of respirators made it difficult for workers to communicate with each other, often resulting in users breaking the face seal to talk
  - Turnout gear (the common protective garments used by firefighters) increased heat stress and physical fatigue
  - At the WTC, the rubble pile was so hot in places that it melted the soles of workers' boots; providing wash stations to cool the boots resulted in wet feet and serious blisters for many workers; some 440 WTC disaster response workers sought treatment for blisters
  - Steel-reinforced boots (soles and toes) protected against punctures by sharp objects but conducted and retained heat, which contributed to blisters and burns
  - Structural firefighting gloves worked well until they got wet and hardened, reducing their dexterity
  - WTC disaster response workers did not consistently protect their hands against potential hazards such as human remains and bodily fluids
  - Safety glasses were readily available but often were open at the sides and did not offer adequate protection against airborne particles
  - Goggles were uncomfortable, hindered peripheral vision, tended to fog, and did not fit well in conjunction with half-face respirators
  - Many disaster response workers at the WTC (especially law enforcement officers) did not consistently use hearing protection, even around heavy machinery, because they needed to hear their radios and voices and listen for tapping when they were searching for survivors
- Most volunteers at the WTC, Pentagon, and Oklahoma City did not receive pre-event training on PPE and hazardous materials
- Although firefighters generally received detailed pre-event training, this was less true for law enforcement officers
- Accurate "real-time" hazard information was not readily available, especially during the anthrax incidents
- Protection from falls was available at some sites (in the form of ropes and harnesses) but was inconsistently used

not be able to provide treatment in a "warm zone" (i.e., the area of reduced contamination outside of the immediate release zone) depending on their training. Non-fire based EMS personnel may require PPE to triage and treat victims in the warm zone. In the event of a mass chemical exposure, victims will likely self-refer to visible ambulances, call 911 from sites removed from the site of release, or make their way to hospitals, by-passing organized EMS and fire services. This movement of contamination on the bodies of patients essentially causes a "migrating" warm zone, causing contamination of previously clean ("cold") areas. This migrating contamination may require protective equipment for EMS responders, and appropriate plans and equipment should be in place. The roles and responsibilities of the responders, as well as the equipment required, need to be defined and drilled in advance of an incident.

Hospitals, until very recently, usually relied on fire services for patient decontamination at the hospital. These resources, however, are often deployed to the scene of the event and are thus unavailable to support the hospital. Most hospitals have now recognized the need for at least some internal capacity for patient decontamination and are equipping their teams with PPE appropriate for decontaminating self-referred contaminated patients. A few hospital teams integrate with community HazMat teams, necessitating additional training and equipment as the mission then changes from a defensive decontamination response to an offensive response at the scene of release.

Risks to Providers

HazMat releases seldom cause serious injury, but the potential exists for both scene responders and hospital receivers to suffer serious consequences of exposure. The Agency for Toxic Substance and Disease Registry (ATSDR) maintains a multistate voluntary accounting of hazardous substance releases, excluding petroleum-related incidents. The Hazardous Substances Emergency Events Surveillance (HSEES) database currently involves 15 states.[11] From 1993 to 2001, 44,015 events were recorded: 3455 (7.8%) of the incidents caused injuries, and 74% of victims were transported to a healthcare facility.[4] In another analysis of HSEES data, only 5% of victims required admission to a healthcare facility.[12] The vast majority had self-limited respiratory symptoms. In 2001, the chemicals with highest potential for injury were chlorine (injury occurred in 18.8% of releases), ammonia (18.2%), acids (14.2%), and pesticides (17%).[13]

HSEES data from 1996 to 1998 show 348 responder injuries in 126 incidents out of a total of 16,986 incidents (0.7%). Law enforcement officers and firefighters accounted for the vast majority of responder injuries, which usually consisted of nausea and respiratory irritation. Hospital admission occurred in 6.6% of cases. No deaths were reported in this 3-year period.[4]

Hospital personnel were injured in 0.3% of the total HazMat events and represented 0.1% of the victims.[4] Six events involved emergency department staff contact with contaminated patients, and five events were HazMat releases at the healthcare facility itself. No provider required hospital admission, and no chemical PPE was used. Other reports of emergency department evacuation and/or provider illness due to off-gassing from contaminated patients have been summarized.[14-19] The most serious of these incidents involve patients with suicidal ingestions of organophosphate pesticides.[14-16] Exposures to these patients caused at least one provider to require intubation and receive aggressive antidotal therapy due to contact with pesticide in emesis and vapors during patient resuscitation.[14] Patients who have ingested organophosphate may off-gas for days and present an ongoing risk to healthcare workers.[16] NIOSH has documented 46 healthcare worker injuries from pesticide agents between 1987 and 1998.[14] In conjunction with the information from the Tokyo subway sarin attack and the chemical terrorism risk posed by these agents, it is clear that these pesticides present a substantial risk of toxicity from secondary exposures.

Limited research is available to document the degree of the off-gassing that occurs from the bodies and clothing of contaminated patients.[20,21] Clothing removal and control may be expected to remove 90% of the contaminant and thus should be a priority.[21,22] Ideally, this should take place in an open-air environment.

Chemical Protective Equipment

Providers may not initially recognize a chemical release when they arrive at a scene. Even though structural firefighting ensembles with self-contained breathing apparatus (SCBA) offer some chemical protection that may be sufficient for victim rescue,[23] the incident commander must determine what actions are appropriate for the situation. Protective suits, gloves, and boots and appropriate respiratory protection must be donned as soon as possible when a chemical threat is recognized.

The Occupational Safety and Health Administration (OSHA) and Environmental Protection Agency define four basic levels of PPE for HazMat scene responses (Table 36-1 and Fig. 36-1) (OSHA standard 29 CFR 1910.120, Appendix B). Generally, as the level of protection increases (A being the highest level), so do the weight, cost, and physiological burden. Increasing protection also generally means decreasing mobility, dexterity, and scope of vision. Inherent risks to PPE include trip and fall hazards; a reduced ability to complete tasks; heat stress[19,24-27]; anxiety[28]; and seizures, which, although rare, have been reported.[19] Cardiovascular demand is dramatically increased as ensemble weight and heat retention increase. PPE must be selected on the basis that it does not impose unnecessary risks on the provider while at the same time offering an appropriate margin of safety against the chemical hazard. Because the selection of PPE usually revolves around the selection of the respiratory component, various types of respirators must be reviewed. Each respirator has an assigned protection factor that reflects the degree of protection afforded to the user. Simply put, 1/protection factor equals the amount of exposure for the wearer. For example, a provider wearing a powered air-purifying respirator (PAPR) with an assigned protection factor (APF) of 1000 is exposed to 1/1000 the level of contaminant as compared with wearing no protection.

TABLE 36-1 CATEGORIES OF PPE

LEVEL	BRIEF DESCRIPTION	ADVANTAGES	DISADVANTAGES
A	Completely encapsulated suit and SCBA	Highest level of protection available for both contact and vapor hazards	• Expense and training requirements typically restrict use to HazMat response teams • Lack of mobility • Heat and physical stresses • Limited air supply • Fit-testing requirements
B	Encapsulating suit or junctions/seams sealed, and supplied-air respirator (SAR) or SCBA	High level of protection adequate for entry into unknown environments	Same as for Level A • SAR hose may pose a trip hazard or become dislodged
C	Splash suit and air-purifying respirator (APR) (note APR and PAPR considered equivalent in classification despite significant difference in protection)	• Significantly increased mobility • Less physical stress • Extended operation time with high levels of protection against certain chemical hazards • No fit-testing required for hood type	• Not adequate for some high-concentration environments, less-than-atmospheric-oxygen environments, or high levels of splash contamination • Expense and training moderate
D	Usual work clothes	• Increased mobility • Less physical stress • Extended operation time • More fashionable	• Offer no protection against specific hazards • Expense and training minimal

Atmosphere-Supplying Respirators

Atmosphere-supplying respirators provide breathable fresh air to the user *independent of the environment* via an air supply hose and/or tank and thus offer a high level of respiratory protection. This type of respirator is required for entry into environments where the identity of and/or the potential quantity of a hazardous substance are unknown or where the quantity of oxygen in the air is unknown.

SCBA is the most common atmosphere-supplying respirator for emergency responses. It provides air via a tank, usually worn on the back. The operational time is limited by the capacity of the tank (usually less than 1 hour). Fire services personnel routinely use this form of respiratory protection, and fire-based EMS services personnel generally incorporate this PPE into their chemical protection planning. Limitations include the equipment's weight (approximately 25 to 30 pounds), cost, need for fit-testing, duration of air supply, and need to refill air bottles. Even though SCBA provides excellent protection, its limitations make it inappropriate for many situations (e.g., caring for a patient with an infectious disease, providing hospital-based decontamination, or securing a perimeter in the warm zone). SCBA has an APF of about 10,000, the highest of any type of respirator.[29]

Supplied-air respirators (SARs) provide air via a hose line from a nearby clean air source (e.g., compressor or hospital supply line). To meet OSHA requirements for level B, respirators must have a tight-fitting face piece and an emergency supply of air in case of line failure or problems.[30] Loose-fitting hoods with a supplied air source do not meet level B standards but are used by some decontamination teams when an additional level of protection is desired due to institutional preference or local hazard profile. Advantages include a potentially unlimited supply of fresh air and longer duration of use. Limitations are primarily mobility and thus flexibility of response. These respirators are best suited to healthcare provider use in a decontamination room or a well-defined area in which the air lines are unlikely to be tangled, stretched, or a tripped hazard. The APF of a typical tight-fitting face piece SAR is 1000, although there may be variability among models and types (e.g., tight-fitting mask versus loose-fitting hood).[29]

Air-Purifying Respirators

Air-purifying respirators (APRs) have cartridges that filter the air *in the user's environment* to remove particulate matter and specific chemicals that the filter is designed to capture. These filters do *not* affect the oxygen concentration of the ambient air and thus cannot be used in potentially oxygen-deficient environments. Only those chemicals for which the filter is designated are removed. Also, the capacity of the filter can be exceeded by large amounts of contaminant, thus these respirators are designed for situations in which the concentration of the agent is either established to be or assumed to be below the threshold for the canister.

Nonpowered APRs use the wearer's work of breathing to pull ambient air through the filter. Examples include dust masks and military and civilian "gas masks." The APF of a nonpowered full face piece APR is 50 when appropriate *quantitative* fit-testing is performed.[29] Of note, this type of mask is used by the military for battlefield protection against lethal levels of nerve and other chemical agents. Advantages include low cost and long duration of use. Disadvantages include increased work of breathing and physiological stress, mask fogging, and the need for fit-testing.

A PAPR uses a motor to pull air through the filter canisters, thus decreasing the work of breathing and the risk of air entrainment around the respirator face piece. PAPRs are often supplied with a loose-fitting disposable or reusable hood that eliminates the need to perform fit-testing and allows use by a broad range of individuals. Hooded PAPRs with "stacked" canisters that offer protection against com-

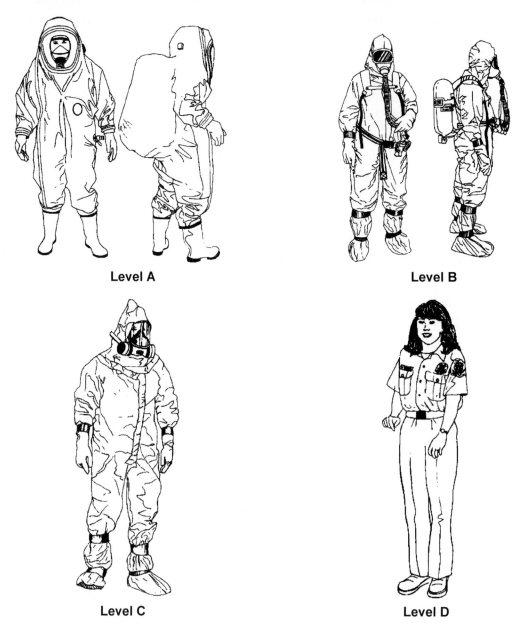

Level A

Level B

Level C

Level D

FIGURE 36–1. Levels of PPE. (From Agency for Toxic Substances and Disease Registry. Emergency Medical Services Response to Hazardous Materials Incidents. Available at: http://www.atsdr.cdc.gov/mhmi-v1-2.pdf.)

mon hazardous chemical and biological agents encountered by first responders and hospital personnel are in widespread use due to their relatively low cost, weight, and the increased flexibility of response allowed. Dependence on battery power, shelf life of the filters, and the need to be able to match the filter to the agent are limiting factors. The currently proposed APF for a PAPR is 1000.[29] Directions for use must be carefully followed; one particular model provides a protection factor of 20,000 when properly donned, but when the inner hood is not tucked in, the protection level declines to 1000 and less[31,32] (personal communication, 2001). Battery packs are usually either single-use or rechargeable. Rechargeable battery packs require ongoing attention to ensure a proper charge, but they offer the flexibility of allowing PAPR re-use during an infectious disease event.

Particulate filter masks such as those commonly used for patient care to protect against tuberculosis and other organisms are also considered APRs. Masks are classified N (not oil resistant), R (oil resistant), and P (oil proof). N95 refers to a filter (the entire mask) that removes 95% of a particulate challenge in the 3- to 5-µm range. N100 respirators filter 100% of the same challenge, yet simple half-face respirators offer an APF of only 10 due to the entrainment of air around the mask and other factors; therefore, changing from an N95 to an N100 offers little additional protection unless a more robust mask ensemble, rather than a simple half-face mask, is used.[33,34]

Respiratory protection technologies are rapidly evolving, and respiratory program administrators should make sure they are familiar with the available options and their relative advantages/disadvantages. Regional cooperative planning and purchases may be helpful to allow for sharing of resources during an incident.

Chemically protective suits must be tailored to the type of use. Suits for hot zone entry where direct contact with a hazardous material is likely must be much more robust than suits for patient decontamination activities. Selection should be guided by National Fire Protection Association (NFPA) standards 1992 and 1994 for site-of-release response activities and by recent OSHA guidance for hospital decontamination activities.[35,36] Chemicals commonly found in local transit, agriculture, or industrial use should also guide selection. Appropriate PPE for perimeter control and EMS warm zone operations remain topics of debate at this time. Generally, suits should be sized far more generously than standard work clothing to prevent tearing during squatting and other activities (e.g., an average 70-kg man should plan to wear a size XXL suit). Many suit configurations are possible, and the optimal configuration will depend on the mission and other equipment in the ensemble. For example, suits without "feet" are preferred when worn with boots (to allow taping over the boot) but those with integrated bootie "feet" are preferred when pull-on "sock" type butyl booties are to be used. These integrated feet should *not* be used as primary footwear at any time because they have poor abrasion resistance.

Boots supplied in sizes medium, large, and extra large rather than fitted sizes may be preferred when equipment is purchased for a group (e.g., hospital decontamination team) rather than being purchased for an individual responder (e.g., firefighter). Butyl or other rubber boots probably afford appropriate protection for warm zone operations. Butyl "sock" type booties may be used on very low abrasion surfaces (e.g., internal hospital decontamination room) but are not generally appropriate for outside use.

Nitrile undergloves with butyl overgloves provide protection against a broad range of hazards for warm zone activities. Silver Shield gloves are more expensive but may be better suited for particular compounds when the agent is known. Overglove selection should balance the need for abrasion resistance with dexterity required to perform tasks (e.g., to administer intramuscular antidotes). The U.S. Army Center for Health Promotion and Preventive Medicine (USACHPPM) recommends 14-mm thickness butyl gloves (standard examination gloves are 4 mm) as a minimum for working with patients contaminated by chemical warfare agents or toxic industrial chemicals.[37]

Biological Protective Equipment

Very few situations require physical decontamination of patients exposed to biological agents. An exception would be patients who present after contamination with biological agents (e.g., anthrax spores) from a dissemination device. PPE for decontamination should consist of the same chemical protective suit and high level of respiratory protection, including a high-efficiency particulate (HEPA) or SAR, that would be used for chemical decontamination activities. PPE for biological agents

in relation to care of patients who are already infected and symptomatic is discussed in the following.

Categories of PPE for biological agents include[38]:

1. *Standard precautions:* Use of gloves and proper hand hygiene to prevent disease transmission for any potentially infectious patient. Gowns and eye protection are added only when patient care activities are likely to result in splashing or soiling.
2. *Contact precautions:* Standard precautions *plus* use of barriers during *all* patient care activities to protect face, arms, and front torso to prevent contact with secretions, emesis, feces, etc. (e.g., enteric infections, many hemorrhagic fever viruses).
3. *Droplet precautions:* Standard precautions with the addition of a droplet respirator (e.g., surgical mask) when working within 3 feet of the patient to prevent transmission of infectious agents that travel by large droplet spread (e.g., cirborne precautions are used against plague); may not be protective against all droplet nuclei.
4. *Airborne precautions:* Standard precautions with an N95 or higher protection respirator to prevent transmission of infectious agents that are spread by aerosols (e.g., airborne precautions are used against chickenpox, smallpox, and tuberculosis).
5. *"Special pathogen precautions":* Based on the SARS experiences, a high-risk pathogen with respiratory spread probably requires greater levels of protection than previously recommended. Constant use of both contact and airborne precautions has generally been advised with the optional use of a PAPR rather than an N95 mask during "high-risk" interventions likely to generate aerosols or provoke coughing (e.g., suctioning, intubation, positive pressure ventilation).[6,7] These precautions are the subject of current discussion.

Patient care providers should have routine access to nonsterile examination gloves, barrier gowns that protect the arms and front torso, standard surgical (droplet) masks, and a face shield that provides adequate splash protection (which may be integrated with the mask, a separate face shield, or goggles) according to the OSHA bloodborne pathogens standard.[39]

Providers should have ready access to higher levels of protection when needed. "Bad bug bags" may be assembled with appropriate gowns, gloves, face shields/goggles, N95 or PAPR respirators, and other supplies so that healthcare providers do not have to assemble the recommended components. Instruction sheets for donning/doffing and disinfection procedures can be included in the bag.[40]

Practitioners fitted for N95 respirators may use these for patient care, and others should have access to a PAPR until they are fitted for an N95 respirator. Plans to rapidly fit-test additional employees during an event that might require prolonged use of airborne precautions (e.g., SARS) should be in place.

Regulations and Training

All PPE must be part of an ongoing program of respiratory protection and HazMat/decontamination response within the agency or institution to ensure that employees who are expected to use these protections are competent and comfortable with the indications, use, and limitations of their equipment. Numerous regulations apply to the selection and proper use of PPE. All persons using PPE must conform to OSHA standards on respiratory protection (29 CFR 1910.134), PPE (29 CFR 1910.132), eye and face protection (29 CFR 1910.133), hand protection (29 CFR 1910.138), hazard communication (29 CFR 1910.1200), and bloodborne pathogens (29 CFR 1910.1030). State OSHA agencies may have stricter requirements than the federal standards. Most occupational or employee health services of agencies/facilities where PPE is used are very familiar with these standards and their application to employees.

The NFPA has numerous standards for the training and equipping of responders (including EMS personnel) to a HazMat incident (e.g., NFPA standards 471, 473, 1981, 1992, 1994, and 1999). Specific guidance is also provided for urban search and rescue teams (NFPA standard 1951).[35] Responders to HazMat releases are covered by OSHA's HAZWOPER (Hazardous Waste Operations and Emergency Response) standard 29 CFR 1910.120, which is perhaps the most comprehensive standard guiding hazardous materials responses.

OSHA requires use of a minimum of level B equipment (i.e., an atmosphere-supplying respirator and chemically protective suit with sealed seams) during a response into a contaminated environment until the concentration of the agent is shown via air monitoring to be below the threshold required for the safe use of an APR or other lesser degree of protection.[41] This requirement presents difficulty for EMS and hospital providers because the agent is often unknown at the time that medical care is provided in the warm zone (i.e., an area where the level of contamination is minimal and controlled). Particularly for hospitals, confusion existed as to what constituted appropriate protection for decontamination team members who provide medical care for contaminated patients and to what degree the HAZWOPER standard applied to community responders geographically separate from the site of release.

OSHA clarified this issue for healthcare facility providers in two letters of interpretation[42,43] and a comprehensive guidance document on PPE and training released in 2004.[36] In this document, OSHA codifies use of PAPRs as the minimum level of respiratory protective equipment for hospitals under certain conditions:

- The facility acts as a "first receiver" for self-referred contaminated casualties, *not* as a responder to a release zone.
- The facility itself is not the site of the hazardous substances release.
- An HVA has been conducted to identify specific hazards to the community and facility.
- The victims must present at least 10 minutes after exposure (to allow time for some of the contaminant to evaporate or dissipate). It will usually take at least this long to get personnel into PPE at the facility.
- The victims' clothing must be rapidly removed and contained.
- Decontamination must occur in a well-ventilated area, preferably outdoors.

When these conditions are met, and absent any particular threats within the community that require higher levels of protection (such as close proximity to a specific chemical production, storage, or disposal site), the minimum level of respiratory PPE is a PAPR with a protection factor of 1000 or greater, which filters organic vapor, acid gas, particulate matter, and biological agents (at the HEPA level).[36]

HAZWOPER also defines training requirements for responders.[44] The application of these regulations to hospital decontamination teams was also clarified in recent OSHA guidance.[36] Awareness training is required for individuals involved in a HazMat response who will not be using PPE or taking actions beyond recognizing and reporting an incident (emergency department staff, law enforcement officers).[43]

At a minimum, all responders who will use chemical PPE must be trained to the operations level (8 hours or to competency)[43] so that each responder can:

- Understand his or her role in the response and the emergency response plan.
- Identify the presence of a hazardous substance through signs and symptoms of exposure.
- Assess site safety, including risks to self.
- Select and safely use appropriate PPE.
- Understand decontamination procedures.

HazMat awareness educational competencies must also be met by providers trained to the operations level. The awareness competencies may be included in the 8 hours of operations training or conducted separately.[36]

In addition, any personnel using respiratory protective equipment must be in compliance with OSHA's respiratory protection standard (29 CFR 120.134). Key features of this standard are:

- Respirator selection procedures.
- Proper use of respirators in routine and reasonably foreseeable emergency situations.
- Medical clearance before use (at minimum, a screening questionnaire; see Appendix C of the standard).
- Fit-testing before use and annually thereafter (see Appendix A and B1 of the standard).
- Inspecting, cleaning/disinfecting, storing, repairing, and maintaining the equipment.
- Training and education on topics such as the types of respiratory hazards they might be exposed to, proper use (including donning and doffing), limitations, and maintenance.

Most medical facilities and response agencies have a respiratory protection program in place. This existing foundation and the subject matter experts in occupational safety and health, infection control, or other related disciplines can assist with implementation of new technologies and protocols.

PITFALLS AND ONGOING CHALLENGES

PPE technology continues to change rapidly. Hopefully, technologies that are lighter weight, less expensive, and less heat-retaining can be developed. Technology change is occurring far more rapidly than the current approvals process and new standards that have arisen in the wake of the events of 2001. Clear guidance on appropriate technologies for warm zone activities is lacking at this time. This can lead to confusion and difficult choices for agencies and facilities, knowing that their PPE selection may be either too much or too little to satisfy future standards. Currently, there is no recommendation or consensus on the level of PPE that is required for hospital-based personnel, much to the consternation of hospital preparedness leaders. Some have proposed a PPE level "H" to meet this need. More research is clearly needed regarding safe but comfortable PPE, methods of decontamination, modeling of airborne concentrations of specific agents, and PPE selection.

Further, detection technologies are needed that can provide better environmental screening for a wide range of hazardous substances and quantitative assessment of agent concentration. Currently, incident commanders may remain confused about appropriate PPE, and this may result in PPE selection that is overly conservative (which risks provider noncompliance and adverse effects from the PPE) or overly liberal (which risks provider injury from the contaminant).

Finally, providers need to be educated about the consequences of not using PPE appropriately, including acute chemical effects and delayed pulmonary effects.

In general, communities and regions can help to reduce issues of PPE interoperability by planning, purchasing, and training together whenever possible. This also allows for caches of materials to be deployed that are true replacements for usual materials and thus will be better accepted and require minimal training.

For too long, jurisdictions have been reluctant to share their problems, issues, and roadblocks in the area of PPE, lest the agency be seen as having problems protecting its responders. Better dialogue and sharing of best practices and lessons learned are of immense value to better HazMat response planning and should be encouraged. The recent NIOSH/RAND report[8] and release of select after-action reports are welcome changes in this history.

Defining hazards in this age of potential chemical terrorism is fraught with peril because we are unable to truly assess the scope of the threat. Thus, PPE must be chosen that will protect appropriately against a broad range of threats without being so restrictive that in the heat of the moment, the provider decides to forgo the PPE and is at risk of becoming a casualty of the event. Balancing cost, ease of use, and scope of protection concerns are delicate decisions with few answers at this time, particularly for those who may have long-duration job tasks in a warm zone environment.

We can only hope that we are not forced to learn too many more harsh lessons about PPE use in the future. In the meantime, however, we should strive to prepare our communities by selecting appropriate protective technologies in relation to perceived threats and practicing our responses so that our personnel are comfortable using their PPE and understand the consequences of not doing so.

REFERENCES

1. Okumura T, Suzuki K, Atsuhiro F, et al. The Tokyo subway sarin attack: disaster management, part 1: community emergency response. *Acad Emerg Med*. 1998;5:613-17.
2. Okumura T, Suzuki K, Fukada A, et al. The Tokyo subway sarin attack: disaster management, part 2: hospital response. *Acad Emerg Med*. 1998;5:618-24.
3. Nozaki H, Hori S, Shinozama Y, et al. Secondary exposure of medical staff to sarin vapor in the emergency room. *Intensive Care Med*. 1995;21:1032-5.
4. Horton DK, Berkowitz Z, Kaye WE. Secondary contamination of emergency department personnel from hazardous materials events, 1995-2001. *Am J Emerg Med*. 2003;21:199-204.
5. Svoboda T, Henry B, Shulman L, et al. Public health measures to control the spread of the severe acute respiratory syndrome during the outbreak in Toronto. *New Engl J Med*. 2004;350:2352-61.
6. Cluster of severe acute respiratory syndrome cases among protected healthcare workers—Toronto, Canada, April 2003. *Morb Mortal Wkly Rep*. 2003;52:433-6.
7. Centers for Disease Control and Prevention. Public Health Guidance for Community-Level Preparedness and Response to Severe Acute Respiratory Syndrome (SARS) Version 2: Supplement I: Infection Control in the Home, Healthcare, and Community Settings. Atlanta: Centers for Disease Control and Prevention; 2004. Available at: http://www.cdc.gov/ncidod/sars/guidance/i/pdf/i.pdf.
8. Jackson BA, Peterson DJ, Bartis JT, et al. *Protecting Emergency Responders: Lessons Learned from Terrorist Attacks*. Santa Monica, CA: RAND Corporation; 2002.
9. Physical health status of World Trade Center rescue and recovery workers and volunteers—New York City, July 2002-August 2004. *Morb Mortal Wkly Rep*. 2004;53(35):807-12.
10. Joint Commission on Accreditation of Healthcare Organizations. *The 2001 Joint Commission Accreditation Manual for Healthcare Facilities EC 1.4 and 1.6 (rev)*. Oakbrook Terrace, IL: Joint Commission on Accreditation of Healthcare Organizations; 2001.
11. Agency for Toxic Substances and Disease Registry. Hazardous Substances Emergency Events Surveillance. Available at: http://www.atsdr.cdc.gov/HS/HSEES.
12. Burgess JL. Risk factors for adverse health events following hazardous materials incidents. *J Occup Environ Med*. 2001;43(6):558-66.
13. Agency for Toxic Substances and Disease Registry. Hazardous Substances Emergency Events Surveillance (HSEES) Annual Report 2001: Victims. Available at: http://www.atsdr.cdc.gov/HS/HSEES/annual2001.html#victims.
14. Centers for Disease Control and Prevention. Nosocomial poisoning associated with emergency department treatment of organophosphate toxicity—Georgia, 2000. *Morb Mortal Wkly Rep*. 2001;49(51):1156-8.
15. Merritt NL, Anderson MJ. Malathion overdose: when one patient creates a departmental hazard. *J Emerg Nurs*. 1989;15:463-5.
16. Merril D. Prolonged toxicity of organophosphate poisoning. *Crit Care Med*. 1982;10:550-1.
17. Thanabalasingham T, Beckett MW, Murray V. Hospital response to a chemical incident: report on casualties of an ethyldichlorosilane spill. *BMJ* 1991;302:101-2.
18. Nocera A, Levitin HW, Hilton JMN. Dangerous bodies: a case of fatal aluminum phosphide poisoning. *Med J Aust*. 2000;173:133-5.
19. Hick JL, Hanfling D, Burstein JL, et al. Personal protective equipment for healthcare facility decontamination personnel: regulations, risks, and recommendations. *Ann Emerg Med*. 2003;42:370-80.
20. Schultz M, Cisek J, Wabeke R. Simulated exposure of hospital emergency personnel to solvent vapors and respirable dust during decontamination of chemically exposed patients. *Ann Emerg Med*. 1995;26:324-9.
21. Fedele P, Georgopolous P, Shade P, et al. Technical report: In-hospital response to external chemical emergencies: Personal protective equipment, training, site operations planning, and medical programs (final draft). Washington, DC: Joint publication of the U.S. Army Soldier and Biological Chemical Command, Environmental and Occupational Health Sciences Institute, and Veterans Health Administration (VHA); 2003.

22. Macintyre AG, Christopher GW, Eitzen E, et al. Weapons of mass destruction events with contaminated casualties: effective planning for healthcare facilities. *JAMA*. 2000;4:261-9.

23. U.S. Army Soldier Biological and Chemical Command. Guidelines for incident commander's use of firefighter protective ensemble with self-contained breathing apparatus for rescue operations during a terrorist chemical agent incident. Aberdeen Proving Ground, MD: U.S. Army Soldier Biological and Chemical Command; 1999.

24. King JM, Frelin AJ. Impact of the chemical protective ensemble on the performance of basic medical tasks. *Mil Med*. 1984;149(9):496-501.

25. Hendler I, Nahtomi O, Segal E, et al. The effect of full protective gear on intubation performed by hospital medical personnel. *Mil Med*. 2000;165(4):272-4.

26. Carter BJ, Cammermeyer M. Emergence of real casualties during simulated chemical warfare training under high heat conditions. *Military Med*. 1985;150(12):657-63.

27. Carr JL, Corona BM, Jackson SE, Bochovchin V. The effect of chemical protective clothing and equipment on Army soldier performance: A critical review of the literature. Technical Memoranda 12080. Aberdeen Proving Ground, MD: U.S. Army Human Engineering Laboratory; 1980.

28. Carter BJ, Cammermeyer M. Biopsychosocial responses of medical unit personnel wearing chemical defense ensemble in a simulated chemical warfare environment. *Military Med*. 1985;150(5):239-49.

29. Occupational Health and Safety Administration. 29 CFR Parts 1910, 1915 1926: Assigned Protection Factors; Proposed Rule. Available at: http://www.osha.gov/FedReg_osha_pdf/FED20030606.pdf.

30. Occupational Health and Safety Administration. Hazardous waste operations and emergency response. Code of Federal Regulations 1910.120(g)(3)(iii). Available at: http://www.osha.gov/pls/oshaweb/owadisp.show_document?p_table=STANDARDS&p_id=9765.

31. Campbell LE, Lins R, Pappas AG. Domestic preparedness: sarin vapor challenge and corn oil protection factor (PF) testing of 3M BE10 powered air-purifying respirator with AP3 cartridge. Aberdeen Proving Ground, MD: U.S. Army Soldier Biological and Chemical Command; 2001.

32. 3M Corporation. Technical Data Bulletin #155: Test criteria for the 3M cartridge FR57 against various military and industrial chemical agents. Available at: http://multimedia.mmm.com/mws/mediawebserver.dyn?fffffff5myruf_3GfT3GfffVNYRAj&egO-.

33. Weber A., et al. Aerosol penetration and leakage characteristics of masks in the health care industry. *Am J Infect Control*. 1993;21:167-73.

34. Chen CC, Willeke K. Characteristics of face seal leakage in filtering facepieces. *Am Ind Hyg Assoc J*. 1992;53(9):533-9.

35. National Fire Protection Association. Codes and Standards. Available at: http://www.nfpa.org/Codes/codesandstandards/hazmat/hazmat.asp.

36. Occupational Safety and Health Administration. *OSHA Guidance for Hospital-Based First Receivers of Victims from Mass Casualty Incidents Involving the Release of Hazardous Substances (Final Draft)*. May 18, 2004.

37. U.S. Army Center for Health Promotion and Preventive Medicine. Personal protective equipment guide for military medical treatment facility personnel handling casualties from weapons of mass destruction and terrorism events. Technical guide 275. Aberdeen Proving Grounds, MD: U.S. Army Center for Health Promotion and Preventive Medicine. Available at: http://chppm-www.apgea.army.mil/documents/TG/TECHGUID/TG275new.pdf.

38. Garner JS. Guideline for isolation precautions in hospitals. The Hospital Infection Control Practices Advisory Committee. *Infect Control Hosp Epidemiol*. 1996;17(4):53-80.

39. Department of Health and Human Services, Department of Labor. Respiratory protective devices: final rules and notice. *Federal Register*. 1995;60(110):30336-30402.

40. Minnesota Department of Health Chapter Association for Practitioners of Infection Control. Personal Protective Equipment for Smallpox and Viral Hemorrhagic Fever Patient Care. Available at: http://www.health.state.mn.us/divs/idepc/dtopics/infectioncontrol/ppe/ppen95.pdf.

41. Occupational Health and Safety Administration. Hazardous waste operations and emergency response. Code of Federal Regulations 1910.120(q)(3)(iii-iv). Available at: http://www.osha.gov/pls/oshaweb/owadisp.show_document?p_table=STANDARDS&p_id=9765.

42. Occupational Health and Safety Administration. Standard interpretations. Training and PPE requirements for hospital staff that decontaminate victims/patients. Available at: http://www.osha.gov/pls/oshaweb/owadisp.show_document?p_table=INTERPRETATIONS&p_id=24523.

43. Occupational Health and Safety Administration. Standard interpretations. Respiratory protection requirements for hospital staff decontaminating chemically contaminated patients. Available at: http://www.osha.gov/pls/oshaweb/owadisp.show_document?p_table=INTERPRETATIONS&p_id=24516.

44. Occupational Health and Safety Administration. Hazardous waste operations and emergency response. Code of Federal Regulations 1910.120(q)(6). Available at: http://www.osha.gov/pls/oshaweb/owadisp.show_document?p_table=STANDARDS&p_id=9765.

chapter 37

Surveillance

P. Gregg Greenough and Frederick M. Burkle, Jr.

The World Health Organization (WHO) defines *surveillance* as "the ongoing systematic collection, analysis, and interpretation of data in order to plan, implement and evaluate public health interventions."[1] The key elements are its continuous nature and its linkage to particular actions. Surveillance is repetitive, ongoing, and tied to operational activity and action-oriented policy, unlike rapid assessments and field surveys, which occur sporadically during a disaster by disparate organizations and institutions and provide a "snapshot" of a particular health issue because they are "one-off" type events. As the emergency phase of a disaster transitions into rehabilitation and development, surveillance data provide a trend analysis to detect successes or failures in policy, programming, and disaster management.

Surveillance also encompasses the "comparison and interpretation of data in order to detect possible changes in the health and environmental status of populations."[2] Data collected and collated as the result of an event undergo timely analysis, interpretation, and distribution to all parties involved in the response and who have a stake in improving the population's health. Thus, surveillance is a cyclical exercise that moves forward in time.[3] In so doing, surveillance tracks the burden of disease on healthcare systems, identifies continuing health problems, and monitors the response to specific interventions. No other means of tracking health trends has this capability during a disaster.

HISTORICAL PERSPECTIVE

Historically, surveillance has been practiced in some form during the development of public health in the Western world. Beginning in the 17th century, Leiniz in Germany and Graunt in England advanced the notion of applying numerical value to disease and death counts. At the same time, Sydenham developed a classification for diseases on which a uniform understanding of its statistical analysis could be understood. By the 19th century, efforts were being made to nationalize health information, collect vital statistics, perform analysis, and initiate a reporting mechanism. In particular, the work of Farr in England and Shattuck in Massachusetts advanced these concepts, applying them to socioeco-

nomic conditions and public health practice. By the turn of the century, all states and most European countries required reporting of specific infectious diseases. In the United States, the great influenza pandemic of 1918-1919 prompted a national mortality reporting requirement.[4]

Events during the 1950s and 1960s helped define the term surveillance and elucidate its role in public health practice. Langmuir at the U.S. Centers for Disease Control and Prevention (CDC) emphasized the systematic collection of pertinent data and its timely analysis and dissemination to policy makers; Raska at WHO stressed that surveillance should apply to prevention as well as control of communicable diseases. In 1968, the World Health Assembly broadened the role of surveillance beyond the realm of communicable diseases. Since then, surveillance has been applied to lead poisoning, injury, drug abuse, congenital malformations, behavioral risk factors, and disasters, as well as many other public health issues.

The routine use of surveillance in humanitarian relief emerged with the development of standards for field operations. Before the 1990s, the profession of humanitarian relief, with its wide range of agencies working at all levels of capacity and often with poorly trained workers and volunteers, was not held accountable for its own work. In 1996, a group of experts from 228 humanitarian organizations began fashioning minimum technical and ethical standards in all sectors—food, nutrition, water, sanitation, and health services. Titled the Sphere Project, it has become the consensus opinion on how humanitarian professionals should operate during conflicts and disasters. According to Sphere, the design and development of health services should be "guided by the ongoing coordinated collection, analysis and utilization of relevant public health data."[5]

Perhaps the most poignant example of the use of surveillance and its immediate ramifications took place in Goma, Zaire, in 1994. Weeks after a sudden massive movement of refugees went to Goma, a land ill-equipped to sustain them and where public health infrastructure was lacking, an epidemic of cholera resulted that was soon followed by dysentery, killing 50,000. During the first month of the epidemic, an emergency surveillance mechanism recorded crude mortality rates of 20 to 35 deaths per 10,000 population per day. Rapidly acquired surveillance data guided relief efforts and targeted interventions to decrease the death rates to 5 to 8 per 10,000 per day by the second month of the crisis.[6] The role of ongoing, pertinent health information in the settings of humanitarian crises that is iterative and available to those who must intervene is now a widely accepted component of disaster response and rehabilitation.

CURRENT PRACTICE

The first order is to establish objectives for the surveillance system. WHO outlines six objectives of surveillance applicable in emergencies: identify public health priorities, monitor the severity of the emergency by collecting and analyzing mortality and morbidity data, detect outbreaks and monitor the response to the outbreak, monitor trends in incidence and case-fatality from major diseases, monitor the impact of specific health interventions, and provide information to the Ministry of Health in the affected area.[7] To achieve these objectives, the surveillance system should be simple and clear in its focus, easily understood by all who receive its information, and flexible to respond to new health problems and program activities.

The next step is to define the population of interest and its relationship to the health sector in the disaster area. What is the demographic makeup of the population (age, sex, ethnicity, etc.)? A discussion of establishing baseline population figures is found in Chapter 52. Where do people live both before and after the disaster? Where do people access health services, if at all? Where do health events occur? What is the structure and capability of the national health information system, and what government, nongovernment, and international agencies are working in the health sector?

To answer these questions, surveillance systems track *indicators*—qualitative or quantitative outcome measures that describe the state of the population in terms of health and the process and outcome of health services; they may correlate or predict the value or measure of a program, system, or organization. Their inherent value in a surveillance system is their ability to be tracked over time and compared with a baseline. Incidence, prevalence, mortality rates, and morbidity rates are the most common quantitative indicators during the emergency phase (Box 37-1).

BOX 37-1 DEFINITIONS OF QUANTITATIVE INDICATORS

- Incidence: The number of new cases of a disease that occur in a specified time period.
- Prevalence: The number of affected persons present in the population at a specified time divided by the population at that time.
- Morbidity rate: The number of persons who develop disease (incidence) or are affected (prevalence) during a specified time period divided by the number of people in the total population.
- Mortality rate: The number of deaths occurring in a population during a specified time divided by the number of people at risk for dying during that period.

A surveillance mechanism is built on the initial rapid assessments during the immediate disaster response. The outputs of those assessments should focus on the health problems that produce the highest morbidity and mortality, especially if the population affected is displaced. Mortality rates are the most important indicator for identifying a population under stress. Most commonly, the crude mortality rate (CMR) is used in emergencies to track the effects of disaster-generated infectious disease or injury. The practical initial quantitative baseline data captured at the onset of the disaster should include:

- Population size, specifically the total population affected; the population of vulnerable groups, including women, elderly, and children younger than 5 years old; and the influx and efflux of persons
- CMR (for calculation, see Chapter 52)
- Mortality rate for children younger than 5 years old (for calculation, see Chapter 52)
- Case-specific mortality and morbidity rates (for calculations, see Chapter 52)
- Nutritional status, specifically weight-for-height ratios of children ages 6 to 59 months

In the emergency phase, diseases most likely to cause death or significant morbidity, such as diarrheal illness (especially in a malnourished displaced population), acute respiratory infection, measles, and meningitis, should be the focus of surveillance. As the emergency evolves into the postdisaster setting, HIV/AIDS, tuberculosis, and sexually transmitted disease rates; chronic disease management; injury; immunization coverage (e.g., the Expanded Program on Immunization); and longer-term healthcare access should be included in ongoing surveillance efforts. Surveillance for the displaced disaster-affected population should eventually be integrated into the national health information system of the country, which is discussed later in this chapter.

Initial qualitative indicators will provide a basis for the needs of the population, especially the state of access to water, sanitation, and health services. Early qualitative critical indicators include:

- Immunization coverage
- Access to sanitation services and ample supplies of potable water
- Access to healthcare services
- Capacity or level of function of healthcare services
- Food distribution

As the disaster response becomes established and transitions into a postdisaster phase, qualitative indicators that examine the relief effort will guide resources and programming. Postemergency phase qualitative indicators may include:

- Ongoing access to healthcare services (the proportion of the population that can use the health service or health facility)
- Availability (the amount of services and resources compared with the total population)
- Health coverage (the proportion of the population that has received a given service)
- Quality of services (a measure of actual services

received compared with standards and guidelines)

- Equity in distribution of health resources (may explain why one subgroup of the population fares worse than another)
- Main program activities (for individual or groups of relief agencies involved in the delivery of care)

In terms of program performance, field epidemiologists recommend that indicators have SMART attributes, an acronym for "*s*pecific, *m*easurable, *a*ccurate, *r*ealistic, and *t*ime-bound."[8] Indicators must be sensitive enough to monitor the impact of relief on the health problems and determine whether the effort is either having a tangible effect on the population or whether new strategies are needed.

Data Collection

The method by which data are collected is wholly dependent on the type of surveillance used. *Active* surveillance system data require a proactive seeking of cases through some type of sampling mechanism, usually direct reports from households or, more commonly, health facilities. Active surveillance is used more during the emergency phase. *Passive* surveillance systems rely on reports from the data sources, typically as cases present themselves. Passive systems lend themselves to long-term ongoing surveillance during the postemergency phase once health services are restored. Both have practical pros and cons. Active surveillance provides more accurate data but is far more labor intensive and thus more costly to implement. The need for accurate mortality rates and incidence of critical diseases justifies its cost and effort during the emergency phase. Passive systems by definition represent a self-selected population and may not accurately represent the greater population. Because passive systems are less costly and require less training, they are more practical for long-term surveillance. In either case, a surveillance system should have high sensitivity, that is, the ability to detect "true" cases of illness or injury.[3]

Often, one may hear the term *sentinel surveillance*. In such a system, selected data collection points (e.g., designated health facilities within the system) will be responsible for identifying and reporting specific diseases or health events. Specific segments of the population or specific locales in the disaster-affected population may be specially chosen for monitoring (e.g., the parameter weight for height in ages 6 to 59 months). Sentinel health events refer to a condition that has the potential to affect the health stability of the population—often a warning signal that the current level of preventive and curative care needs attention—and that should prompt immediate action. One case of meningitis presenting in a crowded displaced persons camp demands an immediate response from health agencies to avert an epidemic catastrophe.

Data collection tools, especially in the emergency phase, should be short, easy to use, readily understandable, and remain consistent over time. These tools should be designed to collect only the minimal, most essential information in a clear and unambiguous fashion. The use of simple uniform case definitions for communicable diseases is critical. All health providers involved in surveillance should know, for instance, that a generalized rash of greater than 3 days' duration *and* a temperature greater than 38°C *and* one or more symptoms of cough, rhinorrhea, or red eyes define a case of measles. Common diarrhea is classified as three or more liquid stools per day and duly recorded. In countries endemic for malaria, a temperature greater than 38.5°C in the absence of other infection is indeed malaria for data purposes. From these simple, yet sensitive, definitions, trends can be followed. Epi Info software, available free of charge from the CDC's Web site, assists in generating data forms and in analyzing the data.

Data sources are most often health facilities, specifically health providers and hospital, emergency department, and clinic records. In displaced populations living in temporary camps, registration systems provide demographic data. Household surveillance may be necessary to identify basic needs. Other sources of demographic and health data include vaccination cards (often carried by mothers), burial records, networks of home visitors, and nongovernment agencies responsible for other sectors of the disaster response (e.g., water, sanitation, food, nutrition). Nontraditional sources of information may be useful, including police, fire, aid agencies, pharmacies, grave-diggers, and others. Abdullah and Burnham[9] elucidate specific indicators with their relevant sources in Table 37-1. In settings in which the health services infrastructure may be destroyed by the disaster, government and nongovernment relief agencies—local and international—need to step in and establish a surveillance system in the course of providing preventive and curative care. The use of standardized patient data collection based on the CDC data classifications improves accuracy.[10]

Surveillance systems should be judged by their simplicity. Data collection should be an easy process and follow a logical format. Indicators should be representative of the population relevant to the disaster and the disaster phase (e.g., diarrhea is more likely to be a problem than hookworm infestation in an emergency). Data outputs should be timely to identify outbreaks and should be reliable (using standard case definitions, for example). Data collection must occur in an ongoing fashion at regular intervals but be flexible to adapt to new health problems or sudden program changes.

Analysis, Interpretation, and Dissemination

During the emergency, data should be collected daily and reported weekly to all government and nongovernment relief agencies working in the health sector. Postemergency phase data may likely be recorded daily but collated monthly for analysis. During all phases, surveillance data should be sent in either paper or digital form to a central location at the field level for analysis. Most countries have some type of ongoing surveillance mechanism to track the burden of disease. Usually, this is a component of a broader health information system housed within a Ministry of Health and has some means

TABLE 37-1 SURVEILLANCE INDICATORS AND SOURCES OF INFORMATION

SURVELLIANCE	INDICATORS	SOURCES OF INFORMATION
Demographic	• Total population • Population structure (age, sex) • Rate of migration (new arrivals, departures) • Identification of vulnerable groups • Births	Registration records, Population census, CHW reports
Mortality[+]	• Crude mortality rate (CMR) • Age-specific mortality rate (<5, >5) • Cause-specific mortality • Case fatality rate (CFR)	Hospital death registers, Religious leaders, Community reporters (including CHWs). • Burial shroud distribution, Burial contractors, Graveyards, Camp administration
Morbidity 1. Routine 2. Outbreaks (daily)	• Incidence rate (new cases) • Prevalence rate (total existing cases) • Age-sex-specific morbidity rate • Proportional morbidity rate	Outpatient and admission records, Laboratories Feeding centre(s) records, Community health worker records
Nutrition (frequent surveys while malnutrition rate is high)	• Global malnutrition rate • Severe malnutrition rate • Rate of weight gain/loss in MCH clinics • Incidence of micro-nutrient deficiency disorders • Incidence of low birth weight • Average daily ration • Delayed age of menarche	Nutrition surveys MCH clinic records Feeding center records Birth registers Camp administration
Program process	• Feeding center enrollment and attendance • Water and sanitation (quantity, quality, access) • Immunization coverage • Maternal health coverage (ANC, assisted deliveries, PNC) • Outpatient and inpatient attendance • ORS distribution	Facility records, Immunization surveys (annual), Traditional birth attendant records

From Abdallah S, Burnham G, eds. *The Johns Hopkins and Red Cross/Red Crescent Public Health Guide for Emergencies.* Baltimore: Johns Hopkins University; 2000.

for data analysis (in the United States, state and local public health offices and the CDC). A country's health information system, assuming it remains intact after the disaster, should provide baseline predisaster health information on communicable and noncommunicable diseases. From this, one may see background health information, such as seasonal variability in endemic diseases, the burden of chronic disease, patterns of injury, and other periodic health trends, from which to evaluate newer surveillance data.

The analysis of surveillance data should focus on the clustering of events over time or the clustering of events within specific subgroups of the population.[11] To that end, the analysis should emphasize trends in time, place, and person. The interpretation should highlight the needs and priorities and, where possible, be referenced against "normal" values or indicator thresholds. What matters most is how indicators change over time and how these changes may be linked to programming.[12] The use of graphs and maps using geographic information system (GIS) software makes interpretation more meaningful to stakeholders. The flow of surveillance data must be coupled with an action-oriented information system whose primary task is to get information to those who need to know and can act.

PITFALLS

A surveillance system must have high sensitivity—that is, the ability to detect true cases of a given health problem

of interest within the population. The greatest enemy of an effective surveillance system is underreporting by those tasked to collect the data for a variety of reasons.

First, surveillance depends on a flow of information; during a disaster, established systems of information flow are easily disrupted (e.g., a health center is destroyed, the population migrates, communications and transportation networks are damaged). Also—and this is true especially of passive type systems—if health providers lack interest, do not see the value in the iterative data collection process, or feel overworked and have limitations on their time due to patient care to report data, the incentive to find and report cases will diminish. Lack of interest is often due to health providers not being provided the analyzed information in the dissemination process and thus not able to appreciate its beneficial effect on the health of the population. Underreporting as a consequence of any these reasons undermines the strength of a surveillance system.

Another concern is the source of information. Relying on health-facility–based surveillance information if the population does not have adequate access to formal healthcare raises the question of whether a health-facility–based surveillance system accurately represents the health needs of the population.[13] This typically means that emergent and urgent health issues are not reliably captured and appreciated by those who could make a difference.

Finally, meaningful analysis and interpretation capacity does not exist in many countries. Despite readily accessible tools, such as Epi Info, and the presence of computer-savvy technical staff who can manage data, there is often a need for personnel with public health understanding and backgrounds to interact with the data to explain its significance to disaster managers and other key stakeholders, who may have only a nominal understanding of the ramifications of public health data for a population.

REFERENCES

1. World Health Organization. Communicable Disease Surveillance and Response. Available at: http://www.who.int/csr/en.
2. Eylenbosch WJ, Noah ND, Foldspang A, et al. The surveillance of disease. In: Eylenbosch WJ, Noah ND, eds. *Surveillance in Health and Disease*. Oxford: Oxford University Press; 1998.
3. Wetterhall SF, Noji EK. In: Noji EK, ed. *The Public Health Consequences of Disasters*. New York: Oxford University Press; 1997:37-64.
4. Thacker SB. Historical development. In: Teutsch SM, Churchill RE, eds. *Principles and Practice of Public Health Surveillance*. New York: Oxford University Press; 2000:1-16.
5. The Sphere Project. *Humanitarian Charter and Minimum Standards in Disaster Response*. Oxford: Oxfam Publishing; 2004:270.
6. Goma Epidemiology Group. Public health impact of Rwandan refugee crisis: what happened in Goma, Zaire, in July, 1994? *Lancet*. 1995;345:339-44.
7. World Health Organization. Surveillance. In: *Communicable Disease Control in Emergencies*. Geneva: World Health Organization; 2003.
8. Bradt DA, Drummond CM. Rapid epidemiological assessment of health status in displaced populations—an evolution toward a standardized minimum essential data set. *Prehospital Disaster Med*. 2003;17(4):178-85.
9. Abdallah S, Burnham G. Disaster epidemiology. In: Abdallah S, Burnham G, eds. *The Johns Hopkins and Red Cross/Red Crescent Public Health Guide for Emergencies*. Baltimore: Johns Hopkins University; 2000.
10. Leonard RB, Stringer LW, Alson R. Patient-data collection system used during medical operations after the 1994 San Fernando Valley-Northridge earthquake. *Prehospital Disaster Med*. 1995;10(3):178-83.
11. Rowley E, Robinson WC. Surveillance and registration systems. In: Robinson WC, ed. *Demographic Assessment in Disasters: A Guide for Practitioners*. Baltimore: Center for International Emergency, Disaster and Refugee Studies, Johns Hopkins Bloomberg School of Public Health; 2002.
12. Médicins Sans Frontiéres. *Refugee Health*. London: Macmillan Education Ltd; 1997.
13. Roberts L, Hofmann CA. Assessing the impact of humanitarian assistance in the health sector. *Emerging Themes Epidemiol*. 2004;1(3):1-9.

chapter 38

Management of Mass Fatalities

Nelson Tang and Chayan Dey

Modern complex disasters have the ever-increasing potential for creating large numbers of deceased, the management of which is of specific importance to the planning and operational response to such events. Historically, disaster consequence management with regard to large numbers of deceased human beings has been a relatively poorly contemplated aspect of response and recovery. Current concepts of operations in disaster medicine place increased emphasis on the management of mass fatalities.

A *mass fatality incident* is generally defined as one in which the numbers of deceased overwhelm the capabilities of local jurisdictions, including the coroner and medical examiner, to appropriately deal with them. Consistent with broader disaster response mechanisms, the management of fatalities resultant from a disaster, whether natural or manmade, requires the effective coordination and deployment of multiple tiers of resources and trained personnel. The timeliness of response to large numbers of fatalities becomes further significant when considered in the context of the families of victims and their need for the identification, documentation, and disposition of the remains of their kin.[1]

In the United States, there are specific federal resources that may be made available to local jurisdictions for the response to mass fatalities in certain circumstances through the Department of Homeland Security (DHS) and the Federal Emergency Management Agency (FEMA). Today, increased awareness exists with regard to the effects of managing large numbers of deceased on rescue and healthcare workers.

HISTORICAL PERSPECTIVE

Conventional paradigms in disaster medicine dictate that the deceased or unsalvageable victims of catastrophic events are to be triaged as expeditiously as possible to a morgue, away from patient care and medical response activities. It is reasonable to expect, however, that local morgue facilities will be quickly overwhelmed by the sheer number of deceased in the aftermath of a large-scale disaster. The increased likelihood of terrorist-instigated disaster scenarios and the potential use of weapons of mass destruction further complicate the

management of the deceased. Concerns for decontamination before disposal and, additionally, the criminal investigation and evidence collection requirements of the law enforcement response to such events make the prospect of removing large numbers of deceased individuals a highly complex undertaking.

In contrast to the earliest notions of mass burials or cremations, more recent event-based disaster experiences have demonstrated that fatalities numbering in the hundreds can be effectively managed, including the organized transportation, processing, identification, and disposition of all bodies recovered. Much of this experience has been derived from civilian and military aviation disasters.[2,3]

Two fundamental assets of forensic medicine—radiographic and dental investigation—have proven to remain essential in mass fatality management. Radiographic screening for foreign bodies, personal effects, dental and surgical artifacts, and occult skeletal injury are well-established techniques in modern forensics. In addition, positive radiographic identification of casualty victims by comparison with available individual antemortem records is similarly effective.[4,5] The evaluation of dental evidence and comparative data for disaster fatality identification are essential tools, and the role of forensic dentists and dental professionals has been described in mass fatality events.[6,7] Such conventional forensic approaches have direct application to mass fatality events, although the technical and operational aspects of such efforts would appear to remain logistical challenges.

CURRENT PRACTICE

In the United States, under the National Response Plan, the National Disaster Medical System (NDMS) is tasked to provide victim identification and mortuary services in declared disasters (Box 38-1).[8] To accomplish this mission, the concept of the Disaster Mortuary Operational Response Team (DMORT) was developed in the early 1990s. Directed by the NDMS under FEMA, DMORTs are composed of medical and forensic volunteers who are activated in the event of a disaster and have specific training and skills in victim identification, mortuary services, and forensic pathology and anthropology methods (Box 38-2).[9] Often, disaster medical assistance team components are co-deployed with DMORT personnel to provide maintenance and emergency healthcare to personnel involved in mass fatality operations. These operations may involve a large number of personnel working in austere conditions for a prolonged period, necessitating medical care maintenance.

DMORT members are required to maintain appropriate and current certifications and licensure within their respective disciplines. During an actual emergency response, DMORTs work under the guidance of local authorities by providing technical assistance and personnel to recover, identify, and process deceased victims.[10] At least one of these teams has expertise in handling contaminated or infected remains.

The Response Division of FEMA currently maintains two Disaster Portable Morgue Units (DPMUs) that may be deployed to support an NDMS DMORT response (Fig. 38-1). The DPMU is a depository of equipment and supplies for deployment to a disaster site. It contains a complete morgue with designated workstations for each processing element and prepackaged equipment and supplies. Both DPMUs are staged at FEMA Logistics Centers, one in Rockville, Md., and the other in San Jose, Calif.[10]

The U.S. military maintains rapidly deployable multidisciplinary resources capable of the rapid recovery, examination, identification, and return of physical remains in response to mass fatality disasters. In 1997, the U.S. Army Europe developed the Disaster Mortuary Affairs Response Team (DMART), patterned after the civilian DMORT concept. This is the only team in the military that combines Mortuary Affairs with forensic personnel to support the combatant commander.[11]

Disaster victim identification (DVI) is a term that has been applied to procedures used to positively identify deceased victims of a multiple casualty incident. Positive identification is required for both legal considerations and for the peace of mind of the families of victims. In general, DVI should not begin until all of the survivors have been identified and transported from the scene. The goal of DVI is to identify all victims by matching antemortem and postmortem data.

The International Criminal Police Organization (Interpol) has developed a system of standard procedures for DVI. Written procedures of the Interpol system exist within the *Disaster Victim Identification Guide*.[12] Although guidelines for DVI must be adapted to individual circumstances, this general approach may be implemented in a variety of disaster settings. Regardless of the actual methods used, it is imperative that DVI be conducted in a timely, accurate, and thorough manner and in keeping with international standards.

The increasing complexity and scale of modern disasters, further amplified by terrorist-orchestrated disasters, have driven the technological advancement of forensic investigation of mass fatality incidents. The development of forensic bioinformatics and high throughput DNA analysis techniques as means for victim identification have been reported as a specific outcomes driven by the immediacies of the Sept. 11, 2001, terrorist attack on the World Trade Center in New York City.[13,14] The future of disaster consequence management is likely to demonstrate the further proliferation of such technically—advanced procedures for ultra-rapid, mass-scale disaster victim identification.

PITFALLS

Recent historical experience with regard to major disasters has demonstrated that effective response to mass fatalities is a distinct possibility. Nevertheless, it would be erroneous to conceptualize such responses without the skills and intervention of dedicated professionals with pre-existing expertise in forensic medicine, pathology, mortuary services, and deceased identification and processing.

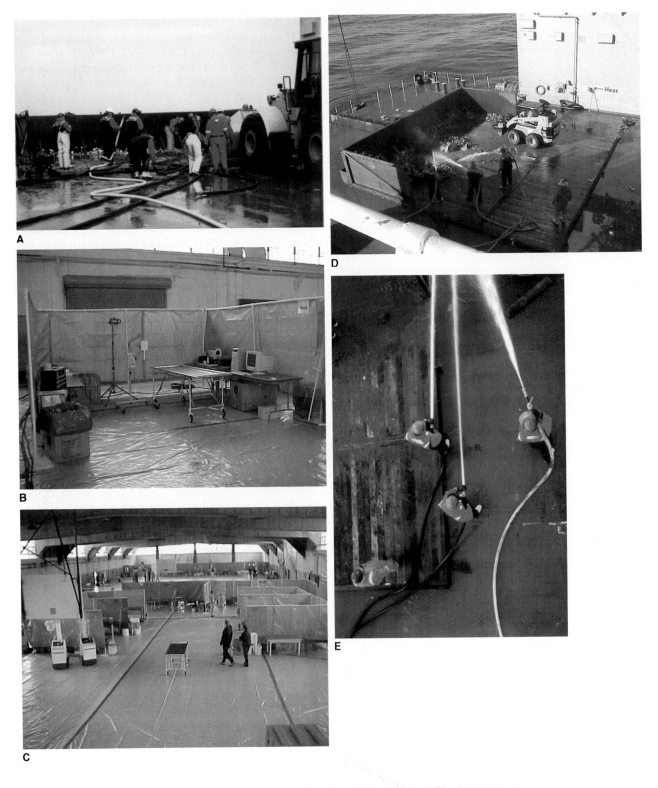

FIGURE 38–1. **A-E,** EgyptAir crash mass fatality recovery operations. **B** and **C** show the DPMU in its setup stage.

Reliance on local resources is unlikely to be sufficient. Coordination of efforts by local authorities with federal specialty teams is essential for the timely and successful completion of mass fatality operations. Disaster planning and response must include appropriate thresholds for activating available mechanisms and deployment of specific dedicated resources for mass fatality management.

Effective postmortem identification of disaster victims has both pragmatic and psychosocial significance an may no longer be considered a luxury but rather a necessity. For legal, ethical, religious, and financial purposes, successful identification of the deceased has considerable significance. The timely issuance of death certificates may have direct import for the registration of the dead and for use in insurance and other possible death benefits claims and is likely to be a requirement for final disposition of individual remains.[15] Definitive victim identification and the expeditious release of physical remains allow bereaved families of victims to make funeral and burial arrangements consistent with religious and individual beliefs. In addition, in the event of multinational disaster scenarios, transport considerations may create additional urgency and pressure for the early release of remains.

The infectious risk of handling corpses is not well understood or quantified. Conventional wisdom dictates that disaster victim recovery, whether living or deceased, be performed with universal adherence to communicable disease protection. Infectious pathogen precautions should be maintained throughout fatality recovery, processing, forensic examination, and disposal. If the disaster event holds the possibility for a chemical or biological weapons attack, workers must have access to personal protective equipment commensurate with the threat. Most disaster sites will present multiple physical and environmental dangers, including debris, hazardous materials, and structural instability. Fatality management workers must be briefed appropriately of such hazards and not be placed in unnecessary risk of physical injury.

The actual scope and extent of the impact of confronting and managing mass fatalities on healthcare and rescue workers are not completely known. There is evidence to suggest that medical training and clinical experience may not provide the needed degree of emotional and psychological protection, as has been previously believed. Instead, it is plausible to expect that significant variability with regard to emotional reactions and psychological vulnerabilities exists among disaster responders before, during, and after exposure to mass fatality events.[16] Prior study in this area suggests that the adverse psychological effects, although not permanent, of disaster victim body handling and identification work are not necessarily correlated with lack of experience or training.[17] It is increasingly common for modern disaster response plans to provide for debriefing and poststress exposure psychological support for responders. It is prudent to consider additional focused support services for those directly tasked with handling and identifying physical remains of disaster fatalities.

CONCLUSIONS

Disasters that engender mass fatality conditions are likely to overwhelm local and even regional resources and the capacity to effectively deal with such contingencies. Analysis of consequence management demonstrates that an integrated, coordinated approach to response can effectively manage large numbers of fatalities. Specific federal assistance is available to augment local resources in the response to mass fatality situations. Through the NDMS, DMORT specialist personnel and DPMU facilities may be deployed under certain circumstances.

Although generally contemplated as a second-tier response consideration, after the management of living victims, the appropriate handling, identification, and disposition of the deceased nevertheless have specific importance. Vigilance must be maintained for the physical safety of personnel managing disaster fatalities, and provisions must be made for appropriate personal protective equipment. The handling of human remains, particularly in a mass fatality disaster, may have a variable but significant emotional and psychological impact on personnel responding to these events.

REFERENCES

1. Hooft PJ, Noji EK, Van de Voorde HP. Fatality management in mass casualty incidents. *Forensic Sci Int.* 1989;40(1):3-14.
2. Clark MA, Clark SR, Perkins DG. Mass fatality aircraft disaster processing. *Aviat Space Environ Med.* 1989;60:64-73.
3. Ludes B, Tracqui A, Pfitzinger H, et al. Medico-legal investigations of the Airbus, A320 crash upon Mount Ste-Odile, France. *J Forensic Sci.* 1994;9(5):1147-52.
4. Lichtenstein JE, Madewell JE. Role of radiology in the study and identification of casualty victims. *Radiologe.* 1982;22(8):352-7.
5. Warren MW, Smith KR, Stubblefield PR, et al. Use of radiographic atlases in a mass fatality. *J Forensic Sci.* 2000;45(2):467-70.
6. Fixott RH, Arendt D, Chrz B, Filippi J, McGivney J, Warnick A. Role of the dental team in mass fatality incidents. *Dent Clin North Am.* 2001;45(2):271-92.
7. Brannon RB, Connick CM. The role of the dental hygienist in mass disasters. *J Forensic Sci.* 2000;45(2):381-3.
8. Disaster Mortuary Operational Response Team. Available at: http://www.dmort.org/DNPages/DMORTHelp.htm.
9. Federal Emergency Management Agency. Resource: Disaster Mortuary Operational Response Team (DMORT). Available at: http://www.fema.gov/preparedness/resources/health_med/dmort.htm.
10. Federal Emergency Management Agency, National Disaster Medical System. What Is a Disaster Mortuary Operational Response Team (DMORT)? Available at: http://www.ndms.fema.gov/dmort.html.
11. Labovich MH, Duke JB, Ingwersen KM, et al. Management of a multinational mass fatality incident in Kaprun, Austria: a forensic medical perspective. *Mil Med.* 2003;168(1):19-23.
12. International Criminal Police Organization (Interpol). Disaster Victim Identification. Available at: http://www.interpol.int/Public/DisasterVictim/default.asp.
13. Cash HD, Hoyle JW, Sutton AJ. Development under extreme conditions: forensic bioinformatics in the wake of the World Trade Center disaster. *Pac Symp Biocomput.* 2003;638-53.
14. Holland MM, Cave CA, Holland CA, et al. Development of a quality, high throughput DNA analysis procedure for skeletal samples to assist with the identification of victims from the World Trade Center attacks. *Croat Med J.* 2003;44(3):264-72.
15. Busuttil A, Jones JSP. The certification and disposal of the dead in major disasters. *Med Sci Law.* 1992;32(1):9-13.
16. Keller RT, Bobo WV. Handling human remains following the terrorist attack on the Pentagon: experiences of 10 uniformed health care workers. *Mil Med.* 2002;167(4):8-11.
17. Taylor AJW, Frazer AG. The stress of post-disaster body handling and victim identification work. *J Human Stress.* 1982;6:4-12.

chapter 39

Disaster Management of Animals

James M. Burke

The current geopolitical climate has forced the United States to explore contingency plans for future environmental disasters. Although most of the research along these lines is focused on human safety, the animal and agricultural aspects of disaster management also need to be explored. Since natural disasters are a more frequent risk to animal populations than possible biological or terrorist threats, the protection of these resources demands proper consideration.

U.S. Agriculture, a $100 billion business, is an important nutritional source and helps sustain our economic growth and military readiness.[1] Concentrating animals into larger facilities to provide abundant food sources increases the agricultural impact of a biological disaster or terrorist threat. The large numbers of companion animals in urban areas, meanwhile, should also be considered during an evacuation, since most disaster shelter facilities do not accept animals. Overall, a large number of animals—both livestock and pets—are likely to need care during a disaster.

Analysis of past disasters highlights some mistakes, but lessons may be learned from them. Large-scale natural disasters, such as hurricanes Andrew and Floyd in 1999, may be viewed as test scenarios from which future contingencies can be developed. Evaluating the mobilization, transportation, and housing of displaced companion animals and livestock helps prepare pet owners and animal producers for future events. Not all contingency factors can be addressed in every disaster plan, and for this reason, a flexible, well-thought-out plan is necessary.

According to the National Academies Board on Agriculture and Natural Resources' report, "Countering Agricultural Bioterrorism," not only is America vulnerable to terrorist attacks against agriculture, but insufficient plans are in place to defend against such attacks.[2] The crippling effects of the foot-and-mouth disease epidemic of 2001 illustrate the local economic disruption and global impact such events entail.[3] Although biological attacks will not cause widespread famine, they could have a direct effect on the national economy, pubic health, and the public's confidence in the food system. Plans need to be drafted now to provide a framework in which a safe, continuous supply of food can be guaranteed, epidemic disease outbreaks can be prevented, and proper care for injured animals can be ensured.

HISTORICAL PERSPECTIVE

As some of history's most recent disasters show, animal healthcare, veterinary infection control, control of stray animals, and the revival of veterinary infrastructures are the primary areas that need to be addressed in effective implemental models developed for the future.

On Aug. 24, 1992, hurricane Andrew ripped through southern Florida, leaving thousands of animals injured, abandoned, or dead. Relief efforts became hampered as organizations and volunteer groups lacked a central command structure. These groups, though well intentioned, were unable to coordinate the necessary supplies and medical resources in a cohesive effort to help those areas most devastated by the hurricane.

On Sept. 16, 1999, hurricane Floyd devastated North Carolina, affecting poultry, pork, and cattle production, as well as horses, cats, dogs, and other pets. North Carolina residents, due to unsubstantiated, predicted dangers in previous media-hyped disasters, ignored calls for evacuation. The lack of pet-friendly evacuation shelters, in addition to the lack of public preparedness, contributed to evacuation failures. Such failures endanger not only animals but their human owners as well. North Carolina State University's College of Veterinary Medicine was able to re-establish a veterinary infrastructure, contributing to the success of the disaster management operation. With its large number of trained personnel, resources, and medical supplies, the college was able to immediately take charge of animal care and control issues, organizing volunteers. In addition to a large number of volunteers, enormous amounts of food and medical supplies were donated, and transportation was made available to help agencies contend with the disaster.

During the hurricane Floyd disaster, medical care for animals was administered through a three-tier system. Tier 1 consisted primarily of vaccinations for cats. Tier 2 included the testing of animals for heartworm infection, and other diagnostic tests. Tier 3 treatments included surgical and medical stabilization of injuries.[3]

On April 25, 1994, a tornado struck West Lafayette, Ind., destroying 67 homes and 60 mobile homes. The civic response to this incident is an example of a lack of evacuation procedures that resulted in massive pet abandonment by individuals in an urban location. Pet abandonment is a consequence of unplanned or poorly executed evacuations. Human-animal bonds are strong, and during a disaster, such bonds may influence one's decision to re-enter a disaster area to retrieve a family pet. Such decisions may pose significant risks not only to individuals and families, but also to emergency personnel, who may need to become involved in rescue efforts.[4] Statistically, owners who regularly visit their veterinarians are less likely than those who do not to lose their pets during evacuations. Individuals with weak or poor human-animal bonds, who have low levels of disaster preparedness, or who own many animals are more prone to leave their animals behind during a disaster.[5] Although pet abandonment is common during disasters, in a national survey the proportion of animals abandoned during disasters was similar to the proportion of animals relinquished to 12 U.S. animal shelters.[5] Pet evacuation failures generally result from low levels of pet care. Promoting responsible pet ownership that includes planning for emergencies, both natural and manmade, is a logical strategy to make owners more responsible for the evacuation of their pets.

On March 4, 1996, a train derailed near Weyauwega, Wisc., causing a fire to erupt in the train's propane-filled cars. Local residents were asked to evacuate due to fears of a major explosion. Risk factors influencing the failure of owners to evacuate the area's cats and dogs included a weak human-animal bond, logistical challenges, and generally low levels of disaster preparedness. During the Weyauwega disaster, 15% of all pet owners were at work and unable to evacuate their pets. The most common reasons for failing to evacuate pets included owners thinking that they would not be gone long and that the evacuated areas were safe for pets.[6] Outdoor cats were at higher risk of evacuation failure since they are more difficult to catch and transport. The higher incidence of the failure to evacuate cats compared with the failure to evacuate dogs likely reflects the greater ease with which dogs can be caught, restrained, and transported. It could also reflect the assumption that cats can "fend for themselves" if left outdoors. Interestingly, households with a high number of cats are more likely to leave a dog behind during evacuation procedures.[6]

In November 1990, western Washington experienced severe flooding. Dairy farmers who were surveyed were asked to evaluate the amount of equipment and personnel available to evacuate cattle, numbers of cattle evacuated, time required for evacuations, and the destination and care of the animals. Financial loss from cattle deaths, illnesses, and halts in production was estimated at $2,786,629.[7] Help for evacuation was readily available from family members, employees, and friends. Because of adequate notice, 5000 animals were evacuated in 20 hours. Evacuated cattle were housed at neighbors' farms, at friends' homes, on high ground, and at a vacant dairy. Not one cow went more than 2 days without fresh water or normal rations. Unfortunately, however, most of the farmers did not plan in advance on where to evacuate and how to care for their animals. In hindsight, farmers said they could have sheltered all of their animals if necessary. Overall, however, it was adequate time that led to the successful evacuation of a large number of animals to safe locations. On shorter notice, such a successful evacuation may not have been achievable.

Horse owners typically treat their animals differently than owners treat general livestock, and they usually have been able to move most, if not all, of their horses within 90 minutes. Data suggest that the relatively small number of horses kept on a farm and the high emotional bond between owners and horses increase their chance of being evacuated in a timely manner. A large number of cattle, by contrast, is not suitable for quick evacuation, and horses are easier to find and transport. According to horse owners in Madison County, Ky., 100% of the horse population could be evacuated if a 12-hour evacuation notice were given.[8]

CURRENT PRACTICE

The first priority in disaster relief is protecting and saving human lives. Animals have traditionally been viewed by emergency management officials as property, and therefore, they receive much less attention than humans. Animal owners, on the other hand, consider animals either as an important source of income or as part of the family. Animal management during natural disasters is best accomplished with a plan created by state and local officials that provides a detailed framework in which to implement care during evacuations. Such a plan's objective should be to bring some type of logistical structure to the chaos that occurs during and after a disaster. As part of this plan, it is essential that veterinarians understand disaster preparedness so that they can integrate themselves more effectively into national, state, and local disaster management systems.

The first step in an adequate disaster plan is denoting a clear chain of command that includes the delegation of responsibility. Without such a framework, independent groups may unintentionally direct resources away from needed areas. State veterinary agencies and practitioners will need to take responsibility for assuming leadership roles to organize animal professionals and lay volunteers. These roles may include developing liaisons with representatives from the Department of Homeland Security (DHS), Department of Health and Human Services, the American Red Cross, National Urban Search and Rescue Response System, and the U.S. Army Veterinary Core at the Department of Defense. The U.S. Army Veterinary Core is activated at the request of a state's governor via the president of the United States. DHS provides Veterinary Medical Assistant Teams (VMATs) to assist local authorities during a federal emergency. VMATs provide care to injured animals and assist with preventative measures to maintain human health and safety. The U.S. Department of Agriculture is responsible for assessing food supply safety issues during disaster situations.[9]

Once a command structure is in place, pet owners need to identify the types of disasters for which they are at risk. To assist pet owners in this process, it is recommended that veterinarians promote the creation of individual household disaster plans. Farms and large agricultural centers with a large number of animals will need to provide an equally detailed evacuation plan that ensures the appropriate feeding, sheltering, and burial of livestock.

VMATs should be called into emergency situations to augment state and local veterinary resources until a self-sufficient response solution is reached in the disaster area. VMATs should be available immediately after a disaster, slowly tapering off as local needs decrease and local resources expand to meet the needs of the victim population. VMATs consist of two veterinarians, four veterinary technicians, and one to three logistical support personnel.[9] The director of the Offices of Emergency Response within DHS and the American Veterinary Medical Association should activate VMAT intervention in an emergency. With necessary medical equipment and supplies at their disposal, these teams will operate as mobile units in disaster areas, responding to advice from regional veterinary activities commanders.[10]

Identifying potential problems in a disaster begins with the process of eliminating any mitigating hazards that may be present on a farm or in an animal-impacted area. Alternative housing and shelter locations, clean food and water access, and accessible transportation must be designated before successful egress can occur. Repairs to barns and buildings will help to decrease the number of potential dangers during evacuation procedures. Most farms have the manpower and resources to move a large number of animals.[7] Farm cats and dogs should be placed in a disaster-proof location, or, because they generally stay close to their homes, turned loose. If shelter cannot be found for aggressive animals, euthanasia is the most humane method of treatment.

Animals that are important to agricultural production or have sentimental value need to be identified ahead of time so they can be transported rapidly. Large animal transports may present a problem to human evacuation, clogging already busy exit routes; therefore, alternative evacuation routes need to be considered in advance. In the event that animal evacuation is not possible, sources of shelter, food, and water will need to be designated, and a plan that addresses how best to re-enter the disaster area to attend to the animals needs to be in place.

It is important that local kennels and pet shelters are able to accommodate the influx of small animals during a disaster. Veterinarians are the best channels for communicating with local pet owners about the safe evacuation of their pets. The American Red Cross, although it does not shelter animals, should also be able to provide information, in coordination with local animal shelters, on how to care for pets in evacuation areas.

Veterinarians play an important role during disasters. Their primary responsibilities include control of disease factors and disease transmission, herd management, animal healthcare, search and rescue operations, animal control, and disaster assessment. Even though it is important that veterinarians have the resources available to locate and call on appropriate experts during a disaster, they also will need to address the proper sheltering of animals, provide advice to animal owners on nutritional requirements, care for sick and injured animals, tend to the proper disposal of carcasses, provide housing to animals, and manage food safety. Veterinarians should have detailed maps of animal centers in their areas, such as

veterinary hospitals, boarding kennels, fairgrounds, racetracks, and other evacuation locations, including slaughterhouse facilities. Veterinarians should also organize therapeutic intervention methods, systems, procedures, and processes to prevent potential illnesses.

Industrial livestock production facilities, as well as home farms, may see a large number of animal habitats destroyed during a disaster, jeopardizing vital food stores. Diseases, exacerbated by impaired food and water supplies, could lead to outbreaks of food poisoning, typhoid, cholera, infectious hepatitis, and gastroenteritis. Removal of fences and enclosures results in the release of animals that subsequently roam unrestricted, increasing their interaction with wildlife, domestic animals, and human populations, providing vectors for potential disease transmission.[11] Veterinarians with training in food and meat hygiene should decide which foods (e.g., milk or meat products) are potentially unsafe and which foods are acceptable for human consumption in the given disaster circumstances.

The American Veterinary Medical Association has created a disaster preparedness series, which is included on its Web site, designed to educate both pet owners and the large industrial animal producers on the natural and technological aspects of disaster preparation.[12] The University of California-Davis Veterinary School also provides online information for facilities planning to offer animal care during evacuations. Animal care operations can find additional printable forms online to help organize the influx of evacuated animals.

Disasters may occur when owners are away from home. In such instances, stickers placed around the homeowner's property in advance can aid rescue personnel. These stickers should contain information pertaining to the types of animals located on the property, the location of the animals, their possible hiding spots, and the location of evacuation supplies. Owners should designate a neighbor familiar with their animals and evacuation plans to be responsible for the animals in the event that they are not at home when a disaster occurs. Identification tags, including rabies and license tags, will help reunite owners with their pets after a disaster. Identification should include the owner's name, home address, phone number, and an out-of-state phone number of someone who can be contacted in the event of an emergency. Suggested methods for identifying large and small animals are included in Box 39-1.

During an evacuation, it is best to separate animals into individual evacuation areas—based on household location and species—to decrease disease transmission.

Large animal evacuations are more difficult to manage than small animal evacuations. Specifically, animals unfamiliar with trailers provide a unique handling and capture challenge. A key recommendation for evacuating larger animals it to acclimate the animals to transportation equipment and the evacuation process in advance.

The evacuation of exotic animals, such as birds, amphibians, and reptiles, can be equally challenging. Birds are best transported in small, securely covered containers to prevent injury. Cages should be covered and placed in quiet locations to decrease the stress of evacuation. Amphibians can be transported in watertight plastic bags and plastic containers, one species per container. Small pet reptiles can be transported effectively in pillowcases, sacks, or transfer carriers. Using the same water that an amphibian inhabited before the evacuation will help minimize physiological stress. All exotic animals should be provided with clean food and water every day, including dietary supplements unique to that animal. Once animals arrive at evacuation facilities, special care must be taken to monitor water and air temperature, humidity, and lighting.

After intake areas at evacuation sites are established (Box 39-2), animals need to be secured in cages or on leashes and properly identified. Identification includes taking a picture of the animal with the owner, if the owner is available. Intake information should include a unique number for the animal and its date of birth, sex, and breed. Bite alert badges, if relevant, should be placed on cages or on the animals' collars. Unless the animal is injured and needs to see a veterinarian, shelter personnel should then take the animals to their perspective housing areas. Injured animals should be taken to a triage area. Intake for dead animals (including strays) should be handled in much the same manner, except that carcasses should be placed in properly designated areas or disposable containers.

The treatment of injuries and infectious diseases needs to occur before an animal is transferred to an intake area and placed among other evacuated animals. Triage sites are to be used as temporary holding facilities where veterinarians can determine whether an animal is stable enough to be transferred to a housing facility. Animals determined to be in life-threatening situations with reasonable prognosis of a full recovery should be triaged to one area, animals with nonlife–threatening injuries should be triaged to a second area, and uninjured animals should be transferred to a third area.

Information on housed animals should include the following:

1. What food and what quantity of food the animal should be fed (Table 39-1)
2. Whether, and how much, the animal is eating
3. Whether the animal is drinking its water
4. Whether the animal is defecating in the cage, and whether stools appear normal
5. Whether the animal appears mentally or physically well

Sheltered animals need to be walked for a total of 3 hours per day, no longer than 15 minutes per walk. Information regarding larger animals needs to be noted, such as their movements or lactations. Abnormalities or unusual behavior occurring in either large or small animals, when properly recorded, will alert veterinary and housing personnel of a potentially sick animal.

Once a disaster is declared over, all animal habitats used before the disaster need to be cleaned and cleared of potential hazards before animals are released back into those environments. Areas surrounding buildings and facilities need to be cleared of any sharp objects, dangerous materials, and wildlife. Large animals should be released into safe, enclosed outdoor areas. Because small animals may encounter dangerous wildlife and other debris if allowed outside unsupervised and unrestrained, they should be released indoors. Animals that may have been left behind without food sources should be reintroduced to food in small servings, gradually working up to full portions. Uninterrupted rest and sleep will help the animals to recover from trauma or stress.[12]

PITFALLS

Traditionally, veterinary public and animal health concerns in disaster management have focused primarily on food safety and supply, injury, and treating infectious diseases. Data, however, suggest that it is equally important to focus on the animals left behind by their owners. In preparation for future events, the evacuation of pets along with human household members must be prioritized.

In surveys of previous disasters, most pet owners proved self-reliant, requiring no public services. Such self-reliance should be encouraged. Unfortunately, however, owners who evacuate pets can hinder the efforts of

TABLE 39-1 HOUSED ANIMALS' FOOD AND WATER REQUIREMENTS

ANIMAL	WATER PER DAY	FEED PER DAY
Cat/dog	1-3 quart per animal	Varies
Cows/horses	7-9 gallons	8-20 lb hay
Poultry	0.5-1.5 gallons per 10 birds	2-4 lb per 10 birds
Sheep/swine	1-4 gallons	3-8 lb hay or grain

Adapted USDA Animal Welfare Information Center Newsletter. Available at: http://www.nal.usda.gov/awic/pubs/awicdocs.htm.

emergency management officers, who are primarily focused on evacuating people. In New York City, after a scaffolding collapse, emergency management personnel initially told people to leave their animals, and several days passed before pet owners were allowed to tend to their animals. Later, emergency management officials were prosecuted for preventing pet rescue.[5] Better coordination with local animal health officials may prevent such problems.

Thirty percent of respondents in one city suggested that they would not evacuate with their pets in an emergency because they would not be able to catch or transport them.[12] Pet evacuation failures occur independently of geographic location and weather conditions at the time of the disaster. Sociodemographic risk factors of pet abandonment, however, are usually present before disasters strike. They include low pet attachment, dogs living outdoors, and owners not having carriers for cats. Therefore, to promote solid animal evacuation practices, animal owners require education by local animal health personnel. In addition, emergency medical systems somewhat promote negligence by pet owners by forcing them to keep their pets at home during an emergency. Further, local emergency shelters do not provide suitable housing for people and their animals. In some instances, individuals abandon evacuation shelters because they are afraid their pets will be jeopardized. Most shelters do not provide any means of animal support because they do not want, or cannot afford, the liability involved in housing both humans and pets. One solution would be to create pet-friendly shelters where humans can evacuate with their animals. Unfortunately, at present, the American Red Cross only has rooms and resources to manage the large number of displaced people and not their pets.[4]

Farms, which usually have large numbers of animals of different species, present unique evacuation planning problems. Most farmers are middle-aged, well-educated individuals living in rural areas. These individuals tend to be somewhat skeptical about evacuation orders delivered through radio and television and instead rely heavily on themselves and their neighbors for information. In one survey, farmers prioritized their evacuation plans by placing family safety first, farm and home security second, and animal concerns third.[13] If cattle needed to remain on the farm, most farmers suggested that 3 days of feed and water would be available. A majority of the farmers surveyed agreed that within 2 weeks, additional feed and water would be needed.[13] Further complicating matters, few areas in disaster situations [SW1]are big enough to accommodate a large number of animals from multiple farms. Therefore, preplanned evacuation areas to corral valuable herd animals need to be identified in advance. Farms can use numerous individuals, family members, employees, and friends to help transport herds of livestock, provided that adequate notice is given. The sheer amount of work necessary to transport agricultural animals necessitates a larger timeframe, allowing greater compliance and removal of animals to safety.[7] The difficulty of gathering a large number of animals, both agricultural and domestic, suggests that animal control personnel need to be more centrally included in evacuation planning and assistance teams.

REFERENCES

1. Adams J. The role of national animal health emergency planning. *Ann N Y Acad Sci.*1999;894:73-5.
2. Moon H, Kirk-Baer C, Ascher M, et al. US agriculture is vulnerable to bioterrorism. *J Am Med Vet Assoc.* 2001;218:96-104.
3. Gibbs P. The foot-and-mouth disease epidemic of 2001 in the UK: implications for the USA and "war on terror." *J Vet Med Educ.* 2003;30:121-31.
4. Heath S, Champion M. Human health concerns from pet ownership after a tornado. *Prehospital Disaster Med.* 1996;11(1):79-81.
5. Heath S, Beck A, Kass P, et al. Risk factors for pet evacuation failure after a slow-onset disaster. *J Am Med Vet Assoc.* 2001;218(12):1905-9.
6. Heath S, Voeks S, Glickman L. Epidemiologic features of pet evacuation failure in a rapid-onset disaster. *J Am Med Vet Assoc.* 2001;218:1898-1904.
7. Linnabary R, New J. Results of a survey of emergency evacuation of dairy cattle. *J Am Med Vet Assoc.* 1993;202:1238-42.
8. Linnabary R, New J, Vogt B, et al. Emergency evacuation of horses—a Madison County, Kentucky survey. *J Equine Vet Sci.* 1993;13:153-8.
9. Heath S, Dorn R, Linnabary R, et al. Integration of veterinarians into the official response to disasters. *J Am Med Vet Assoc.* 1997;210:349-52.
10. Anderson R, Tennyson A. AVMA emergency preparedness planning. *J Am Med Vet Assoc.* 1993;203:1008-10.
11. Moore R, Davis Y, Kaczmarek R. The role of the veterinarian in hurricanes and other natural disasters. *Ann N Y Acad Sci.* 1992;653:367-75.
12. American Veterinary Medical Association. *Saving the Whole Family: Disaster Preparedness Series.* Schaumburg, IL: American Veterinary Medical Association; 2004.
13. Linnabary R. Attitudinal survey of Tennessee beef producers regarding evacuation during an emergency. *J Am Med Vet Assoc.* 1991;199:1022-6.

chapter 40

Urban Search and Rescue

Gregory Ciottone

Urban search and rescue operations are an integral part of the response to disaster. Advances in the recovery of victims trapped for days in the aftermath of a catastrophic event have been some of the most significant improvements in disaster response over the past 25 years. Unlike the disasters of old, recovery of victims now may occur days after the event, resulting in significant changes in the duration of the search and rescue phase of the response. In addition, the emergence of confined space medicine (CSM), the medical care of victims trapped in very small areas, has brought a level of sophistication to the search and rescue operation not previously seen. The study of CSM defines the unusual entrapment situations and unique medical scenarios encountered when caring for victims in collapsed structures.[1] Although there are varying circumstances under which search and rescue may be deployed, in most cases the Urban Search and Rescue (US&R) Task Force (TF) model has been used to safely recover victims of disaster trapped under rubble. The nature of the disaster dictates the techniques and equipment that US&R TFs bring to bear, along with the expertise and experience required to locate and recover trapped victims.

Even though a discussion of the specific techniques used by US&R TFs is beyond the scope of this book, it is essential for any disaster responder to have an understanding of the role of US&R in the overall response. It is very likely that during disaster medicine operations, significant overlap will occur with US&R TF operations. It may be that disaster medicine specialists are called on to provide medical support for specific US&R missions or that these specialists are faced with providing patient care to the victims rescued by US&R personnel. In either case, understanding the basic principles of urban search and rescue, such as the extrication of victims with crush syndrome, is necessary.

HISTORICAL PERSPECTIVE

Search and rescue operations have been a part of disaster response from the earliest recorded events. A report of the attempted rescue and recovery of victims from under the soot caused by the Mount Vesuvius eruption of 79 AD by Pliny the Younger stands as one of the earliest descriptions of search and rescue in a disaster. In virtually all disasters, either natural or manmade, there has been some attempt to rescue victims lost and presumed trapped. The desire to rescue others stricken by disaster crosses cultural bounds and is ingrained in all of us. Until recently, that recovery process typically involved actions by lay people in close proximity to the disaster scene. Formal search and rescue concepts did not develop in the United States until the 1980s. Before that time, any search and rescue activities were typically unorganized and lacked formal training and guidelines. In 1988, after the Office of Foreign Disaster Assistance (OFDA) established teams that responded to several international earthquakes, the Robert T. Stafford Disaster Relief and Emergency Assistance Act of 1988 and the Federal Response Plan (FRP) outlined a specific need for search and rescue as part of the response to disasters.[2] The Federal Emergency Management Agency (FEMA) then created the National Urban Search and Rescue Response System for the rapid deployment of specialized teams on a national level.[1,3] Homeland Security Presidential Directive 5 later mandated the creation of a new National Response Plan. As a result the Department of Homeland Security (DHS) created the National Response Plan of 2004, in which 15 areas are named as Emergency Support Functions (ESFs) required for disaster response, with urban search and rescue being one of them (Box 40-1). This organizational configuration remains today, with USAR teams ultimately falling under FEMA and DHS.

CURRENT PRACTICE

USAR TF Composition

Currently there are 28 US&R TFs in the United States, all under the direction of the DHS.[4] Each TF is designed to be rapidly deployed to disaster sites anywhere in the country, with a goal notification to departure time of 6 hours. Each is equipped and trained to be completely self-sufficient for 72 hours in a disaster zone, and each includes four categories of personnel: search, rescue, medical, and technical. There are 38 specialized positions on the TF, each filled with at least two people. TF Medical Team personnel are physicians and paramedics.

BOX 40-1 EMERGENCY SUPPORT FUNCTIONS

ESF 1	Transportation
ESF 2	Communications
ESF 3	Public works and engineering
ESF 4	Firefighting
ESF 5	Emergency management
ESF 6	Mass care, housing and human services
ESF 7	Resource support
ESF 8	Public health and medical services
ESF 9	Urban search and rescue
ESF 10	Oil and hazardous materials response
ESF 11	Agriculture and natural resources
ESF 12	Energy
ESF 13	Public safety and security
ESF 14	Long-term community recovery and mitigation
ESF 15	External affairs

Within each category, positions are filled with personnel possessing specific specialty training. These include specialists in lifting structures, bracing structures, use of dogs, and use of listening devices and hazardous materials specialists and communications specialists, to name a few.[3] The search team members' responsibility is the location of trapped victims, whereas the rescue team's responsibility is to remove them. Rescue team members also assist with the shoring up of the structure. The technical team manages the liaison with local resources, evaluates and shores up the structure, provides hazardous material identification and management, and manages communications. They are the logistical arm of the TF. The medical teams provide emergency medical care to victims and injured TF members throughout the duration of the operation. They may also be counted on to provide prolonged medical care to victims trapped in the rubble and initial emergency search canine care. The advent of CSM has resulted in an increase in the sophistication of medical care provided by the US&R medical teams.

US&R personnel use personal protection equipment (PPE) specific to the work they must do. The use of respiratory protection in the form of either a mask or self-contained respirator is almost always necessary. There are often hazardous material problems within a work site that may cause the release of noxious gases. At a minimum, dust is always a factor when working under the rubble. Lighted helmets are also required to protect against falling debris, along with some form of eye protection, such as safety goggles. Protective coveralls made of a strong material, such as polyethylene (Tyvek), are used, along with elbow and knee padding. Latex gloves should always be used under leather ones as barrier protection against hazardous materials or bodily fluids. Search and rescue personnel also carry an assortment of equipment necessary, including a safety rope, for the location and extraction of trapped victims. Safety lines are used during the penetration of the rubble and are overseen by the TF safety officer.

US&R Task Force Deployment

The US&R TF is designed to optimize the search and rescue capability of a disaster response operation. To achieve that goal, the team must be rapidly deployable, self-sufficient on arrival and for 72 hours, and possess specialized personnel and equipment. During a deployment, the TF will operate 24 hours a day, rotating its personnel in 12-hour shifts. The 28 US&R TFs in existence are regionally dispersed so that the likelihood of one or more TF being in close proximity to a disaster and able to be on-scene as quickly as possible is increased. Table 40-1 shows the distribution of these teams by state.

On arrival, the TF integrates into the ongoing response operation and into the Incident Command System. Because US&R TFs are rapid-deployment assets, they do not carry heavy machinery to the site. Initially, engineers on the team will assess the site and make determinations as to the equipment and specialty needs. If there is a requirement for heavy equipment, such as ground-moving bulldozers or heavy cranes, the logistics officers, who are a part of the technical team, will begin to liaison with local vendors of such equipment. These same logistics officers, much like in other specialized disaster response teams, will look for caches of food, water, fuel, and other essential supplies to maintain the team on site beyond the initial 72-hour supply the team carries with it.

Each disaster is unique, and the availability of resources is equally different. In urban settings, there is a higher likelihood of obtaining necessary supplies in a timely manner, whereas in more rural settings this task may be a complicated one. The enormity of the tsunami that struck the vast area around the Indian Ocean in 2004 demonstrates the potential difficulties faced by search and rescue teams. The logistics of obtaining necessary equipment and supplies in very rural settings, such as those areas struck by the tsunami, can be an extremely difficult and mission-limiting process. Conversely, after the 2001 WTC attacks, there was a tremendous outpouring of food and supplies into the

TABLE 40-1 DISTRIBUTION BY STATE OF URBAN SEARCH AND RESCUE TASK FORCES

NO. OF USAR TFs	STATE
1	Arizona
8	California
1	Colorado
2	Florida
1	Indiana
1	Maryland
1	Massachusetts
1	Missouri
1	Nebraska
1	Nevada
1	New Mexico
1	New York
1	Ohio
1	Pennsylvania
1	Tennessee
1	Texas
1	Utah
2	Virginia
1	Washington

site. This overabundance of resources can create a logistical problem as well, simply due to the effort required to manage them. There were incidents weeks into the WTC disaster response in which large food stores were becoming rancid, causing a risk of rodent infestation and subsequent infectious disease outbreak. In addition, large numbers of supplies and resources can strain an Incident Command System in a large-scale disaster that is already having difficulties controlling the extent of the response.[5,6] In such scenarios it is important for US&R logistics personnel to ensure that appropriate equipment and supplies specific to the disaster are being obtained and that those supplies are being managed effectively throughout the duration of the deployment.

Search and Rescue Operations

There are five stages to a US&R operation: reconnaissance, assessment of any victims present, detailed search of areas with higher probability of live victims, guided small-scale debris removal, and large-scale debris removal. The first two stages are surface operations only designed to gain knowledge about the rubble pile and to look for victims lying on or near the surface. The last three stages involve penetrating the pile; locating, treating, and removing victims; and removing debris.

Immediately on arrival, as the logistical operation to maintain a safe and self-sufficient presence is under way, the search and rescue stages of operation begin. The search and rescue specialists obtain blueprints of any involved structures from local resources (before arriving on-scene if possible) and begin to devise an approach into the collapsed structures. These blueprints can be invaluable for determining where the rubble may require shoring up and where the potential collapse hazards exist. In addition, it may be possible to identify safe havens where trapped victims may have congregated.

Soon after arrival, a preliminary search by search and rescue specialists takes place. This involves a cautious probing of the surface of the structure and is designed to both develop a working knowledge of the details of the collapsed structure and to attempt to quickly identify trapped victims so that rescue can be accomplished as early as possible. This initial search is typically not done with cameras or dogs and is a relatively superficial one. After the initial search, more formal search and rescue operations begin. During this part of the operation, all resources available to the team are brought into use. The process is much like peeling an onion. The teams must probe and remove debris from the top of the rubble pile down, thereby minimizing the possibility of further collapse. An area to be searched will be identified and the parameters of the search determined. As US&R specialists probe the rubble, "bucket brigades" are set up to remove debris from the area. This is a slow process but is necessary because heavy machinery may disrupt an area and possibly cause secondary collapse onto workers or trapped victims. As an area is searched and the presence of live victims is ruled out, heavy equipment can replace bucket brigades so that rubble can be removed more rapidly. Care still must be taken with the heavy equipment because unexpected live victims may be encountered. The safe removal of rubble from a search and rescue scene by heavy equipment is one of the most difficult operations faced by the task force.

As victims are located, a series of steps is taken to assess their medical condition, ensure their safety, and effect their extrication from the structure. A rapid triage-like assessment will be made of the victim's condition. If possible, vital signs will be taken and the victim will be asked a series of question concerning the extent of his or her entrapment and level of pain and the possible presence of other survivors. Treatment may be started while the victim is being extricated from the structure.

Confined Space Medicine

The medical care of victims entrapped in debris has become an area of great advancement in search and rescue technique over the past decade. With improved search and rescue capabilities came the discovery of victims still alive for days, and rarely more than a week, after a disaster event. This led to the development of an area of medicine studying the care of these victims while still trapped in the rubble and immediately thereafter.

Victims trapped in small, confined spaces pose a considerable challenge to the rescuer. Such spaces are prone to threats affecting both the victim and the rescuer, such as collapse, hazardous materials and gases, temperature extremes, electrocution, and lack of oxygen.[7] These inherent hazards make the extrication and medical care of victims difficult and dangerous operations. Care must be taken initially to ensure that there is no risk of collapse of the space. A determination is made by rescue personnel as to the stability of the structure and the need for shoring up. All hazardous materials in the area must also be identified. Carbon monoxide is a common hazard in spaces where there may be fire, smoke, and operating equipment nearby. Detection of high carbon monoxide levels must be made early, and breathing equipment must be used by both rescuers and victims. Flammable gases also pose a significant threat in closed spaces. The likelihood of fire or explosion with flammable gases present is greatly increased in these spaces, where equipment such as welders and generators may be used. The presence of a flammable gas must be quickly recognized and appropriate steps taken to secure the safety of the area.

Once scene safety has been established and all hazards addressed, the rescuer will implement CSM techniques to care for the trapped victim. Concurrently, efforts will be made to extricate the victim from the scene. Initial assessment and treatment follow standard emergency care procedures, with the victim resuscitated if necessary and the most life-threatening injuries addressed first. The airway may be a difficult management concern for the medical team. Depending on how the victim is trapped and what kind of access there is to the victim, the rescuer may be forced to use unusual airway techniques, such as blind nasal intubation, digital intubation, or cricothyrotomy in suboptimal conditions. It is important, therefore, for the medical personnel to be trained and proficient in many different airway procedures. Clearly there are no medical procedures that should significantly delay the extrication of the patient from the rubble, save for emergent airway intervention. During extrication, as in the management of any trauma patient, strict cervical spine and back immobilization is practiced.

Trapped victims may have a myriad of injuries secondary to the initial trauma or as a result of the prolonged stay beneath the rubble. In addition, infectious disease and hazardous materials exposure issues may arise as well. Each victim must be assessed and treated based on the unique circumstances to which he or she has been exposed.

Crush Injury and Crush Syndrome

One of the more common injury patterns seen in CSM is the crush-injured patient. These injuries are often present in victims of building collapse and earthquakes, in particular, and result from initial trauma and then prolonged time beneath heavy rubble. There are many similarities in both injury patterns of the victims and the immediate layperson response seen in building collapse and earthquake disasters.[8] In each type of scenario, the lay public in the immediate area often attempts to rescue trapped victims. Meanwhile, victims in both building collapse and earthquake scenarios who are trapped beneath heavy rubble for long periods can manifest crush syndrome.

Extrication of victims trapped under heavy rubble is a very difficult task that requires precision logistical planning for shoring up and evaluating the collapsed structure. Victims run the risk of further time beneath rubble, as well as the ongoing risk of secondary collapse. During the extrication of crush-injured patients, there is a period of high risk for sudden death when the heavy material is lifted off the patient. Known as the "smiling death," the victim is typically awake and alert before extrication and then dies within minutes of the heavy material being removed.[9]

Crush injury and crush syndrome are two different entities. Crush injury is the result of direct trauma to a limb and the resultant injury to muscle, soft tissue, and bone. Crush syndrome is secondary to muscle death and the subsequent electrolyte fluxes, third spacing of fluid, and rhabdomyolysis that occur.[10] Death of limb musculature can occur as early as 1 hour after significant trauma or hours later. This leads to necrosis and subsequent breakdown of muscle, causing a release of intracellular contents into the plasma. Therefore, the extent of crush syndrome is directly related to the amount of musculature injured and the time spent under the rubble.[11] These intracellular contents remain localized and build along with lactic acid as more and more muscle dies. The release of these substances into the bloodstream when the limb is freed results in their recirculation. The rapid death seen in some of these cases is thought to occur from cardiac arrhythmia induced by high concentrations of intracellular electrolytes, such as potassium, suddenly bathing the heart.[12] In addition, rhabdomyolysis, which is seen in crush syndrome, often leads to acute renal failure. In both the Armenia and Marmara earthquakes, crush syndrome and acute renal failure were seen in a large number of victims who were rescued alive from the rubble.[13,14]

The treatment of crush syndrome involves intravenous hydration, early hemodialysis, and supportive care. The victim will require large amounts of intravenous crystalloid; this therapy should be started as early as possible. If the victim is trapped and unable to be removed immediately, he or she should have an intravenous line placed while in the rubble, if possible, and rehydration should begin before extrication. Early administration of crystalloid will minimize the occurrence of acute renal failure. The victim's limb must also be monitored for the development of compartment syndrome secondary to limb swelling. Some suggest performing fasciotomy if compartment syndrome is suspected.[15]

Field limb amputation has long been a hotly debated topic in the search and rescue literature. The need for such drastic action is rarely ever considered and has as its only real indication the inability to remove a victim from entrapment when either the scene is becoming unsafe or the patient's medical condition is rapidly deteriorating. The decision to perform field amputation of a limb is one made by the medical team, as part of the US&R TF, under consultation with the rescue personnel. If done, attention must be paid immediately to the control of blood loss and the quick removal of the patient to more definitive care.

Confined Space Medicine Injuries

There are a number of other injury patterns typical in CSM and, therefore, seen in US&R operations. These also present unique obstacles to the US&R medical teams, and the care of such victims requires specialized knowledge and skills. The cause of a building collapse may dictate the type of injures seen. For instance, a collapse due to loss of structural integrity during an earthquake is quite different from a collapse secondary to an explosion. With the heightened concern of terrorist events today, the latter is more and more a possibility.[16] As an example, in the WTC and Pentagon attacks of Sept. 11, 2001, airliners acting as flying explosive devices assaulted the towers. The airplanes exploded on impact. Victims in the immediate area were first traumatized by the explosion and subsequent blast effect, fire in and around the impact zone, and finally the collapse of the structure. Had there been survival of victims from within the collapsed structures, multiple injury patterns would have been seen.

It is not uncommon for victims trapped under rubble to have experienced blast injury from the initial event.[17] Blast injury results from differing effects caused by varying features of the explosion. Blast injury can be divided into four phases: primary, secondary, tertiary, and quaternary. Primary injury pattern is a result of the blast wave created by a high-order explosive, such as ammonium nitrate, creating a super-sonic explosion. This is an overpressurization wave and causes injury and rupture of hollow, air-filled organs, such as lungs, abdominal luminal organs, and eyes. Secondary blast injury occurs from the flying debris generated by the explosion and can injure any part of the body with shrapnel. Tertiary blast injury is the result of the victim being thrown by the explosion and subsequent blunt and penetrating trauma. Finally, quaternary blast injury is "everything else" and includes such things as structure collapse.[18] An understanding of these stages of blast injury and their causes enables the US&R medical teams to predict injury patterns and treat them more effectively.

Prolonged entrapment under rubble may also cause a number of syndromes similar to those seen in patients suffering from exposure. Depending on the amount of time and the conditions under the rubble, victims may have a myriad of exposure syndromes such as hypothermia or hyperthermia, dehydration, starvation, or infection.[19] These syndromes should each be addressed based on their presence at the scene as early as possible. If possible, intravenous lines should be placed and crystalloid hydration begun vigorously if the victim is entrapped and accessible. Warm air and space blankets can be used to counter hypothermia, and nourishment in the form of portable foodstuffs can be administered. The greatest obstacle to the care of these victims is not anticipating the occurrence of these injury states.

PITFALLS

1. It is essential for disaster response specialists to have a working knowledge of the US&R TF makeup and procedures. Not doing so may cause a breakdown in the incident command and disaster response systems.
2. Understanding the pathophysiology of crush syndrome is paramount to the care of entrapped victims. The disaster medical specialist working with US&R assets should be prepared to care for victims with crush syndrome both at the scene and in emergency departments
3. Having a working knowledge of the myriad of injuries that result from structure collapse and victim entrapment will allow the disaster medical specialist to align resources and prepare to receive such casualties. This will, in turn, result in better outcome through more efficient care.

REFERENCES

1. Federal Emergency Management Agency, National Urban Search and Rescue Response System. Medical Specialist Training Manual. Available at: http://www.fema.gov/usr/medmanual.shtm.
2. Cone D. Rescue from the rubble: urban search and rescue. *Prehosp Emerg Care*. October-December 2000;4(4):352-7.
3. Barbera JA, Lozano M Jr. Urban search and rescue medical teams: FEMA Task Force System. *Prehospital Disaster Med*. October-December 1993;8(4):349-55.
4. Federal Emergency Management Agency, National Urban Search and Rescue Response System. Available at: http://www.fema.gov/usr/nusrs.shtm.
5. Romundstad L, Sundnes KO, Pillgram-Larsen J, Roste GK, Gilbert M. Challenges of major incident management when excess resources are allocated: experience from a mass casualty incident after roof collapse of a military compound. *Prehospital Disaster Med*. April-June 2004;19(2):179-84.
6. Pesik N, Keim M. Logistical considerations for emergency response resources. *Pac Health Dialog*. March 2002;9(1):97-103.
7. National Institute for Occupational Safety and Health. *Worker Deaths in Confined Spaces*. Washington DC: US Department of Health and Human Services; January 1994. Publication 94-103.
8. Crippen D. The World Trade Center attack. Similarities to the 1988 earthquake in Armenia: time to teach the public life-supporting first aid? *Crit Care*. December 2001;5(6):312-4.
9. Moed JD. Medical aspects of urban heavy rescue. *Prehospital Disaster Med*. 1991;6:341-8.
10. Odeh M. The role of reperfusion-induced injury in the pathogenesis of the crush syndrome. *New Engl J Med*. 1991;324:1417-22.
11. Sever MS, Erek E, et al. Lessons learned from the Marmara disaster: time period under the rubble. *Crit Care Med*. November 2002;30(11):2443-9.
12. Michaelson M. Crush injury and crush syndrome. *World J Surg*. 1992;16:899-903.
13. Demirkiran O, Dikmen Y, et al. Crush syndrome patients after the Marmara earthquake. *Emerg Med J*. May 2003;20(3):247-50.
14. Klain M, Ricci E, et al. Disaster reanimatology potentials: a structured interview study in Armenia. *Prehospital Disaster Med*. 1989;4:135-52.
15. Resi ND, Michaelson M. Crush injury to the lower limb: treatment of local injury. *J Bone Joint Surg Am*. 1986;68:414-18.
16. Kluger Y, Kashuk J, Mayo A. Terror bombing-mechanisms, consequences and implications. *Scand J Surg*. 2004;93(1):11-4.
17. de Ceballos JP, Turegano-Fuentes F. 11 March 2004: the terrorist bomb explosions in Madrid, Spain—an analysis of the logistics, injuries sustained and clinical management of casualties treated at the closest hospital. *Crit Care*. February 2005;(9)1:104-11.
18. Langworthy MJ, Sabra J, Gould M. Terrorism and blast phenomena: lessons learned from the attack on the USS Cole (DDG67). *Clin Orthop Relat Res*. May 2004;(422):82-7.
19. Kazancioglu R, Cagatay A, et al. The characteristics of infections in crush syndrome. *Clin Microbiol Infect*. April 2002;8(4):202-6.

chapter 41

Medical Care in Remote Areas

Thomas P. LeBosquet III and David E. Marcozzi

Webster's Dictionary offers one definition of "remote" as simply "out-of-the-way." This clarifies the feelings we have connected to this word, but it does not provide an adequate definition in relation to modern medical care. The reality is that "remoteness" covers a vast spectrum. Traditionally, emergency medicine has come to define remoteness as being linked to the time to care. Concepts such as the "golden hour" have sprung from this.[1] In other words, an hour is entirely too long without care to save a patient in need of certain care such as airway management or defibrillation. Over 222 million of the current U.S. population lives in urban areas, whereas only 59 million (21%) live in rural areas.[2] Because of this and the increasing centralization of medical centers within the United States, there has been an increasing need to provide methods of stabilization and transport to patients in remote areas.

HISTORICAL PERSPECTIVE

Medicine has followed the continuum of society from agrarian, rural-based communities, with health care practiced by those indigenous to the area, to a technology-driven, urban-based society with health care dependent on major medical centers whose locations and practitioners remain remote to many people. Indeed, Mott and Roemer[3] preface their 1948 work by stating: "The forces of social organization necessary to bring the average citizen the benefits of applied medical science have been strongest in the cities; the country dweller is last to be served."

Rosenblatt and Moscovice[4] describe a five-step process in the evolution of rural health within the United States. The first, and longest, period covers Colonization to Industrialization (1620-1850). The need for healthcare beyond basic treatment was largely delivered by midwives, men with other professions (such as farmers, who would truly "moonlight" by doctoring on a part-time basis), or clergy devoted to their sect. The second period, Industrial Growth to the "Pre-Flexner Era" (1850-1910), marks the incorporation of science into medicine. The Civil War, advent of anesthesia, and development of sterile technique brought medicine to the point where general practitioners alone could no longer

master the entire scope of medicine. The third period stretches from the publication of the Flexner Report to World War II (1910-1940). The Flexner Report revolutionized the practice of medicine by shifting physician education from a venture to an academic affair.[5] The fourth period moves toward the War on Poverty (1940-1970). Government programs aimed to increase hospital and medical care access. Hospital beds in rural areas were increased, but overall access to care changed little. The last, and current, period is the "Technological Era" (1970-present).

Current Practice

Physician distribution perhaps best illustrates the problems unique to remote areas. Metropolitan areas with populations greater than 1 million have 304 physicians per 100,000 population, whereas rural towns with populations below 2500 have an average of only 53 physicians per 100,000 population. Physician specialty largely determines the type of area chosen for practice. The greater the degree of subspecialization, the larger the area needed to support a practitioner. A family practitioner can run a viable practice with a patient base of 2000, but a single neurosurgeon requires a patient base of 100,000 to remain viable.[6] Because of the need for 24-hour care and cross-coverage, it is impractical for those practitioners who are unable to treat both adults and children to work in certain areas. A population of greater than 10,000 patients, or at least five physicians, is needed before internists and pediatricians can be used well.[6] Not only are generalists more likely to be found in rural areas, they are more able to fit the needs of those areas.

Over the past 50 years, a nationwide system of Emergency Medical Services (EMS) has developed. In 1966 the National Highway Safety Act brought structure to emergency care with the creation of the Emergency Medical Technician (EMT). These providers were trained to assess patients rapidly and transport them to a higher level of care. EMS has now evolved into a large network of systems designed to receive, stabilize, transport, and transfer patients to any level of care required. EMS transport systems allow major medical centers to expand their patient catchment area. For example, at

Duke University, the Life Flight system, a network of ambulances and several helicopters, allows expansion of a large tertiary care center to cover areas of North Carolina, South Carolina, Virginia, West Virginia, and Tennessee.[7]

Many organizations have developed specific criteria for transportation to a hospital for definitive care.[8] When the decision to transfer is contemplated, the practitioner may use a two-step planning process. First, the patient's need for the services of medical and surgical specialties unavailable at the remote center must be assessed. Second, a prognostic view of the patient's overall condition and vital functions is made. The practitioner must ask: "Will this patient's airway deteriorate? Does he need to be intubated now to pre-empt complications in transport? Does he need a chest tube? Does he have sufficient IV access in case resuscitation is needed? Does he need any cardiovascular drips? What if he starts to bleed?" Anticipation of future complications is both the key criterion and caveat when preparing a patient for transport.

Practicing in remote areas means that preventive medicine is vital. Injury prevention can start simply and progress to the more complex. In an area with the potential for delayed access to medical care, injuries handled easily in one locale can become complicated in another. In many remote places, especially those with poor roads or no vehicular access, ambulation remains the main form of transportation. A simple ankle sprain, limiting the ability to walk, hinders activities of daily living and makes extraction to medical care tedious compared with vehicular transport. Minimizing risk is the important consideration of preventive health. Greater caution must also be taken with activities in remote areas. The healthcare practitioner must anticipate specific problems related to the environment that will be encountered.

Williams et al[9] explain the realities of emergency medicine as it is applied in rural and remote settings. They first underline the point that rural emergency medicine is not exclusive to those trained as emergency physicians. Most small, rural emergency departments employ physicians who are neither residency trained in emergency medicine nor board certified in emergency medicine. Many emergency departments make use of family practitioners who practice exclusively in the emergency department or log extra hours outside their normal practice. Upward of 50% of emergency departments across the United States employ either nurse practitioners or physician assistants. Use of these resources may not be a negative. Because emergency medicine residencies are centered in urban areas, it is necessary to have training institutions make available resources for further education in emergency medicine such as publications for nonspecialists and online continuing medical education.

Adaptability to unique situations and conditions is key to optimizing care in remote environments. The number of providers available and the experience of providers often vary. The healthcare team may consist solely of an individual with first-aid training who happens upon the victim, or it may be a complex web of physicians, nurses, rescue workers, and paraprofessionals working together in a preorganized manner. For this reason the concept of a laterally moving hierarchy allows efficiency. In this structure a direct care provider may assume one or multiple patients. A team leader provides direction to providers so care may be coordinated between patients or that critical care may be provided to one patient. Support workers then help with both primary goals such as medical procedures and secondary goals such as reconnaissance of data and equipment, communication, and patient transport. This structure overlaps because the same individual, over time, may act as team leader, direct care provider, and support provider. Also, this structure may allow multiple leaders at multiple levels to provide coordination of care when a larger event occurs and multiple teams are needed (Fig. 41-1).

When preparing to work in a remote area for a significant time, adequate preparation is important. This mostly depends on the length of stay, the type and number of patients being seen, and the area. It may be as simple as a first-aid kit or as elaborate as a busload of supplies. One of the most challenging decisions is which pharmaceutical arsenal to bring. The World Health Organization (WHO) has labeled drug access, as well as the appropriate use, as a major priority. WHO has clearly defined a list of essential medications that "satisfy the priority healthcare needs of the population."[10] These medicines are chosen because of the diseases they treat, their availability, and their prices.

Pitfalls

Several models have been attempted to bring healthcare to truly remote areas, such as rural areas in developing nations. When the population of an area exceeds the need for multiple physicians or is lower than needed to support one physician, a traveling clinic may be one solution. The government of Uttaranchal, India successfully launched such a program. They use a 26-foot mobile clinic created from a mobile home that brings physicians to different areas 4 days a week with return visits monthly. This mobile clinic contains the diagnostic equipment to perform EKGs, some basic laboratory testing, radiographs, and even ultrasound.[11] It is unique in that it provides general healthcare; previous mobile clinics in that area provided only specialty care. It serves as a model for an expanding program. Similar mobile clinics have been started in Central America and have also found success.[12]

Unusual troubleshooting is necessary in remote areas. For example, a high percentage of visitors to New Hampshire's White Mountains seek outdoor recreation. A 25-year-old female takes advantage of a warm winter day and, with one of her college friends, hikes 4 miles inward on Mount Washington to get in some great ice climbing in the Tuckerman Ravine area. After several hours of easy climbs she decides to lead a challenging route by early afternoon. Unfortunately, with her last piece of protection 15 feet below, she realizes the afternoon ice has become soft. Now 30 feet above her belayer, she loses the grip with her crampons, slips and falls that distance to land feet first, and shatters both of her ankles. Upon impact she bounces backward and

Team Members: Experienced Physicians, Newer Physicians, Nurses and Nurses Aides, Paramedics, Emergency Medical Technicians, First Responders, Military, Police, Rescue Workers, Bystanders		
Team Leader:	**Direct Care Providers:**	**Support Workers:**
Responsibilities:	*Responsibilities:*	*Responsibilities:*
• Coordinate care of one or many patients.	• Provide first- and second-degree survey and assessment	• Assist team to prepare necessary resources at the correct time
• Direct activities of group	• Continue provision of ongoing care	• Facilitate activity not directly related to patient care

FIGURE 41–1. Proposed laterally moving structure for care provision in remote areas. It is important to recognize team members can play different roles depending on the situation, location, total number of workers available, and the acuity of the patient. This pattern may also be used in a repeating structure when multiple teams are needed.

thrusts the pick of her ice ax through the left lateral aspect of her chest wall. Within seconds she is now immobile and has a pneumothorax. She was wearing her climbing helmet and is conscious. Her climbing partner, who took an EMT class, knows how to assess her ABCs. He does not have a stethoscope or blood pressure cuff, but he is able to measure that her heart rate is 95. He uses the sling in his first-aid kit and extra clothing in her backpack to stabilize the wound from the ice ax. A climber with another group, who has run over to help, runs to the hut halfway up the trail to use the radio that is there because his cellular phone is not receiving any signal. She has begun complaining that her foot is starting to hurt, but also that it is "falling asleep." Now, what to do with this patient? There are several details of her situation that could compromise her care. She is now sitting, with multiple life- and limb-threatening injuries, in cold snow. Although it is a warm day at 40°F, it is 2 PM and the sun will be going down at 4:15 PM. If the wind picks up, the temperature could easily drop to –10°F overnight. Not only is the stationary patient, whose sweat-soaked clothing will freeze when the temperature drops, at risk, but any potential rescuers would also be at severe risk of hypothermia and cold injuries. It would take hours for the 18 or so people who would be needed to litter out this patient to arrive. She will need to be airlifted; however, she has a pneumothorax. If she did not have a chest tube placed before being carried in the aircraft, her stable pneumothorax could rapidly expand to become a tension pneumothorax. When the helicopter arrived, the rescue team would need the supplies, as well as a capable practitioner, to place the chest tube. Where would this patient need to be transported? The nearby community hospital has amassed an excellent collection of orthopedists because of the local ski areas and their associated injuries. They could handily repair her fractures and relieve her compartment syndrome. However, there is no thoracic surgeon nearby to remove the ice ax perched dangerously close to her pulmonary vasculature. She would need to be transported to a large medical center, which by land would be 2 hours east, 2 hours west, or 3 hours south. Assuming good weather, airlift would reduce these times because much of the land transport time is exacerbated by small rural roads.

This example should illustrate that providing medical care in remote areas requires the coordination of both practitioners and resources. The needs for these are unique and dynamic, and they depend on patient, disease, and location.[13, 14]

SUMMARY

The main points of this chapter are as follows:

1. Healthcare has long been practiced in remote areas.
2. Those traveling through or living in remote areas ultimately will receive care from someone.
3. The practitioner must appropriately mix technology-based care and more traditional physical examination and observation-based techniques when technologies are not available.

4. Each remote setting and situation is different. Care must be tailored to the patient, disease, environment, and resources.

REFERENCES

1. Cowley RA. The resuscitation and stabilization of major multiple trauma patients in a trauma center environment. *Clin Med.* 1976;83:14-22.
2. U.S. Census Bureau. Census 2000 Summary File 2 (SF 2) 100-Percent Data: Urban vs. Rural. 2000. Available at: http://www.census.gov/Press-Release/www/2001/sumfile2.html
3. Mott FD, Roemer MI. *Rural Health and Medical Care.* New York: McGraw-Hill; 1948.
4. Rosenblatt RA, Moscovice IS. *Rural Health Care.* Indianapolis: John Wiley & Sons; 1982, 24-54.
5. Flexner A. *Medical Education in the United States and Canada.* Stanford: The Carnegie Foundation for the Advancement of Teaching; 1910.
6. Ricketts TC. *Rural Health in the United States.* Oxford: Oxford University Press; 1999, 40-41.
7. Duke University. Emergency Medicine Response System. 2004. Available at: *http://www.dukehealth.org/emergency_services/lifeflight.asp*
8. American College of Surgeons Committee on Trauma. *Advanced Trauma Life Support for Doctors. Student Course Manual.* American College of Surgeons; 2001.
9. William JM, Ehrlich PF, Prescott JE. Emergency medical care in rural America. *Ann Emerg Med.* 2000;38:323-7.
10. World Health Organization. 2003. Available at: http://www.who.int/druginformation.
11. Taking Medical Care to Remote Areas. *The Hindu Business Line.* October 30, 2002. <http://www.thehindubusinessline.com/bline/2002/10/30/stories/2002103000901900.htm>
12. Small World Foundation. Fort Lauderdale. Available at: *http://www.smallworld.org/mobilehospital.cfm.*
13. Werner D. *Where There Is No Doctor: a Village Healthcare Handbook* Berkeley: The Hesperian Foundation; 1996.
14. Whitlock W. et al. *Special Operation Forces Medical Handbook.* Teton NewMedia; 2001, 1-12–1-21.

chapter 42

EMS Beyond the Barricade

Louis N. Molino, Sr.

The title of this chapter refers to the EMS operations on the "hot side" of a barricade in response to incidents that involve hazardous materials (also referred to as *HazMat incidents*). The single best working definition of HazMats is when materials released from their containers can and do cause harm to both humans and the environment.[1]

WHERE HAZARDOUS MATERIALS INCIDENTS OCCUR

The more times a hazardous material is handled or manipulated, the more opportunity for an incident to occur. Because of public opinion, legal pressure, and potential litigation, the chemical manufacturing and transportation industries have recognized the need for due diligence in care of these materials throughout the chemical life cycle (see following text). These societal pressures and industry responses have decreased the number of incidents over the past several years.[2]

Responders are often surprised with the numbers and types of chemical operations present in the community.[3] HazMat incidents can occur at every stage of the chemical life cycle, and emergency response forces must be ready to respond to each of these stages[4]:

- Research and development
- Site of manufacture
- Storage (at site of manufacture)
- Transportation
- Storage (at site of use)
- Site of use
- Disposal of waste product

Research and Development

The research and development phase of chemical operations is often one of the most dangerous and is generally undertaken only under extreme safety procedures. Most of the research conducted in the United States is in an academic setting or at dedicated research facilities. These facilities often have their own emergency response capability on-site.[5]

Communities hosting such facilities often meet with the management of the facility to understand the nature of the on-site research. This may conflict with legitimate concerns of industrial espionage. Although chemical producers would be willing discuss any of their work, they may not be willing to discuss details of their ongoing research. These facilities often have plans that are integrated with the local response community to manage emergencies.[5]

Manufacture

The manufacturing process presents the greatest bulk hazard because materials are stored, handled, and mixed at the facility throughout the process. This is also where industry has focused their prevention efforts. Billions of dollars are spent by the chemical industry to prevent incidents or to limit the incident to the plant itself.

In many manufacturing plants, the hazardous materials response capability may be more robust than the local public capability. The local community may be able to draw on these abilities to augment its own response for off-site accidents that occur. This requires preplanning with the plant to determine how the plant can support the public sector response forces and vice versa.[5,6]

Storage (at Site of Manufacture)

Many manufacturing sites store quantities of materials prior to shipment on the same sites as their manufacturing operations. A complete understanding of the nature of the products stored and their associated storage systems for each facility is necessary for emergency response forces. Preplanning is essential for the successful response and operations at bulk storage sites of any type.[5,6]

Transportation

Ultimately all products that are manufactured will be moved to their end users. During transportation, the chemical industry has less control and oversight because of road, weather, and other conditions. Because the incident may occur at any point of the transportation phase, available resources from the chemical company may be far removed from the incident.[5,6]

Storage (at Site of Use)

The nature and types of risks at this point are wholly dependent on the quantity of materials stored and how they are stored. If a quantity of materials is stored on-site, which could present a serious response problem for local emergency forces, preplanning and mutual aid as well as preincident interaction with the chemical producer and user is paramount in order to ensure that all safety precautions are in place.[5,6]

Use

In the use phase, the element of human error predominates. The unintentional or even intentional misuse of chemicals has always plagued emergency response forces. The threat of the intentional misuse of chemicals as "agents of opportunity" is something that emergency planners should consider.[5,6]

Disposal of Waste Product

The final phase of the chemical life cycle is the disposal phase. The disposal phase has an increased potential for a serious incident. With some materials the breakdown products may be more hazardous than the original product itself. In these cases disposal procedures may become complicated.

For most wastes, specific regulations exist to ensure the proper disposal of such products. In the past, large hazardous waste dumps could be found all over the United States. Many have lingering health effects that have plagued the host communities for decades. Cleanup for these sites may cost millions of dollars. Emergency response may be initiated for a previously unknown site when its effects are noticed.[5,6]

HOW HAZARDOUS MATERIALS HARM HUMANS

The three main mechanisms of harm in the case of chemical emergencies are as follows[3,7-10]:

- Flammability: Causing thermal injury such as burns and scalds
- Reactivity: Causing a rapid release of energy when a chemical reaction occurs
- Health effects: Causing the disruption of normal bodily functions

These mechanisms can lead to severe physical trauma (e.g., burns, penetrating and blunt force trauma from the resultant fires, explosions, and other physical means). These injuries are often complicated by the toxic properties of the chemical

Hazardous chemicals can interact with the human body in four routes of exposure:

- Inhalation
- Absorption
- Ingestion
- Injection

HAZMAT BEHAVIOR

Hazardous materials are chemicals that follow the laws of physics and have generally easily predictable properties. By understanding the laws of chemistry and physics, responders can avoid exposure and effectively respond to and mitigate the hazardous materials emergency.[1,6]

Accidental HazMat incidents occur because of one or more of the following initiation events[1]:

- Human error
- Environmental conditions
- Container failure
- Equipment failure

When one or more of these initiators occurs, the hazardous material is released into the environment. A sequence of events known as the Six-Step General Events Behavior Model occurs, which was first described by Ludwig Benner, Jr. in his classic 1978 work, "A Textbook for Use in the Study of Hazardous Materials Emergencies."[11] These six steps are repeated in every incident in which hazardous materials are released into the environment. The six steps are:

- Stress: Something stresses the container
- Breach: The container is breached
- Release: The material in the container is released into the environment
- Engulfment: The material spreads into the environment
- Impingement: The material that has spread comes into contact with people or other exposures to which harm may occur from the resultant contact with the HazMat
- Harm: Harm comes to the living things from the hazardous material

Each of these events must occur in the order described; however, they can occur in rapid succession. The time depends on the nature of the event and the materials and containers involved in the incident.[11]

HISTORICAL PERSPECTIVE

Hazardous materials are among the tools that allow us our modern life. Use of hazardous materials in construction, manufacturing, and fabricating predates the Roman civilization.[5] Since their first use there have been incidents that have caused harm to both humans and to the environment. During the 1960s a number of significant hazardous materials incidents focused public attention on the problems associated with the manufacture, storage, transportation, use, and disposal of such materials.[5] Until the late 1970s, few training courses were offered to the fire, police, and EMS community.[12] Most incidents were managed by the local authorities as best as possible, frequently (and poorly) by EMS teams.[13,14] Several incidents made the EMS community painfully aware of the need for both special training and tactics for response to these types of incidents.[5] There was also the need for special care for the victims of these incidents.[3,7-10]

Training courses on handling of hazardous materials at all levels of proficiency are readily found throughout the United States.[14,15]

Most EMS agencies are ill equipped and poorly trained to respond to HazMat incidents. Even those that may be a part of the fire department system in their community often lack the level of training or the level of preparedness. With the recent influx of funding for local agencies to prepare for weapons of mass destruction (WMD) on a national level, the proficiency of many local fire and EMS agencies to manage "everyday" HazMat incidents has also improved.

CURRENT PRACTICE

All responders are required to meet or exceed the training recommendations of the Occupational Safety and Health Administration (OSHA) regulations found in 29 CFR 1910.120 (q) (6)[12] the standard for HazMat responders. Furthermore, all responders should strive to meet all of the requirements at a minimum of the Operations Level of the National Fire Protection Association (NFPA) 472,[17] the Standard for Professional Competence of Responders to Hazardous Materials Incidents. Doing so ensures that the responders have acquired the necessary knowledge, skills, and abilities needed for a safe response to incidents involving hazardous materials.

Hazardous Materials Incident Response

A hazardous materials response may be initiated for any incident that has a HazMat presence. Incidents resulting in small spills of common hazardous materials are not likely to initiate a HazMat response in most jurisdictions. If the quantity of a hazardous chemical exceeds the local response capability, a HazMat emergency may be declared.[17]

It is difficult to describe a typical HazMat response in the United States as various jurisdictions have established procedures that vary as widely as the response community itself. Until recently ambulances would be dispatched in the course of HazMat response, but the responding personnel would have little or no specialized training and no protective equipment. That has changed significantly over the past decade.[4]

All personnel who may respond to a HazMat incident require training. The level to which personnel are trained may vary within an agency based on assignment and expected duties, but, by federal law, all training must meet certain levels of knowledge and skills as set forth in OSHA 29 CFR 1910.120 (q) (16) as well as NFPA 472. The levels are referred to as Awareness, Operations, Technician, Specialist, and Incident Commander as defined below[16]:

Awareness Level

First responders at the awareness level are individuals who are likely to witness or discover a hazardous substance release and who have been trained to initiate an emergency response sequence by notifying the proper authorities of the release. They take no action beyond notifying the authorities of the release.

Operations Level

First responders at the operations level are those who respond to releases or potential releases of hazardous substances to protect persons, property, or the environment from the effects of the release. They are trained to respond in a defensive fashion without attempting to stop the release. They will attempt to contain the release from a safe distance, keep it from spreading, and prevent exposures.

Hazardous Materials Technician

Hazardous materials technicians respond to releases or potential releases to stop the release of the hazardous material. They approach the point of release in order to plug, patch, or otherwise stop the release of a hazardous substance.

Hazardous Materials Specialist

Hazardous materials specialists respond with and provide support to hazardous materials technicians. Their duties parallel those of the hazardous materials technician, although those duties require a more directed or specific knowledge of the various substances they may be called on to contain. The hazardous materials specialist would also act as the site liaison with federal, state, local, and other government authorities in regard to site activities.

Hazardous Materials Incident Commander

Incident commanders, who assume control of the incident at the scene, receive at least 24 hours of training equal to the first responder operations level and are able to implement the incident command system and the appropriate site, local, regional, and federal emergency response plans.

Once trained, the maintenance of that training and the exercising of both the knowledge and skill components of the training become paramount to ensure competence and the ability to respond both safely and effectively. The incident commander is ultimately responsible for the safety of all responders and victims on the incident scene.

Decontamination

If the contaminant is such that the rescuers could become harmed by the substances that are on the patient, the treatment of that patient should be delayed until the threat is neutralized. In all other cases, the patient's care becomes the first priority.

The generally accepted method of decontamination for most substances is water. Although many types of homemade and commercially available decontamination formulas and units are available, the nozzle of a fire hose is generally the fastest means of delivering the water to the victim and is generally the most rapid form of decontamination available.

Assessment of the HazMat Victim

The assessment of a HazMat victim begins with the rapid and accurate identification of the substances involved in the incident. A methodical assessment of the patient should take place.[4,8,10]

HazMat Physiology and Treatment Protocols[10]

Many antidotes and specific treatment protocols exist for the treatment of chemical exposures. Some are appropriate for prehospital use, whereas others will be performed only in the clinical setting.

Some of the chemicals with specific antidotes or treatment protocols include:

- Cyanide and cyanide compounds
- Hydrofluoric acid
- Aniline dyes
- Nitrites
- Nitrates
- Nitrobenzene
- Nitrogen dioxide
- Organophosphates
- Carbamates
- Phenol
- Chlorine
- Chloramine
- Common lacrimators such as OC spray and mace

Many HazMat teams and their medical personnel carry a HazMat drug box containing medications beyond the normally carried ALS drugs. Some medications in the HazMat ALS drug box may include the following[10]:

- Adenosine
- Metaproterenol (inhaler/nebulizer package)
- Amyl nitrate perles
- Atropine sulfate (often as prepackaged auto injectors)
- Esmolol (Brevibloc)
- Calcium gluconate
- Dextrose 5%
- Dextrose 50%
- Diazepam
- Dopamine
- Epinephrine
- Methylene blue
- Naloxone
- Albuterol
- Pontocaine hydrochloride
- Pralidoxime (2-PAM often carried as prepackaged auto injectors)
- Sodium bicarbonate
- Sodium nitrite
- Sodium thiosulfate

- Thiamine
- Morgan irrigation lens

The specific concentrations and quantities carried vary based on local medical direction and/or state protocols.

Responder Protection for HazMat Response

The most important factor in response to HazMat incidents is self-protection.[17,19,20] The first principle is to avoid contact with any hazardous materials.[17] This requires basic understanding of the chemical and physical properties of the materials involved in the incident. Further protection is provided by wearing specific personal protective equipment (PPE).

There are four recognized levels of personal protection for HazMat incidents.[16] These four levels of protection are based on the following concepts:

- No one glove, boot, or splash suit is omnipotent in protection qualities
- The ensemble is selected based on an analysis of the work to be performed and the hazards likely to be encountered.

The levels of PPE are known as Level A, B, C, and D, and they are described in OSHA, EPA, and NFPA standards in the following basic terms[17]:

- Level A: Full-body vapor proof suits with self-contained breathing apparatus (SCBA) for respiratory protection
- Level B: Full-body protection that is splash resistant with SCBA for respiratory protection
- Level C: Splash protection with chemical-resistant boots and gloves and use of an air-purifying respirator for respiratory protection
- Level D: Normal work uniform

OSHA mandates that training be given to any responder who will be operating in any level of protection. OSHA further mandates that those with the responsibility of determining what specific PPE is to be used on a given response be specifically trained in both the selection process and risk analysis.[16]

PPE usage is a skill that must be practiced. Classroom training alone is not sufficient to ensure that a responder has the skills to use PPE in the hazardous environment found in a HazMat response. Only training and practice can ensure that this skill set will be available during an actual emergency.

Medical Support of the HazMat Team in Incident Operations

One role for the HazMat medical personnel is to support the efforts of the HazMat team as it operates. The use of PPE alone is potentially dangerous, particularly in hot climates. Therefore, even in drills or exercises the availability of HazMat-trained medical personnel ensures the safety of the responder.[6]

PITFALLS

The hazards are based on the chemicals encountered. This can present a problem where the chemicals are not immediately known. In such circumstances the incident commander determines what level of protection and what components of the PPE ensemble are to be used by responders.

CONCLUSION

HazMat operations are rife with risk, but, with proper training and equipment, HazMat teams are able to manage the hazards presented by such incidents on a daily basis. When people are harmed by these materials, EMS beyond the barricade is often the difference between life and death.

REFERENCES

1. Noll GG, Hildebrand MS, Yvorra JG. *Hazardous Materials, Managing the Incident*. Oklahoma City: Oklahoma State University; Fire Protection Publications; 1988.
2. Reinhold VN. *Emergency Responder Training Manual for the Hazardous Materials Technician*. New York: Center for Labor Education and Research; 1992
3. Fire F. *The Common Sense Approach to Hazardous Materials*. New York, NY: Fire Engineering Books and Videos; 1986.
4. New Jersey State Police OEM, DP/HM, and ERPU. *New Jersey HAZMAT Emergency Response Course: Emergency Department Operations Hazmat /WMD Hospital Provider*. New Jersey: New Jersey State Police; 1988.
5. Cashman J. *Hazardous Materials Emergency Response and Control*. Lancaster, PA: Technomic Publishing; 1995.
6. Hawley C. *Hazardous Materials Incidents: Second Edition*. Clifton Park, NY: Delmar/Thomas Learning; 2004.
7. Bevelacqua AS. *Hazardous Materials Chemistry*. Albany, NY: Delmar/Thomas Learning; 2001.
8. Stilp R, Bevelacqua AS. *Emergency Medical Response to Hazardous Materials Incidents*. Albany, NY: Delmar/Thomson Learning; 1997.
9. Bronstein AC, Currance PL. *Emergency Care for Hazardous Materials Exposure*. St Louis: CV Mosby; 1988.
10. Borak J, Callan M, Abbott W. *Hazardous Materials Exposure*. Englewood Cliffs, NJ: Brady/Prentice Hall; 1991.
11. Benner L, Jr. *A Textbook for Use in the Study of Hazardous Materials Emergencies,* 1978.
12. United States Occupational Safety and Health Administration, Code of Federal Regulations (CFR) Title 29 CFR 1910.120 (q) (6).
13. Tokle G. *Hazardous Materials Response Handbook*. Quincy, MA: NFPA; 1993.
14. National Institute for Occupational Safety and Health (NIOSH), Occupational Safety and Health Administration (OSHA), United States Coast Guard (USCG), and United States Environmental Protection Agency (EPA). *Occupational Safety and Health Guidance Manual for Hazardous Waste Site Activities*. U.S. Department of Health and Human Services, 1985.
15. International Association of Fire Fighters. *Training for Hazardous Materials Team Members*. Washington, D.C.: IAFF; 1991.
16. International Society of Fire Service Instructors. *Hazardous Materials Technicians Program*. Ashland, MD: ISFSI; 1993.
17. National Fire Protection Association. NFPA 472 Standard for Professional Competence of Responders to Hazardous Materials Incidents. Quincy, MA: NFPA; 1992.
18. Hawley C. *Hazardous Materials Response & Operations*. Albany, New York: Delmar/Thomas Learning, 2000.
19. National Fire Protection Association. NFPA 471 Recommended Practice for Responding to Hazardous Materials Incidents. Quincy, MA: NFPA; 2002.
20. National Fire Protection Association. NFPA 473 Competencies for EMS Personnel Responding to Hazardous Materials Incidents. Quincy, MA: NFPA; 2002.

chapter 43

Triage

Andrew Reisner

"The train was cut open like a can of tuna. We didn't know who to treat first. There was a lot of blood, a lot of blood."

Enrique Sanchez, Madrid EMS, of simultaneous commuter train bombings, March 2004[1]

Triage is the utilitarian sorting of patients into categories of priority to rationally allocate limited resources; it is, proverbially, to do "the greatest good for the greatest number." Triage fails in one of two ways: undertriage and overtriage. Undertriage represents a failure to identify the casualties who could benefit from scarce medical resources, such as the serious casualty whose life would be saved decisively with rapid evacuation and prompt emergency surgery. In terms of test characteristics, undertriage means poor sensitivity to those who would get the most benefit from the medical resources available. On the other hand, overtriage occurs when casualties who, relatively speaking, do not benefit from a scarce resource nonetheless receive that resource. Overtriage signifies a sorting system with low specificity. Noncritical patients who receive immediate care even though they could safely wait (at the expense of more serious, savable casualties) constitute one form of overtriage. It can also occur when expectant patients, so sick with little chance of treatment success, are provided with precious medical resources.

Triage following disaster is not a single processing step; rather, triage underlies all aspects of the response, including on-site rescue, evacuation, receiving hospital activities, decontamination, and so on. Because the response resources available, the clinical conditions of casualties, and the information available all evolve throughout the time-course of the response, response priorities do so as well. Triage is a dynamic process.

Disaster responses have been suggested to match normative practice as much as practically possible,[2,3] and that, of course, would apply to triage methods. On the other hand, normative practice could pose a liability for massive disasters, in which a set of reflexes could interfere with the truly rational allocation of resources. This trade-off is discussed throughout this chapter. As noted in the following section, many recent disaster responses have been characterized by a general lack of meaningful triage.

HISTORICAL PERSPECTIVE

The roots of disaster triage stretch back to at least eighteenth-century military casualty care. Baron Larré, a surgeon with Napoleon's army, was utilitarian in his methods of managing multiple battlefield casualties, as was the American John Morgan during the U.S. Revolutionary War.[4] Military triage evolved sporadically, but by World War II a hierarchical structure for combat casualty care had been developed. In WWII, the average time from injury to definitive care was 12 to 18 hours. By the Vietnam War, improved triage and air-ambulance capabilities reduced this time to less than 2 hours.[5] This early military history of triage was reviewed nicely by Kennedy.[4]

In the 1980s, civilian prehospital systems became interested in trauma triage for the individual trauma casualty; West[6] showed that serious trauma casualties had superior outcomes when cared for at specialized trauma centers. There were investigations of prehospital criteria for differentiating individual casualties that should be taken to major trauma centers and those that could receive care safely at community medical centers (to avoid overburdening trauma centers with non-serious casualties). Trauma registries enabled the development and validation of various field triage decision-rules, although such criteria have proven problematic (see the Triage Scoring System section). Such civilian trauma scoring in turn influenced modern military triage. In the 1991 Persian Gulf War, Burkle et al.[7] explored the use of Champion's revised trauma score[8] for triage of 461 combat casualties. Triage classification schemes for military and civilian mass casualties, to a large extent, have converged. Both military (e.g., NATO) and civilian (e.g., color coding) triage systems make use of comparable levels of acuity, and the Trauma Sieve and START, which are similar triage decision systems, are used by both civilian EMS as well as British Army soldiers.[9]

Regarding civilian triage, the past 25 years have seen a long litany of horrible events in industrialized countries, including bombings, fires, shootings, and plane crashes.[10] These events show a consistency of scale, with immediately surviving casualties numbering in the dozens or hundreds. Too many retrospective reports noted unsatisfactory execution of triage, particularly prehospital triage, for these events. In the mid-1980s, Vayer et al.[3] cited Butman's analysis of 51 mass-casualty incidents (MCIs) that identified a universal failure to execute proper triage. Inadequate prehospital triage continues to be reported following MCIs: an aircraft crash in Singapore in 2000,[11] the Tokyo Sarin attacks,[12] and the Gothenburg fire disaster.[13] Typically, documentation of prehospital triage during an MCI is quite poor, so retrospective analysis of field triage is simply not feasible, as was the case for the Oklahoma City bombing.[14]

The urban community in a developed country may very well possess the necessary resources to treat dozens or even hundreds of casualties, provided the resources are mobilized and the patients in need of immediate care are identified in a timely fashion. Yet suboptimal use of available community resources is the rule rather than exception; for instance, most casualties self-transport to the closest hospital and leave distant facilities underused.[15] Community resources such as urgent care centers and outpatient clinics, capable of treating the majority of casualties with relatively minor issues, are almost always underused. Almogy et al.[16] reported on the Israeli response to the Jerusalem Sbarro pizzeria bombing in 2001, and observed "in these circumstances [e.g., a mass casualty incident such as a suicide bombing], ordinary hospital resources are heavily burdened, yet delivery of efficient medical treatment is possible by recruitment of all available personnel and resources." In contrast to the many reports of poor triage after disasters, exemplary responses to MCIs have stemmed from exemplary mobilization of resources. After the bombing at Atlanta Centennial Olympics, 30 EMS units evacuated all 111 casualties to area hospitals within 32 minutes. The vast majority of serious casualties were taken to Grady Memorial Hospital where "at one point, there were more physicians than victims in the emergency care center"[17] Those casualties all had good or excellent outcomes. After the Jerusalem Sbarro pizzeria bombing the prehospital response was largely "scoop-and-run." The Ein Kerem Campus, receiving 132 surviving casualties, performed two ED thoracotomies, with no apparent shortage of resources available for those less-critical casualties.[16] Almogy's dictum pertains to most recent disasters in developed countries, which have been limited to dozens or hundreds of casualties. Popular field triage systems (see the Triage Scoring Systems section) are most appropriate for such scale of events.

On the other hand, such triage systems are less applicable to disasters with enormous scales. Counting the 1918 Influenza Pandemic and Hurricane Katrina in 2005,, there have been only nine non-military disasters in the entire history of the United States that resulted in more than 1000 deaths. Internationally, massive disasters have produced tens or hundreds of thousands of dead and injured, such as earthquakes in Tangshan (1976), Armenia (1988), Hanshin-Awaji (1995), and Iran

(2003), as well as the Indian Ocean tsunami (2004). Field triage systems tend to be sensitive and not specific, leading to overtriage. More importantly, they may be too unwieldy to triage massive numbers of casualties. Moreover, they are tailored to traumatic pathology, although broad medical pathology (e.g., infectious disease, metabolic disarray) occurs in the aftermath of these massive disasters and baseline medical emergencies (e.g., heart attacks, tubal pregnancies) continue to occur unabated. Only a minority of emergency department patients were trauma victims following disasters such as the Loma Prieta earthquake and Hurricane Gloria.[18,19]

To the extent that one seeks historical guidance when planning for the future, the emphasis that should be given to preparing for enormous-scale disasters in the United States is unknowable. Such events are so rare that we have little experience to guide us. (Traditionally it has been difficult to find the resources—funding, time, materials—to develop and maintain extensive skills and preparedness.) Similarly, respected authorities have suggested that too much attention has been paid to the unprecedented scenario of weapons of mass destruction (WMDs). Frykberg[10] wrote: "We must resist our current tendency to become overly enamored with the 'weapons of mass destruction' of biologic, chemical and radiologic attacks, in terms of funding priorities and resource allocations that are wholly disproportionate to the clear reality of the terrorist bombing threat." History shows that smaller, more mundane mass casualty incidents must be anticipated, although arithmetic shows how one single WMD event could dwarf the sum of preceding MCIs in morbidity and mortality. In support of Frykberg's position, until emergency systems prove capable of triaging events with dozens or hundreds of casualties, does it make sense to prepare for an unprecedented event with thousands of casualties?

CURRENT PRACTICE

This section offers a technical framework for triage following a disaster. The issues discussed here are important to consider for disaster planning and training (and real-time execution), but the reader must always bear in mind those sobering limitations of triage systems detailed in the previous section. All the same, triage should be carried out to the extent possible at the scene and at every facility and site providing disaster care. Box 43-1 lists considerations that should be made in advance of any disaster. Box 43-2 lists details that need to be determined in real time after a rapid survey of the

---

BOX 43-1 TRIAGE PLAN PREPARATION (TO BE DETERMINED BEFORE ANY DISASTER)

- What triage classification is used, if any (e.g., four or five levels of severity)?
- Will a formal triage scoring system be used?
- What on-site/hospital documentation will be used?

disaster and the scope of casualties. Triage training is specifically discussed at the end of the chapter.

What Triage Classification Is Used? There are several issues to consider for planning a disaster response. First, will a multiple-level triage classification system be used? As noted in the previous section, there are precedents for responses to MCIs with over 100 casualties that consist of prehospital "scoop and run." Then, rather than a rigid triage scheme outside of normative practice, casualties were in essence sorted into one of two categories using clinical judgment: OR or no OR[14,16] These events were notable for a lack of clinically significant bottlenecks in field evacuation and hospital capacity, thus reducing the importance of triage.

In planning for a disaster, it hardly seems prudent to assume such ample evacuative and hospital-based resources would be available, but it does speak to the importance of mobilizing maximum resources. This is the impetus for a more formal triage scheme, such as a four- or five-level classification. In the common four-level system, such as the well-known civilian START system,[20] the categories are: (1) those who will get immediate priority (color-coded red), (2) those casualties who must wait (color-coded yellow), (3) those with the least severe injuries (often referred to as "walking well," color-coded green), and (4) those casualties whose prognosis is so poor that there is no justification for spending limited resources on them (color-coded black). Military triage hierarchies have a similar four- or five-level structure, although the nomenclature is different. For instance, color code green is equivalent to NATO level T3. People responding to international disasters should be aware of all of the triage classifications used by the host country and by the other responding agencies. A slightly more complicated five-level system makes a distinction between patients who will not survive

(color-coded black) and those too gravely injured to receive limited resources (sometimes color-coded blue). But if enough resources become available, blue-coded casualties can then receive care. It has been argued that the option for an intermediate level such as blue may actually produce superior triage decision-making. Given a stark choice between red and black for gravely injured patients who are not yet dead, it might be emotionally difficult for responders to apply a black tag, even though resources would be wasted on the casualty with a very poor prognosis.

When a tiered triage system is to be used, the most complicated issue is selecting the formal criteria to use for assigning each acuity level. This is discussed in detail in the "Will a formal triage scoring system be used?" and "Are normative overtriage and undertriage rates acceptable?" sections. Most triage plans assume, and rightly so, that a casualty who can ambulate (i.e., the "walking wounded") is truly low risk. In a review of nearly 30,000 routine civilian trauma casualties, Meredith[21] find that the ability to follow commands (i.e., GCS motor = 6) upon arrival to an emergency department is an outstanding positive predictor of patient survival. Still, these casualties do require medical attention at some point; head or extremity hemorrhage, open fractures, or penetrating abdominal trauma are injuries that might be present in ambulating patients, which are manageable conditions that become dangerous if not treated within an appropriate timeframe. In Meredith's study, the patients with GCS motor of 6 and outstanding prognoses received normative medical care, not indefinite neglect.

Will a Formal Triage Scoring System Be Used? A formal scoring system can help categorize casualties by objective criteria. Reliance on EMS subjective assessments of severity has been studied as an independent predictor of acuity in routine trauma patients (e.g., not disaster casualties). EMS judgment has been found to be better,[22] equal,[23,24] and worse[25,26] than formal triage scoring. There is evidence that EMS judgment complements objective triage scoring.[23,25,26] Also, these prehospital triage systems are tailored to traumatic pathology, not squeezing chest pain nor focal pain at McBurney's point. The Glasgow Coma Scale (GCS), published in 1974, offered a historic means of stratifying prognosis after head injury.[27] Triage scores for individual trauma patients (see the Historical Perspective section) arose from the need to decide if individual trauma casualties should be transported to specialized trauma centers. The best known are Champion's Trauma Score and Revised Trauma Score (RTS). The original Trauma Score used capillary refill and respiratory expansion, which were felt to be too unreliable. The RTS uses GCS, systolic blood pressure, and respiratory rate, and it yields a score between 0 and 12.[8,28] An RTS of 12 predicts mortality of less than 1% (when given routine clinical care). Mortality of roughly 50% is predicted by an RTS of 5. In general, the use of physiologic criteria tends to be specific, but not as sensitive, for predicting critical injury. Other notable triage scores include the CRAMS and Triage Index, which have also shown suboptimal test characteristics.[29-34] The advantage of a scoring system is that no particular physiologic state preordains a specific triage category; rather, scores for "black" and "red" and "yellow" can be established in real time, based on the perceived balance of casualties and medical resources. Triage scoring offers a flexible, sophisticated approach to triage. However, in the chaos and uncertainty of a disaster—a high-acuity, low-probability event—"sophisticated" can become "complicated" and "flexible" can become "uncertain." If formal triage scoring is to be of benefit, emergency responders must be extremely facile with its use if the benefits are to outweigh the costs. For triage of pediatric casualties, neurologic, cardiovascular, and respiratory triage criteria should be different from those for adults because of the differences in physiology and recuperative capabilities. This motivated the development of specialized pediatric triage criteria, including the pediatric trauma score[35,36] and, more recently, the pediatric triage tape.[37] The former instrument did not prove superior to adult triage scoring systems,[38-40] and the latter has not been extensively validated.

A far simpler alternative to triage scoring is a "cookie-cutter" triage algorithm such as the START system. This system, for example, assigns "red" based on a rigid set of criteria (if airway is compromised, if minute respiratory rate is over 30, if capillary refill is over 2 seconds, or if simple commands cannot be followed).[20] The Triage Sieve is another similar example of an inflexible assignation algorithm; it includes an upper and lower limit for "red" respiratory rate, as well as a fixed upper limit for heart rate (unlike START, it does not use capillary refill).[41] The advantage of such rigid systems is the simplicity to teach and learn and the appropriateness for typical MCIs with dozens or hundreds of casualties. The disadvantage, the inflexibility, is discussed further in the Acceptable Overtriage and Undertriage Rate section.

What On-Site Documentation Will Be Used? The triage tag, a minimal document that can be attached to each casualty, might be the only practical method of communicating findings, interventions, and so on, as countless casualties are passed through a chain of emergency care. However, it has been argued that triage tags are impractical to use, and geographic triage (see later) can obviate the need for tags.[3] In a disaster, hundreds or thousands of tags for each triage category must be immediately available to the responders, who need to be exceptionally familiar with the tags to use them properly under trying circumstances, and frenzied casualties may not take proper care of the tags. After an enormous disaster (thousands of casualties), tags might be especially challenging to use properly, although they could also be especially useful.

Consideration of the use of triage tags requires some research on the part of the customer, since there are over 120 triage label systems in use internationally.[41] Hogan and Burstein[42] suggested the following criteria for the optimal triage tag: (1) It must attach securely to each casualty's body, (2) it must be easy to write on, (3) it must be weather-proof, and (4) it should permit the documentation of the patient's name, gender, injuries, interventions, care-provider IDs, casualty triage score, and an easily visible overall triage category. It must also permit changes to be made, because triage is always dynamic. A detailed graduate thesis with a wealth of detail about this subject is presently posted on the Internet.[43]

Who Will Be the Triage Officer(s)? There must be a major first-pass to establish which casualties can wait, which are top priority, which are expectant, etc. This can occur in the field and/or receiving hospital, but the designated triage officer needs a deep understanding of emergency medical treatments, what outcomes are likely for various casualties, and what resources are necessary for treatments. It may be advantageous to have a physician in this role. In Israel, the role is taken by the surgeon-in-charge, since the emergency care bottleneck following a suicide bombing MCI typically occurs in determining operative priority after rapid evacuation to a receiving hospital.[16] Among multiple important traits, a triage officer needs the experience, disposition, and judgment to act as an able leader under incredible pressure.[42,44]

Who Will Collect Vital Signs for the Triage Officer(s)? The measurement of vital signs should be delegated to assistants to the triage officer. Unfortunately, even in routine clinical conditions, vital sign measurements are confounded by human error and poor technique.[45,46] Retraining improves the accuracy of vital signs[47]; this is important, because during the chaos and stress of an MCI, an accurate set of vital signs determines the fate of an individual (e.g., placement in a triage category).

Physically, Where Will Casualties from Each Triage Category Be Cared for (and Who Will Staff Each Area)? Geographic triage means assigning casualties to different physical locations based on severity. Initially, casualties can be brought to a collection point. From there, the triage officer can determine the appropriate triage category (e.g., red, yellow, black, possibly blue), and then the casualty can be moved to a triage category–specific collection point for further on-site treatment and/or transportation. The walking wounded (green) are readily separated from more seriously injured casualties through good crowd communication and control; most of these casualties could be taken care of in an urgent care center, clinic, or private physician offices, and having some mechanism for directing these casualties away from larger medical centers may be valuable. It has been suggested that dead victims should be moved to an isolated location.[42] Briggs[48] suggests the following are desirable characteristics for on-site triage and treatment locations: (1) proximity to the disaster site, (2) safety from hazards, (3) location upwind when contamination is an issue, (4) protection from climactic conditions, (5) easy visibility, and (6) convenient access for air and land evacuation. No ideal location may be available and the on-site collection point may of mixed utility. For example, during the Sept. 11 World Trade Center attack, only 6.8% of the victims who went to the hospital arrived by ambulance.[49] Quarantelli,[50] in a classic study of EMS in 29 U.S. disasters, noted that most casualties are not transported by a properly staffed ambulance, but by private cars, buses, taxis, and even on foot. Field triage and first aid stations are often bypassed, either because their location or existence is unknown, or because they are considered an "inferior" level of care compared with hospitals. Left to their own, minor or even critical casualties will evacuate themselves to a nearby hospital.[3,42]

Following the Centennial Olympics bombing, ample EMS resources allowed rapid, complete evacuation of casualties, so on-site geographic triage was unnecessary.[17] In small or large disasters, it may be preferable for the triage officers and litter-bearers to circulate and directly move casualties from the scene to appropriate treatment locations, eliminating any collection point. In extremely large disasters, several collection areas might be useful. Vayer[3] cited a number of MCIs, including the Hyatt Regency skywalk collapse and the IBM shooting incident, in which a collection point for triage was useful. It is important to consider the manner and degree to which geographic separation will be enforced. The bigger the disaster, the more crowd control is an issue. For receiving hospitals, crowd control is a must and an unstructured influx of casualties should be anticipated, with most casualties ending up at the closest hospitals while those farther away will await casualties that never arrive. Following the Tokyo subway sarin attack, the St. Luke's emergency department was deluged with 500 patients in the first hour alone.[51] At the scene, crowd control is a more complicated issue. Einav[52] described how Jerusalem EMS evacuates casualties so rapidly that only minimal medical interventions are performed, and no crowd control at all is attempted. Crowd control requires emergency resources and may eliminate the assistance by untrained local citizens who constitute the majority of the response resources after disasters. Regarding crowd control on scene, Vayer[3] suggested that "if patients are medically and emotionally stable and choose to leave, they should be allowed to do so."

What Overtriage and Undertriage Rates Are Acceptable, and What Level of Casualty Gets "Black-Tagged"?

Investigations of trauma triage rules (the prehospital decision of whether or not a patient's severity warrants transport to a specialized trauma center) suggest that overtriage of 50% to 60% is necessary to achieve undertriage rates around 10%.[4,25,26,31,42,53] It has also been noted that the four-tiered START triage algorithm leads to substantial overtriage of disaster casualties.[9,42] This might be acceptable in a response to an MCI with a few hundred surviving casualties. Consider Table 43-1: After a hypothetical terrorist bombing with 100 to 200 surviving casualties, conventional triage practice might overtriage 50% of the intermediate "true yellow," increasing the number of total red. Would it be worth attempting a dramatic departure from normative triage to attempt to reduce the 10 or 20 "false reds"? Routine rates for trauma overtriage and undertriage may be ten-

able for incidents on this scale. It is worth examining other scenarios that suggest how overtriage and undertriage goals must be adapted to the scale of the disaster. An event with 1000 to 2000 surviving casualties would yield 100 to 200 "false-reds," in addition to the 200 to 400 "true-reds," if triage criteria were not appropriately adjusted (see Table 43-1). Such numbers of red critical casualties would likely overwhelm even a large urban area's facilities; therefore the rate of overtriage should be lowered even if that means increasing rates of undertriage (this is the classic sensitivity/specificity trade-off embodied by receiver-operator curves). There are in fact diverse options to how to define "black" casualties, who are considered so sick (e.g., pulselessness, apnea) that resources are wasted on them: An Israeli EMS protocol for MCIs is more specific, considering as dead those with amputated body parts who are not showing signs of movement, as well as those who are pulseless with dilated pupils.[16] In published reports, there is mixed evidence that the overtriage of excessively sick casualties (e.g., the failure to apply a black tag to unsavable survivors) has been an issue. One retrospective analysis of seven separate terrorist bombings noted a correlation between high mortality rates for hospitalized casualties *with* critical injuries and the fraction of casualties hospitalized *without* critical injuries.[55] One explanation would be that overtriage of noncritical casualties cost the truly critical casualties the medical attention they required. On the other hand, the paper did not describe other characteristics of the casualties, such as the age of victims, the distribution of injury severity, and the incidence of head injury. These factors might suggest alternative explanations. Historically, resuscitation of moribund casualties following MCIs offers dismal outcomes[14,56,57] and such heroic measures are generally discouraged. Failure to triage the unsavable as "black" (a form of overtriage) will produce "false reds" who will pointlessly be given precious medical resources (see Table 43-1). Indeed, in designing a response to an earthquake with many thousands of casualties, it has been suggested that casualties with a likelihood of survival less than 50% may need to be "black-tagged."[58] If so, a revised trauma score of 5 or less would be an appropriate criterion.[8]

Undertriage of the critically injured may be just as much of a problem, historically. Following the Oklahoma City terrorist bombing, 100% of the 72 casualties admitted to hospitals survived.[14] Only 3 of the 167 fatalities were even transported from the scene, and those 3 were dead on arrival to the emergency department. Is it possible that

TABLE 43-1 SPECTRUM OF CASUALTIES FOR DIFFERENT SCALES OF DISASTERS (HYPOTHETICAL)

SURVIVING CASUALTIES	TRUE GREEN ~60%*	TRUE RED~20%*	TRUE YELLOW ~20%*	TOTAL RED TRUE RED + 50% OVERTRIAGE OF TRUE YELLOW†	EXPECTANT ~2%
100	60	20	20	30	NA
200	120	40	40	60	NA
1000	600	200	200	300	20
2000	1200	400	400	600	40

*Based on typical distributions of injury severity,[54] for illustrative purposes only.
†Based on typical rates of overtriage of less severely injured casualties, see text for details.

there had been savable casualties at the scene who never received needed care in time? It is important to not reflexively deprive serious casualties of the intensive care they may need when resources are available. Pepe and Kvetan[2] propose a scenario in which "there are 40 patients, 39 of whom are 'walking wounded' and one patient ... is in a state of cardiopulmonary arrest." In such circumstances, standard resuscitation, or at least a "quick look" with a defibrillator, may be appropriate for patients who are moribund. Indeed, for both the Centennial Olympics bombing[17] and the Israeli Sbarro bombing,[54] the balance between the spectrum of casualties and the available medical resources was sufficient that CPR and emergency department thoracotomies were attempted, respectively.

Ideally, triage criteria would be calibrated, using a severity score such as the RTS, to balance the scope of resources available with the scope of casualties. An ideal method would further consider not only mortality, but other issues such as functional outcomes or years-of-life saved. Realistically, however, it does not make sense to expect that the triage method can be tailored so carefully to a given disaster in real-time. Most disaster experiences suggest tremendous uncertainty exists about the extent of the casualties during the initial response[10,54]; when extrications are necessary, the sickest patients are usually last to arrive.[3,14] The "fog of war" complicates the initial responses to any disaster. At the same time, it seems prudent to prepare different triage plans for different scales of disaster (e.g., for dozens versus hundreds versus thousands of surviving casualties).

Assuming 10 Patients in 20 Minutes per Triage Officer,[20], Are There Enough Officers? Are There Enough Other Personnel to Keep up with the Triage Team (e.g., Litter Bearers, Care Providers). If not, Is the Triage Team too Big? In general, the litter bearers, triage officers, and other care providers will not always operate in perfect synchronicity, since there will be irregular hold-ups for various activities. Responders may need to briefly change roles during operations (i.e., a triage officer may hold pressure on a compressible site of hemorrhage for a few moments until someone else becomes available to take over). If any specific activity becomes truly rate-limiting (triage, stretcher transport, etc.), personnel should be reassigned to balance the response. Also, if extrication from the site is the rate-limiting step, triage can be moved to the site itself, so that extrication efforts themselves are triaged, with consideration given to both medical severity and the difficulty of extrication.

Are Resources Being Used Appropriately, Including (a) On-Site Medical Interventions, (b) Evacuation Resources, and (c) Hospital-Based Resources (e.g., Emergency Department Care, Operating Room)? This chapter on triage refers to "response resources" and "emergency care" in rather abstract terms. Detailed discussion gets into the excessively broad subject of trauma management and critical care. Yet, to understand and perform triage, one must understand the costs (in terms of time and materials) and benefits of the emergency care. For instance, putting pressure on an extremity hemorrhage or dressing an open chest wound should be high priority for any responder, since such simple measures can

save a life (assuming the casualty doesn't have additional ominous injuries, such as a massive head injury). Other high-value on-site interventions can include splinting and, if critical care resources are permitting, airway support for decompensating patients. If the balance of responder resources to casualties is permitting, on-site intervention may even include some resuscitation (i.e., quick look with a defibrillator), although attempting such heroic interventions always runs the risk of using up precious responder resources. When neither evacuation nor hospital resources are bottlenecked, on-site interventions should be kept to a minimum. For those casualties evacuated by ambulance, consideration might be given to bypassing the closest hospitals. Also, casualties transporting themselves to the hospital could be advised which hospitals are not getting very many patients and therefore will have shorter waiting times. When evacuation from the scene is a bottleneck, common sense dictates that evacuation priority is for patients who would most benefit from timely hospital care. Suspected abdominal hemorrhage thus precedes compressible extremity hemorrhage, since the former requires an operating room while the latter can be treated initially in the field. A lucid but hypotensive patient with penetrating abdominal trauma should precede penetrating head injury with altered mental status, since the former has a better prognosis if prompt operative care is provided. At the receiving hospital, too, resources (operating room, blood cell transfusions, ventilators) should be triaged. One of the important and often overlooked issues in triage is redistributing the patient load. Receiving hospitals may reevaluate appropriate casualties to remote hospitals with available capacity. Some have argued for turning the closest hospital into a triage center and redistributing the casualties to other facilities from there. However, federal patient transfer regulations (EMTALA) do not make this easy.

After Casualties' Initial Triage, Who Reevaluates the Patient, and How Often? After Each Reassessment, has the Triage Plan been Communicated to All Active Rescuers, Including Victims and Participating By-standers, as is Appropriate? A patient's apparent clinical condition will evolve, as will the available resources. After an initial triage, a formal mechanism for ongoing reevaluation of casualties is necessary for all triage categories (with the possible exception of black). These clinical reevaluations can also establish treatment priorities within various triage groups, since, for instance, red casualties will have intracategory variation in terms of severity and the specific management they require. In some cases, conditions will worsen, and a yellow designation may become red (e.g., evolution of blast lung injury) or red designation may become black (e.g., hypovolemic arrest). In other circumstances, new resources may permit more aggressive care, and a blue or even black designation may be upgraded to red (discussed in the What Triage Classification Is Used? section). Even some of the walking wounded may have conditions that require timely intervention, in case an excellent prognosis is threatened. To effectively re-triage requires updated knowledge of the spectrum of casualties and the resources available; there should be a formal mechanism for such updates.

Focus: Training/Planning Specific Issues

This chapter described options for disaster triage. From a training perspective, the bottom line is this: more sophisticated systems may enable optimal triage, but one must fully commit to training and mastery of any system for it to be of value in the chaotic aftermath of a disaster. Therefore, a system such as START, with its straight-forward four levels and rigid criteria for each category, may be better than a fully improvisational approach that relies on clinical judgments, but not unless it is mastered in training. A five-level system may offer even better triage than a four-tiered system,[4] but it is all the more complicated to learn and execute. Triage tags may offer better record-keeping and patient care, but they will prove simply burdensome if they are unfamiliar to the caregivers dealing with a major crisis. Finally, formal trauma scoring, such as Champion's RTS, might enable the most sophisticated triage, but not if the responders are struggling to properly compute the revised trauma score.

One suggestion for planning a triage response to a disaster is this: Select the most flexible methodology of which your training resources will permit mastery. Rehearsal is crucial, so that the principle of "normative practice" (see the opening paragraphs in this chapter) can be followed in an actual disaster. Authors have suggested the need for weekly practice for proper maintenance of disaster-response skills (e.g., "Triage Tuesday").[3,42] Many triage systems rely on measured vital signs, but as noted, vital signs are often measured poorly even under normative clinical conditions; retraining such skills can be very useful. Formal triage scoring, such as the RTS, can also be used in *designing* simulations so that the survival rate of the hypothetical casualties can be computed and the performance of triage during the exercise can be evaluated objectively. Finally, there may be use to simple table-top simulations as an inexpensive, undemanding complement to full-scale rehearsals.

PITFALLS

- Ineffective triage after unexpected disasters has been the historical norm.
- Effective responses have used exceptional mobilization of prehospital and hospital resources, making triage easier.
- For planning, realize that disasters with dozens or hundreds of casualties have been the norm in developed countries.
- Don't assume that the triage plan for dozens or hundreds of casualties will be suitable for disasters of all scales and conditions.
- Don't assume that the majority of healthcare emergencies following large disasters will be traumatic in nature. Just because there is a disaster, people do not stop having coronary ischemia, asthma attacks, or miscarriages.
- Appreciate the enormous training requirements for any triage plan that deviates from normative health delivery practice.
- Appreciate trade-offs between utility and complexity (four versus five triage levels, rigid "cookie-cutter" triage criteria versus flexible criteria using severity scores, triage tags versus geographic triage, etc.)
- Realize that vital sign measurement technique must be addressed in training.
- Select appropriate, safe locations on-scene and plan for crowd control.
- In real time: reevaluate, reassign, and relate updates to responders.

REFERENCES

1. *Boston Metro*. 2004;3(221):2.
2. Pepe PE, Kvetan V. Field management and critical care in mass disasters. *Crit Care Clin*. 1991;7(2):401-20.
3. Vayer JS, Ten Eyck RP, Cowan ML. New concepts in triage. *Ann Emerg Med*. 1986;15(8):927-30.
4. Kennedy K, Aghababian RV, Gans L, Lewis CP. Triage: techniques and applications in decision making. *Ann Emerg Med*. 1996;28(2):136-44.
5. Eiseman B. Combat casualty management in Vietnam. *J Trauma*. 1967;7(1):53-63.
6. West JG, Trunkey DD, and Lim RC. Systems of trauma care. A study of two counties. *Arch Surg*. 1979;114(4):455-60.
7. Burkle FM Jr., Newland C, Orebaugh S, Blood CG. Emergency medicine in the Persian Gulf War—Part 2. Triage methodology and lessons learned. *Ann Emerg Med*. 1994;23(4):748-54.
8. Champion HR, Sacco WJ, Copes WS, et al. A revision of the Trauma Score. *J Trauma*. 1989; 29(5):623-9.
9. Hodgetts TJ. *Triage: a position statement*. European Union Core Group on Disaster Medicine, 2002, 1-15.
10. Frykberg ER. Principles of mass casualty management following terrorist disasters. *Ann Surg*. 2004;239(3):319-21.
11. Lee WH, Chiu TF, Ng CJ, Chen JC. Emergency medical preparedness and response to a Singapore airliner crash. *Acad Emerg Med*. 2002;9(3):194-8.
12. Okumura T, Suzuki K, Fukuda A, et al. The Tokyo subway sarin attack: disaster management, Part 1: Community emergency response. *Acad Emerg Med*. 1998;5(6):613-7.
13. Gewalli F, Fogdestam I. Triage and initial treatment of burns in the Gothenburg fire disaster 1998. On-call plastic surgeons' experiences and lessons learned. *Scand J Plast Reconstr Surg Hand Surg*. 2003;37(3):134-9.
14. Hogan DE, Waeckerle JF, Dire DJ, Lillibridge SR. *Emergency department impact of the Oklahoma City terrorist bombing. Ann Emerg Med*. 1999;34(2):160-7.
15. Auf der Heide E. *Disaster Response: Principles of Preparation and Coordination*. St. Louis: Mosby; 1989.
16. Almogy G, Belzberg H, Mintz Y, et al. Suicide bombing attacks: update and modifications to the protocol. *Ann Surg*. 2004;239(3):295-303.
17. Feliciano DV, Anderson GV Jr, Rozycki GS, et al. Management of casualties from the bombing at the Centennial Olympics. *Am J Surg* 1998;176(6):538-43.
18. Thompson F. Hurricanes and hospital emergency-room visits - Mississippi, Rhode Island, Connecticut. *MMWR*. 1986;34(51&52):765-770.
19. Pointer JE, Michaelis J, Saunders C, et al. The 1989 Loma Prieta earthquake: impact on hospital patient care. *Ann Emerg Med*. 1992;21(10):1228-33.
20. Super G. *START: a Triage Training Module*. Newport Beach, CA; Hoag Memorial Hospital Presbyterian; 1984.
21. Meredith W, Rutledge R, Hansen AR, et al. Field triage of trauma patients based upon the ability to follow commands: a study in 29,573 injured patients. *J Trauma*. 1995;38(1):129-35.
22. Ornato J, Mlinek EJ Jr, Craren EJ, Nelson N. Ineffectiveness of the trauma score and the CRAMS scale for accurately triaging patients to trauma centers. *Ann Emerg Med*. 1985;14(11):1061-4.
23. Hedges JR, Feero S, Moore B, et al. Comparison of prehospital trauma triage instruments in a semirural population. *J Emerg Med*. 1987;5(3):197-208.

24. Emerman CL, Shade B, Kubincanek J. A comparison of EMT judgment and prehospital trauma triage instruments. *J Trauma*. 1991;31(10):1369-75.
25. Esposito TJ, Offner PJ, Jurkovich GJ, et al. Do prehospital trauma center triage criteria identify major trauma victims? *Arch Surg*. 1995;130(2):171-6.
26. Simmons E, Hedges JR, Irwin L, et al. Paramedic injury severity perception can aid trauma triage. *Ann Emerg Med*. 1995;26(4):461-8.
27. Teasdale G, Jennett B. Assessment of coma and impaired consciousness. A practical scale. *Lancet*. 1974;2(7872):81-4.
28. Champion HR, Sacco WJ, Carnazzo AJ, et al. Trauma score. *Crit Care Med*. 1981;9(9):672-6.
29. Gormican SP. CRAMS scale: field triage of trauma victims. *Ann Emerg Med*. 1982;11(3):132-5.
30. Knudson P, Frecceri CA, DeLateur SA. Improving the field triage of major trauma victims. *J Trauma*. 1988;28(5):602-6.
31. Baxt WG, Berry CC, Epperson MD, Scalzitti V. The failure of prehospital trauma prediction rules to classify trauma patients accurately. *Ann Emerg Med*. 1989;18(1):1-8.
32. Baxt WG, Jones G, Fortlage D. The trauma triage rule: a new, resource-based approach to the prehospital identification of major trauma victims. *Ann Emerg Med*. 1990;19(12):1401-6.
33. Bever DL, Veenker CH. An illness-injury severity index for non-physician emergency medical personnel. *EMT J*. 1979;3(1):45-9.
34. Kilberg L, Clemmer TP, Clawson J, et al. Effectiveness of implementing a trauma triage system on outcome: a prospective evaluation. *J Trauma*. 1988;28(10):1493-8.
35. Tepas JJ 3rd, Mollitt DL, Talbert JL, Bryant M. The pediatric trauma score as a predictor of injury severity in the injured child. *J Pediatr Surg*. 1987;22(1):14-8.
36. Tepas JJ 3rd, Ramenofsky ML, Mollitt DL, et al. The Pediatric Trauma Score as a predictor of injury severity: an objective assessment. *J Trauma*. 1988;28(4):425-9.
37. Hodgetts TJ, et al. Paediatric triage tape. *Pre-hospital Immediate Care*. 1998;2:155-59.
38. Kaufmann CR, Maier RV, Rivara FP, Carrico CJ. Evaluation of the Pediatric Trauma Score. *JAMA*. 1990;263(1):69-72.
39. Eichelberger MR, Gotschall CS, Sacco WJ, et al. A comparison of the trauma score, the revised trauma score, and the pediatric trauma score. *Ann Emerg Med*. 1989;18(10):1053-8.
40. Nayduch DA, Moylan J, Rutledge R, et al. Comparison of the ability of adult and pediatric trauma scores to predict pediatric outcome following major trauma. *J Trauma*. 1991;31(4):452-7; discussion 457-8.
41. Hodgetts TJ, Brett A. Triage. In: Greaves I, Porter K, eds. *Pre-Hospital Medicine*, London: Arnold Publishers; 1999.
42. Hogan DE, Burstein JL. Triage. In *Disaster Medicine*. Philadelphia: Williams & Wilkins, 2002, 10-15.
43. Pyrros DG. The current state of affairs regarding triage tags in the European Union. In *Disaster Medicine*. Republic of San Marino European Centre for Disaster Medicine; 2001, 88. Available at: http://europa.eu.int/comm/environment/civil/prote/pdfdocs/disaster_med_final_2002/d8.pdf.
44. Burkle FM Jr. *Disaster Medicine: Application for the Immediate Managment and Triage of Civilian and Military Disaster Victims*. New Hyde Park, NY: Medical Examination Publishing; 1984
45. Jones DW, Appel LJ, Sheps SG, et al. Measuring blood pressure accurately: new and persistent challenges. JAMA. 2003;289(8): 1027-30.
46. Edmonds ZV, Mower WR, Lovato LM, Lomeli R. The reliability of vital sign measurements. Ann Emerg Med. 2002;39(3):233-7.
47. The sixth report of the Joint National Committee on prevention, detection, evaluation, and treatment of high blood pressure. *Arch Intern Med*. 1997;157(21):2413-46.
48. Triage. In Briggs SM, ed. *Advanced Disaster Medical Response Manual for Providers*. Boston: Harvard Medical International, 2003.
49. Guttenberg MG, Asaeda G, Cherson A, et al. Utilization of ambulance resources at the World Trade Center: Implications for disaster planning. *Ann Emerg Med*. 2002;40(4).
50. Quarantelli EL, *Delivery of Emergency Medical Care in Disasters: Assumptions and Realities*. New York: Irvington Publishers; 1983.
51. Okumura T, Suzuki K, Fukuda A, et al. The Tokyo subway sarin attack: disaster management, Part 2: Hospital response. *Acad Emerg Med*. 1998;5(6):618-624.
52. Einav S, Feigenberg Z, Weissman C, et al. Evacuation priorities in mass casualty terror-related events: implications for contingency planning. *Ann Surg*. 2004;239(3):304-310.
53. Wesson DE, Scorpio R. Field triage—help or hindrance? *Can J Surg*. 1992;35(1):19-21.
54. Peleg K, Aharonson-Daniel L, Stein M, et al. Gunshot and explosion injuries: characteristics, outcomes, and implications for care of terror-related injuries in Israel. *Ann Surg*. 2004;239(3):311-318.
55. Frykberg ER, Tepas JJ 3rd. Terrorist bombings. Lessons learned from Belfast to Beirut. *Ann Surg*. 1988;208(5):569-576.
56. Boehm TM, James JJ. The medical response to the LaBelle Disco bombing in Berlin, 1986. *Mil Med*. 1988;153(5):235-238.
57. Brown MG, Marshall SG. The Enniskillen bomb: a disaster plan. *Brit Med J*. 1988;297(6656):1113-1116.
58. Schulz LH, DiLorenzo RA, Koenig KL. Disaster medical direction: a medical earthquake response curriculum. *Ann Emerg Med*. 1991;20:470-471.

chapter 44

Patient Tracking Systems in Disasters

Charles Stewart

Recent acts of mass terrorism have called attention to the urgent need to improve response during mass-casualty incidents.[1] The risk of these mass-casualty incidents appears to be increasing as a result of population growth, industrialization (and concomitant use of high-energy chemicals and sources), and the threat of terrorism.[2]

One consistent challenge during the disaster response is communication and information management from the field to the care facilities. A critical interdependence exists: accurate information from the field about the incident, medical needs at the scene, numbers and types of patients and their injuries, and patients triaged and treated will affect the demand and use of resources such as ambulances, emergency departments, surgical suites and specialists, and intensive care units. Similarly, information on the availability of ambulances and hospital resources will alter the management and disposition of the victims at the scene.

Following the initial impact of the disaster, the casualties generated by this disaster must be determined. Relatives of patients will want to know where their loved ones are being treated, law enforcement officials may want to interview survivors and suspects, and public health officials will want summaries of patient conditions and dispositions. To respond effectively to inquiries about the missing, victim data *may* have to be collected not just from hospitals, but also from shelters, jails, and morgues. However, most disaster evacuees do not stay in public shelters, but rather seek refuge with family, friends, and neighbors. Therefore, they will need to be contacted via the mass media and encouraged to register via telephone hotlines or Web sites. Victim information should be collected at a central location and be made available via telephone hotlines or web sites distant from the impact area. (In very large disasters, the numbers of inquiries about the missing can exacerbate local telephone and cellular circuit congestion and shut them down momentarily.) Hospitals, concerned about Health Insurance Portability and Accountability Act (HIPAA) regulations and patient confidentiality, may be reluctant to provide patient information to the Red Cross or local authorities. HIPAA regulations do allow the release of information on patient names, locations, and general status for the purposes of notifying patients' next of kin. (See www.hhs.gov.ocr/hipaa)

Patient tracking is the art (and science) of determining which patient with which condition went to which destination (and where they are presently). This includes identification of the patient and identification of the patient's destination. Ideal practice would have the patient's medical records included with this tracking information.

HISTORICAL PERSPECTIVE

If the disaster happens in an isolated area, such as a recent complex multi-vehicle accident along I-80 in Wyoming, tracking of patients is relatively easy; most (if not all) casualties will be taken to one or two facilities.[3] The major casualty tracking problem generated during this disaster was identification of victims who were burned beyond recognition. In most disasters, casualties may have multiple potential destinations.

Complicating the patient-destination match is the large number of patients who will take available transportation to a medical facility without involving EMS workers. For example, during the response to the Sept. 11 World Trade Center attack, only 6.8% were transported by ambulance.[4] In addition, emergency response units from surrounding jurisdictions will often self-dispatch to the disaster.[5,6] Accordingly, they may not be aware of existing local victim tracking system(s). Further complications include air evacuation to remote destinations, transfers to higher levels of care for patients with more complex conditions, and switch of destination during EMS transport.

CURRENT PRACTICE

There are two general types of tracking systems in current use: (1) paper tags, cards, and charts and (2) bar codes and Wi-Fi networks. A third type is currently in development.

Paper Tags, Cards, and Charts

Although separate from triage, the tracking process starts with triage. As patients are categorized by the triage officer and assistant triage officers, they are tagged with a visible indicator of their priority (triage tags) or grouped with similar types of patients in a geographic area (geographic triage). Tracking starts with the recording of these patients (and as much data as time and condition permits) as they enter the medical care system.

When a triage or medical documentation tag is applied to the patient, the preassigned number on the tag is the patient's first identification in the system. In some systems, this tag may be the only reported identification and documentation of medical care of the patient until the patient is taken to the hospital.

The triage officer can rapidly prepare a patient tracking list containing the patient's identification number, sex, apparent age, triage condition, destination, and the time the patient left the scene. The receiving hospital prepares a similar list with identification number, sex, apparent age, triage condition, disposition, and time of disposition (Fig. 44-1).

Several commercially available tag systems can be purchased (Fig. 44-2). These include the METTAG and the Multi-Tag. These tags are preprinted with a unique number to facilitate patient tracking during an incident. Each contains a section for patient information and a section with tear-off strips to categorize the patient's condition.

These tags are advocated by multiple incident training programs such as the Major Incident Medical Management and Support training program.[7,8] In these systems, either tags or a substitute such as pieces of colored aluminum, colored chemical light sticks, or surveyor's tape in multiple colors (red, green, yellow, black, or white) are used to tag each patient.[9,10]

Other examples of medical documentation cards designed to travel with the patient include the NATO military "casualty cards" and the International Committee of the Red Cross casualty card.[11] Documentation cards that are attached to the patient in some form are more likely to remain with that patient and document recent medical interventions to the receiving hospital.

There are several disadvantages to the use of paper tags and cards for patient tracking purposes.

- Application of tags takes time. There is only a single accident where triage tags have been described as being of benefit and this was limited to 22 live casualties.[12] Indeed, multiple casualties have been managed without triage tags and significant time was thought to have been saved in the Sioux City, Iowa DC-10 plane crash.[13] (The alternative to triage tags was a geographical system of triage and sorting.)
- Triage tags are not weather resistant and may be destroyed or mutilated easily.[14] Water can smudge and render illegible data on triage tags.
- Triage tags provide no advance information to the destination. (The information provided is also unavailable to other sites.)
- When patient information such as vital signs, condition, or even destination changes, it may be difficult to change the card/tag. Tear-off triage tags allow only unidirectional changes in the patient's condition.
- Tear-off triage tags may be changed easily by patients or family members in an effort to upgrade the triage classification and expedite medical care or evacuation.
- There is little limited paper "real-estate" space for continuation of vital signs and additional information. On the way to the hospital, the EMS provider can often obtain quite a bit of additional information, such as co-morbid factors like diabetes and heart disease, allergies, and current medications. The usual tag does not provide space for this information to the treating physician or medical provider.
- Triage tags are often discarded, even though they should be part of the medical record. They are

Hospital	Triage Tag Number	Hospital ID Number	Last Name	First Name	Sex	Age	Status	Initials

FIGURE 44–1. Sample patient tracking form.

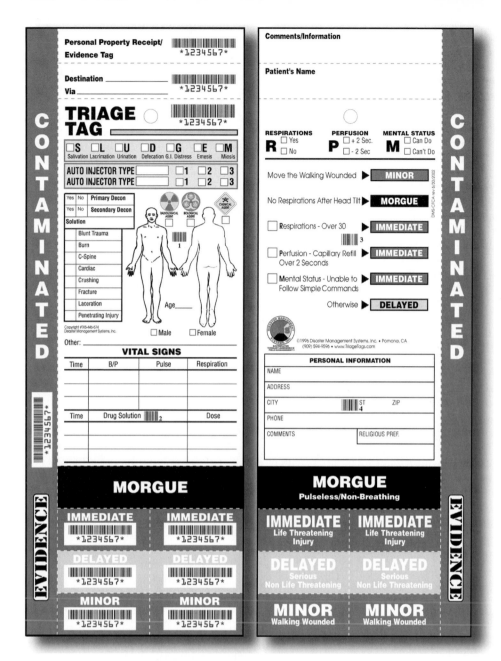

FIGURE 44–2. Sample triage and tracking tag. Please note the following color coding in the tag: Morgue-Black, Immediate-Red, Delayed-Yellow, Minor-Green. (Courtesy of Disaster Medicine Systems, Inc., Pomona, CA.)

often an awkward shape to put into the medical record and may not be recognized by the medical records clerks as part of the medical record.
- There are multiple tag and card formats available and these may be used in the same disaster by different teams. These may generate identical patient numbers for different patients as well as create confusion for medical providers receiving patients with different charting systems.
- When a destination is overwhelmed and the ambulance is diverted to a different destination, the paper triage tag does not reflect a new destination back to the triage officer.

- One of the factors that complicates the use of tracking systems (e.g., triage tags) is the tendency in disasters to abandon paperwork in favor of treating patients.[15]
- In some disasters, triage tags have not been available where needed.[16]

Triage tags do have significant advantages:

- They are cheap and simple to use.
- They are widely used, so many prehospital providers are familiar with their use and layout.
- They require little financial outlay for the disaster response team prior to the accident.

Bar Codes and Wi-Fi Networks

Recent advances in commercial package tracking as used by Fed Ex and UPS allow customers to find the shipping status and location of bar-coded packages and envelopes online. Extension of this technology to triage tracking remedies most of the faults of the paper system and allows the hospital, EMS dispatcher, triage officer, and other appropriate parties to track the human package from triage site to final destination. Alternative schemes with Palm collection devices to supplement basic triage tag data collection have added additional medical information and linked this to the triage tag and the medical record (Fig. 44-3).

By scanning a unique patient wristband at any location (disaster site, site treatment center, emergency department, and hospital ward, operating suite, or ICU), the system can track and provide the last known location of patients.[17-24] These systems have been tested in simulated disaster drills in the United States and Europe with good efficacy.

The addition of a Wi-Fi network collection point and compatible bar-code readers that upload to the network will allow real-time tracking, dispatch, and diversion updates to all participating hospitals and agencies. This gives any participating agency the ability to direct family members to the last known location of the patient.

Similar systems using a radio-frequency identification chip (RFID) can allow remote query of the triage tag or band.[25,26] Marathon runners at large races are tracked during the race with similar technology, which can provide an accurate location of each runner during the race.

Bar-coded tags with Wi-Fi network do have some significant disadvantages, however.

- The technology requires a Wi-Fi network infrastructure to be set up at the disaster. This requires a substantial hardware and software outlay for all participating agencies and hospitals.
- The overall security of Wi-Fi networks is open to much question. Both modification of data and compromise of patient medical data can occur with Wi-Fi networks.
- The system may be unavailable if any electromagnetic jamming occurs and will be destroyed by any EMP effect, which is significant in the case of a nuclear weapon explosion.
- Each bar-code system represents a proprietary software system that may be incompatible with another similar system. This may have significance in adjoining city/county/state governments and some mutual response agreements.
- Bar-code systems require the presence of providers with scanning devices to obtain the tracking data. Keyboard entry of data can occur, but it is much slower and requires a computer with attendant power supply.

Use of barcode readers and networked computers has significant advantages to all parties, including the patient:

- Information about prospective patients is readily available to the receiving hospital. (Information about final destination is available to the dispatch officer for further transportation planning.)
- Information about patients at one facility is readily available to other participating hospitals and agencies.
- Information entered travels with a casualty and can be cross-referenced to medical history, when available. Allergies, medications, and co-morbid factors can be entered by participating sites at any point in the evacuation process. This information can follow the casualty through all levels of medical treatment and be concisely printed for the patient's final chart.
- Information is not limited to a small amount of paper "real estate." This information can even include pictures of the patient and identifying personal effects.
- Entry of initial data and identification of patients in a selected area are both rapid as the barcode is scanned with a reader.

THE FUTURE

The next stage in patient tracking is a wireless communication network to capture and display real-time casualty data, including continuous monitoring of vital signs. The U.S. Navy is investigating the use of a wearable plastic tag with an imbedded electronic chip that stores individual medical data, a palm-sized scanner that electronically reads and writes to the chip, and a central server that collects the database.[27] These smart-card "dog tags" allow data to be carried with the patient, rather than as a network. Use of small automated patient monitoring devices such as the Mobile Medical Monitor (M3) can provide automated data transmission of vital signs, linked to the patient's RFID.[28]

Addition of global positioning data to the electronic tracking record will assist researchers in determining the

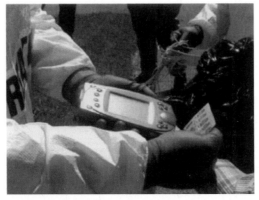

FIGURE 44-3. Bar code reader used in St. Louis County bar code tracking system. (Reproduced from Hamilton J. Automated MCI patient tracking. *JEMS* 2003;28(4):52-56, with permission.)

spot where a specific patient was found during the disaster for later incident reconstruction.

PITFALLS

- When there isn't a means of identification of patients/casualties with a unique identification number, tracking systems either lose all possible privacy and security or become quite difficult.
  - Surveyor's tape, light sticks, and aluminum tags do not allow the triage officer a ready system of counting patient numbers nor allow for numbered patient tracking. Another mechanism will be needed to provide this information.
  - Insufficient tracking tags or supplies for the mass casualty. This occurred during the early phases of both the Tokyo sarin attack and the Sept. 11 World Trade Center attack.
- Multiple entry points exist for casualties into the system. As was apparent in the Tokyo sarin attack, casualties often don't wait for a triage officer and ambulance before they seek medical care. The robust tracking system must be able to account for these patients as they progress through the system.
- Multiple triage tag designs may be used in the same incident, resulting in confusion for providers at all levels.[29,30] This can occur when different agencies respond to the disaster and bring their own tags.
- Numbering systems or tag numbers may be duplicated. This can also occur when different agencies respond to the disaster and bring non-unique numbered tags to the disaster. This will totally confuse efforts at tracking patients.
- Failure to update the tracking model to reflect a changed destination can occur, which happens when ambulances are diverted from one facility to another. When this occurs, finding a patient can become quite difficult if multiple hospitals/receiving facilities are involved in the disaster.
- Inability to gracefully degrade or back-up an electronic system can occur. Battery life for electronic devices is limited. When power supplies and batteries run out, electronic systems will fail. Tracking officers should have a current paper back-up system readily available and should have hard-copy printouts of the current patient load prepared at set intervals. When power supplies fail, these hard-copy editions can gracefully assume the load without complete degradation of the tracking system.
- Given the difficulties ensuring that victim destinations are recorded during transport to hospitals, it is likely in many cases that these data will have to be collected *retrospectively* after transport has occurred.
- Several systems discussed in this chapter use electronic communications on radio frequencies that are easily jammed or use the Internet for communication. Since communications in a disaster is often a casualty of the disaster, the wise tracking officer must plan for this contingency and have a simpler back-up system available.

REFERENCES

1. Wackerle JF. Domestic preparedness for events involving weapons of mass destruction. *JAMA*. 2000;283:252-54.
2. Noji EK. Disaster epidemiology. *Emerg Med Clin North Am*. 1996;14:289-300.
3. Big highway accident occurs on I-80. *Casper Star-Tribune* August 20, 2004. Available at: www.casperstartribune.net/articles/2004/08/20/news/wyoming/66d90603688312ce87256ef5006ea5b7.txt
4. Guttenberg MG, Asaeda G, Cherson A, et al. Utilization of ambulance resources at the world trade center: implications for disaster planning. *Ann Emerg Med*. 2002;40(4):s92.
5. Auf der Heide E. Principles of Hospital Disaster Planning. In: Hogan D, Burstein Jl, eds. *Disaster Medicine*. Philadelphia: Lippincott Williams & Wilkins; 2002, 57-89.
6. Auf Der Heide E. *Disaster Response: Principles of Preparation and Coordination*. St. Louis: CV Mosby; 1989. (Full text available at no charge for noncommercial use at: http://orgmail2.coe-dmha.org/dr/index.htm.)
7. Hodgetts TJ, Mackaway-Jones K, eds. *Major Incident Medical Management and Support, the Practical Approach*. Plymouth, UK: BMJ Publishing Group; 1995.
8. Dernocoeur K. Disasters: Tag, You're It! Available at: http://www.merginet.com/operations/field/DisasterTriageTags.cfm.
9. Vayer JS, Ten Eyck RP, Cowan ML. New concepts in triage. *Ann Emerg Med*. 1986;15:927-30.
10. MacMahon AG. Sorting out triage in urban disasters. *South African Med J*. 1985;67:555-56.
11. Coupland RM, Parker PJ, Gray RC. Triage of war wounded. The experience of the International Committee of the Red Cross. *Injury*. 1992;8:507-510.
12. Beyersdorf SR, Nania JN, Luna GK. Community medical response to the Fairchild mass casualty event. *Am J Surg*. 1996;171:467-470.
13. Kerns DE, Anderson PB. EMS response to a major aircraft incident: Sioux City, Iowa. *Prehospital Disaster Med*. 1990;5:159-166.
14. Plishke KH, Wolf TL, Pretschner DP. Telemedical support of prehospital emergency care in mass casualty incidents. Eur J Med Res 1999;4:394-398.
15. McKinsey & Company. The McKinsey Report—Increasing FDNY's Preparedness. *McKinsey & Company* [Internet]. Available at: www.nyc.gov/htm/fdny/htmlmck_report/toc.html, p. 53.
16. Orr SM. The Hyatt Regency skywalk collapse: An EMS-based disaster response. *Ann Emerg Med*. 1983;12(10):601-605.
17. Bouman JH, Schouwerwou RJ, VanderEijk KJ, et al. Computerization of patient tracking and tracing during mass casualty incidents. *Eur J Emerg Med*. 2000;7:211-216.
18. TracerPlus/Palm OS data collection used for disaster relief management in Michigan and Iowa. Available at: http://www.prweb.com/releases/2003/12/prweb93918.htm.
19. Noordergraaf GJ, Bourman JH, van den Brink EJ, et al. Development of computer-assisted patient control for use in the hospital setting during mass casualty incidents. *Am J Emerg Med*. 1996;14:257-261.
20. Plishke KH, Wolf TL, Pretschner DP. Telemedical support of prehospital emergency care in mass casualty incidents. *Eur J Med Res*. 1999;4:394-398.
21. St. Louis region metropolitan medical response system. Available at: http://mmrs.fema.gov/PublicDocs/NDMS/Showcase/St.Louis/slide01.aspx.
22. Raytheon News Release. Raytheon's Emergency Patient Tracking System component of mutual aid agreement signed by St. Louis-area hospitals. Available at: http://www.raytheon.com/newsroom/briefs/031003.html.
23. Emergency Patient Tracking System found at Newsgram, City of St. Louis. Available at: http://stlouis.missouri.org/citygov/newsgram/volume5/emergencysystem.htm.
24. Hamilton J. Automated MCI patient tracking. *JEMS* 2003;28(4):52-56. Available at: www.JEMS.com
25. Berman J. Exclusive: center to test RFIDs to track patients, equipment. *Health IT World News*. June 29, 2004. Available at: http://www.health-itworld.com/emag/060104/index.html.

26. Achieving better patient care through supply management technology. *Urgent Matters Newslett.* 2003;1:1. Available at: http://www.urgentmatters.org/enewsletter/vol1_issue1/demonstrating_emerging_technology.asp.

27. Ryan D. FH-3 tests patient tracking system in Iraq. *Navy Newstand.* Available at http://www.news.navy.mil/search/display.asp?story_id=7590.

28. Deniston WM, Konoske PJ, Pugh WM. Mobile medical monitoring at forward areas of care (report). San Diego, CA: Naval Health Research Center Medical Information Systems and Operations Research Department, 1998.

29. Paschen HR, High speed train crash at Eschede. *Trauma Care.* 1999;9:68-89.

30. Staff of the accident and emergency departments of Derbyshire Royal Infirmary Leicester Royal Infirmary, and Queen's Medical Centre, Nottingham. Coping with the early stages of the M1 disaster: At the scene and on arrival at hospital. *BMJ* 1989;298:651-654.

chapter 45

Tactical EMS

Jeffery C. Metzger and David E. Marcozzi

The earliest form of our current Emergency Medical Service (EMS) system emerged in the late 1700s from the need to transport and care for patients wounded in military operations. During the intervening 200 years, this early improvisation developed into the civilian EMS system that exists today. In recent years, with law enforcement focusing on covert and tactical operations, it has become evident that specialized medical support is necessary both to decrease the rate of morbidity and mortality and to increase the success rate of missions undertaken.

Tactical Emergency Medical Support (TEMS) refers to medical support for law enforcement operations. It has been defined by the National Association of EMS Physicians (NAEMSP) as "the spectrum of services necessary to establish and maintain the health, welfare, and safety of special operations law enforcement providers."[1,2] The term *emergency medical support* was intentionally chosen in place of *emergency medical services* to convey the wide range of functions beyond simple care for acute injuries during the operation. TEMS entails an overall contribution to mission success and the preservation of life and safety of all persons involved in a mission, including members of the tactical team, suspects, hostages, and civilian bystanders.

TEMS incorporates all levels of medical providers, including law enforcement officers with basic medical training; EMTs, paramedics, or physicians with basic law enforcement training; and dual-trained specialists with backgrounds in law enforcement and medical care. The inclusion of law enforcement duties by the TEMS providers should be limited as much as possible, regardless of the amount of training and experience the provider has. This allows the medical officers the ability to focus on medical duties, reduces the risk of role confusion, and decreases their risk of injury.

TEMS is not military medicine, although it does incorporate many of the rescue and treatment methods and the equipment used in modern military medicine. The resources available, types of wounds incurred, locations of operations, and mission objectives create for the TEMS provider a different environment than that of military medicine, requiring a unique approach to medical care.

HISTORICAL PERSPECTIVE

Since the earliest forms of organized warfare, armed forces have faced the challenge of transporting sick and injured combatants. The first methods were as simple as a strip of cloth attached to two poles, carried by other soldiers or livestock, such as camels and mules.[3] The first recorded use of an ambulance was in 1487 during the Siege of Malaga. At this time, carts were used solely to transport wounded soldiers from the battlefield; no medical aid was rendered. Typically, transportation would not occur until after the battle was over, which meant leaving injured soldiers on the battlefield for hours or days. In the late 1700s, Napoleon Bonaparte appointed Dominique-Jean Larrey to develop a medical patient care system for the French army. Realizing that leaving the wounded soldiers on the field for days at a time increased suffering and mortality, Larrey developed a system in which trained medical personnel entered the battlefield to provide early access to medical care. One of Larrey's important innovations was the design of the *ambulance volante*, or flying ambulance, a carriage staffed with medical personnel.[3,4]

During the U.S. Civil War, Dr. Jonathan Letterman further refined the concept of the field ambulance based on the principles set forth by Larrey. Letterman designed special horse-drawn ambulance trains to transport patients from the battlefield to nearby hospitals. Also during the Civil War, Clara Barton recognized that giving medical aid to wounded soldiers on the battlefield as well as during transport improved their survival rate, and she made it a policy to "treat them where they lie." Based on resulting improvements in wartime survival rate because of rapid access to medical care, the first civilian ambulance service in the United States was created in Cincinnati in 1865, instituting the public EMS system as we know it.[3]

A pivotal moment in the creation of TEMS occurred on August 1, 1966 at the University of Texas in Austin when one man, Charles Whitman, climbed the campus clock tower and proceeded to shoot and kill 15 people and wound 31 others.[4] This incident, and the broader civil unrest of the times, prompted law enforcement agencies to create specialized teams to deal with high-risk situations.

As these teams proliferated and their roles became more defined, it became evident that close association with medical support staff with training in law enforcement tactics would enhance law enforcement missions.[4,5]

By the 1980s, many specialized tactical teams were either training their own officers to render basic aid as designated medics or training medics in special tactics and law enforcement. In 1989 and 1990, two successive national conferences brought together experience and expertise of personnel from more than 40 tactical agencies across 10 states with representatives from EMS and emergency medicine with the goal of advancing tactical medicine.[6,7] These conferences allowed for a collaborative effort toward defining goals and specifying minimum guidelines for medical support for tactical operations.

In 1990 the Casualty Care Research Center developed a national database to catalog the injuries sustained by law enforcement officers and civilians for the purpose of training officers and medical support personnel. In that same year, a collaborative effort between the Department of Defense, Department of the Interior, U.S. Park Police, Uniformed Services University, and Casualty Care Research Center led to the development of the Counter Narcotics & Terrorism Operational Medical Support (CONTOMS) course to provide the first comprehensive TEMS curriculum. Additional medical and professional support for TEMS began in 1993 when the California Chapter of the American College of Emergency Physicians organized the Subcommittee on Tactical Emergency Medicine to promote the availability of emergency physicians to tactical teams throughout California, with the eventual goal of expanding to the national level. Also during this year, the National Tactical Officers Association published a position paper supporting the idea of specialized medical support for tactical operations.[8] In 1999, the National Association of EMS Physicians formed a task force to look at issues surrounding TEMS, and in 2001 it published another supportive position paper. More recently, the American College of Emergency Physicians added a Tactical Emergency Medicine section to further promote the subspecialty and serve as a resource for physicians interested in TEMS. In addition, discussion boards, web sites, and organizations for every level of provider have been developed and are available.

CURRENT PRACTICE

A number of models of emergency medical support for tactical units are currently in use (Table 45-1).[9,10] One common version is the "tactical 911" model, in which EMS is informed that an operation has been planned and is advised to have a unit on stand-by, either at the scene or nearby.[11] Another model involves designating an officer from the tactical unit as the medical officer. One model rapidly increasing in popularity is the "tactically trained medic," with several variations available.

The tactical 911 model consumes the fewest resources and delivers trained medical personnel with a broad range of experience. Potential drawbacks include longer response times, the prospect of medical personnel that have little to no tactical training and are unable to enter the hot zone until the threat is secured, and the possibility of tying up a unit that otherwise could be serving the public. If the unit is pre-staged, the location is often chosen by the commanding officer and is likely to be far from where injuries are expected to occur. This scenario often means a site chosen without regard to the most strategic location for patient access or access to the best evacuation routes. Units are usually not called in for medical care until the scene has been secured.

Some tactical units train a law enforcement officer to provide medical care. This officer usually receives at least basic life support training and sometimes more advanced training such as paramedic or EMT-T training. Although this provides more expeditious access to medical care, the level of training and medical experience is often not as sophisticated as in other models. Another concern with this approach is role confusion (i.e., law enforcement officer versus medical provider). A med-

TABLE 45-1. TACTICAL MEDICAL SUPPORT OPTIONS

	PROS	CONS
Tactical 911	Most economical	Variable levels of experience
	Consumes fewest resources	Unable to enter until threat is secured
	No operational security concerns	
		Takes unit out of service for public
		Staging location concerns
		No medical threat assessment
Law Enforcement Officer with Medical Training	Rapid access to medical care	Variable levels of training and experience
	Access to medical care in the hot zone	
		Possibility of role confusion
	Familiarity with operational tactics	Less familiarity with local medical resources
	Medic provides own security	
	No operational security issues	
Tactically Trained Medic	Rapid access to care	Consumes more resources
	Access to medical care in the hot zone	Potentially not a sworn officer (weapon and arrest concerns)
	More experienced medical support	Operational security issues
	Familiarity with operational tactics	
	Medical threat assessment	

ical officer performing law enforcement duties has an increased risk of direct injury during a mission, potentially jeopardizing medical care for the rest of the team.

A tactically trained medic is a medical provider such as a physician or EMT/paramedic who has received some training in operational tactics and trains directly with the unit.[5,9,11] This allows the medic to operate as an integrated member of the tactical team, with an awareness of the unit's objectives and tactics. It is also important to make clear that the medic's role is primarily medical support and does not include law enforcement duties. The disadvantages associated with this method include liability issues and an increased concern for operational security, especially if the medic is not a sworn officer. This option is also more costly in terms of physical resources and personnel. Variations on this system include on-scene physician medical direction and varying levels of direct medical support in the hot zone. In addition, the medical support provided may be individual (from a single or small group of physicians and EMTs) or agency to agency (integration with the entire EMS system, hospital system, military bases, etc.).

The goal of a medical provider on a tactical team is to keep the team operating at peak performance and to increase the probability of mission success. This includes monitoring the general health of the officers; preplanning operations; monitoring safety measures; and providing medical care during training exercises, the mission, and afterward.

The medical support provided to tactical teams begins well before the start of an operation. Some of the preventive medicine administered by a medical officer may include ensuring that all members are physically capable of performing their duties, checking that necessary vaccinations are up to date, and confirming that thorough medical and psychological assessments have been completed.[1] Depending on the level of the provider, they can either perform these assessments themselves or refer the officers to their primary physicians. Duties may also include training officers in basic first-aid skills.

Training activities account for 24% of all missions that produce casualties.[12] Fortunately, these tend to be less severe than injuries sustained during operations. Medical providers are responsible for the care of these injuries as well as the prevention of injury and illness during training missions, including heat stroke, hypothermia, and hazardous chemical exposure. It is important to plan for necessities such as hydration and nutrition, especially during prolonged training exercises.

Operation preplanning is a crucial duty that greatly affects the safety of the officers and the success of the mission. This involves conducting a complete Medical Threat Assessment (MTA) and examining environmental factors such as weather, terrain, flora and fauna, and potential weapons and hazardous materials, such as those found in drug-manufacturing labs.[13-15] At this point, ailments such as frostbite, heat illness, and dehydration, which may impair the success of the operation, can be foreseen and prevented. The TEMS provider may also play a role in equipment selection based on factors such as duration of the mission, environmental conditions, and

potential presence of hazardous chemicals.[16] During preplanning, it is also important to plan evacuation routes and rendezvous points, anticipate the most appropriate definitive care sites, and calculate the optimal number of ambulances to have on standby.[17] When considering scenarios in which air-evacuation may become necessary, determinations must be made regarding available aircraft, the coordinates of proposed landing zones, and nearby trauma centers with landing zones. Training officers in basic first-aid may also be beneficial. Some agencies issue all members a basic first-aid kit that includes bandages and tourniquets, which may prevent life-threatening exsanguination. Officers must be trained in the use of these devices on themselves and on other team members. Communication methods must be outlined, especially in cases involving potential periods of radio silence. The TEMS providers must also serve as advisors to the tactical commander, which means that recommendations should be offered but the tactical commander will make the final decisions regarding the medical logistics of an operation.

The team's medical equipment should be tailored to its specific needs, depending on factors such as team size, operational environment, mission objectives, and the training of the medical personnel. Factors such as noise and light discipline must also be considered, since bright lights or loud equipment can jeopardize a covert operation. Plans for managing an airway or placing an IV in low- or no-light situations must be considered prior to mission deployment. Portability is another important factor in equipment selection. For example, an extended operation with little opportunity for replenishment of supplies would likely require different equipment than one dealing with a barricaded suspect in a rural area. In any case, a basic kit would include bandaging supplies, gloves, tourniquets, airway supplies (possibly including surgical airway adjuncts), splints, IV kits, fluids, and medications. Those serving with K9 units will also want to keep a kit specifically for their dogs, including special airway equipment, bandages, a muzzle, and gloves.[18] Extended operations will probably require supplies such as food, water, personal medications, and shelter, depending on the environment. Other potentially important elements include planning a rotation of personnel to allow for rest as well as determining the availability of other outside resources that may help the team maintain operational efficiency.

Medical care during the operation is divided into three stages: care under fire, tactical field care, and combat casualty evacuation care. These can also be thought of as care in the hot zone, warm zone, and cold zone, respectively. Traditional EMS teaching begins with scene safety. TEMS also incorporates scene safety, but with a slightly different emphasis. TEMS providers learn how to operate safely in a dangerous environment. Although the environment in which a TEMS provider operates is not always "safe," certain precautions can be taken to minimize risk. A major principle in TEMS is to provide only the necessary care while still in the hot zone before moving to the warm zone, and then to the cold zone. Determining the amount of care needed in the hot zone is often done with remote assessment methodology.

The patient is assessed without direct physical contact, such as the use of binoculars or some other communication system. This allows the medical team to determine the best approach to the patient and to plan strategies for intervention and evacuation before entering the hot zone. The best method of evacuation is self-extraction. When this is not feasible, the team must approach the patient and perform a rapid extraction (Fig. 45-1).

The amount of care provided prior to moving the patient depends on the severity of the injury, the degree of threat, and the transit risk (Fig. 45-2). The transit risk is comprised of three components. The first is the duration of transit. If the transit time will only be a few seconds, most treatments can be delayed until the patient has been moved to a more secure area. The second component is the route of travel. If the evacuation route crosses through the hot zone, it may be safer to stay in one place and begin providing care. The third component of transit risk is the ability to deliver care during transit. This becomes more of an issue the longer the transit time. If care will not be performed during transit, it may be beneficial to perform more care prior to transport to stabilize the patient. As a general rule, only the most critical interventions should be performed in the hot zone. Once in the warm zone, a rapid primary survey may be conducted to identify any immediately life-threatening injuries.[19] This survey would include c-spine precautions, hemorrhage control, airway management, cardiopulmonary resuscitation, initiation of fluid resuscitation, and possibly administration of emergency medications such as analgesics. Consideration may also be given to splinting fractures and dressing wounds depending on the threat level. Attention must then be turned to moving the patient to the cold zone and finally to an appropriate definitive care site. Often there is no strict delineation between hot, warm, and cold zones. In a dynamic environment, such as that of a tactical operation, continuous reassessment of the risk-benefit ratio between medical treatment and extraction must be undertaken.[20]

Care for the team may also involve caring for injured K9 officers.[18] Treatments such as bandaging may help prolong the life of the dog until it can get definitive medical care at a veterinary hospital. Other treatments such as intubation, thoracostomy tubes, and CPR may also be useful, but this may expend valuable resources. A dog with trauma leading to cardiac and/or respiratory arrest is unlikely to survive, even with aggressive field care.

Medical aid for suspects must be performed with caution. They must be searched and any weapons found on their person must be safely disarmed and secured. It is also critical to keep in mind contingencies such as booby traps or other suspects hiding nearby. The most commonly reported type of injury sustained by suspects is gunshot wounds, followed by contusions and abrasions. Other possible types of suspect injuries include blunt injuries from less-lethal weapons such as bean bags and rubber pellets, flash-bangs, as well as the effects of chemical munitions. Flash-bangs have been reported to start fires and cause severe injuries, and even death, to suspects. Lacerations, sprains, and strains are also common injuries seen during the course of an operation.[12]

It may become necessary to treat civilian bystanders or hostages. Injury patterns for civilian bystanders are similar to those for suspects, with ballistic wounds being the most common injury.[12] Syncope from emotional stress may also be seen, but causes such as hypoglycemia or other preexisting medical conditions must be considered. Hostage care may be necessary and could include anything from blunt and penetrating trauma to psychological trauma or injury caused by the rescuing team as seen in Russia in October 2002. During this raid, a sedative gas was used to subdue the captors, but inadvertently killed over 100 hostages and hospitalized hundreds more.

The preservation of forensic evidence is of great importance during tactical operations.[21] Evidence may play a critical role in subsequent legal proceedings and

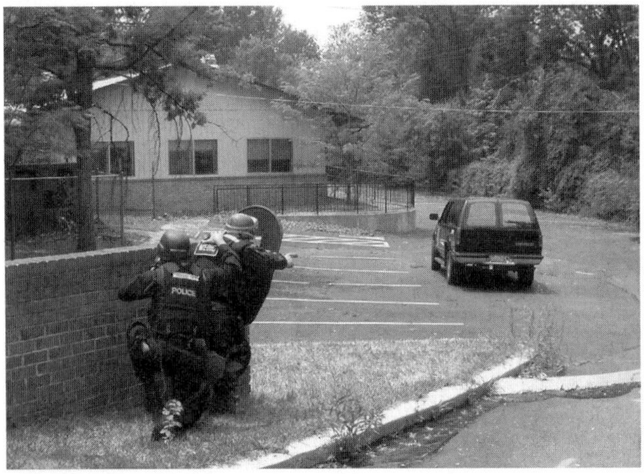

FIGURE 45–1. Medic team advancing on a vehicle. A medic trained in operational tactics can provide medical support in a hostile environment.

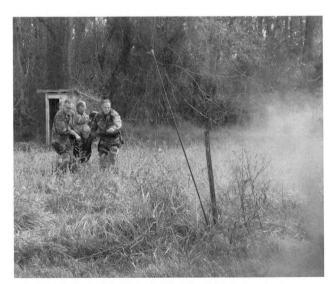

FIGURE 45–2. Simulated wounded officer rescue. Tactical members rescue a wounded officer during a training exercise.

so must be handled properly to avoid altering crucial information or making it inadmissible in court. TEMS providers must have knowledge of what items constitute evidence and how to simultaneously perform their duties and secure evidence without disturbing it. Some examples include how to avoid bullet holes when cutting off clothing and how to handle weapons to avoid disturbing fingerprints.

Barricaded suspects and injured hostages present a unique challenge to the TEMS provider.[22] "Medicine across the barricade" involves communicating with barricaded suspects or hostages to determine what injuries have occurred, the severity of the injuries, and what treatments can be applied. This is the subject of more detailed discussion in another chapter.

After the conclusion of an operation, the TEMS provider may be needed to clear the suspect for incarceration.[23] Providing a screening examination and treatment on-scene may prevent the suspect from requiring transport to an emergency department and the associated risks involved. The purpose of the screening examination is not to identify all medical problems, but to identify any life-threatening emergency conditions likely to require treatment. Although acute trauma certainly needs to be evaluated, other conditions such as bronchospasm from CS (tear gas) exposure and chest pain need to be assessed and treated. For serious injuries, transport may be required. The TEMS provider must have intimate knowledge of local regulations and policies for clearing a suspect in the field and must also be aware of the medical facilities available at the detention facility. If there are ever any questions, the provider should always err on the side of patient safety.[23]

PITFALLS

Several issues surround the provision of medical support in hostile environments. One issue is the law enforcement status of the medical provider. TEMS providers may have the need for self protection and are sometimes armed during an operation. There are many legal and statutory implications involved with carrying and using a firearm in a tactical situation.[24] A provider may be open to civil liability should a weapon discharge and injure or kill a suspect or bystander during an operation. Further, the provider may not have recourse to the same protections as a sworn law enforcement officer. This may be resolved by having the TEMS provider become a reserve officer or deputy sheriff's officer, or, more commonly, by having them remain unarmed but with an escort.

A similar issue involves the power of arrest and whether or not a TEMS provider can detain a suspect. These issues must be addressed on a team-by-team basis prior to initiating an operation.

Medical liability is another issue that surrounds TEMS.[24] Although full-time municipal medics may be covered under their agency's policy, provided they follow established protocols, this must be confirmed in writing and they must still act in accordance with the protocols of their department. All of this should occur under the medical direction of a physician. Physicians who participate in operations should protect themselves with liability insurance, which may or may not be included in their hospital policy. Insurance status and the details of coverage should be documented in writing prior to providing any care in this environment.

REFERENCES

1. Heck JJ, Pierluisi G. Law enforcement special operations medical support. *Prehospital Emerg Care.* 2001;5(4):403-6.
2. Heck JJ, Kepp JJ, Walos G, Vayer J. *CONTOMS Emergency Medical Technician—Tactical Provider Program Student Manual.* Bethesda; Casualty Care Research Center.
3. Blackwell T. Principles of Emergency Medical Services Systems. In Rosen P, Barkin R, eds. *Emergency Medicine Concepts and Clinical Practice.* St. Louis: Mosby; 2002, 2616-2625.
4. Heiskell LE, Carmona RH. Tactical emergency medical services: an emerging subspecialty of emergency medicine. *Ann Emerg Med.* 1994;23:778-85.
5. McArdle DQ, Rasumoff D, Kolman J. Integration of emergency medical services and special weapons and tactics (SWAT) teams: the emergence of the tactically trained medic. *Prehosp Disast Med.* 1992;7:285-8.
6. Rasumoff D. EMS at tactical law enforcement operations seminar a success. *Tactical Edge.* Fall 1989;25-9.
7. Carmona R, Brennan K. Tactical emergency medical support conference a successful joint effort. *Tactical Edge.* Summer 1990;7-11.
8. National Tactical Officers Association. Position statement on the inclusion of physicians in tactical law enforcement operations in the USA. *Tactical Edge.* Spring 1994;86.
9. Lavery RF, Addis MD, Doran JV, et al. Taking care of the "good guys:" a trauma center-based model of medical support for tactical law enforcement. *J Trauma.* 2000;48:125-9.
10. Sharma N. Vancouver police deploy SWAT-Tactical EMS. *Tactical Edge.* Spring 2000;35-38.
11. Jones JS, Reese K, Greg K, et al. Into the fray: integration of emergency medical services and special weapons and tactics (SWAT) teams. *Prehosp Disast Med.* 1996;11:202-6.
12. Casualty Care Research Center. Injury Data Collection Project. Available at: http://www.casualtycareresearchcenter.org/data_injury_page.htm.
13. Carmona R. Inside the perimeter: TEMS and emerging WMD threats. *Tactical Edge.* Fall 2000;70-2.
14. Heck JJ, Byers D. Chemical and biological agents: implications for TEMS. *Tactical Edge.* Winter 2000;52-5.
15. Heiskell LE, Tang D. Medical aspects of clandestine drug labs. *Tactical Edge.* Summer 1994;51-4.
16. Rasumoff D, Carmona R. Inside the perimeter: understanding the risks and benefits in selection of mission-specific personnel protective equipment. *Tactical Edge.* Winter 1993;68-70.
17. McCarthy PM. MEDEVAC operations: a tactical consideration. *Tactical Edge.* Winter 2001;20-2.
18. McDevitt I. *Tactical Medicine: An Introduction to Law Enforcement Emergency Care.* Boulder, CO: Paladin Press; 2001.
19. McCarthy PM. Rapid medical assessment. *Tactical Edge.* Winter 2000;52-5.
20. Rinnert KJ, Hall WL. Tactical Emergency Medical Support. *Emerg Med Clin North Am.* 2002;20(4):929-52.
21. Rasumoff D, Carmona R. Inside the perimeter: forensic aspects of tactical emergency medical support. *Tactical Edge.* Summer 1992;54-5.
22. Greenstone JL. The role of tactical emergency medical support in hostage and crisis negotiations. *Tactical Edge.* Winter 2002;33-5.
23. De Lorenzo RA, Porter RS. *Tactical Emergency Care: Military and Operational Out-of-Hospital Medicine.* Upper Saddle River, NJ: Prentice-Hall; 1999.
24. Greenberg MJ, Wipfler EJ. Administrative considerations for tactical emergency medicine support. *Tactical Edge.* Fall 2000;64-8.

Infectious Disease in a Disaster Zone

Richard A. Tempel and David E. Marcozzi

Recent literature and media have raised the possibility of infectious diseases being used as weapons of mass destruction. Although bioterrorism certainly merits discussion, such as the anthrax incident of October 2001, there have been very few documented cases of such occurrences. This chapter focuses on postdisaster infection. The lack of clean drinking water, proper waste disposal, and the inability to receive prompt medical care all contribute to postdisaster morbidity and mortality. The worst of these scenarios tend to play out in Third-World countries, where densely populated regions are already barely sustaining their people. Programs such as the International Red Cross and Doctors Without Borders often place physicians in these impoverished regions. Identifying, controlling, and treating an epidemic in the setting of a natural or manmade disaster has challenged the knowledge and ingenuity of many physicians and will continue to do so in the future. The goal of this chapter is to provide a framework to assist physicians in the diagnosis and control of infectious disease in a disaster area and to explain where additional resources can be found.

The term *disaster zone* can be applied to a multitude of situations. Some examples of natural and manmade disasters include war, overcrowded refugee camps, industrial accidents, and bioterrorism. With increasing globalization and millions of international travelers and goods, we must also be aware that the victims of a disaster may turn up in emergency departments hundreds of miles from their original site.

The World Health Organization has defined a disaster as *a sudden ecological phenomenon of a sufficient magnitude to require external assistance.*[1] There are no specifics given pertaining to damages or fatalities. This is due to the fact that certain countries have disaster management plans established and may be able to contain an epidemic that may run rampant elsewhere in the world. The capability of a health system to tackle such situations can be defined by its *vulnerability*, which reflects the level of exposure to risk, shock, and stress.[2] A system may be more vulnerable due to poverty, gender, age, ethnicity, comorbid conditions such as HIV/AIDS, or religious identity. Exposure to warfare, destruction of property, and direct attempts to undermine care to the afflicted may also make a system less functional. The ability to handle such factors may be referred to as *resilience*, or the ability to recover from adversity.[3] Resilience can be increased, and vulnerability lessened, with proper planning and well-designed external support.

Recent estimates suggest that 65% of all infectious disease epidemics occur in countries deemed unstable.[4] Forums established by the World Health Organization have noted that only 10% of global spending on health research is devoted to health conditions accounting for 90% of the global disease burden (the 10/90 gap), and that by 2020 the contribution of war and disasters to the global disease burden should increase from 12th to 8th.[5] These numbers are troubling, especially when considering the rankings are based only on immediate morbidity and mortality, and not the long-term, indirect effects of disasters. The upheaval of health systems, access to quality food and sanitation, and economic decline undoubtedly heavily contribute to the total number of deaths due to infection and malnutrition.

HISTORICAL PERSPECTIVE

Historical literature abounds with examples of both war and natural disasters resulting in widespread infection and mortality, directly influencing the direction of human civilization. Although such catastrophes may have been simply part of life in the preindustrialized world, the implementation of sanitation and modern medicine provides the tools to prevent such epidemics today. Nevertheless, hundreds of thousands still die in Third-World countries annually due to the lack of preparation and inability to provide needed resources during and after major disasters.

In 31 BC, while preparing for his invasion of Italy, Marc Antony stationed his army estimated at 30,000 men on the hills above the marsh-bound city of Actium, Greece. Octavian, his rival, quickly encircled the city and camp on both land and sea, preventing supply wagons from entering, and even diverting the city's only supply of freshwater. Such tactics sent the soldiers and the people of Actium into the mosquito-infested swamps to find nourishment. Within 30 days, Antony had lost more than one-third of his army to disease and malnutrition, and Octavian soon became Augustus Caesar. Until the end of the civil war, commanders expected to lose more soldiers from disease than from combat. The first military force to apply successfully all the technology of bacteriology, vector control, immunization, modern surgery, and echeloned care was the Japanese army in 1904-1905 during the Russo-Japanese War. It was the first army to suffer more deaths from enemy action than from disease.

In the sixth century of the Common Era, Hindu doctor Susrata suspected malaria epidemics to be related to seasonal mosquito infestations.[6] The bark of the Peruvian quina-quina tree has been used for the treatment and prevention of malaria since at least the seventeenth century. However, it was not until 1897 that Sir Ronald Ross, using a microscope, deduced that the *Anopheles* mosquito was the vector for transmitting the *Plasmodium* parasite to its human host. This discovery, along with new methods to control the mosquito population, assisted in the expansion of the British Empire throughout the tropics.

Identifying the route of transmission for yellow fever has led to control measures in most developed countries. After the 1793 outbreak of yellow fever in Philadelphia, several physicians attributed its origin to be putrid coffee discharged by a shipping vessel.[7] Construction of the Panama Canal started in 1880 by a French company and failed after 52,816 of its 86,800 men contracted yellow fever, and 5627 of these later died. In 1900, Maryland bacteriologists James Carrol and Jesse Lazear managed to prove an *Aedes* mosquito to be the vector for yellow fever, not by the microscope like Ross, but by inoculating themselves (Lazear later died of the infection). Directed by Major Walter Reed and General William Gorgas, this discovery led to the utter annihilation of mosquito populations (and forest) surrounding the canal. The Panama Canal opened in 1914, and the death rate surrounding the canal was half that of the United States at the time.[6]

In Angola, a 27-year civil war often applying "scorched-earth" strategies ended in a cease-fire on April 4, 2002. A large survey was conducted to evaluate mortality from June 2001 through August 2002 in parts of the region among displaced families.[8] Estimates of crude mortality before the cease-fire reached 10 times that of other developing countries and up to 4 times greater among postwar, displaced populations, in part due to poorly funded United Nations assistance. Both before and after the cease-fire, malaria and other febrile illnesses remained the second leading cause of mortality in the study population. Also, a 23% mortality rate for infants was documented during this period. Examples such as this are evidence of the havoc that disaster can still inflict on humanity and the importance of the developed world to assist in times of need.

Children are often the most vulnerable immediately after a disaster. In developing regions, children are often fully dependent on their care-takers for both food and safety. Even those children who may appear well during a crisis period may fall prey to malnutrition and infection postdisaster, as evidenced by the survey in Bangladesh following its worst flood of the century in 1998.[9] Such fragility requires serial evaluations of populations during and after a disaster so that those initially well may still have access to care if needed.

A recent epidemiologic study by the Japan Disaster Relief Medical Team in Mozambique noted the incidence of malaria increasing four to five times directly after a flood disaster in 2000.[10] Water analyses noted an immediate deterioration in the quality of drinking water. This, combined with an increase in population density and food shortages, no doubt contributed to the 85% infectious disease rate among the patients receiving medical care. Notably, there was a lack of cholera or dysentery infection, which had previously been linked to similar disasters in the region.

In August 1999, the Kocaeli Province of Turkey was struck with a devastating earthquake.[11] An infectious disease surveillance system collected 1468 stool cultures over a 33-day period. The analysis revealed a multifocal, multiclonal increase in diarrheal disease, in particular, distinct *Shigella* serotypes and clones. The reasons why only this infectious agent showed such expansion is unknown, but it demonstrates the need for monitoring systems to better recognize infectious diseases after disasters and to initiate proper treatment.

In 1992, the Cerro Negro volcano erupted near the city of Leon, Nicaragua, and the health effects upon the 300,000 residents were assessed using routine data by the national epidemiologic surveillance system.[12] Healthcare visits for both respiratory and acute diarrheal illnesses increased up to six times when compared with pre-eruption data. Most of these visits were for children younger than 5 years old. Such results indicate the need to assess both air and water quality before and after an eruption and to provide data to better target at-risk persons. This type of data and response development would not be possible without Nicaragua's national epidemiologic surveillance system.

On October 26, 1998, Hurricane Mitch became, at that time, the Atlantic's fourth strongest hurricane ever and wreaked havoc in Central America, resulting in over 10,000 deaths by November 2. International and local medical teams responded, reviewing files from the region of Villanueva, Nicaragua, during a 3-month relief operation.[13] The 30-day postdisaster incidence of acute diarrhea, respiratory tract infections, and malaria was estimated and compared with non-crisis data. The incidence of acute diarrhea doubled, and acute respiratory tract infection was four times more frequent. However, there appeared no significant changes in the incidence of malaria.

Although diseases such as malaria may become more frequent in disaster regions where resistance is already high, exposure to new diseases in more vulnerable populations is also of concern. In 1997 a severe, prolonged drought struck the Australasian region of Indonesia. During this time, more than 550 deaths due to "drought-related" disease occurred in the central highland district.[14] Irian Jaya is home to both coastal lowland and shifting highland populations. The highland populations are known to have a low level of naturally acquired immunity to *Plasmodium falciparum*. On further study, microscopic evidence implicated malaria as the principal cause of death. A retrospective investigation revealed that increased standing water and food shortages resulted in a substantial demographic movement, thus exposing the highland population to malaria. In

October 1997, the rapid evaporation of stream beds and mass antimalarial drug distribution resulted in a precipitous decline in mortality. Examples such as these indicate the risks of population shifts associated with disasters and the need for continued health resource access.

CURRENT PRACTICE

The identification, treatment, and prevention of infectious disease has come a long way since Dr. Lazear's death from inoculating himself with yellow fever in 1900. Robert Koch identified *Bacillus anthracis* over 125 years ago, and Louis Pasteur developed an anthrax vaccine shortly thereafter.[6] Nonetheless, October 2001 found the U.S. Postal Service in a crisis due to the spread of anthrax spores in the mail. Although it resulted in only 22 diagnosed cases (11 inhalation and 11 cutaneous) and only 5 deaths, the outbreak sent shockwaves through the American population. Such an event occurring in an industrialized country with a highly advanced medical system revealed our vulnerability to such incidents and sparked a revolution in infectious disease preparation, for both disaster and nondisaster areas.

The Centers for Disease Control and Prevention (CDC) serve as the lead agency in the United States for disease surveillance and have founded several global initiatives to battle infectious diseases.[15] The CDC represents the lead federal agency for bioterrorism and epidemic response. Globalization has led to foreign diseases arriving on American soil, such as the 1999 outbreak of dengue fever in Texas, where 56 people were afflicted. The CDC has determined that it is far more effective to assist in the control and prevention of infectious disease outside of the country rather than to only attempt to prevent the importation. It would be impossible to examine all persons and goods entering the United States, and those who are asymptomatic would likely still be missed.

Several departments within the CDC work together to quickly assess an outbreak once identified and assistance is requested. The Health Alert Network was established to provide Internet and other forms of communication for local agencies to get advice and assistance from the CDC in an expedient fashion. A rapid response team is sent to investigate, confirm the presence of infectious disease, and assist in the control of the outbreak.[16] The Laboratory Response Network provides laboratory testing, identifying the cause and determining effective treatment protocols. In 2001, the National Electronic Disease Surveillance System (NEDSS) was initiated for entering, updating, and electronically transmitting demographic disease data.[17] This will allow rapid reporting of disease trends to control outbreaks and to monitor for bioterrorist attacks.

Although the location of the next infectious disease outbreak or bioterrorist attack cannot be predicted, a well-prepared disaster plan should be able to provide large quantities of medical supplies in an expedient fashion. The Strategic National Stockpile (SNS) program provides this resource for the entire country.[18] It is a repository of antibiotics, antidotes, antitoxins, life support medications, and other medical/surgical supplies that may supplement and supply state and local health agencies in the event of an infectious disease outbreak. The SNS may be deployed once the affected state has requested assistance from the CDC. Initial deployment consists of "push packages," which are caches of pharmaceuticals, antidotes, and medical supplies designed to address a variety of agents and ready for delivery anywhere in the continental United States within 12 hours. Although not a first-response tool, the National Pharmaceutical Stockpile (NPS) will help augment state and local agency supplies. If additional resources are needed, follow-up vendor-managed inventory supplies can be provided within 24 to 36 hours and can be tailored to the specific needs of the state.

The CDC also works by invitation outside the United States. During a civil war and famine in southern Sudan, a hemorrhagic fever had affected 20,000 people and resulted in 2000 deaths.[15] The CDC assisted the World Health Organization (WHO) in identifying the causative spirochete and implemented measures for disease control. In 2000, the CDC joined a WHO-led investigation of a tularemia outbreak among 500 to 1000 displaced persons returning to damaged homes and farms in rural Kosovo.[15] It became clear that there had been an explosion in the rodent population due to unprotected stocks of food and crops, and the refugees returned home and ingested the contaminated food or water. This epidemic was halted by simple sanitation measures.

Several global health initiatives have recently been initiated by the CDC, including the following:

- Roll Back Malaria: Designed to reduce deaths from malaria by increasing access to prompt and effective treatment, as well as protective intermittent therapy for pregnant women, barrier prevention techniques, rapid response to outbreaks, and new products for prevention and treatment.
- Stop TB: Includes several objectives including the implementation of the directly observed therapy short-course strategy.
- International Partnership Against AIDS in Africa: A Joint United Nations Programme on HIV/AIDS–led effort assisted by the Leadership and Investment in Fighting an Epidemic initiative, providing support to countries hit heaviest by HIV/AIDS.
- Global Alliance for Vaccines and Immunization: Program to strengthen childhood immunization programs in foreign countries.

In addition to the CDC, the WHO provides immediate care anywhere in the world where disaster and infectious disease have overrun the local resources of a country. As an operational organization of the United Nations, the WHO acts as the directing and coordinating authority on all international health activity.[19] On December 26, 2003, a devastating earthquake shook the city of Bam in Iran, killing as many as 30,000 people. With most hospital and health centers destroyed, and approximately 80% of all buildings damaged, local and neighboring health facilities were overwhelmed with the needs of the 100,000 residents of the Bam area. The WHO completed a rapid health assessment on

December 27 and immediately became involved in the provision of food, clothing, sanitation, and medical supplies.[20] Their surveillance systems have also documented all infectious disease and further morbidity and mortality in the area. Weekly assessments available to the public on the WHO Web site allow for identification of potential outbreaks and better allocation of resources to prevent further misery from befalling the people of Bam. Three weeks after the earthquake, there were no new outbreaks of disease and the incidence of diarrhea and other infectious diseases has remained at pre-disaster levels.

In 1859, during the War of Italian Unification, Henry Dunant witnessed the suffering of 9000 wounded troops in the small town of Solfernino, Italy. This experience led him to initiate the groundwork for both the Red Cross and the Geneva Conventions. In 1863, the International Committee of the Red Cross (ICRC) was established. Comprised of both private and public funding, the mission of the ICRC is to "protect the lives and dignity of victims of war and internal violence and to provide them with assistance."[21] National Red Cross societies exist in 178 countries, providing local care and international aid if requested by the ICRC. The concerns of the ICRC often overlap that of the WHO, providing additional support in regions of violent conflict.

In 1971, Doctors Without Borders, or Médecins Sans Frontières (MSF), was established to provide international emergency medical care.[22] Volunteers are sent to the most remote and unstable parts of the world to provide emergency medical care to victims of both man-made and natural disasters. They can provide medical or surgical care, nutrition, sanitation, and local health training quickly and efficiently throughout the world, often working together with the United Nations and the WHO. MSF has been awarded the Nobel Peace Prize for its efforts in emergency medical care.

Local and regional agencies are still required, and essential, as the first responders to a disaster zone. Proper planning and practice have been shown to lead to less confusion and fewer deaths after catastrophic events. Both the NEDSS established by the CDC and the surveillance system in place in Nicaragua provide essential demographic information and the ability to locate disease outbreaks, quickly mobilizing resources for immediate care. The Demographic Surveillance System of the International Centre for Diarrheal Diseases Research, Bangladesh, was used to determine the effectiveness of flood-control embankments in disease prevention in children aged 0 to 4 years.[23] Crude child mortality was reduced by 29% in areas of embankment, but also of importance was the overall 40% reduction in all causes of childhood death due to increased health interventions.

In 1999 the city of Spokane, Washington, experienced a local scare involving anthrax. Deaconess Medical Center, in conjunction with the city, developed a program for obtaining information and antidotes for a variety of biologic agents. Within a year of the incident, a cooperative citywide response to a bioterrorist strike had been implemented. The roles of emergency personnel, hospital physicians, risk-management personnel, and law enforcement have been clearly delineated, and Spokane's local agencies are now more prepared for such an event.[24]

The importance of informing and mobilizing the public cannot be overemphasized. Television, radio, and the Internet can provide vital information from local, state, and federal agencies to large numbers of people in a short amount of time. A recent survey examining the public perception of information sources during a bioterrorist event noted the importance of both local and national spokespersons and periodic updates in maintaining public confidence and security.[25] Faced with a disaster, the local and neighboring populations often provide the most immediate life-saving resources, as evidenced most recently by the overwhelming response to the World Trade Center disaster of September 11, 2001. Blood donations tend to greatly increase during times of crisis, and a study evaluating the safety of blood donations after the 1989 San Francisco earthquake revealed these donations to be as safe as routine donations before the disaster.[26]

The incidence of infectious disease in the disaster settings can be curtailed by implementing local surveillance systems to monitor for outbreaks and encouraging early vaccination as needed. Rapid disaster response strategies that provide survivors with immediate shelter, supplies, and clean drinking water have already contributed to fewer deaths and less suffering in developing countries.

Providing clean water and proper waste disposal are of utmost importance after a natural disaster. Large, displaced populations short on supplies often become fertile ground for diarrheal diseases. It is often difficult to supply remote areas with large tankers of clean water in the midst of violent conflict or natural disaster. Studies have shown simple water sanitation techniques such as heating, agitation, or exposure to sunlight may greatly decrease the incidence of these diseases.[27] A controlled field trial in 1996 showed a 26% decrease in diarrheal disease among Masai children in Kenya using solar radiation alone.[28]

A developed country with proper disaster management strategies in place is likely to be the most resilient when faced with a disaster, both during and immediately after. When a flash flood occurred in the region of Nimes, France, in 1988, 45,000 people had their homes damaged or destroyed, yet only 3 severe injuries and 9 deaths were reported. No new infectious disease epidemics were noted afterward.[29] Results such as this are undoubtedly due to the immediate response of well-trained personnel and distribution of supplies to the victims of the disaster.

In conclusion, infectious diseases in disaster zones have often accounted for greater morbidity and mortality than the disaster itself. Diarrheal and respiratory diseases tend to be the primary culprits, targeting the infirm and the young. Developing countries are often more vulnerable to these afflictions due to the lack of available resources. Both in the United States and abroad, efforts are being made to control unnecessary postdisaster suffering. By installing effective surveillance systems to track infectious disease incidence, and rapid response personnel who are both well-trained and well-equipped, we can improve the resilience of a region. Yet until all human life is considered worth saving, and the 10/90 gap is corrected, it will not be possible to reach this goal. Nevertheless, as evidenced most recently by the WHO response to the earthquake in Iran and the overwhelming response to the 2004 Tsunami in the Indian Ocean, steady progress is being made toward controlling disease in areas where this was once considered an impossibility.

PITFALLS

Although many local and international agencies are available to respond to disasters with strategies to quickly bring personnel and stockpiled supplies, limitations still exist. Remote locations in heavily forested or mountainous regions may lack roads or landing sites from which to deploy large-scale response services. Warring factions often prevent aid from reaching their rivals, or more frequently, the suffering civilians are caught in the cross fire. Some areas may be so dangerous that international agencies will not deploy relief workers, or they may be recalled for fear of injury or death, as seen recently with MSF withdrawal from the Darfur region of Sudan. Specific governments may even refuse help when offered due to political or personal motives.

The fall of the Soviet Union and unmonitored biologic weapons programs in unstable countries may provide terrorists with weapons ranging from anthrax to genetically engineered recombinant microbes. These weapons may be intentionally released anywhere in the world.

In 1975, the Biological and Toxin Weapons Convention was signed by 144 countries, yet it has been shown to be an inadequate control mechanism.[30] Most countries lack the laboratory safety requirements, necessary highly trained personnel, and ability to mass quarantine in the event of a microbial terrorist attack.[31] Although the vaccination of United States emergency personnel to smallpox was deemed a success, it is yet to be determined whether there was an actual need or whether it will be effective should such a catastrophe occur.

Strategies are being devised worldwide, yet at this time few countries are prepared to handle a widespread attack with a contagious pathogen. This correlates to the rarity of these events in recent history because it is difficult to prepare for an event that has only been theorized.

REFERENCES

1. World Health Organization. Emergency Health Training Programme for Africa. Available at: *http://www.who.int/disasters/repo/5506.pdf.*
2. Chambers R. 1989 Vulnerability, coping and policy. IDS Bulletin 20. 1989.
3. Moser CO. The asset vulnerability framework: reassessing urban poverty reduction strategies. *World Dev.* 1998;26(1):1-19.
4. World Health Organization/Communicable Diseases (WHO/CDS). 2000 WHO/CDS/CSR Global outbreak alert and response: report of a WHO meeting. Geneva, Switzerland, April 26-28, 2000:7. Available at: *http://www.who.int/emc-documents/surveillance/docs/whocdscsr2003.pdf.*
5. Griekspoor A, for the Focal Point for Research in Emergencies, Department of Emergency and Humanitarian Action, World Health Organization. The 10/90 gap in health research: assessing the progress: Health effects of conflicts and disasters; where is the evidence? Forum 5 conference of the Global Forum for Health Research, Geneva, Switzerland, October 9-12, 2001. Available at: *http://www.globalforumhealth.org/Non_compliant_pages/Forum5/abstracts/conflictsgriekspoor.html.*
6. Gordon R. *The Alarming History of Medicine.* New York: Richard Gordon, Ltd.; 1993:19-29.
7. Woodward TE. *Research on Infectious Disease at The University of Maryland School of Medicine & Hospital: A Global Experience 1807-2000.* Baltimore: The University of Maryland School of Medicine and the Medical Alumni Association of the University of Maryland, Inc; 1999:7-20.
8. Grein T, et al. Mortality among displaced former UNITA members and their families in Angola: a retrospective cluster study. *BMJ.* 2003 Sep 20;327(7416):650-9.
9. Hossain SM, Kolsteren P. The 1998 flood in Bangladesh: is different targeting needed during emergencies and recovery to tackle malnutrition? *Disasters.* 2003 Jun;27(2):172-84.
10. Kondo H, et al. Post-flood infectious diseases in Mozambique. *Prehospital Disaster Med.* 2002 Jul-Sep;17(3):126-33.
11. Vahaboglu H. Transient increase in diarrheal diseases after the devastating earthquake in Kocaeli, Turkey: results of an infectious disease surveillance study. *Clin Infect Dis.* 2000;31:1386-89.
12. Malilay J, et al. Public health surveillance after a volcanic eruption: lessons from Cerro Negro, Nicaragua, 1992. *Bull Pan Am Health Organ.* 1996 Sep;30(3):218-26.
13. Campanella N. Infectious diseases and natural disasters: the effects of Hurricane Mitch over Villanueva municipal area, Nicaragua. *Public Health Rev.* 1999;27(4):311-9.
14. El Nino and associated outbreaks of severe malaria in highland populations in Irian Jaya, Indonesia: a review and epidemiological perspective. *Southeast Asia J Trop Med Public Health.* 1999 Dec;30(4):608-19.
15. National Center for Infectious Disease. Protecting the Nation's Health in an Era of Globalization: CDC's global infectious disease strategy. 2002:1-9. Available at: *http://www.cdc.gov/globalidplan/4-introduction.htm.*
16. Centers for Disease Control and Prevention. Public health emergency preparedness response, bioterrorism: what has the CDC accomplished? Available at: *http://www.bt.cdc.gov/Documents/BTInitiative.usp.*
17. Centers for Disease Control and Prevention. Programs in brief: research, technology, & data—National Electronic Disease Surveillance System. Available at: *http://www.cdc.gov/programs/research12.html.*
18. Centers for Disease Control and Prevention. The public health response to biological and chemical terrorism: interim planning guidance for state public health officials, appendix II: National Pharmaceutical Stockpile Program, July 2001. Available at: *http://www.bt.cdc.gov/Documents/Planning?PlanningGuidance.pdf.*
19. World Health Organization. Basic texts: Constitution of the World Health Organization. 2004. Available at: *http://policy.who.int/cgi-bin/om_isapi.dll?hitsperheading=on&infobase=basicdoc&record={9D5}&softpage=Document42.*
20. World Health Organization. Rapid health assessment form Iran earthquake, 27 December 2003. Available at: *http://www.who.int/disasters/repo/11635.pdf.*
21. International Committee of the Red Cross. Mission Statement. Available at: *http://www.icrc.org/HOME.NSF/060a34982cae624ec12566fe00326312/125ffe2d4c7f68acc1256ae300394f6e?OpenDocument.*
22. Doctors Without Borders. What is Doctors Without Borders/Médecins Sans Frontières? Available at: *http://www.doctorswithoutborders.org/aboutus/index.cfm.*
23. Myaux JA, et al. Flood control embankments contribute to the improvement of the health status of children in rural Bangladesh. *Bull World Health Organ.* 1997;75(6):533-9.
24. Terriff CM, Tee AM. Citywide pharmaceutical preparation for bioterrorism. *Am J Health Syst Pharm.* 2001 Feb 1;58(3):233-7.
25. Pollard WE. Public perceptions of information sources concerning bioterrorism before and after anthrax attacks: an analysis of national survey data. *J Health Commun.* 2003;8 Suppl 1:93-103; discussion 148-51.
26. Busch MP. Safety of blood donations following a natural disaster. *Transfusion.* 1991;31(8):719-23.
27. McGuigan KG. Solar disinfection of drinking water contained in transparent plastic bottles: characterizing the bacterial inactivation process. *J Appl Microbiol.* 1998;84:1138-1148.

28. Conroy RM, Elmore-Meegan M, Joyce T, McGuigan K, Barnes J. Solar disinfection of drinking water and incidence of diarrhea in Maasai children: a controlled field trial. *Lancet*. 1996;348:1696-97.

29. Duclos P, et al. Flash flood disaster: Nimes, France, 1988. *Eur J Epidemiol*. 1991 Jul;7(4):365-71.

30. Roffey R, Lantorp K, Tegnell A, Elgh F. Biological weapons and bioterrorism preparedness: importance of public-health awareness and international cooperation. *Clin Microbiol Infect*. 2002 Aug;8(8):522-8.

31. Ongradi J. Microbial warfare and bioterrorism [Hungarian]. *Orv Hetil*. 2002 Aug 18;143(33):1935-9.

chapter 47

Pharmaceuticals and Medical Equipment in Disasters

Nicki Pesik and Susan E. Gorman

Disasters can affect a community in many ways, ranging from the destruction of communication and transportation systems, to the loss of personal property, to overwhelming the capacity of medical and health systems. Most natural disasters create a predictable pattern of public health consequences.[1] Emergency health planners can use this knowledge to plan for the needs of a community in terms of resources such as medical and health supplies, communication equipment, and other materials. In addition to natural or technologic disasters, the threat of domestic and international terrorism involving weapons of mass destruction has become an increasing public health concern in the United States and abroad.[2] The medical supplies and equipment used to address events involving weapons of mass destruction often differ from those needed in response to a natural disaster.

Vulnerability assessments and hazard analyses are methods of identifying the hazards and vulnerabilities present and for determining their effect on a community. The vulnerability of a community results from factors that limit its ability to absorb and manage an emergency or disaster.[3-4] Regardless of the disaster, vulnerability assessments should occur continuously throughout the event to determine the ever-changing needs and priorities of the community as the event evolves.[4-5] Particularly in the case of deliberate acts of terrorism, epidemiologic and surveillance information is critical in helping to determine the current and predicted numbers of casualties and to provide emergency planners with critical information regarding the amounts and specific types of medical supplies or equipment required.[6]

Resources are required that most immediately address critical medical needs of the affected victims. Water, food, shelter, and equipment are needed next.[1] Effective resource management requires several basic actions: (1) determining specific resources and the amounts, (2) procuring the resources, (3) preparing an organized and secure area for storage with an inventory tracking system, (4) preparing to receive large amounts of unrequested medical assets, (5) identifying a means to transport and distribute resources where they are needed, (6) identifying locations for dispensing pharmaceuticals or other medical assets, and (7) developing the system for dispensing the medical assets.[7]

Equipment and supplies that are essential to the response capacity of a community can be generally categorized into several areas: direction and control, communications, mass care, and health and medical supplies. Equipment and supplies for health and medical care may be divided into two broad categories. The first category includes the drugs, medical equipment, and supplies that are necessary for direct patient care. This also should include provisions for maintaining primary care services in addition to the medical and health needs created by the disaster. Many patients will seek medical care for chronic conditions because their pharmacies and primary clinics have been destroyed or have become nonoperational.[1] Primary care medicines are often required.[8-9] The second category includes the logistical and occupational health supplies used to support the emergency caregivers and facilities. Some examples include portable shelters, tents, portable water containers, patient stretchers, and personal protective equipment.

Initial steps should be taken during a vulnerability assessment to identify and inventory existing resources, equipment, and supplies that are essential to health and disaster management.[10] Although the federal government may provide a variety of assistance, including medical assets and equipment, it is not expected that this assistance will arrive until 12 to 24 hours after a formal request.[11] International aid often does not arrive for 48 to 72 hours.[1,7] International requests for field hospitals should consider the World Health Organization–Pan American Health Organization (WHO-PAHO) Guidelines for the use of foreign field hospitals. As demonstrated in Bam, Iran, in December 2003 following an earthquake, field hospitals should be operational within the first 24 hours to be useful and should remain on-site for a minimum of 15 days.[12,13]

Determining the quantities of medical supplies and pharmaceuticals needed will depend on several factors, including (but not limited to) the specific threat or disaster, availability of medical assets within the community, extent of disruption of the medical and health systems, number of patients, clinical treatment or prophylaxis protocol, and time to the recovery phase of the disaster response.

Attempts have been made to quantify pharmaceutical stockpiling or evaluate preparedness of emergency departments for an event involving a chemical nerve agent. Resource needs have been estimated for 50 to 500 casualties exposed to chemical agents during one event.[14,15]

HISTORICAL PERSPECTIVE

The Homeland Security Act of 2002 and Homeland Security Presidential Directive (HSPD)-5 required the creation of the National Response Plan (NRP), which will supersede the Federal Response Plan. The NRP outlines and describes the federal resources available to augment or support incident management. The NRP applies to incidents of national significance such as threats or acts of terrorism, major disasters as defined under the Robert T. Stafford Disaster Relief and Emergency Act, and catastrophic incidents defined as those events that result in extraordinary levels of mass casualties, damage, and disruption affecting the population or environment of a community. The NRP will contain a Catastrophic Incident Annex that establishes the coordinated strategy for delivery of applicable federal resources and capabilities that will address mass care, search and rescue, decontamination, medical support, and medical equipment.[16]

In 1998, the Centers for Disease Control and Prevention received funding under an Anti-Bioterrorism Initiative to develop the Strategic National Stockpile (SNS) program to assist states and communities in responding to public health emergencies, including those resulting from terrorist attacks and natural disasters.[6] The SNS program ensures the availability of medicines, antidotes, medical supplies, vaccines, and medical equipment necessary for states and communities to counter the effects of biologic pathogens, chemical nerve agents, radiologic events, and explosive devices. The SNS program is designed to deliver medical assets to the site of a national emergency within 12 hours of a federal decision to deploy medical assets. Medical assets available within the SNS program include antibiotics, chemical nerve agent antidotes, intravenous fluids, intravenous administration supplies, bandages, burn ointments, analgesics, antiemetics, sedatives, antiviral medications, antitoxins, and vaccines.

A 12-hour response time for delivery of chemical nerve agent antidote is not optimal for the initial care of casualties. In addition, many hospitals carry only limited stocks of chemical nerve agent antidotes.[14-17] These antidotes have variable shelf lives, and replacing them is costly and may impact a community's ability to respond. Therefore, the SNS program is currently executing a nationwide forward deployment of chemical nerve agent antidotes under its CHEMPACK project. Through this project, emergency medical services and hospitals will have access to chemical nerve agent antidotes for immediate use during an event.

CURRENT PRACTICE

There are multiple sources for clinical recommendations with regard to the treatment of casualties of events involving biologic, chemical, or radiologic weapons.[18-22] Recommendations regarding personal protective equipment have been hampered by limited regulatory guidance and lack of focused research on personal protective equipment for use in healthcare facilities. However, the current consensus appears to support the use of Level C personal protection (e.g., splash suits, gloves, boots, air-purifying respirators) in most healthcare settings.[23,24] The public health consequences of disasters should also guide emergency planners in assessing the pharmaceutical and medical equipment needs of their communities.[1] Several medical equipment and supply lists exist and can provide examples from which emergency planners may select and begin developing an inventory that is appropriate for their populations and threat analysis.

An international resource is the WHO's *New Emergency Health Kit*.[25] This publication offers a standard list of essential emergency health supplies that are widely accepted internationally. Contents are calculated to meet the needs of 10,000 persons for 3 months. The kit inventory is divided into 10 identical units that would treat 1000 persons, so it is scalable to need. It is designed to meet the needs of a refugee camp and the priorities associated with austere conditions in developing nations.[25] In addition, the WHO has published and developed an essential drug list that identifies those pharmaceuticals that should be available at any given time in appropriate amounts and formulations. The WHO essential drug list has been adopted by numerous international agencies that supply pharmaceuticals within their healthcare programs and is being used to evaluate the appropriateness of drug donations.[26,27]

The SNS program's formulary is directed at biologic, chemical, radiologic, and explosive weapons. Table 47-1 is an overview of the pharmaceuticals used against a variety of agents or events that are contained within the SNS program's formulary. Table 47-1 is not a comprehensive list, but rather, represents categories of medical supplies that can be used to respond to different threats.

A list of medical supplies for healthcare personnel responding to victims of earthquakes has been recommended by emergency medicine faculty at the University of California, Irvine, Medical Center. This list is intended for incorporation into medical backpacks and would be kept with specially trained medical personnel in the trunks of their cars at all times.[28]

Centralized or decentralized stockpiles of medical supplies and equipment may be considered as an option for disaster preparedness. Certain biologic threat agents will require prophylaxis of persons responding to the event. Prepositioned stockpiles can reduce the time to prophylaxis for first responders and provide a sense of security for their welfare. Medical stockpiling may be one option for treatments that must be given within minutes to hours after an event and often much sooner than federal assistance can arrive. Communities with specific technologic risks, such as chemical storage depots or nuclear power plants, may consider the stockpiling of specific antidotes or treatments as part of their disaster plan.

Stockpiling medical assets is an expensive disaster response option.[7] Costs are not only associated with the

TABLE 47-1 PHARMACEUTICALS AND MEDICAL EQUIPMENT IN THE SNS FORMULARY

GENERAL MEDICAL ASSETS	CATEGORY A AGENTS	CHEMICAL NERVE AGENTS	RADIOLOGIC EVENT	CONVENTIONAL WEAPONS
Emergency airway equipment	Ciprofloxacin	Mark 1 Kits	Prussian blue	Suture material
Analgesics	Doxycycline	Atropine	Ca DTPA	Laceration repair kits
Antiemetics	Gentamicin	Pralidoxime	Zn DTPA	Burn ointments
Sedatives	Amoxicillin	Diazepam	Potassium Iodide (KI)	Burn bandages
Intravenous fluids	Rifampin	Pediatric atropine	Cytokine	
Intravenous administration kits	Vaccines	autoinjectors		
Bandages	Antitoxin			
Emergency resuscitation medications				
Ventilators				

initial purchase of pharmaceuticals or equipment, but budgetary considerations must be in place to replace products as they near expiration. Equipment must be maintained and quality assurance provided. Equipment may also need to be replaced as newer models become available. There may be significant logistical costs associated with maintenance, storage, and transportation of the inventory.

Beyond the financial concerns of stockpiling medical supplies and assets, there are multiple logistical and clinical considerations for states, communities, or hospitals to consider. A major component of stockpiling medical assets is determining the storage locations. Pharmaceuticals should be stored in a secure and temperature-controlled environment. An inventory system should be incorporated into any stockpiling program that allows for up-to-date access on available products, notice of impending expiration of product, controlled access to restricted pharmaceuticals such as narcotics, and tracking of distributed products or assets. A centralized storage system of medical assets must be combined with an efficient and secure distribution system. Medical assets should be considered that have longer expiration dates and require no specialized storage needs or ancillary supplies.

Clinical considerations include assessing products for duplicity of use. Products that can be used to respond to multiple agents or events can reduce the number of pharmaceuticals purchased. For example, doxycycline has a Food and Drug Administration (FDA)-approved indication to treat multiple biologic agents including, anthrax, tularemia, and plague. Decisions regarding the formulations of products should consider special populations such as antibiotic suspensions for children or those persons who cannot swallow pills. Appropriate sizes of medical equipment for children should be considered.[15,29] Planners should also recognize that the use of certain medical equipment, such as personal protective equipment, may pose a risk to their healthcare workers. Appropriate training for the use of all stockpiled equipment should be considered.[23] Medical personnel in charge of stockpiles used to address biologic, chemical, or radiologic agents will need to regularly review their formularies for inclusion of improved vaccines, newer treatment modalities, and changes to a drug's approval status by the FDA.

PITFALLS

Problems in disaster resource management can result from insufficient information or assessment of a community's health and other needs. There are countless examples of useless medical supplies and consumables sent to a disaster site, such as drugs labeled in a foreign language, expired drugs, or drugs not commonly used in a particular country.[7,30-33] Most unsolicited medical supplies arrive unsorted, unlabeled, mislabeled, or not intended for emergency use. Time and effort must be expended to determine which resources are needed and which must be discarded. During the 1988 earthquake in Armenia, the donation of tons of pharmaceuticals and other medical supplies overwhelmed the local capacity to store and inventory the donations. At least 50% of medical assets donated to Bosnia and Herzegovina between 1992 and 1996 were considered inappropriate.[32,34-35] Pharmaceutical donations sent to southern Sudan and Lithuania contained potentially dangerous drugs of which at least one, closantel, resulted in adverse side effects.[36,37] The WHO has prepared general guidelines for pharmaceutical donations that include the selection of drugs, quality assurance and shelf life, packaging and labeling, and information and management of pharmaceuticals.[27,33,36] Other examples include specialized external medical teams that arrive too late or are inappropriate for the response. These personnel then require food, shelter, and transportation.[38] Inappropriate and unrequested aid can cost a community money in the storage, handling, and destruction of medical assets. The cost of handling the drugs often exceeds the actual value of the pharmaceuticals themselves.[33,35,39-40]

During international aid response, inappropriate, unneeded, or excess aid can arrive for a variety of reasons, including the belief that any type of international assistance is useful and the affected community is incapable of handling the response themselves.[30,40] This may be the result of lack of communication between the donor and recipient, which leads to unnecessary donations.[33] Assigning personnel to be responsible for inventory control and assessing the overall response needs is often not done.[39] In an effort to provide nations with a supply management system, the WHO developed a system known as the Supply Management Project (SUMA).

The purpose of SUMA is to assist nations in categorizing and inventorying donations supplied during relief efforts.[40] Finally, unrequested and inappropriate donations have occurred because donors may want to receive tax deductions or avoid the costs associated with the destruction of medical supplies with short expiration dates, a practice that has been referred to as "drug dumping."[35]

SUMMARY

The types and amounts of medical equipment and pharmaceuticals required to respond to disasters will be determined by the disaster itself, the response capability of the community, and existing resources within the community. There is no specific list of pharmaceuticals or medical assets that apply to all communities or for all types of disasters. United States federal assistance is, in many cases, designed to augment the community and state response to disasters. It is therefore imperative that communities preidentify the medical resources available for a disaster response such as through the Metropolitan Medical Response System program, SNS program, Department of Veterans Affairs, and regional pharmaceutical caches that may be approved through Health Resource Services Administration grants. Preidentification of available assets will help to avoid duplication of efforts. Communities should closely coordinate the arrival of federal assistance with a distribution system that can efficiently transport critical medical assets where they are most needed. Predisaster preparations may include stockpiling of pharmaceuticals and equipment to respond to a variety of disasters. Although the financial implications of medical stockpiling should be addressed, there may be several reasons to consider stockpiling as an option in pre-disaster preparedness. Stockpiling or forward placement of pharmaceuticals may be considered when the timing of their administration requires that the product be given within minutes to hours to maximize their effectiveness, when limited supplies are generally available within a community, and when hazard assessments indicate a technologic risk to a community. Understanding the pharmaceuticals and medical equipment needed for a disaster should, at a minimum, include taking an inventory of community assets and considering the federal resources that may be requested.

REFERENCES

1. Noji EK. The public health consequences of disasters. *Prehospital Disaster Med.* 2001;5(4):147-57.
2. Sidel VW. Weapons of mass destruction: the greatest threat to public health. *JAMA* 1989;262:680-2.
3. World Health Organization. *Community Emergency Preparedness: A Manual for Managers and Policy Makers.* Geneva, Switzerland: WHO-OMS; 1999;141-160.
4. Lillibridge SR, Noji EK, Burkle FM. Disaster assessment: the emergency health evaluation of a population affected by a disaster. *Ann Emerg Med.* 1993;22:1715-20.
5. Guha-Saphir D, Lechat MF. Information systems and needs assessment in natural disasters: an approach for better disaster relief management. *Disasters.* 1986;10(3):232-7.
6. Rotz LD, Koo D, O'Carroll PW, et al. Bioterrorism preparedness: planning for the future. In: Novack LF, ed. *Public Health Issues in Disaster Preparedness Focus on Bioterrorism.* Gaithersburg, Md: Aspen Publications; 2001:99-103.
7. Pan American Health Organization. Natural Disasters: Protecting the Public's Health. Public. No. 575. Washington, DC: PAHO-OPS; 2000.
8. Henderson AK, Lillibridge SR, Graves RW, et al. Disaster medicine assistance teams: providing health care to a community struck by Hurricane Iniki. *Ann Emerg Med.* 1994;23:726-30.
9. Alson R, Alexander D, Leonard D. Analysis of medical treatment at a field hospital following Hurricane Andrew, 1992. *Ann Emerg Med.* 1993;22:1721-8.
10. Pesik N, Keim M. Logistical considerations for emergency response resources. *Pac Health Dialog.* 2002;9(1):97-103.
11. Manning FJ, Goldfrank L, eds. *Preparing for Terrorism: Tools for Evaluating the Metropolitan Medical Response System Program. Committee on Evaluation of the Metropolitan Medical Response System Program, Board on Health Sciences Policy.* Washington, DC: National Academy Press; 2003:1-332.
12. World Health Organization–Pan American Health Organization. Guidelines for the use of foreign field hospitals in the aftermath of sudden-impact disasters. Washington, DC: WHO-PAHO; 2003:1-20.
13. Plutt I. Field hospitals arrive in Iran following December earthquake. *Disasters: Preparedness and Mitigation in the Americas.* Geneva: WHO-PAHO; 2003:94.
14. Wetter DC, Faniell WE, Treser CD. Hospital preparedness for victims of chemical or biological terrorism. *Am J Publ Health.* 2001;91(5):710-6.
15. Henretig FM, Cieslak TJ, Madsen JM, et al. The emergency department response to incidents of biological and chemical terrorism. In: Fleisher GR, Ludwig S, eds. *Textbook of Pediatric Emergency Medicine.* 4th ed. Philadelphia: Lippincott, Williams and Wilkins; 2000:1763-84.
16. US Department of Homeland Security. National Response Plan, Draft #2, April 28, 2004, Washington, DC: US Department of Homeland Security; 2004.
17. Keim M, Pesik N, Twum-Danso N. Lack of hospital preparedness for chemical terrorism in a major US city: 1996-2000. *Prehospital Disaster Med.* 2003 July-Sept;18(3):193-9.
18. Henderson DA, Inglesby TV, O'Toole T, eds. *Bioterrorism: Guidelines for Medical and Public Health Management.* Chicago: American Medical American Press; 2002:1-244.
19. Jarrett DG, ed. *Medical Management of Radiological Casualties Handbook.* Bethesda, Md: Armed Forces Radiobiology Research Institute; 1999:1-141.
20. *Medical Management of Chemical Casualties Handbook.* 3rd ed. Aberdeen Proving Ground, Md: Chemical Casualty Care Division, United States Army Medical Research Institute of Chemical Defense; 2000:1-290.
21. Kortepeter M, ed. *Medical Management of Biological Casualties Handbook.* 3rd ed. Frederick, Md: United States Army Medical Research Institute of Infectious Diseases; 1998:1-121.
22. National Academies of Science. *Distribution and administration of potassium iodide in the event of a nuclear incident.* Washington, DC: National Academies Press; 2004:1-239.
23. Hick JL, Hanfling D, Burstein JL, et al. Protective equipment for health care facility decontamination personnel: regulations, risks, and recommendations. *Ann Emerg Med.* 2003;42:370-80.
24. Macintyre AG, Christopher GW, Eitzen E, et al. Weapons of mass destruction events with contaminated casualties: effective planning for health care facilities. *JAMA.* 2003;283:242-9.
25. World Health Organization. *The New Emergency Health Kit.* Geneva: World Health Organization; 1990.
26. *The Use of Essential Drugs: Eighth Report of the WHO Expert committee.* Geneva: World Health Organization; 1998.1-77.
27. Lacy E. Pharmaceuticals in disasters. In: Hogan DE, Burstein JL, eds. *Disaster Medicine.* Philadelphia: Lippincott, Williams and Wilkins; 2002:34-40.
28. Schultz CH, Koenig KL, Noji EK. Current concepts: a medical disaster response to reduce immediate mortality after an earthquake. *N Engl J Med.* 1996;334(7):438-44.
29. American Academy of Pediatrics Committee on Environmental Health. Chemical-biological terrorism and its impact on children: a subject review. *Pediatrics* 2000;105: 662-70.

30. de Ville de Goyt C. Stop propagating disaster myths. *Lancet* 2000;356:762-4.

31. de Ville de Goyt C, del Cid E, Romero A, et al. Earthquake in Guatemala: epidemiological evaluation of the relief effort. *Pan Am Health Organ Bull*. 1976;10:95-109.

32. Autier P, Ferir M, Hairapetian A, et al. Drug supply in the aftermath of the 1988 Armenian earthquake. *Lancet* 1990;335:1388-90.

33. World Health Organization. *Guidelines for Drug Donations*. 2nd ed. Geneva:World Health Organization; 1999:1-20.

34. Pan American Health Organization. *Disasters Preparedness and Mitigation in the Americas*. Washington, DC: PAHO-OPS; 1984:1-8.

35. Berckmans P, Dawans V, Schmets G, et al. Inappropriate drug donations in Bosnia and Herzegovnia, 1992-1996. *N Engl J Med*. 1997;18:1842-5.

36. Hogerzeil HV, Couper MR, Gary R. Guidelines for drug donations. *BMJ*. 1997;1082:737-40.

37. Cohen S. Drug donations to the Sudan. *Lancet* 1990; i:745.

38. de Ville de Goyet C. Offers and requests for external medical teams. *Pan Am Health Organ Epi Bull*. 2001;21:4.

39. Auf der Heide E. Resource management. In: Auf der Heide E, ed. *Disaster Response: Principles of Preparation and Coordination*. St Louis: Mosby; 1989:103-32.

40. de Ville de Goyet C, Acosta E, Sabbat P, et al. SUMA (Supply Management Project), a management tool for post-disaster relief supplies. *World Health Statistics Quarterly-Rapport Trimestriel de Statistiques Sanitaries Mondiales*. 1996;49(3-4):189-94.

41. Seaman J. Disaster epidemiology, or why most international relief is ineffective. *Injury* 1990;21(1):5-8.

chapter 48

Displaced Populations

John D. Cahill

Displaced populations have occurred throughout the history of mankind. A large population can be displaced by a multitude of disasters. These include, but are not limited to, natural disasters (e.g., floods, famine, earthquakes, hurricanes, monsoons, and volcanoes), persecution, conflict, and war. As seen in the Hurricane Katrina disaster in 2005, populations that are displaced face many difficult challenges. They are forced to leave their home, possessions, and occupations and be separated from their family and friends. Effects from these disasters can have direct impact on these populations' physical and mental health. There is fear of the unknown and loss of control and self-identity. These populations are vulnerable to abuse on many levels, including human rights and gender-based crimes. Although the burdens of a displaced population may be similar, generally they fall into one of two broad groups: refugees or internally displaced populations.

REFUGEES

The United Nations High Commission of Refugees (UNHCR) estimates that there are approximately 12 million refugees worldwide. The role of this commission is to protect and act as an advocate for this population. The UNHCR defines a *refugee* as a person who has a "well-founded fear of being persecuted for reasons of race, religion, nationality, membership of a particular social group or political opinion, is outside the country of his nationality and is unable or, owing to such fear, is unwilling to avail himself of the protection of that country; or who, not having a nationality and being outside the country of his former habitual residence as a result of such events, is unable or, owing to such fear, is unwilling to return to it."[1] For a person to be considered a refugee, he or she must cross a border into another country. Certain persons are not considered refugees: war criminals, persons who commit acts of terrorism, criminals who have a fair trial and seek refuge to avoid incarceration, soldiers, and economic migrants (those who leave their country on their own will to better their life).

An important principle of refugee law is non-refoulement, which is "a concept which prohibits States from returning a refugee or asylum-seeker to territories where there is a risk that his or her life or freedom would be threatened on account of race, religion, nationality, membership of a particular social group or political opinion."[2]

Refugee status is often considered to be a temporary matter, when in reality it can go on for years to decades. Whole new generations have been born in refugee camps, having no identification with their original country. Generally there are three options for a refugee's destiny: to repatriate to his country, to resettle in the country where he has sought refugee status, or to be resettled to a third country.

INTERNALLY DISPLACED PERSONS

Internally displaced persons (IDPs) may be defined as persons who have been forced to flee their homes to escape armed conflict, generalized violence, human rights abuses, or natural or manmade disasters. They differ from refugees in that they stay within the borders of their home country. It is estimated that the number of IDPs is at least twice the number of refuges worldwide, conservatively being at least 25 million.[3] Because they exist within the borders of a potentially hostile home country, they lack the services and protections available to refugees.

PRIORITIES FOR A DISPLACED POPULATION

Although events that lead up to a movement of a large population may differ, there are certain principles that generally apply. Many different actors may be involved in these movements: governments (including multiple countries, states, or localities), military units, and nongovernmental organizations. Whenever possible, members of the local community should be involved in the decision to move. This includes government officials, professionals (e.g., public health, healthcare providers, engineers), and the local workforce. These groups can be an invaluable resource in understanding the population needs, potential challenges, infrastructure, and cultural issues. Box 48-1 lists the top priorities of a displaced population. The remainder of this chapter will go through the priorities of the initial management of a displaced population.

INITIAL EVALUATION

There should be a clear understanding of the context and what event led to the movement of the population being evaluated. The effects of a war or genocide will require very different resources and management than those of a hurricane. Although it can be difficult in the initial assessment, one should try to consider the potential length of time that this population may be displaced. Historically, the timeframe is often much longer that one would expect. Remember that there are refugees who have been displaced for decades from their original home, and two-thirds of refugees are still living in camps 5 years later. The security of both the population and those responding to the situation needs to be of utmost importance. Unfortunately, at times, this important concept has gone underappreciated or poorly understood.

It is of tremendous value to understand the demographics of the population that has been displaced. This information can be obtained by initial registration of the population, census information, health records, sample surveys, and speaking with local authorities. Basic essential data includes the size, sex, and age distribution of the population; family members; cultural makeup (e.g., religion, ethnicity); medical health, disease prevalence, and vaccine status; and the identification of potential vulnerable groups.

The region where the population is relocating to needs to be well understood. What resources are available to the population? Is there an adequate water supply, and to what extent can it be used? Will proper sanitation be available, and for how long? What amount of food is available locally, and what kind of stores are available? Is the land suitable for living on? What local supplies are available for constructing shelter? What medical care and provisions are available locally? Is there appropriate sanitation? How secure are all these items? What infrastructure is available to bring in further supplies? Are there suitable roads? What size vehicle can the roads accommodate? Are there facilities to repair vehicles that encounter mechanical problems? Are there train stations in close proximity? Where is the closest landing strip, and what is the maximum size aircraft that can land there? Where is the nearest port? If goods are to be shipped in, where can they be stored, and can these items be secured? What are the options to distribute water, food, and supplies in an orderly and safe manner?

Measles

Many healthcare providers are often very surprised to learn that measles continues to be a major cause of morbidity and mortality throughout the world. The pediatric population is at highest risk, and mass vaccination should be highest priority in children from 6 months to 15 years of age.[4] Measles is a RNA paramyxovirus that is highly contagious and is spread through secretions in the respiratory tract. Approximately 90% of susceptible persons will contract the disease after exposure to an infected person.[5] It should be remembered that vitamin A deficiency can cause more severe and complicated cases of measles. All refugee populations should be vaccinated for measles; vitamin A should be distributed when vaccinating.

Water

Water should be top priority in any disaster situation. It is the cornerstone of the foundation for an emergency response. Not only is water a necessity for life, but also for basic hygiene. In the initial response, the quantity of water is more important than the quality. The absolute minimum requirement of water is 5 liters/person/day; this should be increased as soon as possible to reach a level of 15 to 20 liters/person/day. Other things to consider about water include the source, accessibility, location, availability of carrying containers, and security considerations.

Water can be a source of disease on many different levels. Contaminated water, as shown in Table 48-1, contributes significantly to global morbidity and mortality. Freshwater can act as the home for the intermediate hosts that cause schistosomiasis and guinea worm infection. These infections commonly occur when a person stands in water as he or she is collecting it. A lack of water or contaminated water can also contribute to trachoma, which is a major cause of blindness and skin infections. Finally, water can act as the home to insect vectors that cause malaria, dengue fever, filariasis, onchocerciasis, and African trypanoso-miasis.[6] Adequate ways to filter and purify water should be made available.

Sanitation and Hygiene

Besides water, sanitation and hygiene are of top priority in the emergency response. These measures are the first barrier to preventing the spread of fecal/oral disease. On average, humans produce 0.25 liters of stool/day and 1.5

TABLE 48-1   WATERBORNE DISEASES FROM CONTAMINATED WATER INGESTION

DISEASE	MORBIDITY PER ANNUM	MORTALITY PER ANNUM
Diarrhea	1000 million	3.3 million
Typhoid	12.5 million	>125,000
Cholera	>300,000	>3000
Ascaris infection	1 billion	

liters of urine/day. One can easily see how quickly proper disposal and management of waste can become a problem. When considering a sanitation system, one needs to be culturally sensitive to the population that is being served. It is a futile effort to set up a sanitation system if no one is going to use it. Therefore, it is a good idea to involve local residents in setting up a system. Environmental implications should be considered as well: what impact may it have, how long is it going to be used, and is there any potential to contaminate the water supply? Sanitation systems come in two forms, which are listed in Table 48-2.[7]

Food and Nutrition

The demand for food may lead to displacement. This may occur from a natural disaster or from the effects of conflict and war. Malnutrition is a significant cause of morbidity and mortality in many disasters. It is important to not only remember the direct complications of malnutrition and disease states (Table 48-3), but to understand that many diseases are accelerated or severe secondary to malnutrition—particularly in the pediatric population, where the main causes of death go hand and hand with malnutrition. The following are strongly tied to malnutrition: diarrhea, pneumonia, HIV, tuberculosis, malaria, measles, hypoglycemia, and hypothermia.

The daily minimum nutritional requirement should be 2100 kilocalories/person/day. At least 10% of the calories in the general ration should be in the form of fats, and at least 12% should be derived from proteins.[8]

The caloric demand may be higher based on shelter, environment, burden of disease, and underlying nutritional status of the population. Distributing food equitably is an important aspect of feeding large populations. Ideally, this should be done in a community-based setting in an organized and secure manner. Otherwise, food stores will not be distributed equally. Feeding centers should be established for the severely malnutritioned.

A food basket for distribution may include wheat flour, rice, sugar, vegetable oil, salt, and possibly local fish or meat. Other supplements may be included for additional nutritional benefit. It is preferable to use local food when available and to encourage the planting of vegetables. Seeds and other equipment can be distributed to the population. Cultural practices and diet also need to be considered. Utensils and fuel for cooking need to be supplied, depending on the food being distributed. Breast-feeding should be encouraged and bottle feeding avoided.

TABLE 48-3 DISEASE STATES ASSOCIATED WITH MALNUTRITION

DISEASE	DEFICIENCY
Anemia	Iron/vitamin B_{12}
Goiter/cretinism	Iodine
Scurvy	Vitamin C
Rickets/osteomalacia	Vitamin D
Beriberi	Vitamin B_1 (thiamine)
Pellagra	Niacin
Ariboflavinosis	Vitamin B_2 (riboflavin)
Night blindness/xerophthalmia	Vitamin A
Kwashiorkor	Protein

Nutritional screening of the population should be performed to assess particular needs. In general, the incidence of malnutrition in children younger than 5 years of age is used as the general indicator of malnutrition for the population. The weight-to-height index (ideally used), evidence of edema, and the mid-upper arm circumference are means to do a nutritional survey.[9]

Shelter

Depending on the size of the displaced population, several different options may be considered for shelter. With small populations, an attempt may be made to house them with the local population in their homes. As the size grows, this is not possible. Another shelter option is to use existing structures that are already available (e.g., schools, factories, warehouses, and public buildings). Finally, camps can be established for the population to live in. When a camp is being established, considerations on shelter and the site will be based on a number of factors, including type of disaster, size and demographics of the population, anticipated time of displacement (although this is often underappreciated), environmental health risks, terrain, accessibility, available existent structures and infrastructure, climate, security (ideally away from borders), local building materials, and cultural considerations. Table 48-4 lists some general guidelines that are used for site planning.[10]

TABLE 48-2 SANITATION SYSTEMS

WET	DRY
Water seal latrines	Trench
Aquaprives	Pit latrines
	VIP latrine
OXFAM Sanitation Unit	Bore holed
	Composting

TABLE 48-4 RECOMMENDATIONS FOR SHELTER

CONSIDERATION	SPACE
Area available per person	30 m^2
Shelter space per person	3.5 m^2
Number of people per water point	250
Number of people per latrine	20
Distance to water point	150 m, maximum
Distance to latrine	30 m
Distance between water point and latrine	100 m
	75 m every 300 m
Firebreaks	2 m, minimum
Distance between two shelters	

Medical Care

Medical needs may be anticipated based on the circumstances of the event leading to the displaced population. There are some general principles in responding to the acute medical needs of a displaced population. The goals of the healthcare system should be to treat the common communicable diseases (i.e., diarrhea, respiratory tract infections, measles, and malaria), reduce the suffering from debilitating diseases, afford easy access to the necessary care for the population, deal with the majority of diseases at the basic level, and carry out public health surveillance.

Whenever possible, local healthcare facilities and professionals should be used. A large population can quickly overburden the local system, and often a parallel system needs to be developed. A four-tier model for the levels of healthcare managing the initial acute phase has been repeatedly used with success in reducing excess mortality. The levels include a referral hospital (preferably an already functioning local hospital), a central health facility, a peripheral health facility, and home visits/assessments. A referral hospital is used for more specialized care such as major surgery, obstetric emergencies, and more elaborate laboratory and diagnostic facilities. Patients should be referred to this facility only by one of the other tiers, preferably from the central health facility. Depending on the situation, one central health facility should be present for every 10,000 to 30,000 persons in a camp. This facility should include triage, an outpatient clinic (including minor surgical procedures), simple inpatient services (including uncomplicated deliveries), a pharmacy, and simple laboratory facilities. A peripheral health facility should be established for every 3000 to 5000 persons. Here a simple outpatient clinic or department can treat basic health needs (e.g., dehydration, dressing changes) and refer patients to a higher level of care. At all levels, public health surveillance should be conducted.[11]

Based on disease prevalence in the population or region, certain medications may be required. In general, "essential" medical kits have been developed and are available from a number of government and nongovernmental organizations. Ideally, healthcare treatment protocols should be established for the more common illnesses. This affords easier management and better treatment when dealing with large populations. It also allows for the anticipation of necessary supplies and medications.

REFERENCES

1. United Nations High Commission of Refugees. *Convention and Protocol Relating to the Status of Refugees*. Geneva: UNHCR; 1951:16.
2. United Nations High Commission of Refugees. *The Scope and Content of the Principle of Non Refoulement*. Geneva: UNHCR; 2001:5.
3. Norwegian Refugee Project. *Internal Displacement: A Global Overview of Trends and Development in 2003*.
4. Médicins Sans Frontières. The emergency phase: the ten top priorities. In Hanquet G, ed: *Refugee Health: An Approach to Emergency Situations*. London: Macmillan; 1997:39.
5. Cutaneous viral diseases. In: Cook GC, Zumla A, eds. *Manson's Tropical Disease*. 21st ed. Philadelphia: WB Saunders; 2003:842.
6. International emergency medicine. In: Cahill J, ed. *Updates in Emergency Medicine*. New York: Kluwer Academic Publishing; 2003a, 131-3.
7. Eade D. *The OXFAM Handbook of Development and Relief*. Oxford, UK: OXFAM; March 1994:22-23.
8. Famine-affected, refugee, and displaced populations: recommendations for public health issues. *MMWR*. 1992;41(RR-13).
9. Médicins Sans Frontières. *Clinical Guidelines*. Paris: Médicins Sans Frontières; 2003.
10. United Nations High Commission of Refugees. *Handbook for Emergencies*. Geneva: UNHCR; 1982.
11. Médicins Sans Frontières. Health care in the emergency phase. In Hanquet G, ed: *Refugee Health an Approach to Emergency Situations*. London: Macmillan; 1997:125-32.

chapter 49

Rehabilitation and Reconstruction

Elizabeth Temin

There are four phases of emergency management:

1. Preparedness: Planning a response to a disaster.
2. Response: Activities that occur immediately after a disaster. These actions are designed to provide emergency assistance to victims. This phase usually lasts a few days to a few weeks.
3. Recovery: Returning the community to normal or near normal. This phase may last for many years.
4. Mitigation: Preventing or reducing the effects of a disaster. This phase should be integrated into the other three.[1]

This chapter discusses the third and least understood[2] phase of emergency management: recovery. There are many factors that go into recovery, for example, the physical reconstruction of homes and public buildings, transportation, and basic services infrastructure, as well as psychological mending of the community and economic recovery of lost time and resources. This stage cannot be considered in isolation because mitigation, the fourth phase, must be integrated into recovery for it to be sustainable.

In 1977, Haas et al[3] became the first group to identify and describe the recovery process. They listed recovery as a sequential four-stage model of emergency, restoration, replacement, and development. Current models describe a more fluid recovery process with these stages overlapping and potentially occurring simultaneously.[4] For example, replacement reconstruction may occur in some locations while at the same time debris clearance occurs elsewhere. Recovery currently focuses on the idea of *sustainable development,*[4] a concept created by a United Nations Commission in 1986, which refers to recovery as a way to improve the quality of lives and durability of communities.[5] This has been defined in the World Commission on Environment and Development as "meeting the needs of the present without compromising the ability of future generations to meet their own needs."[6] In the short run, it may cost more; better materials may be used, houses and businesses may be relocated, and more stringent building codes and zones laws may be implemented. In the long run, its goal is to protect and strengthen key social and economic infrastructure before disasters strike so as to reduce the likelihood of loss of life and assets[7] and ultimately improve the community and save money.[5]

There is a vast spectrum of disasters, and the process of disaster recovery can adapt the available tools to fit the specific situation. It is useful to apply a framework in thinking about the similarities and differences in disasters. They can be categorized as natural or manmade, sudden onset or slow onset. Examples of natural disasters that are slow onset are droughts or epidemics such as severe acute respiratory syndrome (SARS); sudden onset examples are floods, hurricanes, and earthquakes. Examples of manmade disasters that are slow onset are wars such as the war in Iraq, and sudden onset examples are bombings or terrorist activities such as the Sept. 11, 2001, attacks and the Exxon Valdez oil tanker spill in 1989. In general, the important differences are the duration of the impact and the severity of direct and indirect effects. *Direct effects* are defined as the physical destruction and lives lost as a result of the disaster. *Indirect effects* are the work time lost, jobs lost, and the change in spending in the community involved.

There is also a framework in which to categorize recovery; it can be designated as vertically or horizontally mediated. *Vertical mediation* recovery refers to the hierarchy of local communities, the state government, and the federal government. *Horizontal mediation* refers to the network of groups within a community. Every recovery and management process needs a balance of both vertical and horizontal mediation.

The next three sections of this chapter discuss how certain communities and countries have handled disaster recovery historically, how the United States currently handles disaster recovery, and finally, pitfalls that are common in recovery efforts.

HISTORICAL PERSPECTIVE

The literature on disaster recovery discusses both manmade and natural disasters but has primarily been only descriptive. When the Tsarist regime in Russia was overthrown in 1917, there was an almost complete nullification of all property rights, and the black market became the form of informal barter. Industrial production fell to 20% of pre-war levels by 1920.[8] Hyperinflation occurred, impeding the ability to rebuild the country.

In Hamburg, a series of raids over a period of 10 days in 1943 destroyed almost half the buildings in the city.

In the aftermath, there were as many injured as fatalities, and over two thirds of the city's hospital beds had been destroyed. Over a period of months, 300,000 refugees were rehoused and 500,000 permanently evacuated. Adequate water supply was a problem even though wells had been dug prior to the event. Yet within 5 months, Hamburg had recovered up to 80% of its former productivity.[8]

In 1945, the atomic bomb was dropped on Hiroshima. Deaths were estimated at 80,000, and almost 70% of buildings were destroyed. In this case, recovery took much longer. It was only by 1949, 4 years later, that the population had recovered to its former numbers and 70% of the destroyed buildings had been reconstructed.[8]

In 1982, Marin County experienced continued floods and mudslides until finally a presidential disaster was declared. Federal teams had trouble appropriately identifying local public priorities from the myriad of recovery issues. As an example, the Intelligence Hazard Mitigation Team identified two sites for priority attention. County officials indicated that those were not the priorities they would have selected.[1] Damage survey reports were begun in over 300 sites, and many were held up by disagreements over the definition of a *mudslide* versus a *landslide* and how to define *repair* versus *permanent restoration*. Each of these occurrences receive different levels of funding.[1] On the positive side, Marin County actively included mitigation into recovery efforts. They created landslide-protection zones and required that prospective home buyers receive mandatory notification of stability problems.[1]

In 1988, Jamaica was hit with Hurricane Gilbert. This was the first direct hit with a hurricane in more than 35 years. As a result, Jamaica had been in a period of complacency with a low sense of preparedness and concern for mitigation. Nineteen of the 33 watershed areas had been eroded by deforestation and the expansion of agriculture onto high-slope areas. When Hurricane Gilbert struck, there occurred not only the destruction from the hurricane but also subsequent significant flooding and landslides. Many Jamaicans lived in highly vulnerable locations. The low-income housing in the area that was not built up to the housing codes, and those in floodplains and gullies suffered predominantly.[9] It was estimated that 20% of all housing was damaged and 2% destroyed.[9]

In 1989 when the Loma Prieta earthquake hit Santa Cruz County, the local community was strong. When the Federal Emergency Management Agency (FEMA) came and set up a disaster assistance center (DAC) in the city of Santa Cruz, the citizen leaders requested a satellite DAC to support the rural population. FEMA accepted the request after determining that a significant number of families had been overlooked in their initial assessment. By working together, the community and the federal government were able to adequately support the victims of this disaster.[2]

CURRENT PRACTICE

In the United States, recovery planning started in 1803 when local resources were overwhelmed during a fire in Portsmouth, New Hampshire. The local government asked Congress for help, creating the first legislative act for federal resources. In 1950 the first permanent and general legislation, the Federal Disaster Act, came into existence. This was revolutionary because it was the first Act to create a general response to all disasters. Before this, each disaster resulted in Congress passing a new localized piece of legislation. In 1979, President Carter pulled all the distinct response groups together along with the military resources to create FEMA.

In 1988 Congress passed the Stafford Act, which focused FEMA toward hazard mitigation and coordination of disaster recovery programs. The Disaster Mitigation Act of 2000 established specific requirements for hazard mitigation planning, and grants became available to allow local and state governments to use mitigation funds for predisaster planning.[6] In 2001 the actions of Sept. 11 pushed Congress to create the Department of Homeland Security, which was the largest reorganization of federal agencies since the Great Depression.[6]

The magnitude of disaster recovery depends on the magnitude of the destruction. In a small local disaster, volunteer organizations such as the Red Cross and private insurers may be enough to aid victims. When a disaster overwhelms the recovery forces of a community, that community can turn to the state government, and ultimately to FEMA, for resources. Within the first 48 hours of a disaster, an assessment team should provide an initial assessment of the damage. This includes identifying immediate needs such as food, shelter, and infrastructure. A preliminary damage assessment by the local government will determine whether federal aid may be needed and should be requested. Once the immediate needs are identified, and if federal aid is requested, a second, more in-depth survey should be done by FEMA. This second survey should include asking the plans of the displaced citizens: Do they plan to move, or rebuild in the same spot? Public infrastructure, sewers, and storm drains should be examined. What about the town? What was there before the disaster? What currently exists? Were there any existing plans for expansion of the area that could be used for rebuilding? What are opportunities looking at the long term?[10]

Every U.S. state maintains an Emergency Management Agency (EMA) and an Emergency Operations Plan. Their role is to establish and maintain an emergency program concerned with preparedness, response, mitigation, and recovery; to coordinate and train state and local governments; to recommend whether federal aid is needed in the case of a disaster; and to coordinate state and federal resources and act as an intermediary between local and federal groups.[6] In the past, the majority of these plans have been concerned primarily with the short-term response.[2] Recently many states have been trying to adapt to a more long-term response.

When a disaster, whether natural or manmade, strikes a community in any part of the United States, including the Virgin Islands, Guam, U.S. Samoa, and the commonwealth of the Northern Mariana Islands,[11] if that state is overwhelmed and state resources are not enough to provide aid, the federal government may declare a disaster under the Robert T. Stafford Disaster Relief and Emergency Assistance Act.[11] In 2000 there were 45 major disaster declarations made in 31 states and the District of Columbia.[12] These disasters ranged from tornadoes to wildfires to winter storms. Initial response resources include food, water, emergency generators, and the mobilization of specialized teams (e.g., search and rescue, medical assistance, damage assessment, and communications). For more long-term relief, there are loans and grants to repair or replace housing and personal property, roads, and public buildings. There is also assistance for mitigation opportunities, counseling, and legal services. These services are outlined in the Federal Response Plan (FRP), which describes the policies and plans of 25 federal departments and the U.S. Red Cross.[11] The FRP can be implemented in conjunction with other specialized groups including plans for telecommunications support, the National Oil and Hazardous Substances Pollution Contingency Plan, the Federal Radiological Emergency Response Plan, and the Terrorism Incident Annex.[11] In addition to the FRP, some federal agencies have the authority to provide disaster aid even when the magnitude is not sufficient for the president to declare a federal disaster, including the Department of Agriculture, Department of Commerce, Department of Housing and Urban Development, and the Small Business Association (SBA). The FRP employs a multiagency operations structure based on the Incident Command System (ICS). (See Chapter 30, The Incident Command System.) Disaster Field Offices under the Department of Homeland Security may be created along with a national emergency response team. Recovery efforts are the responsibility of logistics and administration teams within the disaster field offices.

The first source of insurance for all homeowners, businesses, and towns is private insurance. If that is not adequate or not available, the next action should be to register with FEMA by the stated deadline, usually within 2 months of the disaster. After individual private insurance carriers, the SBA provides the next largest portion of aid. All those above a minimum income are referred to SBA and should apply for SBA loans.[10] The loans must be repaid, but they carry low interest rates. These loans include:

1. Home disaster loans to homeowners or renters to repair personal property;
2. Business physical disaster loans to businesses to repair or replace property including real estate, equipment, and inventory (not-for-profit organizations are also eligible);
3. Economic injury disaster loans to small businesses and agricultural cooperatives to replace working capital.[10]

FEMA also offers three types of assistance:

1. Individual and family grants: These loans are granted to persons with needs not met by private insurances, SBA, or volunteer organizations. These grants are for basic needs only, not to return life to normal. Costs can include medical and counseling assistance, housing repair, funeral expenses, and insurance premiums.
2. Public assistance: This program gives aid to local governments for emergency services and the repair or replacement of public facilities, for example, the removal of debris, repair of infrastructure, or emergency protective measures. It is often the most costly element of recovery, and typically the cost is shared with the state in a 75%/25% split.[6]
3. Hazard mitigation grant program[10]: These grants are used by the federal, state, and local governments to incorporate mitigation into the recovery process. Actions may include acquisition of homes, public education, and retrofitting structures to better resist subsequent disasters such as floods and hurricanes. Cost will be shared between federal and state resources.[6]

Businesses have special considerations in light of a disaster. The primary objective of recovery planning is to enable an organization to survive a disaster and to continue normal business operations. To survive, the organization must ensure that critical operations can resume/continue normal processing and minimize the duration of a serious disruption to operations and resources (both information processing and other resources); a premade contingency plan is the best method of accomplishing this.[13] Specific measures may include having an alternate site of operations if the current facility is damaged, storing vital documents off-site, and having an alternative energy source such as a generator. Larger businesses may be better able to withstand a disaster because assets and the workforce may be dispersed across a wider geographical area.[6]

A disaster is a life-altering event. Survivors share an enormous experience and come to view the world around them in new and different ways. Seeking help from the government, voluntary agencies, and insurance companies can be long and frustrating, which may only compound the feelings of helplessness. Anger and further despair are common. Mental health staff may assist persons by reassuring them that this "second disaster" is a common phenomenon[14] and that they are not alone in their frustration. Many people may not want to seek formal counseling, either because of the stigma some still associate with psychiatric help or because they are unwilling to take time away from putting their lives back together or helping others. Very effective mental health assistance can be provided while the worker is helping survivors with concrete tasks. The "over a cup of coffee" method of informal intervention may be the best method to help. For example, a mental health worker can use skilled but unobtrusive interviewing techniques to help a survivor sort out demands and set priorities while they are jointly sifting through disaster rubble.[14]

Although having community involvement is beneficial to the process of recovery, it is also very important for the mental well-being of the community. Failing to involve the community can lead to resentment and fragmentation. The inhabitants may be unhappy when aid is not appropriate to the community's perceived needs, and this insult may be compounded if they are then labeled unappreciative of the federal help. When people have a hand in their own recovery, they feel empowered and will increase their involvement. This leads to a stronger community network that in turn increases the ability to provide self-help.

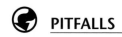

In general, there are two broad problems with disaster recovery: too little horizontal planning or too much dependence on vertical aid. The pitfalls occur when the horizontal and vertical planning are not balanced.

In the case of too much dependence on vertical planning, the community does not contribute anything to the recovery process and the government organizations and nongovernmental organizations dictate the recovery plans. In the past, these groups have come in with the intention of "fixing" the situation. This is referred to as "top down" theory.[9] In addition to not providing the optimal care, this may impede the self-sufficiency of these disaster-struck areas. Assumptions may be made, including the following: (1) the victims are a burden; (2) the host government is weak and cannot manage alone; (3) foreign aid organizations don't require accountability; (4) aid for the victims reflect the defined needs of the victims (when, in fact, the aid reflects the projected need by the donor).[9] An example of this last point was when Hurricane Hugo struck Montserrat in 1989. Ninety-eight percent of all homes were affected, 50% severely and 20% completely destroyed.[9] The Peace Corps brought in large numbers of prefabricated housing to replace all the destroyed homes. Although they were able to help a lot of people numerically, the homes they provided had two-sided pitched roofs instead of the typical Caribbean four-sided roofs that were better able to withstand tropical winds. They also did not have an interior design to allow for cross ventilation. The early recipients of the homes reported this finding to the Peace Corps, but the Peace Corps was unable to change the design. Though well intentioned, the Peace Corps was predominantly meeting the need projected by the donors instead of the actual needs of the victims.[9]

Overdependence on vertical planning can also result in a lack of accountability and thus uneven recovery results. In Jamaica, after Hurricane Gilbert, the primary housing aid program was the Building Stamp Programme, which was set up by the Jamaican government, the World Bank, Canada, Germany, Japan, OPEC, and the United States. Homeowners were issued building stamps based on the extent of damages and financial need. These stamps would then be redeemed only at building supply stores who were members of the Jamaican Hardware Merchants Association for building materials, including zinc sheets, nails, and lumber. Squatters and renters were not eligible for stamps and were left without any recourse for finding aid. People who were not at home during the time of the survey were not listed as needing aid.[9] Additionally, it was found that the stamps were distributed unequally. As a result, many needy people were left without any support.

There is always the risk of creating a "dependency syndrome" by not thinking of sustainable development when investing money and effort into the recovery process.[9] This occurs by the replacement of homes and infrastructure that are likely to be destroyed by subsequent disasters or that do not benefit the town, resulting in the need for continued care for each disaster. Instead of being able to learn from prior occurrences and create a more resilient

town/infrastructure, the same mistakes are repeated over and over again. For example, Jamaicans used the stamps to fulfill daily needs such as mattresses and utensils and did not spend time reinforcing their homes against further hurricanes or floods. When the next hurricane hits, these people will have the same destruction to their homes as occurred with Hurricane Gilbert.[9]

In the case of too little horizontal planning, the results may be a chaotic lack of cooperation between groups and potential leaders. Studies have shown that many community plans focus primarily on the emergency period and do not give adequate attention to recovery and reconstruction. If there is a plan, it often exists on paper only and in the case of an actual disaster it is not used. In fact, many officials are not aware that a plan exists.[4] These flaws lead to chaotic implementation of an ad hoc recovery. The community lacks the ability to work together and thus fragments and cannot unify to control its own affairs. As a result, the redevelopment is likely to be inadequate to fulfill the needs of the community. If there is aid from government and nongovernmental groups, they are sometimes uncoordinated, either duplicating actions, leaving areas without any aid,[4] or giving aid that is inadequate for the needs of the area. In Saragossa, Texas, a small isolated community that was devastated by a tornado in 1987, there was no local government in place at all. When a disaster advisory board was created, it was done without any input from the local inhabitants. The outcome was that the Saragossans considered themselves worse off 2 years after the tornado than they had been beforehand, both because of the quality of the rebuilt neighborhoods and because they felt they were looked on as helpless and ungrateful.[2]

Studies in the Caribbean have shown that the different power levels in an uncoordinated community may lead to powerful interest groups pressuring public authorities to rebuild first in areas in which they have the greatest interest. Poorer neighbors with weaker ties to public authorities will get delayed care.[2]

In the United States, vertical planning predominates because few communities have detailed plans in place and because they may not have the financial reserve to pay for the recovery. When a plan is in place before a disaster, it allows for a strong horizontal network. Then, when a useful vertical element is added, the results can work wonders. By 1975 recurrent floods had repeatedly decimated the town of Soldiers Grove, Wisconsin. Each time they rebuilt. At one point they added a dam, and they planned for a levee but were unable because of financial restrictions. They decided they would take the funds allocated for the levee and use it to plan for town relocation. Although federal funds were slow in coming, they did create a plan. In 1978, when the largest flood in the history of the area occurred, they were ready with a fully written strategy. When they were granted funds for reconstruction, they put their plan into effect. Not only did they relocate out of the flood plain to prevent reoccurrence of this destruction, but they decided to create a town that was 75% solar powered.[5] Because they had had the luxury of time in the planning stage, they had asked each business owner where they wanted to be located and how they wanted their business to be built.

As a result, the town became not only exactly what the community wanted, but its creation instilled a great sense of pride and satisfaction in its citizens, thus creating a happier community as well.

REFERENCES

1. Drabek T, Hoetmer G. *Emergency Management: Principles and Practice of Local Government*. International City Management Association: Washington DC; 1991.

2. Berke P, Kartez J, Wenger D. Recovery after disaster: achieving sustainable development, mitigation and equity. *Disasters*. 17(2):93-109.

3. Haas E, Kates R, Bowden M. *Reconstruction Following Disaster*. Cambridge, Mass: MIT Press, 1977.

4. Petterson J. *A Review of the Literature and Programs on Local Recovery from Disaster*. Natural Hazards Research and Applications Information Center, Institute of Behavioral Science, University of Colorado; 1999.

5. Smart Communities Network. Rebuilding for the future: a guide to sustainable redevelopment of disaster-affected communities, September 1994. Available at: http://www.sustainable.doe.gov/articles/RFTF1.shtml.

6. Emergency Management Institute. Holistic disaster recovery: creating a more sustainable future [online course]. Available at: http://www.training.fema.gov/emiweb/edu/sdr.asp.

7. World Bank Finances Emergency Recovery and Disaster Management Program for the Caribbean. News release no:99/2035/LAC.

8. Hirshleifer J. *Economic Behavior in Adversity*. Brighton: Wheatsheaf Books Ltd; 1987.

9. Berke P, Beatley T. *After the Hurricane*. Baltimore: The Johns Hopkins University Press; 1997.

10. Minnesota Homeland Security and Emergency Management. Recovery from Disaster Handbook. Available at: http://www.dps.state.mn.us/dhsem/Hsem_ view_Article.asp?docid=313&catid=4.

11. Department of Homeland Security. National Response Plan 2004. Available at: http://www.dhs.gov/interweb/assetlibrary/NRPbaseplan.pdf.

12. FEMA News. FEMA hails 2000 as year of major gains in disaster prevention, December 22, 2000. Available at: http://www.fema.gov/news/newsrelease. fema?id=9993.

13. Disaster Recovery Journal. DRJ's Sample DR Plans and Outlines. St. Louis, Mo. Available at: http://www.drj.com/new2dr/samples.htm.

14. Myers D. Psychological recovery from disaster: key concepts for delivery of mental health services. *NCP Clinical Q* 1994;4(2). National Center for Post-Traumatic Stress Disorder, US Department of Veterans Affairs. Available at: http://www.ncptsd.org//publications/cq/v4/n2/myers.html.

chapter 50

Disaster Education and Research

Kenneth A. Williams, Leo Kobayashi, and Marc J. Shapiro

Disaster education, regardless of the audience, has two goals: (1) prevention of disasters, and (2) mitigation of disaster effects, including improved outcome for victims and safety for responders.

Disaster education should be based on principles of adult education and valid research. Education competencies and design should go hand in hand with the design and implementation of disaster research. Unfortunately, most current disaster research is descriptive and not relevant for education planning.

For the general public, disaster preparedness once consisted of personal knowledge. People tended to know their limitations and had familiarity with the risks inherent in local activities and trades. Technological advances have both protected the population in developed countries and increased the risk of extraordinary catastrophe. Disaster research and education must address these changes in order to remain relevant.

HISTORICAL PERSPECTIVE

Various public health triumphs mitigated epidemics and disasters through the years. Dr. John Snow,[1] after brilliant but straightforward epidemiologic investigation, mitigated a cholera epidemic in 1855 by simply removing the handle from the contaminated pump. Hygiene, antibiotics, and field medicine saved countless lives. However, disaster response remained largely an uncoordinated humanitarian effort.

The dictum that there were "no rules" in a disaster became an excuse for response failures and deficient education and planning. Although disasters overwhelmed local response capability, certain types of disasters recurred, and response strategy could therefore be formulated. Subsequent efforts to plan for disaster response were well intentioned but failed because they diverged from daily practice. Complex plans involving communication,[2] patient identification and documentation, and command systems that were literally pulled from cabinets or trailers only for annual drills failed in actual events. The military has learned that soldiers "fight like they train," and they train frequently. Disaster responders need to learn this lesson; disaster response paradigms fail in proportion to their deviation from daily practice.

CURRENT PRACTICE

Education

Adequate disaster education should include age-appropriate guidelines and must follow a basic format for training that allows evaluation of effectiveness. One recommended format is the establishment of clearly stated objectives (e.g., "The children will be evacuated from the school in under 5 minutes," or "The physicians will properly recognize nerve agent exposure from symptoms presented during simulation."). These objectives are next used to develop evaluation tools (e.g., a timed drill for the school, written testing or observed performance for the physicians). Training curricula are then developed to achieve the desired objectives as measured by the evaluation tool. The students, for example, may need little more than general principles ("Follow the teacher's instructions in an emergency") and awareness that the alarm bell signals such an emergency; therefore occasional drills may suffice to maintain the needed level of training. Physicians treating patients exposed to chemicals may be trained using a variety of adult learning techniques.

Target audiences for disaster education include the general public, nonmedical responders, and medical responders. The same principles of effective education apply. General public topics include general disaster readiness, sheltering, evacuation, and first aid. Such education can reduce panic, minimize load on evacuation or shelter systems, and mitigate illness and injury. Nonmedical responder topics vary with the type of responder but should include awareness of medical response issues and plans. Nonmedical responders may include those who provide shelter, evacuation, security, law enforcement, administration, logistics, food and water supply, sanitation systems, transportation, and structural engineering, among many others. Medical responders should improve their readiness through training; including knowledge of education provided to the general public and nonmedical responders. This inclusive and coordinated approach will optimize readiness, prevention, and mitigation.

Readiness is the ability to perform, on request, a specific action in the allotted time. To improve readiness, an agency may work on communication essential to notify personnel of a request for service and coordinate their actions, optimal performance of specific tasks, or means to increase the efficiency of performance. Each of these areas can be the subject of a variety of types of research and training and can apply to the general public and non-medical responders as well as medical responders. For example, is a population ready to evacuate? Are the regional water suppliers ready to secure their facilities and prevent an effort to contaminate public drinking water? A variety of research exercises linked to training programs can improve readiness in such areas.

Communication, a common challenge in disaster response, can be improved with use of robust and redundant technology that is familiar to all users. Practical research can assist agencies in the selection and adoption of flexible communication systems likely to remain functional during disaster events. Research parameters for such systems might include features such as interagency interoperability, simplicity and flexibility of use, sufficient power source and range for anticipated events, and the ability to move data between variable system elements. Drills, technical demonstrations, and prospective data-gathering during real events are some research methods for the evaluation of communication systems.

Similar to readiness, prevention may encompass public health, engineering, zoning, security, or other measures that trap errors that would otherwise, in certain circumstances, lead to disaster. In some cases, a disaster (defined as "an overwhelmingly damaging event") may result in few if any medical casualties. Loss of computer data, defective products, and financial crisis are a few events that can have disastrous results without illness or injury, depending on those affected. Nevertheless, "atraumatic" disasters should be considered in disaster planning, education, and research alongside casualty-producing disasters, at least for healthcare systems if not for all community entities. The disruption caused by a loss of computer data, by revelations of administrative scandal, or by bankruptcy of a relied-on local service can be significant and can create stress and damage comparable to an event that causes injury or illness.

There are many models of adult education that can be used to train disaster responders: self study, distance learning, direct education, hands on learning, drills and exercises, and, most recently, simulation labs. The types of education must be matched to the audience as well as the task to be taught and must also take into account available resources. For example, although the best method of teaching personnel how to do a particular skill may be intensive hands-on experience, there may not be the time or money for large audience training of this type. Types of education include the following:

- Self-study: Involves self-paced learning, either from a text or Internet source. This kind of learning lends itself well to those with limited downtime during their workdays and with time to study that may be off shift or off hours.
- Distance learning: Currently well used by the U.S. Centers for Disease Control and Prevention, this type of learning is often accomplished by a satellite broadcast. It allows many to be trained in a "live environment" where their questions and issues can be addressed.

- Direct education: This involves a lecturer delivering content to a reasonably sized audience. Although this type of education facilitates questions and feedback to participants, it requires a ready pool of expert educators that may not exist in a particular subject or geographic area.
- Hands-on learning: Particularly suited for teaching skills, such as the wearing of protective equipment, this training is labor and time intensive and requires the use of local expertise and small class size–to–instructor ratio.
- Drills and exercises: Although the full-scale exercise with its cast of thousands is usually seen as the ultimate training experience, much can be accomplished by specific, task-oriented drills. Drills and exercises are an excellent place to solidify training, identify future needs, and conduct research.

Simulation Training

Human patient simulation is reaching a larger audience as the technology has improved and become more accessible. Distinct from the training offered by cardiopulmonary resuscitation manikins or personal computer–based multimedia software, high-fidelity medical simulation features integrated life-sized "patients" with programmable, reproducible, and physiologic response capabilities. Interactive communication, the ability to undergo procedural interventions, and real-time recording of events are key features. The application of these tools and techniques to disaster medicine education is now taking place.

Both manikin and virtual reality (VR) simulated patients have been implemented to train healthcare personnel in various fields. Detailed patient presentations in realistic treatment settings, accurate modeling of human physiology, and dynamic changes in response to interventions are contributing to unique educational experiences. Otherwise unachievable training is being made possible for clinical events and care settings that harbor significant risk and enormous consequences. Difficult medical resuscitation and intraoperative crisis management are representative subject areas.

Manikin-based systems such as those using the Laerdal SimMan and METI HPS models are becoming widespread due to the relative ease of setup and maintenance compared to VR counterparts. Expanding from their original role in anesthesia and resuscitation instruction, these manikins are being applied to disaster training in an ongoing exploration of their capabilities. Re-creation of the physical barriers and material impediments to patient care at disaster scenes is a prime area of inquiry. For example, practicing of intravenous access, medication administration, and endotracheal intubation while garbed in personal protective equipment (PPE) is currently being investigated on manikins.[3-6]

Total-immersion virtual reality (TIVR) and associated technologies are also starting to be used for disaster education.[7] Featuring fully computer-generated environments and patients with multisensory interactivity (i.e., visual, auditory, haptic), TIVR advances the "perceptual illusion of non-mediation."[8] This capacity to seamlessly establish the presence of participants within the TIVR-constructed world hints at the potential for tremendously flexible and virtually unlimited simulations for training. A case study in this endeavor is the University of Michigan 3D Lab, where researchers have implemented a disaster scenario inside a Cave Automated Virtual Environment.[9,10] Additional examples are present at the University of Missouri–Rolla[11] and the University of Padova.[12] Lack of standardization and significant startup requirements limit TIVR's accessibility for the time being.

Civilian and Commercial High-Fidelity Simulation Applications in Disaster and Weapons of Mass Destruction Education

With the increasing number of civilian sites featuring various forms of patient simulators, training courses have begun to earnestly delve into disaster-specific content. The fundamentals of disaster medical response, such as situational and hazard assessment, triage, patient examination and treatment, decontamination/provider protection, and evacuation are being addressed.[13] Focused task training as well as exercises fostering specific cognitive processes and teamwork behaviors[14,15] is being undertaken.

Increased funding for disaster and weapons of mass destruction (WMD) training has helped prehospital systems in several states experience sophisticated disaster exercises employing advanced medical simulation. These efforts in Florida, Maryland,[16] and Rhode Island[17] have been primarily based at university-affiliated academic simulation centers receiving state and/or federal support. Significant use of high-fidelity simulation technology for nuclear, biological, and chemical preparedness is most apparent internationally in the Israel Center for Medical Simulation's activities. Their programs address the preparation of physicians, nurses, and paramedics for the casualties of nonconventional warfare.[18-20]

In the commercial sphere, at least two U.S. centers are offering courses using high-fidelity manikin patient simulators for training in WMD and hazardous materials (HazMat). Simulation Training in Emergency Preparedness courses[21] supported by the Health Resources and Services Administration are in progress at the Rhode Island Hospital Medical Simulation Center. The Texas Engineering Extension Service provides another WMD-focused prehospital operations and planning curriculum.[22] These courses for the emergency medical service (EMS) community contain assorted applications of patient simulation, ranging from isolated patient care duties to full-scale multi-manikin disaster drills.

Military high-fidelity simulation applications in disaster and WMD education military forces have routinely been involved in training for disasters, either in support roles for natural calamities or in combat preparation duties. Consequently, many of the issues raised by terrorism and WMDs have been addressed by the military in their established training. Troops engaging in combat have been expected to encounter weaponized chemical toxins, bioweapons, explosives, and radioactive hazards. Whereas the settings in which such exposures can occur have changed, the knowledge and techniques involved in responding to them remain mostly unaltered.

The U.S. military is developing and running training programs focused on the healthcare services specialist, known as a "91W," with a particular interest in chemical, biologic, radioactive, nuclear, and explosive qualifications.[23] Component modules include personal computer–based Simulation Technologies for Trauma Care (STATCARE)[24] and Nuclear Biological Chemical Casualty Training System (NBCCTS)[25] software. Advanced patient simulation within the various project efforts features prominently under the Medical Simulation Initiative. Several hundred high-fidelity manikins in on-site and distance-learning settings have already been integrated into 91W training at various locations.[26-28] WMD-specific applications are being phased in. Additionally, logistical simulation of the mechanics and delivery of medical care at multiple levels in a realistic and complete battlefield environment is progressing with the Combat Trauma Patient Simulator program.[29]

Future Directions in Simulation

Numerous simulation experts and groups are pursuing scientific validation of simulation techniques in healthcare education. The disordered environment of a true disaster make prospective, controlled, and objective studies of educational content transfer difficult. Retrospective analyses may have a role, whereas surrogate markers of training efficacy and improvement in emergency preparedness could serve to demonstrate simulation utility in the interim.

Enhancement of independent disaster response abilities can be individually assessed at "skill stations" akin to those in advanced cardiac life support courses. Global rating scales have surfaced as potential indicators of overall learner competence in educational settings using high-fidelity simulation.[30] Such instruments, using properly defined scoring systems, should help in investigating basic disaster response competencies in conjunction with fully immersive multiple-manikin disaster drills.

Development and testing of tools to demonstrate improved medical responder preparedness with proper disaster training are taking place through federally and state-funded projects. Extensively incorporated into these activities, high-fidelity simulation has already allowed objective examination of EMS providers' scene hazards assessment, triage decision-making, use of novel interventions,[31] and resuscitative actions[13] in PPE. Continued work through such ventures is hoped to establish causal associations between high-fidelity simulation training, enhanced responder readiness training, improved disaster medical response, and ultimately, better patient outcomes.

The greatest challenge for disaster trainers is to maintain the training competencies and certifications initially acquired and to work on continual skill development in an environment where little is changing, and the next disaster may seem far away.

CATEGORIES OF RESEARCH

Disaster research can be categorized and associated with educational objectives. Categories include after-action report/case studies; aftermath epidemiology; discussion of planning, training, and mitigation techniques; trials of specific techniques or equipment; organizational or analytical schemes; and randomized controlled trials.

After-Action Report/Case Studies

A description of the first 10 cases of anthrax in the United States caused by a terrorist event[32] provides an example of the after-action report/case study. These data are useful in planning response magnitude and type. Recurring failures in response are well elucidated in this type of report. While cogently documenting the events surrounding various natural and manmade tragedies, these papers also often report shockingly similar response failures, including those involving communication, logistics, clothing, equipment, interagency cooperation, perimeter control, patient care delays, and suboptimal distribution of casualties.[33] Although various nonmedical entities such as the Federal Aviation Administration and National Transportation Safety Board have implemented various regulatory and technology improvements during the past few decades, reducing the incidence of manmade disasters and mitigating their severity, medical responders often face the same challenges reported 25 years ago.

Aftermath Epidemiology

Descriptions of the delayed effects of a disaster point out needs for subsequent responders and planners. The need to rapidly reestablish infrastructure, to attend to chronic healthcare needs and sanitation, to distribute medications, etc., can all be noted in a review of these research papers. Additionally, descriptions of lingering effects, such as the description of eye injuries following the Tokyo sarin attack, can be illuminating. Cultural diversity may alter the expression of disaster effects, but awareness that disasters have long-lasting and significant effects can be important for planners and educators seeking to address these concerns.

Discussion of Planning, Training, and Mitigation Techniques

A discussion of planning, training, and mitigation techniques might include a survey and discussion related to bioterrorism training for emergency medicine residents.[34] These papers document current education and planning methodologies and are useful in two ways. First, they provide a benchmark for the schemes in place that can be compared with outcome when an event occurs. If a system has a plan in effect, with specific training methods and specific techniques, readiness (as measured in a well-run drill or an actual event) can be compared with alternative systems. Second, these papers serve to distribute the ideas, good and bad, that others have developed. Planners should be familiar with this literature and should seek to learn from the mistakes and brilliant insights of others as they design training and response plans.

Trials of Specific Techniques or Equipment

Although fairly rare in the disaster research literature, trials of specific techniques or equipment present various methodologies for care and use of equipment. Topics such as triage technique, categories of patient condition, patient identification tags, communications equipment,

training programs in specific scenarios or problems, and command structures fall into this literature category. A weakness of many of these papers is failure to document use of the topic item (method, equipment, etc.) in a real event or in a controlled series of drills where it can be realistically compared with an alternative. Papers that tout the utility of an item and offer only a single drill designed to showcase the item should be scrutinized carefully and critically.

Organizational or Analytical Schemes

Organization and analytical schemes discuss progress in disaster management, or lack thereof, and offer schemes or suggestions to improve international coordination, planning focus, funding allocation, etc.[35] They often report the collective wisdom of a group of experts, but occasionally offer the scheme of a single person. In either case, this body of literature should be familiar to all disaster researchers and educators because a certain level of standardization and commonality in definitions and language is essential to collaborative effort.

Randomized Controlled Trials

Vanishingly rare in disaster research, randomized controlled trials are nonetheless very important. The potential to perform research on recurring disasters (e.g., floods, earthquakes, certain transportation disasters) exists, and a few researchers have attempted to gather data comparing use of techniques or equipment with some degree of randomization.

Currently, the most feasible option is the use of recurring drills to conduct research. The Rhode Island Disaster Initiative (RIDI), a federally funded disaster research project that began in 1999, included a series of disaster drills performed in a high-fidelity multiplace simulation center. The ability to accurately reproduce a disaster drill allowed the RIDI team to compare training and equipment practices between randomized responder groups. Future initiatives should move this type of research into formal research formats, such as crossover control or randomized trial models.

REFERENCES

1. Snow J. *On the mode of communication of cholera.* London: John Churchill, 1855:38-55. Available at: http://www.ph.ucla.edu/epi/snow/snowbook2.html.
2. Yoho DR Jr. Wireless communication technology applied to disaster response. *Aviation Space Environ Med.* 1994 Sep;65(9):839-45.
3. Vardi A, Levin I, Berkenstadt H, et al. Simulation-based training of medical teams to manage chemical warfare casualties. *Isr Med Assoc J.* 2002;4(7):540-4.
4. Berkenstadt H, Ziv A, Barsuk D, et al. The use of advanced simulation in the training of anesthesiologists to treat chemical warfare casualties. *Anesth Analg.* 2003;96(6):1739-42.
5. Rhode Island Disaster Initiative Web site. Available at: http://www.ridiproject.org.
6. Kobayashi L, Shapiro MJ, Suner S, et al. Disaster medicine education: the potential role of high fidelity medical simulation in mass casualty incident training. *Med Health RI.* 2003;86(7):196-200.
7. Beier K, Freer JA, Levine H, and the Medical Readiness Trainer Team. An immersive virtual reality platform for medical education: intro-

duction to the Medical Readiness Trainer. *Proceedings of the 33rd Hawaii International Conference on System Sciences (HICSS-33)*, 2000. Available at: http://csdl.computer.org/comp/proceedings/hicss/2000/0493/05/04935025.pdf.

8. Lombard M, Ditton T. At the heart of it all: the concept of presence. *J Computer-Mediated Commun*. 1997;3(2). Available at: http://www.ascusc.org/jcmc/vol3/issue2/lombard.html.

9. University of Michigan 3-D Lab. CAVE Technology Demonstration Disaster Scenario Web site. Available at: http://um3d.dc.umich.edu/index.html.

10. University of Michigan Virtual Reality Laboratory at the College of Engineering. Medical Readiness Trainer Web site. Available at: http://www-vrl.umich.edu/mrt.

11. Leu MC, Hilgers MG, Agarwal S, et al. Training in virtual environments for first responders. *Proceedings of the 2003 ASEE Midwest Section Meeting*. Rolla: University of Missouri–Rolla, 2003. Available at: *http://campus.umr.edu/venom/publications/Leu_ASEE_midwest_meeting'03_paper_(TACOM).pdf.*

12. Gamberini L, Cottone P, Spagnolli A, et al. Responding to a fire emergency in a virtual environment: different patterns of action for different situations. *Ergonomics* 2003;46(8):842-58.

13. Suner S, Williams K, Shapiro M, et al. Effect of personal protective equipment (PPE) on rapid patient assessment and treatment during a simulated chemical weapons of mass destruction (WMD) attack [abstract]. *Acad Emerg Med*. 2004;11(5):605.

14. Kyle RR, Via DK, Lowy RJ, et al. A multidisciplinary approach to teach responses to weapons of mass destruction and terrorism using combined simulation modalities. *J Clin Anesth*. 2004;16(2):152-8.

15. Kobayashi L, Shapiro M, Hill A, Jay G. Creating a MESS for enhanced acute care medical education and medical error reduction: the multiple encounter simulation scenario [abstract]. *Acad Emerg Med*. 2004;11(8):896.

16. Kyle RR, Via DK, Lowy RJ, et al. A multidisciplinary approach to teach responses to weapons of mass destruction and terrorism using combined simulation modalities. *J Clin Anesth*. 2004;16(2):152-8.

17. Kobayashi L, Shapiro M, Hill A, Jay G. Creating a MESS for enhanced acute care medical education and medical error reduction: the multiple encounter simulation scenario [abstract]. *Acad Emerg Med*. 2004;11(8):896.

18. Vardi A, Levin I, Berkenstadt H, et al. Simulation-based training of medical teams to manage chemical warfare casualties. *Isr Med Assoc J*. 2002;4(7):540-4.

19. Berkenstadt H, Ziv A, Barsuk D, et al. The use of advanced simulation in the training of anesthesiologists to treat chemical warfare casualties. *Anesth Analg*. 2003;96(6):1739-42.

20. The Chaim Sheba Medical Center at Tel Hashomer. Israel Center for Medical Simulation Web site. Available at: http://eng. sheba.co.il/main/siteNew/index.php?page=45&action=sidLink&stId=435.

21. Rhode Island Hospital Medical Simulation Center. Simulation Training in Emergency Preparedness (STEP) course Web site. Available at: http://www.lifespan.org/services/simctr.

22. Texas Engineering Extension Service Emergency Services Training Institute (TEEX-ESTI). EMS operations and planning for weapons of mass destruction course Web site. Available at: http://www.teex-esti.com/course_catalog_course.cfm?courseID=159&cid=535&pid=505,535.

23. U.S. Army. 91W Healthcare Specialist Web site. Available at: http://www.cs.amedd.army.mil/91w.

24. RTI International. Simulation Technologies for Advanced Trauma Care (STATCare) Web site. Available at: http://www.rti.org/page.cfm?objectid=3F6A5676-FEF7-423F-92479553E912FB73.

25. U.S. Army Medical Department. Nuclear Biological Chemical Casualty Training System (NBCCTS) software Web site. Available at: http://www.cs.amedd.army.mil/simcenter/NBCCTS.htm.

26. U.S. Army. Camp Shelby Medical Company Training Site Chemical, Biological, Radioactive, Nuclear & Explosive (CBRNE) Training Web site. Available at: http://www.ngms.state.ms.us/mcts/page9.html.

27. MedSMART Inc. International and Distance-Enabled Offerings: U.S. And Global Range Operations. Available at: http://www.med-smart.org/services.html.

28. Research, Development and Engineering Command (RDECOM) Web site. Available at: http://www.globalsecurity.org/military/agency/army/rdec.htm.

29. U.S. Army Program Executive Office for Simulation, Training, and Instrumentation. Combat Trauma Patient Simulator (CTSP) program Web site. Available at: http://www.peostri.army.mil/products/CTPS.

30. Gordon JA, Tancredi D, Binder W, et al. Assessing global performance in emergency medicine using a high-fidelity patient simulator: a pilot study [abstract]. *Acad Emerg Med*. 2004;10(5):472.

31. Vardi A, Berkenstadt H, Levin I, et al. Intraosseous vascular access in the treatment of chemical warfare casualties assessed by advanced simulation: proposed alteration of treatment protocol. *Anesth Analg* 2004;98(4):1753-8.

32. Jernigan J, Stephens D, Ashford D, et al. Bioterrorism-related inhalational anthrax: the first 10 cases reported in the United States. *Emerg Infect Dis*. 2001;7(6):933-44.

33. Williams A. Lessons learned from transportation disasters [unpublished thesis, MPH program] Cambridge, Mass: Harvard University; 1995.

34. Pesik N, Keim M, Sampson TR. Do US emergency medicine residency programs provide adequate training for bioterrorism? *Ann Emerg Med*. 1999;34(2):173-6.

35. Sundnes KO, Adler J, Birnbaum ML, et al. Health disaster management: guidelines for evaluation and research in the Utstein style: executive summary. *Prehospital Disaster Med*. 1996;11(2):82-90.

chapter 51

Practical Applications of Disaster Epidemiology

P. Gregg Greenough and Frederick M. Burkle, Jr.

Regardless of whether a prolonged heat wave hits Europe, a spate of hurricanes occur in the southeastern United States, a volcano erupts in the Philippines, or a complex humanitarian emergency continues in Sudan, each type of disaster has a unique epidemiology. Broadly, *epidemiology* refers to the study of the distribution and determinants of health-related states or events in specified populations and the application of this study to managing and controlling health problems. In essence, epidemiology uncovers the way in which specific disasters generate specific predictable patterns of public health effects, usually disease or injury, in dimensions of time, space, or subgroup within a population.[1]

Disaster epidemiology has a role in every aspect of the disaster cycle, including the development of prevention strategies, the assessment of need and targeting of resources during the impact phase, and the measurement of the effectiveness of the disaster response. Every type of disaster can be classified both as a "disease process" and as a "disease generator." Knowing the types of public health effects of a given disaster can guide disaster preparedness efforts. For instance, a population prone to earthquakes will present acutely en masse to emergency departments with fractures, closed head injury, lacerations, and soft tissue injury. Within days, patients may be at risk for complications such as renal failure and wound infection. Long-term effects such as mental health issues and disability will be public health problems well after the event itself. Advanced understanding of a specific disaster's epidemiology can assist disaster managers and organizations in planning for a disaster response and directing critical resources before, during, and after the event. More importantly, disaster mitigation efforts guided by epidemiology can reduce the number of deaths and minimize the burden of disease caused by a given disaster.

Epidemiology plays a role in the developing world where basic healthcare is lacking, preventable infectious diseases are endemic, famine is recurrent, and subsistent-level poverty the norm. High mortality rates can be expected in places where disasters are superimposed on a baseline poor public health infrastructure. Populations displaced by natural or human-generated disasters are at risk for health, food, water, and shelter insecurities.

HISTORICAL PERSPECTIVE

Epidemiology, which once simply concerned itself with infectious diseases and their relation to a population, has evolved over the years to comprise all hazards that affect the public health, including natural and human-generated disasters. The practical application of epidemiology began with the humanitarian assistance during the Nigerian (Biafran) War of the late 1960s and a variety of natural disasters in the 1970s (e.g., Bangladesh cyclone, 1972; Guatemala earthquake, 1976) and 1980s (e.g., Armenian earthquake, 1988).[2,3,4] These events showed that epidemiologic methods could measure and minimize risk, assess the relief effort, describe patterns of morbidity and mortality, and suggest prevention and intervention strategies. To that end, the Center for Research on the Epidemiology of Disasters (CRED) at the University of Louvain in Belgium was created in the early 1970s; today it maintains a global emergency events database (EM-DAT) that provides information on the effects of the nearly 13,000 mass disasters since 1900. The existence of such a database allows for donors, disaster managers, researchers, and policy makers to make comparisons across disaster type and place and analyze vulnerability factors.

Historically, large numbers of humanitarian relief and multilateral agencies with varying degrees of expertise in humanitarian response did not approach the humanitarian response in a unified, coordinated fashion. However, with the advent in the late 1990s of the Sphere Project, a collective effort of humanitarian nongovernmental organizations (NGOs) and the International Federation of the Red Cross and Red Crescent Societies to reach consensus on minimum standards in health, food, nutrition, shelter, water, and sanitation, a common understanding of the role of epidemiology in supporting the public health in disasters emerged.[5]

CURRENT PRACTICE

Epidemiologic studies in disasters need to be proactive, timely, well-designed, and widely disseminated to all organizations involved in all phases of the disaster cycle.

In addition, the epidemiologic method used should be appropriate for the public health issue in question. The following field methodologies are the keys to critical information during all phases of the disaster.

Vulnerability Analyses

The key purpose of vulnerability analyses is to identify populations at risk in an effort to implement preparedness and mitigation efforts as well as establish a baseline from which rehabilitation efforts can be measured. Thus, a variety of stakeholders—from disaster managers to urban planners to insurance representatives—find such information vital to their respective tasks. A more detailed discussion can be found in Chapter 17; the brief mention here is to highlight the role of epidemiology in the analysis.

Vulnerability is defined as the degree to which one's life and livelihood (or that of a population) is at risk by an encounter with a given hazard. The hazard is the potential for a specific harm-causing event which may directly or indirectly affect the population.[6] Vulnerability is not only measured by degree of exposure of the hazard but also by the level of sensitivity and resilience of the population's environment, or what is increasingly being referred to as the *coupled human-environment system*.[7] Changes in a population's environment affect its ability to absorb the shock of the hazard. Factors inherent in the system's ability to absorb the shock and stresses of a given hazard or combination of hazards may include the level of environmental degradation and deforestation present, the degree of urbanization, the population's socioeconomic status, and the types of livelihoods on which the population depends. On a macro level, transnational factors such as global climate change and debt-relief policies or national factors such as types of national land use planning and degree of communication and transportation infrastructure, degree of governmental stability, and adherence to the rule of law all directly contribute to a given population's vulnerability. All of these factors are potential epidemiologic markers in a vulnerability analysis.

Risk perception—the way a population understands the hazards it may be exposed to, its vulnerability related to that hazard, and the probability of a hazard occurring—may require a qualitative study to determine how a population is likely to prepare for and react to such an event. For instance, using a mental model with respondents affected by flooding, researchers from Carnegie-Mellon University found that most knew very little about the direct causes of flooding and how to protect themselves, and they perceived mitigative efforts such as flood insurance to be unwarranted despite a government effort to address those issues.[8] Such methods provide the ability to get at the underlying thought processes of an at-risk population. Qualitative techniques bring other disciplines into the discourse, such as anthropology, sociology, communications, and social sciences, thus enabling researchers to gain insight into how and why things work in a population and to improve the ability of the population to address its own problems.

Vulnerability analyses can draw from "lessons learned"-type studies in the postdisaster phase. A cohort study of the deaths following the Taiwan earthquake of 1999 showed that people with mental disorders, moderate physical disabilities, or recent hospitalization were the most vulnerable.[9] Similarly, women and elderly groups were found to be at higher risk of injury during the 1994 earthquake in Northridge, California. Those who lived in mobile homes during the 1978 Wichita Falls, Texas, tornado had a significantly higher risk of injury or death.[10] In populations at high risk for a given hazard, applied quantitative epidemiology can identify vulnerable groups for targeted interventions before the next disaster.

Rapid Assessments and Needs Evaluations

The cornerstone of epidemiology's role in disasters is during the response itself. The epidemiologic methods of rapid assessments, surveys, and surveillance should parallel the emergency response. The outcome measures of these methods are termed *indicators*—the quantitative or qualitative criteria used to correlate or predict the value or measure of a program, system, or organization—tools used to inform and guide decision-making during the crisis and beyond.[11] A few examples of general indicators are listed in Box 51-1.

BOX 51-1 COMMON INDICATORS IN RAPID ASSESSMENT

Demographics
- Vulnerable group identification

Health
- Morbidity and mortality rates
  - Crude mortality
  - Under-5 mortality
  - Cause-specific attack
    - Diarrheal illness
    - Acute respiratory infection
    - Malaria (in non-immune)
    - Measles
- Measles immunization coverage

Nutrition
- Global acute malnutrition ($-2\ z$ score weight for height)
- Macronutrient intake
  - Energy (kcal/day)
  - Protein (% of total energy)

Food Security
- Household access

Water and Sanitation
- Quantity (liters/person/day)
- Quality (fecal coliforms/100 ml)
- Household access
  - Distance to source
  - Source/population

Shelter
- Area per person
- Fuel availability (kg/household/day)

Rapid assessments answer the primary questions of "what has happened" and "what is needed"?[12] In the chaos of the moment, multiple agencies will be attempting to get solid information for decision-making and coordination, and information sharing among various agencies will be critical. Often these assessments out of necessity will be "quick and dirty," depending on the nature and timing of the disaster and the need to have information readily available. More important is for public health providers with expertise in field epidemiology to be able to use the right type of epidemiologic tool for the right information. A variety of sources from a variety of methods will allow for the triangulation of data, where multiple sources of information can lend verification to each other—a "cross-checking" reference point. Bradt and Drummond[13] propose an assessment tool containing a "minimum essential data set" of health information that will be uniformly understood and used by all stakeholders partially or entirely. Similar assessment indicators can be found in a number of field-tested resources (Box 51-2).

Rapid assessments are used to examine the situation and the needs, ideally within the first several days of the impact. In so doing, public health providers determine the magnitude of the emergency by characterizing and quantifying the affected population; they identify existing and potential public health problems; they measure present and potential impact, especially health and nutritional needs; they assess resources needed, including availability and capacity of a local response; they aid in planning and guiding an appropriate external or international response; they identify vulnerable groups; and they provide baseline data from which the public health system can be restored.[14] Often it is the *indirect* effects of a disaster, the subsequent migration of populations, separation from food supplies, and destruction of public health infrastructure that eventually cause the greatest mortality and morbidity. After the Asian tsunami of December 26, 2004, a rapid assessment in the six affected provinces of Thailand identified a 1.7 times greater increase in the incidence of diarrheal illness and a significant increase in wound infections compared with normal.[15] Because Hurricane Charley in August 2004 devastated several counties on Florida's Gulf Coast having a large concentration of older adults, the U.S. Centers for Disease Control and Prevention (CDC) and Florida Department of Health performed a rapid assessment of households with adults over 60 years of age who were found to have disruption in medical care for chronic medical conditions.[16]

Rapid assessments and their interpretations critically depend on reliable population denominators. The *count* refers to the absolute number of a population in a specific area in a specific period of time. First-world countries will have background demographic statistics of the population before the disaster strikes, but less developed places or areas with migrating populations may have inexact or nonexistent numbers. Global sources such as the World Health Organization, CRED, Epicentre, or the CDC are sources of information and publications that include *baseline data* on endemic diseases, baseline mortality rates, morbidity incidence rates, nutritional status, sources of healthcare, and the level of health service disruption by past disasters (Table 51-1). Other non-health sources of population data include the U.S. Central Intelligence Agency (CIA)'s *World Factbook,* which provides individual country profiles on infrastructure and government, maps, and census data.

In almost all cases, an effort at population reconnaissance must be made to determine the numbers of affected persons relative to the entire population. Fly overs using aerial photography, satellite images linked to geographic information systems, mapping strategies, or drive- or walk-throughs using handheld global positioning system receivers are typically done to get a rough idea of absolute numbers and degree of devastation. Using multiple approaches allows for the triangulation of population numbers.

Denominators are necessary to calculate a *rate*, the frequency of an event (usually morbidity or mortality) in a population in a specific period of time. Crude rates are calculated for an entire population, whereas specific rates are computed for a specific subgroup of the population. Specific rates highlight vulnerable groups and may be age specific, sex specific, occupation specific, and so on. Death rates are one of the most sensitive indicators of the success (or failure) of emergency relief efforts. Crude mortality rates (CMR), also known as crude death rates (CDR), reflect deaths within a population over a period of time:

$$\text{CMR} = \frac{\text{Number of deaths in time period}}{\text{Total population at mid-period}} \times \frac{K}{\text{Number of days in time period}}$$

where K is a uniform constant by which rates or proportions can be multiplied for purposes of comparison and easy understanding—usually a multiple of 10 (such as 1000, 10,000, or 100,000). CMRs are usually expressed during the emergency phase in deaths per *10,000* population per *day*. CDRs are employed after the health crisis of the impact has passed and are expressed as deaths per *1000* population per *year*. For either figure, the formula for calculation is the same and the underlying rate does not differ.

The consensus among humanitarian agencies is that successful humanitarian relief programs should aim for a

BOX 51-2 RESOURCES FOR ASSESSMENTS

WHO, 1999	Rapid Health Assessment Protocols for Emergencies
UNHCR	*Handbook for Emergencies,* 2nd ed
Médicins Sans Frontiéres, 1997	Refugee Health
Sphere Project, 2004	Humanitarian Charter and Minimum Standards in Disaster Response
Office of Foreign Disaster Assistance	Field Operations Guide
EpiCentre	Rapid Health Assessment of Refugee or Displaced Populations

WHO, World Health Organization; *UNHCR,* United Nations High Commission for Refugees.

TABLE 51-1 RESOURCES FOR BASELINE PUBLIC HEALTH INDICATORS

ORGANIZATION	WEB SITE	MISSION
Center for Research on the Epidemiology of Disasters	http://www.cred.be	• Maintains the EMDAT disaster database • Promotes disaster education and training activities through applied research • Links disaster epidemiology with policy and programming
U.S. Centers for Disease Control and Prevention	http://www.cdc.gov	• Publish Morbidity and Mortality Weekly Reports • Research and document emerging infectious diseases
World Health Organization	http://www.who.int	• Monitor disease burden • Provide tools for research and assessment • Maintain mortality database • Offer geographic information tools
Pan American Health Organization	http://www.paho.org	• Provide baseline health indicators (Western Hemisphere)
EpiCentre	http://www.epiet.org/institutes/Epicentre.htm	• Monitor health trends • Maintain CRID (Regional Disaster Information Center) disaster database
Measure DHS	http://www.measuredhs.com	• Provide National Demographic and Health Surveys
U.S. Central Intelligence Agency World Factbook	http://www.cia.gov/cia/publications/factbook	• Document population and environment data • Monitor governmental structures, communications, transportation • Monitor current political issues

CMR at or below twice the population's baseline (pre-disaster) CMR. A doubling of the baseline rate defines a humanitarian disaster and immediate response. The average baseline CMR in the least developed countries is 0.38 deaths/10,000 persons/day; in developed countries it is 0.25 deaths/10,000 persons/day.[17] A robust system of recording births and deaths as well as a registration system for displaced populations are needed for accurate denominators. This baseline will serve as the foundation by which agencies and disaster managers can follow the trends of mortality and morbidity over time, the function of a surveillance system (see Chapter 37).

Age- and sex-specific death rates—the under-age-5 mortality rate (U5MR) is a frequently used example—are used in emergencies to identify subgroups particularly at risk during the disaster and to further clarify the information buried in the CMR figures. Because young children are a vulnerable group in a disaster, a rise in death rates among children younger than 5 years of age is a warning indicator of significant public health disturbance. Similar to the CMR calculation, the U5MR uses the number of deaths in children younger than 60 months of age over a time interval divided by the total population of children younger than 5 years at the middle of that time period:

$$\text{USMR} = \frac{\text{Number of U.S. deaths in time period}}{\text{Total U.S. population at mid-period}} \times \frac{K}{\text{Number of days in time period}}$$

This is expressed in terms of under 5 deaths per 10,000 population per day (during the emergency phase) or per 1000 population per month (in the postemergency phase). U5MR and CMR are the most commonly used mortality indicators during a disaster.

The causes of specific mortality rates can identify the common causes of death during the emergency. Aside from the mortal injury caused by the disaster itself, the developing world often suffers mortality from diarrheal diseases, measles, acute respiratory infections, malnutrition, and malaria. To be rapid and efficient while maintaining accuracy, uniform simple case definitions (as opposed to laboratory confirmations) should be used in such settings to classify cases. Cases classified by standard case definitions are the numerator with the other components of the formula similar to the previous mortality rate calculations:

$$\text{Cause-specific MR} = \frac{\text{Number of deaths from specific cause in time period}}{\text{Total population at mid-period}} \times \frac{K}{\text{Number of days in time period}}$$

Cause-specific mortality rates can target interventions: if the incidence of deaths from diarrheal illness is high, then a focus on water, sanitation, and hygiene will be most important.

Various causes of injury morbidity vary according to the disaster type. However, infectious diseases are common in all disasters that disrupt the public health infrastructure. The five diseases mentioned above, along with meningitis, should not be missed during a rapid assessment. Interviewing health workers, reviewing clinic records, or directly observing households are techniques to determine the incidence and prevalence of a disease. *Incidence* refers to the number of new cases of a disease that occur during a specific time period; *prevalence* is the number of cases present in the population at the time of assessment.[18] As the emergency phase passes into the postemergency phase, secondary wound infections, acute exacerbations of chronic diseases, and mental health issues add to the burden of the disease in the disaster-affected population.

Participatory Appraisals

In an effort to enhance the role of the affected population in the decision-making process during the response and reconstruction, researchers use participatory methods. Typically these are qualitative unstructured interviews with key informants, persons specifically selected because of their unique role in the community. Such respondents provide insight into the dynamic of the affected community or group, its interpretation of its environment, level of migration, needs, behaviors, and attitudes. Mental health issues require this kind of participatory ethnographic approach. Assessment teams take a listener/observer role. Relatively simple, inexpensive, and fast, participatory appraisals provide subjective nongeneralizable data that often require alternative methods for confirmation. Group interviews can generate "problem trees," a participatory exercise that identifies problems and their root causes.

Surveys: In-Depth Sectoral Assessments

A survey involves a more in-depth study compared with a rapid assessment, usually by means of a detailed study design that employs a sampling methodology and relies on observations, interviews, or questionnaires to yield data on a specific aspect of the disaster. That data undergoes a formal analysis and interpretation. Surveys are used for "one-off" assessments of a given sector (e.g., shelter), subpopulation (e.g., children younger than 5 years), or public health problem (e.g., acute malnutrition). In general, a survey should be used when greater precision is needed to make informed decisions.

Nutritional surveys are the common example. Since undernutrition rates are associated with *excess mortality* from complications of preventable illnesses such as diarrhea, measles, malaria, and acute respiratory infections, it is imperative to determine the level of acute malnutrition within the disaster-affected population. The severity of acute malnutrition in young children is expressed as a *z* score—that difference between the weight-for-height ratio for an individual child and the median value of the population of children divided by the standard deviation of the population. The measure of greatest interest is that segment of the population below −2 *z* score termed *global acute malnutrition,* or *wasting.* Finding the prevalence of wasting within the population of children requires the systematic measuring of weight and height—in essence, a probability sample.

A *sample* is that subset of a population that represents the population well enough to make inferences about it. A sample may be one of two types: a probability sample or nonprobability sample. The former uses random selection to minimize inherent bias, ensuring that each person within the population has an equal chance of being selected; the latter implies that samples are chosen subjectively by the researcher. Nonprobability sampling is quick and easy because it does not require a full listing of the population. If a public health worker wanted to know the prevalence of crush injury after an earthquake to determine the amount of supplies needed, he could visit clinics. However, this nonprobability sample would miss those in the population who still may suffer crush injury but could not make it to a health facility. Thus, nonprobability sampling makes it difficult to measure the level of uncertainty of the results. More often, a probability sample complete with a sampling frame is needed to answer the research question appropriately. *Sampling frames* are full listings of the population as persons or households arranged in units of analysis. Invariably such sample surveys are more expensive (and may be prohibitive in the setting of low resources), demand time (when often an answer is needed immediately), and require a certain level of training (often not found in developing countries).

In addition to nutritional indicators, surveys are commonly used in disasters to measure level of food security, immunization coverage, prevalence of mental health problems, access to clean water, household use of water, hygiene practices, level of infrastructure damage, shelter density, and livelihood disruption, among many other areas of interest. Because they require expertise, planning, and time, surveys are done on any given area of interest usually as a "one-off" event, a snapshot in the disaster response continuum. To adequately follow indicators of interest in real time, a more flexible, rapid, and simple tool should be used.

Surveillance

Monitoring the mortality and morbidity indicators mentioned above, observing for epidemic outbreaks, and monitoring trends in endemic diseases is the role of surveillance in the emergency phase. As the disaster response transitions from the emergency phase to the postemergency and rehabilitation phases, trends in key indicators will measure the effectiveness of the relief efforts. The role of a surveillance system and its applications are discussed in Chapter 37.

PITFALLS

Each epidemiologic method has its drawbacks. Vulnerability analyses fail when they don't take into account all the factors that contribute to the structure of the human environment, particularly the knowledge, attitudes, and behaviors of the population at risk. Rapid needs assessments continue to suffer from lack of common shared indicators between donor agencies, NGOs, and international organizations. Mortality rates may be inappropriately inflated or deflated if the population estimates are not accurate. Respondents may easily introduce biases in participatory appraisals, for example, exaggerating the needs of the community knowing that the interviewer will likely have access to outside resources or, because of mistrust or pride, will minimize the needs. Bias is also inherent in nonprobability sample surveys; critical errors can result when such samples are generalized to a population. Since the humanitarian response depends on each of these methods, it is critical that they are used correctly and appropriately.

REFERENCES

1. Binder S, Sanderson LM. The role of the epidemiologist in natural disasters. *Ann Emerg Med.* Sep 1987;16:1081-84.
2. Sommer A, Mosley WH. East Bengal cyclone of 1970: epidemiological approach to disaster assessment. *Lancet* 1972;1(7759):1029-36.
3. deVille deGoyet C, del Cid E, Romero A, et al. Earthquake in Guatemala: epidemiologic evaluation of the relief effort. *Bull Pan Am Health Organ.* 1976;10(2):95-109.
4. Armenian HK, Melkonian A, Noji EK, et al. Deaths and injuries due to the earthquake in Armenia: a cohort approach. *Int J Epidemiol.* 1997;26:806-13.
5. The Sphere Project: Humanitarian Charter and Minimum Standards in Disaster Response. Available at: http://www.sphereproject.org.
6. World Health Organization. *Community Emergency Preparedness: A Manual for Managers and Policy-makers.* Geneva: World Health Organization; 1999.
7. Turner BL, Kasperson RE, Matson PA, et al. A framework for vulnerability analysis in sustainability science. *Proc Natl Acad Sci U S A.* 2003;100(14):8074-9.
8. Lave TR, Lave LB. Public perception of the risks of floods: implications for communication. *Risk Analysis.* 1991;11(2):255-67.
9. Chou YJ, Huang N, Lee CH, et al. Who is at risk of death in an earthquake? *Am J Epidemiol.* 2004;160(7):688-95.
10. Glass RI, Craven RB, Bergman DJ, et al. Injuries from the Wichita Falls tornado: implications for prevention. *Science* 1980;207:734-8.
11. Spiegel PB, Burkle FM, Dey CC, et al. Developing public health indicators in complex emergency response. *Prehospital Disaster Med.* 2001;16(4):281-5.
12. Robinson WC. *Demographic Assessment in Disasters: A Guide for Practitioners.* Baltimore: Center for International Emergency, Disaster & Refugee Studies, Johns Hopkins Bloomberg School of Public Health. In press.
13. Bradt DA, Drummond CM. Rapid epidemiological assessment of health status in displaced populations: an evolution toward standardized minimum data sets. *Prehosp Disast Med.* 2003;17(4):178-85.
14. Burkle FM. The epidemiology of war and conflict. In: Cahill JD, ed. *Bioterrorism and Complex Emergencies.* New York: Springer Press; submitted for publication.
15. Centers for Disease Control and Prevention. Rapid health response, assessment, and surveillance after a tsunami—Thailand, 2004-2005. *MMWR.* Jan 2005:54(3):61-4.
16. Centers for Disease Control and Prevention. Rapid assessment of the needs and health status of older adults after Hurricane Charley—Charlotte, DeSoto, and Hardee Counties, Florida, August 27-31, 2004. *MMWR.* 2004:53(36);837-40.
17. The Sphere Project. *The Humanitarian Charter and Minimum Standards in Disaster Response.* Geneva: 2004.
18. Gordis L. *Epidemiology.* 2nd ed. Philadelphia: WB Saunders; 2000.

chapter 52

Measures of Effectiveness in Disaster Management

Frederick M. Burkle, Jr. and P. Gregg Greenough

Measures of effectiveness (MOEs) are operationally quantifiable management tools that provide a means for measuring effectiveness, outcome, and performance (including success or failure) of disaster management.[1,2] The foundation units or elements for developing MOEs are found in indicators used to assess, monitor, and evaluate services provided by disaster relief agencies and organizations.[3] Most importantly, MOEs have the capability to serve as an integration performance tool that speaks to the disaster timeline or critical pathway and allows for the horizontal crossing of sector and professional boundaries that may influence both policy decisions and the operationalizing of policy.[4]

HISTORICAL PERSPECTIVE

MOEs were first used in industry to measure the performance of products.[2] Disaster research and application of MOEs were directed primarily toward disaster sector-specific indicators, such as mortality rates, under-age-5 mortality rates, case fatality rates, and water requirements per person per day, to name but a few.[1] Eventually, multiple indicators were studied to determine the influence of multiagency and multisectoral indicators on overall performance. For example, in Somalia, the military developed over 500 security-related indicators, only a small number of which actually were essential to assessing the success or failure of security on the mission. By applying these security indicators against other humanitarian indicators used by relief agencies and logisticians, a clearer picture was gained as to what might be contributing to or detracting from the performance of the mission. For example, failures to adequately mitigate malnutrition in some geographic sectors were found by MOE analysis to be more related to lack of security and access to aid for the intended recipients of care rather than lack of supplies delivered to the local warehouses.[2]

CURRENT PRACTICE

Currently, MOEs are used as combined "essential indicators" to gain an overview of management performance and to help define critical pathways (e.g., the multisectoral/agency organizational response), to assess performance, and to define the end state or sustainability of operations. Essential indicators are MOEs as they subsume the essential indicators, often from each sector, into a definable horizontal measure of overall disaster management. As such, they are the quantifiable language of a critical pathway that disaster managers follow, initially on an hourly and subsequently daily basis, to ensure that management requirements are being met.[3] If expected requirements are not met across the management timeline, this becomes a *negative variance* that must be investigated as to the cause and solved as soon as possible. Also, there may be an unexpected improvement or acceleration of the disaster response timeline that becomes a *positive variance,* which may eventually alter the way the timeline process of management will be defined in future disasters.

Most critical is that MOEs have the capability to unify the language of the disaster event, thereby bringing together the strange bedfellows made up of the varied disaster response agencies and organizations. If disaster organizations agree to share information and work for a common goal, MOEs are a priority in management, evaluation, and monitoring for all concerned, especially the beneficiaries of relief and development.

Whereas MOEs must be quantifiable in nature, this does not exclude semiquantitative or -qualitative indicators that often successfully provide a reliable measure of social, cultural, behavioral, and mental health disaster-related services. To be useful, indicators and the MOEs they support must be defined as precisely as possible, easily understood, reliable, valid, simple, and informative. MOEs must be consistently measurable, cost-effective, sensitive, timely, mission related, and appropriate to the developed critical pathway followed by disaster managers. The key to understanding MOEs and the process by which they are generated lies in (1) the recognition of which indicators are considered essential measures of sector performance; (2) the assessment of the applicability and reliability of these essential indicators and whether they meet usefulness criteria; and lastly (3) the ability of these essential indicators to provide the coordinating language of the timeline or critical pathway specific to the disaster event (Fig. 52-1).

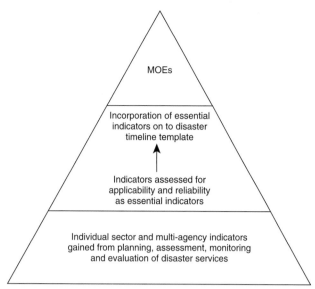

FIGURE 52–1 Measures of effectiveness are based on essential indicators.

MOEs have been applied to complex humanitarian emergencies to study complex multiagency performance as well as in narrowing the field of multiple available indicators in a large-scale bioterrorism event to a workable number of essential indicators that will readily weather management success.[1,2,5] Here the essential indicators that make up the operational MOEs include:

- Measuring response capacity of deployed biologic sensor devices linked to a real-time public health surveillance system;
- Measuring how rapidly a full-coverage health information system is mobilized with timely dissemination of accurate information;
- Measuring variance compliance to a bioagent-specific management timeline;
- Measuring decline in mortality and morbidity;
- Measuring control of transmission rate (Ro) in communicable outbreaks; and
- Measuring management resource distribution across the entire cohort of a vulnerable population.

In this regard, indicators for education of suspected or exposed victims may indeed be useful but may contribute more critically to the knowledge base of more essential indicators such as health information system and decline in mortality and morbidity. If mortality and morbidity is not declining as expected, then the contributing indicators are analyzed for cause.

PITFALLS

The main pitfalls of MOEs are organizational ones. In the heat of a disaster event, they are often neglected or forgotten. It takes some agency leadership to organize a multiagency effort, and although the United Nations (UN) includes MOEs as a need in peacekeeping missions, this is often left to the discretion of the mission commander. That said, the after-action report for UNPRO-FOR, the UN mission to the Former Yugoslavia, criticized the lack of MOEs in the mission planning. The inherent verticality of agencies and organizations in disasters prohibits the horizontal cooperation needed to get MOEs operational. Timelines or critical pathways, although available for natural and chemical disasters management, have not been developed for complex emergencies and large-scale bioterrorism events, the two disasters where they are most needed.

REFERENCES

1. Burkle FM. Complex, humanitarian emergencies: III. measures of effectiveness. *Prehospital Disaster Med*. 1995;10(1):48-56.
2. Dworken JT. *Measures of effectiveness (MOEs) for humanitarian intervention: Restore hope and beyond. Working paper 27.* Washington DC: Center for Naval Analyses; 1993.
3. Spiegel PB, Burkle FM, Dey CC, Salama P. Developing public health indicators in complex emergency response. *Prehospital Disaster Med*. 2001;16(4):281-5.
4. Burkle FM. Complex emergencies: measuring effectiveness across a multitude of indicators. Standardized monitoring and assessment of relief and transition (SMART) workshop. Washington, DC, 26 July 2002. Available at: http://www.smartindicators.org/workshop/agenda2.htm.
5. Burkle FM. Measures of effectiveness in large-scale bioterrorism events. *Prehospital Disaster Med*. 2003;18(3):258-62.

chapter 53

Lessons Learned as a Result of Terrorist Attacks*

Mark E. Keim

The threat of terrorism is a high-priority national security and law enforcement concern in the United States. Modern policy on combating terrorism against the United States has been evolving over the past 30 years. A series of presidential decision directives, implemented guidance, executive orders, interagency agreements, and legislation now provide the basis for counterterrorism programs and activities in more than 40 federal agencies, bureaus, and offices.

Unfortunately, societal reactions and public policy regarding disasters do not always translate into effective outcomes of "lessons learned." Traditionally, after-action studies and reports have been composed of largely anecdotal observations offered by relatively small consensus groups. Although helpful, these methods frequently lack scientific validity. Since most responders (and political policy makers) do not experience a statistically significant number of disaster events themselves, so-called lessons learned often represent the same redundant themes and epiphanies of a relatively novice cohort. In one 2-year comparative study of catastrophes in disaster-prone India, many of the same problems listed as "lessons learned" from one national disaster were only to be repeated just 2 years later and, ironically, were again listed as *lessons learned* in yet another after-action report (Giannone P., personal correspondence, 2004). As another example, remarkable parallels may also be drawn between lessons learned at the Pan American Health Organization Meeting on Evaluation of Preparedness and Response to Hurricanes Georges and Mitch (held over a decade ago)[1] and recent U.S. Government Accountability Office (GAO) reports involving federal and state efforts related to terrorism preparedness.[2-5]

Unfortunately, it has also been the case that even when sound findings are identified within an after-action review, these lessons are "learned" by the group but not implemented into an effective policy. New policies may even become implemented but never validated by real-world experience. And finally, even the best-validated public policies may not be maintained in the absence of an ongoing risk-reduction program.

Terrorism itself has been an age-old threat to the public health and security of many populations throughout the world. During the past three decades, terrorist attacks against the United States have led to a significant number of legislative, regulatory, organizational, and programmatic actions associated with very comprehensive and ambitious expectations. More study is needed before we can conclude to what extent these major changes will have a lasting and significant impact on capacity and capability to deal with future disasters or the practice of disaster medicine as a health science.

Even though the extent of long-term impact remains uncertain, two major accomplishments have become realized: (1) national capacity of emergency management appears to have been increased, and (2) awareness and possibly even commitment to the issue of emergency preparedness also appear to be greater.[6] It would appear that the information and knowledge about what to do in response to the terrorist threat already existed before September 11, 2001. What was lacking was the political backing for change and the political will to act. A rapid series of events involving emergency management and protection of critical infrastructure then followed.

This chapter identifies recent terrorist events that have had a significant impact upon U.S. society and public policy. The discussion correlates these policies with widely accepted doctrines of incident management and disaster risk reduction. From this perspective, these lessons learned represent a recent trend for implementation of what may be more accurately described as already well-established doctrines of disaster medicine and emergency management.

HISTORICAL PERSPECTIVE

Development of Modern U.S. Emergency Management Policy

Modern emergency management policy in the United States began with the "Unlimited National Emergency"

*The material in this chapter reflects solely the views of the authors. It does not necessarily reflect the policies or recommendations of the Centers for Disease Control and Prevention or the U.S. Department of Health and Human Services.

(Proclamation 2487 of May 27, 1941) immediately before World War II. Over three decades later, out of concern for a catastrophic earthquake predicted to occur in the central United States, the Earthquake Hazards Reduction Act of 1977 mandated the development of a Federal Response Plan for a Catastrophic Earthquake. In July 1979, Executive Order 12148 delegated authority to the U.S. Federal Emergency Management Agency (FEMA) to establish federal policies and to coordinate all civil defense and civil emergency planning, management, mitigation, and assistance functions of executive agencies. At this time, FEMA was also assigned the lead responsibility for response to consequences of terrorism. The Robert T. Stafford Disaster Relief Act PL 100-707 was enacted in 1986 to formalize a coordinated federal policy. In 1990, FEMA issued the Federal Response Plan to establish a process for coordinated delivery of federal disaster assistance. After significant criticism of the response to Hurricane Andrew in 1992, Congress adopted a formal *all-hazards approach* to emergency management in the National Defense Authorization Act of 1994, PL 103-160.

In June 1995, President Clinton issued Presidential Decision Directive 39 (PDD 39), the central blueprint for the U.S. counter-terrorism strategy. PDD 39 elaborated a strategy for combating terrorism consisting of three main elements: (1) reduce vulnerabilities and prevent and deter terrorist acts before they occur, (2) respond to terrorist acts that do occur, including managing crises and apprehending and punishing terrorist perpetrators, and (3) manage the consequences of terrorist attacks. All three elements of the strategy include terrorism involving weapons of mass destruction.[7] Emergency managers will recognize these elements as phases of the risk reduction cycle including disaster prevention, mitigation, and response.

The Defense Against Weapons of Mass Destruction Act of 1996, Public Law 104-201, September 23, 1996 (also known as the Nunn-Lugar-Domenici Act), drew on the convergence of federal assets at the Atlanta 1996 Olympic Science and Technology Center[8,9] and directed this momentum to set in place a long-term effort to prepare domestic response for terrorist threats.

Development of Incident Management Systems

The Incident Command System (ICS) was conceptualized more than 30 years ago, in response to a devastating wildfire in California. As a result, Congress mandated that the U.S. Forest Service design a system that would improve wildland fire protection agencies to effectively coordinate interagency action and allocate suppression resources in dynamic situations. This system became known as FIRESCOPE (FIrefighting RESources of California Organized for Potential Emergencies) ICS. Although FIRESCOPE ICS was originally developed to assist in the response to wildland fires, it was quickly recognized as a system that could help public safety responders provide effective and coordinated incident management for a wide range of situations, including

floods, hazardous materials accidents, earthquakes, and aircraft crashes. In 1982, all FIRESCOPE ICS documentation was revised and adopted as the National Interagency Incident Management System (NIIMS). In Homeland Security Presidential Directive-5 (HSPD-5), President Bush called on the Secretary of Homeland Security to develop an NIMS to provide "a consistent nationwide approach for federal, state, tribal, and local governments to work together to prepare for, prevent, respond to and recover from domestic incidents," regardless of cause, size, or complexity.[10]

On March 1, 2004, after close collaboration with state and local government officials and representatives from a wide range of public safety organizations, Homeland Security issued the NIMS guidelines.[10] These incorporate many existing best practices into a comprehensive national approach to domestic incident management and are applicable at all jurisdictional levels and across all functional disciplines or public sectors.

Development of Disaster Risk Reduction Strategies

In 1994, the States Members of the United Nations, having met at the World Conference on Natural Disaster Reduction in the city of Yokohama, Japan, in partnership with nongovernmental organizations and with the participation of international organizations, the scientific community, business, industry, and the media affirmed that "Disaster prevention, mitigation, and preparedness are better than disaster response in achieving the goals and objectives of the Decade. *Disaster response alone is not sufficient, as it yields only temporary results at a very high cost.* We have followed this limited approach for too long. This has been further demonstrated by the recent focus on response to complex emergencies, which, although compelling, should not divert from pursuing a comprehensive approach. *Prevention contributes to lasting improvement in safety and is essential to integrated disaster management*" [emphasis added].[11]

Development of Disaster Medicine

During the late 1980s, disaster medicine began to develop in the United States as a subspecialty of emergency medicine.[12,13] In the 1990s, several disaster medicine fellowships were established and graduated at least six disaster medicine subspecialists. None of these programs received earmarks for federal or state support of disaster medicine. All were closed by the end of the decade.

Recent Terrorist Events That Have Influenced U.S. Policy

The development of new disaster policy is dependent on a society's perception of risk. Public perception of risk is known to be higher immediately after the occurrence of a major disaster. During this time there is a notable window of opportunity for change in disaster-reduction policy. Table 53-1 is a listing of recent terrorist events and their corresponding influence on resultant U.S. policy.

TABLE 53-1 RECENT TERRORIST EVENTS THAT HAVE INFLUENCED U.S. POLICY

DATE	EVENT	DESCRIPTION	SIGNIFICANCE
1984	Bhagwan Rajneesh Salmonella Release	• Salmonella bacteria released in 10 Dalles, Oregon, restaurants • Outbreak linked to Bhagwan Rajneesh religious cult years later • No deaths, over 800 infected	• This was the first large-scale biologic attack in the United States with a high morbidity rate. • For years, this outbreak went largely unrecognized as an intentional event.
1988	Bombing of Pan Am Flight 103	• Parcel bomb detonated on plane while en route from London to New York, explodes over Lockerbie, Scotland • Linked to Libyan Militant Islamic Extremist (MIE) terrorist cell • Killed 270	• In 1989, President George H. W. Bush issued Executive Order 12686, which formed the Presidential Commission on Aviation Security and Terrorism. • President George H.W. Bush signed the Aviation Security Improvement Act of 1990.
1993	World Trade Center (WTC) Bombing	• Truck bomb detonated in the WTC parking garage • Linked to MIE including multiple Arab nationalities. • Killed 6, wounded 1042	• Congress enacted the "National Defense Authorization Act for Fiscal Year 1995, which directed FEMA to: (1) Prepare federal response plans and programs for the emergency preparedness of the United States; and (2) Sponsor and direct such plans and programs to coordinate such plans and programs with state efforts.
1994-1995	Aum Shinrikyo Sarin Attacks	• 1994: Japanese religious cult, Aum Shinrikyo, released sarin nerve agent in a residential area of Matsumoto, Japan. This event killed 7 and injured 500. • 1995: Same group released sarin in the Tokyo subways, killing 12 and injuring hundreds.	• This was the first time that a nonstate group used a chemical weapon against civilians. • Demonstrated how terrorist groups could recruit scientists, obtain deadly chemical or biologic agents, and put plans into action. • President Clinton released PDD 39. • The 1996 Nunn-Lugar-Domenici Act (a.k.a., Defense Against Weapons of Mass Destruction [WMD] Act of 1996) was passed. • In 1997, the Terrorist Annex to the Federal Response Plan was adopted by FEMA. • These events provided evidence of extensively coordinated planning and execution.
1995	Bombing of the Murrah Federal Building in Oklahoma City	• Truck bomb detonated near the Alfred P. Murrah Federal Building in Oklahoma City, Oklahoma. • Linked to U.S. right-wing extremists • Killed 169, injured more than 500	• This was the first instance of large-scale bombing caused by U.S. domestic terrorists. • This was the first use of the President's authority under the Stafford Act to "self-initiate" an emergency declaration for emergencies with federal involvement. • Experts other than foreign policy and security specialists became more involved in terrorist preparedness and response (most notably, disaster medicine). • This event initiated increased awareness of occupational health concerns among disaster responders (most notably, behavioral health).
1995	Chechnyan Threaten to Use Radiologic Dispersion Device (RDD)	• Chechnyan separatists direct news reporter to Moscow park where cesium-137 RDD weapon is found	• First credible threat for use of an RDD (a.k.a. "dirty bomb") by a sub-national group.
1996	Bombing of Lebanon Marine Barracks	• Truck bomb detonated near U.S. military barracks in Lebanon • Linked to MIE	• This event was an asymmetric attack on U.S. military facility by MIE.
1996	Bombing of Khobar Towers	• Truck bomb detonated near U.S. military barracks in Dhahran, Saudi Arabia • Linked to MIE • Killed 19 Americans, injured 500	• This was an asymmetric attack on U.S. military facility by MIE.
1996	Crash of TWA Flight	• Explosion of airliner during takeoff in New York. • Initially believed to be result of a terrorist attack using surface-to-air missile • Later ruled to be accidental	• There was an unprecedented state and federal preparedness activities related to the 1996 Olympic games. • In 1997, the White House Commission on Aviation Safety and Security (Gore Commission) issued a report recommending that "The federal government should consider aviation security as a national security issue and provide substantial funding for capital improvements." • The Department of Homeland Security 2005 budget includes $61 million for the research and development of countermeasures to protect commercial aircraft from shoulder-fired, surface-to-air missiles.

(Continued)

TABLE 53-1 RECENT TERRORIST EVENTS THAT HAVE INFLUENCED U.S. POLICY—Cont'd

DATE	EVENT	DESCRIPTION	SIGNIFICANCE
1996	Bombing of Atlanta Olympic Games	• Occurred within days of the start of the 1996 Olympics • Shoulder-fired surface-to-air missiles were used by MIE to attack aircraft in Kenya, Saudi Arabia, and Iraq during 2003-2004 • Pipe bomb explodes at Centennial Olympic Park, in Atlanta, Georgia, during the ninth day of the 1996 Summer Olympics • Killed one, injured 112	• This bombing occurred during first interagency coordination of federal WMD response teams. • Title XIV of the Defense Authorization Act of 1996, The Defense Against WMD Act (a.k.a. Nunn-Lugar-Domenici Act) was adopted. • The Terrorist Annex to the Federal Response Plan was adopted by FEMA.
1998	U.S Embassy Bombings in Kenya and Tanzania	• Truck bombs detonated simultaneously near U.S. embassies in Nairobi and Dar es Salaam • Linked to MIE, Al-Qaeda terrorist network • Killed 280, injured over 5000	• The first forward staging of a medical stockpile in preparation for WMD casualties was created. • This was the first large-scale attack on U.S. embassies or consulates caused by MIE terrorists. • The event provided evidence of extensively coordinated planning and execution. • The United States responded with cruise missile strikes in Afghanistan and Sudan. • U.S. policy shifted focus toward proactive and global policy that is less constrained about targeting terrorists, their bases, and their infrastructure. • First HHS public health and medical response to overseas terrorism
2000	Attack of the U.S.S. Cole	• Explosion occurred on the destroyer U.S.S. Cole docked at the harbor in Aden, Yemen • Linked to MIE, Al-Qaeda terrorist network • Killed 17, injured 39	• This was the first asymmetric attack on a U.S. naval warship perpetrated by MIE. • The Department of Defense subordinated its terrorism analysis capability under the Joint Chief of Staff/Intelligence. This reduced confusion and clarified responsibility for warning.
2001	WTC and Pentagon Attacks	• Hijacked airliners deliberately flown into WTC towers in New York City and the Pentagon in Washington, DC • Linked to MIE, Al-Qaeda terrorist network • Killed over 3000, injured hundreds	• This attack has had a significant long-term economic impact as well as symbolic significance. • U.S. response included at least 10 pieces of national legislation, two Executive Orders, one Homeland Security Decision Directive, one new federal department (i.e., Department of Homeland Security), and several significant reports. • There was unprecedented speed in the passage of major federal legislation, in absence of Congressional hearings or task forces. • A major reorganization of U.S. intelligence organizational structure occurred in 2004 consistent with recommendations of the 9/11 Commission report.
2001	Anthrax Letter Attacks	• Letters containing anthrax spores mailed to news media personnel and Congress • Leads to the first cases of intentional anthrax infection in the United States • Infections follow a 3-year history of over 1500 anthrax letter hoaxes. • Perpetrators remain at large • Killed 5, infected 18	• This event was the second-largest-scale biologic attack in the United States and had the highest mortality rate. • Reports cited speculation regarding U.S. domestic origin of terrorism. • The challenges and shortcomings facing the nation's public health system were revealed. • The Federal Concept of Operations Plan (CONPLAN) for responses to terrorist attacks was not used. • The FBI did not exercise its crisis management authority, nor did FEMA exercise consequence management authority as called for by PDD 39. • The Federal Response Plan was never activated.
2002-2004	Bombings and attacks in Russia, Indonesia, Philippines, Kenya, Saudi Arabia, Afghanistan, Iraq, and Spain	• A series of terrorist bombings and attacks involving numerous nations • Most attacks are linked to MIEs and some to national separatist movements • Most events kill a few to several hundred victims	• These events illustrated MIE tactics for attacks against broader pro-Western interests. • Events related to national separatist movements revealed a growing level of sophistication in coordination and execution of attacks. • Nations other than the United States became frequent targets.
2004	Attack on US Consulate in Jeddah, Saudi Arabia	• A car bomb detonation and subsequent small arms attack of the US consulate in Jeddah, Saudi Arabia. • Linked to MIE, possibly Al-Qaeda	• Recent U.S. activities resulting in hardening and increasing security of U.S. embassies and consulates proved valuable in mitigating the impact of the attack

CURRENT PRACTICE AND LESSONS LEARNED

Lessons learned as result of recent terrorist attacks can be divided into two main categories: those involving a trend toward a more comprehensive disaster risk reduction strategy (Table 53-2), and those building capacity for more effective models of incident management (Table 53-3).

PITFALLS

Homeland Security and Emergency Management Remain Poorly Defined

Although a new homeland security emphasis is under way throughout the federal government, the process is still evolving. Additional actions to clarify missions and activities will be necessary, and some agencies will need to determine how best to support both homeland security and nonhomeland security missions.[14] Many people are not clear on just what homeland security is and how it is in fact quite different from all-hazard emergency management. People tend to use the terms *homeland security* and *emergency management* synonymously.

The extent to which the homeland security mission is displacing the natural and technologic disaster function is also an important question. Related to this question is the degree to which extensive experience in natural hazards has been leveraged (or ignored) in the new reality of homeland security.

The Need for an All-Hazard Strategic Approach and National Strategy

According to WL Waugh in 2000, "For the most part, policies and programs have been instituted and implemented in the aftermath of a disaster, based almost solely on that disaster experience, and with little investment in capacity building to deal with the next disaster."[15]

After the events of September 11, 2001, national legislation was enacted and organizational changes occurred in the absence of any hearings or studies being ordered to determine what went wrong and what remedies were needed. Another unusual characteristic of the aftermath of this disaster was the speed with which the major federal organizational and coordination changes occurred, even before Congressional hearing or special task forces were formed.[16]

Because the drafters of Public Health Security and Bioterrorism Preparedness Act (June 12, 2002), Public Law 107-188, "did not have detailed information as to how other federal response plans operated or were designed to operate, the statute tends to encourage stove-piping of information, planning and response by the medical community." Additionally, the principal assets of the medical community, including personnel and institutions, are private; therefore, statutory mandates are difficult to apply.[16]

The first step toward disaster risk reduction involves adopting a strategic national approach. The first annual Gilmore report (REF) to the President and the Congress of the Advisory Panel explored a broad range of issues regarding weapons of mass destruction and details of actual terrorist attacks. The report formulated several initial policy recommendations, one of which included "the need for a national strategy to address domestic response to terrorism."[17] The second annual Gilmore report re-sounded the alarm in 2000, stating, "The United States needs a functional, coherent national strategy for domestic preparedness against terrorism."[18]

Comprehensive disaster risk-reduction measures include prevention, mitigation, response, and recovery phases. Recent terrorist attacks have driven emergency management policy toward prevention, preparedness, and mitigation as the most cost-effective interventions. However, these three pre-event disaster risk-reduction activities and programs remain underdeveloped for natural disasters in the United States.

The Need for National Threat and All-Hazard Risk Assessment

According to a Government Accountability Office report in 2001, "The first step toward developing a national strategy is to conduct a national threat and risk assessment."[2] By 1999, a national-level risk assessment of potential chemical and biologic terrorist incidents had not yet been performed.[19]

A *risk assessment* is a decision-making process that is used to estimate risk and then to establish requirements and priorities. The components of risk assessment include asset and loss impact assessment, threat assessment, and vulnerability analysis.[20] Comprehensive risk management strategies involve risk assessment, cost-benefit analysis, risk communication, and risk-reduction activities.

The Department of Justice and the Federal Bureau of Investigation (FBI) have collaborated on such an assessment, but as of September 2001, they had not formally coordinated with other departments and agencies on this task.[2]

Many conflicting statements have been made in public testimony before Congress and in the press concerning the risk of dissemination of a chemical or biologic agent on U.S. soil.[6] The Centers for Disease Control and Prevention (CDC), in partnership with other military and civilian federal governmental organizations, has developed a list of priority agents for biologic warfare.[21] The intelligence community has recently produced National Intelligence Estimates and other high-level analyses of the foreign-origin terrorist threat that include judgments about the more likely chemical and biologic agents that would be used.

In the Homeland Security Act of 2002, Congress required the Homeland Security Department to implement a system for analyzing information on terrorist threats. The Terrorism Threat Integration Center was announced in February 2003 and is housed within the Central Intelligence Agency, serving as a central repository for all government intelligence information. However, this repository does not integrate significant

TABLE 53-2 DISASTER RISK REDUCTION LESSONS LEARNED AS A RESULT OF RECENT TERRORIST EVENTS

LESSON	REPORTS AND FEDERAL ACTIONS
Need for a comprehensive and coordinated disaster risk-reduction strategy	**REPORTS AND RECOMMENDATIONS** • Seiple C. Consequence management: domestic response to weapons of mass destruction. *Parameters.* 1997;Autumn:119-34. • Gilmore Report I: Identified as the "need for national strategy to address domestic response to terrorism." December 15, 1999. • GAO-01-14, *Combating Terrorism: Federal Response Teams Provide Varied Capabilities; Opportunities Remain to Improve Coordination.* November 30, 2000. • Gilmore Report II: Restated "The US needs a functional coherent strategy for domestic preparedness against terrorism." December 15, 2000. • U.S. Commission on National Security/21st Century. Seeking a National Strategy: A Concert for Preserving Security and\Promoting Freedom: The Phase II Report on U.S. National Security Strategy for the 21st Century. April 15, 2000, 17 pp. • GAO-01-822, *Combating Terrorism: Selected Challenges and Related Recommendations,* September 20, 2001. • GAO-01-915, *Bioterrorism: Federal Research and Preparedness Activities,* September 28, 2001. • Gilmore Report III: "Recommended clarifying the role of the military for domestic preparedness against terrorism." December 15, 2001. • GAO-02-893T, *Homeland Security: New Department Could Improve Coordination but May Complicate Priority Setting.* June 28, 2002. • GAO-02-924T, *Homeland Security: New Department Could Improve Biomedical R&D Coordination but May Disrupt Dual-Purpose Efforts.* July 9, 2002. • GAO-02-954T, *Homeland Security: New Department Could Improve Coordination, but Transferring Control of Certain Public Health Programs Raises Concerns.* July 16, 2002. • GAO-03-260, *Homeland Security: Management Challenges Facing Federal Leadership.* December 20, 2002. • GAO-04-100, *Homeland Security: Effective Regional Coordination Can Enhance Emergency Preparedness.* September 15, 2004. • Burkle F, Noji E. Health and politics in the 2003 war with Iraq: lessons learned. *Lancet.* 2004;364(9442):1371; criticized U.S. military-led humanitarian efforts. **FEDERAL ACTIONS** • <THSPD-3: Homeland Security Advisory Supplement, March 2002. • The National Strategy for Homeland Security, July 2002. Available at: http://whitehouse.gov/homeland/book/. • National Security Strategy of the United States, September 2002. Available at: http://whitehouse.gov/nsc/nss.html. • Homeland Security Act, November 2002
Need for a comprehensive analytical risk assessment	**REPORTS AND PUBLICATION** • Gilmore Report I. December 15, 1999. • GAO/NSIAD-98-74, *Combating Terrorism: Threat and Risk Assessments Can Help Prioritize and Target Program Investments.* April 9, 1998. • GAO/NSIAD-99-163, *Combating Terrorism: Need for Comprehensive Threat and Risk Assessments of Chemical and Biological Attacks.* September 7, 1999. • GAO-01-822, *Combating Terrorism: Selected Challenges and Related Recommendations.* September 20, 2001. • Keim M, Intentional Chemical Disasters. In: Hogan D, Burstein J, eds. *Disaster Med.* Philadelphia, Pa: Lippincott, Williams & Wilkins; 2002. **FEDERAL ACTIONS** • Requirement that Department of Homeland Security assess vulnerabilities to and risk of terrorist attacks, promulgated March 2003.
Importance of prevention as a critical component of risk reduction	**REPORTS** • Report of the White House Commission on Aviation Safety and Security (Gore Commission), February 12, 1997. • Gilmore Report III. December 15, 2001. • Report of the 9/11 Commission July 25, 2004. **FEDERAL ACTIONS** • Presidential National Security Decision Directive 138, *Preemptive Strikes Against Terrorists.* April 3, 1984. • Aviation Security Improvement Act of 1990, Public Law 101-604. November 16, 1990. • Cruise missile strikes against Al-Qaeda site in Afghanistan and Khartoum chemical factory, August 1998. • Airport Security Improvement Act of 2000, Public Law 106-528. November 22, 2000. • The U.S.A. Patriot Act, Public.Law 107-56. October 26, 2001. • Authorization for Use of Military Force Against Iraq Resolution of 2002. October 2002. • Enhanced Border Security and Visa Entry Reform Act, Public Law 107-173. May 14, 2002. • Maritime Transportation Security Act, Public Law 107-295. November 25, 2002. • Homeland Security Act of 2002, Public Law 107-296. November 25, 2002. • CIA Terrorism Threat Integration Center. Announced in February 2003. • HSPD-10: Biodefense for the 21st Century. April 28, 2004, initiates U.S. Bioshield program

(Continued)

TABLE 53-2 DISASTER RISK REDUCTION LESSONS LEARNED AS A RESULT OF RECENT TERRORIST EVENTS—Cont'd

LESSON	REPORTS AND FEDERAL ACTIONS
Importance of mitigation as a critical component of risk reduction	**REPORTS** • Critical Foundations: Protecting America's Infrastructure, President's Commission on Critical Infrastructure Protection, 1997. • Gilmore Report III. December 15, 2001. • GAO-01-822, *Combating Terrorism: Selected Challenges and Related Recommendations.* September 20, 2001. • GAO-030165, *Combating Terrorism: Interagency Framework and Agency Programs to Address the Overseas Threat.* May 23, 2003. **FEDERAL ACTIONS** • Presidential Decision Directive/NSC-63, May 22, 1998. • Executive Order 13130, National Infrastructure Assurance Council, 3 CFR, 1999 Comp., p. 203, July 14, 1999. • Executive Order 11211, Critical Infrastructure Protection in the Information Age, 3 CFR, 2001 p. 805, October 16. 2001. • National Strategy for Protection of Critical Infrastructure and Key Assets, February 2003. • National Strategy to Secure Cyberspace. April 2003. • HSPD-7: Critical Infrastructure Identification, Prioritization, and Protection. December 2003.
Importance of preparedness as a critical component of risk reduction	**PUBLICATIONS AND REPORTS** • Sharp T, Brennan R, Keim M, et al. *Medical preparedness for a terrorist incident during the Atlanta Olympics. Ann Emerg Med.* 1998;32:214-23. • GAO/HEHS/AIMD-00-36, *Combating Terrorism: Chemical and Biological Medical Supplies are Poorly Managed.* October 29, 1999. • Gilmore Reports I-IV. December 1999 – December 2002. • GAO-02-141T, *Bioterrorism: Public Health and Medical Preparedness.* October 9, 2001. • GAO-02-149T, *Bioterrorism: Review of Public Health Preparedness Programs.* October 10, 2001. • GAO-03-373, *Bioterrorism: Preparedness Varied across State and Local Jurisdictions.* April 7, 2003. • GAO-03-924, *Hospital Preparedness: Most Urban Hospitals Have Emergency Plans but Lack Certain Capacities for Bioterrorism Response.* August 6, 2003. • Keim M, Pesik N, Twum-Danso N. Lack of hospital preparedness for chemical terrorism in a major US city: 1996-2000. *Prehospital Disaster Med.* 2003;18(3):193-9. • GAO-04-152, *Bioterrorism: Public Health Response to Anthrax Incidents of 2001.* October 15, 2003. • GAO-04-360R, *HHS Bioterrorism Preparedness Programs: States Reported Progress but Fell Short of Program Goals for 2002.* February 10, 2004. • A National Public Health Strategy for Terrorism Preparedness and Response 2003-2008 prepared by the Centers for Disease Control and Prevention, the Agency for Toxic Substances and Disease Registry, and the Department of Health and Human Services. March 2004. **FEDERAL ACTIONS** • HSPD-3: Homeland Security Advisory System, March 2002. • HSPD-5: Management of Domestic Incidents, March 2003. • National Strategy for Integrated Public Warning Policy and Capacity, May 2003. • HSPD-8: National Preparedness, December 2003. • Reorganization of the CDC, 2003-2004.
Importance of response and recovery as a critical component of risk reduction	**REPORTS** • GAO/NSIAD-97-254, *Combating Terrorism: Federal Agencies' Efforts to Implement National Policy and Strategy.* September 26, 1997. • Gilmore Reports I-IV. December 1999 – December 2002. • GAO-01-822, *Combating Terrorism: Selected Challenges and Related Recommendations.* September 20, 2001. • GAO-03-578, *Smallpox Vaccination: Implementation of National Program Faces Challenges.* April 30, 2003. • GAO-04-239, *U.S. Postal Service: Better Guidance Is Needed to Ensure an Appropriate Response to Anthrax Contamination.* September 9, 2004. • GAO-04-152, *Bioterrorism: Public Health Response to Anthrax Incidents of 2001.* October 15, 2003. **FEDERAL ACTIONS** • PPD 67 of October 21, 1998, Ensuring Constitutional Government and Continuity of Government Operations. • CDC Public Health Bioterrorism Preparedness Cooperative Agreement, 2002-2004. • HRSA National Hospital Bioterrorism Preparedness Cooperative Agreement, 2002-2004. • Homeland Security Act, November 2002. • HSPD-5: Management of Domestic Incidents, March 2003.

TABLE 53-3   INCIDENT MANAGEMENT LESSONS LEARNED AS RESULT OF RECENT TERRORIST EVENTS

INCIDENT MANAGEMENT FUNCTION	REPORTS AND FEDERAL ACTIONS
Command and control	**REPORTS** • Gilmore Report I. December 15, 1999. **FEDERAL ACTION** • Presidential National Security Decision Directive 30, Managing Terrorism Incidents, April 10, 1982. • Executive Order 12656 of November 18, 1988, Assignment of Emergency Preparedness Responsibilities, 3 CFR, 1988 comp. p. 585. • HSPD-5: Management of Domestic Incidents, March 2003.
Logistics	**PUBLICATIONS AND REPORTS** **Supply Chain Management** • GAO/HEHS/AIMD-00-36, *Combating Terrorism: Chemical and Biological Medical Supplies are Poorly Managed.* October 29, 1999. • GAO-02-141T, *Bioterrorism: Public Health and Medical Preparedness.* October 9, 2001. • GAO-02-149T, *Bioterrorism: Review of Public Health Preparedness Programs.* October 10, 2001. • GAO-03-924, *Hospital Preparedness: Most Urban Hospitals Have Emergency Plans but Lack Certain Capacities for Bioterrorism Response.* August 6, 2003. **Communications** • Executive Order 12472 of April 3, 1984, Assignment of National Security and Emergency Preparedness Telecommunications Functions, 3 CFR, 1984, comp. p. 193. • Gilmore Report I. December 1999. • GAO-03-139, *Bioterrorism: Information Technology Strategy Could Strengthen Federal Agencies' Abilities to Respond to Public Health Emergencies.* May 30, 2003. • Executive Order 13311 of July 29, 2003, Homeland Security Information Sharing. **Occupational Safety and Health** • New York Department of Health, Data Snapshot: Understanding The Health Impact Of 9/11. Available at: http://www.nyc.gov/html/doh/downloads/pdf/wtc/wtc-report2004-1112.pdf. New York, 2004. • Centers for Disease Control and Prevention. Self-reported increase in asthma severity after the September 11 attacks on the World Trade Center—Manhattan. MMWR. *2002;51(35):781-4.* • GAO-04-239, *U.S. Postal Service: Better Guidance Is Needed to Ensure an Appropriate Response to Anthrax Contamination.* September 9, 2004. • GAO-03-578, *Smallpox Vaccination: Implementation of National Program Faces Challenges.* April 30, 2003. • Lillibridge SR, Sidell FR. *A report on the casualties from the Tokyo subway incident by the US medical team.* Atlanta, Ga: Centers for Disease Control and Prevention; 1995. • Okumura T, et al. Report on 640 victims of the Tokyo subway sarin attack. *Ann Emerg Med.* 1996;28(2):129-35. **FEDERAL ACTIONS** • CDC National Pharmaceutical Stockpile Program established in 1998. Changed to DHS Strategic National Stockpile in 2002 • HPSD-8: National Preparedness; supported ongoing development and adoption of appropriate first responder equipment standards that support nationwide interoperability. • DHS Launches Office of Interoperability and Compatibility in 2004. • OSHA Best Practices for Hospital-Based First Receivers of Victims, December 2004. Available at: http://www.osha.gov/dts/osta/bestpractices/html/hospital_firstreceivers.html.
Operations	**PUBLICATION AND REPORTS** • Pesik N, Keim M. Do emergency medicine residency training programs provide adequate training for bioterrorism? *Ann Emerg Med.* 1999;34(2):173-6. • Keim, M, Kaufmann A. Principles of emergency response to bioterrorism. *Ann Emerg Med.* 1999;34(2):177-82. • GAO-01-14, *Combating Terrorism: Federal Response Teams Provide Varied Capabilities; Opportunities Remain to Improve Coordination.* November 30, 2000. • Gilmore Report III. December 2001; reinforced the need to support medical first responders. **FEDERAL ACTIONS** • In 1996, Department of Health and Human Services establishes Metropolitan Medical Response System (MMRS). • MMRS moved to Department of Homeland Security in 2003. • In 2004, Department of Homeland Security awards American Medical Association $1 million grant for development of Disaster Life Support training for medical professionals.

(Continued)

TABLE 53-3 INCIDENT MANAGEMENT LESSONS LEARNED AS RESULT OF RECENT TERRORIST EVENTS—Cont'd

INCIDENT MANAGEMENT FUNCTION	REPORTS AND FEDERAL ACTIONS
Intelligence/Planning	**REPORTS** • Report of the 9/11 Commission, July 25, 2004. **FEDERAL ACTIONS** • Intelligence Authorization Act for Fiscal Year 2003, Public Law 107-306. November 27, 2002. Administration/Finance • Reorganization of US Intelligence Community, 2004. **REPORTS** • GAO-03-170, *Combating Terrorism: Funding Data Reported to Congress Should Be Improved.* November 26, 2002. **FEDERAL ACTIONS** • Emergency Supplemental Appropriations: Response to Terrorist Attack on September 11, 2001, Public Law 107-38. September 18, 2001. • In August 2002, the Supplemental Appropriations Act for Further Recovery from and Response to Terrorist Attacks in the U.S. contained grant requirements for funding at the state and local levels. • Department of Defense and Emergency Supplemental Appropriations for Recovery from and Response to Terrorist Attacks on the United States, Public Law 107-117, January 10, 2002,. • 21st Century Department of Justice Appropriations Authorization Act, Public Law 107-273. November 2, 2002. • Terrorism Risk Insurance Act, Public Law 107-297. November 25, 2002. • Department of Homeland Security Appropriations Act, Public Law 108-90. October 1, 2003.

information regarding natural and technologic disaster hazards, other than terrorism.

The Need for Improved Coordination Among Federal Agencies

Beyond a national strategy, substantial progress has been made in completing operational guidance and related plans to coordinate agencies. Congress and the President both have recognized the need to review and clarify the structure for overall leadership and coordination.[2] A number of previous GAO recommendations that the federal government complete interagency operational guidance have been implemented. Progress also has been made by some individual agencies that have completed or are developing internal plans and guidance.[2]

According to a 2001 Government Accountability Office report, "However, coordination of federal terrorism research, preparedness, and response programs is fragmented, raising concerns about the preparedness of states and local units to respond to a bioterrorist attack."[22] Concerns also include insufficient state and local planning and a lack of hospital participation in training on terrorism and emergency response planning.[22]

Inherent challenges remain in managing federal programs and resources to combat terrorism. First, numerous federal agencies have some role in combating terrorism. Second, these federal agencies represent different types of organizations, including those involved in intelligence, law enforcement, military matters, health services, environmental protection, emergency manage-

ment, and diplomacy. Another challenge in coordinating budgets to combat terrorism is that funding for these programs is also used for missions unrelated to terrorism.[23]

The Need for Improved Civilian-Military Coordination

PDD 39 of 1995 established an early model for what would become the watershed event for U.S. federal coordination of civilian and military counter-terrorism efforts during the 1996 Atlanta Olympics.[9,24] The 1996 Defense Against Weapons of Mass Destruction Act provided that after 3 years the function could be transferred from the U.S. Department of Defense to some other lead agency with the President's approval. The transfer was made to the Department of Justice in 1999, and the Office of State and Local Domestic Preparedness became the lead. Both FEMA and this organization are now part of the Department of Homeland Security.

In 2000, the second annual Gilmore report recommended clarifying the role of the military in domestic terrorism response.[18] In 2004, Burkle and Noji[25] also cited difficulties involving coordination of civilian and military assets during war in Iraq.

The Need for Improved Regional Coordination

Strategic plans developed by regional organizations can be effective tools to focus resources and efforts to address problems. Given the important role that regional planning and governance can play in improving national preparedness, these developments warrant continuing Congressional oversight.[26]

Occupational Health and Safety Are Critical to Effective Disaster Response

During the anthrax emergency of 2001, nine postal employees associated with two postal facilities that processed tainted letters contracted anthrax, and two employees died. According to a 2004 Government Accountability Office report, "The response to anthrax contamination revealed several lessons, the most important of which is that agencies need to choose a course of action that poses the least risk of harm when considering actions to protect people from uncertain and potentially life-threatening health risks."[27] The World Trade Center attack of 2001 also resulted in a very high occupational health risk to workers.[28,29]

Coordination of Public Information Is a Formidable Challenge

During the anthrax emergency, from October 8 to 31, 2001, the CDC's emergency response center received 8860 telephone inquiries from a wide cross section of society in all 50 states, the District of Columbia, Puerto Rico, Guam, and 22 foreign countries. While local and state officials reported that the CDC's support of their responses to the rapidly unfolding anthrax incidents at the local and state levels was generally effective, the CDC acknowledged that it was not fully prepared for the challenge of coordinating the public health response across the federal agencies. The CDC experienced difficulty serving as the focal point for communicating critical information during the response, and spokespersons for the agency described having to create an ad hoc emergency response center in an auditorium from which to manage the federal public health response, which involved numerous agencies. The CDC also had difficulty managing the influx of information to produce and disseminate guidance rapidly and had difficulty conveying information to the media and public.[5]

Interoperability and Robust Methods of Communication Are Difficult to Maintain

The need for common, agreed-upon standards is widely acknowledged in the health community, and activities to strengthen and increase the use of applicable standards are ongoing. Despite ongoing efforts to address information technology (IT) standards, many issues remain to be worked out, including coordinating the various standards-setting initiatives and monitoring the implementation of standards for healthcare delivery and public health. An underlying challenge for establishing and implementing such standards is the lack of an overall strategy guiding IT development and initiatives.[30]

U.S. Preparedness Varies from State to State

The anthrax incidents during the fall of 2001 raised concerns about the nation's ability to respond to bioterrorist events and other public health threats. Several months after the incidents, the U.S. Congress appropriated funds to strengthen state and local bioterrorism preparedness. However, preparedness varies significantly from state to state.[31]

In 2002, the U.S. Department of Health and Human Services' CDC and Health Resources and Services Administration distributed US$1 billion in funds through two cooperative agreement programs with state, municipal, and territorial governments. States reported progress toward the CDC programs' goals of strengthening public health preparedness but identified factors that hindered them from meeting all of the CDC's 2002 cooperative agreement requirements. All states reported progress in developing the capacities the CDC considers critical for public health preparedness, but no state completed all program requirements.[32]

Disaster Policy and Plans Are Not Always Followed

The anthrax incidents of 2001 required an unprecedented public health response. These biologic attacks on the nation not only affected our government, but also revealed the challenges and shortcomings facing the nation's public health system.

It is important to note that during the anthrax emergency, neither the Federal Response Plan nor the federal Concept of Operations Plan (CONPLAN) for responses to terrorist attacks was used. Under the CONPLAN, the FBI and FEMA play major roles as the lead agencies for crisis management and consequence management, respectively. Although the FBI was very heavily involved in the source letter investigations, the FBI did not exercise its crisis management authorities. FEMA did not serve as the federal lead for consequence management.[6]

New Policies May Result in an Infringement of Civil Liberties of U.S. Citizens

The mandate of increased intelligence gathering and surveillance of U.S. citizens has been met with concerns regarding civil rights, and privacy rights in particular. Some aspects of the USA Patriot Act of 2001 have also been criticized for infringement on civil liberties. Another controversial action of the post-9/11 era was the so-called Carnivore program to intercept cell-phone and Internet transmissions, which still exists in some form despite Congressional efforts to limit or end it.

Repeated Threat Advisories May Result in "Warning Fatigue"

HSPD-3: Homeland Security Advisory System was designed to provide an effective means to disseminate information regarding the risk of terrorist acts to federal, state, and local authorities and the American people by providing warnings in the form of a graduated set of "Threat Conditions" that change as the risk changes. Federal departments and agencies implement their "Protective Measures" when there is a change in the status of the warnings.

The warning system has been criticized regarding both its cost and effectiveness. Most importantly, the Threat Condition assignment from the beginning was designed to be based on a qualitative assessment, not quantitative calculation. Higher conditions are to reflect both probability and consequences.

Lack of Hospital Preparedness and the Myth of Surge Capacity

Despite large expenditures to promote hospital preparedness over the past 8 years, there remain significant gaps in surge capacity as well as basic capabilities related to bioterrorism.[33,34]

The Science and Practice of Disaster Medicine Remain Underdeveloped

Despite all of the recent sociopolitical awareness of the unique and critical mix of disaster management and emergency medicine, disaster medicine remains to date largely underdeveloped as a medical subspecialty. Increased awareness and extensive federal funding for public health and medical preparedness and response have translated into a broadened involvement of postgraduate academia. But, disaster medicine has not matured into subspecialty board or certification status of medicine or public health.

REFERENCES

1. *Meeting on Evaluation of Preparedness and Response to Hurricanes Georges and Mitch, 16-19 February 1999, Santo Domingo, Dominican Republic. Conclusions and Recommendations,* Washington, DC: Pan American Health Organization; 1999.
2. Government Accountability Office. *Combating Terrorism: Selected Challenges and Related Recommendations (GAO-01-822).* Washington, DC: GAO; 2001.
3. Government Accountability Office. *Homeland Security: Management Challenges Facing Federal Leadership (GAO-03-260).* Washington, DC: GAO; 2002.
4. Government Accountability Office. *Homeland Security: New Department Could Improve Coordination but May Complicate Priority Setting (GAO-02-893T).* Washington, DC: GAO; 2002.
5. Government Accountability Office. *Bioterrorism: Public Health Response to Anthrax Incidents of 2001 (GAO-04-152).* Washington, DC: GAO; 2003.
6. Rubin C, Cumming W, Tinmalli R, et al. *Major Terrorism Events and Their U.S. Outcomes (1998-2001).* Arlington, Va: Claire Rubin & Assoc.; 2003.
7. Government Accountability Office. *Combating Terrorism: Federal Agencies' Efforts to Implement National Policy and Strategy (GAO/NSIAD-97-254).* Washington DC: GAO; 1997.
8. Ember LR. FBI takes lead in developing counter terrorism effort. *Chemical & Engineering News.* November 4, 1996:10-16.
9. Sharp T, Brennan R, Keim M, et al. Medical preparedness for a terrorist incident during the Atlanta Olympics. *Ann Emerg Med.* 1998;32:214-23.
10. Homeland Security Presidential Directive 5: Management of Domestic Incidents. February 28, 2003. Available at: http://www.whitehouse.gov/news/releases/2003/02/20030228-9.html.
11. Yokohama Strategy and Plan of Action for a Safer World: Guidelines for Natural Disaster Prevention, Preparedness and Mitigation. World Conference on Natural Disaster Reduction Yokohama, Japan, 23-27 May 1994. Available at: http://www.unisdr.org/eng/about_isdr/bd-yokohama-strat-eng.htm.
12. SAEM Disaster Medicine White Paper Subcommittee. Disaster Medicine: Current Assessment and Blueprint for the Future. *Acad Emerg Med.* 1995;(2)12:1068-76.
13. Waeckerle JF, Lillibridge SR, Burkle FM, Noji EK. Disaster medicine: challenges for today. *Ann Emerg Med.* 1994;23:715-8.
14. Government Accountability Office. *Homeland Security: Management Challenges Facing Federal Leadership. 20 Dec. 2002 (GAO-03-260).* Washington, DC: GAO; 2002.
15. Waugh WL. *Living with Hazards, Dealing with Disasters: An Introduction to Emergency Management.* Armonk, NY: ME Sharpe; 2000.
16. Rubin C, Cumming W, Tinmalli R, et al. *Major Terrorism Events and Their U.S. Outcomes (2002-2003).* Arlington, Va: Claire Rubin & Assoc.; 2004.
17. Gilmore JS, et al. First Annual Report to The President and The Congress of the Advisory Panel To Assess Domestic Response Capabilities for Terrorism Involving Weapons Of Mass Destruction—I. Assessing The Threat, December 15, 1999. Available at: http://www.rand.org/nsrd/terrpanel/terror.pdf.
18. Gilmore JS, et al. Second Annual Report of the Advisory Panel to Assess Domestic Response Capabilities for Terrorism Involving Weapons of Mass Destruction—II. Toward a National Strategy for Combating Threat. December 15, 2000. Available at: http://www.rand.org/msrd/terrpanel/terror2.pdf.
19. Government Accountability Office. *Combating Terrorism: Need for Comprehensive Threat and Risk Assessments of Chemical and Biological Attacks (GAO/NSIAD-99-163).* Washington, DC: GAO; 1999.
20. Keim M. Intentional chemical disasters. In: Hogan D, Burstein J, eds. *Disaster Medicine.* Philadelphia: Lippincott, Williams & Wilkins; 2002.
21. Centers for Disease Control and Prevention. Biological and chemical terrorism: strategic plan for preparedness and response. Recommendations of the CDC Strategic Planning Workgroup. *MMWR.* 2000;49(RR-4):5-6.
22. Government Accountability Office. *Bioterrorism: Federal Research and Preparedness Activities (GAO-01-915).* Washington DC: GAO; 2001.
23. Government Accountability Office. *Combating Terrorism: Funding Data Reported to Congress Should Be Improved (GAO-03-170).* Washington DC: GAO; 2002.
24. Seiple C. Consequence management: domestic response to weapons of mass destruction. *Parameters.* 1997;Autumn:119-34.
25. Burkle F, Noji E. Health and politics in the 2003 war with Iraq: lessons learned. *Lancet.* 2004;364(9442):1371-75.
26. Government Accountability Office. *Homeland Security: Effective Regional Coordination Can Enhance Emergency Preparedness. (GAO-04-1009).* Washington DC: GAO; 2004.
27. Government Accountability Office. *U.S. Postal Service: Better Guidance Is Needed to Ensure an Appropriate Response to Anthrax Contamination. (GAO-04-239).* Washington DC: GAO; 2004
28. New York Dept of Health. Data Snapshot: Understanding the Health Impact of 9/11. Available at: http://www.nyc.gov/html/doh/downloads/pdf/wtc/wtc-report2004-1112.pdf.
29. Centers for Disease Control and Prevention. Self-reported increase in asthma severity after the September 11 attacks on the World Trade Center. *MMWR.* 2002;51(35):781-4.
30. Government Accountability Office. *Bioterrorism: Information Technology Strategy Could Strengthen Federal Agencies' Abilities to Respond to Public Health Emergencies (GAO-03-139).* Washington, DC. GAO; 2003.
31. Government Accountability Office. *Bioterrorism: Preparedness Varied across State and Local Jurisdictions (GAO-03-373).* Washington, DC: GAO; 2003.
32. Government Accountability Office. *HHS Bioterrorism Preparedness Programs: States Reported Progress but Fell Short*

of Program Goals for 2002 (GAO-04-360R). Washington, DC: GAO; 2004.

33. Keim M, Pesik N, Twum-Danso N. Lack of hospital preparedness for chemical terrorism in a major US city: 1996-2000. *Prehospital Disaster Med*. 2003;18(3):193-9.

34. Government Accountability Office, *Hospital Preparedness: Most Urban Hospitals Have Emergency Plans but Lack Certain Capacities for Bioterrorism Response (GAO-03-924)*. Washington, DC: GAO; 2003.

chapter 54

The Psychology of Terrorism

Robert A. Ciottone

Terrorism is an elusive term to define, one that seems "far too nimble a creature for social science to be able to pin it down in anything like a reliable manner...."[1] Experientially, however, terror has a shared and familiar meaning within everyone's frame of reference. The origins of those feelings may be recent or they may be remote and only dimly recalled under the usual conditions of everyday life. Nevertheless, every individual within a population either is or has been the child who fears monsters lurking in places that cannot be seen clearly. Because of the universality of such experiences, feelings of terror remain potentially resurgent for every person.

Terrorists seek to destabilize population groups by a variety of means. One method is to resurrect through their actions the primitive and enveloping fears associated with the sense that "monsters" may act unpredictably and with impunity. Further, terrorists seek to imbue the destabilizing impact of such events for both individuals and for societal institutions with sustained, destructive energy. Although terrorist-driven occurrences are temporally circumscribable, the psychological effect of terrorism is more a process than an event. A host of factors conspire to perpetuate the psychologically destabilizing effect of terrorism long after a focal event has occurred. These include uncertainty about the potential for and the possible timing of renewed attacks, disruption of infrastructure upon which many have relied, fears that health services may become overtaxed and unavailable when they are most needed, and concern about loved ones in areas presumed to be particularly vulnerable.

Problematic psychological reactions to destructive terrorist-driven occurrences are not restricted to individuals who directly witness the event or who are affected by it in a relatively direct manner. Indeed, "media coverage of major terrorist events tends to be intense, capturing acute suffering and vulnerability. Unlike fictional stories, it portrays actual events and is sometimes unedited. And it produces the images of death and destruction that instill fear and intimidation in the larger public."[2] At the very least, the psychological effects of disastrous events can severely tax the ability of those affected to function with a level of efficiency that characterized their pre-event baseline.[3] Moreover, erosion of that efficiency may persist for many months and perhaps much longer, particularly with regard to incidence rates of psychiatric dysfunction and/or of stress-related physical illness within an affected population.

HISTORICAL PERSPECTIVE

Terrorism has been defined as violence involving attacks on a small number of victims in order to influence a wider audience.[4] Much that has been written about the psychology of terrorism has centered on the emotions, motivations, cognitions, and other aspects of the psychological profile of those who would perpetrate such violence. As Cooper[5] noted, "The true terrorist must steel himself against tender-heartedness through a fierce faith in his credo or by a blessed retreat into a comforting, individual madness." If the presumed gift of a wooden horse that secretly held in its belly attackers who were bent on surprise and violence qualifies by this definition, the roots of terrorism stretch back through antiquity. More recently, in the centuries from the Middle Ages to the Industrial Revolution, warfare was conducted according to an implicit code of rules that sought in its most caricatured instances to render military conflict a "civilized affair," however much of an oxymoron that phrase might have been even in days past. Eventually, international organizations such as the League of Nations and later the United Nations came about in part out of a need to hold conflict within some bounds, even if it could not be eliminated entirely. Further, the Geneva Convention sought explicit agreement to rules of conduct on the part of potential adversaries before conflict had even emerged.

The goals underlying such efforts have proved elusive at best. As Crenshaw[6] noted, "Significant innovations" in terrorism occurred in 1968 with the onset of relatively routine diplomatic kidnappings and hijackings involving extortion or blackmail. The pattern of increase in terrorist activity since that time, and to the present has been all too familiar. Silke[1] has strongly argued the importance of researching this phenomenon with all of its implications. Having reviewed the literature, however, Silke,[7] like Merrari[8] before him, found that systematic inquiry by psychologists and psychiatrists fell short of what seemed to be needed.

Notwithstanding the importance of inquiry into factors related to the development of individual and group manifestations of terrorism, the focus here is on its psychological effect on the affected population who will look to emergency medicine for care. The goal of this chapter is to consider psychological factors related to the effect of terrorism on a population. Although some specific guidelines may be derived from a conceptualization of that sort, the purpose is rather to develop an awareness of psychologically contextual issues that may productively inform, although not necessarily direct, the judgments and decisions of service providers functioning in a terrorist-driven circumstance.

CURRENT PERSPECTIVES

First responders and caretakers are clearly among those in the population who can be affected most directly by terrorist events. Not only do they share in the danger of feeling overwhelmed and in the risk for problematic reactions, they also bear the expectations of others to remedy what might seem to be an impossible situation at times. Further, they share with those to whom they provide services the need that the toll taken by terrorism upon them be monitored and managed. The alternative—of implicitly adopting the false notion that first responders and medical practitioners are somehow above the psychologically harmful effect of terrorism or immune to it—invites multiple problems that have the potential of proliferating because of their effect on the service function. Accordingly, in the context of responding to terrorism, one of the imperatives for emergency medicine personnel must be to attend to the psychological needs of peers and of subordinates. For them, the sustained nature of the problem can exact a toll far exceeding the accustomed demands of providing emergency care.

Although the psychological effect of terrorism for both individuals and societal institutions can be considered in its various aspects, an over-arching concept would provide coherence to considerations that might otherwise seem scattered. One such conceptually unifying theoretical perspective is the *orthogentic principle*, a holistic developmental notion first articulated by Werner[9] and later by Wapner and Werner.[10] Essentially a *meta-theoretical* notion, the orthogenetic principle was subsequently elaborated by Wapner,[11-13] and by Kaplan, Wapner, and Cohen.[14] Briefly stated, that principle holds that *all that occurs through development proceeds from the global and diffuses through increasing states of differentiation and hierarchic integration*. In this context, "development" is not temporally defined nor is it tied to chronometry. Instead, the principle applies to any developmental phenomenon ranging, for example, from the microgenesis of thought behind each word spoken to the experience of an overall self-world relationship throughout the life span.

Through the prism of the orthogenetic principle, the developmental continuum from diffuse through integrated is conceived of as a dynamic one within the context of which is the potential for developmental advance (toward increased integration) and/or de-differentiation (regression to a more primitive developmental level). Movement forward (developmental advance) and/or movement backward (developmental regression) is not a discrete event but an ongoing process. Each advance in the direction of increasing differentiation brings with it the requirement that the parts of experience be hierarchically integrated (i.e., subordination of the differentiated parts to the whole) in a yet more refined fashion. Conversely, de-differentiation leads to a less integrated experience with a correspondingly less refined sense of part-whole and of means-ends relationships and of the instrumentalities available for transacting with the environment thus construed. Developmental advance along that continuum brings with it an increasing sense of mastery, whereas de-differentiation or regression to a more developmentally primitive level invites a growing sense of feeling overwhelmed.

Within that frame of reference, terrorism can be seen as an effort to bring about de-differentiation and correspondingly more developmentally primitive functioning within populations and among the individuals that comprise them. Accordingly, interventions intended to address terrorism and its effects can be characterized as more or less facilitative of developmental advance and, correspondingly, of some increased level of mastery.

Acts of terrorism result psychologically in both direct and indirect destructive consequences of the sort that bring about developmental regression to a relatively less differentiated sense of one's relationship with the surroundings. The direct consequences typically have a powerful immediacy in their effect on the consciousness of affected segments of the population. Those consequences may well prove precipitously de-differentiating in their assault on the sensibilities of those persons who are affected. Indirect effects, on the other hand, can be less apparent, particularly in the immediate aftermath of the disaster, but their destructive influence on the population and upon its institutions may be equally, if not more, disruptive to the functioning of the society.

The orthogenetic principle provides, in effect, a reference point by which to gauge and monitor the psychological harm done by terrorism as well as the potential efficacy of efforts intended to mollify the psychological impact of sudden and disastrous terrorist-driven events. Initially, consideration must be given to the psychological vulnerabilities of individuals and/or of groups with regard to the risk of developmental regression. In other words, what has been the effect of trauma and of related fears upon individuals' cognitive, emotional, and valuative perceptions of and transactions with the physical, interpersonal, and sociocultural aspects of their surroundings? Stated differently, what changes have occurred with regard to what those affected by terrorism know with some confidence about the objects and places in their surroundings, how have their feelings about them changed, and what shifts have occurred in their attaching relative importance or unimportance to those objects and places? Likewise, how have knowing, feeling, and valuing shifted with regard to the interpersonal environment and in relation to their perceived environment of customs, responsibilities, and expectations? Second, how might a particular effort foster developmental advance in these areas? In other words, what is the best way to facilitate movement toward an approximation of pre-event psychological baseline?

The direct effects of terrorism are closely linked to the physical realities of the event (explosions, collapse of buildings or other structures, infectious outbreaks, etc.). According to Shalev,[15] however, traumatic events such as acts of terrorism can also be described according to their psychological dimensions. The two are obviously intertwined. Indeed, as Shalev has also noted, "Shortly after exposure, the traumatic event ceases to be a concrete event and starts to become a psychological event."[15] Physical injuries, often of a mangling and grotesque sort, together with the tragic loss of lives, typically become the signature of the event in the popular mind. Those images serve as a reference both for on-site survivors and, as a result of media coverage, for those who learn of the disaster from a distance. Moreover, such images can quickly become an experiential template onto which both proximate and remote observers project their own sense of vulnerability and/or that of their loved ones. In the context of responding to terrorism, therefore, emergency interventions on behalf of victims as well as the ancillary and administrative procedures established to support them should emphasize not simply the reactive measures taken, but proactively oriented steps as well. The goal is to impart the promise of mastery of the circumstance by conveying some sense that those acting as agents for the well-being of the affected remain able to act on their behalf. By the very nature of terrorism, some of those efforts may have to be shaped on an *ad hoc* basis. Even in that circumstance, however, it is important to establish and maintain an approach that is consistent in both appearance and substance with a relatively differentiated response, rather than one that conveys a global, diffuse, and relatively undifferentiated quality.

The destruction of property and infrastructure, the limits imposed on transportation, and the disruption of communication typically serve to further compound the effect of terrorism on the accustomed behavior patterns of those sectors of society that have been affected directly. In effect, individuals as well as groups and organizations may be severely limited in the use of accustomed instrumentalities that they have habitually used as a means of transacting with their surroundings. Regression to developmental primitivity is a distinct risk for those persons and institutions thus deprived of the tools by which to manage ongoing experience and to meet needs that have been readily satisfied in the past.

Developmental de-differentiation in the wake of terrorist-driven events and the resulting increase in stress that may in turn compromise health can also result from sociological factors. In the past, populations could be expected to unite when confronted with a common foe. Attacks or states of siege were typically seen as the work of "outsiders." As a result, those who comprised the population attacked were the "insiders," united at least to that degree and able to take some measure of comfort from the availability and presumed good will of neighbors. In a terrorist environment, however, there is the distinct danger that neighbors may seem suspect. "Cells" of ter-

rorists may operate anywhere and, as a result, danger may be perceived as potentially stemming even from those who seem to be "insiders" or members of the same targeted population. As a result, the cohesiveness that usually occurs within a population on the heels of an attack may be severely compromised. Further, anyone exhibiting characteristics similar to those associated with the assumed perpetrators of the terrorism may become the object of suspicion, if not attack. Backlash effects can then lead to divisiveness and thereby compound the resulting stress experienced by individuals within the population. Given the demonstrable relationship between stress and health, it is incumbent upon caretakers and service providers to remain mindful of this potential psychosocial complication and to temper their interventions with sensitivity.

These and other direct effects of terrorism can severely tax and compromise the psychological resources and abilities required to cope with the demands of daily living. The resulting de-differentiation would be further compounded if some semblance of pre-disaster infrastructure and service capability is not restored relatively soon after the focal event or if no believable estimation is issued as to when such restoration will occur. Accordingly, an important part of an effective emergency response includes providing accurate information regarding system level plans and prospects for returning to a pre-event baseline of service delivery. Although meeting this requirement of comprehensive care might be subsumed under the principle of providing reassurance, it is important from a developmental perspective that it not be trivialized. Further, it is important that information provided not be false or contrived, particularly since subsequent determination of intentionally misleading facts having been provided would probably compound the psychological damage it may have been intended to relieve.[16] Instead, a straightforward acknowledgement that information is not available is much more helpful, particularly when accompanied by an indication that facts will be sought out and shared when they become known.

Offering reassurance without misleading patients is a concern that applies to all aspects of clinical care. Providing services in response to terrorism is no exception. In fact, by virtue of the sense of the potentially overwhelming danger that seems to linger in the wake of terrorist-driven events, that requirement, particularly when viewed from a developmental perspective, becomes a salient one. To err by presenting patients with excessive ambiguity invites the projection of fears that might be much more extreme than the reality, however harsh. Such projections could well prompt developmental regression in the experience of self-world relationships. On the other hand, the other extreme of seeking to reassure patients by straining the limits of believability cannot only destroy trust and encourage regression, but can also render its future restoration difficult at best. Accordingly, patients' psychological well-being and developmental advance are best served by clinicians relating with honesty tempered by empathic consideration for patients' subjective experience.

Observable instances of terrorism differ in terms of the degree and extent of their physical destructiveness. More circumscribed acts of terrorism such as a bomb being detonated outside a police station or a polling place would obviously have a correspondingly less pervasive and/or less extensive impact on infrastructure and on the operation of societal institutions. Developmental regression, however, remains a danger. Those individuals upon whom the event directly impinges by its actual occurrence or by the fear that its having been threatened was intended to cause might well experience a disruption in their perception of "self–world relationships" and in their ability to manage themselves productively. Their reaction, in other words, could prove analogous to that which would likely occur on a larger scale in the wake of more extensive incidents. Moreover, even those not directly affected by the event could well come to experience themselves as operating in a context of potentially sudden and unexpected hazard such that their actions might well become more tentative and fearful and less purposefully goal oriented.

Indirect, destructive effects of manmade disasters are often subtle and insidious in their erosive effect on the developmental level of functioning of societal institutions as well as on that of the individuals within them. The frequent absence of immediate and overt indications of those effects notwithstanding, disruptions in cognitive, emotional, physical, and behavioral functioning in significant segments of the population can be anticipated in the aftermath of a terrorist event.[16] These may be sustained by lingering (if not growing) fear, and by feelings of helplessness in the face of an unseen and perhaps unidentified perpetrator who may strike again with no warning. The resulting perception of risk represents a strong challenge to the capacity of individuals and of groups to cope with the demands of everyday life with the same level of efficiency that characterized their pre-event behavior. As a result, clinicians may well note that lapses will occur in patients' (as well as in peers' and subordinates') previously accustomed patterns of judgment, decisiveness, establishing and maintaining priorities, and other related psychological functions.

Organizations as well as individuals are likely to experience these changes to varying degrees. Such effects may very well linger for a significant period after the terrorist event. For those in authority to provide supportive oversight of groups assigned various responsibilities therefore takes on an even greater importance than usual.

Indirect effects of a manmade disaster also include a significant increase of pressure upon public health systems for resources and services. Those demands typically occur in two phases. First is an obvious requirement to respond to direct casualties of the disaster. It is necessary, however, to also anticipate a predictable increase in stress-related illness that typically follows such events. In addition to psychiatric reactions such as depression and posttraumatic stress disorder, rates of physical stress-related illnesses also rise when the psychological resources of a population are taxed by trauma.[17] Psychiatric problems, not restricted in their increased incidence to the immediate aftermath of focal terrorist events, tend to increase within a traumatized population about 3, 6, and 18 months after the event. The increased incidence rates of these and of stress-related physical illnesses in particular may well extend much further.[18]

Accordingly, planning for health care within a population exposed to a man-made disaster must adopt a long-term view that takes the continuing effect of trauma on the health of an exposed population into account.

When negligence or incompetence results in death and/or destruction, those who perceive themselves as being at risk from its recurrence are likely to experience emotions ranging from fear and anger to distrust of societal institutions and their stewards. Intentional events of destruction such as acts of terrorism, however, may well have even more disruptive psychosocial effects, both immediate and delayed. Similarly, the devastation wrought by a naturally occurring disaster may be greater in terms of casualties and damage to infrastructure, yet the psychological impact of the terrorist-driven may still prove more extensive. Why is this the case? One reason has to do with perceived intentionality on the part of the potential causal agent of the danger.

A central tenet of most teleologically oriented theoretical perspectives in psychology (including the holistic developmental system of conceptual constructs) is that individuals impose meaning upon their experience and that they transact with the surroundings thus construed.[19] When the source of a seemingly amorphous but apparently present danger is perceived as intentionally malevolent, the safety of self and of others feels particularly at risk. When that potential source of danger is hidden from view and perhaps anonymous as well, feelings of fear and helplessness are further compounded. Moreover, locations usually perceived as safe provide little comfort and do not satisfy the wish to hide in protected places.

It is important to recall that problematic reactions to destructive occurrences are typically not restricted to individuals who directly witness the event. As previously noted, media coverage of events may in some ways leave those who are more distant with an even broader and potentially more de-stabilizing view than is available to those who are closer to the event but whose view of it is less expansive. In either case, the psychological effects can severely tax the ability of those affected to function with a level of efficiency that characterized their pre-event baseline. Further, persons affected by virtue of their relatedness to victims of a disaster and/or by disruption of their relationship with societal systems affected by the disaster (e.g., supply systems for food, water, medical services) may be at extreme risk for problematic reactions. Specifically, they may well be left in an ego-dystonic state of perceived inefficacy, vulnerability, and dysphoria.[20] Those effects can be profound. Indeed, those who remain thus affected for 1 year may not recover.[21]

As noted previously, one consequence of the de-differentiating effect of exposure to critical events upon perception is to reactivate developmentally primitive perceptual tendencies and to vaguely recall fears that were prominent during childhood. The reasons for that frequently evident phenomenon are straightforward. Every individual has, at some time in her or his life, experienced a profound and panic triggering sense of helplessness in the face of what seems to be overwhelmingly threatening. Given the continuing availability of that frame of reference, terrorists who are intent on wreaking havoc and who seem to strike without warning may recall the feelings that perhaps long ago were as overwhelming as they might to the child who was fearful of monsters in the shadows. Just as the child looked to a parent to "put on the light" and check for danger, those affected by a terrorist event look to authorities for reassurance. They seek to put aside their feelings of terror, and, to some degree, to master the ongoing experience to some degree. Moreover, just as the child needed reassurance on more than one occasion, populations look to perceived authorities such as service providers for repeated signals that problems are being addressed.

PITFALLS

Clinicians are, by the nature of their responsibilities, obliged to remain alert to the signs that pressures are giving rise to stress that has the power to potentiate physical illness and/or to retard healing. To be sure, "pressure" and "stress" are often used as interchangeable terms as if they were fully synonymous. To say "I am under stress" carries that implication. In one sense, however, pressure differs from stress in that pressure impinges on people. Stress, on the other hand, can be seen as a quality of the response that is made by individuals trying to manage pressure. The distinction is more than semantic; it is an important one because it implies that some measure of control over stress is possible, independent of the pressures that may operate outside of one's control. The psychological pressures associated with terrorism can obviously be extreme, but an effort needs to be made nonetheless to intervene in ways that, to the extent possible, minimize the extent to which those pressures are translated into stress and thereby into increased vulnerability to related illness.

What might be anticipated when the pressures related to terrorism become pathogenic sources of stress? Among the most frequently occurring, posttraumatic stress disorder (PTSD) represents one very prominent problematic sequellum associated with exposure to terrorism.[22] Those who have been directly exposed to traumatic events are at greatest risk for developing PTSD, particularly if they have experienced physical immobility and/or helplessness while trying to escape; or if they have first-hand experience of the sounds, smells, and images; or if their lives have been permanently altered by the death or injury of a loved one.[23] Among those working in concert with emergency medicine providers, even the anticipation of handling of bodies and body parts after violent death can foreshadow PTSD.[24,25]

The signs of PTSD may include excessive excitability and arousal, emotional numbing, repetitive intrusive memories of the trauma, and a general inability to function with the efficiency that was typical prior to the trauma. From a diagnostic standpoint, PTSD is evident when these and related symptoms persist for at least 1 month and when significant distress results from them (DSM IV). The persistence of symptoms differentiates PTSD from acute stress disorder (ASD), which involves a clinically significant response to trauma similar to that seen in longer-term stress disorders (i.e., at least 2 days but no longer than 4 weeks.[26] The most recent revision

of that diagnostic reference allows for a kind of second-order effect by including affected family members of those who suffered the event directly and emergency workers who responded to their needs as being among those considered potential victims of PTSD.

According to Muldoon,[27] some studies suggest that the distress that foreshadows the development of PTSD in fact may be cumulative in a trans-generational sense. Israeli soldiers for whom one or both parents were holocaust survivors, for example, showed a higher incidence of PTSD.[28] In a potentially related way, children of Vietnam veterans who had experienced particularly high levels of stress in that conflict showed higher levels of behavioral disturbance.[29]

Early warning signs of PTSD include memory disturbances that may involve even previously automatized means-ends and part-whole perceptions and behavior sequences. Additional indicators may include flashbacks and traumatic dreams, episodic presentation of a seemingly dissociated or dazed appearance (e.g., the "thousand mile stare"), the emergence of panic attacks, fears, irritability, and tendencies to "self medicate" (i.e., substance abuse).

Developmental regression as a function of the effect of terrorism may first emerge as somewhat less specific antecedents to the symptoms associated with PTSD and/or with other problematic sequelae. As outlined by the Critical Incident Stress Foundation,[16] the tendencies that become evident when stress begins to take a toll will most likely include disruptions in *cognitive functioning*, such as confused thinking, disorientation, indecisiveness, and difficulty establishing priorities. Difficulties with *emotional functioning* that will most likely become evident may include feeling overwhelmed and unable to manage, extreme anger and/or grief, a pervasively and persistently depressed mood, etc. *Physical functioning* may well reflect problems that include increased blood pressure, increased heart rate, dizzy spells, rapid breathing, etc. Adverse effects on *behavioral functioning* may lead to changes in eating and sleep patterns, interpersonal withdrawal, changes in behavior patterns associated with the activities of daily living, etc.

What are the implications of this aspect of a patient's problematic psychological response for clinicians trying to address the consequences of terrorism? How might the lingering perception of continuing risk from recurrent events be managed? How best to mobilize and direct patients' energies to facilitate recovery rather than to allow those energies to be spent in diffuse anger or transformed into feelings of helplessness? In addressing these and related matters, clinicians' efforts should be shaped by an ongoing monitoring of the extent to which developmental de-differentiation is being averted and developmental advance is instead being fostered.

From the outset, clinicians must adopt a manner, particularly in communication, that conveys a determination to focus on resolving the problem. It is also important to "put on the light," as it were, to offset the potential for resurgence of archaic fears that monsters lurk in the shadows. This can be accomplished in part by providing information that does not compromise honesty but which nevertheless conveys the message that gains are being made. At a systematic level as well (and with particular reference to the needs of peers and subordinates), the efforts made by emergency medicine personnel would be well supported by encouraging that information about perpetrators to be made public once some reasonable level of certainty about its accuracy can be assumed. As van der Kork[23] has noted, "After safety is assured, psychological intervention may be needed. People have to learn to put words to the problems they face, to name them and to formulate appropriate solutions."

When ambiguity persists and rumor holds sway, fears can be projected that are so extreme as to invite re-traumatization. The importance of dispelling ambiguity notwithstanding, however, identification should not be made in ways that might encourage wariness and distrust because of reliance on categories such as ethnicity, religious affiliation, etc. Such groupings do little or nothing to assuage anxiety and may, in fact, lead to its exacerbation because of their infusing potential alarm into categories that have been otherwise relatively benign within the population affected by terrorism. Instead, citing the allegiance of terrorists groups to shared goals of de-stabilization and to the use of terrorist methods in the service of a specified cause might be a useful supplement to providing the names of perpetrators if available in the process of identification. By this means, stress is less likely to be compounded by the relatively undifferentiated formlessness of those who would do harm.

To label that which is unknown is to impart some sense of mastery and control. Those who might otherwise be immobilized to some degree by fear can then use the label to perceive an otherwise amorphous threat as one that at least has a name and, thereby, some boundaries and limits to its potential malevolence. Fear then takes on a more circumscribed and seemingly more manageable form. Conversely, in the absence of a name for the potential danger, the sense of jeopardy and the stress-inducing need for sustaining a state of heightened vigilance increases.

Not all victims of terrorist-driven events suffer developmental de-differentiation resulting in stress-related dysfunction or physical disease. According to van der Kork,[23] however, "almost everyone is perturbed during the aftermath of a trauma, and everyone experiences a degree of intrusiveness and sadness." Many others, however, have a much more difficult time "getting over it." In addition to PTSD, consequences of exposure to such events can include depression and disabling, treatment-resistant symptoms of fear and anxiety as well as marital crises and other relationship problems.[17] Accordingly, "Understanding the mechanisms of mental traumatization is extremely important when seeking to evaluate and assist the recent survivor."[30]

To rely primarily on the verbal re-framing of experience in an effort to provide psychological assistance in the wake of trauma may well prove less than productive, particularly in the early stages of intervention.[31] In fact, studies have shown that high levels of arousal, such as those associated with trauma, result in frontal lobe functions being suppressed,[32,33] as are Broca's area functions, which are needed to put feelings into words.[34] Subcortical centers, on the other hand, have been impli-

cated as more prominent in the neuropsychological mediation of trauma, particularly with regard to the limbic system.[35,36] Accordingly, Shalev[15] has noted that soothing bodily contact with the recently rescued is often helpful, but gender and social boundaries must be respected. Bringing in relatives of victims and others close to them may be especially helpful in this regard with caregivers serving as coaches. By these means, a relatively more differentiated and integrated sense of the relationship between the self and the physical, interpersonal, and socio-cultural aspects of the environment can be fostered and maintained. For this reason, "The first role of a therapist is to assess the strengths and weaknesses of the survivor's immediate supporters"[15] and to provide them with the support needed. Thereafter, interventions derived from the principles of cognitive-behavioral therapy have been shown to be of more benefit than supportive counseling alone during the post acute phase of early syndrome formation.[37]

Having particular relevance to the challenge of precluding developmental regression in the wake of exposure to traumatic events, approaches referred to as "debriefing" involve semi-structured group interventions geared toward alleviating potentially de-differentiating distress and thereby preventing pathological reactions. Two approaches, one introduced by Mitchell[38] and another by Dyregov,[39] have had relatively extensive application. The first, subsequently advanced through the *Critical Incident Stress Foundation*, has been presented as a training program for volunteers who might be mobilized for service in the wake of a disaster, whether naturally occurring or terrorist driven. The process involves several phases, beginning with an introduction during which personal identification takes place along with a definition of expectations, a setting of limits, and an explanation of confidentiality. There follows a "fact stage" during which each participant is asked to describe the event from his or her own perspective and a "thought stage" during which each participant is asked to recall first thoughts as the event occurred. In the "reaction phase" each person is asked to identify the worst part of the experience, one that she or he would erase from memory if possible. During the "symptom phase" that follows, each person is invited to explain how he or she is different because of the incident and to describe how life has been since the event. A teaching phase then takes place during which debriefing team members seek to "normalize" reactions by explaining their predictability as extraordinary characteristics of the circumstance rather than of the experiencing individual. The team also gives suggestions intended to aid recovery (e.g., relaxation and deep breathing exercises). Finally, during a "re-entry phase," team members provide a summarization and encourage cognitive re-framing of the experience to include some positive outcomes (e.g., lessons learned, insights achieved).

Some studies[40-42] have failed to show that debriefing prevents stress disorders. Those same studies, however, indicate that most participants recall the sessions as helpful and satisfying. Moreover, Shalev et al.[43] found that debriefing significantly reduces concurrent distress and enhances group cohesion.

CONCLUSION

By way of summary, it is important to recall that terrorists seek to de-stabilize individuals and societal organizations by undermining the cognitive, affective, and valuative perspectives that individuals and societal organizations have of the physical, interpersonal, and socio-cultural aspects of the world. In other words, terrorists seek to re-shape the frame of reference by which people know about, have emotional reactions to, and attach relative importance to the world of objects and places, of people and of laws, and of rules, customs, and expectations. To the extent that they succeed, terrorists can compromise the psychological and physical health of individuals and thereby undermine the strength of a society. Accordingly, those in authority, and in particular the health service providers within a society, must make decisions and initiate efforts with judgment that is informed by sensitivity to the importance of both avoiding developmental de-differentiation and of fostering developmental advance.

REFERENCES

1. Silke A. Preface. In: Silke A, ed. *Terrorists, Victims and Society*. West Sussex, England: John Wiley and Sons; 2003, xv-xxi.
2. Pfefferbaum B. Victims of Terror and the Media. In: Silke A, ed. *Terrorists, Victims and Society*. West Sussex, England: John Wiley and Sons; 2003, 175-87.
3. Spurrell M, MacFarlane A. Posttraumatic stress disorder and coping after a natural disaster. *Soc Psychol Psych Epidemiol*. 1993:28;194-200.
4. Crenshaw M. How terrorists think: what psychology can contribute to understanding terrorism. In: Howard L, ed. *Terrorism, Roots, Impact, Response*. London: Praeger; 1992.
5. Cooper H. The terrorist and the victim. *Victimology* 1993: 1(2);229-39.
6. Crenshaw M. The logic of terrorism: Terrorist behavior as a product of strategic choice. In: Reich W, ed. *Origins of Terrorism*. Washington DC: The Woodrow Wilson Center Press; 1998.
7. Silke A. The road less travelled: trends in terrorism research 1990-1999. Paper presented at the International Conference on Countering Terrorism through Enhanced International Cooperation, September 22-24, 2000, Courmeyeur, Italy. Cited in Silke A, ed. *Terrorists, Victims and Society*. West Sussex, England: John Wiley and Sons; 2003.
8. Merrari A. Academic research and governmental policy on terrorism. *Terrorism Political Violence*. 2001:3(1);88-102.
9. Werner H. *The Comparative Psychology of Mental Development*. New York: International Universities Press; 1948.
10. Wapner S, Werner H. *Perceptual Development*. Worcester, MA: Clark University Press; 1957.
11. Wapner S, Kaplan B, Cohen S. An organismic-developmental perspective for understanding transactions of persons-in-environments. *Environ Behav*. 1973:5;255-89.
12. Wapner S, Kaplan B, Ciottone R. Self-world relationships in critical environmental transitions: childhood and beyond. In: Liben L, Patterson A, Newcomb N, eds. *Spatial Representation and Behavior Across the Life Span*. New York: Academic Press; 1981.
13. Wapner S. Transitions of persons-in-environments: Some critical transitions. *J Environ Psych*. 1981:1;223-39.
14. Kaplan B, Wapner S, Cohen S. Exploratory applications of the organismic-developmental approach to man-in-environment transactions. In: Wapner S, Cohen S, Kaplan B, eds. *Experiencing the Environment*. New York: Plenum; 1976.
15. Shalev A. Treating survivors in the acute aftermath of traumatic events. In: Chu J, ed. *Terror in the Nation: The Mental Health Clinician's Role*. Publication prepared as part of a conference sponsored by McLean Hospital, Boston, MA, April 12, 2002.
16. Everly G, Mitchell J. *Critical Incident Stress Management: Advanced Group Crisis Interventions—A Workbook*, ed 2. Ellicott City, Md: Critical Incident Stress Foundation; 2000.
17. American Psychological Association. "When disaster strikes . . . ." In: Terror in the Nation: The Mental Health Clinician's Role. Publication prepared as part of a conference sponsored by McLean Hospital, Boston, MA, April 12, 2002.
18. Volkman P. Presentation of the basic critical incident stress management course and the advanced critical incident stress management course. Brattleboro Retreat, Brattleboro, VT, Sept. 30–Oct 4, 2002.
19. Wapner S, Kaplan B, Cohen S. An organismic developmental perspective for understanding transactions of man-in-environment. *Environ Behav*. 1973;5:200-89.
20. Everly G. Emergency mental health: an overview. *Int J Emerg Ment Health*. 1999;1:1.
21. Freedman S, Peri T, Brandes D, et al. Predictors of chronic PTSD: a prospective study. *Br J Psych*. 1999;174:353-59.
22. Shalev A, Freedman S, Peri T, et al. Prospective study of posttraumatic stress disorder and depression following trauma. *Am J Psych*. 1998;155(5):630-7.
23. van der Kork B. The assessment and treatment of complex PTSD. In: Yehuda R, ed. *Psychological Trauma*. New York: Academic Press; 2002.
24. McCarroll J, Ursano R, Wright K, et al. Handling bodies after violent death: Strategies for coping. *Am J Orthopsych*. 1993;63(2):209-13.
25. McCarroll J, Ursano R, Fullerton C. Symptoms of PTSD following recovery of war dead: 13-15 month follow-up. *Am J Psych*. 1995;152:939-41.
26. Sprang G. The psychological impact of isolated acts of terrorism, In Silke A, ed. *Terrorists, Victims and Society*. West Sussex, England: John Wiley and Sons, 2003.
27. Muldoon O. The psychological impact of protracted campaigns of political violence on societies. In: Silke A, ed. *Terrorists, Victims and Society*. West Sussex, England: John Wiley and Sons, 2003.
28. Solomon Z. Does the war end when the shooting stops? The psychological toll of war. *J Appl Social Psych*. 1990;20/21:1733-45.
29. Rosenbeck R, Fontana A. Transgenerational effects of abusive violence on the children of Vietnam combat veterans. *J Trauma Stress*. 1998;11(4):731-42.
30. Shalev A, Ursano R. *Mapping the Multidimensional Pictures of Acute Response to Traumatic Stress*. London: Oxford University Press; 2001.
31. van der Kork B. Beyond the talking cure: somatic experience, subcortical imprints and the treatment of trauma. In: Shapiro S, ed. *EMDR: Toward a Paradigm Shift*. New York: APA Press; 2001.
32. Arnsten A. The biology of being frazzled. *Science* 1998;280:1711-2.
33. Birnbaum S, Gobeske K, Aurbach J, et al. A role for norepinephrine in stress-induced cognitive deficits: alpha-1-adrenoceptor mediation in the prefrontal cortex. *Biol Psych*. 1999;46:1266-74.
34. Rauch S, van der Kork B, Fisher R, et al. A symptom provocation study of posttraumatic stress disorder using positron emission tomography and script-driven imagery. *Arch Gen Psych*. 1996;53:380-7.
35. van der Kork B. The body keeps the score: Memory and the evolving psychobiology of posttraumatic stress. *Harv Rev Psych*. 1994;1:253-65.
36. van der Kork B, van der Hart B, Marmar C. Dissociation and information processing in posttraumatic stress disorder. In: van der Kork B, McFarlane A, Weisaeth L, eds. *Traumatic Stress: The Effects of Overwhelming Experience on Mind, Body and Society*. New York: Guilford Press; 1996.
37. Bryant R, Harvey A. Relationship between acute stress disorder and posttraumatic stress disorder following mild traumatic brain injury. *Am J Psych*. 1998;155:625-9.
38. Mitchell J. When disaster strikes . . . *J Emerg Med Services*. 1983;8:36-9.
39. Dyregov A. Caring for helpers in disaster situations: Psychological de-briefing. *Disaster Manag*. 1989;2:25-30.
40. Bisson J, Jenkins P, Alexander L, et al. Randomised controlled trial of psychological debriefing for victims of acute burn trauma. *Br J Psych*. 1997;171:78-81.
41. Deahl M, Gilham A, Thomas J, et al. Psychological sequelae following the Gulf War: Factors associated with subsequent morbidity and the effectiveness of psychological debriefing. *Br J Psych*. 1994;165:60-5.
42. Shalev A, Freedman T, Peri T, et al. Prospective study of posttraumatic stress disorder and depression following trauma. *Am J Psych*. 1998;155:255-61.
43. Shalev AY, Peri T, Rogel Fuchs Y, et al. Historical group debriefing after combat exposure. *Mil Med.*, 1998;163(7):494-8.

chapter 55

Medical Intelligence*

Mark E. Keim

DEFINITION

Medical intelligence can be defined as "that category of intelligence resulting from collection, evaluation, analysis, and interpretation of foreign medical, bio-scientific, and environmental information which is of interest to strategic planning and to military medical planning and operations for the conservation of the fighting strength of friendly forces and the formation of assessments of foreign medical capabilities in both military and civilian sectors."[1]

Medical intelligence related specifically to the threat of terrorism has obvious applicability to civilian sectors as well. It involves information as applied to the identification, characterization, and management of the risk as applied to both military and civilian countermeasures against terrorism.

Collection of medical intelligence may include both classified and open sources. Evaluation may involve preexisting publications or ongoing public health surveillance, and it may also include analysis and/or interpretation of well-established or newly gained data. Characterizations may include situational awareness of current events[2] as well as descriptions of both foreign and domestic medical and public health capabilities and capacity.

HISTORICAL PERSPECTIVE

The Importance of Medical Intelligence

The greatest threat to military forces is often not enemy guns but rather the type of casualty referred to as a disease and non-battle injury (DNBI). The statistics regarding the effect of disease on military operations are remarkable. During the Civil War, an estimated 414,152 deaths were a result of disease, outranking battle deaths by a ratio of over 2:1.[3] In his Civil War memoir, then Major Jonathan Letterman—father of modern U.S. military operational medicine—wrote the following passage[4]:

A corps of medical officers was not established solely for the purpose of attending the wounded and sick.... The leading idea, which should be constantly kept in view, is to strengthen the hands of the Commanding General by keeping his army in the most vigorous health, thus rendering it, in the highest degree, efficient for enduring fatigue and privation and for fighting.

The following statistics reveal that the threat of disease during military operations had not ceased by the twentieth century:

- Influenza killed 43,000 U.S. military personnel in World War I. In the U.S. Army, influenza accounted for 80% of all casualties during the war.
- 50% of the U.S. marines deployed to Lebanon in 1958 were incapacitated with severe diarrhea.
- 80% of the U.S. sailors deployed in the Suez in 1975 were stricken with dysentery.
- 30% of the U.S. soldiers deployed to the Sinai in 1982 became dehydration casualties.
- 30% of the U.S. soldiers participating in a combined exercise in Botswana in 1992 returned home with spotted fever rickettsiosis.[4]

Clearly, Major Letterman understood that one of the keys to a successful military campaign is the implementation of preventive procedures to reduce DNBI rates. More recently, two widely recognized authorities in military preventive medicine—Llewellyn Legters and Craig Llewellyn of the Uniformed Services University of the Health Sciences (USUHS)—highlighted the four main objectives of a successful preventive medicine program[4]:

- To determine the nature and magnitude of the disease and injury threats in the planned area of operations before deployment
- To identify the principal countermeasures that must be emphasized to reduce the threats to acceptable levels
- To train individuals in the use of these countermeasures
- To rigorously enforce these countermeasures in the operational area

These measures correspond well with processes of analytical risk management, including risk assessment,

---

*The material in this chapter reflects solely the views of the author. It does not necessarily reflect the policies or recommendations of the Centers for Disease Control and Prevention nor the U.S. Department of Health and Human Services.

countermeasure determination, risk communication, and countermeasure implementation.

The Development of Modern Medical Intelligence in the United States

During World War II the U.S. Army Medical Intelligence Office (under the Army Surgeon General) was responsible for medical intelligence for the U.S. military. In 1963, the Defense Intelligence Agency (DIA) Medical Intelligence Division assumed this mission. In 1973, the DIA underwent a significant reduction in force; the Medical Intelligence Division was abolished and the U.S. Army Surgeon General then assumed the entire medical intelligence mission. In 1982, the Armed Forces Medical Intelligence Center (AFMIC) was officially established as a tri-service intelligence activity. The Army Surgeon General was designated as Executive Agent. In 1992, AFMIC became a "DIA Field Production Activity."[5]

CURRENT PRACTICE

Military Medical Intelligence

The primary source of military medical intelligence in the United States is the DIA's AFMIC now located at Fort Detrick, Maryland. The AFMIC produces finished, all-source medical intelligence in support of the Department of Defense (DoD) and its components, national policy officials, and other federal agencies. Assessments, forecasts, and databases are prepared on worldwide infectious disease occurrence, global environmental health risks, foreign military and civilian health care capabilities and trends, and militarily significant life science technologies.

Infectious disease and environmental health components of AFMIC focus on those infectious diseases and environmental health factors that could degrade the effectiveness of military forces deploying worldwide for contingency, humanitarian relief, and peacekeeping operations. In addition, these worldwide infectious diseases and environmental degradation have national security and policy implications.

Foreign medical capabilities are assessed to include a country's ability to provide medical services and support to its military forces and civilian population. Key elements include foreign military and civilian medical capabilities (e.g., treatment facilities; medical personnel; treatment capability; training, emergency, and disaster response; logistics; medical and pharmaceutical industries; and research and production facilities).

AFMIC's life sciences and biotechnologies components address foreign basic and applied biomedical and biotechnological developments of military medical importance, including biological, chemical, psychological, and biophysical factors. In addition, key areas of interest include foreign civilian and military pharmaceutical industry capabilities and innovations as well as foreign scientific and technological medical advances for defense against nuclear, biological, and chemical warfare.

Medical intelligence is prepared under the DoD Intelligence Production Program (DoDIPP) and managed by the DIA's Directorate for Analysis and Production. To meet the needs of a diverse consumer group, AFMIC has created a product line providing intelligence via various media: electronic message, CD-ROM, hard copy, and Intelink.

AFMIC's assessments are consulted before troops are deployed to foreign areas for combat, peacekeeping, or humanitarian operations. AFMIC assessments of potential health risks and foreign health care capabilities allow the medical community to plan for the proper prophylaxis (preventive measures such as providing safe water and food and protective measures against insects), health care support, and medical personnel support. AFMIC also provides time-sensitive, finished medical intelligence in response to direct requests from consumers at the national, departmental, or operational and/or tactical levels. Table 55-1 represents a comprehensive listing of traditional sources of military medical intelligence available in the United States.[4-7]

Civilian medical intelligence

Any small or large outbreak of disease should be evaluated as a potential bioterrorist attack. The cause of a disease or even the occurrence of something unusual may be very difficult to determine, especially if the initial cases are few. Surveillance needs to be more than routine. Infectious disease criteria for differentiation of bioterrorism from natural outbreaks have been well defined in the literature, as well as within Section 6 of Part I of this textbook.[8,9,11,13] This initial investigation does not always have to be time consuming or involve law enforcement. Simply looking the facts surrounding the outbreak to determine if anything seems unusual or indicates bioterrorism will suffice in most cases.[8]

The most important factors affecting early detection of a bioterrorist event are likely to be the rate of accrual of new cases at the outset of the epidemic, geographic clustering, the selection of syndromic surveillance methods, and the likelihood of making a diagnosis quickly in clinical practice.[12]

National, regional, and local public health departments must be linked in a network of real-time communication with the medical response community, public safety, regional poison control centers, and regional laboratory capacities for integration of information management, passive and active surveillance systems, and epidemiologic investigation. In 1998, Keim, Kaufmann, and Rodgers[14] were the first to propose development of such a comprehensive system as part of the U.S. Public Health Service.

The primary source of civilian medical intelligence in the United States is the Centers for Disease Control and Prevention (CDC). (Table 55-2 represents a comprehensive listing of traditional sources of civilian medical intelligence available in the United States.)[15-19]

The role of the U.S. public health system has evolved significantly since September 11 and the anthrax attacks of late 2001. The public health threat associated with the release of chemical, biological, and radiological/nuclear agents has drawn the CDC and the entire public health system into a national security role. The safety and health of people across the United States and around

TABLE 55-1 MILITARY SOURCES OF MEDICAL INTELLIGENCE

SOURCE	PRODUCT	DESCRIPTION
Armed Forces Medical Intelligence Center (AFMIC), Ft. Detrick, Maryland.	Urban Medical Capabilities Study	Includes a map of the urban area, general health information, and locations, descriptions, and imagery of key medical treatment facilities
	Medical Capabilities Studies (MEDCAP)	Comprehensive evaluation of a country's civilian and military healthcare systems
	Quick Response Tasking (QRT)	A way of asking AFMIC for answers not found in published studies. Their phones are secure via STU-III through the TS-SCI level.
	Joint Worldwide Intelligence Communication System (JWICS)	Secure telecommunications system, which links sites throughout the intelligence and operations communities. It allows, among other things, secure teleconferencing.
	Medical Intelligence Imagery Brief (MIIB)	Annotated imagery with derived text describing and analyzing a significant medical event of current interest
	Medical Intelligence Note (MIN)	Provides a brief assessment of important medical developments to meet time-sensitive requirements for support to medical planning and decision-making as well as material research, development, and acquisition
	Life Sciences and Biotechnology	Assesses foreign basic and applied biomedical and biotechnological developments of military medical importance, foreign civilian and military pharmaceutical industry capabilities, and foreign scientific and technological medical advances for defense against CBRNE warfare.
	Medical, Environmental, Disease Intelligence and Countermeasures (MEDIC)	Provides worldwide infectious disease and environmental health risks hyperlinked to the Joint Service–approved countermeasure recommendations, military and civilian health care delivery capabilities, operational information, disease vector ecology information, and reference data
	Health Services Assessment (HSA)	Provides bottom-line assessment of a country's health services capability
	Infectious Disease Risk Assessments (IDRA)	Pre-deployment force protection planning guidance that assesses the baseline risk from infectious diseases of operational military importance on a country-by-country basis worldwide
	Disease Occurrence WorldWide (DOWW)	Short, timely alerts that assess risk to U.S. forces from foreign disease outbreaks that may affect military operations and forecast disease risks associated with recent environmental disasters
	Environmental Health Risk Assessments (EHRA)	Assesses environmental health risks of operational military significance on a country-by-country basis worldwide
	Industrial Facility Health Risk Assessment (IFHRA)	Assesses health risk associated with potential exposure to toxic industrial chemicals at specific industrial facilities worldwide
	Industry Sector Profile (ISP)	Assesses potential environmental and human health impacts related to routine emissions and large-scale chemical releases from industrial activities by industry sector
	Toxic Industrial Chemical Risk Assessment (TICRA)	Provides a country-by-country prioritization of industrial facilities based on the potential exposure to toxic chemicals and expected adverse health effects
	AFMIC Wire	A periodic message update that provides analysis of newly reported information of immediate interest to deployed or deploying forces
Defense Pest Management Information Analysis Center (DPMIAC)	Disease Vector Ecology Profiles (DVEP)	Information regarding disease risks, infectious agents, modes of transmission, geographic and seasonal incidence, and prevention and control recommendations
Navy Environmental Health Center	Navy Preventive Medicine Information System (NAPMIS)	A computerized information system designed to support the Fleet and Fleet Marine Force with consistently updated preventive medicine and vector-borne disease profiles of countries of military importance
Walter Reed Army Institute of Research (WRAIR)	Communicable Disease Report	Identifies disease outbreaks worldwide. In addition, WRAIR quickly responds to ad hoc queries and provides timely regional medical information.
U.S. Army Research Institute of Environmental Medicine (USARIEM)	Deployment Manuals	Address soldier health and performance in a wide variety of environments
All national-level intelligence organizations	INTELINK	Described as the "classified on-ramp to the information superhighway." All national-level intelligence organizations have home pages on INTELINK, including AFMIC. In addition, each of the Unified Command Joint Intelligence Centers has a home page.
Assistant Secretary of Defense for Health Affairs (ASDHA) with support from Armed Forces Research Institute of Medical Sciences (AFRIMS)	DoD Global Emerging Infections System (GEIS)	Serves as the focal point for DoD efforts to address emerging infectious diseases. The Military Health System network of clinical and laboratory resources provides infrastructure for GEIS. The emphasis of GEIS is on the strengthening of laboratory-based surveillance, particularly for influenza and other respiratory illnesses, for reportable illnesses, for changes in antibiotic resistance patterns, and for other evidence of emerging infections. DoD overseas laboratories provide forward sentinel surveillance sites for GEIS activities.

TABLE 55-2 CIVILIAN SOURCES OF MEDICAL INTELLIGENCE

SOURCE	DESCRIPTION
Centers for Disease Control and Prevention (CDC) Public Health Information Network (PHIN)	A public health architecture that will coordinate existing and new public health information systems for interoperable use of information technology across public health. PHIN is composed of five key components: detection and monitoring, data analysis, knowledge management, alerting, and response. PHIN will integrate and build on the technical standards and infrastructure established through other CDC/ATSDR initiatives, including EPI-X, NEDSS, and PULSENET.
CDC Epidemic Information Exchange (EPI-X)	A secure web-based communications network for public health officials. Using advanced Internet and communications technologies, EPI-X provides 24 hours a day, 7 days a week (24×7) emergency alerts and creates a protected forum to share important disease information nationwide positioning public health officials to detect and respond accordingly to suspect terrorism emergencies. EPI-X is used as a communication tool by DHHS and CDC/ATSDR emergency operations centers and state terrorism coordinators to exchange routine and emergent public health information with state and CDC/ATSDR public health professionals rapidly and securely.
CDC PULSENET	An early warning system for outbreaks of foodborne disease consisting of a national network of public health laboratories that performs DNA "fingerprinting" on bacteria that may be foodborne. The network identifies and labels each "fingerprint" pattern and permits rapid comparison of these patterns through an electronic database at CDC/ATSDR to identify related strains. PULSENET participants include all 50 state public health laboratories, 5 local public health laboratories, 7 FDA laboratories, the USDA food safety and inspection laboratory, 7 Canadian laboratories and participation from a variety of nations across Europe, the Middle East, Latin America, and the Pacific rim.
CDC Nationwide Chemical Poisoning and Radiological Illness Monitoring System	Working to develop standard protocols to identify and respond to events while enhancing communications among local, state, federal, and other partners, including poison control centers. This early warning system will be sensitive and specific enough to identify cases associated with chemical and radiological exposures. It will include long-term follow-up of potentially exposed subjects and an automated tracking system that provides daily incidence data on symptoms and syndromes that may indicate chemical and radiological exposure.
CDC Biowatch	Assisting the Department of Homeland Security and the Environmental Protection Agency (EPA) to perform 24×7 environmental surveillance using existing EPA and Department of Energy (DOE) air quality–monitoring systems. Air samples will be tested in cities for the presence of biological pathogens to generate early warnings of possible attacks. Implementation consists of three primary components: field (sampling devices, collection, transport, and verification), laboratory (processing and polymerase chain reaction, PCR analysis), and consequence management. Laboratory response network confirmatory-level labs will conduct the necessary laboratory analyses.
CDC Laboratory Response Network (LRN)	A consortium of laboratories comprised primarily of state, local, and federal public health laboratories, each with different capabilities and levels of expertise. As a network, it provides immediate and sustained laboratory testing and communication in the event of public health emergencies, particularly in response to acts of terrorism. Members belong to different agencies and jurisdictions but are unified by a common system of operations.
CDC Health Alert Network (HAN)	An e-mail messaging and distribution structure that ensures local health departments have timely and rapid access to emerging health information in order for the frontline professionals to effectively translate the data into health action. HAN provides three primary capacities: (1) high-speed internet connectivity, (2) broadcast capacity for emergency communication, and (3) distance-learning infrastructure for real-time training.
CDC National Public Health Information Coalition (NPHIC)	Activities include scheduling routine teleconferences to discuss and coordinate communication about specific agents currently or potentially of concern, establishing a secure section of the NPHIC website to allow members to post and exchange information about communication needs and resources around specific events, and providing input to such emergency response planning efforts as the ASTHO anti-terrorism task force.
CDC Emergency Communications System (ECS)	Ensures rapid, effective, and consistent CDC/ATSDR communication response to the news media, the public, and key stakeholders in the event of terrorism or a national public health emergency.
CDC Early Aberration Reporting System (EARS)	A widely used syndromic surveillance tool. City, county, and state public health officials in the United States and abroad currently use EARS on syndromic data from emergency departments, 911 calls, physician office data, school and business absenteeism, and over-the-counter drug sales. The EARS program presents its analysis in a complete HTML website containing tables and graphs linked through a home page.
CDC Health Information for International Travel	A document often referred to as the "Yellow Handbook," which identifies current vaccination requirements, immunization and prophylaxis recommendations, and regional health hazards.
CDC Morbidity and Mortality Weekly Report (MMWR)	Contains data on specific diseases as reported by state and territorial health departments and reports on infectious and chronic diseases, environmental hazards, natural or human-generated disasters, occupational diseases and injuries, and intentional and unintentional injuries.
US Department of State Country Background Notes	Provides information on geographic entities and international organizations. It is updated periodically.
World Health Organization (WHO) Vaccination Certificate Requirements and Health Advice for International Travel	Identifies current vaccination requirements, immunization, and prophylaxis recommendations as well as regional health hazards.
WHO Weekly Epidemiological Record (WER)	Instrument for the rapid and accurate dissemination of epidemiological information on cases and outbreaks of diseases under the International Health Regulations and on other communicable diseases of public health importance, including newly emerging or reemerging infections.

TABLE 55-2 CIVILIAN SOURCES OF MEDICAL INTELLIGENCE—Cont'd

SOURCE	DESCRIPTION

iJET Travel Risk Management
  1. Travel Intelligence
     Services
  2. Worldcue Risk
     Management System
  3. GlobalGuardian
	1. Provides corporate staff and employees tactical information and reports for more than 180 countries and 260 cities to help travelers avoid disruptions and to stay safe, healthy, and productive.
	2. Provides corporate security, travel, and human resource personnel the ability to track, locate, and communicate with travelers at all times, anywhere in the world.
	3. Provides both response capability and proactive risk mitigation services, such as consulting, contingency planning, training, and intelligence.

the globe demands the best science, immediate public health service, and a sound strategy to prepare for and respond to terrorist threats.

With the realization that the threat of bioterrorism was increasing, the CDC developed a strategic plan for preparedness and response to terrorism. The CDC centers, institutes, and offices contribute their expertise toward this effort, by improving[15]:

- Detection and investigation
- Prevention programs
- Worker safety
- Laboratory sciences research
- Communication
- Workforce development
- Long-term consequence management

Terrorism-preparedness activities described in CDC's strategic plan include the development of a public health communication infrastructure, a multilevel network of diagnostic laboratories, and an integrated disease surveillance system.[20] These are remarkably similar to the 1998 recommendations of Keim, Kaufmann, and Rodgers.[14] Surveillance systems collect and monitor data for disease trends and/or outbreaks so that public health personnel can protect the nation's health. CDC now maintains several effective surveillance tools and systems that can be used to gain medical intelligence for the detection and characterization of terrorism. CDC is also now working with state and local health departments and information system contractors to develop real-time special event syndromic surveillance and analytical methods. Throughout the planning documents developed for bioterrorism response, veterinarians are also considered as a key part of the disease surveillance system.[21]

Methods for conducting public health surveillance may differ considerably by program and disease. Regardless of these differences, however, all surveillance activities share many common practices in the way data are collected, managed, transmitted, analyzed, accessed, and disseminated. CDC's long-term vision is that of complementary electronic information systems that automatically gather health data from a variety of sources on a real-time basis, facilitate the monitoring of the health of communities, assist in the ongoing analysis of trends and detection of emerging public health problems, and provide information for setting public health policy.

Currently there are multiple systems in place that support communications for public health labs, the clinical community, and state and local health departments. Each has demonstrated the importance of being able to exchange health information. However, many of these systems operate in isolation, not capitalizing on the potential for a cross-fertilization of data exchange. CDC is working to provide a cross-cutting and unifying framework to better monitor these data streams for early detection of public health issues and emergencies. Ensuring the security of this information is also critical, as is the ability of the network to work reliably in times of national crisis.

A bioterrorist attack, like other health threats, would be detected first at the local level. Health departments throughout the nation must be prepared to detect and respond to those threats. CDC has established a communications, information, distance-learning, and organizational infrastructure in partnership with the National Association of County and City Health Officials (NACCHO), the Association of State and Territorial Health Officials (ASTHO), and other health organizations for a new level of defense against health threats, including the possibility of bioterrorism. CDC officials, state and local health departments, poison control centers, and other public health professionals can now access and share preliminary health surveillance information quickly and securely. Users can also be notified actively of health events as they occur.

Most biological agents can be diagnosed at standard hospital clinical laboratories.[22] CDC has established a consortium of laboratories comprised primarily of state, local, and federal public health laboratories, each with different capabilities and levels of expertise.[23] National laboratories, including those operated by the CDC and the U.S. Army Medical Research Institute of Infectious Diseases (USAMRIID), are responsible for specialized strain characterizations, bioforensics, select agent activity, and handling of highly infectious biological agents and toxic chemicals. Reference laboratories are responsible for investigation and/or referral of specimens. They are made up of more than 100 state and local public health, military, international, veterinary, agriculture, and food- and water-testing laboratories. In addition to laboratories located in the United States, facilities located in Australia and Canada serve as reference laboratories. Sentinel laboratories are hospital-based, clinical institutions, and commercial diagnostic laboratories. These sentinel laboratories now play a key role in the early detection of biological agents. Sentinel laboratories provide routine diagnostic services, rule-out, and referral steps in the identification process.[15]

Integration of Civilian and Military Medical Intelligence

In order to investigate unusual epidemics, we require information about the ecological and biologic characteristics of the pathogen, the natural routes of infection, the pathogenesis, the clinical picture and immunology of certain diseases, the epidemic foci, and the special characteristics of an artificial dissemination of this pathogen. It is also essential that there is an adequate and efficient field analysis of the epidemic, an examination of the clinical picture and the epidemiologic situation, and a collection of representative samples and data for statistically sound epidemiologic, epizootiologic, medical, and laboratory analysis. This necessitates properly trained mobile investigation teams with appropriate technical equipment. In order to be the most effective, these teams must include both civilian and military forces.[10]

There is now a growing integration of civilian and military medical intelligence systems. One example is the DoD laboratory-based global influenza surveillance system. Military global influenza surveillance began in 1976 as an Air Force program.[24] In 1996, President Clinton issued Presidential Decision Directive NSTC-7, which formally expanded the mission of the DoD to support global surveillance, training, research, and response to emerging infectious disease threats.[25] As a result, the efforts of national surveillance programs, overseen by the World Health Organization (WHO) and administered by institutions such as the CDC, the U.S. armed forces and 60 to 70 collaborating laboratories annually culminate in the development of effective influenza vaccines.[26]

Another indication of further integration of U.S. civilian and military medical intelligence systems is that of the U.S. military officer participation in the CDC Epidemic Intelligence Service (EIS). Although the EIS was born in 1951 (in part because of a perceived biological warfare threat), the U.S. military did not participate actively in EIS

until 1994. Since then, military officers have had a growing presence in EIS and the DoD has a permanent liaison stationed at CDC. From a national perspective, this collective benefit in epidemiological judgment and networking will specifically contribute to the execution of various national plans to defend against biological attacks.[27]

Medical Intelligence and Risk Management

Risk assessment is a systematic process for quantifying the likelihood of adverse health effects in a population following exposure to a specified hazard. A risk assessment is a decision-making support tool used to establish requirements and prioritize program investments. Analytical risk management is the process of selecting and implementing prevention and control measures in order to achieve an acceptable level of that risk at an acceptable cost (Table 55-3).

It is impossible to avoid all possible risk of terrorism. Compared with risk avoidance, which seeks to counter all possible vulnerabilities, risk management instead weighs the risk of loss against the cost of control measures. Risk management is composed of three main elements: risk assessment, cost-benefit analysis, and risk communication. The components of analytical risk assessment with regards to terrorism include asset and loss impact assessment, threat assessment, and vulnerability analysis.[28]

Accurate threat assessment can only come from the military and intelligence community. Thus, well-integrated medical intelligence provides the preexisting public health and intelligence systems with the ability to recognize and characterize a population's risk for terrorism in advance of any subsequent countermeasures in the form of prevention and control. Soundly performed risk assessments help ensure that specific programs and

TABLE 55-3 ELEMENTS OF ANALYTICAL RISK MANAGEMENT

PROCESS	ACTIVITIES
Impact assessment	• Determining critical assets (i.e., a population)
Asset assessment	• Identifying undesirable events and expected loss or damage.
Loss assessment	• Prioritizing assets based on consequence of loss
Threat characterization	• Identifying indications, circumstances, or events with the potential to cause the loss of or damage
Hazard identification	to an asset.
Adversary intent	• Assessing intent and motivation of each adversary
Adversary capability	• Assessing capabilities of each adversary
Adversary history	• Determining frequency of past events
	• Estimating threat relative to each critical asset
Vulnerability analysis	• Identifying potential weaknesses that may be exploited by an adversary to gain access to an asset
Potential vulnerabilities	• Identifying existing countermeasures and their level of effectiveness, which may be used in reducing
Existing countermeasures	vulnerability
	• Estimating degree of vulnerability to each asset and threat
Countermeasure determination	• Identifying potential actions that may be taken or physical entities that may be used to eliminate or
Prevention	lessen one or more vulnerabilities
Control	
Cost-benefit analysis	• Identifying countermeasure costs and benefits
	• Conducting cost-benefit and tradeoff analyses
	• Prioritizing options
Risk communication	• Preparing a range of recommendations for decision-makers and/or the public

related expenditures are justified and targeted according to the threat and risk of validated terrorist attack scenarios generated and assessed by a multi-disciplinary team of experts.[29]

Intelligence and law enforcement threat information is a key input into a risk assessment process. Risk assessments are widely recognized as valid decision-support tools to establish and prioritize program investments and are grounded in risk management

Medical intelligence may be applied within the process of analytical risk management in an effort to better protect and defend both civilian and military populations against terrorism. The intelligence community has produced National Intelligence Estimates (NIE) and other high-level analyses of the foreign origin terrorist threat that include judgments about the more likely chemical and biological agents that would be used. An NIE is intended to help decision-makers think through critical issues by presenting the relevant key facts, judgments about the likely course of events in foreign countries, and implications for the United States.

A threat analysis—the first step in determining risk—identifies and evaluates each threat on the basis of various factors such as its capability and intent to attack an asset and the likelihood and the severity of the consequences of a successful attack. Valid, current, and documented threat information, including NIEs, in a risk-assessment process is crucial to ensuring that countermeasures or programs are not based solely on worst-case scenarios and therefore out of balance with the threat. Risk-management principles acknowledge that (1) although risk generally cannot be eliminated, it can be reduced by enhancing protection from validated and credible threats, and (2) although many threats are possible, some are more likely to be carried out than others. Risk assessments form a deliberate, analytical approach that results in a prioritized list of risks (i.e., threat-asset-vulnerability combinations) that can be used to select countermeasures to create a certain level of protection or preparedness. Because threats are dynamic and countermeasures may become outdated, it is generally sound practice to periodically reassess threat and risk. To perform a realistic risk assessment of terrorist threats, a multidisciplinary team of experts would require several inputs, including written foreign and domestic threat analyses from the intelligence community and law enforcement as well as civilian public health and medical intelligence.

PITFALLS

Less-than-Complete Integration of Veterinary Medicine into Medical Intelligence Systems

Although recent reports have emphasized the need for improving the ability to detect a biological terrorist attack on human populations, the use of veterinary services in this effort and the potential for the targeting of livestock (e.g., horses, cattle, sheep, goats, swine, and poultry) have been addressed only briefly. Improving

surveillance for biological terrorist attacks (that target livestock) and improving detection and reporting of livestock, pet, and wild animal morbidity and mortality are important components of preparedness for a covert biological terrorist attack. Although veterinarians have been mentioned as an integral part of biological terrorism preparedness planning, the importance of improving surveillance among livestock, pet, and wild animal populations has not been emphasized. Any improvement in detection of a covert biological terrorist attack should be a goal of human and veterinary health programs. Although a system for detecting and reporting nonendemic or foreign animal diseases exists in the United States, the system needs strengthening to increase the likelihood of detecting a covert biological terrorist attack on humans or other mammals. Following a covert bioterrorist attack with an agent targeting livestock or human populations, the front line of practicing human and veterinary healthcare providers will be essential for detection, reporting, and response.[30]

Inherent Difficulties in the Natural Course of Bioterrorism-Related Illness

Inherent difficulties in the natural course of bioterrorism-related illness may limit the use of medical intelligence to rapidly recognize the clues of a bioterror attack. In one example, the steep epidemic curve expected in a bioterrorism attack is similar to that expected with other point source exposures, such as foodborne outbreaks.[8]

Even in the presence of known indicators of bioterror attack, it may not be easy to determine that an attack occurred through nefarious means. For example, in spite of a CDC-led investigation, it took months to determine that an outbreak of salmonellosis in Oregon was caused by intentional contamination of salad bars.[31] Other naturally occurring outbreaks such as the hantavirus outbreak in the Four Corners area of the United States[32] and the tularemia outbreak in Kosovo, have been mistakenly thought of as possible results of intentional contamination.[10]

Lack of Clinical Training Among Medical Personnel

Lack of clinical training among medical personnel with respect to illness related to chemical and biological terrorism may limit the timeliness of medical intelligence. Even emergency medicine residency training programs have exhibited a less-than-optimum capability for training physicians to diagnose and treat these rarely seen maladies.[33]

Challenges Involving Integration of Civilian and Military Medical Intelligence

There may also be challenges involving the integration of civilian and military medical intelligence. This first became obvious with respect to national terrorism response during the 1996 Centennial Olympic Games in

Atlanta, Georgia, when unprecedented preparations were undertaken to cope with the health consequences of a terrorist incident involving chemical or biological agents.[34,35] Local, state, federal, and military resources joined to establish a specialized incident assessment team and Science and Technology Center.[35] Before the Atlanta Olympic Games, however, only certain specialized units within the military and the law enforcement communities were prepared to cope with chemical or biological agents. The literature that dealt with protecting the public health at large events did not address terrorism or these agents in any detail. There was no single plan or organization to guide response preparations. The city of Atlanta had little indigenous capability to recognize or deal with terrorism involving chemical or biological agents. Efforts undertaken to cope with chemical or biological terrorism for the Olympic Games were therefore the result of the federal plan plus the diverse initiatives of many organizations and agencies from both within and outside of the city.

A Science and Technology Center was created at the CDC, which was conveniently located in Atlanta, to provide emergency public health, medical, toxicologic, forensic, and scientific consultation after a suspected terrorist event involving chemical or biological agents. The Science and Technology Center was closely linked with the FBI assessment team and included representatives from a number of the environmental and infectious disease laboratories at CDC, the Agency for Toxic Substances and Disease Registry, and the military.[35]

The Center also had representatives from the local public health and emergency medicine community. Almost all of the major federal and military organizations in the United States that would have had a role in responding to a chemical or biological terrorist incident were deployed to Atlanta during the Olympic Games. Before this time, few of these organizations had ever collaborated to respond to a terrorist action, nor had many worked with local emergency response personnel. The Games served as an unprecedented opportunity to develop and realign integrated response plans through daily interactions, formal planning sessions, tabletop exercises, conferences, and field exercises. The event also served as a precedent for the integration of civilian and military assets within the context of Presidential Directive 39[36] into a configuration that would later evolve into the current National Response Plan.[37] Subsequent reviews of this historic benchmark event have described challenges involving the integration of civilian and military medical intelligence.[34,35] The issue of coordination was again encountered during the anthrax mail attacks of 2001.

Inherent Difficulties of Syndromic Surveillance

Inherent difficulties of syndromic surveillance may limit usefulness of early warning of outbreaks related to a bioterror attack. Passive disease-reporting systems not directly linked to the laboratory could result in delays in the recognition of disease outbreaks. Other difficulties with current surveillance systems include: incomplete data capture; inaccurate data; gaps in provider appreciation for the importance and usefulness of surveillance activities, data, and information; difficulty in geographic localization of an outbreak and tracking geographic locations of patients; inadequate indicators to serve as triggers for a response; limited surveillance of response personnel; limited feedback to reporting installations; and suboptimal laboratory integration.[6]

The signs of terrorist attack may also appear insidiously, with primary-care providers witnessing the first cases. However, it may not even be emergency room personnel who first detect a problem. The first to notice could be a hospital laboratory seeing unusual strains of organisms, a county epidemiologist keeping track of hospital admissions, a pharmacist distributing more antibiotics than usual, a 911 operator noticing an increase in respiratory distress calls, or a funeral director with increased business.[8]

Despite the small number of patients, the published descriptions of 11 persons with inhalational anthrax in the United States may offer four lessons for detecting a bioterror epidemic.[12] First, a key objective of syndromic surveillance is to detect early-stage disease, but fewer than half of these patients sought care in the early stage of illness before hospitalization was necessary. Second, emergency room data are a common source for syndromic surveillance, but detecting an increase in visits coincident with hospital admission may not provide an early warning because the time needed to process surveillance data and investigate suspected cases would be at least as long as the time for admission blood cultures to be positive for *Bacillus anthracis*. Third, the four patients who received early care and were discharged to home were assigned three different diagnoses, which suggests that syndromic surveillance systems must address the potential variability in how patients with the same infection may be diagnosed during the prodrome. Finally, rapid diagnosis after hospitalization was possible only in those patients who had not received antibiotics before cultures were taken.

REFERENCES

1. U.S. Military Glossary. Available at: http://usmilitary.about.com/library/glossary/blglossary.htm.
2. Walden J, Kaplan EH. Estimating the size of bioterror attack. *Emerg Infect Dis*. 2004;10(7):1202-5.
3. Casualties in the Civil War. Available at: http://www.civilwarhome.com/casualties.htm.
4. Sanftleben K. Medical Planners Resource Center: Medical intelligence and preventive medicine. Available at: http://www.geocities.com/CapitolHill/7533/hb-2.htm.
5. Armed Forces Medical Intelligence Center. Available at: http://mic.afmic.detrick.army.mil.
6. Kortepeter MG, Pavlin JA, Gaydos JC, et al. Surveillance at U.S. military installations for bioterrorist and emerging infectious disease threats. *Mil Med* 2000;165:238-9.
7. Medical Intelligence Resources for the CATF Surgeon. Surface Warfare Medicine Institute. Available at: http://www.vnh.org/FleetMedPocketRef/FleetMedicinePocketRef2001.doc.
8. Pavlin JA. Epidemiology of bioterrorism. *Emerg Infect Dis*. 1999;5(2):528-33.
9. Noah DL, Sobel AL, Ostroff SM, et al. Biological warfare training: infectious disease outbreak differentiation criteria. *Mil Med*. 1998;163(4):198.

10. Grunow R, Finke EJ. A procedure for differentiating between the intentional release of biological warfare agents and natural outbreaks of disease: its use in analyzing the tularemia outbreak in Kosovo in 1999 and 2000. *Clin Microbiol Infect.* 2002;8(8): 510-21.

11. Treadwell TA, Koo D, Kuker K, Khan AS. Epidemiologic clues to bioterrorism. *Public Health Reports.* 2003;118:92-8.

12. Buehler JW, Berkelman RL, Hartley DM, Peters CJ. Syndromic surveillance and bioterrorism-related epidemics. *Emerg Infect Dis.* 2003;9(10):1197-1204.

13. Walden J, Kaplan EH. Estimating the size of bioterror attack. *Emerg Infect Dis.* 2004;10(7):1202-5.

14. Keim M, Kaufmann A, Rodgers G. Recommendations for Office of Emergency Preparedness/CDC Surveillance, Laboratory and Informational Support Initiative. Centers for Disease Control and Prevention, National Center for Environmental Health. Atlanta: May 4, 1998. Available at: http://www.cdc.gov/nceh/ierh/Publications/*default.htm#Emergency%20Health%20Management.

15. Centers for Disease Control and Prevention. Biological and Clinical Terrorism: Strategic Plan for Preparedness and Response. Recommendations of the CDC Strategic Planning Workgroup MMWR 2000;49(RR-4):5-6.

16. Centers for Disease Control and Prevention. Emergency preparedness and response. Available at: http://www.bt.cdc.gov/.

17. iJET Travel Risk Management. Available at: http://www.ijet.com/services/intelligence.html.

18. World Health Organization. Available at: http://www.who.int/en/.

19. U.S. Department of State Country Background Notes. Available at: http://www.state.gov/r/pa/ei/bgn/.

20. Biological and chemical terrorism: strategic plan for preparedness and response. Recommendations of the CDC Strategic Planning Workgroup. *MMWR.* 2000;49(RR04):1-14.

21. Noah DL, Crowder HR. Biological terrorism against animals and humans: a brief review and primer for action. *J Am Vet Med Assoc.* 2002;221(1):40-3.

22. Pavlin JA. Bioterrorism and the importance of the public health laboratory. *Mil Med.* 2000;165(Suppl 2):25-7.

23. Lillibridge SR. Testimony presented to the Government Reform and Oversight Committee, Subcommittee on National Security. Washington, DC, Sept. 22, 1999.

24. Williams JR, Cox NJ, Regnery HL. Meeting the challenge of emerging pathogens: The role of the United States Air Force in global influenza surveillance. *Mil Med.* 1997;162(2):82-6.

25. National Science and Technology Council Presidential Decision Directive (NSTC-7): Emerging Infectious Diseases. Washington, DC, The White House, 1996.

26. Canas LC, Lohman K, Pavlin JA, et al. The Department of Defense laboratory-based global influenza surveillance system. *Mil Med.* 2000;165(2):52-6.

27. Noah DL, Ostroff SM, Cropper TL, et al. U.S. military officer participation in the Centers for Disease Control and Prevention Epidemic Intelligence Service. *Mil Med.* 2003;168(5):368-72.

28. Keim M. Intentional chemical disasters. Hogan D, Burstein J, eds. *Disaster Medicine.* Philadelphia: Lippincott, Williams & Wilkins; 2002.

29. Combating Terrorism: Need for Comprehensive Threat and Risk Assessments of Chemical and Biological Attacks. NSIAD-99-163 (28 pp. plus 3 appendices), Sept. 7, 1999. Available at: http://www.gao.gov/archive/1999/ns99163.pdf.

30. Ashford DA, Gomez TM, Noah DL, et al. Biological terrorism and veterinary medicine in the United States. *JAMA.* 2000;217(5):664-7.

31. Torok TJ, Tauxe RV, Wise RP, et al. A large community acquired outbreak of salmonellosis in Oregon caused by intentional contamination of salad bars. *JAMA* 1997;278:389-95.

32. Horgan J. Were Four Corners victims biowar casualties? *Sci Am* 1993;269:16.

33. Pesik N, Keim M. Do US emergency medicine residency programs provide adequate training for bioterrorism? *Ann Emerg Med.* August 1999;34(2):173-6.

34. Seiple C. Consequence management: domestic response to weapons of mass destruction. *Parameters* Autumn 1997:119-34.

35. Sharp TW, Brennan RJ, Keim M, et al. Medical preparedness for a terrorist incident involving chemical or biological agents during the 1996 Atlanta Olympic Games. *Ann Emerg Med.* August 1998;32: 214-23.

36. Office of the Press Secretary, White House, U.S. Policy on counterterrorism. *Presidential Directive.* Annapolis, MD, June 21, 1995. Unclassified version available at: http://www.fas.org/irp/offdocs/pdd39.htm.

37. Initial National Response Plan, 2004. Available at: http://www.nemaweb.org/docs/national_response_plan.pdf.

chapter 56

Thinking Outside the Box: Health Service Support Considerations in the Era of Asymmetrical Threats

Pietro D. Marghella and Duane C. Caneva

When the Cold War effectively ended in the early 1990s, it marked the passing of an era in warfare. For generations, we had become used to viewing the spectrum of warfare from a traditional and symmetrical linear perspective. As events progressed in intensity, so did the population-at-risk (i.e., those involved with the prosecution of a battle) and the level of expected casualty production. In the linear threat environment (which traditionally constitutes force-on-force engagements), where casualty models based on reliable sources and a similar historic event could be used to determine scope, scale, and timing of expected casualties, medical planning simply involved constructing an adequate health service support architecture to support the population-at-risk based on the level of intensity they expected to incur in the operational environment.

The last quarter of the twentieth century bears witness to a shift in the prosecution of warfare away from those traditional linear events to one dominated by the threat of asymmetrical attacks. As the balance of power shifted to a sole-surviving global hegemon (the United States), rogue nations and nonstate actors wishing to influence world affairs or advance their political or religious goals realized that the only way to strike at their enemies was through the use of terrorism, which by definition is non-linear or asymmetrical in its approach. A further evolution of this strategy, termed *fourth generation warfare,* postulates that the driving factors of this global transition are more than the progression from the industrial age to the information age, but include political, social, and economic factors. The threat consists of an enemy made up of loosely associated groups or franchises of cells that are bound by common goals, if not ideology. They leverage various networks available in the information age to attack our new center of gravity—political will. They are skilled in using to their advantage the endless news cycles, legitimate-appearing organizations, lobbying efforts, support and encouragement from useful idiots, and even political donations or lobbying to peddle influence, sway public opinion, and effect outcomes favorable to their cause. The tactics result in an increased risk of asymmetrical attack in the face of partisan discord in the political arena and divided public opinion.[1]

To complicate matters even further, chemical, biologic, radiologic, nuclear, and high-yield explosive (CBRNE) weapons of mass destruction (WMD) have entered the scene as the potential "weapon of choice" for terrorist organizations, which seek to inflict the greatest possible damage on their targets in hopes of creating large-scale conflagrations that cause second-, third-, fourth-order, or even higher, cascading effects (e.g., medical, political, economic, international events) and unintended consequences. It appears that the most fervent hope of terrorist organizations is to create so significant a set of ripples as to upset the very order and stability of our society, to the point of bringing us to the very precipice of collapse.

In the new generation of warfare, our planning for emergency management will prove challenging for several reasons:

1. CBRNE agents can cause incidents that cross the linear spectrum of casualty production relative to agent used. Terrorist organizations and rogue nonstate actors now have access to improved weapons technology and weapons with the potential for far greater impact that have been developed outside the control of state-sponsored programs through the targeting of increased population densities and by our own increased reliance on critical infrastructures in our society. Further, some terrorist groups no longer seek to cause terror as the sole end, but seek to kill as many people in their target population as possible.
2. There are no useful casualty rates to extract from CBRNE environments, hence no empirical data to determine what the event will look like relative to casualty production.
3. CBRNE mass casualty incident requirements (e.g., "detect to determine work environment") differ from military nuclear, biologic, and chemical defense conducted on the battlefield ("detect to avoid") and from hazardous materials response ("detect to contain").

4. The very nature of terrorism will mandate that emergency response measures will always be conducted in "crisis mode." Concepts like "graceful" or "managed" degradation of the standards of care that should be addressed in preincident planning will most certainly have to be considered under the constraints of the crisis, when there is little room for thoughtful consideration. Self-organization of response components will need to occur in response to chaotic conditions set by the incident.

5. The potential for catastrophic casualty events will be high, especially if nuclear or biologic agents are employed. As terrorists become emboldened—or desperate—the very fact that the majority of their potential targets live in free and open societies only enhances the opportunity to create such nightmarish scenarios, especially as access to increased weapon technology progresses and our population densities remain static in high-threat locations. Given these assumptions, emergency planning should assume that response and support infrastructure would be significantly stressed from the onset of an attack.

From here on in, we enter into a new set of assumptions about the world we live in and how we intend to prevent, prepare for, and mitigate the threats we now face. First, it is important for us to accept what we would have previously considered absurd in terms of threats is now entirely possible. In the post-9/11 era, we face scenarios that could make the events of *that* fateful day pale in comparison. Second, we have to recognize that another attack (or attacks) could occur at any time, anywhere around the world. Indeed, intelligence services tell us (in open-source literature) that one of the preferred methods of inciting terror and mass panic is multinodal, simultaneous targeting against multiple sectors of critical infrastructure to enhance the systemic impact of the event and maximize the stress on our collective response network. And third, we have to recognize that we are just not collectively prepared to deal with a high-end attack. Disaster management for high operational to strategic level events is simply too immature to assume that we would capably and adequately handle an event that has few, recent U.S. historical precedents.[*] Hence, there is a pressing mandate for us to consider alternative strategies for complex emergency and disaster management, strategies that move away from the traditional, linear, and symmetrical approaches we have historically employed in the emergency response arena. It's time to enter the environment "outside the box."

WHAT'S OUTSIDE THE BOX?

The phrase "thinking outside the box" has long been a mantra of the business community to discourage managers and executives from becoming too lock-step (or

linear) in their approach to standards of acceptable business practices. Above all, thinking outside the box promotes the notion of the paradigm shift, which seeks to break away from a standards-based approach in which rigorous statutes are followed without deviation. Performing qualitative and quantitative risk assessments, leveraging the collective experience and expertise of the emergency management community, and demonstrating a willingness to take greater risk for potentially much greater benefit, indeed, operating on the edge of chaos,[2] is clearly the order of the day in the new threat environment in which we now find ourselves. It also represents an opportune time to identify—indeed create, if necessary—the unrecognized dimensions and disciplines (the "unknown unknowns") that may prove to provide the solution sets we need to assuage these threats. To this end, the following out-of-the-box strategies are offered for consideration.

Be Practical

Our approach to complex disaster and emergency management has to be pragmatic. As a human species, we have a nearly reflexive way of ignoring the potential for staggering calamity. Maintaining a mental attitude of "If I don't think about it, perhaps it will go away!" is indeed a dangerous perspective to keep when there is more than sufficient evidence that our enemies wish to do us great harm. A common progressive rationalization process is thinking that "It won't happen; or, it won't happen to me; or, it will happen to me but won't be severe; or, it will happen to me and be severe, but somebody else will rescue me." It is equally dangerous to engage in a pessimistic approach when planning for catastrophic attacks that produce strategic-level casualty streams. If we simply assume that our collective response resources are going to implode under the weight of an event, we ignore the opportunity to take qualitative measures to improve our level of preparedness through pre-event (deliberate) planning and resource building—the greater the effort made in developing response capabilities, the higher the threshold at which the system fails.

The public health, medical, and emergency response communities that will bear the most weight of the emergency management mission must ignore the tendency to view the world through rose-colored glasses. Certain scenarios that are deemed plausible *are* indeed chilling to think about. An improvised nuclear weapon detonation in a major metropolitan area, or the dissemination of a biologic agent that causes a widespread outbreak of a highly lethal disease, are incredibly frightening to consider, but consider them we must because these scenarios are entirely plausible in today's threat environment. Plausibility—no matter how extreme—must drive what we prepare for, and facing the threats head on will be the only way we are able to increase our level of preparedness.

Be Proactive

Homeland Security Presidential Directive 5 mandated that the U.S. Department of Homeland Security (DHS) develop the National Incident Management System

---

[*] Catastrophic Casualty Events (CCE) are stratified at three levels: Level I, up to 1000 casualties; Level II, up to 10,000 casualties; and Level III, above 10,000 casualties. For the purpose of this discussion, the authors argue that any attack at Level II or above will tax our emergency response systems to the point of corruption.

(NIMS) and designated the DHS as the primary agency for homeland security issues. The NIMS has established pillars of emergency management and disaster preparedness as preparedness, prevention, mitigation, response, and recovery, and mandates that the DHS develop an NIMS Integration Office to coordinate and integrate across these pillars nationally. It follows, then, that our planning be proactive versus reactive, with much to do preincident. Proactivity in the complex emergency and disaster management arena equates to considering the notion of deliberate planning as a very important tool in the planner's kitbag. Deliberate planning before an event allows us the time to expend intellectual capital on the various scenarios of concern on the CBRNE WMD threat environment. It provides us with an opportunity to consider how the complex mix of response assets and protocols, equipment, and logistical resources can all be coordinated to be in the right place at the right time to help facilitate response. Done right, deliberate planning flows directly into crisis action planning as soon as either an event trigger is noticed or an actual event occurs. Skilled emergency planners and managers recognize that once an actual situation develops, planning becomes fluid, and in some cases, many of the response accommodations made in the deliberate phase may no longer be applicable. As is often stated, it is not so much the plan that is important but the planning process; however, it is far easier to flex an existent plan to an unfolding event than it is to develop a plan from scratch the moment an attack or complex emergency occurs. Simply being reactive to an emergent event is a recipe for disaster, since disasters are multidimensional and create far too much "fog" to ever sort out in a sufficient period to effectively mitigate the impact.

Avoid Duplicating Efforts

The previous point leads to the issue of economy of effort. Justifying the resources required to prepare against terrorist attacks can be a challenge in appropriating the capital, time, and other scarce resources. However, numerous arguments and examples exist that support such efforts being a routine part of strategic planning for any business, sector, enterprise, or agency as well as identifying funding sources for capabilities.[3,4]

Such topics as continuity of operations, critical infrastructure protection, or protection of mission-critical resources are just as important in government, military, or business sectors, although the economic benefit derived by these practices may not be initially obvious. Identifying these benefits and recognizing the randomness of complex emergencies and the unintended consequences that can snowball or cascade into second-, third-, or higher-order effects of catastrophic event requires significant insight, experience, and expertise but represent good and necessary business practices. Developing and maintaining a robust medical system able to sustain an adequate response capability represents a benefit to society at large, and funding and support sources should reflect this.

Disperse Resources

From a logistical perspective, it further follows that we consider moving away from centralized resource management to dispersed resource management relative to catastrophic emergency response. Former Commander of the United States Pacific Command Admiral Joseph Prueher wrestled with the challenges of having the largest geographic combatant command area of responsibility of all of the U.S. Combatant Commanders. To describe the challenges he faced in theoretical terms, he coined the notion of the "tyranny of distance" relative to the rapidity of response. Simply put, the farther your response resources are from the event, the longer it will take to get those resources to an affected population; hence, your ability to adequately respond will be proportionately diminished.

The dispersed prepositioning of the Strategic National Stockpile (SNS) is an excellent demonstration of how to overcome the challenges to rapid response. The DHS and the Department of Health and Human Services recognized that a centralized location of the stockpile could be detrimental to rapid response distribution to an affected locale. To better facilitate distribution, the stockpile was broken down into 12 geographically disparate locations around the United States, with organic movement resources to facilitate distribution in the wake of an event. Following suit by prepositioning other response assets (including stockpiles of minimal care beds and healthcare staff to support large populations affected by an attack or disaster) would help in minimizing the impact of the tyranny of distance and would improve overall response capabilities. The SNS "ChemPack" program illustrates this principle even further for the example of a chemical attack, placing time-critical supplies closer to where they might be needed.

Expand the Medical Infrastructure

In formulating plans for managing catastrophic casualty events, it will be necessary to break the medical paradigm that relies on hospitals for the management of casualties and constitutes a rigid standard of care. With the advent of managed care in the last quarter of the twentieth century as a nearly universal approach to the provision of hospital-based medicine in the United States,[5] the notion of "available beds" for disaster and emergency situations has dissolved. It should now be considered a false expectation that hospitals (as finite physical structures) will be capable of taking on casualties from an event that could produce sudden spikes of thousands, if not tens of thousands or more, victims. In all likelihood, these resources would collapse under the weight of even a moderate event, essentially eliminating the most important resource of an affected area's medical infrastructure—its cadre of trained professional healthcare providers. Efforts made using a multidisciplinary approach have afforded excellent guiding and design principles for hospital-based mass casualty care in response to CBRNE incidents, including issues of surge capability, optimizing productivity, leveraging on technology, and managing a degradation of capability.[4]

The solution for catastrophic-scale incidents again lies in the deliberate planning before an event occurs, when regional planners can identify "locations of opportunity" that can be used as alternate care facilities. Any physical structure that offers large open space where casualties can be directed to obtain support is a candidate for this designation; gyms, schools, shopping malls, and sports arenas all represent excellent locations for use under emergency conditions. Similarly, if basic utilities remain intact, hospitals could be established in select neighborhoods where a house serves as a ward and a block or street serves as the "hospital." The trained professional staffs of regional medical facilities can then be used to triage patients to these sites and oversee the provision of minimal care support through the use of community-based care by family and noninjured survivors. Limited staff capabilities would be addressed through various mechanisms, such as national credentialing or emergency credentialing procedures allowing for rapid credentialing of professionals provided from outside the affected region, temporary extension of current privileges under innovative supervision, longer hours, and cancellation or postponement of routine medical care. Use of paramedical or lay personnel with on-the-job training, and again, innovative supervision, could also provide additional caretakers. Coupled with the prepositioning of minimal care beds as mentioned above, this strategy could be useful in preserving the community's medical infrastructure while still offering a viable way of handling potentially catastrophic casualty streams. Such "off-site" care facilities would require additional, complex coordination with the regional healthcare community through critical functions including information and communications, transportation, logistics and supply, government services, mortuary affairs, and a host of public health services making for an extremely challenging situation. Although degradation in the standard of care would be anticipated and difficult to determine ahead of time, this issue, as well as credentialing and privileging issues, should be addressed as part of a national strategy.

Network Multidisciplinary Resources

Identifying not only the multiple disciplines necessary in developing response capability, but also the multiple dimensions and layers of planning required across preparedness, prevention, mitigation, response, and recovery phases of emergency management must be explored. Response occurs not only within the wire diagram framework of the Incident Command System, but, depending on size and scope, occurs functionally across sectors, critical infrastructures, industries, and complexes in conjunction with government agencies, nongovernmental organizations, and the citizenry. Perhaps the greatest asset in industrialized nations is industry itself, with its innovators and entrepreneurs. Table 56-1 compares various emergency management functions, emergency support functions, and critical infrastructures likely to form the complexes with a role in emergency management. Such complexes overlap and must be networked.

Within the medical complex are different dimensions such as emergency medical services; the medical treatment infrastructure; public health departments; the pharmaceutical industry; the diagnostic equipment industry; the laboratory, medical logistical, and supply industry; and care providers and technicians. In its entirety, the med-

---

TABLE 56-1 COMPARISON OF EMERGENCY MANAGEMENT FUNCTIONAL AREAS, EMERGENCY SUPPORT FUNCTIONS, AND CRITICAL INFRASTRUCTURE SECTORS

EMERGENCY MANAGEMENT FUNCTIONAL AREAS*	NRP EMERGENCY SUPPORT FUNCTIONS†	CRITICAL INFRASTRUCTURE SECTORS (PDD-63)‡
Command staff	Transportation	Information and communications
Fire and emergency services	Information technology and communications	Banking and finance
Emergency medical services	Infrastructure	Water supply
Security/law enforcement	Firefighting	Transportation (aviation, highways, mass transit, rail, waterborne, pipelines)
Explosives ordnance disposal	Information and planning	Emergency law enforcement services
Public works	Mass care, housing, human services	Continuity of government services
Public affairs	Resource support and logistics management	Emergency fire services
Mass care	Public health and medical services	Public health
Health service support	Urban search and rescue	Energy (electric power, oil, and gas production and storage)
Occupational safety and health	Hazardous materials response	Special functions
Industrial hygiene	Food and agriculture	Law enforcement and internal security
Meteorology and oceanography	Energy	National defense
Supply and logistics	Law enforcement	Foreign affairs
Mortuary affairs	Economic stabilization, community recovery, and mitigation	Foreign intelligence
Emergency response teams	Emergency public information and external communications	

*Adapted from U.S. Navy Emergency Management Program.
†NRP, National Response Plan, Final Draft, June 30, 2004.
‡PDD-63, Presidential Decision Directive-63, May 22, 1998.

ical complex represents a powerful capability if it is coordinated across public, private, and government assets at local, regional, state, and federal levels; however, it must also network with other complexes including security/law enforcement, emergency and fire services, government, supply and logistics, the general public, media, and transportation, and it must do so with the right processes, disciplines, and specialists in all five phases of emergency management. As an example, medical syndromic surveillance must be integrated with surveillance in other areas such as law enforcement, intelligence, food, water, transportation, education, and the public and private sectors, and how these sectors interrelate needs to be explored.

Explore Capabilities to Handle Mass Casualty

One area of discipline that needs further development is the study of mass casualty care. Development, evaluation, and validation of tactics, techniques, and procedures used for the triage and treatment of mass casualty victims in chaotic, perhaps even contaminated environments needs to be done using the scientific method, and progression from consensus-based guidelines to evidence-based practices must be made a priority. Such issues as triage, mass casualty airway management, or mass casualty decontamination techniques, and the ability to correlate response requirements with resources and capabilities in real time, represent some of the areas in need of further study.

Provide Emergency Management Training

We need to identify standard training requirements and positional competencies for key roles in our emergency management programs. This would include training for emergency response personnel tailored to their specific needs but standardized for that sector or industry, and this must be affordable and available locally. Required sustainment training should include practical application of skills in evaluated exercises and not just training on individual response equipment. Advanced training should be developed for a portion of those (perhaps 20%), advancing their skills and enabling them to act as "force multipliers" or "self-organizers" during practical application exercises and enabling them to lead squad-level teams in the Incident Command System in the response phase. Expert-level "train the trainer" training for a select number should include advanced "live fire"–type training and enable these responders to lead at the group, departmental, or division level in the Incident Command System during the response phase. Finally, and most importantly, this training should be institutionalized and incorporated into academic curricula using national standards.

Educate the Populace

Taken one step further relative to training, there is a need to train or, at least, sensitize the population on how complex emergencies and disasters will be managed, including where to access medical care after an event has occurred. It will require a significant, national-level effort to set an initiative of this level in motion. At the height of the Cold War, our national civil defense program was the mechanism by which we educated, trained, and sensitized our nation to the omnipresent threat of nuclear attack. Many of us who came of age in this era can well remember the authoritative voice over the radio announcing "THIS IS A TEST OF THE EMERGENCY BROADCAST SYSTEM"; the sound of the weekly civil defense siren; and the ubiquitous duck-and-cover drills requiring us to dive under our school desks at a moment's notice. Although to some a wistful memory of their youth and a bygone era, these now represent a "back-to-the-future" concept of emergency preparedness we must embrace if we are to prepare our citizenry for the inevitability of a calamitous event, whether it is natural or manmade. Our national leadership has to lean forward to reinvigorate a civil defense program that provides education, training, and substantive direction on how to enhance our individual survivability. They should leverage the proliferation of media platforms that can carry the preparedness message, including television, radio, and the World Wide Web. Civil defense preparedness has to be reinculcated into our population, lest we again be caught off guard the next time an attack or disastrous event occurs.

Develop the Preparedness Architecture

Finally, we need to take the steps necessary to complete the national response and preparedness architecture. When DHS Secretary Tom Ridge announced the increase in the national threat level on December 21, 2003, it set into motion a unique and historically unprecedented planning evolution that culminated in the fielding of the Catastrophic Incident Response Annex Supplement (CIRAS) of the National Response Plan (NRP). This plan now describes how the collective federal partner agencies will respond to assist state and local authorities with the management of a catastrophic casualty event. Although significant as a first-order effort to put our collective arms around newly emerging threats, there are still overall gaps in our planning architecture due to the fact that the state and local strata of response have not yet developed supported and/or supporting plans to the national-level initiatives of the CIRAS/NRP. To help enhance the effectiveness of our response and preparedness efforts, there needs to be as seamless an architecture as possible between those three levels of response. Failing to coordinate our consequence management strategy is a recipe for chaos and failure at the moment of execution, and it should at all costs be avoided.

CONCLUSION

Prior to September 11, 2001, using phrases like "thinking outside the box" would have been considered trite by any standard and would likely have relegated the writer to the ranks of the new-idea and catch-phrase challenged. Since that time, America's perception of the world has changed in a way so dramatic that even the most prescient prognosticators of global events could not have possibly predicted. Given that fact, any decision on how to approach these dramatic shifts that doesn't rely on thinking outside of the box dooms us to failure from the start for one glaringly simple reason: all of the strategies developed for complex emergency and disaster management in the pre-9/11 era would never have offered useful solution sets for the scope and scale of events that we believe will now have reasonable expectation to occur. The challenge is to develop adequate policy, doctrine, and strategy for the conduct of our crisis response and consequence management efforts in the face of the present threats. Emergency preparedness professionals must consider adopting new approaches to the management of these events if we are ever to achieve success in the new threat environment.

REFERENCES

1. Hammes TX. The evolution of war: the fourth generation. *The Marine Corps Gazette*. September 1994.
2. Koehler GA. What disaster response management can learn from chaos theory. Conference Proceedings, May 18-19, 1995. Available at: http://er1.org/docs/references/General%20Articles/Chaos%20 and%20Disaster%20Planning/index.html.
3. Barbera JA, Macintyre AG, DeAtley CA. Ambulances to nowhere: America's critical shortfall in medical preparedness for catastrophic terrorism. BCSIA Discussion Paper 2001-15, ESDP Discussion Paper ESDP-2001-07. Cambridge, Mass: John F. Kennedy School of Government, Harvard University; October 2001.
4. All-Risks-Ready Emergency Department. Project ER One. Available at: http://er1.org.
5. Tufts Managed Care Institute. A Brief History of Managed Care. 1998. Available at: http://www.tmci.org/downloads/BriefHist.pdf.

chapter 57

Accidental Versus Intentional Event

Joanne Cono

Not all disasters are easily recognized in their early stages. Although disasters caused by weather events (e.g., tornadoes, hurricanes, lightning), geologic events (e.g., earthquakes, volcanic eruptions), and some technologic events (e.g., bomb explosions, nuclear reactor accidents, structural failures) are quickly attributable to a physical source, other disasters such as acts of biologic, chemical, or radiologic terrorism may not be readily recognized or characterized.[1] Recognizing and responding to these types of disasters requires patience, a high index of suspicion, clinical astuteness, and rapid epidemiologic assessment and response. Disasters that manifest with physical illness in a population may go unrecognized over a period of time and not become apparent until many persons become ill or die, or the contaminating or infectious agent is identified as one that does not commonly occur or does not appear to be a plausible natural finding.

When an illness is attributed to an unexpected biologic, chemical, or radiologic agent, information from a detailed patient clinical and epidemiologic history is the most effective tool to distinguish "accidental" or "natural" outbreaks from "intentional" or "terrorism-related" outbreaks. Local and state public health authorities should be notified when a patient is diagnosed with an unusual illness or syndrome. Public health authorities will begin the larger-scale epidemiologic investigation and the public health response necessary to control disasters caused by biologic, chemical, and radiologic terrorism. When an intentional terrorist event is suspected, public health authorities also will engage law enforcement agencies to begin concurrent criminal investigations.

HISTORICAL PERSPECTIVE

Biologic, chemical, or radiologic terrorism is the deliberate use of any of these agents against people, animals, or agriculture to cause disease, death, destruction, or panic for political or social gains. The only factor differentiating an accidental event from a terrorist event may be the malicious intent.[2] Historically, there have been serious outbreaks that have been mistaken for intentional terrorist attacks and serious outbreaks for which terrorism was quickly ruled out.

Two naturally occurring infectious disease outbreaks in the United States were initially feared to be the result of terrorist attacks: the hantavirus pulmonary syndrome outbreak of 1994[3] and the West Nile fever outbreak of 1999.[4] Both were caused by newly emergent infectious diseases and required careful evaluation of clinical and epidemiologic data to assign causality. In each case, a new viral pathogen was identified that was not endemic to the United States. Both outbreak investigations yielded reasonable alternative explanations that refuted the terrorism hypothesis.

The smallpox outbreak of 1978 in Birmingham, England, is an example of an accidental outbreak that today might raise suspicions of a terrorist attack. The last case of naturally occurring smallpox anywhere in the world was diagnosed in Somalia in 1977, and endemic smallpox had not been seen in England since 1975. Ten months after the world's last case, a 40-year-old woman in Birmingham, England, was found to have smallpox.[5] She died 3 weeks later, but not before infecting her mother (who recovered) and perhaps her father (who, though febrile, died of myocardial infarction within the incubation period of disease). Prompt vaccination of contacts and isolation of febrile contacts quickly extinguished the outbreak. Public health investigators concluded that source of the outbreak was most likely the smallpox laboratory at University of Birmingham. The index case patient was a medical photographer who worked in an office immediately above the laboratory. Matching strains of smallpox confirmed the source, although the route of virus transmission is less certain. This was the last outbreak of smallpox in the world. In 1980, the World Health Assembly declared smallpox to be eradicated from the planet. Any smallpox outbreaks that occur posteradication most likely will be first investigated as a terrorist event.

During the anthrax attacks of 2001, the first case of anthrax was initially suspected to be a naturally occurring case.[6-8] The index patient, a resident of Florida, traveled through rural North Carolina 3 days prior to becoming ill with inhalational anthrax, an uncommon diagnosis even in animal handlers, and an even more unusual diagnosis in an office worker. Since anthrax spores are regularly found in soil and cases can occur among persons who are exposed to animal products that have been contaminated by soil, this particular case was investigated for sources of animal exposure. None was found. When further epidemiologic investigation revealed anthrax spores in the patient's workplace and a coworker became ill with inhalational anthrax, terrorism was recognized. In this attack, 21 persons were infected via the postal system. This case study illustrates the importance of considering terrorism when investigating outbreaks that occur in unusual geographic locations (e.g., anthrax in urban/suburban Florida), among unusual populations (e.g., office workers with no animal contact), and in clusters (e.g., more than one person in the same office).

CURRENT PRACTICE

Disease outbreaks have occurred and been investigated for many years. However, recent events such as the 2001 anthrax attacks and the 1994 and 1995 sarin gas attacks make it necessary to consider terrorism when evaluating outbreaks of infectious and noninfectious disease. A terrorist agent may be a very common organism, such as influenza or *Salmonella*, or may be a more exotic organism such as Ebola virus or variola virus.

Unusual clusters of illness may signal terrorist events that require prompt public health and law enforcement responses. Although most clusters of disease will have a source other than a deliberate act of criminal intent, terrorism should be considered in the differential diagnosis. Each situation must be evaluated based on its specific context.

As noted above, today a single case of smallpox would be immediately investigated as a case of biologic terrorism; however, some events may be more subtle. When investigating a disease outbreak, there are a number of clues that should heighten the suspicions of the clinician and epidemiologist that a terrorist attack has occurred.[9-15] Because no list of clues can be all-inclusive, all healthcare providers should be alert for the possibility that a patient's condition may not have occurred through natural means.

Although terrorist attacks could ultimately affect large numbers of people, disease in a single patient may be the first clue. Disease caused by an uncommon organism, such as smallpox, anthrax, or viral hemorrhagic fever, may signal a bioterrorism event. Suspicion may be further heightened by a less common presentation of one of these organisms. For example, whereas a small number of cases of cutaneous anthrax occur naturally each year in the United States, cases of inhalational anthrax are highly unusual. Furthermore, should a disease present in a geographic location where it is not usually seen, such as anthrax in a nonrural area or plague in the northeastern United States, further investigation for the possibility of bioterrorism is needed. Unexpected seasonal distribution of disease, such as influenza in the summer or antiquated, genetically engineered, or unusual strains of infectious agents may also be clues. Multiple unusual or unexplained diseases in the same patient may indicate that multiple organisms or substances were used in an intentional act, as could disease presenting in an atypical age-group or population, such as anthrax in children or varicella-like rashes in adults.

When a disease strikes more than one person, additional clues may arise. Large numbers of cases of unexplained disease or death may signal bioterrorism, as may an unexplained increase in the incidence of an endemic disease that previously had a stable incidence rate. If an unusual condition strikes a disparate population, such as respiratory illness in a large population, this may signal the release of a biologic agent, as would a large number of people seeking medical care at a particular time, signaling they may have been present at a common site when an agent was released. Likewise, large numbers of persons presenting with similar illnesses in noncontiguous regions may be a sign that there have been simultaneous releases of an agent. Finally, animal illness or die-off that precedes, follows, or occurs simultaneously with human illness or death may signify the release of an agent that affects both animals and humans.

When there is no other explanation for an outbreak of illness, it may be reasonable to investigate terrorism as a possible source. Common sources of exposure to an agent may include food and water that has been deliberately contaminated, respiratory illness due to proximity to a ventilation source, or the absence of illness among those in geographic proximity but not directly exposed to the contaminated food, water, or air.

Each event must be evaluated in context. Terrorism is still the least common explanation for disease, and other more common explanations should be evaluated and ruled out. Clues that may raise the suspicion that an intentional event has occurred can be broken down into some general categories: epidemiologic, unusual variations in disease outbreaks, unusual characteristics of disease, and animal signals.

Epidemiologic Clues

- A single case of an unusual disease, such as plague, smallpox, or anthrax, without an acceptable epidemiologic explanation
- Illness among persons with exposure to a common ventilation source and absence of disease among persons not exposed to that ventilation source should raise suspicions of an intentional aerosol release of an agent
- Large numbers of persons seeking care for a similar condition at the same time, which may indicate a point source
- Clusters of similar disease outbreaks in noncontiguous geographic locations, indicating multiple attacks
- Large numbers of cases of unexplained diseases or deaths

Unusual Variations in Disease Outbreaks

- Unexplained increases in an endemic illness, such as an increase in plague case in the southwest United States
- Disease occurring outside of its usual seasonal cycle, such as an influenza outbreak during the summer
- Disease occurring outside of its usual geographic distribution, such as plague or hantavirus occurring in the northeastern United States

- Disease that appears to be transmitted via common exposure to an aerosol, food, or water that may have been intentionally contaminated

Unusual Characteristics of Disease or Agents

- Isolation of a genetically engineered, antiquated, or laboratory-manufactured strain of organism
- Isolation of a weapons-grade form of an agent
- Isolation of a known organism with an unusual antibiotic-resistance pattern
- Unusual presentations of clinical disease, such as pneumonic plague (rather than bubonic plague usually caused by bites from infected fleas) or inhalational anthrax (rather than the more common cutaneous presentation)
- Common disease with a higher than expected mortality, or decreased patient response to usual treatments
- Several conditions or clinical syndromes occurring in the same patient, which may indicate genetically engineered or artificially combined agents
- Disease or syndromes occurring in unusual populations, such as outbreaks of chickenpox-like rash in adults or anthrax among office workers
- Unusual disease outbreaks that occur across a large geographic area, suggesting the aerosol release of an agent
- Similar genetic types of a pathogen identified across disparate geographic locations or at different times in the same location

Other Species Signals

- An unusual pattern of animal disease or death preceding human disease or death, or an unusual pattern of animal disease or death that follows human disease or death; both may indicate a large-scale release of an agent, with differing susceptibilities between animals and humans.
- Insect die-off or plant die-off associated with human illness may indicate an environmental chemical release in which the symptoms of human poisoning syndromes may be nonspecific.
- Physical findings in the environment such as liquid droplets or puddles, powders or dusts, vapors or clouds, or unusual odors in the vicinity of human or animal cases may indicate a release of a biologic, chemical, or radiologic agent.

Radiologic and Chemical Agents

Although these examples focus mostly on biologic terrorism, the tenets presented apply to radiologic and chemical events too. Covert radiologic events, such as intentionally hiding a cobalt or cesium source stolen from a medical facility in a public place, may expose many unsuspecting people.[16] During cases of accidental exposure, involved persons again may not realize that they have been exposed, such as in the 1987 Goiania incident in Brazil, in which a canister of cesium-137 was inappropriately discarded by a cancer treatment facility. One family brought home the sealed radioactive element and unwittingly exposed multiple family members who became ill. Neighboring families came to look at the fluorescent blue substance, some covering their skin with it. Although clinicians did not make the link to radiation exposure in this cluster of illness, the family's grandmother realized that her family became ill shortly after the radioactive canister entered their home. She surrendered the canister to health authorities, though not before an estimated 244 people in the community were exposed.[17]

With sufficient exposure, whether intentional or accidental, multiple persons may present with acute radiation syndrome, which during its prodromal phase is characterized by nausea, vomiting, and diarrhea that last for several days after exposure. This is followed by a latent phase, during which a patient feels well for a few weeks until obvious radiation illness begins.[18] This spectrum of clinical illness can easily be confused with a self-limited gastrointestinal illness, particularly if a number of people attend the same event during which the exposure occurs and then present with gastrointestinal symptoms. A thorough epidemiologic investigation may rule out a common food source. A high index of suspicion for a radiation event should be maintained, especially when an infectious pathogen is not readily identifiable from clinical specimens. Patients with acute radiation syndrome may also experience cutaneous radiation syndrome, a dermatologic condition, consisting of erythema, pruritus, and desquamation. These cutaneous symptoms, accompanied by gastrointestinal symptoms and the absence of an infectious pathogen in a cluster of patients, may indicate a radiation exposure, whether accidental or intentional. Hidden sources of exposure usually lead to diagnostic delays. Again, prompt epidemiologic investigation of unusual cases can hasten the identification of a source, and criminal investigation is needed to determine possible intent.

Likewise, recognizing exposures to chemical agents can be challenging, even though the epidemiologic clues listed above still apply. Chemical exposures may be overt and quickly recognized, like the 1984 industrial accident in Bhopal, India,[19] in which a release of methyl isocyanate killed 2500 people during the first week and an estimated 3500 more over the following 10 years. Or a chemical incident may be covert as in contamination of food, water, or consumer products.[20] Some exposures may cause delayed health effects, making it more difficult to identify an exposure source. Chemical exposures often cause nonspecific illnesses, or syndromes of illness that are less familiar to many clinicians. Additionally, if chemicals are mixed, classic toxicologic syndromes such anticholinergic poisoning may not be apparent because patients may experience a broad array of symptoms rather than a single recognizable syndrome.

There are many case reports that illustrate these diagnostic and investigative challenges of chemical exposures. In the United States, in the Tylenol tampering cases of 1982[21] and other medicine tampering cases like it,[22] otherwise healthy patients who ingested cyanide-laced over-the-counter medications became seriously ill and multiple deaths occurred. In the Tylenol incident, the first two deaths were thought to be due to stroke and myocardial infarction. But an astute clinician linked the unexplained syndromes of hypotension and acidosis in multiple family members of the first victim, and subsequent toxicologic testing revealed cyanide poisoning. This case report demonstrates the importance of considering chemical exposure when a cluster of patients presents with illness that is sudden, unexpected, and without prodrome. When clinical information does not indicate a naturally occurring disease, toxicology screening for poisoning is a reasonable next step.

Similarly, unexplained deaths or serious illness in an otherwise healthy population may indicate a chemical exposure. Over a 6-month period in 1985, 109 children were diagnosed with acute anuric renal failure at a single hospital in Haiti.[23] This condition had not been seen at the hospital in the 5 prior years. A traceback investigation revealed that these children had ingested a locally manufactured acetaminophen syrup preparation that was glycerin contaminated with diethylene glycol, the chemical used as automotive antifreeze. Ninety-nine of the children died. A criminal investigation ensued and determined that the poisoning was not intentional, but rather was caused by a departure from manufacturing quality control measures.

Pesticides are a group of toxic chemicals that are readily available to terrorists and also can accidentally contaminate the food supply, sickening large numbers of people in disparate geographic areas. In Oregon in 1985, a physician reported to the State Health Division 5 cases of organophosphate poisoning, resulting in cholinergic crisis. Epidemiologic investigation revealed that the patients had become ill after eating watermelon. Additional cases were reported in Oregon, Washington, and California.[24] Over 3 months, more than 700 cases were identified in 7 U.S. states, and 483 cases occurred in Canada. The outbreak was linked to aldicarb sulfoxide poisoning, a toxic metabolite of Aldicarb, the systemic pesticide that was used on the watermelons originating from California. The rapid notification of public health authorities led to timely identification of the poison, although the outbreak was protracted due to the far-reaching shipping network of the global food supply. The contamination was not found to be intentional.

In another pesticide-related case, in Michigan in 2003, 92 people became ill and 1700 lb of ground beef were recalled due to nicotine-based pesticide contamination.[25] However, in this case, the epidemiologic investigation identified a single supermarket source of the contaminated meat, and the concurrent criminal investigation led to the arrest of a supermarket employee who intentionally contaminated 200 lb of ground beef with Black Leaf 40 insecticide, which contains nicotine.

These pesticide contamination case studies illustrate the following: (1) clinicians should consider chemical poisoning in outbreaks of unexpected serious illnesses; (2) prompt reporting to authorities can more rapidly initiate public health response activities by linking distant outbreaks to a common source; and (3) accidental and criminal events may involve the same clinical illness but can be distinguished by epidemiologic and criminal investigations.

PITFALLS

There is no one algorithm that can determine whether a biologic, chemical, or radiologic disaster is naturally occurring, accidental, or intentional. Situations in which multiple agents have been used may be more difficult to recognize and may pose a greater diagnostic challenge, but once identified may be more easily characterized as intentional. Certain terrorist events will remain difficult to detect; however, through careful evaluation of all epidemiologic clues and a thorough outbreak investigation, it is possible to make educated decisions that will permit the public health and law enforcement emergency responses necessary to limit the damage caused by an intentional disaster.

REFERENCES

1. Landesman LY. Public health response to emerging infections and bioterrorism. In: *Public Health Management of Disasters: The Practice Guide*. Washington, DC: American Public Health Association; 2001:121-138.
2. Keim M. Intentional chemical disasters. In: Hogan D, Burstein J, eds. *Disaster Medicine*. Philadelphia: Lippincott, Williams & Wilkins; 2002.
3. Centers for Disease Control and Prevention. Outbreak of acute illness: Southwestern United States, 1993. *MMWR* 1993;42:421-4.
4. Nash D, Mostashari F, Fine A. Outbreak of West Nile infection, New York City area. *New Engl J Med.* 2001;344(24):1858-9.
5. Fenner F, Henderson DA, Arita I, et al. *Smallpox and its Eradication.* 1980.
6. Centers for Disease Control and Prevention. Update: investigation of anthrax associated with intentional exposure and interim public health guidelines, October 2001. *MMWR* 2001;50(41):889-92.
7. Maillard JM, Fischer M, McKee KT, et al. First case of bioterrorism-related inhalational anthrax, Florida, 2001: North Carolina Investigation. *Emerg Infect Dis.* 2002;8:1035-8.
8. Traeger MS, Wersma ST, Rosenstein NE, et al. First case of bioterrorism-related inhalational anthrax in the United States, Palm Beach County, Florida, 2001. *Emerg Infect Dis.* 2002;8:1029-34.
9. Treadwell TA, Koo D, Kuker K, et al. Epidemiologic clues to bioterrorism. *Pub Health Rep.* 2003;118:92-8.
10. Centers for Disease Control and Prevention. Recognition of illness associated with the intentional release of a biological agent. *MMWR* 2001;50:893-7.
11. Cono J. Chapter 8: Recognizing Bioterrorism. In: *Bioterrorism Reference for Pediatricians*. American Academy of Pediatrics. In press.
12. Henretig FM, Cieslak TJ, Eitzen EM. Biological and chemical terrorism. *J Pediatr.* 2002;141;311-26.
13. Buehler JW, Berkelman RL, Hartley DM, et al. Syndromic surveillance and bioterrorism-related epidemics. *Emerg Infect Dis.* 2003;9:1197-204.
14. Grunow R, Finke EJ. A procedure for differentiating between the intentional release of biological warfare agents and natural outbreaks of disease: its use in analyzing the tularemia outbreak in Kosovo in 1999 and 2000. *Clin Microbiol Infect.* 2002;8:510-21.
15. Pavlin JA. Epidemiology of bioterrorism. *Emerg Infect Dis.* 1999;5;528-30.
16. Smith JM. Clinician outreach and communication activity conference call summaries and slides: radiation emergencies (February 24, 2004). Centers for Disease Control and Prevention Available at: http://www.bt.cdc.gov/coca/summaries/radiation022404.asp.
17. Neifert A. Case study: accidental leakage of cesium-137 in Goiania, Brazil in 1987. Huntsville, Ala: Camber Corporation. Available at: http://nbc-med.org/sitecontent/medref/online/ref/casestudies/csgoiania.html.
18. Mettler FA, Voelz GL. Current concepts: Major radiation exposure—what to expect and how to respond. *N Engl J Med.* 2002;346(20):1554-61.

19. Dhara VR, Dhara R. The Union Carbide disaster in Bhopal: a review of health effects. *Arch Environ Heal*. 2002;57(5):391-404.

20. Centers for Disease Control and Prevention. Recognition of illness associated with chemical exposure. Broadcast transcript, August 6, 2004. Available at: http://phppo.cdc.gov/phtn/webcast/chemical-exp/8-6editedscript.htm.

21. Wolnik KA, Fricke FL, Bonnin E, et al. The Tylenol tampering incident: tracing the source. *Anal Chem*. 1984;56:466A-8A, 470A, 474A.

22. Centers for Disease Control and Prevention. Epidemiologic notes and reports: cyanide poisonings associated with over-the-counter medication—Washington State, 1991. *MMWR* 1991;40(10):167-8.

23. Centers for Disease Control and Prevention. Fatalities associated with ingestion of diethylene glycol-contaminated glycerin used to manufacture acetaminophen syrup: Haiti, November 1995-June 1996. *MMWR* 1996;45(30):649-50.

24. Centers for Disease Control and Prevention. Epidemiologic notes and reports: aldicarb food poisoning from contaminated melons: California. *MMWR* 1986; 35(16):254-8.

25. Centers for Disease Control and Prevention. Nicotine poisoning after ingestion of contaminated ground beef: Michigan, 2003. *MMWR* 2003;52(18):413-6.

chapter 58

Multimodality, Layered Attack

Nicholas Vincent Cagliuso, Sr.

It is thoroughly conceivable that the next major terrorist incident will include the tactic of coordinated simultaneous attacks in multiple geographic locations, both in the United States and abroad, and employ a combination of conventional and unconventional weaponry that may involve weapons of mass destruction (WMDs; i.e., chemical, biologic, radiologic, nuclear, or explosive [CBRNE] agents and devices) with the intent to kill large numbers of people over minutes, hours, or days. Then again, one need not wait until the *next* attack to witness a similar type of event. Rather, comparable scenarios have been effectively carried out for well over three decades, resulting in both the deaths of thousands and the long-term psychological impacts that terrorists so eagerly desire. Near-simultaneous or simultaneous attacks, as witnessed most recently in the Madrid, Spain, train bombings in March 2004 and on Sept. 11, 2001, when multiple hijacked aircraft were used as missiles in New York, Washington, DC, and Pennsylvania, have been used with great success by terrorists, particularly when conventional tactics (e.g., small arms, incendiaries, and explosives) are used. This chapter takes the notion of near-simultaneous or simultaneous attacks one step further by adding to them the coordinated application of a CBRNE agent in the minutes, hours, or days after the initial attack and applies to them the term *multimodality, layered attack.* Here, instead of the perpetrators targeting locations with a similar threat, they select several types of attack modes. The Iran-Iraq War of the 1980s provides one glaring example of these tactics that illustrates the implications to the both the prehospital and hospital communities.

Given the tactics employed during recent terrorist events and terrorists' drive to continually expose their targets' vulnerabilities, a newly focused attention and need for an intellectual and practical drive toward understanding multimodality, layered attacks more keenly is warranted and is examined here.

The Notion of Terrorism

To understand the concept of multimodality, layered terrorist attacks, a baseline established by an agreed-upon definition of terrorism itself must exist. Although there is no universally accepted definition of *terror-*ism,[1,2] this chapter uses the U.S. Department of State's definition found in Title 22, Chapter 38, Sec. 2656f[3] of the United States Code that states, "the term 'terrorism' means premeditated, politically motivated violence perpetrated against noncombatant targets by subnational groups or clandestine agents." Attention is brought to the terms *premeditated* and *noncombatant targets,* highlighting that events of this kind are not accidental (see Chapter 57, Accidental versus Intentional Event) and are aimed at civilians and off-duty military personnel.

Modes of Attack

Given the variety of motives for and classifications of terrorism, a discussion of which is beyond the scope of this chapter but is treated in other parts of this textbook (see Chapters 55 and 56), a review of the two primary modes of terrorist tactics—conventional and unconventional—follows, with special consideration given to simultaneous deployments within each.

Conventional Tactics

Conventional or traditional attack modes include those attacks that do not involve WMD. Rather, small arms, explosives, and incendiary devices are used, and as recent terrorist events indicate, these devices have had a more significant impact than those that include WMD.[4] As demonstrated by the August 2004 increase in the terror threat level for the financial services sectors in New York, New Jersey, and Washington, DC, intelligence continues to suggest that the use of the tried-and-true conventional weapons (e.g., truck bombs) are likely to remain a favored choice of terrorists. Examples of such incidents include the bombings at the World Trade Center in New York City in 1993 and the Alfred P. Murrah Federal Building in Oklahoma City in 1995, which collectively resulted in the deaths of 174 persons.

Unconventional Tactics

Unconventional or WMD attack modes involve the use of chemical, biologic, radiologic, nuclear, and high-yield explosives (CBRNE) devices.

Chemical attacks (see Section 9) have included the release of the nerve agent sarin in Matsumoto, Japan, in 1994 and again in the Tokyo subway system in 1995 by the Aum Shinri Kyo cult. Despite the cult's considerable financial wealth, the technical expertise that it could call on from its well-educated members, and the vast resources and state-of-the-art equipment at their disposal, the group could not carry out even a single truly successful chemical or biologic attack.[5] Even the sarin attack on the Tokyo subway would be laughable if not for the tragic deaths of 12 persons and the physical and psychological harm caused to many more victims.

Biologic incidents (see Section 10) include the fall 2001 anthrax attacks in Florida, New York City, New Jersey, Washington, DC, and Connecticut where contaminated letters were processed and sent to media outlets and elected officials through the U.S. mail. Although the use of biologic weapons by terrorists has the potential to harm and kill thousands of people,[6] the extent to which incidents involving weapons of this sort, such as the dissemination of anthrax or smallpox, will occur in the future in the United States or elsewhere is unknown. This is in part because terrorist attacks with biologic weapons have been extremely rare.[7] However, when examining multimodality, layered attacks, one must note that the line between chemical weapons and biologic weapons is being blurred by rapid developments in biotechnology and the emergence of a new generation of toxins and bioregulators.[8] As a result, numerous implications in the detection of and response to chemical and biologic incidents are now exacerbated by the already present challenges in dealing with these incidents. Moreover, a follow-up attack that includes, for example, the release of an agent such as smallpox could pose threats to large populations because of the potential for person-to-person transmission, enabling spread to other cities and states and exacerbating what would already be a nationwide emergency.[9] The employment of multiple chemical and biologic agents is a very likely scenario of the future, thereby challenging the medical community to be increasingly proactive in its development of appropriate countermeasures.[10]

Radiologic weapons (see Section 8) or "dirty bombs" (see Chapter 177) disperse radioactive materials in a conventional device such as a bomb or other explosive container. To date, the use of nuclear and related weapons has been the sole purview of nation-states.[11] In 1995, alleged Islamic rebels from Chechnya were reported to have buried, but not to have detonated, a 30-lb box of cesium-137 and dynamite near the entrance of a busy Moscow park. The potential use by terrorists of nuclear, radiologic, and related weapons expands the nuclear weapons threat to new actors with links to the global complex of nuclear weapons and nuclear power facilities.[11]

Nuclear weapons release large amounts of energy and are used for large-scale destruction. A nuclear weapon was first used in warfare on August 6, 1945, when the United States exploded a nuclear weapon over Hiroshima, Japan.[11] There, tens of thousands of deaths were caused by the resultant ionizing radiation. Acute radiation poisoning occurs when a patient absorbs a large amount of radiation over a short period of time, with three specific syndromes associated with radiation absorption: cerebral syndrome, gastrointestinal syndrome, and hematopoietic syndrome.[12] Those not receiving doses high enough to cause acute illness and death are at increased rates of risk for cancer and inheritable genetic damage.[11]

The use of any or all of these attack modes is not the only issue of concern. Rather, the tactics through which they are employed, namely their use in a coordinated matter in conjunction with or following a conventional attack, is the primary issue at hand. As such, a discussion of the use of multiple modes of attack deployed in a simultaneous or near-simultaneous fashion follows.

Categorization of Simultaneous Attacks

It is now well recognized that the nature of global and national affairs dictates that a wide variety of terrorism threats already exist, that others will assuredly emerge and develop, and that the United States homeland will be among the targets of such threats for the foreseeable future.[13] Surely, the most serious concern about terrorism is that terrorists are seeking to kill and injure more and more people. And although this is undeniable, one must remember that the desired effect of terrorism is not only the physical harm to the victims but also the accompanying psychological impact on the target and the society to which it belongs. Surely, mass fatalities have an impact; images and reports of thousands dead or injured are a heinous reality of terrorism. But the concomitant fear and anxiety about one's own safety, concerns about the ability of government to protect its citizens, and the foreboding danger brought about by the potential for future acts of terror are of utmost importance to the terrorist as well. As a consequence, the terrorist's victims must be carefully selected to ensure the maximum possible psychological impact on the target.[14] And while the target selection is important (e.g., urban rail hub versus rural elementary school), the timing with which the attacks are carried out—particularly if in a coordinated, simultaneous manner—is paramount to ensuring desired impacts. On Sept. 11, 2001, 2752 people lost their lives, the most fatalities of any single documented terrorist event,[15,16] and the method of attack selected by the terrorists was one that included coordinated, layered attacks across a variety of geographic areas. Although it was a day of utter devastation, one need only think about the effects had the terrorists added follow-up attacks that included, say, a CBRN event. As such, a discussion of the two main, but certainly not exhaustive, classifications of simultaneous, layered attacks follows.

The first includes *multiple incidents in a single jurisdictional target*. Attacks of this sort may commence as a single incident (e.g., a single suicide bus bombing) but can quickly evolve into an attack against multiple targets, including first responders. For example, the March 2004 bombings in Madrid, Spain, which were the deadliest terror strikes in Europe since the bombing of Pan Am flight 103 over Lockerbie, Scotland, in 1988, killed 270, and were the worst terrorist assault in Spanish history, took place at the height of a weekday rush hour when three separate trains were hit by 10 near-simultaneous explosions before 8 AM. The attacks occurred between 7:39 and 7:54 AM, with multiple explosions at the Santa Eugenia, El Pozo, and Atocha stations. And although three other bombs were found and detonated by police, 192 people were killed and 1800 wounded.

In attacks of this sort, multiple weapons or secondary devices are employed with the intentions not only to kill large numbers, but also to drain the resources of the affected jurisdiction by rendering an area insecure and to hamper both rescue efforts and injury control.[17] In many cases, first responders become victims as well as they attempt to manage the initial incident and fall victim to the follow-up attacks.

Given the sophistication of these types of attacks, improved coordination among the perpetrators is required and will usually involve multiple persons to carry out.[18] Incorporate hypothetically into this scenario the release of a chemical agent, such as the nerve gas tabun, (which is so powerful a poison that even short-term exposure to small concentrations of its vapor results in immediate symptoms and death may result[19]), and the effectiveness of a multimodality, layered attack becomes evident.[20]

The second type of simultaneous attack classification involves *multiple incidents across multiple jurisdictional targets*. Here, too, tactics may begin with one or more concurrent attacks but quickly evolve into an attack against multiple targets, again including first responders, in geographically separated areas with multiple weapons or secondary devices. Attacks of this variety are the embodiment of multimodality, layered attacks. These attacks are aimed at confounding emergency response systems and depleting resources of the local jurisdiction and, in most cases, beyond to the state and federal levels. Although the events of Sept. 11, 2001, exemplify an attack of this type using conventional means, one could not begin to imagine the impacts had the perpetrators (in addition to carrying out the carefully coordinated hijackings of four commercial airliners, each filled with jet fuel, and slamming them into targets), added to their repertoire the release of a CBRN agent later in the day or in the days immediately thereafter, either somewhere in the United States or in its interests abroad. Surely the obvious ramifications, in addition to the physical and emotional trauma already requiring attention, would be further complicated by identification of the agent, an in-depth epidemiologic investigation, extended incident and resource management, and of course, resumption and recovery initiatives.

Multimodality, layered events of the future may be complicated by the use of multiple CBRN agents or the delivery of chemical and replicating agents and/or their toxins that have been carefully matched, based on their ability to generate specific symptoms, resulting in the potentiation of health effects.[10] Accordingly, agent detection requires the availability of rapid diagnostic methods and procedures (e.g., syndromic surveillance) to assess illnesses that will be the result of multiple agents.[10] Given the sophistication required to effectively carry out attacks of this sort, namely increased timing,

organization, and coordination of the perpetrators, and as has become increasingly popular, suicide attacks, several persons would almost certainly carry these out.

The near-simultaneous bombings of U.S. embassies in Nairobi, Kenya, and Dar es Salaam, Tanzania, which resulted in hundreds of deaths coupled with the attacks of Sept. 11, 2001, are clear examples of multiple-incident, multiple-jurisdiction, layered attacks. The demonstration of an operational capability to coordinate two nearly simultaneous attacks on United States embassies in different countries to a large extent influenced U.S. policy.[21]

Although many terrorism experts point to the change in targeting and the style of attack as evidence of a possible broadening of the strategy from mainly guerilla insurgency against U.S. forces to include a coordinated terrorist campaign that includes foreign elements, how the threat will actually evolve is difficult to predict.[22] In all cases, the aim of these attacks was to maximize injury and cause complex trauma, thereby elevating the killing ratio.[23]

Although the ability to conduct multiple, coordinated attacks against several targets is not new for terrorist groups such as Al-Qaeda, (which, to date, is the only organization that has successfully used suicide attacks on U.S. soil[22]), the manner in which these attacks is being conducted indicates refined capabilities and sophisticated tactics,[4] bringing into focus the reality that future terrorist attacks will likely include even greater use of multimodality, layered attack tactics.

HISTORICAL PERSPECTIVE

Until Sept. 11, 2001, a total of no more than perhaps 1000 Americans had been killed by terrorists either in this country or abroad since 1968—the year credited with marking the advent of the modern era of international terrorism because the Popular Front for the Liberation of Palestine hijacked an El Al flight on July 23 of that year.[24]

The significance of the Sept. 11, 2001 incidents from a terrorist operational perspective is that simultaneous attacks, using far more prosaic and arguably conventional means of attack (such as car bombs), are relatively uncommon. For reasons not well understood, terrorists typically have not undertaken such coordinated operations. This was doubtless less of a choice than a reflection of the logistical and other organizational hurdles that most terrorist groups are not able to overcome.[24] In fact, the initial "planes operation" (as it was termed by Al-Qaeda operatives), embraced the idea of using suicide operations to blow up planes as a refinement of the original "Manila" air plot. All of the planes hijacked were to be crashed or exploded at or about the same time to maximize the psychological impact of the attacks.[25]

During the 1990s, perhaps only one other (presumably unrelated) terrorist incident evidenced those same characteristics of coordination and high lethality: the series of attacks that occurred in Bombay in March 1993, where a dozen or so simultaneous car bombings rocked the city and killed nearly 300 persons and wounded more than 700 others.[26] Indeed, apart from the attacks on the same morning in October 1983 of the U.S. Marine barracks in Beirut and a nearby French paratroop headquarters, and the IRA's near-simultaneous assassination of Lord Mountbatten and remote-control mine attack on British troops in Warrenpoint, Northern Ireland, in 1979, it is hard to recall many other significant incidents reflecting such operational expertise, coordination, and synchronization.[26]

That is not to say, however, that similar types of operations have not been planned and foiled. Ramzi Ahmed Yousef, the convicted mastermind of the 1993 New York World Trade Center bombing, and 15 other persons reportedly intended to follow that incident in June 1993 with the simultaneous bombings of the Holland and Lincoln Tunnels and George Washington Bridge (all owned and operated by The Port Authority of New York and New Jersey, the owner of the World Trade Center) that are used daily by thousands of commuters between New Jersey and Manhattan.[27] What's more, the plans also included the simultaneous bombings of 11 U.S. passenger airliners while in flight over the Pacific Ocean in 1995.[28] The importance of simultaneity in attacks is confirmed in these events and, more recently, during the interrogation of Khalid Sheikh Mohammed on August 18, 2003.[25]

CURRENT PRACTICE

Small arms, explosives, and incendiaries are the weapons used in most terrorist acts.[15] Although the use of nonconventional weapons (i.e., WMD) must not be ignored, it is these modes of attack that have had a more significant impact, as recorded terrorist events in recent years demonstrate.[4,15,29]

Al-Qaeda and its affiliates have demonstrated that the organization is highly determined and motivated to conduct high-profile, mass-casualty attacks and, increasingly, it is civilian, noncombatant targets that they select. The 2003 Bali nightclub bombing, Moscow theater siege, and combined Mombasa, Kenya, car bombing and surface-to-air missile attacks are indicative of this emergent and increasingly popular tactic.

It must be noted that although damage to a target—or in a multimodality, layered attack, multiple targets—may be relatively small (e.g., a single suicide bomb in a bus or a single aircraft downed), the political and psychological impacts will be rather large. To wit, the impact of bombs, and for that matter terrorist acts in general, goes beyond mortality and morbidity.[30] It is the creation of psychological terror, which simultaneous attacks produce so readily, that can cause chaos and panic.[31]

Response Strategies

Given the now-ubiquitous threat of terrorist acts coupled with their sudden nature, the most effective response strategy (absent preventing the attack to begin with) is for local, regional, state, and federal partners to develop flexible strategies that can be adjusted quickly and appropriately to the type of incident that occurs. This type of strategy requires management coordination, compatible communication systems, and real-time information feedback to decision-makers that permits near immediate changes in strategy when required.[15] The ability to respond across a broad technologic spectrum of potential adversarial attacks is one of the primary lessons to be learned from all terrorist attacks. Recognizing that the threat of terrorism is comparatively new to the United States and that many dimensions of the initial response to this threat are only now being implemented (e.g., the National Incident Management System and the National Response Plan) with no level of resources able to fully prevent the United States from being attacked in the future,[13] understanding the full range of injuries and disorders, including posttraumatic stress disorder, is critical.[32] Although history does not always repeat itself, it can surely serve as a gauge for what terrorists are at least capable of and how we should respond. Al-Qaeda's strength lies not in geographic possession or occupation of a defined geographic territory but in its fluidity and impermanence. The activities of Ramzi Ahmed Yousef, the reputed mastermind of the first World Trade Center Attack in 1993, involved a grand scheme to simultaneously bomb 12 American commercial aircraft in midflight over the Pacific Ocean (the infamous "Bojinka" plot), which did not require extensive operational bases and command nor control headquarters in an existing country to execute the planning and execution.[33]

The new means of terrorist attacks we are likely to face will involve not only WMDs and weapons of mass disruption, but conventional means to attack critical infrastructure targets such as nuclear and chemical plants, agricultural nodes, and the hearts of the American and world economy, with catastrophic human and economic consequences.[32]

Suicide Attacks

Suicide attacks by terrorist organizations have become more prevalent globally, and assessing the threat of these attacks has therefore gained strategic importance to the United States and its interests at home and abroad.[22] Essentially a punishment strategy, suicide terror has become increasingly prevalent over the past two decades simply because terrorists have learned that attacks of this type work. The success of suicide attacks lies within two primary consequences. First, it inflicts immediate punishment against the target. Second, its success implies a threat for more punishment in the future. Implicit in the act is the powerful message that the attacker(s) could not be deterred and connects the attacker to a broader community, which one would speculate allows for the act of martyrdom. In suicide terrorism, the weaker, usually a person or small group acts as the coercer, with the stronger group (e.g., Western society) serving as the target.

In the case of Al-Qaeda, Osama bin Laden has been characterized as a terrorist CEO, organizing its "spectaculars," or high-visibility, high-casualty operations such as the Sept. 11, 2001 attacks, the bombing of the U.S.S. Cole, and the East Africa embassy bombings.[34] Unlike many other terrorist organizations, Al-Qaeda has no single modus operandi, making it all the more formidable.[34] However, simultaneous attacks using multiple bombs coordinated to explode in several cities across the country at sites such as stores, schools, hospitals, apartment buildings, and gas stations, each vital to the U.S. economy and populace, are not beyond conception.

An innovative use of suicide bombings as a component of multimodality, layered attack methods involves the use of combining its self-destructive tactics with CBRN agents. Suicide tactics could significantly improve the potentiality of a successful CBRN weapons attack itself.[35] Here, the unimportance of being exposed to extremely dangerous materials permits the attacker to carry out increasingly perilous experiments, thereby expanding the chance of generating and using a potent and effective CBRN weapon.[35]

Second, notable tactical opportunities arise for terrorists who are apathetic to making contact with a CBRN agent during delivery. In addition to greater access to the target and enhanced control over the outcome, elimination of shielding measures during the attack such as personal protective equipment decreases the risk of early detection and interdiction of the attack. Again, thinking along the lines of multimodality, layered attacks, the bodies of terrorists could also be used as crude delivery systems, if the perpetrators are infected with a contagious agent and deployed to crowded areas.

It is clear that suicide operations are responsible for a large number of fatalities. Of the 30 single most deadly terrorist incidents carried out to date since 1990, 15 involved suicide bombers, and 7 of the remaining 15 attacks were perpetrated by groups with a record of using suicide bomb delivery.[36] The fact that groups using this tactic are responsible for the majority of high-fatality incidents suggests that they have reached an advanced level of enemy dehumanization and are therefore psychologically closer to perpetrating mass-casualty CBRN attacks.[35]

PITFALLS

Arguably, many people were lulled into believing that mass-casualty, simultaneous attacks in general, and those of such devastating potential as witnessed on Sept. 11, 2001, were likely beyond most capabilities of most terrorists. Yet, the tragic events of that day demonstrate how profoundly misplaced such assumptions were.[24] As such, the significance of past successes (e.g., largely foiling most of bin Laden's terrorist operations during the period between the August 1998 embassy bombings and the November 2000 attack on the U.S.S. Cole) and the terrorists' own incompetence and propensity for mistakes (e.g., Ahmad Ressam's bungled attempt to enter the United States from Canada in December 1999) were likely overestimated.[24] Some experts believe there was significant overlap in the planning for these attacks and the one against the U.S.S. Cole in Aden. Doing so suggests a multitrack operational and organizational capability to coordinate major, multiple attacks at one time.[24]

Preparedness

Much of the terrorism preparedness pre-9/11 focused on the comparatively low-end threat posed by car and truck bombs against buildings or the more exotic high-end threats, involving biologic or chemical weapons or cyber-attack. In many respects, preparedness planning continues to (quite possibly erroneously) assume mass-casualty attacks involving biologic or chemical agents released at key infrastructure (e.g., air and rail terminals). As demonstrated by the attacks of 9/11 and certainly a topic of debate between politicians, homeland security personnel, and emergency management professionals, sizable gaps remain in fortifying plans for a traditional and long-proved tactic such as airline hijackings. Mitigating and preparing for tactics of this sort has been neglected in favor of other, less conventional threats (e.g., chemical, biologic, and radiologic) with the consequences of using an aircraft as a suicide weapon almost completely discounted.[24]

Although so-called WMDs were not used in the Sept. 11 attacks, the destruction was nonetheless "massive."[22] Consequently, the very real prospect of combining modern weapons technology (i.e., CBRN weapons) with an age-old willingness to die in the act of committing an attack could be unprecedentedly dangerous.[22] Furthermore, with increasing numbers of casualties from multiple suicide attacks occurring globally in places such as Israel, Saudi Arabia, Morocco, Russia/Chechnya, and postconflict Iraq, a discourse on the threat of future suicide attacks is warranted.[22] One need only to examine the Department of State's Patterns of Global Terrorism, 1983-2001,[36] to see the efficiencies gained by attacks of this sort. Pape[37] found that, from 1980 to 2001, suicide attacks represented only 3% of all terrorist attacks but accounted for 48% of total deaths due to terrorism.

In retrospect, it arguably was not the 1995 sarin nerve gas attack on the Tokyo subway and nine attempts to use bioweapons by the Aum Shinri Kyo cult that should have been the dominant influence on counterterrorist thinking. More accurately, a 1986 hijacking of a Pan Am flight in Karachi, where the terrorists' intentions were reported to have been to crash it into the center of Tel Aviv, and the 1994 hijacking in Algiers of an Air France passenger plane by terrorists belonging to the Armed Islamic Group, who similarly planned to crash the fuel-laden aircraft with its passengers into the heart of Paris[24] should have served as keen indicators of the type, scope, and overall capabilities of those responsible for events to come.

A long-standing and now proven incorrect notion is that terrorists were more interested in publicity than killing and therefore had neither the need nor interest in annihilating large numbers of people.[24] In 1975, Jenkins[38] noted that, "Terrorists want a lot of people watching and a lot of people listening and not a lot of people dead." Just 10 years later, he reiterated, "Simply killing a lot of people has seldom been one terrorist objective...Terrorists operate on the principle of the minimum force necessary. They find it unnecessary to kill many, as long as killing a few suffices for their purposes."[38] Clearly, the events of Sept. 11 prove such notions now to be wishful thinking, if not dangerously anachronistic.[24]

When speaking to the notion of pitfalls, one must consider the difficult concept of "How do we assess the threat of terrorist events that have not occurred?"[39] Although there is no black-and-white, one-sentence response, we know that today's terrorists are becoming demonstrably more adept in their tradecraft of death and destruction. They are more formidable in their capacity for tactical modification and innovation in their methods of attack (e.g., simultaneous and near-simultaneous deployments), and they have become increasingly competent in operating for sustained periods while avoiding detection, interception, or capture.[40]

Moreover, even attacks that are not successful by conventional measures can nonetheless serve as a success for terrorists provided they are daring enough to garner media and public attention. And given the world's recent hypersensitivity to threats and suspicious incidents, which is the terrorist group's fundamental organizational imperative to act, even if their action is not completely successful but brings them publicity, their tenacious pursuit for fresh ways to overcome, circumvent, or defeat governmental security and countermeasures is fueled. Accordingly, attacks at all points along the conflict spectrum—from the crude and primitive to the most sophisticated—must be anticipated and appropriate measures employed to counter them.[40]

It must be noted that a limited terrorist attack involving, not a WMD per se, but an unconventional chemical, biologic, or radiologic weapon on a small scale, either isolated or as a component of a succession of smaller incidents occurring either simultaneously or sequentially in one or more geographic locations, may yield disproportionately large consequences, generating fear and alarm and serving the terrorists' purpose just as well as a larger weapon or more ambitious attack with massive casualties.[5]

Although many may think of multimodality, layered attacks as restricted to the use of simultaneous suicide attacks, one must examine for example biologic agents, looking specifically at microorganisms, which when used in combination have the potential to create a more severe disease state.[10] Similarly, infection with one agent with a shorter incubation period that may weaken overall resistance may provide easier opportunities for infection with a second organism with greater morbidity and mortality.[10] The ability of multiple organisms with different levels of virulence to confuse medical officers looking for a common etiology accentuates the need for sensitive and specific diagnostic tests to be available in the field setting.[10]

Scenarios of the future may be complicated by the possible use of multiple agents or the delivery of chemical and replicating agents and/or their toxins that have been carefully matched based on their stability and ability to generate specific symptoms. Health effects could be potentiated. Therefore, from a medical perspective, detection requires the availability of rapid diagnostic methods and procedures to assess illnesses that will be the result of multiple agents.[10]

The most widespread and most open use of chemical weapons on a battlefield in recent decades was by Iraq in its conflict with Iran. Undetonated shells were sampled and several laboratories in Europe analyzed their contents. A vesicant or blister agent (mustard) and a nerve agent (tabun) were identified. About 100 Iranian soldiers with chemical wounds were sent to European hospitals for care; their wounds were consistent with vesicant injury. A team appointed by the UN secretariat went to Iranian battlefields and hospitals and found chemical shells and patients with chemical injuries. The public outcry at the use of these weapons was less than overwhelming. Ignoring protests from the world community, Iraq continued to use these agents.[41]

The real issue and the most likely threat may not be the ruthless terrorist use of some weapon of mass destruction, but the calculated, deliberate, and delicately planned use of some chemical, biologic, radiologic, or nuclear weapon[5] in conjunction with conventional means in a simultaneous or near-simultaneous time frame to achieve far-reaching psychological effects.

MEDICAL MANAGEMENT OF MASS-CASUALTY EVENTS

In the 17-minute period between 8:46 and 9:03 AM on Sept. 11, 2001, New York City and the Port Authority of New York and New Jersey had mobilized the largest rescue operation in the City's history.[25] In all, over 25,000 people were rescued from the World Trade Center complex on that day, and although the costs in terms of first responders' lives were great, their selfless acts will never go unnoticed. During mass-casualty events, terror victims often arrive at hospitals in clusters, whereas during more isolated assaults they arrive either as individuals or a few at a time.[42] The medical management of events of this sort, in which the goal is to save as many lives as possible and to decrease morbidity, requires that the most senior clinician assume command of the incident and adjust the available resources optimally to the excessive needs.[42]

Events of this kind require medical management skills, rather than clinical capabilities, to come first. Here, the aims of saving as many lives as possible and decreasing morbidity dictate skillful prioritization of decisions to restore the balance between needs and available resources. To wit, the principles of the medical management of mass-casualty events, where the medical system is overwhelmed and the balance between resources and demands is undermined[43] (namely, those that result from terrorist acts), have been fully described elsewhere.[37,42] Although all terrorist attacks, conventional and unconventional, have the potential to produce significant physical and psychological trauma, simultaneous attacks by their very nature are far more efficient in overburdening medical systems at the local level, and if the nature of the simultaneous attacks is on a large scale, on the regional or national level. Consequently, the success in the management of large-scale medical events comes in extensive early preparation.[43]

An additional contrast between isolated terrorist events and the multimodal, layered sort treated in this chapter lies in the duration of the events. Here, a short-term event such as the bombing of a single bus can be localized in nature, requiring the response of a single jurisdiction's first responders and treatment by a local hospital, and if necessary, specialty centers. Conversely, a multimodal, layered attack may necessitate the national response system in which resources from across the nation are activated and deployed to those areas hardest hit as well as those where intelligence suggests likely near-term attacks. Here, dividing the patient load between community hospitals, large urban medical centers, and specialty-care centers (e.g., trauma, burns, hyperbaric) will help minimize the likelihood that no one facility is overwhelmed by the event.

Use of the National Incident Management System and the National Response Plan, each of which provide for the establishment of an Incident Command System/unified command should be engaged at the beginning of the event by the affected local jurisdiction. An interface between prehospital systems and receiving medical centers is paramount. The different modes of terror currently compose a new field of epidemiology that demands ongoing activities at all levels[43] and place increased and unique demands on first responders and in-hospital clinical, management, and support staff.

Terrorist acts produce more victims and higher mortality rates than is seen from natural disasters and, therefore, medical personnel must ensure that medical protocols exist for both the daily treatment and transportation of patients as well as situations that place unexpected demands on the system.[35]

The current terror wave engulfs the entire world. The greatest threat to U.S. citizens comes from the possibility of further attacks orchestrated or inspired by Al-Qaeda, either in the United States or abroad.[22] Contemporary terrorist behavior and tactics seek to destroy those components of our lives that celebrate the very freedom we enjoy. The reality is that we cannot deny terrorists attractive targets. Rather, through effective programs, stakeholders can make attacks more difficult to carry out and less effective.

The events of Sept. 11, 2001, are an egregious reminder of how terrorists can fulfill their aims of death, fear, and intimidation through conventional means. The terrorism of today wields conventional and nonconventional WMDs—biologic, chemical, and nuclear—that damage the body, the mind, and the soul.[44] One needs only to think of the exponential effects a multilayered, simultaneous attack scenario can have on trust in government, the economy, and national security, as compared with a single isolated attack. These events demonstrate the ability of even one significant, new terrorist incident to instantly reignite worldwide fears and concern.[33]

Israel has long maintained the notion of "mega-terrorism," a concept that embodies the notion of multimodal layered attacks. Here, not only are the obvious terrorist uses of WMDs brought to bear and specific highly symbolic locations (e.g., The White House and New York Stock Exchange) targeted, but the more prosaic types of incidents such terrorist attacks on elementary schools or the assassination of political and business leaders (e.g., mayors, "capitalist" business executives) carried out in a short term (e.g., minutes, hours, or days) in ways that

although not necessarily causing extensive human loss to life (purely in terms of numbers), would nonetheless have profound, far-reaching psychological repercussions on the targeted society.[33]

The fundamental nature and character of terrorism changed with the events of 9/11 and, moreover, has continued to change and evolve since then. Based on the simultaneous attacks carried out on that day, coupled with previous foiled attempts of that sort and the destruction of the Taliban, one can reasonably assume that the multiyear planning period of all previous Al Qaeda spectaculars alone suggest that it is premature to write off Osama bin Laden or his followers.[33] Terrorism is becoming increasingly difficult to characterize as an identifiable phenomenon amenable to categorization or clear distinction. Given the success of the Sept. 11 attacks, it is difficult to make a case against a similar, more devastating attack using multiple modes of attack that may have been set in motion before Sept. 11, 2001, and is only now slowly and inexorably unfolding.[33] The masterminds behind the attack proved the impotence of the mightiest military power to protect its citizens against these kinds of devastating blows. From the terrorists' point of view, the attack on America was a perfectly choreographed production aimed at American and international audiences.[20]

Before Sept. 11, 2001, most, if not all, acts of terrorism resulted in a great deal of publicity in the form of news reporting. But given the multimodal, layered nature of the attacks on that day, the images of commercial airliners crashing as suicide/homicide missiles into the very symbols of America's economic and military might continue to remain almost incomprehensible.[20] Surely the attacks could have been scheduled at night, sparing many lives, and still raked in a great deal of publicity. But the bright daylight of that once-beautiful September morning made certain that the most spectacular of sights and the loss of life would occur. In all these respects, no previous act of terrorism even came close to the events of Sept. 11.[20]

The events of Sept. 11 demonstrated the effectiveness of multimodal, layered attacks within the United States and provide a solemn and serious reminder that this tactic remains a likely means of attack in other democracies as well. Without the capability to track down and capture surviving terrorists, as was the case in the first World Trade Center bombing and the Oklahoma City bombing, the United States (and any target society, for that matter) forfeits its capacity to bring the perpetrators to justice. Concurrently, terrorists and their supporters get the opportunity to idolize those who committed suicide in order to kill and use their examples to recruit more volunteers as human bombs.[20]

Terrorists are well aware of the extreme difficulty, if not impossibility, in altogether preventing suicide terror, both in the example of the traditional single suicide bomber or the more advanced operations, such as those used on Sept. 11, 2001. Although the idea that terrorists may obtain and use WMDs cannot be ignored, the more immediate concern must be the prospect that Sept. 11 might well become the most attractive model for terrorism in the near future.[20]

REFERENCES

1. Long D. *The Anatomy of Terrorism*. New York: Free Press; 1990.
2. Parachini J. Comparing motives and outcomes of mass casualty terrorism involving conventional and unconventional weapons. *Stud Conflict Terrorism*. 2001;24:389-406.
3. Legal Information Institute. U.S. Code Collection, Title 22, Chapter 38: § 2656f. Annual country reports on terrorism. September 20, 2004. Available at: http://www4.law.cornell.edu/uscode/22/2656f.html.
4. U.S. Department of Homeland Security. Statement by the Department of Homeland Security on Continued Al-Qaeda Threats [press release], November 21, 2003. Available at: http://www.dhs.gov/dhspublic/display?content=3017.
5. Hoffman B. Change and continuity in terrorism. *Stud Conflict Terrorism*. 2001;24:417-28.
6. Kuh S, Hauer J. The threat of biological terrorism in the new millennium. *Am Behav Scientist*. 2001;44(6):1032-41.
7. Sidel V, Levy B. Biological weapons. In: Levy B, Sidel V, eds. *Terrorism and Public Health: A Balanced Approach to Strengthening Systems and Protecting People*. New York, Oxford University Press; 2003.
8. Spanjaard H, Khabib O. Chemical weapons. In: Levy B, Sidel V, eds. *Terrorism and Public Health: A Balanced Approach to Strengthening Systems and Protecting People*. New York, Oxford University Press, 2003.
9. Lillibridge SR. Statement on Medical Responses to Terrorist Attacks. Delivered September 22, 1999, before the House Committee on Government Reform, Subcommittee on National Security, Veterans Affairs, and International Relations. Available at: http://www.hhs.gov/asl/testify/t990922a.html.
10. Takafuji E, Johnson-Winegar A, Zajtchuk R. Medical Challenges in Chemical and Biological Defense for the 21st Century. In: Zatjchuk R, Bellamy R, eds. *Textbook of Military Medicine*. Office of the Surgeon General, U.S. Department of the Army; 1996.
11. Sutton P, Gould R. Nuclear, radiological and related weapons. In: Levy B, Sidel V, eds. *Terrorism and Public Health: A Balanced Approach to Strengthening Systems and Protecting People*. New York, Oxford University Press, 2003.
12. Bradshaw R, Cahill J. Radiation and the EMS Responder. *FireEMS* 2004; July/August:22-8.
13. *Forging America's New Normalcy: Securing our homeland, preserving our liberty. The Fifth Annual Report to the President and the Congress of the Advisory Panel to Assess Domestic Response Capabilities for Terrorism Involving Weapons of Mass Destruction*. December 15, 2003. Available at: http://www.rand.org/nsrd/terrpanel/.
14. Boshoff H, Botha A, Schonteich M. Fear in the City: Urban terrorism in South Africa, Monograph 63. Institute for Security Studies. Available at: http://www.iss.co.za/Pubs/Monographs/No63/CONTENT63.HTML.
15. Cukier W, Chapdelaine A. Small arms, explosive and incendiaries. In: Levy B, Sidel V, eds. *Terrorism and Public Health: A Balanced Approach to Strengthening Systems and Protecting People*. New York, Oxford University Press, 2003.
16. McCarthy M. Attacks provide the first major test of USA's national anti-terrorist medical response plans. *Lancet* 2001;358:941.
17. Christen HT, Walker R. Weapons of mass effect: explosives. In: Maniscalco PM, Christen HT, eds. *Understanding Terrorism and Managing the Consequences*. Upper Saddle River, NJ: Prentice Hall; 2002.
18. *Weapons of Mass Destruction Incident Management/Unified Command*. Texas Engineering Extension Service; 2003. Available at: http://teexweb.tamu.edu/teex.cfm?pageid=training&area=teex&Division=ESTI&Course=154217&templateid=14&navdiv=ESTI.
19. Perry-Robinson J, Goldblat J. *Chemical Warfare in the Iran-Iraq War: Stockholm International Peace Research Institute Chemical Weapons Fact Sheet I*. Stockholm, Sweden: International Peace Research Institute; 1984.
20. Nacos BL. The terrorist calculus behind 9-11: a model for future terrorism? *Stud Conflict Terrorism*. 2003;26:1-16.
21. Lilja GP, Madsen MA, Overton J. Multiple casualty incidents. In: Kuehl AE, ed. *Prehospital Systems and Medical Oversight*. Dubuque, IA, Kendall/Hunt, 2002, pp 821-7. Available at: http://www.kendallhunt.com/index.cfm?TKN=A670EE07-306E-01A4-A274E0523817B189&PID=219&PGI=172.
22. Kurth Cronin A. *Terrorists and Suicide Attacks: Congressional Research Service, Report # RL32058*. August 28, 2003. Available at: http://www.fas.org/irp/crs/RL32058.pdf.
23. Mintz Y, Shapira SC, Pikarsky AJ, et al. The experience of one institution dealing with terror: the El Aqsa Intifada riots. *Isr Med Assoc J*. 2002;4:554-6.
24. Hoffman B. Terrorism and counterterrorism after September 11th. *U.S. Foreign Policy Agenda: An Electronic Journal of the U.S. Department of State*. Vol 6, No 3, November 2001.
25. The National Commission on Terrorist Attacks upon the United States. *The 9/11 Commission Report*. Washington, DC, WW Norton; 2004.
26. Dugger C. Victims of '93 Bombay terror wary of U.S. motives. *NY Times*. September 24, 2001. Available at: http://mumbai-central.com/nukkad/sep2001/msg00288.html.
27. Hoffman B. *Responding to Terrorism Across the Technological Spectrum*. Strategic Studies Instate Conference Series. Carlisle Barracks, PA, U.S. Army War College, April 1994.
28. Bone J, Road A. Terror by degree. *Times Magazine (London)*. October 18, 1997.
29. Mascrop A. Mass hysteria the main threat from bioweapons. *BMJ* 2001;323:2-5.
30. Meyer M. The role of the metropolitan planning organization (MPO) in preparing for security incidents and transportation system response. U.S. Department of Transportation, Federal Highway Administration, Transportation Capacity Building Program. Available at: http://www.planning.dot.gov/Documents/Security paper.doc.
31. Stein M, Hershberg A. Medical consequences of terrorism. *Surg Clin North Am*. 1999;79:1537-52.
32. Abenhaim L, Dab W, Salmi LR. Study of civilian victims of terrorist attacks (France 1982-1987). *J Clin Epidemiol*. 1992;45:103-9.
33. Hoffman B. Al Qaeda, trends in terrorism, and future potentialities: an assessment. *Stud Conflict Terrorism*. 2003;26:429-42.
34. Hoffman B. The leadership secrets of Osama bin Laden: the terrorist as CEO. *Atlantic Monthly*. April 2003. Available at: http://www.theatlantic.com/doc/print/200304/hoffman.
35. Dolnik A. Die and let die: exploring links between suicide terrorism and terrorist use of chemical, biological, radiological and nuclear weapons. *Stud Conflict Terrorism*. 2003;26:17-35.
36. U.S. Department of State. *Patterns of Global Terrorism, 1983-2001*, 2002.
37. Pape R. The strategic logic of suicide terrorism [unpublished manuscript]. February 18, 2003.
38. Jenkins B. *The Likelihood of Nuclear Terrorism*. Santa Monica, Calif: The RAND Corporation, P-7119; 1985:6.
39. Lesser I, Hoffman B, Arquilla D, et al. *Countering the New Terrorism*. Santa Monica, Calif: The RAND Corporation; 1999.
40. Hoffman B. Terrorism trends and prospects. In: Lesser I, Hoffman B, Arquilla D, et al, eds. *Countering the New Terrorism*. Santa Monica, Calif: The RAND Corporation; 1999.
41. Sidell FR, Franz DR. Overview: defense against the effects of chemical and biological warfare agents. In Zatjchuk R, Bellamy R, eds. *Textbook of Military Medicine*. Office of the Surgeon General, Washington, DC, U.S. Department of the Army; 1996.
42. Shapira S, Mor-Yosef S. Terror politics and medicine: the role of leadership. *Stud Conflict Terrorism*. 2004;27:65-71.
43. Shapira SC, Shemer J. Medical management of terrorist attacks. *Isr Med Assoc J*. 2002;4:489-92.
44. Shemer J, Shoenfeld Y. Diabolical, haunting terror: here and now. *Isr Med Assoc J*. 2002;4:483-4.

chapter 59

Operations Security, Site Security, and Incident Response

Paul M. Maniscalco, Paul D. Kim, Neil A. Commerce, and Jeffrey A. Todd

In preparing organizations and persons for response to a high-impact/high-yield emergency incident, one of the most often overlooked requirements are operations security (OPSEC) and site security. Bound inextricably with coordination and integration strategies for response, OPSEC and site security are often compromised in the "heat of the battle" as responders with nothing but the best of intentions converge on the scene of the disaster implementing strategies that, pre-event, have failed to address these most important aspects of the incident response and management strategy. The discipline to apply the principles of OPSEC and site security following a preestablished, organized, and well-practiced plan is crucial given the nature of the threat and the variety of conditions that may present themselves. Failing to address OPSEC and site security issues before an event amounts to failing to protect the protectors.

Terrorist attacks present the contemporary emergency services manager or chief officer with more complex challenges and more probable risks. Site Security and OPSEC are multifaceted concepts, bringing together elements as diverse as protecting information concerning an organization's activities, intentions, or capabilities to scene access, traffic control, and evidence protection. Due to the fact that this involves so many different aspects of disaster response, and because it cannot be completely achieved without full integration of each of those aspects, site security is best understood broadly. Robust control of the incident and proximal areas should be the desired goal. This includes holding sway over the human and material flow into, out of, and around the site; providing for the security and safety of responding personnel; providing these responders with the ability to perform their jobs; and ensuring personnel accountability and the fulfillment of performance requirements.

For an OPSEC program to be effective, personnel must be aware of OPSEC concerns, must implement OPSEC countermeasures when appropriate, and must be observant of potential collection activities directed at their organization. This is only possible if the members of the organization understand the range of threats affecting their organization and actively support the OPSEC program.[1]

Under these definitions, the framework that makes for effective and successful deployment of OPSEC/site security strategies is the Incident Management System/unified command structure (IM/UC) as articulated in the National Response Plan (NRP) and the National Incident Management System (NIMS). Many OPSEC and site security issues can be addressed merely by properly applying these disciplined and standard structures, practices, and protocols. For example, interagency integration problems involving the establishment of a chain of command, which produced many of the issues that plagued security at the World Trade Center site in the aftermath of the Sept. 11, 2001, events, could have been significantly ameliorated by the implementation of an effective IM/UC early in the event as well as the requisite immediate establishment of a workable security perimeter. Simply restating the requirement for implementing the IM/UC system, which has already been established with the release of the NRP and the resulting NIMS, is not the purpose here. Moreover, this chapter seeks to address the issue of the role OPSEC and site security play in the response to a terrorist incident within the framework of the IM/UC process.

INCIDENT MANAGEMENT/UNIFIED COMMAND AS THE FOUNDATION

Every person who chooses to devote his or her life's work to responding when others are fleeing must resist the urge to "run in" without fully understanding what he or she faces beyond that door, on the other side of that cloud of smoke, or around the next corner. Although this is easier said than accomplished, in a terrorist event, the survival of these people to fight another day depends on projecting or knowing what threats lay ahead. The organizational protocol that is established by IM/UC is simply the framework by which OPSEC/site security can be efficiently, effectively, and successfully established; in other words, IM/UC is required but not sufficient on its own. Although not a panacea, IM/UC implementation is crucial for us to remediate the hard lessons learned in the recent past, fixing the problems inherent in past responses and implementing standards for OPSEC and site security.

The adoption and implementation of the NIMS–IM/UC framework addresses and corrects a large portion of site security issues by the incorporation of the talents and service provided via the law enforcement community at the command post; it is important to note, however, that not all of these issues are terrorism specific,[2] and the UC concept should be allied at most emergency scenes.

Many of the difficulties inherent in the massive response of multiple agencies are as prevalent in an earthquake as in a dirty bomb attack. What makes the issue of OPSEC/site security so important and unique in the context of terrorism is the particular nature of the threat. The unpredictability of terrorism creates conditions that are fluid, requiring speed and flexibility of thought and action as well as thorough planning and preparation. Furthermore, the targeting of responders and "soft targets" such as healthcare facilities and schools makes this an even more complex matter to address and manage to ensure one's own safety and the safety of those responders that are being coordinated at the scene.

HISTORICAL PERSPECTIVE

In analyzing many major recent terrorist attacks (including and after the 1993 World Trade Center bombing), numerous areas of concern consistently emerge. By identifying each of these and focusing on the pitfalls of the response at the time, as well as stating how response could have been improved, one can hope to draw lessons and establish best practices for future incidents. As just noted, these concerns fall into two general categories. First are those that are potentially present in any sort of disaster and that can be remedied by the proper implementation of IM/UC. These include the following:

- Victim rescue in the immediate aftermath of an incident;
- Personnel needs including work shifts to ensure proper rest, adequate personal protective equipment, continuation of normal emergency medical services (EMS)/law enforcement/fire services over the course of the event;
- Organizational integration /interoperability communication issues;
- Public relations, including that with dignitaries, media, charities, families of victims/missing;
- OPSEC/site security;
- Staffing support for other elements.

Secondly, some concerns are unique to terrorism and cannot be addressed simply by the implementation of IM/UC. These therefore require further attention and creativity and are listed as follows:

- Search for secondary devices and hostile threats to the scene and responders;
- Perimeter establishment and access control;
- Traffic and crowd control;
- Evidence recovery and protection.

CURRENT MEDICINE

OPSEC/SITE Security: Challenges of a General Nature

The importance IM/UC plays in enabling successful OPSEC/site security cannot be overstated. Perhaps the key component in OPSEC/site security is communication and coordination among responders, and the primary focus of IM/UC is just that. The following section addresses each aspect of OPSEC/site security that can be helped by the implementation of IM/UC, including multiple examples from recent terrorist attacks where such implementation would have directly resulted in saved lives or property. Suggestions are then made as to how these issues can be dealt with in future events.

Victim Rescue

The first challenge to OPSEC/site security is victim rescue in the immediate aftermath of an incident. This is the initial and most dramatic problem faced by all responders during and immediately after a terrorist attack. As mentioned briefly before, a driving characteristic that defines all responders is the natural instinct to rush forward, nobly doing whatever one can to quickly save as many lives as possible. However, for both the safety of the responders and the victims, some restraint and organization must be exercised, or the overall incident outcome may become negative and people may die needlessly. Among the lasting images from the events of Sept. 11 are the hundreds of first responder personnel rushing to the scene to help all who were victimized by these horrible attacks. One striking example in a day full of actions hampering, hindering, and preventing all good intentions was the Shanksville, Pa, plane crash site, which on Sept. 11, 2001, was overwhelmed and severely congested because of response units, both on and off duty, making their way to the scene either by self-dispatch or by convincing dispatchers to send more help. The resulting chaos clogged the scene, severely complicating command and control, and confusing perimeter maintenance.[3]

This area of OPSEC/site security primarily deals with ensuring an effective response rather than an unorganized, potentially dangerous, and surely less effective response. Implementation of IM/UC could have diminished the reported congestion because it states that off-duty response personnel should not respond to an event unless directed to do so. Although operational doctrine dictates that you "man your post" until otherwise directed, the reality is that such a situation rarely exists. The instinct to respond is powerful and is complicated by the "*touch the plane*" phenomenon,[4] in which people feel they have to be at the disaster scene so they can tell anyone who will listen that they were indeed there "when it happened." Therefore, it is incumbent on the agency and organizational leaders to stress and practice operational discipline that demands coordination and adherence to strict deployment protocol. Another relevant example is the Bali bombing of October, 2002. As with all responders, the Bali responders rushed in to help victims and save as many lives as possible, and in doing so rendered OPSEC/site security nonexistent and placed many more lives in danger in the event of another coordinated secondary attack. Although it may be difficult to find fault with the selfless actions of such responders, it is crucial that this emotional response be tempered by reason and the knowledge that restraint and discipline are not only necessary, they are required to ensure that the investigation is permitted to bring the perpetrators to justice.

Finally, there is the example of the brave responders to the World Trade Center attacks. In their zeal to charge into the scene and save as many people as possible, the "tunnel vision" they experienced allowed them to neglect properly assessing the danger to their own lives. Although this is a "unique event" in our history with no historical reference point, the fact of the matter is that the multiple planes used in the attack were an effective secondary device of significant proportion.

OPSEC/site security involves understanding the situation to the greatest degree of accuracy possible, including the possibility that attempting to rescue victims immediately may not be the wisest, safest, or most appropriate course of action. Although it may seem that delaying rescue efforts is tantamount to abandonment of our duty to act and is contrary to the oath many of us swear to, in the end lives may be saved by taking the time to fully assess the situation in a coherent fashion before executing operational response.

Personnel Needs

The security needs of response personnel are a major issue to be tackled in planning for response to a high-impact/high-yield emergency incident. These needs are varied and can be very complex, complicated, and resource demanding during and after a terrorist event.[5] These demands are further amplified given the dual threat of the likelihood of hazardous materials being present and the active intent of the terrorist to hurt or kill as many people as possible, including responders.

One very good example of this occurred during the 1997 Tokyo sarin attacks in the subway. Japanese medical personnel lacked proper personal protective equipment; more than 20% of the staff of St. Luke's International Hospital exhibited some sort of detrimental physical effects after treating victims of the attack.[6] Had the hospital planned properly and equipped the facility/personnel, in addition to regularly training all employees, the instances of secondary contamination would have been greatly reduced.

The most recent and well-known example of responders lacking proper personal protective equipment was the Sept. 11, 2001 attacks. Early in the response, heavy particulate asbestos was found at the site, and later Freon, cadmium, and other hazardous materials were identified, yet there were responders without proper protective equipment.[7] This can be attributed to both poor planning and logistics acquisition problems because there was simply not enough equipment to go around. This indicated that planners failed to grasp the scope or even believe that a possible attack could occur, and poor logistics come into play because the equipment that was present was not distributed properly.[8]

Another critical aspect of protecting responders in a traditional sense involves personnel rest and rehabilitation, which are critical to the success and sustainability of an operation. Although responders are often willing to work to the point of exhaustion, this is dangerous to the responders, the victims, and the effectiveness of your operation. Fatigue creates more victims through poor decision-making, increased stress and frustration, and impaired judgment. The medical profession has been and continues to address the effects of sleep deprivation and fatigue due to errors that can be directly traced back to exhausted healthcare providers. Several well-publicized studies that chronicle the effects of long work hours in life-and-death stressful environments reveal errors have produced increased morbidity and mortality in the patients being cared for by these well-meaning professionals. Studies conducted over the last several years reveal that moderate sleep deprivation produces impairments in cognitive and motor performance equivalent to legally prescribed levels of alcohol intoxication.[8]

The last thing any coordinated response should have to deal with is victims among the responding rescue workers and responders. To help prevent and ensure the equitable and safe distribution of personnel, IM/UC has instituted a system by which the Incident Commander assigns shifts to the workers, thereby forcing rest on the weary, whether or not they realize they need it at the time.

The final personnel need addressed in this chapter is that of continuation of public services, including EMS, medical, law enforcement, and fire service, through the end of the incident and into the recovery and mitigation stages. Sustaining 911 response capacities for an entire community should be a significant goal that first responders must strive to achieve. Just because one is being confronted with a large disaster in one's community does not alleviate the obligation to ensure the best possible planning efforts to sustain "all" emergencies in the community are managed appropriately. Clearly, and especially in the case of EMS, the fiscal implications of having a sustainable and robust response system that can handle any and all 911 calls at all times is strictly prohibitive. The burden sharing that has become accepted widely is the use of mutual aid compacts between communities, regions, and now states under the Emergency Management Assistance Compact.[9] The key to successful sustained operation is embracing this concept and employing it, as required, on a regular basis. Furthermore, reviewing response protocols for uniformity, ensuring interoperability, and having a shared vision of application of OPSEC and site security tactics are integral on "game day."

Hospitals share the same concerns for their facilities and staff. During the planning phase for responding to disasters, hospital planners must take the time to consider a number of issues that previously did not require their attention. Such matters include increased security, physical management of patient flow, personnel protective equipment, decontamination strategies, and staff training and support. One hospital failure that resulted in much national media attention occurred in Florida during the hurricane season of 2004. In this case, Florida Hospital Ormond Memorial fired and/or suspended about 25 nurses for not working during Hurricane Frances. The nurses were fired for not calling in, not showing up, or refusing to work, whereas others were suspended for not completing a shift.[10] The hospital stated that critical care employees are required to work during a disaster under hospital policy. Some nurses responded in media accounts alleging that they were not trained to deal with these extreme scenarios and also questioned who would protect their families. In any event, the fact of the matter remains that, in a crisis, staffing rosters that were expected to be populated based on the internal disaster plan were not, leaving the facility in the lurch to cover staff vacancies and sustain operations.

Another unfortunate occurrence in the aftermath of disasters is civil unrest and criminal activity. Police presence is often distracted and concentrated at the site of the disaster, coverage is weakened in the areas where law enforcement officers would normally patrol or deploy, and if the presence is weakened enough, citizens may and have taken to looting nearby houses, commercial districts, and in some cases emergency response equipment. Examples of this can be found in the history of countless disasters, as recently as Hurricane Charley's landfall in Florida in August 2004, and there are even unsubstantiated accusations of looting by the responders themselves in the Sept. 11, 2001 to attacks on New York City.[11]

Community planners, responders, and emergency services personnel must also consider the likelihood of a situation where events have created a large-scale area that is too dangerous for anyone to enter or respond. Responders must ask themselves two questions and must answer them honestly: (1) In such a situation, what are the primary responsibilities of responders in getting people out, keeping people from entering, and making sure that the area remains contained? (2) Are the responders prepared to evacuate, relocate, secure, and effectively close a significant portion or an entire city, as was necessary during the Chernobyl disaster?

Proper and effective deployment of law enforcement officers is a key aspect of the incident management, NIMS, and NRP. With proper law enforcement tactical implementation, the lion's share of criminal activity or any form of civil disorder can be mitigated. The implementation strategy also provides for more effective coordination of responders at the scene, affording a higher level of coherence to ensure security of all personnel, integrated operations, investigatory processes, and sustained evidentiary recovery can all be achieved.

A similar concern exists for fire services in the wake of a disaster, specifically in fire-heavy disasters. The typical response for the fire service is to rush to the scene of a major blaze, such as the World Trade Center, and engage as quickly as possible to control the threat and resolve the problem. One can only imagine the collateral dangers if coincidental fires emerge in other parts of a city, particularly in the event of a secondary terrorist attack. The successes of mutual aid are clearly evident in the various responses to a number of large-scale disasters, but especially on Sept. 11, 2001.

Emergency management professionals often speak of the "secondary" attack, but how many communities, agencies, and/or organizations responsible for response and recovery actually have plans in place for a controlled, coordinated, organized deployment in the face of a growing disaster? Despite what most would believe and as horrible as the Sept. 11 attacks were, the United States has yet to experience a true mass-casualty, mass-fatality event that overwhelms the capabilities of the affected community and the country. We as responders must revisit the pain and shock we all felt on Sept. 11, 2001, when 3000 persons were murdered. Three thousand sounds like an unimaginable number, but to our enemies 3000 is a training exercise.

INTEGRATION

Integration issues are a crucial consideration in any response to an emergency, but they are critical for a large-scale incident. The most obvious example of this is in the immediate aftermath of the Sept. 11, 2001 attacks on the World Trade Center in New York City. Interoperability between fire and police radios was found to be a major problem during the response to the 1993 bombing of the World Trade Center, and unfortunately, the same problem reared its ugly head on Sept. 11, 2001. Because of overloaded radio equipment, firefighters in Tower 1 of the World Trade Center were unaware of reports of the imminent collapse of the tower from an New York Police Department (NYPD) helicopter and therefore did not initiate their own evacuation. This lack of communication resulted in an increased number of casualties that could have been avoided. The proper implementation of IM/UC, which stresses both horizontal and vertical information sharing, would have required interoperable radios, and the NYPD helicopter in the air above the World Trade Center would have been able to relay the information regarding the collapse to the fire department, allowing them to have a fuller understanding of the events and begin evacuating.[12]

The Moscow Theater siege of October 2002 is another tragic example of the cost of lives lost when agencies are not integrated. Chechen terrorists took over the theater, claimed the patrons as hostages, and were killed when Russian commandos pumped a toxic gas into the theater that rendered both terrorists and hostages unconscious, killing some. The refusal and delay by Russian authorities to release information regarding the type of gas used to subdue and incapacitate the Chechen terrorists rendered medical personnel unable to properly diagnose and treat the nearly 650 hostage victims of the gas, 117 of whom perished in the rescue.[13] The unfortunate reality is authorities in the Spetsnaz (Russian Special Forces, who carried out the raid) did not involve the medical community. If the Spetsnaz had coordinated the assault and included a medical component in tactical operations, the critical medical communication and coordination would have positioned the rescue attempt for greater success, saving additional lives because the medical knowledge, treatment, and response capabilities would have been on scene and poised to effectively respond when needed.

THE PRESS AND DIGNITARIES

Public relations is an important aspect of OPSEC/site security because outside factors such as the media and the family of victims can seriously complicate a response. One good example of the lack of OPSEC/site security with respect to the media causing major problems was evident during the "Beltway Sniper" shootings of October 2002 in the Virginia, Washington, DC, and Maryland area. The sniper pair left notes for the police with specific instructions not to be relayed to the press and allegedly made numerous requests for the media not to be involved in the interaction between the snipers and police.[14] The press obtained this information through the notorious "unnamed source" and went public with information that not only jeopardized the investigation, but also put many lives in danger. The resulting lack of trust between the sniper and the police interfered with communication between investigators and the perpetrators and slowed the investigation as authorities shifted focus toward damage control.

The media can be a great asset when responding to an incident, provided relations take place in a controlled, efficient manner. An example of the positive and negative roles the media can play in responding to an event was during the sarin attacks in Tokyo. The most common and frustrating problem during any response is a lack of communication, and the Tokyo incident was no exception. Personnel at local hospitals had no idea what type of hazardous material or contaminant was creating the medical problems they were encountering. The hospital and healthcare personnel dealing with the unknown became aware of the substance from watching the local television broadcasts; coincidentally, physicians who had experience with sarin and the effects on humans had also been watching. The resultant communication between the physicians viewing the news coverage and the hospitals correctly identified the culprit. Concurrently, the media was criticized for filming while people suffered and died instead of helping them to the hospital.[15]

Media coverage of terrorist events can be a double-edged sword, and it is up to planners to ensure that the benefits of having the media present are not outweighed by the disadvantages. This will entail having a public information officer (PIO) who is trained prior to an incident on the successful discharge of the PIO duties. This person is integrated into the command structure to assist with response information dissemination and management of the media.

In the event of a major disaster, it is common practice for officials of all levels to visit the site to offer reassurance, from Governor John Ellis Bush flying in to visit the areas devastated by Hurricane Charley in the summer of 2004 to President George W. Bush visiting New York City after Sept. 11, 2001. It is necessary to have strict OPSEC/site security to maintain the safety of these dignitaries, as well as to ensure they and their entourages do not disturb the scene and hinder the investigation. Although the visit of these dignitaries is important to reassure the public, it must not come at the cost of successfully executing the response plan at a local, state, or national level. As has been stated, planning cannot take place in a vacuum; plans to deal with the onslaught of media and dignitaries must be a part of the ongoing community response to any event that may overwhelm a community's ability to operate under "normal" daily conditions. Therefore, meet-and-greet sessions and planning meetings must be conducted with all involved parties to include the local media, with the primary goal that all participants have a job to do and planning before the worst case scenario occurs will allow for the completion of the mission in a safe and cooperative manner. All egos, preconceived assumptions, and negative relationships must be checked at the door.

OPSEC/SITE SECURITY DEMANDS FOR OFF-SITE OPERATIONS

Finally, there is the issue of security and staffing support for elements of the response not located directly at the event site, such as joint or regional operation centers, joint or regional information centers, multiagency coordination centers, morgues, and food distribution and donation reception sites. Although these sites may not be physically located inside the incident perimeter, they are no less likely to be targeted. These critical areas are all vulnerable to being compromised or attacked by a variety of means including, but not limited to, physical attacks with arms, explosives, criminal acts, and hazardous material dispersal.

Law enforcement officials of some type, be they federal marshals or local police or security forces, must be present to ensure protection and sustained operation of these vital services. It is absolutely vital to the success and continuation of the response that community planners; local, city, and county emergency managers; and all those who will respond (paid and volunteer) meet on a regular basis before a catastrophic emergency to promulgate prudent operational response doctrine, to ensure OPSEC and site security, and to test planning strategies through comprehensive exercising.

OPSEC/SITE SECURITY FOR A TERRORIST INCIDENT

It isn't enough to simply adopt and fully implement the NIMS-IM/UC framework to control and overcome the majority of OPSEC/site security issues, although it is important to note that the majority of concerns, challenges, and problems faced by EMS, medical, law enforcement, security, and fire services are not unique to terrorism/WMD events. The implementation of a plan and/or a system to alleviate identified problems and to avoid new problems is only as good as the training that is provided to familiarize all those who will use the plan and/or system.

It is impossible and may border on negligence to expect that people, agencies, departments, and communities will be able to use plans designed to place everyone on "the same sheet of paper" without coherent, comprehensive, ongoing training and exercising.

In the case of a natural disaster, for example, the difficulties inherent in the massive response of multiple agencies remain. The logistics involved in mobilizing personnel, equipment, and resources coupled with emotional, hungry, tired victims and those nefarious few who are bent on taking advantage of victims in need create circumstances that will derail the best laid plans. Now, add to that a situation in which these very same people are asked to respond, faced with all the normal obstacles, but have had little or no time to be acquainted with the new plan and even less time being trained on the plan's usefulness, purpose, and operational guidance. You now have the current scenario in place; add to this already chaotic, stressful, and incredibly frustrating event the current severity and the particular nature of the threats we face in the post-Sept. 11 era.

The unpredictability of terrorism presents conditions that are highly fluid and subject not only to the whims of nature or the physics of a damaged building but to the advanced plans and suicidal determination of well-trained terrorists. Additionally, your garden-variety terrorist does not have to fear Occupational Safety and Health Administration requirements, does not have to apply for permits, does not have to worry about the adequacy of financial support, does not have labor laws and/or legal restraints preventing action, and the list goes on. The terrorist groups we have identified, and most likely those we have yet to uncover, commit, plan, train, and act in an organized, efficient, and effective manner.

An organizational structure adequate to deal with such an elusive threat, represented by NIMS–IM/UC, only provides the means by which proper measures can be successfully implemented. This, however, is a question not of whether a strategy will be properly followed but of what that particular strategy entails. The plan in no way provides implementation funding avenues, training and educational funding, staffing backfill or overtime funding that will allow comprehensive training and education, equipment acquisition and maintenance, etc. Any plan is only as good as the assumptions it is based on, and a plan certainly is useless when those who are expected to use it have yet to see the plan and have no training in implementing it.

The critical issue that must be addressed is the priority that must be given to OPSEC/site security at all incidents, not just those eventually identified as terrorism/WMD related. This will create a familiarity with OPSEC and site security for all responders and institutionalize these policies into the way we do business at all times.

The after-action reports from numerous major terrorism incidents clearly reveal shortcomings in OPSEC/site security that warrant significant emphasis and close attention by agencies developing their terrorism/WMD response plans in concurrence with NIMS–IM/UC.

There is a striking convergence of properties that characterizes this second grouping of OPSEC/site security concerns: they cannot be solved by organizational reform alone, and they are all particularly pertinent in a terrorist/WMD attack. This highly interconnected list for scene management includes perimeter establishment, access and egress control, personnel accountability, evidence protection and chain of custody, and the search for secondary devices and threats. Solving the inadequacies in these areas requires not just that the organizational structure exist, but that it be imbedded in a prominent position within the Incident Command structure.

ESTABLISHING A PERIMETER

The effective establishment of a perimeter is often a crucial aspect of gaining control over the scene of an attack. Establishing a perimeter has ramifications in all aspects of maintaining OPSEC/site security. Force protection cannot be ensured, evidence cannot be protected, chain of custody cannot be guaranteed, and access to the scene cannot be controlled with a porous or haphazard creation of a perimeter.

The overall response to the 1995 terrorist bombing of the Alfred P. Murrah Building in Oklahoma City, Oklahoma, is an excellent model of what was right and what was wrong. There existed three layers of perimeters, quickly established by morning on the day after the bombing: the inner perimeter was designed to provide limited access to only those personnel authorized to participate in the rescue/recovery work and the criminal investigation, a staging area also served as a buffer for workers, and a cordon limited traffic access.[16] Unfortunately, an effective perimeter was not established immediately, and the site quickly became overwhelmed with hundreds of well-meaning people who wanted to help in any way they could. Because no control existed over any area of the dangerous site, one convergent responder, a nurse, was killed early on due to fallen debris. The eventual establishment of an effective perimeter was accomplished by close coordination of disparate agencies and proper use of their abilities, along with the securing and construction of fencing.[16]

At the World Trade Center site on Sept. 11, in admittedly more trying circumstances, "Perimeter security was not adequately established, allowing large numbers of unnecessary personnel to enter," due in large part to a 5-day delay in the creation of an adequate credentialing system and the construction of a fence.[16] It took an extra 4 days at the World Trade Center to establish security even approaching the perimeter set up at the Murrah building. The potential repercussions of this sort of inattention are massive.

An example of inattention is the case of 1997 bombing of a women's clinic in suburban Atlanta, in which Eric Rudolph allegedly planted a secondary explosive device timed to detonate on the arrival of personnel responding to the initial explosive event. A CNN camera crew filming an interview with a witness of the initial blast caught the nearby second explosion on film; both media and civilians were endangered because they were allowed access to an area surrounding the scene that should have been secured. The uncontrolled scene increases the potential and likelihood that persons not involved in the initial catastrophic event will become victims as a result of a secondary attack, the hazardous material (if present) will be spread to a wider area of the city, and the criminal investigation will be hampered or destroyed. Ground zero of a terrorist attack, therefore, demands special attention to the formation of perimeters as a necessary prerequisite to full OPSEC/site security.

The cooperation and discipline required to ensure security and safety does not and will not happen overnight or because it is the right thing to do. All aspects of scene control must be carefully planned, practiced, and exercised on an ongoing basis. It is impossible to expect two completely divergent disciplines to come together and cooperate without the right training and education. One large group of people is running in to tear the scene apart to look for victims, survivors, and treat the injured. The other large group requires the meticulous preservation of evidence and maintaining the site just as it was found. There is no question that each group has vital and incredibly important roles and responsibilities, and none more important than the other. But it is naïve and irresponsible for any responding person, agency, group, or department to expect these two parallel forces to eventually meet in the middle without long-term focused efforts aimed at settling the differences and ensuring that both jobs are completed efficiently and in a timely manner. This can only be accomplished well before the need through regular meetings, educational sessions, and training. Failure to address this coordination factor before an event will result in a response that resembles a cacophony rather than the desired symphony.

EVIDENCE PROTECTION

As already stated, ensuring the preservation of evidence is another fundamental aspect of OPSEC/site security in the event of a terrorist/WMD attack. Consider the Oklahoma Department of Civil Emergency Management After Action Report, which outlines the problems that presented themselves because of the large number of volunteers who were incorporated into rescue operations without being registered or identified. "Since the site was a crime scene, all our volunteers were required to be critically screened before they could work at the bomb site," the report stated.[16] Fortunately, authorities were able to quickly implement this system to rectify the unimpeded access people had previously been afforded; about 30 unauthorized "convergent responder" volunteers were evicted from one floor alone.

This was not handled as well at the site of the 2002 Bali bombings. There, "the crime scene was seemingly ruined and unprotected" due, in addition to unavoidable circumstances involved in the response, to "the public's curiosity," which was apparently allowed to hinder the investigation despite the fact that a police line had been set up.[18] The removal, addition, destruction, or alteration of material, whether intentional, unintentional, or simply the product of an inexperienced volunteer seeking a souvenir, could prove to be a major hindrance to the proper conduct of the criminal investigation and identification of those responsible. Even the most minute and seemingly unimportant pieces of evidence often prove to be irreplaceable in these situations and cannot afford to be compromised. To the untrained eye, the aftermath of a terrorist attack is a pile of debris or a chaotic mass of

humanity. To the trained criminal investigator, the scene is a road map that tells the complete story of the circumstances leading up to the event and the event itself. As noted above, the control of access to the site of a WMD incident through well-guarded and protected perimeters and a secure credentialing system that does not allow for forgeries is the only way to guarantee the integrity of the crime scene.

INFORMATION SECURITY AND TRAFFIC AND CROWD CONTROL

Information security and dispersal interacts with traffic and crowd control to make up an extremely important aspect of OPSEC/site security in the event of a terrorist attack. In this case, OPSEC/site security takes on a much broader scope because activity elsewhere affects the flow of people and materials in and out of the site itself, as well as the city or general area in which the attack has occurred. The frightening nature of terrorism, especially for cases in which a WMD is implicated either by fact or by speculation, could and will result in mass hysteria and chaos. In the absence of accurate, timely information from authorities, rumor-mongering can take root, leading to potentially disastrous public panic. Something in the vein of an uncontrolled large-scale attempt to flee a city in the midst of reports of a chemical or biologic outbreak would freeze attempts to contain the attack and bring more people into open exposure.

Take the following description of the evacuation of coastal Florida at the approach of Hurricane Floyd in 1999: "Even many of those not in evacuation zones fled at the sight of satellite images on the news, which depicted a monstrous Floyd larger than the entire state of Florida... the result was a transportation nightmare."[19] The Florida public being frightened by memories of 1992's Hurricane Andrew is akin to today's nationwide memory of Sept. 11, 2001; combined with sensationalizing factors such as talk of a hurricane engulfing a state or the imminent citywide release of a chemical agent, they can easily produce wholesale disorder. Full control of the site of a terrorist disaster area requires that the information being disseminated from a scene be released in multiple mediums and methods of communication to dispel rumors and with an eye to directing the public to the proper course of action. Emergency response managers and chief officers cannot lose sight of the fact that our communities are made up of cultures that interpret the same information in different ways. Keeping in mind the cultural, language, and educational barriers that make up each community requires extensive preparations to ensure a complete information-sharing plan of action. Concurrently, traffic and crowd control of the entire surrounding area must be fused with information control to ensure that on-site efforts receive proper support and aid.

Control of human traffic also has great importance in its localized form. In the rush to leave a scene to avoid injury or seek medical attention, it is very possible that citizens may unintentionally carry biologic or chemical hazards with them. Depending on the nature of the agent that has been introduced, the failure to contain contaminated people or other material could lead to secondary infections. The 1995 sarin nerve agent attack on the Tokyo subway system is an example of the difficulties and effects associated with the uncontrolled vector of contaminated victims. In that incident, over 4000 affected, some contaminated and off-gassing victims showed up seeking medical treatment without official transport. This means that a very large number of people who either came into contact or had a good chance of coming into contact with sarin were moving freely throughout the city. It is fortunate that the toxicity of the sarin used in the attacks was not potent enough to kill many more, and the off-gassing that occurred resulted in illness and not death.

Citizens who sought medical assistance were not treated by responders prepared to bring decontamination assets to the scene, causing a high rate of secondary exposure among the medical staff at unspecialized facilities. Containment of the incident area includes, therefore, the ability to bring specialized treatment to the site: "[A]gent absorbed by cloth may be released as a vapor by the cloth for 30 minutes or more after exposure."[6] Again, because the sarin had been put together quickly and was only 30% pure, the agent did not lead to any serious injuries in those who were not in direct contact with the dispersal device.[20] However, it is startling that such an impure chemical mixture was able to affect over 20% of the hospital workers treating victims who hadn't been in direct contact with the sarin dispersal device and had been transported from the scene over an extended period of time.[20] The lesson is clear: in responding to an attack in which biologic, chemical, or radiologic weapons are suspected, establishing control of the traffic of people both in and out of the area is crucial for the protection of the scene victims and those would-be victims in the surrounding communities.

SECONDARY DEVICES OR THREATS

Perhaps the most pressing and worrying element of concern is that of secondary devices and threats targeting responders and evacuating civilians. Terrorism poses a distinct, highly dangerous hazard and challenge in itself, but the potential for secondary attacks and fallout aimed at even more casualties in those responding to assist further complicates the big picture and any attempts to control the aftermath. Terrorism aims in many cases to cause as much damage or harm to as many people as possible, so the use of a "follow-up" attack should not be addressed as merely a marginal possibility but as a primary consideration.

The previously mentioned example of Eric Rudolph and his alleged involvement in abortion clinic bombings is relevant here as well. The detonation of a bomb outside of an Atlanta nightclub 1 week after the women's clinic blast where a secondary attack was successful provided responders with enough warning to suspect such a setup in Atlanta. Fortunately, the responders remained diligent, and the secondary device that Rudolph had allegedly planted was found and disarmed before it could kill or injure any of the responders. Similar terror tactics have been used extensively by several international ter-

rorist organizations, most notably the "Real Irish Republican Army" (IRA) and the Colombian paramilitary guerilla group known as the Revolutionary Armed Forces of Colombia (FARC). IRA guerilla forces "have operated a two-bomb strategy, hoping secondary devices 'catch' security forces rushing to the scene of the first."[21] The adoption of such tactics by the enemies of the United States, given their resourcefulness and excellent access to information, should certainly not be discounted.

Preparation for such a scenario has been found lacking. In the aftermath of the collapse of the World Trade Center towers, the initial rescue phase was followed by a massive recovery effort. Within a day or so after the two towers collapsed, there were already thousands of workers on the scene. Estimates place the number of volunteers and workers at ground zero after the attacks at 30,000 to 40,000.[17] At the same time, however, "risk of secondary attack was not made a priority as the rescue effort was vigorously pursued."[21] The buildings in the immediate vicinity were not searched for 4 days and even then took months to be cleared. There was no standard procedure for obtaining resources such as military aid. Failure to immediately secure a perimeter and control site access, as mentioned above, left avenues open through which to strike.

In addition, the majority of the nation's federal response to the disaster was housed in one Manhattan hotel surrounded by response vehicles brightly decorated with a wide variety of responding agency's logos, decals, and identifying placards. The worst-kept secret in the entire city of New York was where all the federal responders were resting, recuperating, and spending their down time. There is no question that a well-planned or even a last-minute secondary attack could have been carried out that would have produced a very high number of casualties due to the large number of vulnerable personnel in the area. Such an attack would have crippled the New York response, but more importantly, the secondary attack at that particular time would have crippled the nation due to the message it would have sent to those not directly affected by the events in New York and Washington, DC.

Numerous tactics could be applied in a secondary attack. The potential for snipers to receive training and apply it with startling effect was demonstrated by the killing spree undertaken by the Beltway Snipers, John Allen Muhammad and Lee Boyd Malvo. Powerful and accurate weapons such as shoulder-fired rocket-propelled grenade launchers and American-made Stinger missiles, in addition to heavily proliferated small arms, are obtainable through the international black market and have been proved to be deadly in small-scale guerilla conflicts in Africa, the Middle East, and across the globe. Suicide attacks come in many forms, including truck bombs and explosives strapped to the body, and these can also be devastating in effect. It is clear, therefore, that there is both a real threat and a worrisome example in which this threat was not prepared for sufficiently. The NYPD report makes this apparent: "NYPD lacked systematic intelligence and threat assessment function and had difficulty assessing risk of further terrorist attack in weeks after 9/11."[7]

CONCLUSION

OPSEC and site security are the most important concepts that can be engaged through a conscientious, comprehensive effort to protect and secure vital infrastructure before, during, and after a catastrophic event. To ensure that OPSEC/site security is a concept that is embraced and promoted, dialogue with all traditional and nontraditional response agencies should occur on an ongoing basis prior to "game day." These "meet and greet, break bread" gatherings will require the checking of egos at the door and the establishment of a real goal-oriented working session. The creation of Memoranda of Understanding that details the roles, duties, and responsibilities of all agencies and responders will assist in the development of long-term working relationships all aimed at the security, safety, and preservation of life and limb.

REFERENCES

1. Operations security: intelligence threat handbook. Available at: http://www.fas.org/irp/nsa/ioss/threat96/part01.htm.
2. Maniscalco PM, Christen HT. *Understanding Terrorism and Managing its Consequences*, Upper Saddle River, NJ: Prentice Hall; 2001.
3. Federal Emergency Management Agency. *Responding to Incidents of National Consequence: Recommendations for America's Fire and Emergency Services Based on the Events of September 11, 2001, and Other Similar Incidents*. FA-282-May 2004:34. Available at: http://www.usfa.fema.gov/downloads/pdf/publications/fa282.pdf.
4. Federal Emergency Management Agency. *Responding to Incidents of National Consequence: Recommendations for America's Fire and Emergency Services Based on the Events of September 11, 2001, and Other Similar Incidents*. FA-282-May 2004. Available at: http://www.usfa.fema.gov/ downloads/pdf/publications/fa-282.pdf.
5. Maniscalco PM, Christen HT. *Understanding Terrorism and Managing its Consequences*. Upper Saddle River, NJ: Prentice Hall; July 2001:44.
6. Sarin poisoning on Tokyo subway. Southern Medical Association; June 3, 1997. Southern Medical Journal 1997; 90:587–593.
7. McKinsey & Company. *Improving NYPD Emergency Preparedness and Response*. August 19, 2002. Available at: http://www.nyc.gov/html/nypd/pdf/nypdemergency.pdf.
8. Metzgar C. Moderate sleep deprivation produces impairments in cognitive and motor performance equivalent to legally prescribed levels of alcohol intoxication. *Professional Safety* 2001; 46(1):17.
9. Emergency Management Assistance Compact Web site. Available at: http://www.emacweb.org/.
10. The Associated Press. Nurses fired or suspended for not working during Hurricane Frances. *Sun-Sentinel*. Available at: http://www.hirenursing.com/c/nursing/newsdetailx/nurses-fired-for-not-working-hurricane9417.htm.
11. WNBC. Small businesses cry foul after alleged lootings, but Bloomberg denies wrongdoing, plays up heroism of NYPD. November 19, 2002. Available at: http://www.wnbc.com/news/1424628/detail.html.
12. Fire Department of the City of New York. *Increasing FDNY's Preparedness*. McKinsey & Company; August 19, 2002:32. Available at: http://www.nyc.gov/html/fdny/html/mck_report/toc.html.
13. Glasser SB. Russia confirms gas was opiate-based fentanyl. *Washington Post* October 30, 2002. Available at: http://www.washingtonpost.com/ac2/wp-dyn?pagename=article&contentId=A40202-2002Oct30&notFound=true.
14. CNN. Witnesses recall telephone conversations during sniper shootings. October 31, 2003. Available at: http://www.cnn.com/2003/LAW/10/30/muhammad.trial/index.html.
15. Japan-101. Sarin gas attack on the Tokyo subway. Available at: http://www.japan-101.com/culture/sarin_gas_attack_on_the_tokyo_su.htm.
16. The City of Oklahoma City After Action Report: Alfred P. Murrah Federal Building Bombing, July 1996. Available at: http://www.mipt.org/murrahfinalrpt.asp.
17. Federal Emergency Management Agency. *Responding to Incidents of National Consequence: Recommendations for America's Fire and Emergency Services Based on the Events of September 11, 2001, and Other Similar Incidents*. FA-282-May 2004:46-48. Available at: http://www.usfa.fema.gov/downloads/pdf/publications/fa-282.pdf.
18. Pastika MM. Summary of the Bali blast case. *Feral News* Jan 2003. Available at: http://www.asyura.com/2003/war25/msg/494.html.
19. Kriner S. Hurricane Floyd: filled with sound and fury, signifying—traffic? October 12, 1999. Available at: http://www.disasterrelief.org/disasters/990928evacuations/. Nerve Agent: GB (Sarin) Available at: http://cbwinfo.com/chemical/nerve/gb.shtml.
20. Organization for the Prohibition of Chemical Weapons. Chemical terrorism in Japan: the Matsumoto and Tokyo incidents. Available at: *http://www.opcw.org/resp/html/japan.htm*. Sarin poisoning on Tokyo subway. Southern Medical Association; June 3, 1997.
21. CNN. Real IRA guerrillas back to haunt London. March 4, 2001. Available at: http://www.cnn.com/2001/world/ europe/uk/03/04/britain.irish.blast.01.reut/.
22. Senay E. Ground zero workers' health cloudy. September 11, 2003. *The Early Show*. Available at: http://www.cbsnews.com/stories/2003/09/10/earlyshow/contributors/emilysenay/main572586.shtml.

chapter 60

Integration of Law Enforcement and Military Resources with the Emergency Response to a Terrorist Incident

Eric Sergienko

In a terrorist incident, medical and rescue resources will respond to locate, extricate, treat, and transport patients. At the same time, law enforcement resources will respond to investigate, interview, and collect evidence. Medical operations can interfere with the investigation and successful prosecution of terrorist activity. Movement through the scene can disrupt or destroy evidence. At the same time, by limiting access to the scene, law enforcement can have an impact on the ability of medical responders to effectively treat patients and move them from the scene.

Integrating the law enforcement response with the medical response requires cooperation at all levels of the operation: tactically, where individual responders must work side by side; operationally, where a unified command must smoothly coordinate resources at the incident site; and strategically, where resource and response decisions must be made. Emergency medical technicians, nurses, and physicians need to be aware of evidence preservation and crime scene management. Mass fatality management will have to coincide with evidence processing.

Furthermore, in a large-scale incident, regardless of its type, military resources may respond to the scene. The military has unique assets that can respond to a terrorist incident, including weapons of mass destruction (WMD) detection, decontamination, and mitigation. They can serve to augment the medical, rescue, and law enforcement capabilities of the civilian community. However, both the military responder and their civilian requester must understand the processes that allow the use of military resources and the rules under which they function.

The potential conflicts between medical responders and law enforcement officials must be addressed prior to the actual incident. The relation between military assets and the civilian government must be established. By recognizing the distinct roles that each agency plays in responding to the terrorist incident, the responder can better address his mission and the incident commander can better utilize resources.[1,2]

In the wake of the attacks of Sept. 11, 2001 and the anthrax mailing that followed, there is significant flux occurring in the legal and administrative framework that organizes the U.S. federal and state response to terrorist incidents. To better understand these changes, it is helpful to look at the trends in the response to terrorism as a crime and terrorism as a mass-casualty event over the last 25 years.

HISTORICAL PERSPECTIVE

Law Enforcement

Since the 1980s, in differentiating between the roles of rescuers and the roles of investigators, the terms *consequence* and *crisis management* have been used. The Federal Emergency Management Agency (FEMA) defines *consequence management* as the actions taken to protect public health and safety, restore essential government services, and provide relief to governments, businesses, and persons affected by the consequences of terrorism. *Crisis management,* in contrast, is the measures taken to identify, acquire, and plan the use of resources to anticipate, prevent, and resolve a threat or act of terrorism.[3]

Consequence management is maintained at the lowest level of government possible. If the consequences of a terrorist incident can be met with resources from the local level, there should be minimal involvement of state or federal resources. If local government is not able to adequately manage the consequences of the incident, it will turn to the state government for assistance. If the state cannot meet the needs of the incident, it will turn to the federal government. At the federal level, consequence management has been the responsibility of the agency providing civil defense. Since the 1970s, this has been FEMA.[4]

In contrast, crisis management, since its conception, has been felt to be a function of the federal government. The concept of terrorism as a criminal act evolved from the realm of sabotage and espionage where an individual, working as an agent of an enemy state, performs an action that is injurious to the government or its people. Acts of terrorism, by extension, are acts committed by transnational or nonstate organizations. As a result, these are prosecuted in the federal courts under U.S. Code. The Department of Justice was appointed the lead federal agency for crisis management in the 1980s. The Federal Bureau of Investigation (FBI) was then delegated the responsibility for crisis management.[5]

The difficulty with having two different response operations to the same incident was that each entity, rescue, and investigation had a different set of objectives. Neither felt the other had a complete view of the incident. Conflict in managing the incident was a natural outgrowth of these unshared objectives. Furthermore, there was conflict vertically as different agencies with the same function competed for control of the scene.

The Stafford Act was passed in 1974 and amended in 1988 to delineate the federal response to a disaster. The Act was not made with a specific reference to terrorism. It did, however, state that nothing within the Act was to construe an investigatory role for any federal agency other than the FBI.[6]

In 1986, in response to the Vice President's Task Force on Terrorism, President Reagan issued the first guidance on responding to terrorism. Although largely designed to address attacks outside of the United States, it named the FBI as the lead agency for dealing with acts of terrorism. The next administrative guidance on terrorism would not occur until 1996.

The first large-scale act of terrorism on U.S. territory occurred in 1993. The World Trade Center was the site of an improvised explosive device detonation that resulted in 6 deaths and more than 1000 injuries. An area 150 feet wide and 5 stories deep was destroyed. There was minimal conflict between the crisis and consequence functions of this incident. The incident was initially felt to be a transformer explosion with a resultant fire. Because of this, command and control was largely performed by Fire Department of the City of New York (FDNY). Fire ground operations were handled with resources from the FDNY only, with mutual aid being required for the emergency medical services (EMS) response. Only later did it evolve into a crime scene. The area was then processed initially by four FBI evidence technicians and four Bureau of Alcohol, Tobacco, and Firearms evidence technicians working with a local New York Police Department chemist. After-action reports indicated a minimum number of conflicts between federal and local law enforcement officials. These reports attribute this to an already established Joint Terrorism Task Force (JTTF), which had been in existence in New York City since the 1980s.[7-9]

JTTFs have been established in 56 major metropolitan areas that have FBI field offices. Each is made up of FBI special agents and local law enforcement officers. The local officers are made Special Deputy U.S. Marshals. They share in the responsibility of gathering intelligence, investigating, and prosecuting terrorist-related crimes. Funding of the JTTF is largely through the FBI, although the local government continues to pay the salaries of its officers.[10]

In response to the Oklahoma City bombing in 1995, President Clinton signed Presidential Decision Directive 39 (PDD-39). The response required was greater than the resources available to the local or state government. Furthermore, the incident was recognized nearly immediately as a criminal action. Although there was immediate involvement of federal agencies, there was little coordination between the consequences and crisis functions. PDD-39 established guidelines for federal command and control in the event of a terrorist incident. Specifically, it designated the Department of Justice as the lead federal agency for operational response and crisis management. The attorney general delegated this role to the FBI. It designated FEMA as the lead federal agency for consequence management. Furthermore, it specified that crisis management would take precedence over consequence management—the FBI would remain in charge of the scene until the attorney general had turned the scene over to FEMA.[11]

Presidential Decision Directive 62 (PDD-62) directed the federal agencies in their preresponse planning to counterterrorism and consequence management. It established a national level coordinator for security, critical infrastructure protection, and counterterrorism. It provided guidance on the role of the Department of Justice, Department of Health and Human Services, and Department of Defense in preparing the Metropolitan Medical Strike Team (now Metropolitan Medical Response System) in the first 120 cities that established them.[12]

The Concept of Operations Plan (CONPLAN) for terrorism, signed in 2000, reaffirmed the role of the Department of Justice as the lead federal agency, a responsibility that is delegated to the FBI, in the response to terrorism. As such, the FBI remained the on-scene commander until the attorney general relinquished control to FEMA. However, there was much in terms of transitioning from a focus on crisis management to creating an environment that focused on a unified command involving all agencies that had a response. The FBI would establish a Joint Operations Command (JOC) that would serve as a focus for crisis management in the unified response. It was intended to complement and work with the local agencies' Incident Command System.[13]

On Sept. 11, 2001 the World Trade Center was attacked for a second time. In a much larger and clearly more destructive attack, the response was also large and difficult to manage. Again, the JTTF was crucial in providing a guiding framework for the crisis management response. There was a coordinated response to evidence processing that seemed to minimally affect the rescue efforts. The resources of the FDNY and other rescue agencies were continued well past the rescue phase due to their expertise in urban search and rescue. The most serious concern with Sept. 11 was not a conflict between law enforcement and rescue, but the lack of coordinated communications that may have led to unnecessary morbidity and mortality. The police commander ordered the evacuation of his personnel from the building after receiving information pointing to the potential for collapse, but this was not relayed to the firefighters.[14]

The success of the management of the response to the Pentagon attack can largely be attributed to the ability of the first responders, the Arlington Fire Department, to assert themselves as the incident commanders. Until the initial rescue and recovery operations were completed, the command remained with one agency as the lead, while other agencies actively contributed to the management of the incident.[15]

The Initial National Response Plan (INRP) was enacted in September 2003 while a final National Response Plan (NRP) was being developed. The INRP uses existing documents to blend response models to increase the possibility of harmonious relations at the incident site.

When signed, the NRP will become the guiding document for federal response to terrorism, supplanting the Federal Response Plan, the INRP, and the CONPLAN. It delineates the role of the Department of Homeland Security in the response to terrorism. It proposes moving more toward a unified command with a designated Principal Federal Official (PFO) as the overall senior federal official at the scene. Using Homeland Security Presidential Directive 5 as its guidance, it will eliminate the distinction between *consequence* and *crisis* response.[16]

Military

The military has been involved in support to civilian disasters since the inception of the union. The use of the military for non–law enforcement response is legal and well established in both statute and case law. The military has performed *ad hoc* relief missions to natural disasters both as an immediate response to emergencies in adjacent civilian communities (as in the San Francisco earthquake of 1906) or in sustained efforts as approved by Congress. It was not until the Federal Civil Defense Act of 1950 that Congress codified the military's standing role in civilian disasters. This was later expanded in the Stafford Act in 1974 and its amendments in 1988.

However, there is often concern about the use of military in support of civilian law enforcement. Originally, the states were concerned about the federal government maintaining a standing army. In the Reconstruction Era after the Civil War, the Union Army was used to maintain order in the Southern states. The reaction to the conduct of the Army in this time was to limit the use of the Army in civilian law enforcement. Feeling that the Army's enforcement of polling laws led to the party's loss of the presidency, a Democratic Congress passed the Posse Comitatus Act in 1878. A *posse comitatus* (Latin for "power of the county") historically is a collection of able-bodied citizens working under the country sheriff to enforce the laws. Currently, under Title 18 section 1385 of the U.S. Code, the Army and Air Force are prohibited from serving as a posse or other form of law enforcement. By Department of Defense policy, this has been extended to the Navy and the Marine Corps.

Since the passing of the Posse Comitatus Act, the military has continued to respond to natural disasters to support civilian communities. Neither does the Posse Comitatus Act completely eliminate the use of the military as an aid to law enforcement. It does allow for the suppression of riots and controlling of crowds. The last large-scale use of this provision of the U.S. Code was in 1992, when President George H.W. Bush responded to the Los Angeles riots by deploying over 4000 U.S. Army and Marine troops and "federalized" (used as part of the U.S. Army) over 4000 California National Guardsmen. Furthermore, it is important to note that the Coast Guard is excluded from the Posse Comitatus Act. The Coast Guard, part of the Department of Homeland Security, is the United States' leading maritime law enforcement agency. Its duties include drug enforcement, immigration control, and port security.[17]

The Stafford Act identifies the Department of Defense as a resource that may be requested by the state governor from the president. In an incident in which a disaster declaration is expected, the president can direct the secretary of defense to provide military resources to the response for a period of up to 10 days. Once a declaration has been made, the resources are available through the established Joint Field Office. Expenses that the Department of Defense incurs in either of these responses modes are reimbursable.

Additionally, under the concept of *immediate response,* a local commander can use assets available to him to provide aid to an adjacent civilian community. This immediate response is done only to prevent the loss of life or limb or to minimize property damage. Traditionally, the period of time in which an immediate response can be performed is generally considered the first 3 days of a disaster. After that period, it is expected that requests for assistance will come through the channels established for crisis or consequence management (e.g., a state governor will request assistance from the president, then the president tasks the military with providing support). Under the concept of immediate response, the local commander can provide support to law enforcement when there is the possibility of loss of life or wanton property destruction, or to restore the functions of government.[18]

CURRENT PRACTICE

Law Enforcement

Local law enforcement will respond to the scene of a terrorist incident as they would any major crime scene. The concept is to minimize the number of people necessary at the scene so as to keep contamination of the scene to a minimum. An internal and external perimeter will be established. There will be an attempt to track personnel entering and exiting the scene. As with the first World Trade Center bombing, there will be an attempt to process the evidence with as few people as possible.

If it is one of the 56 metropolitan areas that have a JTTF, it is likely that there will be an immediate FBI/local police response aimed at determining the cause of the incident. In the past, the JTTFs have been able to determine that incidents were not terrorist in nature more rapidly than a traditional divided approach to intelligence development.

The initial federal law enforcement response will assess the scene to determine if the event is the result of a terrorist attack. The local FBI special agent in charge (SAC) will typically do this. If the SAC determines that this is likely a terrorist event, he or she will set up a Crisis Management Group. The Crisis Management Group will begin to coordinate the crisis management aspects of a terrorist incident. Initially, they will establish an FBI command post that will coordinate their efforts with the first responders' command post that is addressing consequence management. Ideally, this will evolve into a unified command structure supported by the Department of Homeland Security's Joint Field Office and by local, state, and regional Emergency Operations Centers.[19]

DHS will establish a Joint Field Office within 4 to 12 hours of determining that a terrorist incident has occurred. The Joint Field Office functions in essence as an Area Command as established in ICS, or similar to a regional Emergency Operations Center (Fig. 60-1). It incorporates a coordination group, operations group, administration/finance group, logistics group, and a planning management group paralleling the ICS used at the local level.

The PFO coordinates the efforts of the command group, which incorporates the senior representative from FEMA as the federal coordinating officer and the SAC from the FBI as senior federal law enforcement officer. As well, there are liaisons from all involved federal agencies, as well as state and local representatives.

The Domestic Emergency Support Team (DEST) is a rapidly deployable interagency support team that brings to the on-scene commander the breadth of expertise available from the federal government. Typically, the DEST will deploy immediately to an incident that may require federal support. The DEST may then become the nucleus of the Joint Field Office.[20,21]

The FBI has had a Hazardous Materials Response Unit (HMRU) since 1996 to collect evidence in a hazardous environment. Deployed from FBI headquarters to a hazardous materials release, regardless of accidental or intentional release, the HMRU is capable of operating in a hostile environment to process it as a crime scene. In addition to the HMRU, designated FBI field offices maintain smaller, but similarly equipped Hazardous Materials Response Teams to act as an immediate response resource to local incidents. In addition, the FBI response will include an Evidence Response Team, a team of 8 to 50 members from a local field office that will process evidence from a crime scene.[22]

It is expected that rescuers will need to enter the scene of a WMD release. However, to minimize the risk of contamination of the scene, multiple courses have been developed for the EMS and firefighter communities to recognize a criminal or terrorist incident, to minimize scene contamination, and to relate crime scene information to law enforcement officials.[23]

At the tactical level, local special weapons and tactical teams have the need for integral EMS support. Typically, either SWAT officers are trained to the EMT or paramedic level or an experienced EMS provider is trained to operate in a tactical environment. Training for the medical provider is aimed at providing emergency care in an austere tactical environment. In addition, the EMS provider gives preventive care as well, measuring heat stress and injury potential, and enforcing work/rest cycles. Some agencies have developed a local joint task force to

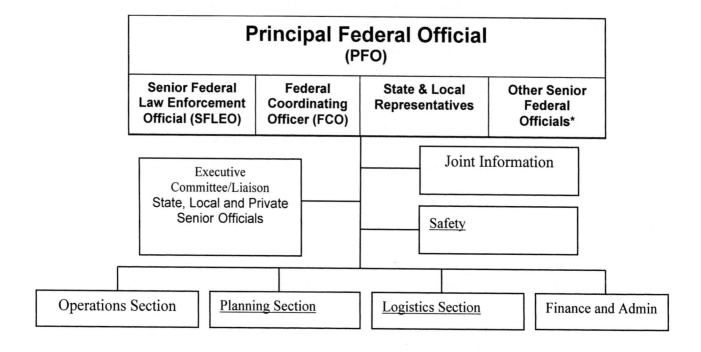

*Includes the Defense Coordinating Officer (DCO)

FIGURE 60–1. Organization of Joint Field Office.

respond to a WMD release. Made up of local fire, EMS, law enforcement, and explosive ordnance disposal personnel, this task force trains personnel to provide a unified initial response within the hot zone. It has many of the capabilities of the National Guard's WMD–Civil Support Team, including agent identification, hazard mapping, and plume modeling.

Military

Civil support is the provision of Department of Defense support to U.S. civil authorities for domestic emergencies and for designated law enforcement and other activities. The Department of Defense undertakes civil support missions when its involvement is appropriate and when a clear end point for the Department of Defense role is defined. A term analogous to civil support is *military assistance to civil affairs* (MACA). This is the broad definition for the use of military resources in responding to a civilian incident.

The commander of any military force is tasked with first protecting his or her resources and personnel, being ready for his or her war-fighting mission, and keeping his or her higher authority aware of the situation. After this, excess resources can be committed to a civilian incident. Within the realm of MACA are several categories that are defined within the U.S. Code. *Military support to civil affairs* is the application of military resources to a civilian emergency or disaster. Another term that is in increasing use is *defense support to civil affairs*. Department of Defense Directive 3025.1 currently guides this.[24]

Military aid to civil disturbance is the use of military force to quell a civil disturbance. The use of federal military assets requires an executive order from the president specifically indicating the location for assets to be deployed. The key to using military forces is retention of command and control of military resources by civilian authority.

Military support to law enforcement agencies is technical assistance rendered to civilian law enforcement agencies. This can include military resources that are not available to civilians such as aerial surveillance, technical assistance with these resources, and tactical advice. It does not include actual law enforcement powers. The Department of Defense also has authority to provide support to the U.S. Secret Service for missions related to the president of the United States. These may include airlift, communications, medical, and explosive ordnance disposal support.

Improvised nuclear device (IND) response is outlined in Department of Defense Directive 3150.5. It assumes that any IND release is an act of terrorism and establishes the FBI as the lead federal agency. It establishes the Army as the lead Department of Defense agency for response to an IND release that is not on property controlled by other Department of Defense assets.

Despite growth in the civilian response to WMD, the Department of Defense, including its Reserve and National Guard components, remains the largest repository of resources to the response to WMD release. For this reason, a response should be expected from the Department of Defense in the case of a WMD release.

However, the response is not automatic and depends on the local military commander having resources that are available to respond. Local governments with adjacent Department of Defense assets should do their best to establish Memoranda of Understanding and Mutual Aid Agreements so that resources used in the immediate response mode can freely flow across territorial boundaries. Requests for support using this mode are made from local or state government to the base commander or regional commander.[25]

The initial pathway to request military resources, other than through immediate response, is through the state governor to the U.S. president. The president will delegate this request to the secretary of defense. The secretary of defense will turn to the director of military support (DOMS). The DOMS oversees an operational staff within the Department of Defense for the coordination of military assets in a civil emergency. Until a Joint Field Office is established with a defense coordinating officer (DCO) in place, the DOMS validates all mission requests, identifies available units, and initiates the deployment orders (Fig. 60-2).

The DCO serves as the senior Department of Defense representative within the Joint Field Office. Typically, the DCO is a senior officer (colonel, captain, or flag rank officer) who is responsible for coordinating all Department of

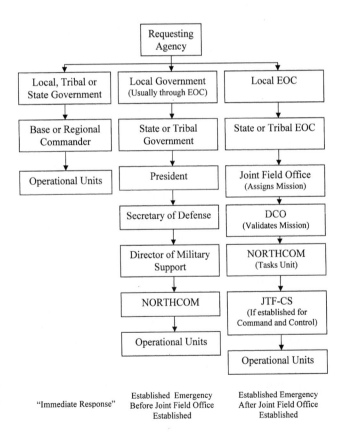

EOC – Emergency Operations Center
NORTHCOM – United States Northern Command
DCO – Defense Coordinating Officer
JTF-CS – Joint Task Force Civil Support

FIGURE 60–2. Pathways for requesting military assistance.

Defense elements at an incident. He or she is responsible for validating any requests made from the federal coordinating officer FCO or PFO. To assist the DCO, there is a defense coordinating element that is composed of an experienced staff of emergency planners and managers.

The emergency preparedness liaison officer (EPLO) is a senior military officer, typically a reservist, who serves to coordinate federal planning with state and local agencies. There is an EPLO associated with each state and with each FEMA region. In a typical tour, they attend planning sessions and tabletop and full-scale exercises. In the event of an actual incident, the EPLO would be activated to continue as a full-time liaison between the local and state response and the Department of Defense response. If a Joint Field Office is established with a DCO in place, the EPLO is attached to continue this role within the organized response under that office.[26]

U.S. Northern Command (NORTHCOM) is the command and control structure for organizing Department of Defense assets into an effective homeland security response. Established in October 2002, it has minimal assets under its operational control; rather, it serves as a clearinghouse for planning and coordinating response. During an incident, NORTHCOM would receive tasking either from DOMS, prior to the establishment of a DCO, or from the DCO after he or she has been activated.

Joint Task Force Civil Support (JTF-CS) is the NORTHCOM command that would provide command and control of Department of Defense assets after a chemical, biologic, radiologic, nuclear, or explosive (CBRNE) incident. It is a standing joint task force located at Fort Monroe, Va, commanded by a "federalized" National Guard general (a guardsman usually works for a state, but when federalized becomes an asset of the regular forces). When directed by the commander of NORTHCOM, JTF-CS would deploy to the incident site and establish command and control of Department of Defense forces to provide military assistance to civil authorities. JTF-CS focuses on consequence management and would report to and work closely with the lead federal agency in this response (either FEMA or, in the case of a foreign incident, the Department of State). Typically, the DCO would be attached to the JTF-CS staff as a special assistant. The DCO would continue his or her focus of validating missions and authorizing the use of Department of Defense assets.

The Marine Corps' Chemical Biological Immediate Response Force (CBIRF) is a battalion-sized unit able to deploy to a WMD scene. It has a large integral medical unit with emergency physicians, environmental health specialists, and medical technicians. Its parent command is the 4th Marine Expeditionary Brigade (MEB), Antiterrorism (AT). The 4th MEB/AT has several other smaller units that may be tasked to a homeland security or defense mission. Currently, CBIRF is based south of Washington, DC. However, it is often staged to support national special security events.

The Army has organized its WMD response into a single organization, the Guardian Brigade. Consisting of a headquarters element, a Chemical Biological Rapid Response Team (C/B-RRT), the Technical Escort Unit (TEU), and the 52nd Ordnance Group, it is located at Aberdeen Proving Grounds in Maryland. It is proposed that the Guardian Brigade will eventually transition to the CBRNE command.

The Army's C/B-RRT is a rapidly deployable asset from the Guardian Brigade to provide assessment of a potential chemical or biologic incident. The mission of C/B-RRT is to coordinate the activities of all Department of Defense assets responding to a CBRNE incident.

The TEU is a battalion-sized active duty Army unit. It has been in existence for over 60 years. Initially formed to provide technical support during the transport of chemical munitions, its mission has expanded to respond to the release or potential release of chemical or biologic agents. The unit's chief focus is to render safe operations of munitions that may be used to disseminate chemical or biologic agents. Typically, the TEU deploys in small teams of fewer than a dozen. Teams from the unit have been extensively deployed overseas, but the unit will also stage for national special security event.

WMD–Civil Support teams (WMD-CST) are full-time National Guard teams that have the operational role of providing an intelligence gathering and reach-back capability for the local incident commander. They are a state asset and report to the governor via the state's adjutant general (the commander of the state's National Guard). The WMD-CST consists of 22 active-duty guardsmen. Each guardsman is extensively trained in various aspects of WMD management. As a team, they can provide identification, threat modeling, mitigation, medical assessments, and recommendations and can communicate this to subject matter experts. The WMD-CST can make recommendations to the incident commander in these areas. Once in place, they can act as the initial liaison between the local incident command structure and arriving Department of Defense resources. However, they lack the depth to provide mass decontamination, treatment, or care.

The Air Force's Radiation Assessment Team is a deployable team from San Antonio, Tex, designed to respond to incidents involving radiation emergencies, from release of radioactive isotopes to WMDs. They perform analytical dosimetry, health physics, and plume modeling.

The Medical Commands of the Army, Air Force, and Navy maintain deployable medical assets. An example is the Air Force's Expeditionary Medical Support (EMEDS). EMEDS is a modular response field hospital that is built around a central resuscitation area, operating room, and intensive care unit module. The basic EMEDS can deploy in hours, is air transportable in a single C-130, can be broken down into backpack-sized loads, and has enough material to do multiple resuscitations and 10 surgeries. Additional beds and ancillary capabilities can be added as needed.

PITFALLS

Law Enforcement

"Who is in charge here?" "Who is in charge of what?" The evolution of command and control at a potential terrorism incident has evolved from divided law enforcement and rescue response and a divided local and federal response to a unified command structure that treats all responding agencies as equals. Under the auspices of a principal federal officer, the command structure should fall out to meet both the crisis and consequences issues of the incident; this is the way it is designed on paper. The pitfall of the current command structure is that it includes people who have always been in charge of their own operations and are now working together.[27]

Patient care versus evidence preservation—this is truly the yin and yang of a terrorist incident. The more we take care of patients, the more likely we are to disturb the crime scene and destroy evidence. When involved in the response to a terrorist incident, the EMS responder must stop to assess the scene not only from a mass-casualty management standpoint, but also from the forensic viewpoint. It is likely that the EMT or firefighter may be the first, and perhaps only, witness to a particular piece of evidence.

Military

The use of the military is a well-described process. For forces that are proximate to an emergency, regardless of whether it involves terrorist activity, the local commander can operate under the auspices of immediate response. These are actions that can be taken to save life or limb or to preserve property. If the event does not fall into either of these categories, the military should not be asked to deploy, nor should they agree to. The duration of response should also be taken into account. Generally, an immediate response is understood to be the first 72 hours or so of an incident.

A concept that needs further clarification is the definition of *proximate*. Can a commander who is distant from a scene, but who is the nearest available source of a scarce resource, dispatch those resources to the incident scene?

One concern of the commander using the immediate response mechanism is whether he will be reimbursed for his actions. All actions taken by the military and all requests made by their civilian cooperators should be well documented, so that later claims for costing can be justified.

Although it is clear that the Posse Comitatus Act does not apply to the use of the military resources in non–law enforcement situations, there will always be a concern expressed that the military is involved in civilian affairs. To minimize these concerns, the military should only be used for validated missions. Furthermore, military assets should not be placed in a potential situation where lethal force may be needed without clear instructions from higher authority.

REFERENCES

1. Anonymous. Preface. In: *National Interagency Management System*. Washington, DC: Federal Emergency Management Agency, Government Printing Office; 2004.
2. Homeland Security Presidential Directive 5: National Strategy for Homeland Security. Washington, DC: Office of the White House; 2002.
3. Anonymous. Appendix A: definitions and acronyms. In: *Regional Emergency Coordination Plan*. Washington, DC: Metropolitan Washington Council of Governments; 2002.
4. Clinton W. *Presidential Decision Directive 39: US Policy on Counterterrorism*. Washington, DC: 1995. Available at: www.fas.org/irp/offdocs/pdd39.htm.
5. Carlson J. Critical incident management in the ultimate crisis: counterterrorism. *FBI Law Enforcement Bull*. 1999;68(3):6-8.
6. Sub Chapter IV: B emergency preparedness. In: *The Robert T. Stafford Disaster Assistance and Emergency Relief Act, as amended, 42 USC 5121, et seq*. 1988:36-46. Available at: www.dem.dcc.state.nc.us/mitigation/Library/Stafford.pdf.
7. Fusco A. Overview: chief of department. In: United States Fire Administration. *The World Trade Center Bombing Report and Analysis*. Emmitsburg, Md: Federal Emergency Management Agency; 1993:1-23.
8. Goldfarb Z, Kuhr S. EMS response to the explosion. In: United States Fire Administration. *The World Trade Center Bombing Report and Analysis*. Emmitsburg, Md: Federal Emergency Management Agency; 1993:92-110.
9. Martin RA. The Joint Terrorism Task Force: a concept that works—FBI–New York City Police Department. *FBI Law Enforcement Bulletin*. 1999;68(3):9-10.
10. Cumming A, Masse T. Intelligence Reform Implementation at the Federal Bureau of Investigation: Issues and Options for Congress. 2005, CRS Report for Congress. Available at: www.fas.org/sgp/crs/intel/RL33033.pdf.
11. The Subcommittee on Economic Development. Public Building and Emergency Management Hearing on Combating Terrorism: Options to Improve the Federal Response. Available at: http://www.house.gov/transportation/pbed/04-24-01/04-24-01memo.html.
12. Anonymous. *White Paper on Presidential Decision Directive 62: Protection Against Unconventional Threats to the Homeland and Americans Overseas*. Washington, DC: 1998. Available at: http://www.fas.org/irp/offdocs/pdd-62.htm.
13. Anonymous. Chapter IV: Concept of Operations. In United States Government Interagency Domestic Terrorism. *Concept of Operations Plan (CONPLAN)*. Washington, DC: 2001: 19-26. Available at: www.fbi.gov/publications/conplan/conplan.pdf.
14. Kean T, Hamilton L, Ben-Veniste R, et al. Chapter 9.2: September 11, 2001. In: *The 9/11 Commission Report*. Washington, DC: Government Printing Office; 2004:285-313.
15. Kean T, Hamilton L, Ben-Veniste R, et al. Chapter 9.3: Emergency response at the Pentagon. In: *The 9/11 Commission Report*. Washington, DC: Government Printing Office; 2004:311-4.
16. Department of Homeland Security. National Response Plan. Washington, DC: Department of Homeland Security; 2004. Available at: http://www.dhs.gov/dhspublic/display?content=3611.
17. Brake JD. *Terrorism and the Military's Role in Domestic Crisis Management: Background and Issues for Congress*. Washington, DC: Congressional Research Service; 2003.
18. Anonymous. Immediate response. In: *Department of Defense Emergency Preparedness Course Handbook*. Fort MacPherson, Ga: Department of Defense; 2004.
19. Rohen G. WMD Response: Integrating the Joint Operating Center and the Incident Command System. *Police Chief Magazine*. 2001. Available at: www.iacptechnology.org/Library/ WMDResponseIntegratingJointOpsandIncidentCommand.pdf.
20. Anonymous. Emergency preparedness and response. In: The National Strategy for Homeland Security. Washington, DC: Department of Homeland Security; 2003:41-5.
21. Anonymous. National Response Plan. In: *Department of Defense Emergency Preparedness Course Handbook*. Fort MacPherson, Ga; Department of Defense; 2004.
22. Fletcher WD, Field VW, Wade C. FBI Laboratory. Available at: http://www.fbi.gov/hq/lab/labhome.htm.
23. Anonymous. *Weapons of Mass Destruction Crime Scene Management for Emergency Responders: Compendium of Federal Terrorism Training Courses*. Washington, DC: Department of Homeland Security; 2004.
24. Atwood DJ. *Military Support to Civil Authorities (MSCA): Department of Defense Directive 3025.1*. Washington, DC: Department of Defense; 1993.

25. Taft WH. *DOD Response to Improvised Nuclear Device (IND) Incidents: Department of Defense Directive 3150.5.* Washington, DC: Department of Defense; 1987.
26. Anonymous. *Army Emergency Preparedness Liaison Officer (EPLO) Program. FORSCOM Regulation 140-12.* Fort Mac-Pherson, GA; Department of Defense; 2001.
27. Smithson A. *Prepared Statement Before the House Committee on Government Reform, Subcommittee on National Security, Veterans Affairs, and International Relations and the House Committee on Transportation and Infrastructure, Subcommittee on Economic Development, Public Buildings, and Emergency Management.* Washington, DC: 2001. Available at: www. house.gov/transportation/ pbed/04-24-01/smithson.html.

chapter 61

Nuclear Disaster Management*

George A. Alexander

The events of Sept. 11, 2001 and the worldwide proliferation of nuclear materials, including theft and smuggling, increase the possibility that a nuclear disaster event may occur from the terrorist use of radiation as a weapon. There are two documented incidents of the threatened use of radiation as a terrorist weapon thus far,[1] both of which occurred in Russia. In 1995, Chechen insurgents buried a cesium-137 "dirty bomb" in a Moscow park and alerted the media before it was detonated. In 1998, a container of radioactive materials was found attached to an explosive mine near a railroad line in Chechnya.

Nuclear disasters can have different scenarios. An extreme situation would be the threat of a terrorist attack using a low-yield 10-kiloton nuclear weapon. The threat of a nuclear terrorist attack with a nuclear device or radioactive materials is not a question of if, but when. Many people have become aware of the threat of such an attack because of increased media attention. Successful planning for a nuclear attack or accident now becomes imperative.

This chapter presents important concepts of nuclear disaster management. The aim is to offer a basic understanding of the threat and effect of nuclear disasters, including accidents and terrorist events. This chapter provides a brief historical overview of the development of the nuclear era, the nuclear arms race, and present concerns. It highlights some basic physical and biologic principles of radiation injury that are commonly misunderstood by healthcare professionals. The chapter reviews various nuclear disaster scenarios, summarizes medical management principles, and underscores obstacles to nuclear disaster management.

HISTORICAL PERSPECTIVE

Following the discovery of radioactivity in 1896, the understanding of atomic physics increased rapidly in the early twentieth century.[2] Ernest Rutherford is recognized as the father of nuclear physics. In 1908 he received the

Nobel Prize for chemistry for his "investigations into the disintegration of the elements, and the chemistry of radioactive substances."[3] He was directly responsible for training many physicists at Cambridge University in England. In the latter capacity, he was also indirectly responsible for much of the nuclear physics research that was being conducted at many universities by his former students throughout the world and for the development of the nuclear era.

In 1938 Hahn and Strassman in Berlin described the phenomenon of nuclear fission.[2] They determined that when uranium was bombarded with neutrons, the nucleus split into two parts of comparable mass with the release of an enormous quantity of energy. This observation would lead to the Manhattan Project and eventually to the production of the atomic bomb (A-bomb).[3] In 1942 Fermi achieved the first controlled self-sustaining nuclear reaction.[3] In August 1945 the first atomic bombs (or fission bombs) were detonated over Hiroshima and Nagasaki, Japan.

The development of the atomic bomb would lead ultimately to the development of the even more devastating hydrogen bomb (H-bomb). In the 1950s, justification of work on the hydrogen bomb (fusion or thermonuclear bomb) was based on the fact that it produced less radioactive fallout and therefore was considered a "cleaner" nuclear weapon.[4] Enhanced radiation weapons (neutron bombs) were later developed to minimize the effects of blast and heat on buildings and to maximize the effects of the neutrons on living organisms (e.g., to kill tank crews without causing much collateral damage).[4]

During the Cold War era, the nuclear arms race between the United States and the former Soviet Union continued for more than 30 years. By the early 1980s the number of nuclear warheads worldwide was estimated to be in excess of 40,000.[5] The explosive power of these warheads ranged from about 100 tons up to more than 200 million tons equivalent of high explosives. During this same time period the total strength of nuclear arsenals was believed to have been equivalent to about 1 million Hiroshima bombs or 13,000 million tons of TNT (trinitrotoluene).

With the end of the Cold War in the late 1980s, the threat of Armageddon—a nuclear war between the United States and the former Soviet Union in which 200

*The views expressed in this chapter are those of the author and do not necessarily represent the official policy or position of the National Cancer Institute, the National Institutes of Health, or the Department of Health and Human Services.

million Americans might not survive the war—was eliminated.[6] However, this apparent relief from the Armageddon syndrome has been short-lived because the twenty-first century now appears to be more dangerous and less predictable. The risk that someone might detonate a nuclear weapon in anger or retribution is probably greater than at any other time since the 1962 Cuban missile crisis.[7] Moreover, nuclear weapons ambitions are spreading not only to states, but also to terrorist groups. Osama bin Laden has talked of acquiring nuclear weapons as a "religious duty."[7]

Today, the most likely threat from nuclear weapons is based on a scenario of a terrorist group or rogue nation using a single, low-yield device, such as a suitcase-size tactical nuclear weapon.[8] The second most likely threat is from an improvised nuclear device (IND) used by terrorists and composed of either weapons-grade (enriched) uranium or plutonium-239. The third most likely terrorist nuclear threat is from a radiologic dispersal device (RDD), also known as a "dirty bomb." (See Chapter 177 for a more complete discussion of the RDD.) Although the detonation of an RDD does not produce a nuclear yield, RDDs are important because of their potential to cause a nuclear disaster using high explosives to disperse very high levels of radioactivity associated with materials from nuclear reactors, spent fuel storage depots, nuclear fuel reprocessing facilities, high-level nuclear waste sites, or transport vehicles.[8]

The development of man-made radioactive isotopes and nuclear weapons during and after World War II was an important factor in the birth of the nuclear weapons industry in the mid-twentieth century. Most of what we know today about nuclear disasters comes from the atomic bomb experience of World War II and from radiation accidents that have occurred over the past 60 years. Information on the effects of nuclear weapons has been obtained from Hiroshima and Nagasaki and from animal experimentation conducted during atmospheric tests of the 1950s.[9] Data on the consequences of radiation accidents have been obtained from the methodical medical and scientific assessments of radiation accident victims. The existence of national and international registries on accidental radiation injuries has helped to characterize the types and patterns of radiation damage and to provide useful information for optimal medical management of victims.[10] The knowledge gained from these experiences serves as the foundation of nuclear disaster management for the twenty-first century.

CURRENT PRACTICE

Nuclear weapons produce their biologic effects through the direct or indirect effects of blast, heat, and radiation.[11-13] The first two effects are fairly simple and the mechanisms of their injury are readily understood. Radiation, on the other hand, is a more complex noxious agent and is generally misunderstood by health professionals. Understanding how radiation interacts with matter provides insights into methods used to detect and measure radiation, reduce the biological hazards, and manage nuclear disasters and their consequences.

Basic Principles

Radiation Physics

After a nuclear weapon detonation, a tremendous amount of energy is quickly released in the form of ionizing radiation. Ionizing radiations are defined as those "types of particulate and electromagnetic radiations that interact with matter and either directly or indirectly form ion pairs."[14] Ionizing radiations can be divided into two categories: directly ionizing and indirectly ionizing. Directly ionizing radiations are charged particles (electrons, protons, beta particles, alpha particles, etc.) that have sufficient kinetic energy to produce ionizations through direct collisions with bound orbital electrons of an atom or molecule. Indirectly ionizing radiations are uncharged particles or photons (neutrons, x-rays, gamma rays, etc.) that can liberate bound orbital electrons, but only indirectly.

Both x-rays and gamma rays are photons, or small quantized packets of pure electromagnetic energy just like light. However, they have a much higher non-visible frequency. X-rays and gamma rays differ only in their origin. X-rays are produced in the outer orbital shells of atom, whereas gamma rays come from within the nucleus of the atoms. X-rays and gamma rays are low linear energy transfer radiations; that is, they deposit relatively low amounts of energy along the track of radiation as they penetrate tissue and deposit energy deep in the body. Many radioactive isotopes decay by emitting several different types of particles. The most common forms of particle radiation are alpha, beta, and neutron.

Alpha particles are massive, charged helium nuclei. Because they deposit all of their energy over a very short distance, alpha particles are classified as high linear energy transfer radiation. Because of their size, alpha particles can easily be stopped using a sheet of paper or light clothing. Beta particles are very lightly charged high-speed electron particles that can penetrate to a depth of a few centimeters. Neutron radiation is an uncharged particle that is emitted during a nuclear detonation almost exclusively from the fission and fusion processes themselves. Important factors that will prevent or minimize the effects of radiation exposure on humans include the principles of time, distance, and shielding. (See Chapter 70 for a discussion of radiation safety.)

Radiation Biology

Radiation biology is the field of study that describes the many changes that radiation produces in biological material. Charged particles (e.g., electrons, protons, beta particles, alpha particles, fission fragments) are directly ionizing because they can disrupt (ionize) chemical bonds and produce chemical and biologic changes.[15] Electromagnetic radiations (e.g., x-rays, gamma rays) are indirectly ionizing because they do not themselves cause any chemical or biologic changes. Instead, they deposit kinetic energy into the material through which they pass and produce secondary charged particles (electrons) that can produce subsequent chemical and biologic alterations. Radiation can damage a cell by indirectly interacting with water molecules in the body. This leads to the creation of unstable, toxic hyperoxide molecules (free radicals) that then damage sensitive molecules and subcellular structures. Ionizing radiations transfer energy to biologic material by two mechanisms: ionization and excitation.[15]

Alpha radiation is fully absorbed within the first millimeter of exposed skin. It is generally not an external radiation hazard. Alpha radiation poses serious health hazards if it is inhaled, ingested, or deposited in an open wound. If an alpha-emitting radioactive material is internally deposited, all of the radiation energy will be absorbed in a very small volume of tissue immediately surrounding each particle of material. The internal deposition of alpha particles can cause radiation injury over a long period. If a beta-emitting radioactive material is on the surface of the skin, the ensuing beta radiation causes damage to the basal stratum of the skin and produces deep "beta" burns—lesions similar to superficial thermal burns. If the beta material is incorporated internally into the body, the beta radiation can cause considerable injury. Gamma radiation is highly energetic and penetrating and therefore is both an internal and external radiation hazard. Gamma rays can cause whole-body injury. Neutron radiation is extremely penetrating and can also result in whole-body irradiation. Compared with gamma rays, neutrons can cause 20 times more damage to tissues.[16]

The sensitivity of cells, tissues, and organs to a dose of ionizing radiation depends primarily on two factors: the rapidity of cell division and the radiosensitivity of the cells.[15] Cells are most sensitive to radiation during mitosis, when DNA is being divided. Rapidly dividing cells are more radiosensitive. Tissues and organs that depend on an active stem cell pool will be more radiosensitive than those tissues and organ systems made up of mature cellular pools with little or no stem cell activity.

Radiation Dose and Units

Quantities of radiation can be expressed in several different ways. The term *radiation exposure* applies to air only and is a measure of the amount of ionization produced by x-ray and gamma radiation in air. It is a measure of how much ionization is produced in air and is measured in coulombs per kilogram (C/kg) of dry air. The roentgen (R) is an older unit of radiation exposure and applies only to x-rays and gamma rays up to energies of about 3 MeV. ($1R = 2.58 \times 10^{-4}$ C/kg.)

The *radiation absorbed dose* is the amount of energy deposited in a given mass of absorbing material. The conventional unit for absorbed dose, the *rad* (radiation absorbed dose), is equal to the absorption of 100 ergs of energy in 1 gm of absorbing medium, typically tissue. (1 rad = 100 ergs/g of medium.) The SI unit of absorbed dose, the gray (Gy), is defined as the absorption of 1 Joule of energy per kilogram of medium. (1 Gy = 1 J/kg = 100 rad and 1 rad = 1 cGy.)

The term *dose equivalent* is necessary because different radiations produce different amounts of biologic damage. It is defined as the product of the absorbed dose and a factor, Q (the quality factor), that characterizes the damage associated with each type of radiation.

In the conventional system, the unit of dose equivalent is the *rem*, which is calculated from the absorbed dose as rem = rad × Q. The SI unit of dose equivalent is the sievert (Sv), or sieverts = Gy × Q.

Radioactivity is the activity level of a radioactive isotope expressed as the number of atoms that will disintegrate (decay) per second. One becquerel (Bq) is equal to one nuclear transformation per second. The unit in the traditional system is curie, where 1 curie (Ci) = 3.7×10^{10} Bq. The term *dose rate* is the dose of radiation per unit of time.

Nuclear Disaster Scenarios

In light of the terrorist attacks of Sept. 11, 2001, it is important to understand possible nuclear disaster scenarios. Sept. 11 was a "day of unprecedented shock and suffering in the history of the United States. The nation was unprepared."[17] The greatest threat we face in the world today is from nuclear terrorism.[18] The vast stockpiles of nuclear weapons and highly enriched uranium and plutonium in Russia are vulnerable to theft and illicit trafficking. Russia remains the most probable source for a terrorist to obtain a nuclear weapon or materials to construct a weapon, followed by Pakistan and North Korea. North Korea is believed to be the world's most promiscuous nuclear proliferator.[18] The leaking of weapons technologies allows smaller terrorist groups to wreak havoc and cause greater destruction. Globalization has made if easier for terrorists to travel, communicate, and transport weapons. There is a burgeoning and well-organized black market for nuclear technologies and arms. Sept. 11 was a wake-up call to America. Americans do fear more terrorist attacks and more Middle East instability.[19] In fact, a recent poll taken in 2003 found that four of every ten Americans say that they "often worry about the chances of a nuclear attack by terrorists."[20] The threats of terrorist attack will be far more serious if North Korea and Iran develop nuclear programs.

DETONATION OF NUCLEAR WEAPONS

Strategic Nuclear Weapons

Strategic nuclear weapons are devices constructed by a government or country. This category of arms made up the main strategic arsenal during the height of the Cold War. These weapons generally had a yield (or size) from 170 kilotons to 24 megatons.[5] Interestingly, the Soviets are reported to have had some warheads with yields as high as 100 megatons. Strategic nuclear weapons could be carried to the intended target by various delivery vehicles including land-based intercontinental ballistic missiles, submarine-launched ballistic missiles, or long-range bombers. The detonation of a strategic nuclear weapon in the United States today is unlikely. However, the risk of such an event would most likely be associated with the accidental launch of a former Soviet Union nuclear weapon resulting from equipment malfunction, warning system failure, or dissidents getting hold of strategic weapons and launching them.

Tactical Nuclear Weapons

Tactical nuclear weapons are also fabricated by a government or country and have yields from less than 0.1 to more than 100 kilotons.[5] These nuclear systems have been designed or could be used by a military organization for employment against, for example, military targets in a theater of war. Such weapons are artillery shells, ground mobile rockets and missiles, and air-launched bombs. Tactical nuclear weapons may be the size of a suitcase or backpack.

Imagine a terrorist scenario in which a 10-kiloton nuclear weapon is stolen from a Russian arsenal and detonated in New York City, San Francisco, Houston, Washington, Chicago, or Los Angeles.[20] If a terrorist group, such as Al Qaeda, was to rent a van and carry this nuclear weapon into the middle of Times Square in New York and detonate it next to the Morgan Stanley headquarters on Broadway, Times Square would vanish within a second.[20] The resulting fireball and blast wave would destroy instantly the theater district, the New York Times building, Grand Central Station, and every other building within a third of a mile from "ground zero." The resulting firestorm would engulf Rockefeller Center, Carnegie Hall, the Empire State Building, and Madison Square Garden. On a typical workday, more than 500,000 people may crowd into an area within one-half mile radius of Times Square. A noon-time detonation could potentially kill all of these people including hundreds of thousands of others who would die from collapsing buildings, fire, and fallout. The electromagnetic pulse from the blast would destroy phones, radios, and other electronic communications. Emergency medical services and hospitals would be overwhelmed by the injured.

Improvised Nuclear Device

An IND is fabricated by a non-governmental organization or terrorist group. It is made up of either highly enriched uranium or plutonium-239. Tens of thousands of potential weapons (softball-size lumps of highly enriched uranium and plutonium) remain today in unsecured storage facilities in Russia, vulnerable to theft by criminals who could sell them to terrorists. Since the collapse of the former Soviet Union, there have been hundreds of confirmed cases of successful theft of nuclear materials. If successful, detonation of an IND could produce a nuclear yield similar to that of Hiroshima with the release of radiation, blast, and thermal pulses with considerable radioactive fallout. Fabrication of such a device would be difficult because of the sophisticated expertise and engineering required. A terrorist organization might be able to produce a partial yield, producing less effect.

Effects of Nuclear Weapons

In this section, the basic characteristics of the effects of nuclear weapons are summarized with an emphasis on the information of greatest use to nuclear disaster managers. There are numerous other references[8,16,21,22] that treat this subject in much greater detail.

The main physical effects of nuclear weapons are blast, thermal radiation (heat), and nuclear radiation. These effects depend on the yield of the weapon, physical design of the weapon, and method of employment.[22] The altitude at which a weapon is detonated will determine the relative effects of blast, heat, and nuclear radiation. Nuclear detonations are usually classified as airbursts, surface bursts, or high-altitude bursts.

The blast and thermal effects of a detonation produce the greatest number of immediate human casualties.[21] Immediately after detonation the temperature at the center of the fireball reaches 1,000,000° C, producing a shock wave traveling at supersonic speeds, followed by hurricane-force afterwinds and an intense flash of thermal radiation. A 5-psi (pounds per square inch) blast wave and 160-mph blast winds associated with the blast wave would destroy a two-story brick house, rupture the human eardrum, or hurl a person against stationary structures.[21] A pressure level of 15 psi could produce serious intrathoracic injuries, interstitial hemorrhage, edema, and air emboli as well as serious abdominal injuries, such as hepatic and splenic rupture.

The thermal radiation is associated with burns, including *flash burns* and *flame burns*, and certain eye injuries, including *flash blindness* and *retinal burns*. Flash burns result from the skin's exposure to a large quantity of thermal energy in a very short time, leaving the affected skin with a charred appearance. Flame burns result from the contact with a conventional fire, such as that on clothing. Flash blindness is a temporary condition; however, a retinal burn that results from looking directly at the fireball causes a permanent blind spot.

Detonation of a nuclear weapon produces a variety of nuclear radiations.[21] Initial radiation consists of neutrons and gamma rays produced within the first minute after detonation. The main hazard from initial radiation is acute external whole-body irradiation by neutrons and gamma rays. Residual radiation is generated beyond the first minute after detonation and includes gamma rays, beta particles, and alpha particles. These radiations are produced as highly radioactive fission fragments and activated weapons material. The main hazard from residual radiation is radioactive fallout, which can remain a significant biologic hazard long after detonation.

ATTACKS ON NUCLEAR REACTORS

The potential of terrorist attack on a nuclear power plant has been mentioned by the media. However, the probability of an attack is low. The low probability is due to the high security surrounding a nuclear reactor and the safety systems incorporated into it. There is extensive shielding around the reactor core and large amounts of explosives would be needed to breach the reactor core. If an accident occurs, reactors are designed to slow down and stop the reaction. A reactor coolant system does contain some radioactivity, which could be released if the coolant system were damaged. Radioactive iodine and noble gases would probably be released. There would be immediate health effects nearby from the release. The release of large amounts of radioactive iodine could have long-term effects such as thyroid cancer in children. It is possible that a jumbo jet could crash into a reactor or adjacent spent fuel storage facilities, but it would be difficult in the latter situation to expose a large population to radiation from "spent" fuel rods. Recent computer modeling and engineering studies suggest that the construction of most reactors could withstand a direct hit from a commercial aircraft flying into a reactor at less than 300 mph. However, some scientists question these findings and believe that penetration of the containment dome could cause the reactor to melt down. The 1986 Chernobyl nuclear power plant accident in the former Soviet Union serves as a harsh reminder of scenarios in which terrorists might possibly cause a nuclear disaster by breaching a nuclear reactor and releasing radioactive materials into the environment.

DETONATION OF A RADIOLOGIC DISPERSAL DEVICE

An RDD is a device that combines radioactive materials with conventional explosives. (See Chapter 178 for a more complete discussion of the RDD.) It may be made from traditional dynamite, TNT (trinitrotoluene), ammonium nitrate, or a variety of other explosive materials.[23] When detonated, an RDD kills or injures through the initial blast, which causes damage from the expansion of hot gases and by dispersing radioactive materials that are highly toxic over a wide geographic area without a nuclear explosion. Some common radioactive sources that have a high probability of being used in an RDD include cobalt-60, strontium-90, cesium-137, iridium-192, radium-226, plutonium-238, americium-241, and californium-252. The dispersal effects of an RDD depend on the amount of explosives, the physical form of the radioactive source, and the atmospheric conditions.[24] RDDs are attractive to terrorists because they are relatively easy to acquire and have the potential of causing casualties, contamination of widespread areas, adverse psychological effects on people, and economic disruption.

SIMPLE DISPERSAL DEVICE

A simple dispersal device (SDD) is a device containing a high-energy source that irradiates people or spreads radioactive material in a populated area, such as an airport, train station, sports arena, or theater. Use of such a device to cause radiation exposure in unsuspecting people is considered a terrorist act. Common radioactive sources that could be used in an SDD are the same as the sources mentioned previously for RDDs. The threat of radiation exposure from an SDD would have the same psychological effect on people as an RDD—instilling fear.

RADIATION ACCIDENTS

Information on radiation injuries has been gathered over a period of 70 to 100 years.[25] Important information obtained from previous worldwide radiation accidents is useful in preparing and planning for nuclear terrorism and/or disasters. Radiation accidents can occur in situations where there are problems with nuclear reactors as well as industrial and medical sources of radiation. From 1946 to 2000, there have been more than 120 documented fatalities resulting from radiation accidents worldwide.[26] Serious radiation accidents in the United States have been rare.[27] From 1944 to June 2000, only 30 lost their lives in 13 separate radiation accidents in the United States. There were 233 other less serious accidents during the same period. In the former Soviet Union 59 deaths occurred from radiation accidents between 1950 and 2000.[28]

There are two categories of radiation accidents.[29] The first category is an *external exposure* accident, that is, external irradiation from a source distant to or in close proximity to the body. Once a person has been removed from the source of radiation or the radiation-producing machine has been turned off, the irradiation stops. This exposed person does not become radioactive and there are no hazards to other people. The second category is a *contamination* accident. A person contaminated with radioactive material will continue to be irradiated until the radioactive material is removed, eliminated, or decays away. Contamination may occur in the form of radioactive gases, liquids, or particles. The contamination can be spread to other parts of the victim's body as well as to others. There is a third category of accident—a combination of the two.

The effects seen in persons who have been exposed in radiation accidents can be categorized as either deterministic or stochastic radiation effects.[30] Direct deterministic effects include the different types of acute and chronic radiation syndromes. The clinical manifestations of radiation injury include the latter as well as characteristic erythema, blistering, and even necrosis caused by local radiation damage. These deterministic effects occur when a specific dose-level threshold has been exceeded. The direct deterministic effects on an individual will depend on the dose of radiation received, the quality or type of radiation, the volume of tissue irradiated, and the time over which the dose is received. The stochastic effects are long-term and include, for example, the induction of cancer and potential genetic abnormalities. More in-depth information on the medical management of radiation accident patients can be found in *Medical Management of Radiation Accidents*.[31]

Principles of Medical Management

The optimal medical treatment for injury following detonation of a nuclear weapon can be found in several valuable sources.[9,16,21,22,32-34] The interested reader is referred to these sources. Other articles[24,33,35-37] have addressed medical treatment of individuals injured by a terrorist act involving radioactive materials.

Conventional injuries should be treated first, since radiation contamination is not a life-threatening medical emergency. Patients with traumatic blast and radiation injury should be resuscitated and stabilized. Airway, breathing, and circulation always take priority. These patients require more specialized treatment. Decontamination of patients should be carried out according to accepted standards of radiation decontamination. (See Chapter 70 for further discussion.) Specialists in hematology, oncology, radiation, and infectious disease should be consulted. Effective treatment of internally contaminated patients requires knowledge of both the radioactive isotope and its physical form. Treatment should be instituted quickly to ensure effectiveness. However, with a terrorist incidence, initially the radioactive source or sources are not known.[33] Several general approaches may be used to treat internal radiation contamination, including reduction of absorption (Prussian blue), dilution (force fluids), blockage (potassium iodide), displacement by non-radioactive materials (oral phosphate), mobilization as a means of elimination from tissue (ammonium chloride), and chelation (Ca-DTPA and Zn-DTPA).[38]

Patients who have received a low whole-body radiation dose may develop gastrointestinal (GI) distress within the first 2 days. Antiemetics may be effective in reducing the GI symptoms. The latter will usually subside within the first day. If not, parenteral fluids should be considered.

The prognosis for patients who have suffered traumatic blast, burn, and radiation injury is worse than for patients with radiation injury alone.[39] A wound that is contaminated with radioactive materials should be rinsed with saline and treated using conventional aseptic techniques.[24] Alpha-emitting radioactive isotopes, for example, that contaminate wounds are usually excised. In patients who receive whole-body doses of radiation greater than 100 cGy, the wound should be closed as soon as possible to prevent it from becoming an entry for lethal infection.

In spite of the wide availability of antibiotics, infections from opportunistic pathogens are a major problem among patients exposed to intermediate and high doses of radiation. In these cases the primary determinants of survival are treatment of microbial infections and aggressive resuscitation of the bone marrow.[39]

PITFALLS

Obstacles to the provision of optimal nuclear disaster management include:

- Lack of adequate preparation of nuclear disaster management planning for possible nuclear terrorism and accidents before they occur
- Lack of coordination with local and state emergency response agencies
- Lack of understanding of the physical and biologic principles or radiation interaction by medical and public health professionals and nuclear disaster managers
- Lack of involvement of behavior and social health professionals to address the psychological consequences of nuclear terrorism and disasters
- Failure to adequately secure sources of highly enriched uranium and plutonium
- Failure to adequately secure nuclear weapons
- Failure to secure industrial and medical radiation sources and radioactive materials that would prevent any loss of control and consequent misuse

REFERENCES

1. Edwards R. Only a matter of time? *New Scientist* 2004;182(2450):8-9.
2. Wilson W. *A Hundred Years of Physics*. London: Gerald Duckworth & Co; 1950.
3. Weber RL. *Pioneers of Science: Nobel Prize Winners in Physics*. London: The Institute of Physics; 1980.
4. Rotblat J. Digest of nuclear weaponry. In: Cassel C, McCally M, Abraham H, eds. *Nuclear Weapons and Nuclear War: A Source Book for Health Professionals*. New York: Praeger; 1984, pp 76-88.
5. Report of the Secretary General. Factual information on present nuclear arsenals. In: Cassel C, McCally M, Abraham H, eds. *Nuclear Weapons and Nuclear War: A Source Book for Health Professionals*. New York: Praeger; 1984, pp 61-75.
6. Gray CS, Payne K. Victory is possible. In: Cassel C, McCally M, Abraham H, eds. *Nuclear Weapons and Nuclear War: A Source Book for Health Professionals*. New York: Praeger; 1984, pp 48-57.
7. A world wide web of nuclear danger. *The Economist*. Feb 28 – March 5, 2004, pp 25-27.
8. National Council on Radiation Protection and Measurement. Management of terrorist events involving radioactive material. Report No. 138. Bethesda, MD: National Council on Radiation Protection and Measurement; 2001.
9. Holdstock D, Waterston L. Nuclear weapons, a continuing threat to health. *Lancet* 2000;355:1544-7.
10. Guskova AK. Medical characteristics of different types of radiation accidents. In: Gusev I, Guskova AK, Mettler FA Jr, eds. *Medical Management of Radiation Accidents*, ed 2. Boca Raton, FL: CRC Press; 2001, pp 15-22.
11. Glasstone S, Dolan P. Biological effects. In: Cassel C, McCally M, Abraham H, eds. *Nuclear Weapons and Nuclear War: a Source Book for Health Professionals*. New York: Praeger, 1984; pp 91-118.
12. Wald N. Radiation injury. In: Cassel C, McCally M, Abraham H, eds. *Nuclear Weapons and Nuclear War: a Source Book for Health Professionals*. New York: Praeger, 1984; pp 121-138.
13. Beebe GW. Ionizing radiation and health. In: Cassel C, McCally M, Abraham H, eds. *Nuclear Weapons and Nuclear War: a Source Book for Health Professionals*. New York: Praeger, 1984; pp 139-158.
14. Sholtis JA Jr. Ionizing radiations and their interactions with matter. In: Conklin JJ, Walker RI, eds. *Military radiobiology*. San Diego, CA: Academic Press, Inc, 1987, pp 55-86.
15. Holahan EV Jr. Cellular radiation biology. In: Conklin JJ, Walker RI, eds. *Military Radiobiology*. San Diego, CA: Academic Press; 1987, pp 87-110.
16. Jarrett D, ed. *Medical Management of Radiological Casualties: Handbook*, ed 1. AFRRI special publication 99-2. Bethesda, MD: Armed Forces Radiobiology Research Institute; 1999.
17. National Commission on Terrorist Attacks Upon the United States. *The 9/11 Commission Report: Final Report of the National Commission on Terrorist Attacks Upon the United States*. New York: W.W. Norton & Company; 2004.
18. Allison G. Nuclear terrorism poses the gravest threat today. *The Wall Street Journal Europe*. July 14, 2003, p A10.
19. Seib GF. As Bush and Kerry focus elsewhere, atomic threats stew. *The Wall Street Journal*. Aug 11, 2004, p 4.
20. Allison G. *Nuclear Terrorism: The Ultimate Preventable Catastrophe*, ed 1. New York: Times Books; 2004.
21. Zajtchuk R, Jenkins DP, Bellamy RF, et al, eds. *Medical Consequences of Nuclear Warfare*, vol 2. Falls Church, VA: TMM Publications, Office of the Surgeon General; 1989.
22. United States Army Center for Health Promotion and Preventive Medicine. *The Medical NBC Battlebook*. USACHPPM Tech Guide 244, 2000.
23. King G. *Dirty Bomb: Weapon of Mass Disruption*. New York: Penguin Group; 2004.
24. Mettler FA Jr, Voelz GL. Major radiation exposure—what to expect and how to respond. *N Engl J Med*. 2002;346:1554-61.
25. Guskova AK. Radiation sickness classification. In: Gusev I, Guskova AK, Mettler FA Jr, eds. *Medical Management of Radiation Accidents*, ed 2. Boca Raton, FL: CRC Press, 2001; pp 23-31.
26. Mettler FA Jr, Guskova AK. Treatment of acute radiation sickness. In: Gusev I, Guskova AK, Mettler FA Jr, eds. *Medical Management of Radiation Accidents*, ed 2. Boca Raton, FL: CRC Press, 2001; pp 53-67.

27. Ricks RC, Berger ME, Holloway EC, Goans RE. Radiation accidents in the United States. In: Gusev I, Guskova AK, Mettler FA Jr, eds. *Medical Management of Radiation Accidents,* ed 2. Boca Raton, FL: CRC Press, 2001; pp 167-172.

28. Soloviev V, Ilyin LA, Baranov AE, et al. Radiation accidents in the Former U.S.S.R. In: Gusev I, Guskova AK, Mettler FA Jr, eds. *Medical Management of Radiation Accidents,* ed 2. Boca Raton, FL: CRC Press, 2001; pp 157-165.

29. Mettler FA Jr, Kelsey CA. Fundamentals of radiation accidents. In: Gusev I, Guskova AK, Mettler FA Jr, eds. *Medical Management of Radiation Accidents,* ed 2. Boca Raton, FL: CRC Press, 2001; pp 1-13.

30. Guskova AK. Medical characteristics of different types of radiation accidents. In: Gusev I, Guskova AK, Mettler FA Jr, eds. *Medical Management of Radiation Accidents,* ed 2. Boca Raton, FL: CRC Press, 2001; pp 15-22.

31. Gusev I, Guskova AK, Mettler FA Jr, eds. *Medical Management of Radiation Accidents,* ed 2. Boca Raton, FL: CRC Press, 2001.

32. Conklin JJ, Walker RI, eds. *Military Radiobiology.* San Diego, CA: Academic Press; 1987.

33. Leikin JB, McFee RB, Walter FG, et al. A primer for nuclear terrorism. *Dis Mon.* 2003;49:479-516.

34. Fong FH Jr. Nuclear detonations: evaluation and response. In: Hogan DE, Burstein JL, eds. *Disaster Medicine.* Philadelphia: Lippincott Williams & Wilkins; 2002, pp 317-39.

35. Waselenko JK, MacVittie TJ, Blakely WF, et al. Medical management of the acute radiation syndrome: recommendations of the Strategic National Stockpile Radiation Working Group. *Ann Intern Med.* 2004;140:1037-51.

36. Moulder JE. Post-irradiation approaches to treatment of radiation injuries in the context of radiological terrorism and radiation accidents: a review. *Int J Radiat Biol.* 2004;80:1-8.

37. Turai I, Veress K, Gunalp B, et al. Medical response to radiation incidents and radionuclear threats. *BMJ* 2004;328:568-72.

38. Voelz GL. Assessment and treatment of internal contamination: General principles. In: Gusev I, Guskova AK, Mettler FA Jr, eds. *Medical Management of Radiation Accidents,* ed 2. Boca Raton, FL: CRC Press, 2001; pp 319-36.

39. Conklin JJ, Walker RI. Diagnosis, triage, and treatment of casualties. In: Conklin JJ, Walker RI, eds. *Military Radiobiology.* San Diego: Academic Press; 1987, pp 231-40.

chapter 62

Chemical Attack

Duane C. Caneva

The rise of the asymmetric threat of terrorist activities combined with the dual-use nature of technology, its rapid advancement, and proliferation of information has made the concern of chemical attack no longer limited to the battlefield. In addition to conventional chemical warfare agents, the threat now includes use of toxic industrial chemicals and materials that, as part of an industrial-based economy, are ubiquitous in much of developed society. Preventing, preparing for, and responding to such an attack requires consideration of a myriad of issues and integration across diverse disciplines to ensure optimal use of limited resources and the development of best practices. Coordination of these efforts into a cogent emergency management program requires levels of integration across communities, jurisdictions, regions, states, agencies, and industries that will also improve our response capability to challenges of all sorts and drive us toward better business practices. This chapter focuses on the basics of preparing for and responding to a chemical attack.

HISTORICAL PERSPECTIVE

Brief History

The history of chemical warfare is rich and fascinating, an excellent summary of which is documented in the *Textbook of Military Medicine*.[1] The "modern era" began during the events leading up to and surrounding World War I. In the United States the Chemical Warfare Service was established on June 28, 1918 as part of the National Army with responsibilities for all chemical weapons research, defense, training, medical treatment, and production facilities. The offensive weapons program was officially terminated by signature to the Chemical Weapons Convention (CWC) on Jan. 13, 1993, with Senate approval on April 24, 1997, and the infrastructure converted to a strictly passive defense program.

Through this infrastructure, the U.S. military has provided valuable input toward preparations for a chemical attack. This, combined with Hazardous Materials (HazMat) Response work statutes from the Occupational Safety and Health Administration (OSHA)[2] and National

Fire Protection Administration (NFPA) Guidelines[3] governing fire and emergency services response have served as the cornerstone for our current doctrine and policy for emergency response requirements in preparing, training for, and responding to chemical attacks in non-combat situations.

The Chemical Weapons Convention

The United Nations Chemical Weapons Convention, formally titled the "Convention on the Prohibition of the Development, Production, Stockpiling and Use of Chemical Weapons and on Their Destruction" opened up for signature on Jan. 13, 1993 after 20 years of negotiation and entered into force on April 29, 1997. Signed by 182 UN member nations to date, it describes the prohibition of use of specific chemical warfare agents, production limits for study, measures to ensure compliance, and destruction of stores of chemical stockpiles. The CWC established the Organization for the Prevention of Chemical Weapons (OPCW), located in The Hague, to serve as its operational arm, conducting verification activities, ensuring implementation of convention provisions, and providing a forum for consultation and cooperation.[4]

Chemical Agents

A chemical attack traditionally involves highly toxic chemical warfare agents that are specifically designed to cause morbidity and mortality, produced in significant amounts with appropriate dispersal technologies, and controlled under the CWC. A chemical attack can also involve toxic industrial chemicals that, while not as toxic as chemical warfare agents, are more readily available in larger quantities and are less tightly controlled. Currently, approximately 125,000 chemicals are designated as a toxic industrial chemical, generally defined as a chemical, excluding chemical warfare agents, that has an LCt_{50} (Lethal Concentration for 50% of a population exposed over a given time, t) less than 100,000 mg-min/m^3 in any mammalian species, and produced in quantities exceeding 30 tons annually at any one production facility. Of these, approximately 4600 are considered "critical"[5] and almost 400 "extremely hazardous."[6]

Agents can be dispersed in various forms—including vapor, aerosols, smokes, liquids on surfaces, or solids—depending on the characteristics of the agent and the intended exposure route. Individual agents, their characteristics, and treatment are covered elsewhere in this section.

CURRENT PRACTICE

Current tactics, techniques, and procedures for emergency management of chemical attack have evolved from a combination of response practices from emergency services, hazardous materials (HazMat) response, and military chemical warfare defense doctrine. Various panels have developed consensus "best practices," reports, and documents, many compiled and available at the Chemical and Biological Defense Information Analysis Center (CBIAC).[7] The National Medical Response Teams (NMRT), part of the National Disaster Medical System (NDMS) under the Federal Emergency Management Agency (FEMA), represent civilian teams charged with responding to CBRNE mass casualties and providing decontamination and medical triage and treatment. The military developed the U.S. Marine Corps Chemical Biological Incident Response Force (CBIRF)[8] to respond to mass casualty CBRNE attacks. Both teams represent model constructs for concepts of operations for their particular missions. The main construct of the response strategy to an incident site discussed here parallels that of CBIRF.

Doctrine and Policy

National Incident Management System (NIMS)

Homeland Security Presidential Directive 5 (HSPD-5) establishes the Department of Homeland Security (DHS) as the primary agency for Federal response to incidents of national significance and directs the DHS to develop a national strategy for management. Promulgated on March 1, 2004, the National Incident Management System (NIMS) defines the comprehensive approach in preventing, preparing for, mitigating, responding to, and recovering from domestic incidents using a standard Incident Command System (ICS) and Unified Command System (UCS) to develop a common operating picture accessible across jurisdictions and functional agencies.[9] The approach is to be used at federal, state, local, and tribal government municipalities. As per HSPD-5, adoption of the NIMS is required at federal levels and is a condition for federal preparedness assistance for state, local, and tribal governments, essentially making it the de facto national standard at all levels of government.

For the medical community incident management, several systems are available. Hospital Emergency Incident Command System (HEICS) provides a consensus incident command system that is readily available from various Internet sources. Another comprehensive approach is the Medical and Health Incident Management (MaHIM),[10] which includes a systems engineering approach in identifying all roles and responsibilities required in a medical and health incident management system.

Emergency Management Programs

HSPD-5 establishes and defines five phases of emergency management as prevention, preparedness, mitigation, response, and recovery around which emergency management programs (EMPs) are built. Variably called Disaster Response Plans or various iterations, programs now encompass "all hazards" approaches to disasters and are more commonly being referred to as EMPs, which include a comprehensive plan or specific plans for various incident types. Hospitals and health system personnel have significant roles and responsibilities in each of these five phases and should coordinate via their incident management system with local and/or regional EMPs via local emergency preparedness committees (LEPCs) or other appropriate mechanisms during all phases.

For chemical attacks, critical actions in pre-incident planning phases include (1) identifying first responders/first receivers for triage as well as treatment and decontamination teams, and (2) establishing appropriate training programs, respiratory protection programs, equipment programs, exercise and evaluation programs, communication plans, evacuation procedures, shelter-in-place procedures, and warning and notification procedures. Conducting hazard and vulnerability assessments will assist in determining personal protective equipment (PPE) requirements and identifying other, specific planning requirements. This should be done in conjunction with local, municipal efforts. Community planning for hospitals should include coordinating with other regional hospitals on all aspects of emergency management programs including communications, mutual aid agreements, specialized treatments, alternate care facilities, cross credentialing, information management, supplies and logistics, and training exercises.

Finally, the critical step may be the networking and information management links that are established during the pre-incident phases; although having a plan is important, having gone through the planning process is the critical step. Such links allow for rapid reorganization or self-organization of response systems under catastrophic duress, but they must be established pre-incident to be effective.

CURRENT STANDARDS AND GUIDELINES

The current operating standards and guidelines applicable in responding to chemical attacks present challenges on several fronts. Statutes established for either the workplace or the battlefield are less than optimal for emergency, life-saving actions in mass casualty responses in an urban setting. The need for multi-disciplinary expertise in developing emergency management programs also requires that various regulatory agencies and professional societies work together in establishing more pragmatic statutes and guidelines. Challenges lie in developing standards around so many unknown entities within the response requirements and the limited real-world experience of large-scale catastrophes. A review of some of the various agencies with statutory authority or interest, or those representing funding resources, reveals the importance of coordination and cooperation in this effort. Further detail is provided elsewhere in this text.

The *Occupational Safety and Health Agency (OSHA)*[11] within the *Department of Labor* serves as an advocate for worker health and safety by developing standards for workers and workplaces. This includes setting exposure levels to hazardous chemicals during work cycles as well as short-term and emergency exposure levels. It also works with the National Institute of Occupational Safety and Health (NIOSH), other federal agencies, and private industry to develop standards for general emergency planning,[12] Hazardous Waste Operations and Emergency Response Standard (HAZWOPER),[13] and personal protective equipment (PPE)[14] for emergency response personnel. More specific information is available in the OSHA Technical Manual.[15] OSHA also participates in the development and evolution of the National Response Plan.

The Code of Federal Regulations serves as the basis for first responder safety in emergency response to chemical attack; however, several observations should be made. OSHA recognizes that statutory code written for emergency first responders at an incident site may be too restrictive for "first receivers,"[16] or those healthcare workers who receive contaminated victims at treatment facilities. Recognizing that, OSHA has promulgated guidelines to provide hospitals with expert consensus of what are reasonably safe response practices.[17] Also, incident commanders may use their expertise and experience to make a "risk assessment" that allows responders under their supervision to deviate from standards in order to save lives.[18]

The *National Fire Protection Association (NFPA)*[19] develops guides and recommends practices, codes, and standards for the protection of firemen and emergency medical technicians. Standards are enforced through OSHA promulgation, such as those that define the PPE levels, with Level 1 being vapor-protective for hazardous chemical emergencies, Level 2 being liquid splash–protective for hazardous chemical emergencies, Level 3 being liquid splash–protective for non-emergency, non-flammable hazardous chemicals, and Level 4 being standard work clothes.[20] These levels correspond closely to OSHA Levels A-D respectively. NFPA also has several guidelines regarding competencies for first responders.[21-23]

The *National Institute for Occupational Safety and Health (NIOSH)*,[24] a division of the Centers for Disease Control and Prevention (CDC), seeks to prevent work-related illness and injury by ensuring the development, certification, deployment, and use of personal protective equipment and fully integrated, intelligent ensembles. Although NIOSH establishes standards, it does not have enforcement authority. The National Personal Protective Technology Laboratory at NIOSH partners with NFPA, OSHA, the Department of Defense (DoD), the National Institute of Standards and Technology (NIST), and the National Institute of Justice (NIJ) in the development of standards for CBRN respirators and their certification. All respirators used for response in a chemical attack must meet NIOSH certification, once those standards have been promulgated. More information is available at the CDC website.[25]

The *Office of Law Enforcement Standards (OLES)*[26] at NIST, part of the NIJ, works with various agencies and partners to establish objective performance standards and equipment testing programs for critical equipment.[27] CBRNE standards development falls under the "Critical Incident Technologies" program area. Applying technical expertise and "gold standard" laboratory capabilities, OLES works with its partners to identify technical issues, develop standard testing protocols, identify testing labs, and develop standards for such things as communications interfaces for the first responder in protective equipment, tracking first responders, and networking sensors. The standards are then issued out through the appropriate agency with statutory authority, such as NIOSH, Environmental Protection Agency (EPA), OSHA, FEMA, NFPA, DoD, or DHS. OLES also partners with the Interagency Board (IAB, see below). PPE Guidelines are promulgated through the U.S. Department of Justice Law Enforcement and Corrections Standards and Testing Program.[28]

The *Interagency Board for Standardization of Equipment and Interoperability,*[29] formed in the late 1990s through a partnership with DoD and FBI, ensures standardization and interoperability throughout the response community in preparing for and responding to weapons of mass destruction (WMDs) incidents. Although it is not a statutory setting agency, it has an expanded stakeholder list of federal and local partners that includes statutory agencies. Its four equipment subgroups—Medical, PPE and Operational Equipment, Decontamination and Detection, and Communications and Information Systems—work through a standards coordination committee, in conjunction with a science and technology committee, to develop, maintain, and update a national standardized equipment list (SEL). This SEL is maintained online at the National Memorial Institute for the Prevention of Terrorism Responder Knowledge Base site.[30] The site links to the current SEL and the Office of Domestic Preparedness (ODP) Authorized Equipment List (AEL), cross-references them with each other, and provides links to appropriate statutes, guidelines, and equipment vendors that have met standards.

Research, Development, and Support

In addition to many excellent academic research centers, the *Technical Support Working Group (TSWG)* conducts the U.S. interagency research and development program for combating terrorism, coordinates research and development requirements, promulgates technology information transfer, and has influence on basic and applied research, with the CBRN Countermeasure Subgroup focusing on chemical incident response issues. The TSWG has broad representation from federal agencies and has international participation. Examples of important projects funded by the TSWG include development and certification of standard drinking tube systems for masks and development of a heat stress calculator for personnel in PPE.

Other Agencies and Departments

Specific roles of federal agencies and departments are covered elsewhere in this textbook; however, some specific agencies merit mention here.

The *Department of Health and Human Services (DHHS)* has several entities with relevance for chemical attack. The *National Library of Medicine (NLM)*, represents a ready, useful resource for information on chemicals.[31] They have also developed a tool, WISER (Wireless Information System for Emergency Responders), to make these data portable and accessible. The mission of the *Agency for Healthcare Research and Quality (AHRQ)* is to improve the quality, safety, efficiency, and effectiveness of health care for all Americans.[32] AHRQ develop models, tools, and other resources to assist hospitals in emergency preparedness that are readily available. They work closely with the Health Resources and Systems Administration (HRSA) to develop standards for providing grants to states to improve readiness.[33] AHRQ has developed several tools, including a vulnerability assessment tool specific for CBRNE for hospitals. The mission of the *Agency for Toxic Substances and Disease Registry (ATSDR)*, as an agency of DHHS, is to serve the public by using the best science, taking responsive public health actions, and providing trusted health information to prevent harmful exposures and disease related to toxic substances.

ATSDR is directed by Congressional mandate to perform specific functions concerning the effect on public health of hazardous substances in the environment. These functions include public health assessments of waste sites, health consultations concerning specific hazardous substances, health surveillance and registries, response to emergency releases of hazardous substances, applied research in support of public health assessments, information development and dissemination, and education and training concerning hazardous substances. ATSDR produces toxicologic profiles for hazardous substances found at National Priorities List (NPL) sites that are ranked based on frequency of occurrence at the sites, toxicity, and potential for human exposure. The profiles for nearly all of the 270 toxic substances on the NPL are available at the ATSDR website.[34]

The DoD is covered in more detail in other chapters of this textbook; however, several agencies play significant roles in preparing for and responding to chemical attacks.

The *Research Development & Engineering Command (RDECOM)*, formerly known as the Soldier Biological Chemical Command (SBCCOM), represents the research and development (R&D) arm of the U.S. Army's chemical corps. RDECOM, with the *Edgewood Chemical Biological Center (ECBC)* applies this R&D effort to develop concepts of operations, training programs (they developed the 120-city Improved Response Program), partnering efforts across the chemical-biologic response paradigm, and providing publications addressing significant, challenging issues in chemical incident response.[35,36] RDECOM also serves as the partnering test facility with NIOSH to perform official testing of mask/filter combinations against chemical weapons for CBRN certification. Applied technology projects include the Automated Decision Aid System for Hazardous Incidents (ADASHI), a "black box" consequence management tool for responding to chemical incidents.

The Army Forces Command *20th Support Command (CBRNE)*, formerly known as Guardian Brigade, includes the former Technical Escort Unit (TEU) and the Chemical Biological Rapid Response Team (CBRRT), and represents an expert team specializing in responding to emergency, non-lifesaving aspects of chemical incidents.

The U.S. Marine Corps' *Chemical Biological Incident Response Force (CBIRF)* is a rapid response, anti-terrorism unit located in Indian Head, MD. Specializing in life-saving aspects of emergency management in contaminated environments, the unit serves as a model for CBRNE response teams around the world. Working closely with partners at the local, state, and federal levels as well as with private industry, CBIRF contributes to development, evaluation, and validation of best practice tactics, techniques, and procedures for "all hazards" emergency management planning, improvement of response equipment, and development of advanced training techniques.

The *U.S. Army Medical Research Institute for Chemical Defense (USAMRICD)* provides the nation's primary medical laboratories charged with identifying chemical weapons threats and developing medical countermeasures, including antidotes, barrier creams, decontamination solutions, and chemoprophylaxis. The training arm of "ICD" develops and provides the chemical portion of the "gold standard" Medical Management of Chemical/Biological Casualties and the Field Management of Chemical and Biological Casualties Courses.

THE RESPONSE

While it is true that many chemicals cause their effects within seconds to minutes after exposure, the efficacy of response actions extends much longer beyond several hours, and planning assumptions should account for this. For example, during the Iran-Iraq war of the 1980s, Iran suffered several chemical warfare mass casualty attacks of nerve agents, mustard agent, or combination of the two (and sometimes in combination with conventional artillery attacks). The Iranian health system responded to these mass casualties, adjusting strategies and procedures over time by providing medical care closer to the incident site, eventually providing mobile medical teams to provide care at the scene. Lessons learned from published exploits of response include the need to treat early and far forward in order to confer maximal patient benefit, the need for an integrated system of care, and a rapid response to antidote therapy and recovery for mild, uncomplicated casualties.[37]

Several factors make it difficult to predict response time requirements. Toxicity and lethality data of specific agents are derived from animal models and are not easily translatable to humans. Toxicity curves are likely affected by extremes of age, confounding medical problems, and concomitant trauma, with unknown effects on the course of poisoning and greater potential for effects of sub-lethal exposures. Finally, the management of large-scale mass casualty incidents is poorly studied as well, particularly in a heterogeneous population. The additional response burden of working in PPE and having an additional decontamination step in the treatment protocol adds another dimension of complexity. The critical point is that response time requirements and treatment outcomes are not known and may be affected by a multitude of factors.

Initial Actions

Recognizing an attack

Indicators of a chemical attack generally occur rapidly. Crude explosive dissemination devices typically use a third of the explosives component as comparable conventional explosive devices in order to minimize consumption of agent and maximize spread. Consequently, improvised explosive devices (IEDs) that seem to have more smoke than blast or fire may indicate a chemical dispersal device. Vapor clouds, smokes without fires, or more sophisticated spray devices or aerosolizers in unusual places may indicate an attack. Multiple, unexplained victims with similar symptom patterns—difficulty breathing (lewisite or mustard agent if onset delayed), tearing, dimmed vision, muscle weakness, nausea (nerve agent symptoms), or burning skin and eyes—or dead animals may indicate a chemi-

cal attack. Any chemical attack is both a HazMat incident and a crime scene, and preservation of crime scene evidence should be considered when practical.

Establishing scene safety

Initial actions on scene should include maintaining a high index of suspicion for the presence of a toxic material and secondary explosive devices. Establishing a safe zone for "cold zone" operations is paramount, with approaches toward the "hot zone" from upwind and upgrade when practical. A "warm zone" or contamination reduction corridor, defines the area that is initially uncontaminated, adjacent to the hot zone where decontamination will occur. Ambulatory victims can be directed toward safe havens to await further directions as the response ensues. The incident commander—the senior, most experienced first responder on scene—determines actions.

Response Capabilities

Effective response to chemical attacks involving mass casualties is best approached by defining the response requirements at the incident site across functional capabilities. Elements will vary in size and capability depending on the requirements defined for the response, resources available, or as per the incident commander. These same elements can be used for defining requirements at remote response sites that may be needed, such as at hospitals or alternate treatment sites preparing to treat victims who were not evaluated or decontaminated at the incident site. Figure 62-1 demonstrates a typical incident site response scheme.

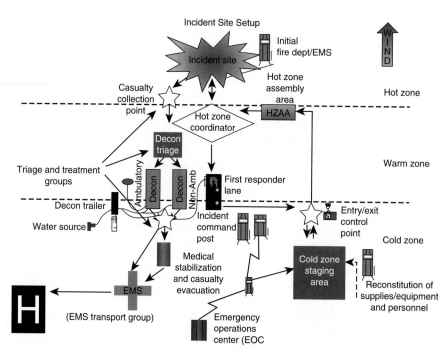

FIGURE 62–1. Typical incident site response scheme.

Command and Control

The incident commander retains not only crisis action planning responsibility, but also accountability of response personnel and liability for actions during the response. As per the NIMS, the incident command system (or unified command system) is the national standard response structure, with the "best qualified" person on scene assuming the role of incident commander, and command switching to a unified command system as soon as reasonably achievable. ICS training and Job Aids listing such things as organizational charts, roles, responsibilities, meetings, Response Action Guides, and sample forms are available from various sources.[38-40] Handheld information technology emergency response tools (e.g., CoBRA, ADASHI, CATS, CAMEO, WebEOC) are also commercially available.

The size and impact of the incident drive the manning of the positions in the ICS, with roles and responsibilities becoming more specific as the size increases. ICS recommends that the "span of control," or the number of personnel under a supervisor, not exceed four to six persons. The incident commander establishes a command post in a safe place near the incident site, analyzes the incident, develops the incident action plan, implements the plan, and evaluates the progress. A hazard and risk assessment allows the incident commander to determine the threats and estimate the potential course and harm in order to develop strategic goals and tactical objectives, determine required protective measures, and assign team tasking goals and missions to the various response squads, teams, or units. The risk assessment also allows the incident commander to use experience and expertise to deviate from statutory regulations, if necessary. Leaders are expected to coordinate and integrate their teams into the incident commander's incident action plan.

Reconnaissance/Hazard Detection and Identification

Describing the environment of the "hot zone" is the role of the reconnaissance team. Merely detecting an agent is insufficient because the incident site becomes a workplace and the working parameters must be defined. Such information as oxygen levels, presence of explosive gases, presence of chemical agents, radioactivity, mechanical hazards, and structural integrity of buildings—as well as reporting on casualty numbers, locations, and conditions—must be relayed back to the incident commander for consideration in the management of the incident. Typically, this team works initially in OSHA Level A (NFPA Level 1) or Level B (NFPA Level 2) suits, since the environment is "undefined," unknown, or levels that are an immediate danger to life and health (IDLH).

Various detection/identification technologies are available and beyond the scope of this chapter. Much research is being conducted in making handheld devices capable of detecting and identifying chemical agents. Technologies range from Drager Tubes to ion mobility spectrometry, flame ionization, surface acoustic wave analysis, and gas chromatography/mass spectrometry (GCMS) in conjunction with solid phase micro-extraction (SPME) fibers. Information provided by the reconnaissance team allows the incident commander to determine the appropriate level of personal protective ensemble for the various other elements of the response team. Because quantitative levels of chemicals are difficult to determine rapidly at an incident site with current technology, exposure levels based on concentration are difficult to use, often driving the decision to use higher levels of PPE.

Casualty Extraction

Casualty extraction is likely the most emotionally and physically challenging of the functional elements because it requires the ability to make life-and-death decisions in chaotic environments while undergoing demanding physical exertion and working in high levels of PPE. Victims that cannot ambulate out of a toxic environment must be carried out in order to optimize outcome. Criteria for determining prioritization of extraction are sorely lacking at this time, and current protocols are not evidence-based or optimized for survivability. Heat stress and heat exhaustion collapse are significant problems for these workers, particularly on warm, sunny days, with work cycles usually limited to 30 minutes or less.

Casualty extraction should include personnel as "victim assist teams" that also protect the response team during the critical initial set-up period when contaminated, ambulatory victims could wander outside of established control zones and decontamination corridors, interfere with set-up efforts of response personnel, or cross-contaminate clean areas. Such teams then assist with patient flow, transport, care, and crowd control.

Medical Triage, Treatment, and Transport

The medical section of the command post oversees the medical triage, treatment, and transport of patients at the incident site, interfacing with other aspects of the ICS/UCS in carrying out the incident action plan. Depending on the size of the response, there may be branches overseeing triage and treatment or transportation groups, divisions, or task forces.

Most triage systems currently in use lack evidence to support their efficacy. Further, it may be that alterations of standards of care may need to be considered.[41] Recently, evidence-based triage systems employing algorithms that consider medical resources, transport times, and predicted survivability have been proposed to optimize overall survivability.[42] Although correlated to trauma databases, it is not clear whether the same criteria used for triage prioritization would correlate to survivability for a chemical incident.

Although dependent on available resources, triage and treatment teams are best placed at naturally occurring "bottlenecks" in processing victims from the incident site "hot zone" through the contamination reduction corridor (e.g., warm zone) to a medical stabilization area in the cold zone in preparation for transfer to the EMS transportation teams. Depending on distances and specifics of the incident site, a casualty collection point might be established at the border between the hot and warm zone where extractors can transfer victims to initial care in a relatively less-contaminated environment. This provides early access to medical attention for initial triage and treatment, such as administration of antidotes, and shortens the extraction cycle for the extraction team. Although it may be beneficial to deploy limited medical personnel into the hot zone to provide limited triage, medical direction, and antidote administration, there is, at this time, little evidence to support this as being the best use of limited medical resources.

Medical treatment teams placed on both ends of the decontamination process will facilitate better prioritization of patients processing through decontamination, provide medical oversight for patients during the formal decontamination process, and facilitate re-triage and treatment in preparation for transfer to emergency medical system transportation units. Naturally occurring bottlenecks in the decontamination process will suggest that a "decon triage" medical treatment area be established on the warm zone end of the decontamination process for non-ambulatory patients. Although little more than the ABCs (airway, breathing, circulation) can be done in the contaminated environment of the warm zone, the results of chemical attacks primarily affect the ABCs, and management of the airway in a contaminated environment should be a primary area of focus for planning and preparation for a chemical attack. Appropriate administration of antidotes is accomplished along the entire medical treatment corridor. Depending on the composition of the medical teams, special protocols requiring specialized training for antidote administration by non-licensed medical responders may be needed. These should be established during the preparation phase of an emergency management program.

PPE requirements for medical providers in the warm zone are an area of interest to OSHA, although the incident commander determines the requirement for the level. For response conducted remote from the incident site, such as at a hospital or alternate care facility, OSHA has promulgated specific guidelines mentioned previously.

Decontamination

Decontamination remains an area of intense research and development. Current best practices rely on physical removal of agents using soap and water. Use of 0.5% bleach solution has fallen out of favor. Several good consensus standards have been promulgated.[43-46] There is evidence, however, to suggest these water-based techniques, if not performed immediately after exposure, may not be effective, and may even cause more harm.[47] Others argue for a more rational approach that considers high molecular weight solutions optimized for specific agent characteristics including solubilities.[48]

For ambulatory patients, most systems essentially represent mass shower sequences through tents for set periods of time, with a range of shower times depending on various factors. Although it is commonly stated that disrobing may provide up to 90% decontamination in and of itself, some care to technique must be applied to prevent cross contamination. Decontamination of non-

ambulatory patients is time and manpower intensive. Even the most elaborate systems and experienced teams do not provide adequate throughput for true mass casualty incidents. Roller systems that allow easier, rapid movement of patients through a "car wash"–like system take more than 2 to 5 minutes per patient. Set-up times for different teams and systems vary and, if not pre-positioned, provide additional challenges because of large footprints and time to set up. In addition, mass casualty decontamination setups pose the inability to move easily if necessary and require a water source.

Several critical issues in the decontamination process are worth mentioning briefly. At least three separate lanes for processing people through should be recognized: a lane for ambulatory patients, a lane for non-ambulatory patients, and a separate lane for responders. Each group will have different decontamination requirements and priorities, and likely utilize different processes. The responder lane becomes especially critical for responders on supplied air who will usually be near the end of their air supply. Cutting clothes with "J knives" versus scissors may enhance the throughput capability and avoid hand fatigue.

Neutralizing solutions such as Reactive Skin Decontaminant Lotion (RSDL) are commercially available and offer significantly more favorable decontamination performance[49]; however, further evaluation needs to be done, including FDA licensing as a medical drug if such solutions are to be used for full-body decontamination. Controlling water temperature during the decontamination process can be a challenge given portability, sourcing, and volume requirements. Decontamination lanes are typically manned with non-medical personnel, so medical oversight during the decontamination process needs to be provided with clear protocols for alerting medical providers of issues in the decontamination process. Finally, the environment in decontamination systems can become very hot and humid. The effect on personnel, as well as filter performance, must be considered.

Scene Security/Explosives Ordnance Disposal (EOD).

Scene security plays several significant roles including maintaining order, controlling and maintaining zone boundaries for contaminated areas and scene perimeters, directing traffic flow, and preventing secondary attacks that might jeopardize the initial response. EOD teams, when available, provide a sweep for secondary devices such as improvised explosive devices (IEDs) that might be targeting responders.

Supplies and Logistics

The role of logistics is to ensure the needed resources—be they supplies, equipment, personnel, or specialized services—get to the proper person or place at the proper time and in the proper amount. Actions range from maintaining and resupplying critical resources such as PPE suits and filters and decontamination supplies, to fluids and food to reconstitute the responders. It is crucial that response teams identify and carry items they will need in a given response and not represent a logistical burden when they present to an incident, and that they be able to provide accurate estimates on the duration of their resources, identify sources to replace consumed supplies, and identify any critical support requirements that the unit might have.

For logistical support of chemical attacks, there are several programs, in addition to the Strategic National Stockpile (SNS), worth mentioning that can provide critical supplies to a response in a more reasonable time frame.

The *Chempack Program*, part of the SNS Program, provides forward placement of supplies and equipment specifically needed in the event of a chemical attack to provide state and local government these critical supplies and improve the response times, spread-loading them across the nation, and placing them closer to large population centers where they might be needed.

The Emergency Management Strategic Healthcare Group, under the Veterans Health Administration (VHA) of the Department of Veterans Affairs, addresses emergency management functions for the VHA including medical support to the DoD, NDMS, and the National Response Plan as needed. VA Medical Centers maintain caches with products to respond to CBRNE incidents for treating veterans, VA staff, and other individuals seeking treatment at a VA facility.

The Department of Justice Office for Domestic Preparedness maintains the *Prepositioned Equipment Program (PEP)*.[50] The PEP sustains a community's response to CBRNE incidents by providing equipment for emergency responders and replenishing assets consumed in the response. The sets are standardized, incorporating lessons learned and experiences into the items containing PPE, detection, communications, medical, technical rescue, and decontamination equipment. Located strategically throughout the United States, they are containerized and palletized and are able to be transported on two tractor-trailers, or by air, to provide nationwide response within 12 hours. They are accompanied by a team of technicians to assist in deployment and operations of the equipment, particularly the communications and detection equipment.

As part of the NDMS, there are four specialized teams for CBRNE response located to respond regionally across the United States, the *National Medical Response Teams (NMRT)*. The teams often pre-deploy to planned events with credible threats, national special security events (NSSEs), after a CBRNE incident has occurred, or anytime the FBI determines a credible threat exists. Each team consists of 56 HazMat medical specialists with extensive training in CBRNE response. In addition to emergency life-saving response capability across the functional elements of CBRNE response, the team carries antidotes for 15,000 chemical nerve agent casualties and can deploy in conjunction with other NDMS units for extended medical treatment capabilities.

Command and Control

The Incident Command System or Unified Command System (ICS/UCS) provides a standard framework for responding to a chemical attack. The incident commander, located at the incident command post, estab-lishes the incident action plan following general incident action guides. The NIMS provides guidance on these activities.

PITFALLS

Integration and Coordination

At the federal level, integration for emergency management response and homeland security is now the responsibility of the DHS, with the NIMS Integration Center established to oversee the process. It is incumbent on responders and managers at every level in the preparedness and response effort to ensure understanding of systems architecture, statutes, procedures, roles and responsibilities that affect them, and the integration into their emergency management program as appropriate and needed. Various tools are available that allow communities of response personnel to coordinate and communicate more efficiently.[51] Use and integration of information management tools is another area undergoing rapid development and should be encouraged with development of standards. Co-operation and compromise are necessary as we identify our requirements and develop capabilities.

Learning Lessons Learned

The Memorial Institute for the Prevention of Terrorism[52] Lessons Learned Information Sharing[53] is designed to capture insights from various levels of government response and share the information appropriately with emergency response personnel and homeland security officials. Active participation with a lessons learned program should be considered part of the professional responsibilities of emergency response personnel. Lessons learned come not only from actual response experiences, but also from standard training, evaluating exercises, and ensuring feedback loops in evolving and improving plans, procedures, and protocols as well as the information shared appropriately.

Standards and Guidelines

Efforts at developing standards, guidelines, and statutes that optimize the risk/benefit ratios for saving lives and property while providing safe practices for emergency response personnel are being made that include multiple disciplines and areas of expertise. The speed at which this occurs is affected by the governmental bureaucratic systems that control such processes, finite fiscal and personnel resources, and operational urgency. Response personnel must actively seek continuing education and training on current status of these as they undergo significant and rapid change.

Non-Traditional Agents

As a parting consideration, it is vital to keep in mind that many of the classical chemical warfare agents about which we learn and train are over 60 years old. With the further progress of technology and science, it is likely that development of weapons of mass destruction will not necessarily require the resources of a state-sponsored program, and that novel agents may be developed with unfamiliar effects and presentations. As part of our preparation, we must foster and maintain our ability for critical reasoning, assessing, adapting, and improvising.

REFERENCES

1. Joy R. Historical aspects of medical defense against chemical warfare. In: Sidell F, Takafuji E, Franz D, eds. *Medical Aspects of Chemical and Biological Warfare, Textbook of Military Medicine, Part I*, 1997. Borden Institute, San Antonio, TX. Available at: http://www.vnh.org/MedAspChemBioWar/
2. 29 CFR 1910 series.
3. National Fire Protection Administration: NFPA 471, 472, 473, 1600, 1994.
4. Organization for the Prevention of Chemical Weapons: Available at: http://www.opcw.org/html/db/cwc/eng/cwc_frameset.html.
5. National Library of Medicine Hazardous Substances Database. Available at: http://toxnet.nlm.nih.gov/cgi-bin/sis/htmlgen?HSDB.
6. Environmental Protection Agency. Alphabetical Order List of Extremely Hazardous Substances (Section 302 of EPCRA). Available at: http://yosemite.epa.gov/oswer/ceppoehs.nsf/Alphabetical Results?openview.
7. Chemical and Biological Defense Information Analysis Center (CBIAC). Available at: http://www.cbiac.apgea.army.mil/
8. U.S. Marine Corps Chemical Biological Incident Response Force. Available at http://www.cbirf.usmc.mil.
9. National Incident Management System, Dept of Homeland Security, 01 Mar 2004. Available at: http://www.fema.gov/nims/
10. Barbera JA, Macintyre AG. Medical and Health Incident Management (MaHIM) System: A Comprehensive Functional System Description for Mass Casualty Medical and Health Incident Management. Washington, DC: Institute for Crisis, Disaster, and Risk Management, The George Washington University; October 2002.
11. Occupational Safety and Health Agency. Available at: www.OSHA.gov.
12. 29 CFR 1910.38, 29 CFR 1926.35.
13. 29 CFR 1910.120, 29 CFR 1926.65.
14. 29 CFR 1910.132 to 137.
15. Occupational Safety and Health Agency. OSHA Technical Manual, Chapter 1, Section VIII. Available at: www.osha-slc.gov.
16. Koenig, KL. Strip and shower: the duck and cover for the 21st century. *Ann Emerg Med.* 2003;42:391-4.
17. Occupational Safety and Health Agency. OSHA Guidance for Hospital-Based First Receivers of Victims from Mass Casualty Incidents Involving the Release of Hazardous Substances. January 2005. Available at: http://www.osha.gov/dts/osta/bestpractices/html/hospital_firstreceivers.
18. 29 CFR 1910.120.
19. National Fire Protection Association. Available at: http://www.nfpa.org/index.asp?cookie%5Ftest=1
20. National Fire Protection Association. NFPA 1990 series.
21. National Fire Protection Association. NFPA 471, Recommended Practice for Responding to Hazardous Materials Incidents. 2002 ed.
22. National Fire Protection Association. NFPA 472, Standards for Professional Competence of Responders to Hazardous Materials Incidents. 2002 ed.
23. National Fire Protection Association. NFPA 473, Standard for Competencies for EMS Personnel Responding to Hazardous Materials Incidents. 2002 ed.
24. National Institute for Occupational Safety and Health. Available at: www.cdc.gov/niosh.
25. Centers for Disease Control and Prevention. Attention emergency responders: how to determine if your SCBA respirator is certified by NIOSH for CBRN environments... Available at: www.cdc.gov/niosh/npptl/cbrncheck.html.
26. Office of Law Enforcement Standards. Available at: www.eeel.nist.gov/oles.
27. Office of Law Enforcement Standards. Equipment Guides Link. Available at: www.eeel.nist.gov/oles/oles_guide_publications.html.
28. National Institute of Justice. NIJ Guide 102-00, Guide for Selection for Personal Protective Equipment for Emergency First Responders (Respiratory Protection), Nov 2002.
29. Interagency Board. Available at: www.iab.gov.
30. National Memorial Institute for the Prevention of Terrorism, Responder Knowledge Base. Standardized equipment list. Available at: http://www2.rkb.mipt.org/
31. National Library of Medicine. NLM information on chemicals. Available at: http://sis.nlm.nih.gov/chemical.html
32. Agency for Healthcare Research and Quality. Available at: http://www.ahrq.gov.
33. Health Resources and Systems Administration. Available at: http://www.hrsa.gov/bioterrorism.
34. Agency for Toxic Substances and Disease Registry. Available at: http://www.atsdr.cdc.gov/about.html.
35. An Alternative Health Care Facility: Concept of Operations for the off-site Triage, Treatment, and Transportation Center. Mass Casualty Care Strategy for a Chemical Terrorism Incident, Chemical Weapons Improved Response Program, SBCCOM, March 2001.
36. Guidelines for Mass Fatality Management During Terrorist Incidents Involving Chemical Agents, SBCCOM, Nov 2001.
37. Newmark J., The birth of nerve agent warfare, Neurology, 2004 May 11; 62(9) 1590-6
38. FEMA Incident Command System Self-study course. Available at: http://www.osha.gov/SLTC/etools/ics/index.html.
39. Occupational Safety and Health Agency. OSHA e-tools: Incident Command System. Available at: http://www.osha.gov/SLTC/etools/ics/index.html.
40. Office of Hazardous Materials Safety. Emergency Response Guidebook. Available at: http://hazmat.dot.gov/pubs/erg/gydebook.htm.
41. AHRQ Publication No. 05-0043, Altered Standards of Care in Mass Casualty Events, April 2005. Available at: http://www.ahrq.gov/research/altstand/altstand.pdf
42. Sacco, J., et. al., Precise Formulation and Evidence-based Application of Resource-constrained Triage, Acad. Emerg. Med., Vol 12, Number 8, 759-770. Available at: http://www.aemj.org/cgi/content/abstract/12/8/759
43. Patient Decontamination Recommendations for Hospitals, Emergency Medical Services Authority, #233, CA, July 2005, Available at: http://www.emsa.ca.gov/aboutemsa/emsa233.pdf
44. Best Practices and Guidelines for CBR Mass Personnel Decontamination, ed 2. Aug 2004, Technical Support Working Group. Available at: http://www.tswg.gov/tswg/cbrnc/MPDPOrder.html
45. NFPA Handbook Supplement 7. Guidelines for Decontamination of Fire Fighters and Their Equipment following Hazardous Materials Incidents, 2002.
46. Guidelines for Cold Weather Mass Decontamination During a Terrorist Chemical Agent Incident, SBCCOM, Jan 2002.
47. Loke, W.-K, et al. Wet decontamination-induced stratum corneum hydration—Effects on the skin barrier function to diethylmalonate, J. Appl. Toxicol. 19:285-290 (1999).
48. Buckley, T.J., et. al., A Rational Approach to Skin Decontamination. Available at: http://www.skcinc.com/CLI/A%20Rational%20Approach.pdf
49. Clawson, R.E., Overview of a Joint US/Canadian Test and Evaluation Program, DECON 2002, San Diego, CA, Oct 2002.
50. Prepositioned Equipment Program. Available at: http://www.ojp.usdoj.gov/odp/equipment_pep.htm.
51. DisasterHelp (DHelp). Available at: https://disasterhelp.gov/portal/jhtml/index.jhtml.
52. Memorial Institute for the Prevention of Terrorism. Available at: http://www.mipt.org
53. U.S. Department of Homeland Security. Lessons Learned Information Sharing. Available at: https://www.llis.dhs.gov/.

chapter 63

Biologic Attack

Andrew W. Artenstein

Bioterrorism can be broadly defined as the deliberate use of microbial agents or their toxins as weapons against noncombatants outside the setting of armed conflict. The broad scope and mounting boldness of worldwide terrorism, exemplified by the massive attacks on New York City and Washington, DC, on Sept. 11, 2001, coupled with the apparent willingness of terrorist organizations to acquire and deploy biologic weapons, constitute ample evidence that the specter of bioterrorism will pose a persistent global threat.

As in other aspects of daily life, and the practice of medicine in particular, the concept of "risk" is germane to considerations regarding an attack using biologic agents. *Risk,* broadly defined as the probability that exposure to a hazard will lead to a negative consequence, can be accurately calculated for a variety of conditions of public health importance (Table 63-1). However, the quantification of risk as it pertains to bioterrorism is imprecise because accurate assessment of exposure depends on the whims of terrorists, by nature an unpredictable variable. Although the probability of exposure to a biologic attack is statistically low, it is not zero; and because the negative consequences are potentially catastrophic, an understanding of biologic threat agents and a cogent biodefense strategy are important components of disaster medicine.

TABLE 63-1 U.S. MORTALITY RISK ANALYSIS*

Heart disease	1 in 397
Cancer	1 in 511
Stroke	1 in 1,699
Alzheimer's	1 in 5,752
Motor vehicle accident	1 in 6,745
Homicide	1 in 15,440
Drowning	1 in 64,031
Fire	1 in 82,977
Bicycle accident	1 in 376,165
Lightning strike	1 in 4,478,159
Bioterrorism (anthrax)	1 in 56,424,800

*U.S. Population divided by the number of annual deaths for 2000.
Source: Harvard Center for Risk Analysis, http://www.hcra.harvard.edu © 2004 CEEP

HISTORICAL PERSPECTIVE

Biologic weapons have been used against both military and civilian targets throughout history. In the fourteenth century, Tatars attempted to use epidemic disease against the defenders of Kaffa by catapulting plague-infected corpses into the city.[1] British forces gave Native Americans blankets from a smallpox hospital in an attempt to affect the balance of power in the eighteenth century Ohio River Valley.[1] In addition to their well-described use of chemical weapons, Axis forces purportedly infected livestock with anthrax and glanders to weaken Allied supply initiatives during World War I. Perhaps the most egregious example of biologic warfare involved the Japanese program in occupied Manchuria from 1932 to 1945. Based on survivor accounts and confessions of Japanese participants, thousands of prisoners were murdered in experiments using a variety of virulent pathogens at Unit 731, the code name for the biologic weapons facility there.[2]

The United States maintained an active program for the development and testing of offensive biologic weapons from the early 1940s until 1969, when the program was terminated by executive order of then President Nixon, although efforts continue with regard to countermeasures against biologic weapons. The Convention on the Prohibition of the Development, Production, and Stockpiling of Biological and Toxin Weapons and on Their Destruction (BWC) was ratified in 1972, formally banning the development or use of biologic weapons and assigning responsibility for enforcement to the United Nations.[1] Unfortunately, the BWC has not been effective in its stated goals; multiple signatories, including the former Soviet Union and Iraq, have violated the terms and spirit of the agreement. The accidental release of aerosolized anthrax spores from a biologic weapons plant in the Soviet Union in 1979, with at least 68 human deaths from inhalational anthrax reported downwind, was proved years later to have occurred in the context of Soviet offensive weapons production.

Recent events have established bioterrorism as a credible and ubiquitous threat. The intentional contamination of restaurant salad bars with *Salmonella* by a

415

religious cult trying to influence a local election in The Dalles, Oregon in 1984[3]; the revelations that Aum Shinri Kyo, the Japanese cult that released sarin nerve agent in the Tokyo subway system in 1995 had unsuccessfully experimented on multiple occasions with spraying anthrax from downtown rooftops before their successful chemical attack; and the findings of the UN weapons inspectors of massive quantities of weaponized biologic weapons in Iraq during the Gulf War and its aftermath[4] served as sentinel warnings of a shift in terrorism trends. The anthrax attacks in the United States in October and November 2001, following the catastrophic events of Sept. 11, elevated bioterrorism to the fore of the international dialogue.

CURRENT PRACTICE

Threat Assessment

Biologic agents are considered weapons of mass destruction (WMDs) because, as with certain conventional, chemical, and nuclear weapons, their use may result in large-scale morbidity and mortality. A World Health Organization (WHO) model based on the hypothetical effects of the intentional release of 50 kg of aerosolized anthrax spores upwind from a population center of 500,000 (analogous to that of Providence, RI) estimated that the agent would disseminate in excess of 20 km downwind and that nearly 200,000 people would be killed or injured by the event.[5] Biologic weapons possess unique properties among WMDs. By definition, biologic agents are associated with a clinical latency period of days to weeks, in most cases, during which time early detection is quite difficult with currently available technology. Yet, early detection is critical because specific antimicrobial therapy and vaccines are available for the treatment and prevention of illness caused by certain biologic weapons; casualties from other forms of WMDs can generally only be treated by decontamination (with antidotes available for only some types), trauma mitigation, and supportive care. Additionally, the specter of a biologic attack provokes fear and anxiety—"terror"—disproportionate to that seen with other threats.

The aims of bioterrorism are those of terrorism in general: morbidity and mortality among civilian populations, disruption of the societal fabric, and exhaustion or diversion of resources. A successful outcome, from a terrorist standpoint, may be achieved without furthering all of these aims. The anthrax attacks in the United States in 2001 evoked fear and anxiety and diverted resources from other critical public health activities despite the limited number of casualties. In many cases, the surge capacity of our public health system was inadequate to deal with the emergency needs.

To be used in large-scale bioterrorism, biologic agents must undergo complex processes of production, cultivation, chemical modification, and weaponization. For these reasons, state sponsorship or direct support from governments or organizations with significant resources, contacts, and infrastructure would predictably be required in large-scale events. However, recent revelations have suggested that some agents may be available on the worldwide black market and in other illicit settings,[6] thus obviating the need for the production process. Although an efficient mode of delivery has traditionally been felt to be necessary, the anthrax attacks in the United States in late 2001 illustrated the devastating results that can be achieved with relatively primitive delivery methods (e.g., high-speed mail sorting equipment and mailed letters).

Numerous attributes contribute to the selection of a pathogen as a biologic weapon: availability or ease of large-scale production; ease of dissemination, usually by the aerosol route; stability of the product in storage, as a weapon, and in the environment (biologic entities differ in their physical properties); cost; and clinical virulence. The last of these refers to the reliability with which the pathogen causes high mortality, morbidity, or social disruption. The Centers for Disease Control and Prevention (CDC) have prioritized biologic agent threats based on the aforementioned characteristics,[7] and this has influenced current preparedness strategies (Table 63-2). Category A agents, considered the highest priority, are associated with high mortality and the greatest potential for major impact on the public health. Category B agents are considered "incapacitating" because of their potential for moderate morbidity but relatively low mortality. Most of the category A and B agents have been experimentally weaponized in the past and are thus of proven feasibility. Category C agents include emerging threats and pathogens that may be available for development.

Another factor that must be addressed in assessing future bioterrorism risk is the historical track record of experimentation with specific pathogens, an area that has been informed from the corroborated claims of various high-level Soviet defectors and data released from the former offensive weapons programs of the United States and United Kingdom.[1,6,8] It is apparent from these sources, combined with the burgeoning fields of molecular biology and genomics, that future risk scenarios may have to contend with genetically altered and "designer" pathogens. To this end, a miscellaneous grouping of potential threat agents is added to the extant CDC categories in Table 63-2. The most cautious approach to assessing risk may be to remain open to additional, novel possibilities.

Bioterrorism Recognition

By definition bioterrorism is insidious; absent advance warning or specific intelligence information, clinical illness will be manifest before the circumstances of a release event are known. For this reason, healthcare providers are likely to be the first responders to this form of terrorism. This is in contrast to the more familiar scenarios in which police, firefighters, paramedics, and other emergency services personnel are deployed to the scene of an attack with conventional weaponry or a natural disaster. Physicians and other healthcare workers must therefore maintain a high index of suspicion of bioterrorism and recognize suggestive epidemiologic clues and clinical features to enhance early recognition and guide initial management of casualties. This remains

TABLE 63-2 AGENTS OF CONCERN FOR USE IN BIOTERRORISM

HIGHEST PRIORITY (CATEGORY A)

Microbe or toxin	Disease
Bacillus anthracis	Anthrax
Variola virus	Smallpox
Yersinia pestis	Plague
Clostridium botulinum	Botulism
Fracisella tularensis	Tularemia
Filoviruses	Ebola hemorrhagic fevers, Marburg disease
Arenaviruses	Lassa fever, South American hemorrhagic fevers
Bunyaviruses	Rift Valley fever, Congo-Crimean hemorrhagic fevers

MODERATELY HIGH PRIORITY (CATEGORY B)

Coxiella burnetti	Q fever
Brucella spp.	Brucellosis
Burkholderia mallei	Glanders
Alphaviruses	Viral encephalitides
Ricin	Ricin intoxication
Staphylococcus aures enterotoxin B	Staphylococcal toxin illness
Salmonella spp., *Shigella dysenteriae, Escherichia coli* 0157:H7, *Vibrio cholerae, Cryptosporidium parvum*	Food- and water-borne gastroenteritis

CATEGORY C

Hantavirus	Viral hemorrhagic fevers
Flaviviruses	Yellow fever
Mycobacterium tuberculosis	Multidrug resistant tuberculosis

MISCELLANEOUS

Genetically engineered vaccine-and/or antimicrobial-resistant category A or B agents
HIV-1
Adenoviruses
Influenza
Rotaviruses
Hybrid pathogens (e.g., smallpox-plague, smallpox-ebola)

(Artenstein AW, Bioterrorism and Biodefense. In: Cohen J, Powderly WG, eds. Infectious Diseases, second edition. Mosby: London, 2003:99-107) Used with permission.

the most effective way to minimize the deleterious effects of bioterrorism on individual patients and on the public health.

Early recognition is hampered for multiple reasons. As discussed above, it is likely that the circumstances of any event will only be known in retrospect, therefore it may prove problematic to immediately discern the extent of exposure. Terrorists have an unlimited number of targets in most open, democratic societies; it is unrealistic to expect that without detailed intelligence data, all of these can be secured at all times. Certain sites such as government institutions, historic landmarks, or large events may be predictable targets, but there are other, less predictable possibilities. In fact, government data support businesses and other economic concerns as the

main targets of global terrorism during the period from 1996 to 2002.[9] Metropolitan areas are considered vulnerable, but owing to the expansion of suburbs, commuters, and the clinical latency period between exposure and symptoms inherent with biologic agents, casualties of bioterrorism are likely to present for medical attention in diverse locations and at varying times after a common exposure. An event in New York City on a Wednesday morning may result in clinically ill persons presenting over the ensuing weekend to a variety of emergency departments within a 60-mile radius. Additionally, modern modes of transportation ensure that there will be affected persons thousands of miles away at both national and international locations related to a common exposure. This adds layers of complexity to an already complicated setting and illustrates the critical importance of surveillance and real-time communication in this setting.

Further hindering the early recognition of bioterrorism is that initial symptoms may be nondiagnostic. In the absence of a known exposure, many symptomatic persons may not seek medical attention early, or if they do, they may be misdiagnosed as having a flu-like illness. Once beyond the early stages, many of these illnesses progress quite rapidly and treatment may be less successful. Most of the diseases caused by agents of bioterrorism are rarely, if ever, seen in clinical practice; physicians are therefore likely to be inexperienced with their clinical presentation. Additionally, these agents by definition will have been manipulated in a laboratory and may not present with the classic clinical features of naturally occurring infection. This was dramatically illustrated by some of the inhalational anthrax cases in the United States in October 2001.[10]

Early recognition of bioterrorism is facilitated by the recognition of epidemiologic and clinical clues. Clustering of patients with common symptoms and signs, especially if these are unusual or characteristic of bioterrorism agents, is suggestive and should prompt expeditious notification of local public health authorities. This approach will also lead to the recognition of outbreaks of naturally occurring disease or emerging pathogens. The recognition of a single case of a rare or nonendemic infection, in the absence of a travel history or other potential natural exposure, should raise the suspicion of bioterrorism and should prompt notification of public health authorities. Finally, unusual patterns of disease such as concurrent illness in human and animal populations should raise suspicions of bioterrorism or another form of emerging infection. An effective response to bioterrorism requires coordination of the medical system at all levels, from the community physician to the tertiary care center, with public health, emergency management, and law enforcement infrastructures.

Threat Agents

This section provides a broad overview of the biologic threat agents thought to be of major current concern—largely, the CDC category A agents. Extensive coverage of specific pathogens can be found in related chapters in this text and in other sources.[11] Data concerning clinical incubation periods, transmission characteristics, and infection control procedures for agents of bioterrorism are provided in Table 63-3. Syndromic differential diagnoses for select clinical presentations are detailed in Table 63-4.

Anthrax

Anthrax results from infection with *Bacillus anthracis*, a gram-positive, spore-forming, rod-shaped organism that exists in its host as a vegetative bacillus and in the environment as a spore. Details of the microbiology and pathogenesis of anthrax are found in Chapter 102. In nature, anthrax is a zoonotic disease of herbivores that is prevalent in many geographic regions; sporadic human disease results from environmental or occupational contact with endospore-contaminated animal products.[12] The cutaneous form of anthrax is the most common presentation; gastrointestinal and inhalational forms are exceedingly rare in naturally acquired disease. Cutaneous anthrax occurred regularly in the first half of the twentieth century in association with contaminated hides and wools used in the garment industry, but it is uncommonly seen in current-day industrialized countries due to importation restrictions. The last known case of naturally occurring inhalational anthrax in the United States occurred in 1976.[13]

It had been previously hypothesized that large-scale bioterrorism with anthrax would involve aerosolized endospores with resultant inhalational disease, but the recent attacks in the United States illustrate the difficulties in predicting modes and outcomes in bioterrorism: the attacks were on a relatively small scale, and nearly 40% of the confirmed cases were of the cutaneous variety.[14] The serious morbidity and mortality, however, were related to inhalational disease, as was the case in the Sverdlovsk outbreak in 1979. Therefore, planning for larger-scale events with aerosolized agent seems warranted.

The clinical presentations and differential diagnoses of cutaneous and inhalational anthrax are described in Table 63-4. The lesion of cutaneous anthrax may be similar in appearance to other lesions, including cutaneous forms of other agents of bioterrorism; however, it may be distinguished by epidemiologic as well as certain clinical features. Anthrax is traditionally a painless lesion (unless secondarily infected) and associated with significant local edema. The bite of *Loxosceles reclusa*, the brown recluse spider, shares many of the local and systemic features of anthrax but is typically painful from the outset and lacks such significant edema.[15] Cutaneous anthrax is associated with systemic disease and its attendant mortality in up to 20% of untreated cases, although with appropriate antimicrobial therapy mortality is less than 1%.[13]

Once the inhaled endospores reach the terminal alveoli of the lungs, generally requiring particle sizes of 1 to 5 fm, they are phagocytosed by macrophages and transported to regional lymph nodes, where they germinate into vegetative bacteria and, subsequently, disseminate hematogenously.[12] Spores may remain latent for extended periods of time in the host, up to 100 days in experimental animal exposures.[14] This has translated into prolonged clinical incubation periods after exposure to endospores; cases of inhalational anthrax occurred up to 43 days after exposure in the Sverdlovsk experience, although the average incubation period is 2 to 10 days, perhaps influenced by exposure dose.[12,14]

Before the U.S. anthrax attacks in October 2001, most of the clinical data concerning inhalational anthrax derived from Sverdlovsk, the largest outbreak recorded. Although there is much overlap between the clinical manifestations noted previously and those observed during the recent outbreak, more detailed data are available from the recent U.S. experience. There were 11 confirmed persons with inhalational anthrax, 5 (45%) of whom died. Although this contrasts with a case-fatality rate of greater than 85% reported from Sverdlovsk, the reliability of reported data from this outbreak is questionable.[14] Patients almost uniformly present an average of 3.3 days after symptom onset with fevers, chills, malaise, myalgias, nonproductive cough, chest discomfort, dyspnea, nausea or vomiting, tachycardia, peripheral neutrophilia, and liver enzyme elevations.[10,16] Many of these findings are nondiagnostic and overlap considerably with those of influenza and other common viral respiratory tract infections. Recently compiled data suggest

TABLE 63-3 INFECTION CONTROL ISSUES FOR SELECTED AGENTS OF BIOTERRORISM

DISEASE	INCUBATION PERIOD (DAYS)	PERSON-TO-PERSON TRANSMISSION	INFECTION CONTROL PRACTICES
Inhalational anthrax	2–43*	No	Standard
Botulism	12–72 hours	No	Standard
Primary pneumonic plague	1–6	Yes	Droplet
Smallpox	7–17	Yes	Contact and airborne
Tularemia	1–14	No	Standard
Viral hemorrhagic fevers	2–21	Yes	Contact and airborne
Viral encephalitides	2–14	No	Standard
Q fever	2–14	No	Standard
Brucellosis	5–60	No	Standard
Glanders	10–14	No	Standard

*Based on limited data from human outbreaks; experimental animal data support clinical latency periods of up to 100 days (Artenstein AW Bioterrorism and Biodefense. In: Cohen J, Powderly WG, eds. Infectious Diseases, second edition. Mosby: London, 2003:99-107). Used with permission.

TABLE 63-4 PRESENTATIONS AND DIFFERENTIAL DIAGNOSES OF BIOTERRORISM AGENTS

CLINICAL PRESENTATION	DISEASE	DIFFERENTIAL DIAGNOSIS
Non-specific flu-like symptoms with nausea, emesis, cough with or without chest discomfort, without coryza or rhinorrhea, leading to abrupt onset of respiratory distress with or without shock, mental status changes, with chest radiograph abnormalities (wide mediastinum, infiltrates, pleural effusions)	Inhalational anthrax	Bacterial mediastinitis, tularemia, Q fever, psittacosis, Legionnaires' disease, influenza, *Pneumocystis carinii* pneumonia, viral pneumonia, ruptured aortic aneurysm, superior vena cava syndrome, histoplasmosis, coccidioidomycosis, sarcoidosis
Pruritic, painless papule, leading to vesicle(s), leading to ulcer, leading to edematous black eschar with or without massive local edema and regional adenopathy and fever, evolving over 3-7 days	Cutaneous anthrax	Recluse spider bite, plague, staphylococcal lesion, atypical Lyme disease, orf, glanders, tularemia, rat-bite fever, ecthyma gangrenosum, rickettsialpox, atypical mycobacteria, diptheria
Rapidly progressive respiratory illness with cough, fever, rigors, dyspnea, chest pain, hemoptysis, possible gastrointestinal symptoms, lung consolidation with or without shock	Primary pneumonic plague	Severe community-acquired bacterial or viral pneumonia, inhalational anthrax, inhalational tularemia, pulmonary infarct, pulmonary hemorrhage
Sepsis, disseminated intravascular coagulation, purpura, acral gangrene	Septicemic plague	Meningococcemia; Gram-negative, streptococcal, pneumococcal or staphylococcal bacteremia with shock; overwhelming postsplenectomy sepsis; acute leukemia; Rocky Mountain spotted fever; hemorrhagic smallpox; hemorrhagic varicella (in immunocompromised patients)
Fever, malaise, prostration, headache, myalgias followed by development of synchronous, progressive papular leading to vesicular and then pustular rash on face, mucous membranes (extremities more than the trunk); the rash may become generalized, with a hemorrhagic component and system toxicity	Smallpox	Varicella, drug eruption, Stevens-Johnson syndrome, measles, secondary syphilis, erythema multiforme, severe acne, meningococcemia, monkeypox, generalized vaccinia, insect bites, Coxsackie virus infection, vaccine reaction
Non-specific flu-like illness with pleuropneumonitis; bronchiolitis with or without hilar lymphadenopathy; variable progression to respiratory failure	Inhalational tularemia	Inhalational anthrax, pneumonic plague, influenza, mycoplasma pneumonia, Legionnaire's disease, Q fever, bacterial pneumonia
Acute onset of afebrile, symmetric, descending flaccid paralysis that begins in bulbar muscles; dilated pupils; diplopia or blurred vision; dysphagia; dysarthria; ptosis; dry mucous membranes leading to airway obstruction with respiratory muscle paralysis; clear sensorium and absence of sensory changes	Botulism	Myasthenia gravis, brain stem cerebrovascular accident, polio, Guillain-Barre syndrome variant, tick paralysis, chemical intoxication
Acute-onset fevers, malaise, prostration, myalgias, headache, gastrointestinal symptoms, mucosal hemorrhage, altered vascular permeability, disseminated intravascular coagulation, hypotension leading to shock with or without hepatitis and neurologic findings	Viral hemorrhagic fever	Malaria, meningococcemia, leptospirosis, rickettsial infection, typhoid fever, borrelioses, fulminant hepatitis, hemorrhagic smallpox, acute leukemia, thrombotic thrombocytopenic purpura, hemolytic uremic syndrome, systemic lupus erythematosus

(Artenstein AW, Bioterrorism and Biodefense. In: Cohen J, Powderly WG, eds. Infectious Diseases, second edition. Mosby: London, 2003:99-107) Used with permission.

that shortness of breath, nausea, and vomiting are significantly more common in anthrax, whereas rhinorrhea is uncommonly seen in anthrax but noted in the majority of viral respiratory infections.[17]

Other common clinical manifestations of inhalational anthrax include abdominal pain, headache, mental status abnormalities, and hypoxemia. Abnormalities on chest radiography appear to be universally present, although these may only be identified retrospectively in some cases. Pleural effusions are the most common abnormality; infiltrates, consolidation, and/or mediastinal adenopathy/widening are noted in the majority. The latter is thought to be an early indicator of disease, but computed tomography appears to provide greater sensitivity than chest radiographs for this finding.

The clinical manifestations of inhalational anthrax generally evolve to a fulminant septic picture with progressive respiratory failure. *B. anthracis* is routinely isolated in blood cultures if obtained before the initiation of antimicrobials. Pleural fluid is typically hemorrhagic; the

bacteria can either be isolated in culture or documented by antigen-specific immunohistochemical stains of this material in the majority of patients.[10] In the five fatalities in the U.S. series, the average time from hospitalization until death was 3 days (range, 1 to 5 days), which is consistent with other reports of the clinical virulence of this infection. Autopsy data typically reveal hemorrhagic mediastinal lymphadenitis and disseminated, metastatic infection. Pathology data from the Sverdlovsk outbreak confirm meningeal involvement, typically hemorrhagic meningitis, in 50% of disseminated cases.[18]

The diagnosis of inhalational anthrax should be entertained in the setting of a consistent clinical presentation in the context of a known exposure, a possible exposure, or epidemiologic factors suggesting bioterrorism (e.g., clustered cases of a rapidly progressive illness). The diagnosis should also be considered in a single individual with a consistent or suggestive clinical illness in the absence of another etiology. The early recognition and treatment of inhalational anthrax is likely to be associated with a survival advantage.[10] Therefore, prompt empiric antimicrobial therapy should be initiated if infection is clinically suspected. Combination parenteral therapy is appropriate in the ill person for a number of reasons: to cover the possibility of antimicrobial resistance; to target specific bacterial functions (e.g., the theoretical effect of clindamycin on toxin production); to ensure adequate drug penetration into the central nervous system; and perhaps to favorably affect survival.[10] In the future, it is likely that novel therapies such as toxin inhibitors or receptor antagonists will be available to treat anthrax.[19] Detailed therapeutic and postexposure prophylaxis recommendations for adults, children, and special groups have been recently reviewed elsewhere.[14] Anthrax vaccine adsorbed has been proved to be effective in preventing cutaneous anthrax in human clinical trials and in preventing inhalational disease after aerosol challenge in nonhuman primates.[20] The vaccine has generally been found to be safe but requires six doses over 18 months with the need for frequent boosting. Its availability is currently limited although it is hoped that second-generation anthrax vaccines, currently in clinical trials, will prove effective.

Smallpox

The last known naturally acquired case of smallpox occurred in Somalia in 1977; the disease was officially certified as having been eradicated in 1980, the culmination of a 12-year intensive campaign undertaken by the WHO.[21] However, because of concerns that variola virus stocks may have either been removed from or sequestered outside of their officially designated repositories, smallpox is considered to be a potential agent of bioterrorism. Multiple features make smallpox an attractive biologic weapon and ensure that its reintroduction into human populations would be a global public health catastrophe: it is stable in aerosol form with a low infective dose; case fatality rates are historically high, approaching 30%; secondary attack rates among unvaccinated close contacts are 37% to 88% and are amplified; and much of the world's population is susceptible, as routine civilian vaccination was terminated more than two decades ago, vaccine-induced immunity wanes over time, and there is no virus circulating in the environment to provide low-level booster exposures.[22] Additionally, vaccine supplies are currently limited, although this problem has begun to be addressed, and there are currently no antiviral therapies of proven effectiveness against this pathogen.

After an incubation period of 7 to 17 days (average, 10 to 12 days), the patient experiences the acute onset of a prostrating prodrome of fever, rigors, headache, and backache that may last 2 to 3 days. This is followed by a centrifugally distributed eruption that generalizes as it evolves through macular, papular, vesicular, and pustular stages in synchronous fashion over approximately 8 days, with umbilication in the latter stages. Enanthema in the oropharynx typically precedes the exanthem by a day or two. The rash typically involves the palms and soles early in the course of the disease. The pustules begin crusting during the second week of the eruption;

separation of scabs is usually complete by the end of the third week. The differential diagnosis of smallpox is delineated in Table 63-4. Historically, varicella and drug reactions have posed the most diagnostic dilemmas.[22]

Smallpox is transmitted person to person by respiratory droplet nuclei and, less commonly, by contact with lesions or contaminated fomites. Airborne transmission by fine-particle aerosols has, under certain conditions, been documented.[22] The virus is communicable from the onset of the enanthema until all of the scabs have separated, although patients are thought to be most contagious during the first week of the rash due to high titers of replicating virus in the oropharynx. Household members, other face-to-face contacts, and healthcare workers have traditionally been at highest risk for secondary transmission. Thus, hospitalized cases are placed in negative-pressure rooms with contact and airborne precautions to minimize this risk, and those not requiring hospital-level care should remain isolated at home to avoid infecting others.

The suspicion of a single smallpox case should prompt immediate notification of local public health authorities and the hospital epidemiologist. Containment of smallpox is predicated on the "ring vaccination" strategy, which was successfully deployed in the WHO global eradication campaign and mandates the identification and immunization of all directly exposed persons, including close contacts, healthcare workers, and laboratory personnel. Vaccination, if deployed within 4 days of infection during the early incubation period, can significantly attenuate or prevent disease and may favorably affect secondary transmission.[22] Because the occurrence of even a single case of smallpox would be tantamount to bioterrorism, an epidemiologic investigation would be necessary to ascertain the perimeter of the initial release, so that tracing of initially exposed persons can be accomplished.

Botulism

Botulism, an acute neurologic disease resulting from intoxication with Clostridium botulinum, occurs sporadically and in focal outbreaks throughout the world related to wound contamination by the bacterium or ingestion of foodborne toxin. A detailed discussion of botulism is found in Chapter 132. Aerosol forms of the toxin, a rare mode of acquisition in nature, have been weaponized for use in bioterrorism.[4] Botulinum toxin is considered to be the most toxic molecule known; it is lethal to humans in minute quantities. It blocks the release of the neurotransmitter acetylcholine from presynaptic vesicles, thereby inhibiting muscle contraction.[23]

Botulism presents as an acute, afebrile, symmetric, descending, flaccid paralysis. The disease manifests initially in the bulbar musculature and is unassociated with mental status or sensory changes. Fatigue, dizziness, dysphagia, dysarthria, diplopia, dry mouth, dyspnea, ptosis, ophthalmoparesis, tongue weakness, and facial muscle paresis are early findings seen in more than 75% of cases. Progressive muscular involvement leading to respiratory failure ensues. The clinical presentations of foodborne and inhalational botulism are indistinguishable in experimental animals.[23]

The diagnosis of botulism is largely based on epidemiologic and clinical features and the exclusion of other possibilities (see Table 63-4). Clinicians should recognize that any single case of botulism could be the result of bioterrorism or could herald a larger-scale "natural" outbreak. A large number of epidemiologically unrelated, multifocal cases should be clues to an intentional release of the agent, either in food or water supplies or as an aerosol.

The mortality from foodborne botulism has declined from 60% to 6% over the last four decades, probably as a result of improvements in supportive care and mechanical ventilation. Because the need for the latter may be prolonged, limited resources (e.g., mechanical ventilators) would likely be exceeded in the event of a large-scale bioterrorism event. Treatment with an equine antitoxin, available in limited supply from the CDC, may ameliorate disease if given early.

Plague

Plague, the disease caused by the gram-negative pathogen *Yersinia pestis*, presents in a variety of forms in naturally acquired disease and is extensively covered in Chapter 103. Plague is endemic in parts of Southeast Asia, Africa, and the western United States. Aerosolized preparations of the agent, the expected vehicle in bioterrorism, would be predicted to result in cases of primary pneumonic plague outside of endemic areas. As was the case with the anthrax attacks in the United States in 2001, however, additional forms of the disease such as bubonic and septicemic plague might also occur.

Primary pneumonic plague classically presents as an acute, febrile, pneumonic illness with prominent respiratory and systemic symptoms; gastrointestinal symptoms, purulent sputum production, or hemoptysis occur variably.[24] Chest roentgenogram typically shows patchy, bilateral, multilobar infiltrates or consolidations. In the absence of appropriate treatment there may be rapid progression to respiratory failure, vascular collapse, purpuric skin lesions, necrotic digits, and death. The differential diagnosis, as noted in Table 63-4, is largely that of rapidly progressive pneumonia. The diagnosis may be suggested by the characteristic small gram-negative coccobacillary forms in stained sputum specimens with bipolar uptake ("safety pin") of Giemsa or Wright stain.[25] Culture confirmation is necessary to confirm the diagnosis; the microbiology laboratory should be notified in advance if plague is suspected because special techniques and precautions must be employed.

Treatment recommendations for plague have been reviewed elsewhere.[25] Pneumonic plague can be transmitted from person to person by respiratory droplet nuclei, thus placing close contacts, other patients, and healthcare workers at risk. Prompt recognition and treatment of this disease, appropriate deployment of postexposure prophylaxis, and early institution of droplet precautions will interrupt secondary transmission.

Tularemia

Francisella tularensis, the causative agent of tularemia, is another small gram-negative coccobacillus that would likely cause a primary pneumonic presentation if delivered as an aerosol agent of bioterrorism. Inhalational tularemia presents with the abrupt onset of a febrile, systemic illness with prominent upper respiratory symptoms, pleuritic chest pain, and the variable development of pneumonia, hilar adenopathy, and progression to respiratory failure and death in excess of 30% of those who do not receive appropriate therapy.[26] The diagnosis is generally based on clinical features after other agents are ruled out. Laboratory personnel should be notified in advance if tularemia is suspected because the organism can be very infectious under culture conditions. This agent is discussed in depth in Chapter 104.

Viral Hemorrhagic Fevers

The agents of viral hemorrhagic fevers are members of four distinct families of ribonucleic acid viruses that cause clinical syndromes with overlapping features: fever, malaise, headache, myalgias, prostration, mucosal hemorrhage, and other signs of increased vascular permeability and circulatory dysregulation leading to shock and multiorgan system failure in advanced cases.[27] Specific agents are also associated with specific target organ effects. These pathogens, discussed in detail in Chapters 118 to 121, include the agents of Ebola, Marburg, Lassa fever, Rift Valley fever, and Congo-Crimean hemorrhagic fever.

Hemorrhagic fever viruses have been viewed as emerging infections in nature due to their sporadic occurrence in focal outbreaks throughout the world, and they are thought to be the results of human intrusion into a viral ecologic niche. They are, however, potential weapons of bioterrorism because they are highly infectious in aerosol form, are transmissible in healthcare settings, cause high morbidity and mortality, and are purported to have been successfully weaponized.[8] Blood and other body fluids from infected patients are extremely infectious, and person-to-person airborne transmission may occur; therefore, strict contact and airborne precautions should be instituted in these cases.[27] Treatment is largely supportive and includes the early use of vasopressors as needed. Ribavirin is effective against some forms of viral hemorrhagic fevers but not those caused by Ebola and Marburg viruses. Nonetheless, this drug should be initiated empirically in patients presenting with a syndrome consistent with viral hemorrhagic fever until the etiology is confirmed.

Management of Special Patient Populations

The approach to the management of diseases of bioterrorism must be broadened to include children, pregnant women, and immunocompromised persons. Specific recommendations for treatment and prophylaxis of these special patient groups for selected bioterrorism agents have been recently reviewed.[13,25,26] A general approach requires an assessment of the risk of certain drugs or products in select populations versus the potential risk of the infection in question, accounting for extent of exposure and the agent involved. The issue extends to immunization because certain vaccines, such as smallpox, pose higher risk to these special groups than to others. This will affect mass vaccination strategies.

Psychosocial Morbidity

An often overlooked but vitally important issue in bioterrorism is that of psychosocial sequelae. These may take the form of acute anxiety reactions and exacerbations of chronic psychiatric illness during the stress of the event, or posttraumatic stress disorder (PTSD) in its aftermath. Nearly half of the emergency department visits during the Gulf War missile attacks in Israel in 1991 were related to acute psychological illness or exacerbations of underlying problems.[28] Data from recent acts of terrorism in the United States suggest that PTSD may develop in as many as 35% of those affected by the events.[29] In the early period after the Sept. 11, 2001, attacks in New York, PTSD and depression were nearly twice as prevalent as in historical control subjects.[30] Although close proximity to the events and personal loss were directly correlated with PTSD and depression, respectively, there was a substantial burden of morbidity among those indirectly involved. The psychological impact of these events and of the ongoing international concern over terrorism can be expected to be significant and sustained for society as a whole.

PITFALLS

The response to bioterrorism is unique among weapons of mass destruction because it necessitates the consequence management that is common to all disasters as well as the application of basic infectious diseases principles: disease surveillance, infection control, antimicrobial therapy and prophylaxis, and vaccine prevention. For these reasons, physicians are likely first responders to bioterrorism and are expected to be reliable sources of information for their patients, colleagues, and public health authorities.[31]

There remain a number of potential pitfalls regarding disasters involving a biologic attack that must be identified and managed to optimize the public health. As alluded to above, the clinical latency period between exposure to an agent and the manifestation of signs and symptoms is on the order of days to weeks with most of the CDC category A, B, or C agents, other than with preformed pathogen-derived toxins. For this reason, early diagnoses of the first cases are likely to prove problematic and require heightened clinical vigilance.[32] Even after early victims have been diagnosed, communications among hospitals and other healthcare institutions on a local, regional, national, and international level will be essential to define the epidemiology and possibly to identify exposure sources. Given the extent and ease of rapid movement within our world, clinical presentations from a point-source biologic attack could occur in widely disparate geographic locations. Additionally, it is likely that a terrorist attack would be multifocal in any case. A similar epidemiologic approach using case definitions, case identification, surveillance, and real-time communications is necessary whether the event is a malicious attack, emergent from nature, or unknown.[33]

Other potential pitfalls reside in the arena of diagnostic techniques, treatment, and prevention of disease related to biologic agents. Although an active area of research, the development of field-ready, highly predictive, rapid screening tests for agents of bioterrorism has not, as yet, progressed to the point at which such assays are approved by the U.S. Food and Drug Administration and available for deployment. Treatment and prevention issues, such as the absence of effective treatments for many forms of viral hemorrhagic fevers; shortages in the availability of multivalent anti-toxin for botulism; projected shortages in the availability of mechanical ventilators to manage a large-scale attack using botulism; lack of human data regarding the use of antiviral agents in smallpox; and the unfavorable toxicity profiles of currently available smallpox vaccines remain unresolved but active areas of research. The fact that modern molecular biologic techniques have been used to produce genetically altered pathogens with "designer" phenotypes, such as antimicrobial or vaccine resistance, adds additional layers of complexity to an already complex problem. Finally, as has been vividly illustrated during the recent epidemic of severe acute respiratory syndrome[34] and had been well recognized when epidemic smallpox occurred with regularity,[22] transmission of infection within hospitals is common. Healthcare workers, our first line of defense against an attack using biologic agents, remain at significant occupational risk.

REFERENCES

1. Christopher GW, Cieslak TJ, Pavlin JA, et al. Biological warfare: a historical perspective. *JAMA* 1997;278:412-7.
2. Harris SH. *Factories of Death: Japanese Biological Warfare, 1932-45, and the American Cover-Up.* New York: Routledge; 1994.
3. Torok TJ, Tauxe RV, Wise RP, et al. A large community outbreak of Salmonellosis caused by intentional contamination of restaurant salad bars. *JAMA* 1997;278:389-95.
4. Zilinskas RA. Iraq's biological weapons: the past as future? *JAMA* 1997;278:418-24.
5. World Health Organization. *Health Aspects of Chemical and Biological Weapons: Report of a WHO Group of Consultants.* Geneva: World Health Organization; 1970:98-9.
6. Miller J, Engelberg S, Broad W. *Germs: Biological Weapons and America's Secret War.* New York: Simon and Schuster; 2001.
7. CDC. Biological and chemical terrorism: strategic plan for preparedness and response. *MMWR* 2000;49(RR-4):1-14.
8. Alibek K. *Biohazard.* New York: Random House; 1999.
9. United States Department of State. *Patterns of Global Terrorism 2001.* Washington, DC: U.S. Department of State; May 2002.
10. Jernigan J, Stephens DS, Ashford DA, et al. Bioterrorism-related inhalational anthrax: the first 10 cases reported in the United States. *Emerg Infect Dis.* 2001;7:933-44.
11. Sidell FR, Takafuji ET, Franz DR, eds. *Medical Aspects of Chemical and Biological Warfare. Textbook of Military Medicine series. Part I, Warfare, Weaponry and the Casualty.* Washington, DC: Office of the Surgeon General, Department of the Army; 1997.
12. Dixon TC, Meselson M, Guillemin J, et al. Anthrax. *N Engl J Med.* 1999;341:815-26.
13. Inglesby TV, Henderson DA, Bartlett JG, et al. Anthrax as a biological weapon: medical and public health management. *JAMA* 1999;281:1735-45.
14. Inglesby TV, O'Toole T, Henderson DA, et al. Anthrax as a biological weapon, 2002: updated recommendations for management. *JAMA* 2002;287:2236-52.

15. Freedman A, Afonja O, Chang MW, et al. Cutaneous anthrax associated with microangiopathic hemolytic anemia and coagulopathy in a 7-month-old infant. *JAMA* 2002;287;869-74.

16. Barakat LA, Quentzel HL, Jernigan JA, et al. Fatal inhalational anthrax in a 94-year-old Connecticut woman. *JAMA* 2002;287:863-8.

17. CDC. Considerations for distinguishing influenza-like illness from inhalational anthrax. *MMWR* 2001;50:984-6.

18. Abramova FA, Grinberg LM, Yampolskaya O, et al. Pathology of inhalational anthrax in forty-two cases from the Sverdlovsk outbreak of 1979. *Proc Natl Acad Sci USA*. 1993;90:2291-4.

19. Friedlander AM. Tackling anthrax. *Nature* 2001;414:160-1.

20. Friedlander AM, Pittman PR, Parker GW. Anthrax vaccine: evidence for safety and efficacy against inhalational anthrax. *JAMA* 1999;282:2104-6.

21. Fenner F, Henderson DA, Arita I, et al. *Smallpox and its Eradication*. Geneva: World Health Organization; 1988.

22. Breman JG, Henderson DA. Diagnosis and management of smallpox. *N Engl J Med*. 2002;346:1300-8.

23. Arnon SS, Schechter R, Inglesby TV, et al. Botulinum toxin as a biological weapon: medical and public health management. *JAMA* 2001;285:1059-70.

24. Artenstein AW, Lucey DR. Occupational plague. In: Couturier AJ, ed. *Occupational and Environmental Infectious Diseases*. Beverly, Mass: OEM Press; 2000:329-35.

25. Inglesby TV, Dennis DT, Henderson DA, et al. Plague as a biological weapon: medical and public health management. *JAMA* 2000;283:2281-90.

26. Dennis DT, Inglesby TV, Henderson DA, et al. Tularemia as a biological weapon: medical and public health management. *JAMA* 2001;285:2763-73.

27. Borio L, Inglesby T, Peters CJ, et al. Hemorrhagic fever viruses as biological weapons: medical and public health management. *JAMA* 2002;287:2391-405.

28. Karsenty E, Shemer J, Alshech I, et al. Medical aspects of the Iraqi missile attacks on Israel. *Isr J Med Sci*. 1991;27:603-7.

29. Yehuda R. Post-traumatic stress disorder. *N Engl J Med*. 2002;346:108-14.

30. Galea S, Ahern J, Resnick H, et al. Psychological sequelae of the September 11 terrorist attacks in New York City. *N Engl J Med*. 2002;346:982-7.

31. Artenstein AW, Neill MA, Opal SM. Bioterrorism and physicians. *Ann Intern Med*. 2002;137:626.

32. Artenstein AW. Bioterrorism and biodefense. In: Cohen J, Powderly WG, eds. *Infectious Diseases*. 2nd ed. London: Mosby; 2003:99-107.

33. Artenstein AW, Neill MA, Opal SM. Bioterrorism and physicians. *Med Health RI*. 2002;85:74-7.

34. Svoboda T, Henry B, Shulman L, et al. Public health measures to control the spread of the severe acute respiratory syndrome during the outbreak in Toronto. *N Engl J Med*. 2004;350:2352-61.

chapter 64

Future Biologic and Chemical Weapons*

James M. Madsen and Robert G. Darling

HISTORICAL PERSPECTIVE

Biologic and chemical weapons have been used throughout history.[1] For millennia, indigenous South American peoples deliberately used plant-derived arrow poisons such as curare and toxins from poison dart frogs, although these preparations were used mainly for hunting. Similar toxins were used in Africa. The ancient Greeks, for whom *toxikon* meant "arrow poison," tipped arrows with winter aconite, and this practice continued into medieval Europe and persisted into the seventeenth century in Spain and Portugal.[2] Soldiers in India used smoke screens, incendiary weapons, and toxic fumes as early as 2000 BCE, and the Sung Dynasty in China employed a wide variety of arsenical smokes and other poisons in battle. The military use of toxins dates from at least the sixth century BCE, when Assyrian soldiers poisoned enemy wells with ergot-contaminated rye. In 423 BCE, during the Peloponnesian War, Thracian allies of Sparta captured the Athenian fort at Delium by using a long tube and bellows to blow a poisonous smoke from coals, sulfur, and pitch into the fort. Greek fire (likely composed of rosin, sulfur, pitch, naphtha, lime, and salt-peter) was invented in the seventh century CE and proved to be a very effective naval weapon. Various poisons saw battlefield use during medieval times, and the use of poisons for murder (including assassinations) became widespread. Other examples before the twentieth century include the contamination of water by dumping the corpses of dead humans or animals into wells, the use of snakes and other creatures as poisonous vectors, and occasionally, fomites to transmit infections such as smallpox to unsuspecting victims. This latter technique was used with remarkable success during the French and Indian War (1754-1767), when Sir Jeffrey Amherst was alleged to have given "gifts" (blankets) harboring the pus and scabs from smallpox victims to unsuspecting Native American Indians. The Indians possessed no immunity against smallpox and thus experienced very high rates of infection and mortality as smallpox swept through the local tribes.[3]

During the late nineteenth and early twentieth centuries, the science and technology necessary for the development of sophisticated biologic and chemical weapons proceeded apace. World War I saw the first large-scale use of "poison gas," including lacrimators, chlorine, phosgene, arsenicals, cyanide, and sulfur mustard. By the end of the war, nearly one in every three rounds was a chemical munition. Dr. Shiro Ishii and other Japanese scientists in the infamous Unit 731 worked on the weaponization of anthrax, plague, smallpox, and tetrodotoxin as well as a variety of chemical agents during World War II. There are even suspicions that the bomb used in the assassination of Reinhard Heydrich in Czechoslovakia in 1942 contained botulinum toxin.[4] After World War II, ricin was used as an injectable assassination weapon, and in the 1970s and 1980s T-2 toxin, a trichothecene mycotoxin, was alleged to have been the toxic component of the "yellow rain" employed against H'Mong refugees from Laos. More recently, Iraq and Iran both used chemical weapons against each other in the Iran-Iraq War of the 1980s, and Iraq had a weapons program that included the development of sulfur mustard, nerve agents, "Agent 15" (an anticholinergic incapacitating agent), botulinum toxin, epsilon toxin from *Clostridium perfringens*, and aflatoxin.[5] Militia groups in the United States and terrorist groups throughout the world have used ricin for political purposes.

American scientists started developing chemical weapons as a response to the use of chemical warfare in Europe during World War I and conducted both offensive and defensive research on biologic and chemical weapons. However, in 1969, the United States unilaterally renounced the first use of chemical agents, halted chemical-agent production, and terminated its offensive biologic weapons program.

In 1972, the Biological Weapons and Toxins Convention was created; it was signed by representatives from 104 nations, including the United States (which ratified the Convention in 1975), the Soviet Union, and Iraq, although many signatories did not consider toxins to be biologic weapons and did not consider the treaty binding on toxin use. Since that time, at least 140 nations have either signed or ratified this treaty.[6] However, the

---

*The views expressed in this article are those of the author and do not necessarily reflect the official policy or position of the U.S. Army, U.S. Navy, any other U.S. military organization, or any of the places where Dr. Darling works, or any governmental organization.

Soviet Union and Iraq began violating the treaty in short order. In the Soviet Union, weapons scientists stepped up research and development of numerous biologic and chemical weapons as part of one of the largest and most comprehensive biologic-weapons programs in history. Soviet scientists created large stockpiles of weaponized anthrax, plague, smallpox, tularemia, nerve agent, mustard, and other biologic and chemical agents.[5]

In 1979, the world was put on notice of the devastating potential that biologic weapons pose to humanity. In that year, a small quantity of weapons-grade anthrax was accidentally released from a manufacturing plant located in the former city of Sverdlovsk (now Yekaterinburg) in Russia. Seventy-seven cases and 66 deaths were reported. Dr. Matthew Meselson, a Harvard scientist, was permitted to study the event many years later and reported the results of his work in a 1979 *Science* article. Meselson determined that the majority of the deaths had occurred among victims living in a narrow 4-km-wide band downwind from the plant. Animal deaths were confirmed as far as 30 km downwind. Meselson further concluded that less than 1 g of weapons-grade anthrax had been released from the plant.[7] If his calculations are accurate, weaponized anthrax possesses staggering potential as a biologic weapon given its stability, its relative ease of production, and its ability to be dispersed in a clandestine manner over great distances.

In March 1995, after having unsuccessfully attempted to deploy biologic agents, members of the Aum Shinri Kyo cult executed a coordinated attack with the nerve agent sarin (GB) on the Tokyo subway system. Over 5500 people sought medical treatment, and a dozen died. The Aum Shinri Kyo had used sarin in Matsumoto 9 months earlier in an attack that had exposed more than 300 people and had killed 7 in an attempt to assassinate judges unfavorable to their cause.[8,9]

The anthrax attacks in the fall of 2001 involved the use of letters containing weapons-grade anthrax mailed through the U.S. postal system. Five people died and 17 became ill with either cutaneous or inhalational anthrax. Buildings contaminated with spores included the Hart Senate Office building and the Brentwood postal facilities in Washington, DC. It cost millions of dollars to rehabilitate these buildings. The anthrax used in the attacks was determined to be extremely potent and could have caused far greater numbers of casualties had it been dispersed more widely.[10,11]

According to Dr. Ken Alibek, former Deputy Director of Biopreparat, the Soviet Union's nominally civilian medical research institute, Soviet scientists and physicians spent large sums of money and manpower during the 1980s and 1990s developing the most lethal and potent biologic weapons known to man. In addition to weaponizing the etiologic agents of anthrax, smallpox, Marburg fever, and others, they created antibiotic-resistant strains of *Yersinia pestis* (plague), *Francisella tularensis*, and other pathogens. Furthermore, by applying genetic engineering techniques, the Soviets are also alleged to have created pathogens with novel characteristics and strains of several organisms capable of defeating certain vaccines.[12]

As we enter the biotechnologic revolution of the twenty-first century, our understanding of molecular biology, genetics, and biochemistry is exploding. The human genome has been sequenced, and it is now possible to manipulate genes from disparate organisms to create new and novel pathogens. Scientists are also able to synthesize and weaponize a number of different endogenous biologic-response modifiers including cytokines, hormones, neurotransmitters, and plasma proteases. But even nature continues to surprise us. New, naturally occurring infections with the potential to cause large-scale human diseases and death continue to emerge at an ever-increasing rate throughout the world, and it is conceivable that these pathogens could also be weaponized by enterprising scientists.

This chapter briefly reviews the future of chemical and biologic weapons as we enter this new era of explosive growth in our understanding of the life sciences. We are presented with an extraordinary opportunity to solve a host of human afflictions or to create new classes of biologic and chemical weapons that have the capacity to destroy our civilization as we know it today.

FUTURE BIOLOGIC WEAPONS

The appearance of a new or reemerging infectious disease has global implications. During the past 20 years, over 30 new lethal pathogens have been identified.[13] A classic example of this emerging threat is pandemic influenza. In 1918, as World War I was coming to an end, the Spanish flu struck with devastating consequences. In less than 1 year, this virus was able to circumnavigate the globe and kill an estimated 40 million people.[14] More recently, the emergence of severe acute respiratory syndrome (SARS) in Southeast Asia resulted from a coronavirus that jumped species from animals to humans and rapidly spread to 29 countries in less than 90 days. Novel and dormant infectious agents such as SARS or influenza appear to be emerging or reemerging with increasing frequency and with greater potential for serious consequences. Many factors contribute to the emergence of new diseases: environmental changes, global travel and trade, social upheaval, and genetic changes in infectious agent, host, or vector populations. Once a new disease is introduced into a suitable human population, it often spreads rapidly and with devastating impact on the medical and public health infrastructure. If the disease is severe, it may lead to social disruption and have a profound economic impact. Outbreaks of emerging or reemerging diseases may be difficult to distinguish from outbreaks as a result of intentional introduction of infectious diseases for nefarious purposes.

As scientists develop more sophisticated laboratory procedures and increase their understanding of molecular biology and the genetic code, the possibility of bioengineering more virulent, antibiotic, and vaccine-resistant pathogens for military or terrorist uses becomes increasingly likely. It is already theoretically possible to synthesize and weaponize certain biologic response modifiers (BRMs) as well as to engineer genomic weapons capable of inserting novel DNA into host cells.

The potential to cause widespread disease and death with any of these weapons is incalculable and concerning. Scientists and policy makers have begun to address the issue with a robust research agenda to develop medical countermeasures.

Selected Emerging and Reemerging Infections with Weaponization Potential

Because emerging diseases are so diverse and endemic to different geographic locations, their complete description is beyond the scope of this chapter. However, some of these infections may become future threats as agents of biologic warfare or terrorism. The most worrisome emerging infectious disease may well be the one we don't know about. Recent experience with HIV, Ebola fever, SARS, monkeypox, West Nile fever, and hundreds of other "new" diseases reveal that we will continue to be surprised.

Avian Influenza

Avian influenza, or highly pathogenic avian influenza, has periodically caused human infections primarily through close contact with avian species, most often through occupational contact at chicken or duck farms in Southeast Asia. As of May 2004, a large outbreak of avian influenza involving the H5N1 strain and human cases has been reported in two countries from this region.[15] Thus far, no human-to-human transmission has been reported, but the potential exists for genetic reassortment between avian and human or animal strains of influenza. A recent report in the journal *Science* linked the influenza virus responsible for the 1918 epidemic to a possible avian origin.[16] If true, avian influenza may pose a much greater danger to human populations than previously reported. The disease presents in humans in a fashion similar to other types of influenza viruses. It usually begins with fever, chills, headaches, and myalgias and often involves the upper and lower respiratory tract with development of cough, dyspnea, and in severe cases, acute respiratory distress syndrome. Laboratory findings may include pancytopenia, lymphopenia, elevated liver enzymes, hypoxia, a positive reverse transcriptase-polymerase chain reaction test for H5N1, and a positive neutralization assay for H5N1 influenza strain. In vitro studies suggest that the neuraminidase (NA)-inhibitor class of drugs may have clinical efficacy in the treatment and prevention of avian influenza infection.[17]

Human Influenza

The threat for pandemic spread of human influenza viruses is substantial. The pathogenicity of human influenza viruses is directly related to their ability to alter their eight viral RNA segments rapidly; the new antigenic variation results in the formation of new hemagglutinin (HA) and NA surface glycoproteins, which may go unrecognized by an immune system primed against heterologous strains.

Two distinct phenomena contribute to a renewed susceptibility to influenza infection among persons who have had influenza illness in the past. Clinically significant variants of influenza A viruses may result from mutations occurring in the HA and NA genes and expressed as minor structural changes in viral surface proteins. As few as four amino acid substitutions in any two antigenic sites can cause such a clinically significant variation. These minor changes result in an altered virus able to circumvent host immunity. Additionally, genetic reassortment between avian and human or avian and porcine influenza viruses may lead to the major changes in HA or NA surface proteins known as *antigenic shift*. In contrast to the gradual evolution of strains subject to antigenic *drift*, antigenic shift occurs when an influenza virus with a completely novel HA or NA formation moves into humans from other host species. Global pandemics result from such antigenic shifts.

Influenza causes in excess of 30,000 deaths and over 100,000 hospitalizations annually in the United States. Pandemic influenza viruses have emerged regularly in 10- to 50-year cycles for the last several centuries. During the last century, influenza pandemics occurred three times: in 1918 ("Spanish influenza," a H1N1 virus), in 1957 (Asian influenza, a H2N2 subtype strain), and in 1968 (Hong Kong influenza, a H3N2 variant). The 1957-1958 pandemic caused 66,000 excess deaths, and the 1968 pandemic caused 34,000 excess deaths in the United States. The 1918 influenza pandemic illustrates a worst-case public health scenario; it caused 675,000 deaths in the United States and 20 to 40 million deaths worldwide.[16] Morbidity in most communities was between 25% and 40%, and the case-mortality rate averaged 2.5%. A reemergent 1918-like influenza virus would have tremendous societal effects, even in the event that antiviral medications were effective against this more lethal influenza virus.

SARS and SARS-associated Coronavirus

SARS-associated coronavirus (SARS-CoV) emerged as the cause of SARS during 2003. That year, SARS was responsible for approximately 900 deaths and over 8000 infections in people from at least 29 countries worldwide. Before a case definition had been clearly established, Chinese authorities reported to the World Health Organization (WHO) over 300 cases of an atypical pneumonia with five related deaths, all originated from Guangdong province in China during February 2003. The infection quickly spread as infected patients traveled to Hong Kong and from there to Vietnam, Canada, and other locations. Only eight laboratory-confirmed cases occurred in the United States, but there is concern that the U.S. population is vulnerable to a widespread outbreak of SARS such as the one that occurred in China, Hong Kong, Singapore, Toronto, and Taiwan in 2003.[18]

A SARS case definition evolved from this initial report to the WHO by Chinese health authorities in February 2003. A case was initially defined by clinical criteria; a suspected or probable case was defined as an illness that included potential exposure to an existing case and fever with pneumonia or respiratory distress syndrome. In April 2003, a confirmed case was defined as a case from which SARS-CoV was isolated from culture.[19] SARS-CoV infections have an incubation period of 2 to 10 days. Systemic symptoms such as fever and chills followed by a dry cough and shortness of breath begin within 2 to 7 days. Patients may develop pneumonia and lymphopenia by days 7 to 10 of the illness. Most patients with SARS-CoV have a clear history of exposure either to a patient with SARS or to a setting in which SARS-CoV is known to exist. Laboratory tests may be helpful but do not reliably detect infection early during the illness. SARS-CoV should be suspected in patients requiring hospitalization for radiographically confirmed pneumonia or acute respiratory distress syndrome of unknown etiology and one of the following risk factors during the 10 days prior to the onset of illness: (1) travel to China, Hong Kong, or Taiwan, or close contact with an ill person having a history of such travel; (2) employment in an occupation associated with a risk for SARS-CoV exposure; or (3) inclusion in a cluster of cases of atypical pneumonia without an alternative diagnosis.

A "respiratory hygiene/cough etiquette" strategy should be adopted in all SARS-affected healthcare facilities. All patients admitted to the hospital with suspected pneumonia should receive the following measures: (1) They should placed in droplet isolation until it is determined that isolation is no longer indicated (standard precautions are appropriate for most community-acquired pneumonias; droplet precautions for non-avian influenza); (2) they should be screened for risk factors of possible exposure to SARS-CoV; and (3) they should be evaluated with a chest radiograph, pulse oximetry, complete blood count, and additional workup as indicated. If the patient has a risk factor for SARS, droplet precautions should be implemented pending an etiologic diagnosis. When there is a high index of suspicion for SARS-CoV disease, the patient should be treated in terms of SARS isolation precautions immediately (including airborne precautions), and all contacts of the ill patient should be identified, evaluated, and monitored.[19] Although ribavirin, high-dose corticosteroids, and interferons have been used in treatment, it is unclear what effect they have had on clinical outcome. No definitive therapy has been established. Empiric antibiotic treatment for community-acquired pneumonia by the current American Thoracic Society/Infectious Diseases Society of America guidelines is recommended pending etiologic diagnosis. Diagnostic tests for SARS-CoV include antibody testing using an enzyme immunoassay and reverse transcriptase-polymerase chain reaction tests for respiratory, blood, and stool specimens.[20] In the absence of known SARS-CoV transmission, testing is recommended only in consultation with public health authorities. Testing for influenza, respiratory syncytial virus, pneumococcus, chlamydia, mycoplasma, and legionella should be conducted, since the identification of one of these agents excludes SARS by case definition. Clinical samples can be obtained during the first week of illness with a nasopharyngeal swab plus an oropharyngeal swab and a serum or a plasma specimen. After the first week of illness, a nasopharyngeal swab plus an oropharyngeal swab and a stool specimen should be obtained. Serum specimens for SARS-CoV antibody testing should be collected when the diagnosis is first suspected and at later times as

indicated. An antibody response can occasionally be detected during the first week of illness, is likely to be detected by the end of the second week of illness, and at times may not be detected until more than 28 days after the onset of symptoms. Respiratory specimens from any of several different sources may be collected for viral and bacterial diagnostics, but the preferred specimens of choice are nasopharyngeal washes or aspirates.[20]

Nipah and Hendra Viruses

The Nipah and Hendra viruses are closely related but distinct paramyxoviruses that compose a new genus within the family Paramyxoviridae. The Nipah virus was discovered in Malaysia in 1999 during an outbreak of a zoonotic infection, now called *Nipah virus encephalitis,* involving mostly pigs and some human cases.[21] Hendra, the causative agent of Hendra virus disease, was identified in a similar outbreak involving a single infected horse and three human cases in Southern Australia in 1994.[22] It is believed certain species of fruit bats are the natural hosts for these viruses and remain asymptomatic. Horses and pigs act as amplifying hosts for the Hendra and Nipah viruses, respectively. The mode of transmission from animal to humans appears to require direct contact with tissues or body fluids or with aerosols generated during butchering or culling. Personal protective equipment including gowns, gloves, and respiratory and eye protection is advised for agricultural workers culling infected animal herds. Thus far, human-to-human transmission of these viruses has not been reported.

In symptomatic cases, the onset of disease begins with flu-like symptoms and rapidly progresses to encephalitis with disorientation, delirium, and coma. Fifty percent of those with clinically apparent infections have died from their disease. There is currently no approved treatment for these infections, and therefore, therapy relies heavily on supportive care. The antiviral drug ribavirin has been used in past infections, but its effectiveness remains unproven in clinically controlled studies.[23] Although no person-to-person transmission is known to have occurred, barrier nursing and droplet precautions are recommended because respiratory secretions and other bodily fluids are known to harbor the virus. The clinical laboratory should be notified before specimens are sent because these may pose a laboratory hazard. Specimens for viral isolation and identification should be forwarded to a reference laboratory. Requests for testing should come through public health departments, which should contact the Centers for Disease Control and Prevention (CDC) Emergency Operations Center at 770-488-7100 before sending specimens.

Biologic Response Modifiers

BRMs direct the myriad complex interactions of the immune system. BRMs include erythropoietins, interferons, interleukins, colony-stimulating factors, granulocyte and macrophage colony-stimulating factors, stem-cell growth factors, monoclonal antibodies, tumor-necrosis-factor inhibitors, and vaccines.[24]

A growing understanding of the structure and function of BRMs is driving the discovery and creation of many novel compounds including synthetic analgesics, antioxidants, and antiviral and antibacterial substances. For example, BRMs are being used to treat debilitating rheumatoid arthritis by targeting cytokines that contribute to the disease process.[25] By neutralizing or eliminating these targeted cytokines, BRMs may reduce symptoms and decrease inflammation. BRMs may also be used as anticarcinogens, with the following goals: (1) to stop, control, or suppress processes that permit cancer growth, (2) to make cancer cells more recognizable, and therefore more susceptible, to destruction by the immune system, (3) to boost the killing power of immune system cells, such as T cells, natural killer cells, and macrophages, (4) to alter growth patterns in cancer cells to promote behavior like that of healthy cells, (5) to block or reverse the processes that change a normal cell or a precancerous cell into a cancerous cell, (6) to enhance the ability of the body to repair or replace normal cells damaged or destroyed by other forms of cancer treatment, such as chemotherapy or radiation, and (7) to prevent cancer cells from spreading to other parts of the body.[26,27]

More of these promising new drugs are currently in development. It can be readily theorized that research to develop various BRMs can be subverted to a malicious end. That is, instead of using BRMs to suppress cancer growth or to decrease disease susceptibility, researchers could develop compounds to cause illness and death. Other drugs could be designed to alter certain metabolic processes or to alter brain chemistry to affect cognition or mood. The opportunity for mischief is limited only by the imagination of the person with ill intent.

Bioengineered Pathogens

The rapid advance of biotechnology has the potential to alter the present and future threat of biologic weapons. Already, complete or partial genomic sequence data for many of the most lethal human pathogens (such as anthrax, plague, and the smallpox virus) have been published and are widely available via the Internet.[28] In addition to the enormous explosion in our knowledge of human pathogens, there is a parallel increased understanding of the complexities of the human immune response to foreign agents and toxins. Such knowledge has led to a deeper understanding of the development of basic immunity to a variety of different human infectious diseases. With this increase in scientific knowledge has come the power to manipulate the immune system at its most fundamental level. As we prepare for future threats, we must not ignore the potential quantum leap that biotechnology offers our enemies in developing new biologic-warfare threats. In fact, there is mounting evidence that new biologic agents have already been produced by former adversaries. Examples of such new threat agents and the potential effects they might have on human subjects have been detailed in the scientific and popular literature. Examples of biologic threats that could be produced through the use of genetic engineering technology include the following: (1) microorgan-

isms resistant to antibiotics, standard vaccines, and therapeutics, (2) innocuous microorganisms genetically altered to produce a toxin, a poisonous substance, or an endogenous bioregulator, (3) microorganisms possessing enhanced aerosol and environmental stability characteristics, (4) immunologically altered microorganisms able to defeat standard threat identification and diagnostic methods, (5) genetic vectors capable of transferring human and foreign genes into human cells for therapeutic purposes,[28] and (6) combinations of these with improved delivery systems.

POTENTIAL FUTURE CHEMICAL WEAPONS

Nature of the Problem

The threats associated with the use of chemical weapons as battlefield or terrorist weapons are not easy to assess.[29,30] Risk assessment of use must take into account national laws, international treaties and conventions, and the likelihood of adherence to these legal obligations. Loopholes in existing agreements can be exploited to develop weapons that are technically not proscribed by international law. Goals and objectives may vary depending on whether military use is planned at the strategic, tactical, or operational level and whether the developer is a national government, a breakaway republic, a kidnapped or recruited scientist, or a terrorist cell. Risk of use may also differ depending on whether the targets are military versus civilian, human versus nonhuman (animals or plants, including livestock and crops), or individual (as in assassinations) versus large groups, and depending on whether the aim is death versus incapacitation. Risk also depends on agent availability and on the technology available for production, storage, and dissemination; current advances in technology are associated with a higher risk of weaponization. The fallibility of intelligence can be illustrated by two examples from the twentieth century and one from the twenty-first:

1. During most of World War II, the Allied perception of risk from possible chemical-agent use by Axis powers focused on those agents, primarily pulmonary agents and vesicants, known from World War I. In fact, Germany had developed a new kind of chemical-warfare agent, the compounds later to be called G-series nerve agents. Their existence came as a complete surprise to Western governments when, in the waning days of the European campaign, Allied soldiers advancing into Germany discovered buried nerve-agent munitions and entire nerve-agent factories. Why these agents were never used on the battlefield is a topic of much speculation, but in retrospect they clearly posed the most lethal, yet unrecognized, threat from Germany.[31]

2. Assessment of the chemical threat posed by Saddam Hussein at the time of the Gulf War of 1991 centered on the known Iraqi use of sulfur mustard and nerve agents during the Iran-Iraq War in the 1980s. It was not until 1998 that Reuters News Agency reported the

discovery by British intelligence that Iraq had stockpiled large quantities of a "mental incapacitant" (incapacitating agent) known as Agent 15.[32]

3. The risk of use of chemical agents by Iraq after 2001 was assessed to be high partly because of the known stockpiles of sulfur mustard and nerve agents (as well as the suspected stockpiles of cyanide and the new revelations about Agent 15) from the time of the 1991 Gulf War. Although a full accounting has yet to be made, allegations have been made that most of the Iraqi chemical stockpile was actually destroyed in 1991 or soon afterward and that the risk of their use was actually very low. Whether those reports are true does not invalidate the argument that the risk from these agents was still very much debatable.

Chemical agents originally used during World War I are sometimes considered obsolete, especially in comparison to the more potent nerve agents and incapacitating agents. However, agent potency is only one part of the story. To deliver the 10 μg that represents a lethal dose for half of an exposed group (LD_{50}) of the nerve agent VX would seem to be easier than delivering the 3 to 7 g that constitute the LD_{50} of sulfur mustard and more difficult than delivering the much smaller lethal doses of toxins such as botulinum toxin. In fact, sulfur mustard is easier to synthesize than is nerve agent and is easy to disseminate in a clandestine manner to create delayed effects. Thus, mustard still lays claim to being the "King of Gases," and it has allegedly been used in a variety of venues since the end of World War II. Most known chemicals with toxicities equal to or greater than that of ammonia could theoretically be used as chemical-warfare or terrorism agents.

Existing Agents and Their Potential for Future Use

Existing chemicals capable of weaponization for military or terrorist use include the following:

1. Battlefield and riot-control agents
   a. Pulmonary agents (see Chapter 93)
   b. Vesicants (see Chapter 92)
   c. Cyanide (see Chapter 94)
   d. Nerve agents (see Chapter 91)
   e. Antimuscarinic agents such as BZ and Agent 15 (see Chapter 95)
   f. Riot-control agents (see Chapter 98)
   g. Defoliants and other herbicides
   h. Novichok
   i. New chemicals employed for physicochemical effects
2. Related compounds
   a. Battlefield incendiary agents, smokes (including standard military white obscurant smoke, or HC smoke), and other combustion products such as oxides of nitrogen and perfluoroisobutylene (PFIB)
   b. Opioids (see Chapter 97) and other anesthetic agents (see Chapter 100)
   c. Cholinergic agents (see Chapter 99)
   d. Psychedelic indoles and other hallucinogens (see Chapter 96)

3. Toxic industrial chemicals or materials (see Chapter 90)
4. Poisons
5. Toxins (see Chapters 131-137)
6. Combination of chemicals

Existing chemicals remain candidate agents for future use. Some compounds not developed to cause injury or incapacitation nevertheless can be very dangerous; HC smoke, for example, can cause the same type of pulmonary damage induced by phosgene. The CDC lists nearly 70 separate chemicals, including a variety of toxic industrial chemicals and poisons, as potential agents for terrorism. These include osmium tetroxide, long-acting anticoagulants, heavy metals, toxic alcohols, and white phosphorus.[33] A recent issue of the *Morbidity and Mortality Report* includes an even longer list.[34] Pyrolysis products from explosions and conflagrations may release large quantities of cyanide and other toxicants that, although different from the original chemicals present, may still cause death. Industrial chemicals are readily available in large quantities as preformed compounds and should be considered high on the list of potential terrorist agents.[35,36] Toxins, which are chemicals produced within biologic organisms, also represent high-threat agents.[37] New chemicals are currently being synthesized on rigid three-dimensional molecular skeletons, the most promising of which are the norbornanes. Building on norbornane geometry allows for a modular enhancement of the number of functional sites on a given molecule. Since many norbornane derivatives, such as the mixture of chlorobornanes known as the toxaphenes, are persistent and have significant acute and chronic toxicity, these derivatives have been considered potential candidates for new agents.[38]

Novichok[39-42] (Russian for "newcomer") refers to the alleged Russian development of a highly toxic binary nerve agent or generation of nerve agents (sometimes called "fourth-generation" agents). Only sketchy and unverifiable information is available in the unclassified literature, but the existence of these agents would demonstrate the possibility of creating new chemical compounds toxic enough to be used as chemical-warfare or terrorist agents. So-called GV analogs combining some of the properties of G-series and V-series nerve agents have also been suggested as potential new agents.[38] The use in 2002 of an incapacitating gas (thought to be an opioid compound derived from fentanyl and possibly mixed with another anesthetic agent) in the siege of a Moscow theater taken over by Chechen rebels was evidence either of the deployment of a preexisting anesthetic agent or of a new anesthetic compound.[43,44] Organofluorines have been investigated because of their reported ability to defeat protective-mask or chemical-filtrations systems.[38] Other incapacitating agents under development exert primarily physical rather than chemical effects and include immobilizing agents ("stickums"), antitraction gels ("slickums"), and malodorants.[45]

Technologic Modifications of Battlefield Chemical Agents and Delivery Systems

Ways in which existing or future battlefield chemical agents and delivery systems could be modified to improve performance must be considered. These modifications include the following:

1. Agent thickening
2. Binarization
3. Micronization: "dusty agents"
4. Developments in delivery systems
   a. Dual-use cyberinsects and biorobots
   b. Nanotechnology

Small quantities of thickening agents, such as acrylates, can be added to chemical agents to increase their viscosity. Thickened agents are more persistent in the environment and in wounds than are nonthickened agents, and they are less easily decontaminated.[46] Although no nation is currently known to stockpile thickened agents, the technology for their production is relatively simple and requires only standard chemical-warfare agents and the right proportion of a thickener.[38a,38b,47] Many industrial chemicals and other poisons could theoretically be rendered more effective as battlefield or terrorist agents by thickening.

In the 1950s, the U.S. Army began to investigate the then-new technology of binarization, although production did not accelerate until the 1960s and deployment was not widespread until the 1980s.[39] A binary chemical weapon did not employ a new kind of agent but rather represented a novel way of producing and storing an already existing type of agent. The idea was to make storage of chemical rounds safer by stopping the production process at the penultimate synthetic step, resulting in two precursor compounds that when mixed would create the desired agent. These two precursors could then be stored separately. Just prior to use, one component could be inserted into a round, where it would be separated from the other precursor by a thin membrane. The impact and momentum of the launch of the projectile would burst the membrane to allow for mixing of the components and in-flight production of the chemical agent. In practice, this process was often not complete, but the 20% or so of ancillary reaction product was often extremely toxic by itself. Binarization or some similar production-arrest method could theoretically be used by a clandestine terrorist cell to help evade detection and to decrease the risks associated with the production, transportation, and use of chemical agents.

Micronization is a type of particularization involving the production of extremely fine particles onto which a chemical agent can be adsorbed. During World War II, Germany explored particularization of sulfur mustard onto small carrier particles of silica (silicon dioxide), although other powdered silicates (talc, diatomite, and pumice) and clays (kaolinite and Fuller's earth) can also be used.[48] The advantages of such "dusty agents" are increased volatility (used to facilitate the movement of relatively nonvolatile agents such as sulfur mustard and the persistent nerve agent VX into the alveoli) and increased penetration of clothing and chemical protective equipment.[49] Iraq used a "dusty mustard" composed of 65% sulfur mustard adsorbed onto silica particles ranging in diameter from 0.1 to 10 microns during its war with Iran. Micronization of a variety of chemical, biologic, and toxin agents requires a certain degree of technologic sophistication that is becoming increasingly easy to acquire.

Agent delivery can potentially be modified in a variety of ways in addition to thickening and micronization. The Jordanian government released a report in 2004 of the discovery of an elaborate plot by Al Qaeda terrorists for a two-stage attack using a massive vehicle-borne improvised explosive device followed by the release of toxic chemicals to include acetones, nitric acid, and sulfuric acid.[50] Similarly, enhanced-fragmentation munitions could be used in combination with chemical agents to drive the agents more effectively into the body.

Innovative new delivery systems taking advantage of advances in robotics include the proposed use of cyberinsects and biorobots to deliver biologic agents, chemical agents, or toxins.[51] Engineering on an even smaller scale is the purview of nanotechnology, also called "micromechanical engineering" and "microelectromechanical systems."[52] Nanotechnology takes advantage of the unique properties of materials on the scale of about a nanometer (10^{-9} meter)[53] and deals with the molecule-by-molecule or even atom-by-atom assembly of materials. Nanoparticles behave in unusual and unpredictable ways, are small enough to enter cells easily, and in fact are being developed to provide not only better storage and dispersal of pharmaceutical products but also more efficient transport of both biologic organisms (such as viruses) and chemical compounds into the body.[52] In some cases they may be surprisingly toxic, partly because of the ease with which they can cross membranes (including the blood-brain barrier) and enter cells.[54] This toxicity could be exploited by governments or terrorist organizations interested not only in small-particle delivery of chemical agents but also in the ancillary and perhaps synergistic effects of the carrier materials themselves.

Nanomaterials can be encapsulation compounds such as *fullerenes*, or buckyballs, which are hollow 60-carbon geodesic shells; *nanoshells* (for example, a gold shell surrounding an inert silica core); a "self-assembled, polyamino acid nanoparticles system" under development in France; or *dendrimers*, which are onion-like layers of shells surrounding a biologically active core.[53] Any of these materials could be used to deliver existing or new chemical agents. Other nanomaterials include self-assembling liquids composed of cylindrical nanofibers (each 6 to 8 nm in diameter) that solidify upon injection to form structured scaffolds capable of presenting ordered peptide signals to cells. A *ferrofluid* such as a colloidal suspension of nanoscale ferrous oxide can be coupled with antibodies in a laboratory to detect and concentrate rare human cells in a diagnostic setting, but this technology could easily be adapted to target those cells in vivo. *Quantum dots* are nanoscale semiconductor crystals that show promise in the in vitro and in vivo diagnosis of a variety of conditions; although their main use is projected to be in the laboratory, animal experimentation involving injected quantum dots has demonstrated successful targeting of lymph nodes and of prostate-cancer xenografts in mice.

Adverse health effects from any of these kinds of nanoparticles could represent a primary goal for military or terrorist operatives in addition to the toxicity of any other chemicals delivered by the nanoparticles. Water-soluble fullerenes have caused brain damage in large-mouth bass,[55] dendrimers can cause osmotic and membrane damage and can activate the clotting and complement systems, and quantum dots composed of selenium, lead, and cadmium can release those metals into cells, depending on the composition of the surface coating of the dots.[53]

"Designer" Chemicals from Biotechnologic Processes

Biotechnology refers to "any technological application that uses biological systems, living organisms, or derivatives thereof, to make or modify products or processes for specific use."[56] Biotechnology includes such time-honored practices as the baking of bread and the brewing of beer, but in the twenty-first century refers in particular to genetic engineering, that is, the artificial transfer of genes from one organism to another and the consequent alteration of the genetic structure of a cell.[57] It is founded on the basic sciences of genomics (the study of the genetic composition of an organism) and proteomics (the study of the expression of the genome by means of protein synthesis). "Designer" chemicals could be produced from biotechnologic processes. These processes include the following: (1) combinatorial chemistry and ligand modification, (2) genomics and target identification, (3) microarrays, proteomics, and rational agent design, and (4) toxicogenomics, database mining, and the prediction of toxicity.[58]

Combinatorial chemistry is the production of complex sets, or so-called libraries, of related compounds, as in the case of the norbornane derivatives previously described. Automated screening techniques to select for library elements with desired toxic effects on specified target organs can process several hundred thousand compounds a day against several dozen different proteins. This obviously accelerates tremendously the development of new chemical agents.

Genomics has benefited enormously from three modern scientific efforts: the Human Genome Project, the Human Genome Diversity Project, and gene therapy.[59] Identification and cataloging of hundreds of single-nucleotide polymorphisms (individual sequence variations) allows for the selection of genomic sequences to be mass-produced for insertion into cells for the creation of a specific effect. Targeting unusual sequences of high prevalence in certain populations raises the specter of genomic, or ethnic, weapons, as previously described. Less appreciated is the potential for genomics to be used to develop drugs, chemical or toxin agents that can also be targeted to specific variants within a population of humans, animals, or crops. The widespread availability of genome libraries on the Internet makes it nearly impossible to control or restrict access to the already published genomic libraries on over a hundred microbial pathogens.[60]

Proteomics complements genomics by characterizing the protein expression of segments of the genome and by making it easier to develop compounds that target or produce a specific protein. Direct gene insertion, genetic delivery via virus or bacteria, or drug tailoring to affect a given protein can all be used. A scorpion toxin has already been successfully engineered into a virus that acts as a pesticide against caterpillars. Protein sequences in toxins are partly responsible for resistance to light, oxygen, moisture, and desiccation; the insertion of genes to create altered proteins or the introduction of chemical agents engineered to cause structural changes in expressed proteins could significantly alter the toxicity of a given compound.[58] Furthermore, the widespread use of DNA microarrays (glass slides or chips imprinted with thousands of specific single-stranded DNA sequences) allows for fast automated screening of candidate compounds.

Scientists involved in the selection and evaluation of specific chemical agents can now use toxicogenomics (the study of genetic variation of response to toxins) and data mining (the computerized analysis of databases of drug and chemical information via sophisticated neural nets) as tools to eliminate less likely candidates and to algorithmically predict compounds with high toxicity or with other desired characteristics relating to environmental persistence, toxicokinetics (absorption, distribution, biotransformation, and elimination), and toxicodynamics (mechanism of action). Such tools will undoubtedly lead to the development not only of new pharmaceutical agents but also of designer toxins for military or terrorist use.[58]

CONCLUSIONS

If history is any guide, new biologic and chemical weapons and novel "mid-spectrum" agents (e.g., toxins, bioregulators, synthetic viruses, and genocidal weapons) will be developed in the future, and new modifications will be found to improve the production, weaponization, storage, delivery, and action of existing agents.[61] Naturally occurring emerging infectious diseases provide examples of newly identified pathogens with weaponization potential, and mid-spectrum agents such as toxins and bioregulators will undoubtedly assume more prominence with the accelerating pace of nanotechnology (for improved delivery and for synergistic toxicity) and biotechnology. Agents of any category can theoretically be engineered to target specific genes or proteins with differential population prevalence to produce genomic or ethnic weapons; and advances in proteomics, toxicogenomics, and computerized database mining could be used for the rapid and efficient development of not only new drugs but also new chemical agents for terrorism.[62] Biotechnology has now advanced to the point that no special equipment is required beyond that available to any modern molecular-biology laboratory, and the scale of operations is also well within the means of governments and terrorist groups.[59] The threats from future modification of existing agents and from the development of new agents, new agent-development technologies, and innovative delivery systems should not and must not be underestimated.

REFERENCES

1. Joy RJT. Historical aspects of medical defense against chemical warfare. In: Sidell FR, Takafuji ET, Franz DR (eds): *Medical Aspects of Chemical and Biological Warfare*. Textbook of Military Medicine, Part I. Washington, DC: Borden Institute; 1997:111-28.
2. Mann J. *Murder, Magic and Medicine*. Oxford, UK: Oxford University Press; 1992:17.
3. Fenn EA. *Pox Americana: The Great Smallpox Epidemic of 1775-82*. New York, NY: Hill & Wang; 2001.
4. Williams P, Wallace D. *Unit 731: Japan's Secret Biological Warfare in World War II*. London, UK: Hodder and Stoughton; 1989.
5. Christopher GW, Cieslak TJ, Pavlin JA, Eitzen EM. Biological warfare: a historical perspective. *JAMA* 1997;278:412-7.
6. Regis E. *The Biology of Doom: The History of America's Secret Germ Warfare Project*. New York, NY: Henry Holt and Company; 1999.
7. Meselson M, Guillemin J, Hugh-Jones M, Langmuir A, et al. The Sverdlovsk anthrax outbreak of 1979. *Science* 1994;266:1202-8.
8. Tucker J. *Toxic Terror: Assessing Terrorist Use of Chemical and Biological Weapons*. Cambridge, Mass: MIT Press; 2000.
9. Noah DL, Huebner KD, Darling RG, Waeckerle J. The history and threat of biological warfare and terrorism. *Emerg Med Clin North Am.* 2002;20:255-71.
10. Fennelly KP, Davidow AL, Miller SL, et al. Airborne infection with *Bacillus anthracis*—from mills to mail. *Emerg Infect Dis.* 2004;10:996-1001.
11. Follow-up of deaths among U.S. Postal Service workers potentially exposed to *Bacillus anthracis*: District of Columbia, 2001-2002. *MMWR* 2003;52(39):937-8.
12. Alibek K, Handelman K. *Biohazard: The Chilling True Story of the Largest Covert Weapons Program in the World—Told from the Inside by the Man Who Ran it*. New York: Random House; 1999.
13. Morens DM, Folkers GK, Fauci AS. The challenge of emerging and remerging infectious diseases. *Nature* 2004;430:242-9.
14. Philips H. *The Spanish Influenza Outbreak of 1918-19: New Perspectives*. London: Routledge; 2003.
15. Centers for Disease Control and Prevention. Avian influenza in humans. Available at: http://www.cdc.gov/flu/avian/gen-info/avian-flu-humans.htm.
16. Stevens J, Corper A, Basler C, Taubenberger JK, Palese P, Wilson IA. Structure of the uncleaved human H1 hemagglutinin from the extinct 1918 influenza virus. *Science* 2004;303: 1866-70.
17. Centers for Disease Control and Prevention. Interim guidance for protection of persons involved in U.S. avian influenza outbreak disease control and eradication activities. Available at: http://www.cdc.gov/flu/avian/protectionguid.htm.
18. Teleman M, Boudville I, Heng B, et al. Factors associated with transmission of severe acute respiratory syndrome among health-care workers in Singapore. *Epidemiol Infect.* 2004;132(5):797-803.
19. Revised US surveillance case definition for severe acute respiratory syndrome (SARS) and update on SARS cases: United States and worldwide, December 2003. *MMWR* 52:1202-6.
20. Centers for Disease Control and Prevention. Severe acute respiratory syndrome: public health guidance for community-level preparedness and response to SARS version 2. Supplement F: Laboratory guidance. Appendix F8—Guidelines for laboratory diagnosis of SARS-CoV infection. Available at: http://www.cdc.gov/ncidod/sars/guidance/f/app8.htm.
21. Centers for Disease Control and Prevention. Hendra virus disease and Nipah virus encephalitis. Available at: http://www.cdc.gov/ncidod/dvrd/spb/mnpages/dispages/nipah.htm.
22. Mackenzie J. Emerging viral diseases: an Australian perspective. Available at: http://www.cdc.gov/ncidod/eid/vol5no1/mackenzie.htm.
23. Snell J. Ribavirin therapy for Nipah virus infection. *J Virol.* 2004;78:10211.
24. Kagan E. Bioregulators as instruments of terror. *Clin Lab Med.* 2001;21(3):607-18.
25. O'Dell J. Therapeutic strategies for rheumatoid arthritis. *N Engl J Med.* 2004;350:2591-602.
26. U.S. Congress, Office of Technology Assessment. *Technologies Underlying Weapons of Mass Destruction*. Chapter 3: Technical Aspects of Biological Weapon Proliferation. OTA-BP-ISC-115. Washington, DC: U.S. Government Printing Office; 1993.
27. Bokan S, Breen J, Orehovec Z. An evaluation of bioregulators as terrorism and warfare agents. Available at: http://www.asanltr.com/newsletter/02-3/articles/023c.htm.
28. Black JL. Genome projects and gene therapy: gateways to next-generation biological weapons. *Milit Med.* 2003;168(11):864-71.
29. Cordesman AH. Defending America: Iraq and other threats to the U.S. involving weapons of mass destruction. Center for Strategic and International Studies; 2001. Available at: http://www.csis.org/burke/hd/reports/iraq_otherthreatsWMD.pdf.
30. U.S. Government Accounting Office. *Combating Terrorism: Need for Comprehensive Threat and Risk Assessments and Chemical and Biological Agents. Report to Congressional requesters. GAO/NSIAD-99-163*. Washington, DC: GAO; 1999:1-36.
31. Sidell FR. Nerve agents. In: Sidell FR, Takafuji ET, Franz DR, eds. *Medical Aspects of Chemical and Biological Warfare*. Textbook of Military Medicine, Part I. Washington, DC: Borden Institute; 1997:111-28.
32. Fitzgerald GM, Sole DP. CBRNE: incapacitating agents, Agent 15. *eMed J*. 9 Sep 2004. Available at: http://www.emedicine.com/emerg/topic913.htm.
33. Centers for Disease Control and Prevention. Chemical agents. 2004. Available at: http://www.bt.cdc.gov/agent/agentlistchem.asp.
34. Centers for Disease Control and Prevention. Biological and chemical terrorism: strategic plan for preparedness and response. Recommendations of the CDC Strategic Planning Workgroup. *MMWR* 2000;49(RR-4):Box 5 (Chemical Agents).
35. Burklow TR, Yu CE, Madsen JM. Industrial chemicals: terrorist weapons of opportunity. *Pediatr Ann.* 2003;32(4):230-4.
36. U.S. Department of Health and Human Services: Agency for Toxic Substances and Disease Registry. Industrial chemicals and terrorism: human health threat analysis, mitigation and prevention. Available at: http://www.mapcruzin.com/scruztri/docs/cep1118992.htm.
37. Madsen JM. Toxins as weapons of mass destruction: a comparison and contrast with biological-warfare and chemical-warfare agents. *Clin Lab Med.* 2001;21(3):593-605.
38. U.S. Army Chemical School. NBC Annex to OE, Version 1.2. July 7, 2005. Available at: http://www.wood.army.mil/cmdoc/WFS/THREAT%20&%20Contemporary%20Operational%20Environment/index.htm.
38a. CBWInfo.com. Blister Agent: Sulfur Mustard (H, HD, HS). 1999. Available at: http://cbwinfo.com/Chemical/Blister/HD.shtml.
38b. CBWInfo.com. Nerve Agent: GD (Soman). 1999. Available at: http://cbwinfo.com/Chemical/Nerve/GD.shtml.
39. Smart JK. History of chemical and biological warfare: an American perspective. In: Sidell FR, Takafuji ET, Franz DR, eds. *Medical Aspects of Chemical and Biological Warfare*. Textbook of Military Medicine, Part I. Washington, DC: Borden Institute; 1997:9-86.
40. Adams JR. Russia's toxic threat. *Wall Street J.* April 30, 1996:A18.
41. Englund W. Ex-Soviet scientist say Gorbachev's regime created new nerve gas in '91. *Baltimore Sun*. 16 Sep 1992; 3A. See http://nl.newsbank.com/nl-search/we/Archives?p_action=list&p_topdoc=11.
42. Sands A, Pate J. CWC compliance issues. In: Tucker JB, ed. *The Chemical Weapons Convention: Implementation Challenges and Solutions*. Washington, DC: Center for Nonproliferation Studies, Monterey Institute of International Studies; 2001:17-22.
43. Coupland RM. Incapacitating chemical weapons: a year after the Moscow theatre siege [commentary]. *Lancet* 2003 Oct 25; 362(9893):1346.
44. Bismuth C, Borron SW, Baud FJ, Barriot P. Chemical weapons: documented use and compounds on the horizon. *Toxicology Letters.* 2004;149:11-8.
45. Jane's Chem-Bio Web. News, US pursues incapacitating agents for military and law enforcement. November 22, 2002. Available at: http://chembio.janes.com [subscription required].
46. Hurst CG. Decontamination. In: Sidell FR, Takafuji ET, Franz DR, eds. *Medical Aspects of Chemical and Biological Warfare*. Textbook of Military Medicine, Part I. Washington, DC: Borden Institute; 1997:351-9.
47. Takafuji ET, Kok AB. The chemical warfare threat and the military healthcare provider. In: Sidell FR, Takafuji ET, Franz DR, eds. *Medical Aspects of Chemical and Biological Warfare*. Textbook of Military Medicine, Part I. Washington, DC: Borden Institute; 1997:111-28.

48. Croddy E. Dusty agents and the Iraqi chemical weapons arsenal. Washington, DC: Center for Nonproliferation Studies, Nuclear Threat Initiative; 2002. Available at: http://www.nti.org/e_research/e3_20b.html.

49. U.S. Congress, Office of Technology Assessment. *Technologies Underlying Weapons of Mass Destruction, OTA-BP-ISC-115.* Washington, DC: U.S. Government Printing Office; 1993:32.

50. Jane's Chem-Bio Web. News: Jordan-based terrorists planned to use vehicle-borne improvised explosive devices (VBIED's), chemicals in two-stage attack. April 28, 2004. Available at: http://chembio.janes.com [subscription required].

51. DaSilva E. Biological warfare, bioterrorism, biodefence and the biological and toxin weapons convention. *Electronic J Biotechnol (EJB).* 1999;2(3):99-128. Available at: http://www.ejbiotechnology.info/content/vol2/issue3/full/2.

52. Jane's Chem-Bio Web. News: Nanotechnology: the potential for new WMD. January 10, 2003. Available at: http://chembio.janes.com [subscription required].

53. Perkel JM. The ups and downs of nanobiotech. *The Scientist.* August 30, 2004;18(16). Available at: http://www.the-scientist.com.

54. Weiss R. Nanotechnology precaution is urged: miniscule particles in cosmetics may pose risk, British scientists say. *Washington Post.* July 30, 2004:A02.

55. Oberdörster E. Manufactured nanomaterials (fullerenes, C 60) induce oxidative stress in the brain of juvenile largemouth bass. *Environ Health Persp.* July 2004;112:1058-62.

56. Wikipedia, The Free Encyclopedia. Biotechnology. Available at: http://en.wikipedia.org/wiki/Biotechnology.

57. Convention on Biological Diversity, United Nations Environment Program. Governments to advance work on Cartagena Protocol on Biosafety [press release]. Available at: http://www.biodiv.org/doc/meetings/bs/iccp-03/other/iccp-03-pr-en.pdf.

58. Wheelis M. Biotechnology and biochemical weapons. *The Nonproliferation Review.* Spring 2002:48-53.

59. Barnaby W. *The Plague Makers: The Secret World of Biological Warfare.* 3rd ed. New York: The Continuum International Publishing Company; 2000:131-48.

60. Russo E. NRC wants genome data unfettered. *The Scientist.* September 10, 2004. Available at: http://www.the-scientist.com. Also available at: http://www.biomedcentral.com/news/20040910/01.

61. Aas P. The threat of mid-spectrum chemical warfare agents. *Prehospital Disaster Med.* 2003;18(4):306-12.

62. Dando MR. The danger to the Chemical Weapons Convention from incapacitating chemicals. First CWC Review Conference Paper No. 4. In: Pearson GS, Dando MR, eds. *Strengthening the Chemical Weapons Convention.* Bradford, UK: University of Bradford Department of Peace Studies; 2003:1-19.

Improvised Explosive Devices

Edward B. Lucci

Improvised explosive devices (IEDs) have become the most common weapons of terrorists. Explosions and bombings remain the most common deliberate cause of disasters involving mass casualties.[1] By definition, an IED is a conventional explosive weapon with fragmentation and blast effect, deployed in an unconventional fashion. It is generally cheap, simple in design, and easy to construct with readily available materials. IEDs vary in size, destructive capacity, and degrees of sophistication. Most are conventional high-explosive charges. However, the threat exists of including chemical, biologic, or nuclear material to improve the destructive power and psychological effect of the device.

The frequency of terrorist bombings using IEDs directed at civilian populations, particularly suicide bombings, has increased worldwide and has resulted in unexpected mass-casualty incidents descending on civilian medical systems. Victims of IEDs will frequently suffer a combination of blast, penetrating, and thermal injuries. The management of these complicated injuries often falls outside the experience of most physicians. An analysis of 220 bombings between 1969 and 1983 revealed an average of 15.3 casualties per incident, 13% of whom died at the scene, and 30% of whom were hospitalized.[2]

Unpredictable in timing and location, a large explosive device with multiple injured could easily strain even the most prepared emergency response systems. To be able to deal effectively with casualties from IEDs, providers must be knowledgeable of the patterns of injury and barriers to care associated with these types of terrorist events. The planning for medical management of bombing victims must revolve around the basic lessons learned from prior bombing disasters. Certain injuries must be recognized as prognostic markers of severity and be selected out for immediate care to optimize survival. Fortunately, the majority of blast victims who survive transfer to the hospital can be successfully treated.[3] The goal of this chapter is to outline broad principles that are generally applicable to the effective delivery of medical care in a sudden-impact disaster resulting from terrorists' use of IEDs.

HISTORICAL PERSPECTIVE

Since the emergence of gunpowder and explosives on the battlefield, victims have been exposed to the blast effects of explosive devices. The history of IEDs is closely tied to the history of terrorists and counter-insurgents who have used them. The first recorded use of a terrorist explosive was in Antwerp, Belgium, in 1585. Seven tons of gunpowder was placed on a river barge and detonated by insurgents to destroy a bridge on the River Schelt.[1,4] The modern era of terrorism began in the late 1960s and has been the most destructive in history.[5] Since then, the number and destructive power of bombings has steadily increased. There was a 10-fold increase in terrorist bombings worldwide between 1968 and 1980. In the United States alone, there were 12,216 bombing incidents between 1980 and 1990, the vast majority of which resulted from pipe bomb–type IEDs.[6]

Terrorist attacks are extremely diverse, particularly with regard to type of explosive device, size of charge, and location of detonation. The medical literature describes various terrorist attacks using IEDs in Great Britain, France, Israel, Italy, Lebanon, Saudi Arabia, South America, Spain, sub-Saharan Africa, the United States, and Yemen.[2,3,7-13]

IEDs have been used against the U.S. military in Vietnam, Lebanon, Saudi Arabia, and most recently in Iraq. In Vietnam, IEDs were more commonly referred to as "booby traps" and usually were concealed to detonate when a nearby "harmless" object was encountered. These IEDs usually consisted of a conventional explosive device such as a grenade, artillery shell, or mine. A common form was the pipe bomb, a length of pipe filled with trinitrotoluene (TNT) and fused with a detonating cord. Fragments such as nails or glass were often added. As many as 14% of U.S. Army casualties in Vietnam were generated by booby trap–type IEDs.[14] Today, pipe-bomb use occurs almost daily worldwide.[15]

Northern Ireland became the scene of an urban terrorist campaign in August 1969. IEDs were deployed against the public and against security forces, and in some cases the bombers themselves became the victims. Multiple studies have characterized the nature of these bombings and examined the casualty profiles. During the period of August 1969 to June 1972, there were at least 1500 hospitalizations in Northern Ireland resulting from terrorist bombings and 117 deaths (most deaths occurred before reaching the hospital).[16-18] Bombs ranged from 2 to 200 lb.[18] A 1978 review of 1532 bombing victims (78 explosions, 13 of which had more than 20 victims transported), revealed 16% were admitted, and less than 1% of those who reached the hospital died. Twenty-five percent required a surgical procedure, most of which were simple wound cleaning and suturing.[16,18]

IED detonations associated with collapsing a structure have had devastating consequences.[19,20] A major loss of American lives from a terrorist bombing with a vehicle-borne IED occurred in 1983 in Beirut, Lebanon. The suicide detonation of a truck packed with ammonium nitrate resulted in an explosive force equivalent to 6 to 12 tons of TNT, the largest deliberate non-nuclear man-made explosion to date. The explosion collapsed the four-story airport terminal building housing U.S. forces. There were 346 casualties with 234 (68%) immediate deaths. Most survivors had noncritical injuries.[1,2]

In the late 1970s and early 1980s, several cities in Israel were victimized by terrorist bombings. The emergence of suicide bombings in the 1990s led to an increase in the magnitude and severity of incidents. Between 1994 and 1998 there were 18 suicide bombings in Israel alone—12 in crowded urban areas and 4 in crowded buses. An in-depth review of 4 bombings in 1996 revealed a total of 297 victims.[8] A 7.8% fatality rate occurred in open-air bombings versus 49% in the confined space of a bus. Victims in buses had a higher incidence of primary blast injury (PBI), which was predominantly lung injury and more extensive burns, but no difference was found regarding number of burns, penetrating injuries, or traumatic amputations when compared with injuries among open-air bombing victims.[7]

In Iraq today, terrorists have integrated pipe-bombs, mortars, artillery projectiles, anti-tank mines, rockets, and other explosive-filled ordnance, into simple command-detonated devices, either hard-wired or radio controlled allowing remote detonation via battery-powered remote car alarm, doorbell, pager, or cell phone[21] (Fig. 65-1). During Operation Iraqi Freedom (OIF), U.S. and Coalition forces experienced 708 incidents of IED attacks during one 90-day period alone.[21]

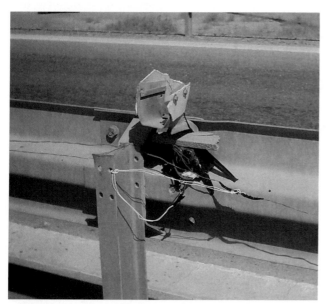

FIGURE 65–1. Garage door opener detonation device (notice wire).

Currently in Iraq, IEDs are being camouflaged to resemble roadside garbage or debris, hidden in roadside abandoned vehicles, or placed in potholes, under rocks, or in animal carcasses, and they are deployed both individually and as "daisy-chained" munitions (i.e., linked munitions exploding in series). They have been most commonly targeted against unarmored vehicles in small convoys or the rear of larger convoys.[21] Roughly 50% of IEDs encountered during OIF failed to function properly. The average IED in Iraq during OIF has been estimated to be 1 to 2 kg; however, large vehicle-borne IEDs (VBIEDs) containing bulk explosives have been detonated with devastating effect.[21]

CURRENT PRACTICE

Clinical Effects of Blast Injury

An IED will create wounds according to several effects: the blast effect from the force of the explosion, the ballistic effect of flying fragments, and the thermal effect from the explosion's heat. These effects will generate casualties according to the victim's distance from the epicenter of the explosion (Fig. 65-2). Persons who are close to the explosion will show evidence of all types of injuries; those farther away will sustain only penetrating injury. Persons receiving combined ballistic, blast, and thermal injuries usually suffer mutilating blast injury and are unlikely to survive. Generally speaking, the closer one is to an exploding device, the less likely one is to survive or even enter the medical treatment system.[22]

High-explosive detonation is a high-speed, almost simultaneous chemical decomposition of solid or liquid explosive into a gas. The result is an expanding sphere of high-pressure, high-temperature gas blast wave propagating radially from the explosion at or above the speed of sound, the magnitude and speed of which is dependent on the type and size of explosive and the surrounding medium.[23] The presence of reflecting surfaces (such as a wall) may magnify the original incident pressure many times, and severe blast injury may be seen in patients thought to be a safe distance from the blast.[13,24] Stress and shear waves, spalling, implosion, and inertia are some of the proposed mechanisms by which the blast wave damages tissue.[25,26]

The ability of a blast to cause damage to the body depends on the blast load, that is, the peak pressure and duration of overpressure produced by the explosion.[27] The three factors that govern the blast load imposed on the body include:

1. The size of the explosion;
2. The medium in which it explodes;
3. The distance from the center of the explosion.

Many factors can reduce the blast loading on the body within confined spaces, such as pillars, furniture, and other victims.[16,17] British research suggests a charge equivalent to 20 kg of TNT that explodes more than 6 m from the body is unlikely to cause severe blast injury to the lungs in an open-space explosion.[28]

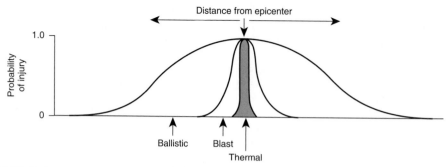

FIGURE 65–2. The probability of sustaining trauma is related to the casualties' distance from the epicenter.

Explosions resulting from IED detonation can cause a great variety of injuries. There are three injury types propagated by an explosive blast: the blast pressure effect, the fragmentation effect, and the impact effect from the victim being thrown against an object, traditionally termed primary, secondary, and tertiary blast injuries, respectively.[2,17,25,26] Studies have suggested that the majority of bombing injuries are from secondary or tertiary blast effect[18,27] and are most often soft tissue, orthopedic, and head injuries.[18-20,29] The head and neck are the areas most vulnerable to injury.[30] Severe head injury is the leading cause of death in blast victims.[3,16,17,20,29,31] Penetrating neck and torso trauma is also a common cause of death.[18]

PBIs are caused by the direct concussive effect of the blast wave on the body, are unique to explosions, and are characterized by damage to air-filled organs. The lungs, ears, and gastrointestinal tract are most susceptible.[25,31] Solid organs are protected from PBI. PBI of the lung is the hallmark of PBI caused by explosions but is not the most common injury.[7] It is essentially manifested as pulmonary contusions.[27,32] Significant blast injury to the lung causes intra-alveolar hemorrhage and edema and a rapid fall in oxygenation.[31] PBI is uncommon in survivors of terrorist bombings; however, it is found to be common in victims who die at the scene, in victims of explosion in an enclosed space, and in patients who are "severely wounded." Investigators report an incidence of 1% to 2% in surviving casualties. A significantly higher percentage of PBIs are reported in the Israeli literature, but the occurrence is still less than 20%.[2,3,7,18,32]

Injury to the lung is the cause of the greatest morbidity and mortality. In lung injury, limited peak inspiratory pressure, volume-controlled ventilation, and permissive hypercapnia have benefited patients. Some advocate the prophylactic placement of chest tube thoracostomy in patients with a deteriorating condition.[25,33]

Tympanic membrane rupture is the least severe form of PBI and another hallmark injury of the blast wave. Tympanic membrane rupture is common and is considered an indication of a patient's exposure to blast.[9] All who were severely injured in a study by Katz et al.[3] had ruptured tympanic membranes.[34] If this structure is clinically intact, serious blast injury is unlikely.[16,30] Spontaneous healing occurs in 50% to 80% of patients, with some permanent hearing loss being reported in up to 100% of victims.[7]

Another hallmark of blast injury is the appearance of air emboli in the pulmonary and coronary vessels.[9,16] For neurologic deterioration attributed to air emboli, some have advocated hyperbaric therapy.[16] Sometimes no distinct injuries are identifiable. In Israel, as many as 30% of fatalities in suicide bombings had no obvious external cause of death.[7] It is postulated that in cases where no visible external injuries exist, cardiac dysrhythmia or air emboli caused cardiac arrest.[9]

Primary blast injury of the bowel is variable in explosions and has more commonly been considered a consequence of underwater explosion only.[3] The colon is the most common site of hemorrhage and perforation. Presentation of this type of injury may be acute or delayed.[3,33]

Secondary blast injury is caused by rapid acceleration of projectiles embedded in the explosive or flying debris caused by the explosion. The resulting ballistic injury patterns will reflect the velocity and shape of the bomb fragments or flying glass, for example. This is the predominant injury among surviving casualties and the critical factor is the anatomic site penetrated.[2,22] In many studies, virtually all injuries seen in survivors were caused by secondary missiles rather than the blast wave itself.[16]

Tertiary blast injuries are a result of the impact of a victim being thrown against an object. These are managed as conventional trauma, either blunt or penetrating if secondarily impaled.

Miscellaneous injuries encompass all other injuries due to the explosive device such as those resulting from fire and heat, including flash burns, smoke inhalation, and crush injury.[16] External burns are usually superficial due to the short duration of the explosive flash, and clothing offers some degree of protection unless the person is caught in a building or vehicle ignited by the explosion.[33]

Civilian bombings usually result in low mortality rates unless there is a structural collapse or a very large explosive charge or an explosion within a confined space occurs.[9,34] On average, about 1% to 5% of victims will die at the scene, 25% to 50% of those transported will need admission, approximately 10% will be seriously injured, and a smaller percentage will require surgery.[3,33,34] The majority of victims seeking medical care will be slightly injured with abrasions, lacerations, and contusions.[34] Fatalities tend to incur multiple injuries: head, blast lung, abdominal, and chest injuries and traumatic amputations.[2,3,8] Injuries most commonly seen in fatalities include head/brain injury (66%), skull fracture (51%), diffuse lung contusion (47%), tympanic membrane rupture (45%), and liver laceration (34%).[30]

Among survivors, soft tissue and musculoskeletal injuries are caused most commonly by secondary and tertiary blast effects. Critical injuries occur infrequently in bombing survivors, and abdominal injury is rare, but may be associated with either the blast wave and hollow viscous perforation or acceleration/deceleration (tertiary blast) injury.[2]

Traumatic amputation is a marker of severe injury not usually associated with survival and is frequently associated with other injuries, such as chest and abdominal injuries.[12,16] Patients may suffer from mangled extremities as a result of an incident involving an IED. Predicting the ultimate viability of a mangled extremity remains a challenge for orthopedic surgeons.[11,30,35]

Factors that correlate with ultimate outcome and optimum survival in victims of blast due to an IED include explosive force, anatomic site of injury, time interval from injury to treatment, and availability of surgeons.[1,2]

Key Management Principles of Victims of IEDs

Triage and Management of the Victims of IEDs in the Field

The goal of field management should be to quickly identify the critically injured patients who need immediate care and to provide them with life-saving procedures, stabilization, and transport to surrounding hospitals as rapidly as possible, avoiding a "second wave" phenomenon. Four phases at the scene have been suggested[7]:

1. A *chaotic phase* lasts 15 to 25 minutes, characterized by the lack of a leader. Victims who can walk will evacuate themselves to the nearest hospital. The first to arrive at the hospital are those with minor injuries, and these victims seldom receive any treatment at the scene.[7]
2. Next comes a *reorganization phase* lasting up to 60 minutes characterized by the leader (usually emergency medical services [EMS] personnel) assuming control at the scene. This is likely the most important management phase.[7] The leader ensures life-threatening injuries are identified and prioritized for evacuation. The goals of medical leadership at the site must include rapidly establishing communication with local EMS and ensuring safety at the scene.[30] The number of casualties and severity of injuries must be accurately communicated to EMS to ensure optimal distribution of patients to receiving facilities. Scene safety remains a paramount concern because both secondary explosive device detonation as an observed tactic of terrorists and hazardous debris in a collapsed structure threaten rescuers.[2,24] At the site, the presence of a crater and building collapse are important observations regarding blast strength.[33]
3. A *site-clearing phase* lasts 1 to 3 hours, depending on the need for extrication.[7] The EMS commander should ensure that no victims are missed. Hospital "exportable" teams, essential in rural mass-casualty scenarios, would arrive on site.
4. The *late phase* is a poorly defined period between when the site is cleared of victims and 24 to 48 hours afterward. Some victims with slight wounds may not acknowledge their injuries for many hours after the event and may seek medical care at this time.[7]

The presence of multiple wounds in the same casualty and the presence of multiple casualties require that treatment be prioritized both in the field and at the hospital. The challenge of field triage in the bombing incident is to identify the minority of casualties who are critically injured and require immediate care among the great majority of less severely injured casualties. U.S. and European data suggest that 85% of surviving victims may be triaged and treated as outpatients.[36] Rapid and accurate triage could significantly reduce mortality among bombing survivors, whereas routine over-triage could result in loss of potentially salvageable lives as nearby medical facilities become overwhelmed.[2] Urban locations are likely to enhance the value of accurate triage. In isolated locations where prolonged transport of critically injured and delayed treatment must be taken into account, over-triage may become a necessity.[2] Victims with no evidence of external trauma and no loss of consciousness can be cleared in the field.[12] The activity level of potential blast-exposed persons should be reduced at the scene because data suggest victims of pulmonary PBI fare poorly when significant physical activity follows blast injury.[37] Occasionally it may be necessary to amputate a mangled extremity to free an entrapped patient. Although this is rarely required in the disaster setting, it should still be performed at the lowest possible level.[30]

No major difference exists between initial care to a patient with blast injury and victims of other more conventional trauma. Definitive care should not occur at the triage area in the field. Basic guidelines should include the following[7]:

1. Victims who are apneic, pulseless, and not moving should be considered dead.[7] Cardiopulmonary resuscitation at the scene is futile and not indicated.
2. Airway management with C-spine control is effective treatment in an unconscious patient with an unsecured airway or inadequate ventilation. Victims with respiratory distress require early advanced life support. Patients who are intubated and ventilated are at high risk for tension pneumothorax. In a suspected pneumothorax in the field under positive pressure ventilation, needle decompression is prudent, particularly if the patient will require air evacuation.[7]
3. Control of hemorrhage in the field is necessary for treatment of external bleeding of the extremities. Application of a tourniquet is appropriate only if direct pressure has failed.[7] Administration of intravenous fluid should not delay transport to the hospital.
4. Fracture alignment is critical and may restore blood flow in the mangled extremity. Because splinting material will be scarce, limb-to-limb and limb-to-body splinting will suffice temporarily.

5. Covering open wounds with dressings is desirable but should not delay transport if not readily available.

Hospital Management of IED Victims

Effective triage by the most experienced hospital provider (often a surgeon or emergency physician) at the hospital unloading point for ambulances should place patients into "urgent" versus "nonurgent" categories, depending on their need for surgery.[7] Nonurgent patients (i.e., those for whom delayed or minimal care is required) are not in need of surgery in the next few hours. Unless a patient dies on arrival, the decision to declare a patient "expectant" (i.e., unsalvageable) should be made in the resuscitation bay only after more thorough evaluation.[7]

Patients categorized as "urgent" should receive resuscitation in accordance with advanced trauma life support protocols. Hemodynamically unstable patients should be transferred to the operating room as soon as possible, for definitive control of bleeding.[7] There is no place for emergency department thoracotomy in traumatic arrest from a terrorist bombing.[7,25] Deteriorating respiratory function is most likely secondary to blast effect; however, bilateral tension pneumothoraces should be ruled out with needle decompression. The minimal acceptable treatment for severe thoracic trauma is empiric chest tube thoracostomy.[7] Due to the high velocity associated with fragments, all penetrating wounds of the chest and abdomen should be explored.[30] PBI should be considered in all persons exposed to blast, although serious PBIs are uncommon in survivors. The immediate management of patients with suspected PBI should include a response tempered with physiologic end points for oxygenation, ventilation, and fluid replacement.[33]

Stable patients with abdominal trauma are managed with nasogastric decompression, intravenous fluids, antibiotics, and analgesia.[7] Focused abdominal ultrasound evaluation, if available, is superior to time-consuming diagnostic peritoneal lavage (DPL). Computed tomography (CT) scans should be performed judiciously in the initial phase when casualties are still arriving. The only mandatory CT scans performed initially are for head injury in patients with altered mental status to rule out intracranial bleeding.[7] Plain radiographs unlikely to affect the immediate management of patients should be deferred, at least until all urgent patients have been evaluated.

Initially, when the ultimate number of casualties is unknown, the hospital capacity must be protected because conservation of critical hospital resources is paramount. Therefore, in the immediate aftermath of the explosion, minimal acceptable care is permitted on a temporary basis, with concentration placed on the maximal number of salvageable patients. Initial surgical procedures may need to be in the form of damage control surgery. When casualties are no longer arriving, optimal care should be the goal.[7]

Nonurgent patients are referred to the predesignated area where they are reevaluated for admission or discharge as soon as possible. Guidelines for the use of blood should be restricted and a preselected upper limit of units to be transfused for individual victims should be determined to avoid premature depletion of resources.[7]

Fragmentation injuries predominate in patients presenting to the hospital. In bombing victims, wound contamination caused by high-velocity fragments is more extensive, and primary closure should not be attempted.

Injury to the lungs will be the greatest cause of morbidity and mortality. Clinically, blast lung presents early. The diagnosis is suspected on clinical grounds and confirmed by chest radiograph. This diagnosis must be excluded in patients who require general anesthesia or air evacuation and prophylactic chest tube thoracostomy has been advocated in PBI under these circumstances due to the risk of tension pneumothorax. When PBI is suspected and operative procedures are required, local, regional, or spinal anesthesia is preferred over general anesthesia.[37] Patients suffering from PBI to the lungs require intensive care unit management. Many casualties will require positive pressure ventilation for a variety of reasons. Pressure-controlled ventilation, high-frequency ventilation, and permissive hypercapnia have been successful modes of respiratory support.[7,33]

Missed injuries after bombings are not uncommon and should be avoided by repeat examinations. For patients in whom PBI is suspected, some period of observation is prudent.[25,33] PBI of the auditory system can be easily overlooked. Isolated tympanic membrane rupture is not a marker for life-threatening PBI, and absence of rupture makes pulmonary PBI unlikely unless the patient was wearing hearing protection.[16] Prior to discharge, all patients must be evaluated for tympanic membrane injury and ocular injuries from flying debris.[7,16]

Following immediate life-saving surgical procedures, nonexsanguinating chest and abdominal injuries that endanger life should undergo operation.[7] After this, surgical treatment of closed-head injuries with intracranial hemorrhage is warranted. Extremity injuries including bone and vascular injury should be stabilized; however, time-consuming vascular and nerve reconstruction is inappropriate at this point. Wound cleansing and debridement are the last group of patients to undergo operation. Secondary distribution of patients in need of orthopedic fixation and debridement to neighboring hospitals for more timely surgical care is appropriate.[7]

Some of the injured as well as some of the rescuers will suffer posttraumatic stress. Staff debriefing sessions should be held immediately after acute events.[38]

Algorithms exist for the management of respiratory distress, neurologic abnormalities, and gastrointestinal injury in a blast casualty.[37]

PITFALLS

Planning in detail for a disaster can be an overwhelming task doomed to incompletion. Planning instead for disasters of moderate size will yield a better chance of succeeding. Ideally, any plan should allow for modular expansion of response.[38] In a similar sense, planning for low-probability events such as a terrorist bombing competes with day-to-day activities.[38] Any opportunity to share intelligence between law enforcement and the medical community that might assist in improving response planning should be exploited.

Communications plans must ensure that communication capability continues after explosion and mass-casualty incident. Effective communication would improve casualty flow from the site to the hospital and ensure optimal distribution of patients and help prevent a second-wave phenomenon at receiving hospitals. Even in the United States, 67% of disasters had no communication existing between the disaster site and the receiving hospitals.[38,39]

A lack of experienced medical leadership at the scene may be a significant impediment to appropriate treatment and medical regulation in evacuation at the site.[10,30] In addition, over-triage is common in both the prehospital and hospital setting.[2,34] In one large study, over-triage averaged 59%, but in many studies it has been considerably higher.[18]

Virtually all blast victims will have some degree of hearing impairment, which will complicate attempts to communicate with survivors but requires no field management.[24,30] Hearing protection can attenuate external overpressure and protect against tympanic membrane rupture.[37,38]

A high index of suspicion is helpful in detecting occult injuries in bombing victims. Arterial air embolism to the brain or heart may be the most common cause of death in immediate survivors and often occurs at the initiation of positive pressure ventilation.[33] Mechanical ventilation should be avoided due to the risk of air embolization and further barotraumas, when possible.[16,37] Bowel perforation, while uncommon, frequently may have a delayed onset of symptoms.[12] In addition, severe injuries to the gastrointestinal tract from blast rarely occur in isolation, and these other injuries may mask the less obvious and subacute bowel injury.[3] Although there are few survivors of blast injury sufficiently severe to cause bowel perforation, isolated abdominal PBI may be clinically silent until complications are advanced.[3,16] Compartment syndrome may be seen wherever limb fractures, vascular injuries, and crush injuries occur in the setting of explosion and collapsed structures. The diagnosis is largely clinical and a healthy index of suspicion is required.

Primary closure of blast wounds have a high rate of secondary infection and should be avoided.[12,16,37] The use of body armor (ballistic vest) offers protection against secondary and tertiary blast effects but may be associated with an increased incidence of PBI.[30,37,40,41]

Lastly, movement on medical evacuation aircraft requires special patient preparation, particularly if concern for pneumothorax or need for mechanical ventilation exists.[42]

CONCLUSIONS

It is clear that terrorism will continue to plague societies in the twenty-first century. It is less clear what form the threat will take. Acts of terrorism in the United States and internationally have grown more destructive during the past decade, and this trend can be expected to continue.[5] As advances in weapons technology present new challenges to the disaster medicine community, success will require further commitment to develop creative ways to meet those challenges.[43]

Terrorist bombings using IEDs, one type of sudden-impact disaster, occur without warning; however, they possess certain predictable characteristics based on historical data. An organized and coordinated response will reduce mortality and preserve resources for patients most in need of care. Medical providers must identify the pattern of primary, secondary, and tertiary injuries associated with IEDs, in addition to recognizing the hallmarks of blast injury and significance of markers of serious injury. Hospital resources must be expended in the optimal manner, to include prudent hospital triage and surgical care, in order to deliver the best possible outcome for victims of terrorist bombings associated with IEDs.

REFERENCES

1. Frykberg E. Medical management of disasters and mass casualties from terrorist bombings: how can we cope? *J Trauma.* 2002; 53:201-12.
2. Frykberg E, Tepas, J. Terrorist bombings: lessons learned from Belfast to Beirut. *Ann Surg.* 1988;208:569-76.
3. Katz E, Ofek B, Adler J, et al. Primary blast injury after a bomb explosion in a civilian bus. *Ann Surg.* 1989;209:484-8.
4. Slater M, Trunkey D. Terrorism in America: an evolving threat. *Arch Surg.* 1997:132:1059-66.
5. U.S. Department of Justice. Federal Bureau of Investigation. Terrorism in the United States 1999: Counterterrorism Threat Assessment and Warning Unit. Washington DC; U.S. Department of Justice, Counterterrorism Division; 1999:1-62.
6. Karmy-Jones R, Kissinger D, Golocovsky M, et al. Bomb-related injuries. *Mil Med.* 1994;159:536-9.
7. Stein M, Hirschberg, A. Medical consequences of terrorism: the conventional weapon threat. *Surg Clin N Am.* 1999;79:1537-52.
8. Leibovici D, Gofrit, O, Stein, M, et al. Blast injuries: bus versus open-air bombings—a comparative study of injuries in survivors of open-air versus confined-space explosions. *J Trauma.* 1996;41:1030-5.
9. Kluger Y. Bomb explosions in acts of terrorism-detonations, wound ballistics, triage, and medical concerns. *IMAJ* 2003;5:235-240.
10. Brismar B, Bergenwald L. The terrorist bomb explosion in Bologna, Italy, 1980: an analysis of the effects and injuries sustained. *J Trauma.* 1982;22:216-20.
11. Hull J. Traumatic amputation by explosive blast: pattern of injury in survivors. *Br J Surg.* 1992;79:1303-6.
12. Langworthy M, Sabra J, Gould M. Terrorism and blast phenomena: lessons learned from the attack on the USS Cole. *Clin Ortho Rel Res.* 2004;422:82-7.
13. Covey D, Lurate R, Hatton C. Field hospital treatment of blast wounds of the musculoskeletal system during the Yugoslav civil war. *J Orthop Trauma.* 2000;14:278-86.
14. Bellamy R, Zajtchuk R. Assessing the effectiveness of conventional weapons. In: Zajtchuk R, Jenkins D, Bellamy R, eds. *Conventional Warfare: Ballistics, Blast, and Burn Injuries.* Textbook of Military Medicine, part I. Washington, DC: Office of the Surgeon General at TMM Publications; 1991:53-82.
15. Gibbons A, Farrier J, Key S. The pipe bomb: a modern terrorist weapon. *J R Army Med Corps.* 2003;149:23-6.
16. Mellor S, Cooper G. Analysis of 828 servicemen killed or injured by explosion in Northern Ireland 1970-84: the Hostile Action Casualty System. *Br J Surg.* 1989;76:1006-10.
17. Cooper G, Maynard R, Cross N, et al. Casualties from terrorist bombings. *J Trauma.* 1983;23:955-67.
18. Hadden W, Rutherford J, Merrett J. The injuries of terrorist bombing: a study of 1532 consecutive patients. *Br J Surg.* 1978;65:525-31.
19. Frykberg E, Hutton P, Balzer R. Disaster in Beirut: an application of mass casualty principles. *Mil Med.* 1987;152:563-6.
20. Mallonee S, Shariat S, Stennies G, et al. Physical injuries and fatalities resulting from the Oklahoma City bombing. *JAMA* 1996;276:382-7.
21. U.S Department of Defense Force Protection Working Group to the Coalition Provisional Authority. Baghdad, Iraq: January 16, 2004:1-5 [unclassified]. Unpublished data.

22. Bellamy R, Zajtchuk R. The weapons of conventional warfare. In: Zajtchuk R, Jenkins D, Bellamy R, eds. *Conventional Warfare: Ballistics, Blast, and Burn Injuries*. Textbook of Military Medicine, part I. Washington, DC: Office of the Surgeon General at TMM Publications; 1991:1-52.

23. Stuhmiller J, Phillips Y, Richmond D, et al. The physics and mechanisms of primary blast injury. In: Zajtchuk R, Jenkins D, Bellamy R, eds. *Conventional Warfare: Ballistics, Blast, and Burn Injuries*. Textbook of Military Medicine, part I. Washington, DC: Office of the Surgeon General at TMM Publications; 1991:241-70.

24. Boffard K, MacFarlane C. Urban bomb blast injuries: patterns of injury and treatment. *Surg Ann*. 1993;25(part 1):29-47.

25. Phillips Y. Primary blast injuries. *Ann Emerg Med*. 1986;15:1446-50.

26. Stapczynski J. Blast injuries. *Ann Emerg Med*. 1982;11:687-94.

27. Sharpnack D, Johnson A, Phillips Y. The pathology of primary blast injury. In: Zajtchuk R, Jenkins D, Bellamy R, eds. *Conventional Warfare: Ballistics, Blast, and Burn Injuries*. Textbook of Military Medicine, part I. Washington, DC: Office of the Surgeon General at TMM Publications; 1991:271-94.

28. Owen-Smith M. Explosive blast injury. *J R Army Med Corps*. 1979;125:4.

29. Hill J. Blast injury with particular reference to recent terrorist bombing incidents. *Ann R Coll Surg Engl*. 1979;61:4-11.

30. Gans L, Kennedy T. Management of unique clinical entities in disaster medicine. *Emerg Med Clin N Am*. 1996;14:301-26.

31. Mellor S. The pathogenesis of blast injury and its management. *Br J Hosp Med*. 1988;39:536-9.

32. Mayorga M. The pathology of primary blast overpressure injury. *Toxicology* 1997;121:17-28.

33. Wightman J, Gladish S. Explosions and blast injuries. *Ann Emerg Med*. 2001;37:664-78.

34. Phillips Y, Richmond D. Primary blast injury and basic research: a brief history. In: Zajtchuk R, Jenkins D, Bellamy R, eds. *Conventional Warfare: Ballistics, Blast, and Burn Injuries*. Textbook of Military Medicine, part I. Washington, DC: Office of the Surgeon General at TMM Publications; 1991:221-40.

35. Lange R. Limb reconstruction versus amputation decision making in massive lower extremity trauma. *Clin Orthop Rel Res*.1989; 243:92-9.

36. Horrocks C. Blast injuries: biophysics, pathophysiology, and management principles. *J R Army Med Corps*. 2001;147:28-40.

37. Phillips Y, Zajtchuk J. The management of primary blast injury. In: Zajtchuk R, Jenkins D, Bellamy R, eds. *Conventional Warfare: Ballistics, Blast, and Burn Injuries*. Textbook of Military Medicine, part I. Washington, DC: Office of the Surgeon General at TMM Publications; 1991:295-335.

38. Leibovici D, Gofrit O, Shapira S. Eardrum perforation in explosion survivors: is it a marker of pulmonary blast injury. *Ann Emerg Med*. 1999;34:168-72.

39. Severance H. Mass-casualty victim "surge" management: preparing for bombings and blast-related injuries with possibility of hazardous materials exposure. *N C Med J*. 2002;63:242-6.

40. Argyros G. Management of primary blast injury. *Toxicology* 1997;121:105-15.

41. Hayda R, Harris R, Bass C. Blast injury research. *Clin Orthop Rel Res*. 2004;422:97-108.

42. Geiling J. Medical support to the Kenya embassy bombing: a model for success or a platform for reform. *USAWC Strategy Research Project*. Carlisle Barracks, Pa: U.S. Army War College; 2000:1-58.

43. SAEM Disaster Medicine White Paper Subcommittee. *Disaster Medicine: Current Assessment and Blueprint for the Future*. 1995;2:1068-76.

chapter 66

Directed-Energy Weapons

M. Kathleen Stewart and Charles Stewart

As new technology becomes available and the military uses become apparent, terrorists will adopt it and often increase its lethality. Directed-energy weapons include microwave-radiation emitters, particle beam generators, and lasers. Directed-energy weapons rely on electromagnetic waves or subatomic particles that impact at or near the speed of light. Several of these weapons have already been tested in combat and are now potentially available to terrorists.

Whatever the form of electromagnetic energy used for the directed-energy weapon, they all share certain characteristics that make them revolutionary weapons:

- They hit a target at the speed of light.
- They are line-of-sight weapons.
- The price of use is typically a small fraction of what it costs to fire a missile or a large gun. Low- and medium-power lasers can be cheaply obtained.
- They are able to engage many different targets because of their instantaneous effects and the ease of re-aiming them.

HISTORICAL PERSPECTIVE

Lasers

Immediately after the development of the first functional laser, the military (and hence terrorist) potential of the laser was apparent. Modern pulsed lasers can reach energy levels of up to millions of watts in a fraction of a second.

Lasers are the only directed-energy weapons currently fielded by both the United States and other military forces. In many cases, the laser is not intended as a weapon, per se, but rather as a targeting device for another weapon such as a missile or a "smart" bomb. The properties of the laser are particularly suited for this purpose. The military in many nations developed lasers for use as range finders and target designators.

Laser light has special qualities, including the following:

- The light released is *monochromatic;* it contains one specific wavelength of light (one specific color). The wavelength of light is determined by the amount of

energy released when the electron drops to a lower orbit. This wavelength depends on the material of the laser and the method by which it was stimulated to emit light.
- The light released is *coherent.* It is "organized"—each photon moves in step with the others (i.e., the waves of the electromagnetic radiation are in phase in both space and time). This means that all of the photons have wave fronts that launch in unison and the beam is parallel.
- The light is very *directional.* A laser light has a very tight beam and is very strong and concentrated. A light bulb, on the other hand, releases light in many directions, and the light is very weak and diffuse.
- Finally, laser light does not disperse over long distances due to this parallel nature (collimation) of the laser beam.

Military laser devices can easily cause retinal injury, even at a distance of many miles. Military planners found that this optical effect can be used as an anti-personnel system to actively disable personnel by blinding or "dazzling" them. By 1985, the British Navy had developed an unclassified weapon that was fitted aboard ships to blind oncoming enemy pilots at ranges up to 3 miles.

Many thousands of target-designation and distance-ranging lasers have been manufactured and sent out with troops of multiple countries. Because of this availability, they may find their way into the hands of terrorists and be used against U.S. civilians. Other civilian lasers can be easily adapted to similar purposes.

Muggers in England have used simple laser pointers to blind victims before robbing them.[1] There have been many anecdotal reports of eye pain and headaches lasting for several weeks after brief ocular exposures to laser-pointer beams.[2] The pathology of this pain is difficult to understand, since lasting pain is not a common consequence of retinal laser treatment for diabetes, when a considerable amount of laser energy is delivered to the retina.[3,4]

Lasers have already been used by terrorists in an attempt to blind helicopter pilots.[5] It would be no great stretch for a terrorist to mount a relatively powerful laser on a truck or within a car and attempt to blind pilots who are landing at a commercial civilian airport.[6] Likewise, simple lasers may destroy vision in law enforcement officers responding to a terrorist attack.

Microwave-Radiation Emitters

Long-term exposure to high-intensity microwaves can produce both physical and psychological effects on humans, including sensations of warmth, headaches, generalized fatigue, weakness, and dizziness. The effect depends on the power output of the weapon and the distance between the generator and the person.

The U.S. Air Force has fielded a microwave system (area denial system, or ADS) that uses the surface heat production of very-high-power microwaves to induce people to leave an area.

Particle Beam Generators

A particle beam is a directed flow of atomic or subatomic particles. These high-energy particles, when concentrated into a beam, can melt or fracture metals and plastics. They also generate X-rays at the point of impact. These weapons are in development stages only and would be quite unlikely to be found in the hands of terrorists.

CURRENT PRACTICE

There is no foolproof countermeasure for a blinding laser. Each of the available protective efforts will hinder a person's ability to see and to carry out activities requiring sight.

Laser radiation does not travel through opaque objects. Any opaque cover will provide protection against all but very-high-power military lasers. Avoid looking directly at any laser beam or its reflection, if at all possible. Reflections off shiny surfaces may cause damage, despite forward cover. Wearing an eye patch on one eye offers partial protection from blinding lasers; unfortunately, it also deprives the wearer of depth perception and peripheral vision. Patching only prevents blinding in the patched eye.

The present method of protection from the laser threat is quite simple: a pair of "protective sunglasses" can be fashioned that reflect the laser light but let other wavelengths through, so that the wearer can see to do other tasks. These helmet visors or goggles would prevent laser radiation from damaging the wearer's eyes. This works well if the laser threat has been previously identified and is limited to one or two wavelengths. However, there are multiple frequencies available in lasers.

The management of casualties from the effects of laser light is discussed later in this chapter. The triage of these casualties can be accomplished by use of the triage algorithm as shown in Figure 66-1.

Casualties from consequent events, such as a blinded driver or pilot crashing his or her vehicle, are managed in the customary fashion covered by trauma protocols. There would be no difference in management of these casualties if they had a concomitant eye injury.

Key Management Issues

Laser Eye Injury

The eye is the part of the body most vulnerable to laser hazards. Eye damage can occur at much lower-power levels than those causing changes to the skin. This damage may be either temporary or permanent, depending on the wavelength and power of the laser. Because the eye is more sensitive and the pupil is larger during darkness, laser weapons have a greater effect at night than during the day. Generally, eye injuries are far more serious than injuries to the skin.

If the person is using a see-through optical device, such as binoculars, the beam strength is magnified and greater injury to the eye can result. Even modestly powered lasers can temporarily blind an unprotected human looking through a telescope or binoculars. Higher-power lasers can be used to destroy objects in flight or on the ground.

The light intensity of the image formed on the retina is 100,000 times greater than the light intensity at the front of the eye. It is this considerable *optical gain* that creates an eye hazard when laser beams enter the eye. When a person is exposed to laser light, they can be temporarily blinded (dazzling), be blinded for a prolonged time (photolysis), or incur permanent changes in visual function from retinal lesions or hemorrhages.

Far-infrared radiation, which ranges from 3000-nm to 1-mm wavelengths, is absorbed primarily by the cornea (Fig. 66-2). A high-energy laser pulse may severely burn or perforate the cornea. Severe burns or perforations should not be patched, and the eye should be protected to ensure that the vitreous humor does not leak out. Minor laser burns to the cornea may be treated with an eye patch and appropriate eye antibiotics.

Some infrared radiation in the IR-A range (700- to 1400-nm wavelength) and the IR-B range (1400 to 3000 nm) is absorbed directly by the lens. Radiation in the 400- to 1400-nm wavelength range (visible light and IR-A) is the most hazardous because it is transmitted by the optical components of the eye. It reaches the retina, where most of the radiation is absorbed in the retinal pigment epithelium and in the choroid, the dark brown layer with exceptionally large blood vessels and high blood flow rate. The infrared spectrum is often used for military target-designation lasers.

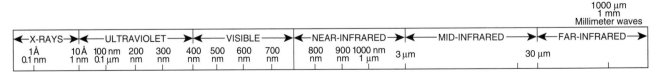

FIGURE 66-1. Steps in laser injury triage.

Damage to the retina or hemorrhaging from retinal damage can cause a complete loss of vision. Persons who see large dark spots at or near the center of their vision, who have a large floating object in their eye, or who have an accumulation of blood in the eye should be promptly evacuated to a hospital with ophthalmologic support. Hemorrhage into the eye should be treated by positioning the patient in a head-up position to allow the blood to settle into the lower part of the eye. Laser burns to the retina do not require an eye patch. Indeed, an eye patch may reduce the person's remaining vision.

There is no currently accepted treatment for laser-or light-induced eye injuries. A laser eye injury can worsen with time, so anyone with a suspected laser eye injury should be both evaluated promptly and again at regular intervals.

Laser Skin Burns

The risk of skin injury is greater than the risk of eye injury by a laser because humans have a lot more skin tissue than eye tissue. However, skin injuries from lasers are much less serious than eye injuries. In part, this is because skin injuries often don't have the dire consequences of eye injuries and partly because the eye concentrates the laser's beam as described above. With enough power and duration, a laser beam of any wave-length in the optical spectrum can penetrate the skin and cause deep internal injury.

The pain from thermal injury to the skin by most targeting lasers is enough to alert a victim to move out of the beam path. Unfortunately, a number of high-power and visible lasers and infrared lasers are now used in industry. These are capable of producing significant skin burns in less than a second.

PITFALLS

Knowing the type of laser involved in an injury may be very valuable. Table 66-1 provides a breakdown of laser type bioeffects. It must be stressed that, to be effective, laser protective goggles or glasses must be donned before exposure to the laser and must have the appropriate frequency rejection characteristics for the laser used. This presents a difficult problem for law enforcement and providers of emergency medical services who may be faced with any of these lasers as a terrorist threat.

It is expected that a tunable (frequency-agile) laser threat will also develop soon. The technical approach used to protect against fixed-frequency lasers cannot be applied to protection from the agile threat or even to protection from a larger number of fixed-frequency threats. As more band-rejection filters are built into a

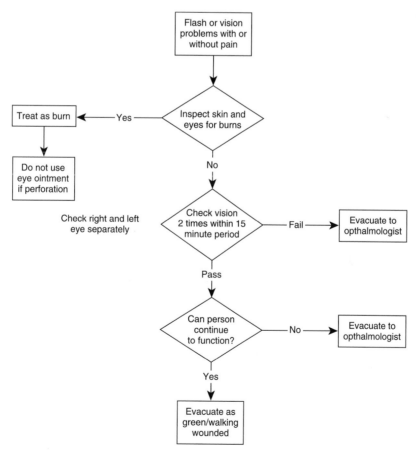

FIGURE 66–2. The patient with a laser eye injury may have sharp eye pain, sudden loss of vision, streaky or spotty vision, or disorientation. The damage to the eye tissue may vary with the wavelength of the laser.

TABLE 66-1 SUMMARY OF BIOEFFECTS OF COMMONLY USED LASERS

LASER TYPE	WAVELENGTH	BIOEFFECT	TISSUE AFFECTED			
	(μm)	Process	Skin	Cornea	Lens	Retina
CO_2	10.6	Thermal	X	X		
HFl	2.7	Thermal	X	X		
Erbium-YAG	1.54	Thermal	X	X		
Nd-YAG*	1.33	Thermal	X	X	X	X
Nd-YAG	1.06	Thermal	X			X
Gas (diode)	0.78–0.84	Thermal	†			X
He-Ne	0.633	Thermal	†			X
Ar	0.488–0.514	Thermal/ Photochemical	X			X‡
XeFl	0.351	Photochemical	X	X		X
XeCl	0.308	Photochemical	X	X		

CO_2, Carbon dioxide; HFl, hydrogen fluoride; YAG, yttrium aluminum garnet; Nd, neodymium; He-Ne, helium-neon; Ar, argon; XeFl, xenon fluoride; XeCl, xenon chloride.
Wavelength at 1.33 nM or more common in some Nd-YAG lasers has demonstrated simultaneous cornea/lens/retina effects in biologic research studies.
†Power levels not normally sufficient to be considered a significant skin hazard.
‡Photochemical effects dominate for long-term exposures to retina (exposure times more than 10 seconds).

sandwich, transmission of light through the visor at other wavelengths decreases also, making it unusable at night and limiting its utility in the daytime.

REFERENCES

1. Anonymous. Killer pens. *Newsweek*. November 24, 1997:8.
2. Seeley D. *Laser Point Causes Eye Injuries?* Orlando, Fla: Laser Institute of America; 1997.
3. Mainster MA, Sliney DH, Marshal J, et al. But is it really light damage? *Ophthalmology*. 1997;104:179-90.
4. Yolton RL, Citek K, Schmeisser E, et al. Laser pointers: toys, nuisances, or significant eye hazards? *J Am Optom Assoc*. 1999;70(5): 285-9.
5. *Daly v Fesco Agencies NA, Inc.* United States District Court, Western District of Washington. Case Number C01-0990C.
6. Anonymous. Russian ship's laser causes eye injury, Navy officer says. Washington, DC: February 12, 1999. Available at: http://www.aeronautics.ru/nws002/ap036.htm.

chapter 67

Emergency Department Design

Robert H. Woolard

In the United States, hospitals build new emergency departments (EDs) every 15 to 20 years. Renovations of existing EDs occur every 5 to 10 years. The main concerns of ED designers are providing efficient spaces for routine care, handling peak volumes, and anticipating future needs. Well-designed EDs accommodate daily, weekly, and seasonal tidal peaks and valleys in patient flow. The variety of high- and low-acuity illnesses and injuries requires EDs to prioritize care into critical, emergent, and urgent treatment. EDs meet community needs for specialized care by providing areas for unique care needs with pediatric, cardiac, trauma, geriatric, or poison centers. Often only as a last thought do EDs include some design features for disaster and mass-casualty response.[1,2] In the wake of terror-related events, such as the New York City World Trade Center disaster on Sept. 11, 2001, many EDs are being designed or renovated to meet new disaster needs. These designs and renovations include decontamination, isolation, and other specialized treatment areas, as well as expanding capacity to treat multiple victims within or next to EDs.

HISTORICAL PERSPECTIVE

In the aftermath of recent terror events and subsequent disaster planning, hospital architects have begun to design EDs to better meet the needs anticipated from a terror attack. Some ED design lessons have been learned from terror events. From the Tokyo sarin gas event and other natural disasters, such as earthquakes, hospitals know they will need to plan for surge capacity. Methods of alerting ED staff early and protecting emergency care providers from contamination are needed, another lesson made clear by the Tokyo sarin gas event in which many emergency providers were contaminated. The New York City World Trade Center event illustrated the need to respond to a disaster scene and continue to treat a sustained increase in ED volume over prolonged periods. In New York, the clean-up phase after the event led to prolonged increased prehospital and ED volume. Most care was provided by emergency personnel working close to ground zero. From the anthrax mailings in the wake of the World Trade Center event, we can learn to anticipate the need for accurate public information.

The ED remains the most available point of access to immediate healthcare in the United States. ED designers are now anticipating increased volumes of patients that might be generated by disaster or a terror event. Although a stressed public needs information and health screenings that perhaps can be met by providers outside the ED, the ED will be accessed for counseling and screening when other services are overwhelmed or delay to access is encountered. In past disasters, shelter needs were met outside the ED. However, needs for quarantine during bioterror events may create shelter needs in EDs.

ED design and response capability after Sept. 11 has become a larger concern for public disaster planners, the federal government, and hospital architects. Two federally funded projects coordinated by emergency physicians, one at Washington Hospital Center (ER1) and another at Rhode Island Hospital (RIDI), have developed and released recommendations. ER1 suggests designs for a new ED that meets any and all anticipated needs of a disaster event.[3] RIDI has developed new disaster-response paradigms, training scenarios, and response simulations that also can be used in ED design.[4]

CURRENT PRACTICE

ED design would be tremendously enhanced if a prototype "disaster-ready" ED such as ER1 could be built. ED designers may not be able to create an "all-risks-ready" ED given financial constraints. However, incorporating disaster-ready suggestions when EDs are renovated or built new will improve our readiness and may be more financially feasible. New building materials, technologies, and concepts will continue to inform the effort to prepare EDs for terror attack. Urban ED trauma centers are attempting to develop capacity to serve as regional disaster resource centers and respond out to a terror event. These EDs are designed to incorporate larger waiting and entrance areas, adjacent units, or nearby parking spaces in their plans to ramp up treatment capacity. More decontamination and isolation capacity is being built to help control the spread of toxic or infectious agents. Information systems are being made available to provide real-time point-of-service information and any needed "just in time" training for potential terror threats. The technology needed to respond to a terrorist event, such as personal protective equipment (PPE), is becoming more widely available and is stored where easily available in EDs. Although mass decontamination can occur close to the disaster scene, EDs are gearing up to decontaminate, isolate, and treat individuals or groups contaminated with biologic or chemical materials. Four elements of ED design are being addressed to prepare EDs for terror events: scalability, security, information systems, and decontamination.

Scalability, Surge, and Treatment Capacity

EDs are generally designed with sufficient, but not excess, space. The number of treatment spaces needed in an ED is usually matched to the anticipated ED patient volume; roughly 1 treatment space per 1100 annual ED visits or 1 treatment space per 400 annual ED hospital admissions is recommended.[1] According to disaster planners, a major urban trauma center ED built for 50,000 to 100,000 visits per year should have surge capacity up to 100 patients per hour for 4 hours and 1000 patients per day for 4 days. One Sept. 11 challenge is to provide "surge capacity" to meet anticipated patient needs. Hospitals are woefully overcrowded, and EDs are routinely housing admitted patients.[5-7]

EDs are now being designed to allow "growth" into adjacent space: a ground level or upper level, a garage, or a parking lot. Garage and parking lot space has been used in many disaster drills and mass exposures. Garages and parking lots are more purposely designed with separate access to streets, allowing separation of disaster traffic and routine ED traffic. Needed terror-response supplies (e.g., antidotes, respirators, personal protective gear) are being stored near or within the ED. The cost of ventilation, heat, air conditioning, communication, and security features often prohibits renovation of garages. More often, tents are erected over parking lots or loading areas. Modular "second EDs," tents or structures with collapsible walls (fold and stack), have been deployed by disaster responders. These can be used near the main ED, preserving the ED for critical cases. Some hospitals are considering beds in halls, patient rooms, and other spaces to increase their ability to generate surge capacity. Hallways can provide usable space if constructed wider and equipped with medical gases and adequate power and lighting. Often only minimal modifications are necessary to make existing halls and lobbies "dual-use" spaces. Some hospitals have increased space by installing retractable awnings on the exterior over ambulance bays or loading docks. Tents are often used outside EDs as decontamination and treatment areas in disaster drills. Tents with inflatable air walls have the added benefit of being insulated for all-weather use.

In the military, the need to provide treatment in limited space has resulted in the practice of stacking patients vertically to save space and to reduce the distances that personnel walk. U.S. Air Force air evacuation flights have stacked critical patients three high. These bed units could be deployed for a mass event. Portable modular units are also available to help EDs address the space needs. Unfortunately, many EDs rely on other facilities in the regional system. In a terror event on a hospital campus, the ED function may need to be moved to a remote area within the hospital. Many disaster plans designate a preexisting structure on campus as the "backup" ED. The area is stockpiled with equipment, and plans for access and patient and staff movement are developed.

Although the capacity to handle patient surges is being addressed regionally and nationally, large events with high critical care volumes may overtax the system of the trauma centers regionally. The National Medical Disaster System can be mobilized to move excess victims and establish field hospitals during events involving hundreds or thousands of victims.

The ED plan to provide treatment during disaster must consider evacuation, since the event may produce an environmental hazard that contaminates the ED. Evacuation of ED patients has been addressed by ED designers. Some EDs have the capacity to more easily evacuate. In better planned EDs, stairwells have floor lights to assist in darkness. Stairways are sufficient in size to allow backboarded patients to be evacuated. The communication and tracking system includes sensors in corridors and stairways. Patient records are regularly backed up to portable disk and available for evacuation.

Security

Securing the function of an ED includes securing essential resources: water, gases, power, ventilation, communication, and information. ED security involves surveillance, control of access and egress, threat mitigation, and "lockdown" capacity. Surveillance exists in almost all EDs. Many ED parking and decontamination areas are monitored by cameras. The wireless tracking system can also be part of the surveillance system. A tracking system can create a virtual geospatial and temporal map of staff and patient movement. Tracking systems have been used in disaster drills to identify threat patterns. Most EDs have identification/access cards and readers. Chemical and biologic sensors for explosives, organic solvents, and biologic agents are becoming available. When selecting a sensor, designers consider sensitivity, selectivity, speed of response, and robustness.[8-12] Sensor technology is an area of active research that continues to yield new solutions that are being incorporated into EDs. In concept, all entrances could be designed to identify persons using scanning to detect unwanted chemicals, biologic agents, or explosives and to detain and decontaminate as needed.

Most EDs have multiple entry portals for ingress of patients, visitors, staff, vendors, law enforcement personnel, and others. EDs are using screening and identification technologies at all entrances in combination with closed circuit video monitoring. Personnel must be dedicated for prompt response when needed. Automation of identification can efficiently allow safe flow of patients, staff, and supplies. Vehicle access has been managed by barcoding staff and visitor vehicles. At some road access points, automated scanners could monitor and control vehicle access. Modern EDs limit the number of entrances and channel pedestrian and vehicular traffic through identification control points. For the most part, points of entrance into the ED can be managed with locking doors, ID badge control points, and surveillance to allow desired access for staff and supplies. Thoughtful planning should facilitate rapid access between the functional areas such as the ED, operating rooms, and critical care units. Movement within and between buildings needs to be controlled and must allow a total lockdown when necessary.

Direct threats to the ED include blasts and chemical, biologic, and environmental contamination. There are several strategies to mitigate blast. Twelve-inch-thick conventional concrete walls, using commercially available aggregates (147 lb per cubic foot) affords reasonable blast protection.[16,17] On some campuses, the space between the ED and the entrance is designed largely to prevent direct attack.[18] However, atriums are terror targets. Although atriums are useful as overflow areas, their windows and glass create hazardous flying debris. Given the threat of blast attack, communication, gas, electric, water, and other critical services should be remote from vulnerable areas and shielded when they traverse roads and walkways. Protection against release of chemical and biologic agents inside or outside the ED requires a protective envelope, controlled air filtration in and out, an air distribution system providing clean pressurized air, a water purification system providing potable water, and a detection system. Better HVAC systems can pressurize the envelope and purge contaminated areas.

Information

Anticipated computing needs for ED operations during disaster events are immense. In most EDs, large amounts of complex and diverse information are routinely available electronically. Overflow patients in hallways and adjacent spaces can be managed with mobile computing, which is available in many EDs. Wireless handheld devices can facilitate preparation for disasters and allow immediate access to information by providers in hallways and decontamination spaces. Multiple desktop workstations are available throughout most EDs. During disaster, displays of information that will aid decision-making include bed status, the types of rooms available, the number of persons waiting, and ambulances coming in. Monitors now display patient vital signs, telemetry, and test results. Significant improvements in efficiency and decision-making can be achieved when more real-time information is available to decision-makers. Multiple computer screens enhance ED readiness.

Clinical decision tools, such as UpToDate,[19] make information readily available to providers. These and other "just-in-time" resources will be needed when practitioners treat unusual or rare diseases not encountered in routine practice. The wide variety of potential disaster scenarios argues for the availability of just-in-time information. Information specific to a disaster event should be broadcast widely on multiple screens in many areas. Cellular links and wireless portable devices should also receive information. Access to information has been enhanced in most EDs through cell phone use, etc. This facilitates making information available to guide each staff member.

Diagnostic decision support systems have been demonstrated to help practitioners recognize symptom complexes that are uncommon or unfamiliar. Information systems should be capable of communicating potential terror event information regularly. Many EDs have log-on systems that require staff to read new information. In a disaster-ready ED, a list of potential threats could be posted daily. However, the utility of computer references or on-call experts is limited by the practitioner's ability to recognize a situation that requires the resource.

Computer-based patient-tracking systems are available for routinely tracking patients in most EDs. Some computer-based tracking systems have a disaster mode that quickly adapts to a large influx of patients allowing for collation of symptoms, laboratory values, and other pertinent syndromic data. In many regions, EDs serve as a terror surveillance network. Routine data obtained on entry are passively collected and transferred to a central point for analysis. In the event of a significant spike in targeted patient symptom complexes, these data can trigger an appropriate disaster response. The capacity for this entry point surveillance should be anticipated and built into any disaster-ready ED information system.[21-23] For example, data terminals allowing patient input data at registration similar to electronic ticketing at airports could passively provide information. This self-service system could add to ED surge capacity. Similarly, real-time bed identification, availability, and reservation systems used to assist patient management in some EDs could aid ED function during disaster. Movement to an inpatient bed is a well-documented choke point recognized nationally during normal hospital operations and becomes an issue during disaster.

Lobby screens can facilitate family access to information during a disaster, displaying information about the event and patient status. During disasters, family members can be given access to screens to query for missing persons. Computers with Internet access that could display event information are available in patient rooms in some EDs.

During the anthrax mailings, public hysteria taxed the healthcare system. Posttraumatic stress, anxiety, and public concern over possible exposure to a biologic or chemical agent may generate a surge of minor patients at EDs. Within some EDs, lecture halls or media centers are available (generally used for teaching conferences) but could provide health information and media briefings during disaster. The media are an important source of public information and must be considered when planning disaster response. Information from a media center in the ED could be released to the Internet and closed-circuit screens. Accurate information can allay public concerns and direct the public to appropriate resources and access points.

Isolation and Decontamination

Many EDs have patient decontamination (DECON) areas. Adequate environmental protection for patients undergoing DECON is necessary and includes visual barriers from onlookers, segregation of the sexes, and attention to personal belongings.[24,25] In many EDs, DECON areas are being added to accommodate mass exposures. EDs have added or augmented DECON facilities. DECON areas should have a separate, self-contained drainage system, controlled water temperature, and shielding from environmental hazards. Exhaust fans are used to prevent the buildup of toxic fumes in these decontamination areas. For most EDs, mass DECON has been accomplished by using an uncovered parking lot and deploying heated and vented modular tent units. Uncovered parking areas adjacent and accessible to the ED have been enabled for disaster response. Other EDs use high-volume, low-pressured showers mounted on the side of a building. Serial showers allow multiple patients to enter at the same entrance and time. However, serial showers do not provide privacy, can be difficult for an ill patient to access, and can lead to recontaminated water runoff. Also, persons requiring more time may impede flow and reduce the number of patients decontaminated. Parallel showers built in advance or set up temporarily in tenting offer greater privacy but require wider space and depth. Combined serial and parallel design allows the advantages of each, separating ill patients and increasing the number of simultaneous decontaminations.[26]

Often built into the ED is another DECON room for one or two patients with the following features: outside access; negative-pressure exhaust air exchange; water drainage; water recess; seamless floor; non-pervious, slip-resistant, washable floor, walls, and ceiling; gas appliances; supplied air wall outlets for PPE use; high-input air; intercom; overhead paging; and an anteroom for DECON of isolated cases. PPE is recommended for use by military and fire departments during events involving hazardous materials. Hospitals use these devices and store a reasonable number of protective ensembles (i.e., gloves, suits, and respiratory equipment) usually near the ED DECON area. DECON areas are built with multiple supplied air outlets for PPE use to optimize safety and maximize work flexibility. A nearby changing area is available in some EDs. The changing area is laid out to optimize medical monitoring and to ease access to the DECON area.[27-31]

Some capability to isolate and prevent propagation of a potential biologic agent has been designed into most EDs. Patients who present with undetermined respiratory illnesses are routinely sent to isolation. A direct entrance from the exterior to an isolation room is not usually available but has been a recent renovation in some EDs. Creation of isolation areas poses special design requirements for HVAC, cleaning, and security to ensure that infections and infected persons are contained. An isolation area should have compartmentalized air handling with high-efficiency filters providing clean air.[32-35] Biohazard contamination is particularly difficult to mitigate. Keeping the facility "clean" and safe for other patients is an extreme challenge. Biologic agents of terrorism may resist decontamination attempts. Infected patients present a risk to staff. Few triage areas and ED rooms have been designed for decontamination. Surfaces must be able to withstand repeated decontamination. Sealed inlets for gases and plumbing have also been considered.[36-38] Patients who are isolated can be observed with monitoring cameras. Some isolation areas include a restroom within their space, which helps restrict patient egress.

General ED areas could have DECON capabilities built in. Floor drains have been included in some ED rooms for easier decontamination. Infection control is improved using polymer surface coatings that are smooth, nonporous, and tolerant to repeated cleaning, creating a virtually seamless surface that is easy to clean. These coatings can be impregnated with antimicrobial properties enhancing their biosafe capability. Silver-impregnated metal surfaces in sinks, drains, door handles, and other locations can reduce high bacterial content. Silver-impregnated metal has demonstrated antimicrobial effects.[39]

Conventional ventilation systems use 15% to 25% outside air during normal operation, thus purging indoor contaminants. Air cleaning depends on filtration, ultraviolet irradiation, and purging. HVAC design should model demand for adequately clean air and also for isolation of potential contaminants.[40] The disaster-ready ED requires protection from external contaminations as well as contagious patients. A compartmentalized central venting system without recirculation has the ability to remove or contain toxic agents in and around the ED. Compartmentalized HVAC systems allow for the "sealing" of zones from each other. More desirable HVAC systems electronically shut down sections, use effective filtration, and can "clean" contaminated air. A compartmentalized system can fail, but it only fails in the zone it is servicing; smaller zones mean smaller areas lost to contamination. These systems are less vulnerable to global failure or spread of contamination. Modular HVAC units developed for field military applications have been added to existing ED isolation areas for use when needed to create safe air compartments.

PITFALLS

Cost may prohibit addressing issues like building more space or better ventilation, decontamination, and isolation facilities. If added space and facilities are not made more available, many lives may be lost during a disaster event. When monies are spent for terror readiness, EDs must continue to function day to day. EDs will be challenged to provide efficient routine care and also handle the consequences of a terror event or natural disaster. These competing functions could result in EDs that cannot handle routine care.

These design efforts could also lead to unnecessary increases in expenditures in anticipation of terror events that never materialize. To the extent that efforts to provide disaster care can be translated into solutions that address other more immediate hospital and ED problems, they will gain support. More access to information systems providing just-in-time training could inform staff not only of terror events but of mundane policy changes and unique patient needs such as bloodless therapy for Jehovah's witnesses, etc. Better information access could also improve routine ED efficiency and communication with patients and families. However, these rationales may not prevail to fund disaster readiness. Decontamination equipment and areas may be used for commercial hazardous materials spills. Isolation areas could be more routinely used in an effort to contain suspected contagions, such as severe acute respiratory syndrome (SARS).

Lack of bed capacity in hospitals leads to ED overcrowding. Scalable EDs may offer temporary solutions in times of over-burdened hospital inpatient services. However, once reserve spaces are used to solve other over-capacity problems, those spaces may no longer be available for disaster operations. Thus, a new facility could "build" the capability of handling large surges of patients into adjacent spaces, only to lose it by filling these spaces with excess patients whenever the hospital is over census.

Finally, a terror event may be different from those for which we prepare. The rarity of terror events creates a need for us to test our disaster plans, skills, and capacities in drills. Drills may uncover design problems that can then be addressed but may only prepare us for anticipated threats.

CONCLUSION

Why pour such resources into building capacity that we hope never to use? Among the lessons learned from past disaster events is the need to develop disaster skills and build a disaster-response system from components that are in daily use. Systems that are used routinely are more familiar and more likely to be used successfully during terror events. Certainly the surge capacity of a "terror-ready" ED would be used for natural disaster response and in disaster drills. The surge space could also be used for over-census times, public health events, immunizations, and health screenings. A modern ED should serve as a community resource, deploy and test capacities regularly in disaster drills, and maintain "readiness" in a post-Sept. 11 world.

REFERENCES

1. Australian College for Emergency Medicine. Emergency Department Design Guidelines. Available at: http://www.acem.org.au/open/documents/ed_design.htm.
2. Emergency department design. Riggs LM, ed. *Functional and Space Programming*. Dallas, Tex: American College of Emergency Physicians; :111.
3. ER One/All-Risks-Ready Emergency Department. Available at: http://www.er1.org.
4. Rhode Island Disaster Initiative. Improving disaster medicine through research. Available at: http://www.ridiproject.org/page_manager.asp.
5. Andrulis DP, Kellermann A, Hintz EA, et al. Emergency departments and crowding in US teaching hospitals. *Ann Emerg Med*. 1991; 20(9):980-6.
6. Meggs WJ, Czaplijski T, Benson N. Trends in emergency department utilization, 1988-1997. *Acad Emerg Med*. 1999;6(10):1030-5.
7. Bazarian JJ, Schneider SM, Newman VJ, Chodosh J. Do admitted patients held in the emergency department impact the throughput of treat-and-release patients? *Acad Emerg Med*. 1996; 3(12):1113-8.
8. Physical Security Equipment Action Group (PSEAG). Department of Defense. Available at: http://www.dtic.mil/ndia/2002security/toscano.pdf.
9. Ellis AB, Nickel AL, Shaw GA, Heirseele KV. Interior/Exterior Intrusion and Chemical/Biological Detection Systems/Sensors. *Proceedings of the Same National Symposium on Comprehensive Force Protection, Charleston, SC*. OPNAVINST 5510.1G, 45B. November 2001.
10. Jurs PC, Bakken GA, McClelland HE. Computational methods for the analysis of chemical sensor array data from volatile analytes. *Chem Rev*. 2000;100(7):2649-78.
11. Kissinger PT. Electrochemical detection in bioanalysis. *J Phar Biomed Anal*. 1996;14(8-10):871-80.
12. Lonergan MC, Severin EJ, Doleman BJ, et al. Array-based vapor sensing using chemically sensitive, carbon black-polymer resistors. *Chem Mater*. 1996; 8(9)2298-312.
13. *Standard of Safety Levels for Human Exposure to Radio Frequency*. ANS/IEEE C95.1-2002. Available at: http://www.osha.gov/sltc/ radiofrequencyradiation/standards.html
14. *Code of Federal Regulations*. 47CFR 15 Available at: www.access.gpo.gov/cgi-bin/cfrassemble.cgi?title-200347.
15. Nuclear Shielding Supplies and Service, Inc, Web site. Available at: http://www.nuclearshielding.com.
16. Heavy Concrete Web site. Available at: http://www.Heavy Concrete.com.
17. Nadel BA. Designing for security. *Architectural Record*. March 2002.
18. Putting Clinical Information into Practice. UpToDate Web site. Available at: http://www.uptodate.com.
19. Bennett NM, Konecki J. Emergency department and walk-in center surveillance for bioterrorism: utility for influenza surveillance [abstract]. ICEID 2002. *Emerg Infect Dis*. 2005; 11(8). Available at: http://www.cdc.gov/ncidod/eid/index.htm.
20. Gunn JE, McKenna V, Brinsfield KH, et al. Boston Æ warning early surveillance system for bioterrorism: September 11-November 11 [abstract]. ICEID 2002. *Emerg Infect Dis*. 2005; 11(8). Available at: http://www.cdc.gov/ncidod/eid/index.htm.
21. Karpati A, Mostashari F, Heffernan R, et al. Syndromic surveillance for bioterrorism New York City, Oct-Dec 2001[abstract]. ICEID 2002. *Emerg Infect Dis*. 2005; 11(8). Available at: http://www.cdc.gov/ncidod/eid/index.htm.
22. Gong E, Dauber W. Policewomen win settlement. *Seattle Times*. July 11, 1996:B1.
23. Stern J. *Fire department response to biological threat at B'nai B'rith Headquarters, Washington DC: report 114 of the Major Fire Investigative Project*. Emmitsburg, Md: US Fire Administration; October 2001.
24. Barbera JA, Macintyre AG, DeAtley CA. *Chemically contaminated patient annex (CCPA): Hospital Emergency Operations Planning Guide*. United States Public Health Service, Washington, DC. March 2001.
25. Burgess JL, Kirk M, Barron SW, Cisek J. Emergency department hazardous materials protocol for contaminated patients. *Ann Emerg Med*. 1999;34(2):205-12.
26. Centers for Disease Control and Prevention. CDC recommendations for civilian communities near chemical weapons depots. *60 Federal Register*. 1995;33307-18.
27. US Department of Labor, Occupational Safety and Health Administration. *Hospitals and Community Emergency Response: What You Need to Know*. Washington DC: Emergency Response Safety Series. OSHA 1997;3152.
28. Macintyre AG, Christopher GW, Eitzen E Jr, et al. Weapons of mass destruction events with contaminated casualties: effective planning for health care facilities. *JAMA* 2000;283(2):242-9.
29. Shapira Y, Bar Y, Berkenstadt H, et al. Outline of hospital organization for a chemical warfare attack. *Isr J Med Sci*. 1991;27(11-12):616-22.
30. *Guidelines for Design and Construction of Hospitals and Healthcare Facilities*. Philadelphia: The American Institute of Architects Academy of Architecture for Health; 2001.
31. Transport Canada. *Emergency Response Guidebook: A Guidebook for First Responders During the Initial Phase of a Dangerous Goods-Hazardous Materials Incident (ERG 2000)*. Washington DC: U.S. Department of Transportation, and Secretary of Transport and Communications of Mexico; 2000.

32. Department of Health and Human Services. *Metropolitan Medical Response System's Field Operation Guide*. Washington DC: Department of Health and Human Services; November 1998.

33. Volume I – Emergency Medical Services: A Planning Guide for the Management of Contaminated Patients, Agency for Toxic Substances and Disease Registry, March 2001.

34. Victorian Government Health information. Infectious Diseases Epidemiology and Surveillance. Victoria, Australia. Available at: http://www.dhs.vic.gov.au/phb/9906058a/9906058.pdf.

35. American Institute of Architects. *Guidelines for Design and Construction of Hospital and Health Care Facilities, 1996-7*. Washington, DC: American Institute of Architects Press; 1996.

36. Barbera JA, Macintyre AG, DeAtley CA. Chemically Contaminated Patient Annex: Hospital Emergency Operations Planning Guide [August 23, 2001, draft]. Washington, DC: George Washington University; 2001.

37. Deitch EA, Marino AA, Gillespie TE, Albright JA. Silver-nylon: a new antimicrobial agent. *Antimicrob Agents Chemother*. 1983; 23(3):356-9.

38. Kowalski WJ, Bahnfleth WP, Whittam TS. Filtration of airborne microorganisms: modeling and prediction. *ASHRAE Transactions*. 1999;105(2):4-17. Available at: http://www.engr.psu.edu/ae/iec/abe/publications/filtration_airborne_microorganism.pdf.

chapter 68

Chemical, Biologic, and Nuclear Quarantine

Patricia A. Nolan

As a society, we in the United States seek protection from harm through the exercise of police power as a basic function of constitutional governments "to provide for the general common defense and promote the general welfare."[1] At the same time, we value individual liberty as the greatest good. This chapter examines the actions we can use to control the spread of a disease or toxin by controlling the movement of goods, animals, and people. These actions are embodied in the term *quarantine*. The emotional power of the term comes from the tension between our competing values of personal liberty and protection from harm. The word quarantine implies coercion, restricted movements, isolation from others, loss of property, and loss of liberty. We quarantine that which we seek to avoid or believe to be contaminated. In our use of police power (i.e., regulations, orders, law enforcement, and similar instruments) to restrict the movement of goods and peoples and to require examination, treatment, and confinement, we must also respect civil protections to limit our improper, excessive, or unethical use of this power.

In a terrorist event or a natural epidemic, principles of control, carefully applied, can reduce the number of casualties by preventing secondary cases. Data obtained through examining and monitoring of exposed persons can be used to identify and respond to subsequent cases, as well as to clarify the initial event.

The purpose of quarantine is to prevent the spread of a contagious disease in a population. Successful quarantine measures are based on the specific features of the biologic agent. Some elements of quarantine action may be appropriate in a terrorism event that involves biologic or chemical toxins or radiologic contamination. Quarantine is a set of legally authorized procedures instituted to accomplish the following:

- Identify what and who have been exposed;
- Determine which exposed people, animals, and/or goods are likely to be contaminated or infected;
- Prevent transmission by managing those who are contaminated or infected;
- Prevent subsequent exposures and contaminations.

Typical quarantine actions include the following:
- Identification of potentially infected or contaminated persons, animals, and goods;
- Initiation of protective measures to prevent further transmission of infectious agents;
- Initiation of protective measures to prevent exposed persons from becoming infected;
- Control of interaction of potentially or actually infected persons, animals, or goods with uninfected populations or goods.

Careful implementation of quarantine measures can assist in controlling fear and panic as well as controlling the spread of infectious agents or contaminants. At the same time, disasters require prompt decision-making and decisive action in the face of limited information. Healthcare personnel making quarantine decisions must have delegated authority from the government to act in ways that restrict liberties or take property. The critical safeguards in a disaster include formal orders for quarantine measures of persons, which are as specific as possible to the circumstances, opportunity for administrative or judicial review, and frequent, timely renewal of the conditions. For the protection of all, there are significant penalties for failure to comply with quarantine orders. These safeguards create a need for adequate records of the decisions made and the evidence used. Physicians should make it a point to know their responsibilities for reporting and controlling infectious diseases in the state in which they practice.

Consultation among law enforcement, emergency management, and public health agents is important in setting priorities among competing disaster management and antiterrorism demands. For example, cordoning off areas of contamination and preventing removal of goods may be less of a law enforcement concern than apprehending terrorists, yet failure to prevent movement of contaminated or infected goods may be devastating from a public health perspective.

QUARANTINE HISTORY

Our modern concepts of protecting society by isolating persons and controlling movement of animals and goods

451

to prevent the spread of contagious diseases can be traced to the Middle Ages. Leprosy was recognized as contagious, and lepers were separated from the community and isolated from society. As early as 583, authorities restricted the association of lepers with healthy people, building on the biblical sources in Leviticus.[2] In the mid-fourteenth century, authorities isolated victims of plague in their homes with their families until all had died or recovered. These periods of isolation varied in length, but a 40-day period became fairly standard.[2]

History is replete with instances of inequitable application of quarantine measures. The poor and the outcast were more likely to be confined, deprived of their livelihoods, and subjected to inhumane treatment as epidemics swept through. Modern epidemics, such as tuberculosis and HIV, reveal that better understanding of contagion does not always result in equitable responses. A preference for voluntary measures does not assure equity, especially if some groups have less access to medical care and other prophylactic measures.

Important elements of quarantine included requirements for the reporting of diseased persons and those in contact with them, civil or religious authorities empowered to decide who and/or what should be quarantined, and criteria for ending the quarantine. Quarantines have been enforced by armed force and imprisonment. As the nature of contagion became better understood, and as treatments and preventives were developed that reduced contagion, the definition of *quarantine* has been modified. Isolation and treatment of the infected; observation and control of movements of the exposed; vaccination and/or prophylactic treatment of the exposed; destruction or disinfection of animals, goods, and premises; extermination of disease vectors; and active case-finding and investigation are all now used to control the spread of contagious diseases.

We use governmental police power to ensure compliance with these control measures. In each state in the United States, specific statutes define the limits of the state's authority. As the views of civil liberties have shifted, the authority to impose quarantine became more limited and procedural safeguards were put in place. Many states revised public health statutes to codify the necessary procedures. In the first 5 years of the twenty-first century, many states revised statutes concerning emergency powers of the state in the event of terrorist attacks. The revision process has brought issues of civil liberties and the use of police powers to control the intentional introduction of infectious disease into sharp relief. Each state resolves the tension a little differently.

CURRENT PRACTICE

Quarantine measures are undertaken to separate sources of infection from susceptible populations. The same measures may be useful when extended beyond infectious agents to radiologic sources and toxic agents in terrorism incidents and mass disasters. Throughout our statutes there is a preference for voluntary cooperation with control measures, coupled with authority to enforce control measures when necessary.

In many statutes and descriptions, the terms *isolation* and *quarantine* are coupled. However, we can distinguish *quarantine* as control measures applying to those exposed to the agent of concern, and *isolation* as control measures applying to those known to be infected and capable of transmitting the agent. Thus, quarantine is the more expansive concept, applying to those who are not sick or even infectious at the outset. Isolation may require the more restrictive measures, since those persons are known to be infectious to others. In a population under quarantine, those who become infected and capable of transmitting disease need to be isolated from those who are exposed but may not be infected. In healthcare institutions, these distinctions become particularly important in sustaining the viability of the institution.

The general measures of quarantine include restriction of movement, periodic examination and testing, requirement of prophylactic treatment, closure of premises, and destruction of animals or goods. These are frightening concepts to many, especially in times of civil disorder related to terrorism or mass disasters. During an epidemic or after a terrorist attack, very large populations or geographic areas could be subject to quarantine measures, adding to fear and panic. Clear communication of the reasons for and the terms of quarantine measures are essential. The goals of actions include establishing trust that healthcare professionals and the government are taking the steps needed and applying them in an equitable manner. The clinician can play a role in controlling panic and gaining cooperation among the public in controlling spread of the agent.

In imposing quarantine in response to a terrorist event or a disease outbreak, we must emphasize voluntary compliance with quarantine measures, and we must use the least restrictive measures likely to be effective. The quarantine actions needed depend on characteristics of the biologic agent, the people and animals at risk, and the local environment. The quarantine officer has to use the best available evidence on the biologic agent; the time, place, and route of exposure; and the resources at hand or en route. The quarantine plan must establish a rapid, safe, and efficient means of determining who has been exposed, when they were exposed, and what their current health status is. The plan must set out the options for control measures and surveillance. The plan must also provide for reassessment and adjustment as new information is acquired.

To initiate quarantine, one must establish that there is a risk of transmission of an infectious agent so significant that liberties must be restricted, and that the specific measures imposed have a likelihood of preventing transmission. In the early stage of responding to a biologic attack, there may be little confirmed data and substantial confusion. The quarantine officer should set the decision parameters for control measures based on what is known and what is suspected. The most restrictive approach is reserved for infectious diseases known to be effectively transmitted from person to person by airborne, droplet, and fomite routes, such as plague, smallpox, severe acute respiratory syndrome (SARS), and measles. If exposure to these is suspected, the initial determinations of exposure and infectiousness should be very sensitive, tolerating a high false-positive rate. As better data are obtained, adjustments in sensitivity follow.

In designing the screening system for determining who is infectious, who has been exposed, when they were exposed, and what their current health status is, consider the number of people to be examined, the time-frame necessary for controlling a particular infectious agent in the circumstances, and the risk that additional exposure to the agent could occur. Choose sites and facilities that can meet the security needs (e.g., access, parking, crowd control, and containment) that will protect vital healthcare assets and that will not interfere with other essential response actions. Consider the relationship between the quarantine functions and the population-wide actions such as mass immunization that may be planned.

The examination area should be set up to provide infection control, confidentiality, personal privacy, good lighting, and efficient movement of subjects and examiners. Design may vary substantially depending on the putative agent (e.g., addressing risks of contagion or dealing with potential symptoms such as vomiting, diarrhea, or skin lesions) and the numbers and skills of examiners. In a setting with few physicians, physician assistants, and nurse practitioners, history-taking and initial examinations may be completed by nurses, with clinician backup when a more detailed examination is required of those with "positive" findings or symptoms. Skilled volunteers, such as retired health professionals or student health professionals, may be recruited as well.

The first step in determining the need for isolation and quarantine is the finding of a history of exposure to an infectious agent that is transmitted from human to human or from animals or goods to humans. The interviewer needs a clear understanding of the parameters of exposure to make a determination that a person or animal is exposed and therefore subject to voluntary or involuntary quarantine measures. Confirmation of movements and actions that place the person or animal in proximity to the infectious agent is particularly important. The likelihood of exposure due to proximity varies with the nature of the agent and the exposing event.

People who are already terrorized will have difficulty determining exposure for themselves, so careful history-taking is essential. More than one question should be planned for each critical item to detect errors and dissimulation. The interviewer should clarify any contradictions and make a decision on what exposure, if any, has occurred for each person or animal. When obtaining information about a third party, such as a child, the interviewer should determine whether another person has information that needs to be considered.

If the putative exposure is to infectious persons or animals, the history must include all interactions within the longest period of infectiousness, not just the most recent interaction or the interactions after symptoms have developed. If the putative exposure is the result of being in a place, exact locations, times, and activities are important facts.

Quarantine measures restrict fundamental liberties. The decision needs to stand up in legal proceedings, yet

be efficient. History-taking forms that facilitate the recording of the key decisions will provide evidence and aid efficiency. The form should ensure that details about the exposure are recorded and that extraneous information is minimized. Recording exact answers enhances both the interviewer's decision record and the interviewee's understanding of exposures.

In attacks with very short exposure-to-symptom times, such as some poisons, toxins, or radioactivity, the history of exposure may be very limited, essentially addressing opportunity. Assessing vital signs and detecting symptoms becomes the central concern in such exposures, with prompt decontamination often the action of choice. Once it is determined that the risk of transmission is minimal, full attention is directed to treatment.

Once it is determined that a person or animal has been exposed to an infectious agent transmissible to others, the next requirement is an initial physical examination. The objectives of the initial examination include the following:

- Establish the current state of health
- Determine whether any symptoms of exposure to the putative agent(s) are present
- Determine a prophylactic management plan
- Establish the baseline for monitoring during quarantine
- Determine the level of restriction necessary to prevent further spread of the disease

Accurate recording is critical because of the legal concerns about quarantine. The administrative or judicial reviewer will need these data in assessing the quarantine measures imposed. Change in health status during prophylactic treatment and quarantine monitoring is critical to decision-making on isolation, further control of movement, and initiation, change, and discontinuation of treatment.

In addition to eliciting the current state of health, the examiner should determine the presence of health factors that increase the risk of infection (e.g., immune compromise, organ transplants, medications) and the presence or absence of symptoms of the putative agent. Allergies, medication use, and other possible contraindications to vaccine or prophylactic treatment should be elicited as appropriate to the circumstances.

The examiner should verify critical vital signs, most importantly the presence or absence of fever. When the putative agent causes shock or collapse, blood pressure should be monitored during the examination process. Determining the presence or absence of specific symptoms indicative of infection or contagion is the first task. This information is critical in protecting all persons being examined as well as examiners. The time of appearance of signs and symptoms of infection is essential in subsequent decisions regarding prophylaxis, immunization, and infection control.

Control of Individual Movement

The actual conditions of quarantine and isolation depend on many factors. The nature of the putative agent, how communicable it is, the initial symptoms of disease, the contagious period, and the routes of transmission all influence the decisions. Ordinarily, these decisions will be made by the local or state public health authority and communicated to all examiners along with specific authorization to make quarantine and isolation decisions. The goal is voluntary compliance with necessary precautions. Many jurisdictions require a court order to initiate or enforce restrictions of movement or confiscation of property. If civil authority is seriously disrupted, local physicians may be faced with making decisions in a vacuum (see Pitfalls section).

The primary purpose of quarantine is to separate the unexposed population from the exposed population to prevent future exposures. The unexposed may be instructed on protective measures. In some circumstances, unexposed persons may be offered immunization or prophylactic treatment. A clinician acting in an individual capacity may be requested to provide vaccines or medications to unexposed persons not subject to past or likely future exposure (see Pitfalls section). For example, in the event of a smallpox outbreak, health authorities could decide to immunize whole populations if the resources were sufficient to do so without jeopardizing the protection of those already exposed or infected. More frequently, healthcare workers, caretakers of animals, and family members of persons under quarantine are candidates for prophylaxis by vaccine or medication.

Exposed persons and animals without signs or symptoms of infection are subject to quarantine. The nature of quarantine measures is dependent on characteristics of the agent and the outbreak, the cooperation and resources of the persons, the ability to confine or control animals, the capacity of the authority to monitor quarantine, and the level of risk of wider infection. For exposed *but not yet infectious* persons who can be monitored, confinement is often unnecessary. This strategy is dependent on early detection of infectiousness. The advantage is that individual liberty is only minimally compromised. The disadvantage is that maximum cooperation and significant monitoring is essential to detect "becoming infectious." The infectious agent involved is critical because a person may be infectious before symptoms appear or during a nonspecific prodrome. Many state quarantine laws prescribe the use of the least restrictive quarantine measures (Box 68-1).

Those who fail to observe the conditions of quarantine are subject to court-enforced orders of confinement and/or treatment. In a large-scale event, quarantine orders may be presented to all persons under observation, all persons receiving vaccines or prophylaxis, or all caregivers of infected persons to secure compliance and to provide the basis for enforcement action in the event that cooperation is lost.

Those who develop evidence of infectivity or contagiousness are subject to isolation and more stringent confinement. Conditions of isolation may include confinement at home (with or without additional precautions); confinement in a particular facility or unit; or restrictions in employment, public activities, etc. The isolation and quarantine of infectious persons must be maintained until the risk of transmission is *de minimus*. Isolation and quarantine may include requirements for treatment or immunization, and compliance with requirements may be relaxed once treatment is under way or immunization is effective.

BOX 68-1 EXAMPLES OF QUARANTINE MEASURES FOR DIFFERENT CIRCUMSTANCES

- Current evidence indicates that SARS is not spread by asymptomatic persons, but once fever develops, transmission may occur. Healthcare workers caring for SARS patients may be allowed to continue working and moving from home to work as long as fever is monitored at every shift. Persons exposed to SARS may be allowed to continue living in the community on daily fever monitoring with no restriction unless fever appears. Quarantine measures requiring confinement are imposed when fever is detected and remain in effect until the person is determined no longer infectious.
- Salmonella can be transmitted by anyone shedding the bacteria in stool. Most people with salmonellosis are advised to use proper hygiene measures to interrupt fecal-oral transmission. Because the interactions of small children increase fecal-oral transmission risks, children may be excluded from daycare settings. Inpatients are subject to enteric precautions to reduce transmission risks in institutions with many vulnerable patients. Because hygiene measures are often not followed, food service, childcare, and healthcare workers with salmonellosis may be excluded from working in food service or with young children or vulnerable patients until two consecutive stool samples collected 24 hours apart test negative for salmonella.
- If a bioterrorist or natural outbreak of severe, febrile respiratory disease is suspected, but no source has been identified, any person with fever and lower respiratory tract disease is suspected as a source of exposure until more information is obtained. Hospital emergency departments are required to set up isolation care sites and conduct any such patient directly to those sites for evaluation. Those requiring admission are isolated with respiratory precautions. Those not requiring admission are ordered into home confinement. All personnel in the chain caring for these patients are using personal protection equipment and are monitored on each shift for fever. Visitors and other staff at healthcare facilities are required to have their temperatures taken prior to admittance to the facility to protect patients and staff.

In a large-scale event, or when travel is interrupted (e.g., an airplane exposure) or people are dislocated (e.g., a flood), quarantine measures must include providing alternate shelter for people in quarantine. Shelter provisions must provide a means to segregate infectious persons under conditions of isolation as required. In planning for a response to a smallpox bioterrorism attack, many communities considered what facilities would be needed to house those being monitored and those being isolated and treated. Recent outbreaks of SARS and monkey pox have demonstrated the need to protect healthcare facilities and healthcare workers and the importance of quarantine measures that allowed early detection of second- and later-generation cases.

We have effective vaccines for some potential agents of bioterrorism and for many epidemic infections. Some vaccines are effective after initial exposure, either preventing or modifying the disease and influencing the potential for contagion. In the case of smallpox, for example, intensive efforts to identify and vaccinate all contacts were the control measures that led to eradication. If a vaccine is available, persons or animals exposed but without active disease should be immunized. Other control measures, such as fever watch, exclusion from school or work, and/or periodic examinations must continue until a vaccine take is evident or a full incubation period has passed (Box 68-2).

Prophylactic treatment is used therapeutically to prevent the appearance of disease in a person or to modify its course. Prophylactic treatment may be effective in controlling the spread of infectious disease by preventing individuals from becoming infectious. If exposed persons receive prophylactic treatment, the quarantine measures should be modified to address any potential for transmitting infection without manifesting signs and symptoms. Surveillance may be directed to determining completion of the prescribed prophylaxis and reinstitution of controls if compliance is incomplete (Box 68-3).

Travel in airplanes, ships, trains, and buses where an infectious agent is thought to have been released or where a person with an infectious disease is identified presents special considerations. In the initial investigation period, groups of people thought to have been exposed to an infectious agent with a short incubation period may be detained for examination. The purpose of the quarantine is to determine whether any others are infected and to initiate surveillance of exposed persons. Attention should be directed toward making a decision about the index case as quickly as possible while the necessary examination of all others is taking place under infection control precautions, reducing both the risk of further exposure among the passengers and the risk of exposing other populations. The responsible jurisdiction may have

responsibility for housing, feeding, and treating persons so detained. Although these are often international quarantines conducted by the U.S. government, not all such instances involve international travel (Box 68-4).

In an unfolding epidemic or outbreak, whether natural or manmade, control of movements of populations is challenging. Restricting the movements of large numbers of persons may quickly defuse an outbreak. However, confining people who will soon become infectious with others who have not yet been infected may increase the opportunities for contagion. A rapid response may encourage compliance with measures to provide large-scale prophylaxis and reduce panic if it is perceived as equitable and reasonable. The same action may interfere with compliance and increase panic if it is perceived as inequitable or poorly understood. Priorities must be set based on local laws and conditions, the infectious agent and modes of transmission, and national and international regulations.

Trust is a vital commodity. If the required restrictions are short term and involve options for treatment and/or immunization, then voluntary compliance is significant. During the 2003 SARS outbreak in Toronto, Canada, only 27 written quarantine orders were required.[3] Even in the face of the unknown, compliance with measures perceived as reasonable can be high. As a situation drags on, issues become more complex, and maintaining compliance with complex regimens of disease control is more difficult.

PROTECTING COMMUNITY ASSETS

Critical issues need to be addressed to protect vital community assets. Key assets among these are healthcare institutions, schools, businesses, and agriculture and food production.

Healthcare Assets

Infected, exposed, and unaffected persons mingle in healthcare settings. In addition to promoting strict isolation of infectious persons and the adoption of stringent

BOX 68-4 EXAMPLES OF TRAVEL-RELATED QUARANTINE MEASURES

- A child on a long airplane trip may develop symptoms suspicious of measles. Data must be collected on the immunization status and current health status of all travelers. Data on the seating arrangements and movements about the plane of the child and other occupants are useful. Immunization can be provided to any unimmunized person. If immunization is unavailable or refused, detailed contact information for the next 3 weeks for any susceptible person is collected, as is precautionary information.
- In a more complex scenario, the diagnosis of measles is made after the debarkation and airline manifests must be used to find and notify fellow passengers.
- Travelers with suspected SARS provide recent examples. Temperature screening at embarkation and debarkation of travelers from areas with reported cases provide an opportunity to detect cases before passengers are dispersed to many destinations. The quarantine officers need data to decide whether to detain any passengers if there is a suspected case. Data are collected on the body temperature, the current health status, the seating arrangements, and movements about the plane of all travelers. Detailed travel plans and contact information for all nonfebrile travelers for the next 10 days are obtained in some instances. Before release from quarantine, travelers receive "fever watch" instructions and directions to report to medical care if fever develops.

infection control measures in emergency departments and hospitals, quarantine measures may include cohorting of patients and healthcare workers among institutions to reduce the introduction of infection into all institutions. Hygiene and barrier protection for staff, patients, and visitors should be considered. If the numbers of infectious patients overwhelm the isolation capacity of hospitals, setting up separate temporary facilities to care for infected persons may be used in outbreak control.

Measures to protect physician offices and clinics are very important. Hygiene (e.g., handwashing, equipment disinfection), barrier protection (e.g., gloves and masks), and isolation spaces (e.g., separate rooms or entrances) can increase safety in the office setting. Some examples of other important protective measures include the following:

- Telephone screening
- Home visiting
- Redirecting symptomatic patients to special facilities
- Reducing waiting times in communal areas
- Isolating symptomatic patients from other patients

Long-term care facilities serving the vulnerable and frail may be required to reduce movement in and out, limiting or prohibiting visitors, or monitoring the health of staff and visitors. Where feasible, long-term care and childcare facilities should immunize new admissions.

Schools

In a crisis, many parents declare that their first action will be to collect their children from school. Schools may be needed as space to provide mass distribution of prophylaxis or shelter for persons displaced by the outbreak or related events. On the other hand, schools provide a structured environment for children where they can be monitored for early signs of infection and receive directly observed prophylaxis. Daycare and alternative childcare arrangements present the same infection control issues as any congregate setting.

School events may involve only the children in a single school, and decisions on cancellation can be based on the health status of children in the school. Other events involve multiple schools, and decisions should be made on the basis of the health conditions in the wider community. We tend to be more ready to restrict school-related events than other mass gatherings, but the same considerations should apply to any mass gathering involving children.

Travel

The travel of infected persons may be governed by international regulations. In the event of a bioterrorism event or a large outbreak, instructions to exposed persons to postpone travel, to report to surveillance authorities, or to undergo directly observed prophylaxis or therapy may provide effective quarantine. Travel restrictions of this type may interrupt travel in mid-journey, creating a necessity for safe shelter and medical supervision. Private vehicle travel from an affected to an unaffected area by potentially infected persons is more difficult to control. If civil authorities are busy with law enforcement investigations and emergency response actions, the work of enforcing a quarantine of individual travelers may be left for the destination jurisdiction.

Mass Gatherings

Organized mass gatherings such as concerts, movies, and athletic events may be canceled based on the health conditions in the community. Conditions to be considered are the infectious agent and expected transmission routes, the number of exposed persons in the community, and the level of response to infection control measures.

Mass prophylactic treatment or immunization clinics present special cases of mass gatherings, where careful attention to identifying and promptly isolating infectious persons is vital. All mass clinics must be designed to reduce the risk of contagion, identifying potentially infectious persons and isolating them at the earliest possible time.

Business

During the SARS outbreaks in 2003, some businesses were closed because of infected workers failing to follow quarantine requirements. A larger number of workers were quarantined and kept from the workplace. In some cases, governments made special arrangements for compensation of those unable to work because of quarantine requirements.[3] The potential for airborne transmission of the virus led to more stringent control measures than would be used if closer contact were required for transmission. Fear of contagion among coworkers may force closures even when exposed persons have followed quarantine instructions.

Individual businesses may be subject to quarantine because of other sources of infection. Warehouses, shipping businesses, and post offices may require quarantine because of contaminated goods. More difficult decisions involve marketplaces where vital goods are procured. In the 2003 SARS outbreak in Singapore, the government closed an entire marketplace because an infected person failed to obey the quarantine order.[3] With airborne infections, transmission can occur in the supermarket or the mall. In general, emphasis on the control of the movements of infected persons may be more effective than closing the marketplace.

Agriculture and Food Production

A number of the important epidemic and bioterrorism agents can compromise food production even without directly affecting humans. Agricultural and food production may be curtailed because of infected or contaminated animals or plants. Animals exposed to infected animals present major quarantine problems. Issues include protection of other animals from direct exposure, prevention of contamination of the environment, protection of agricultural and food industry workers, and protection of the food supply. When domestic animals are involved, agricultural and public health authorities are consulted. Depending on the pathogen, the animals in a herd may be quarantined or destroyed. While decisions are pending, healthy animals need to be segregated from diseased animals. No movement in or out of an exposed herd can be allowed. Movements of people, equipment, vehicles, and other fomites must be controlled.

Destruction of animals can create additional hazards. Worker protection and carcass disposal methods must be designed to minimize exposure to the agent and prevent environmental contamination. Substantial investigation is needed to determine the breadth of quarantine by geography and species. Transport equipment and downstream food products may also be subject to quarantine.

Goods contaminated with transmissible biologic agents must be decontaminated or destroyed. While decisions are made about the actual contamination, quarantine measures to prevent access to or movement of the goods must include protection from human, animal, and environmental exposures, depending on the agent involved. All equipment used must be tracked in the event that destruction or decontamination is required.

Balancing Civil Liberty with Quarantine

Quarantine and isolation restrict our civil liberties. In most healthcare settings, voluntary cooperation is sufficient, particularly when a patient is benefiting from treatment and shares in the effort to protect others from illness. In keeping with civil rights, the principle of "least restrictive measures" to protect the public is used, but the threat of law enforcement underlies these measures.

In the 1980s, the AIDS epidemic occasioned much discussion of the use of quarantine. Procedural changes were made in statutes in many jurisdictions to establish legal process to protect liberties. In the 1990s, concerns about confidentiality and privacy were prominent, placing real and perceived barriers in the way of reporting infectious disease and communicating about contacts to infectious disease. In the first decade of the twenty-first century, concern has turned to recognizing and containing terrorism. The law reflects these competing concerns and continues to change.

Advance planning for quarantine and isolation measures in various situations will help, but the decisions about a specific event are made with limited information under significant pressure. We must initiate action based on a high degree of suspicion and then narrow the response action as data improves. With the media leaning in and the lawyers poised, we still must use the most sensitive indicators available, risking false positives initially. In these circumstances, attention to equity and form is vital. Record-keeping and consistent reevaluation of circumstances, knowledge, and decisions are essential.

Obtaining Compliance

"Quarantine is a preventive measure and not a punishment"[4] is an important reminder. The goal of the effort is to prevent the spread of disease and minimize terror and civil disruption. Good information repeated often is an essential component of the disease control effort. So is the appeal to duty, to concern for the community, and to self-preservation. Issues of compensation for lost wages, care for family members, and similar concerns of persons subject to quarantine cannot be ignored if we are to be successful in meeting the goal. Especially under the pressure of terrorism and demands for action, it is easy to move to coercive measures when appeals to finer instincts would gain much compliance. This can be self-defeating because people fearing confinement go underground and spread disease because they have taken none of the desired prevention measures.

Attention Fatigue

Healthcare professionals are notorious for inattention to infection control. Constant vigilance is necessary to maintain quarantine, isolation, and infection control measures throughout an epidemic. Initial disbelief, even if scientifically justified, can lead to a low index of suspicion. Even when an attack has occurred, attention to infection control wanders. After the first cases of deliberate anthrax infections in 2002, many people took envelopes and packages containing white powders to police stations and emergency departments. Many became complacent after a few negative swabs and a few pranks. If one of those had contained anthrax spores, more people could have been exposed and infected. Hospital emergency departments could have been closed until the spores could be removed.

Communications

Single cases and a few contacts are a familiar problem for clinicians. Whole communities present many new stresses. Healthcare workers become key communicators to keep disease in check without undue disruption of civic and personal life. We are not all comfortable with this role. At the very least, the healthcare professional must be prepared to present findings and their significance for contagion clearly, to convey expectations to patients and those under quarantine, and to negotiate with those enforcing quarantine.

The physician or other healthcare worker making a quarantine decision must have clear authorization from the appropriate jurisdiction to do so. If civil authority is seriously disrupted, local physicians may be faced with making decisions without clear delegation. Consultation with the available law enforcement leadership is essential in such circumstances. The healthcare professional must create a record of data and decisions that will be available for subsequent civil court decisions.

Effective quarantine requires cooperation among the medical community and the affected populations. Clear instructions and information about the options available are essential. Threat of enforcement action provides an incentive to cooperate with restrictions on freedom. In every instance, we need to balance police action with the economic and social consequences. Judicial procedures may be especially important in bioterrorism because of the need to conduct law enforcement investigations and handle potential criminals in the health system.

Quarantine measures include ordered examination, treatment, and vaccination. Healthcare workers may need to be deputized to carry out these functions. Unwilling or uncooperative patients present additional threats. Practitioners need to be prepared to deal with law enforcement officers and to support them in handling difficult, potentially infectious patients.

Physicians, nurses, and other healthcare workers may be called on to put themselves in harm's way by working with infectious persons. Once exposed, healthcare workers may be restricted to working with the infected, or not at all. Developing quarantine health facilities to care for the infected and sick presents an ongoing risk to healthcare workers and their families and may require additional limitations on liberty.

Physicians can expect a lot of questions about protecting self and loved ones from patients and the community. Should I leave the area; keep my kids from school or other activities; go to work? Do I need treatment, vaccines, or a prescription? In an unfamiliar situation, and with personal concerns of a similar nature, physicians need a framework for collecting essential information and providing useful advice.

Conflicting Goals

Physicians are accustomed to placing the needs of each individual patient first. Making decisions to require treatment or to refuse treatment to patients with lower-priority needs places a physician in a new relationship with patients. The new relationship presents ethical dilemmas, yet the pressure of the emergency situation leaves little time for reflection and consultation.

Many of the pitfalls result from this conflict in goals. Difficult decisions in preventing the spread of communicable diseases stem from the need to balance personal liberty and community protection. The decisions are made in the context of uncertainty. A high index of suspicion leads to more prompt decisions and more emphasis on protection of the community. To keep faith with the demand for liberty, quarantine decisions need to be reviewed frequently. Clear expectations of the length of quarantine and the accompanying disease control steps must be explained to the patent. *Maintain trust in the face of insecurity and uncertainty.*

REFERENCES

1. The Preamble of the Constitution of the United States.
2. Rosen G. *A History of Public Health*. New York: MD Publications; 1958.
3. Rothstein MA, Alcalde MG, Elster NR, et al. Quarantine and Isolation: Lessons Learned From SARS. A Report to the Centers for Disease Control and Prevention Institute for Bioethics, Health Policy and Law [unpublished manuscript]. Louisville, Ky: University of Louisville School of Medicine; November 2003.
4. Rhodes JD. Quarantine Law: History and Implementation Today. A SARS case study [unpublished manuscript]. April 25, 2004.

chapter 69

Chemical Decontamination*

Barbara Vogt Sorenson and John Sorensen

Decontamination is defined as the reduction or removal of chemical (or biologic) agents by physical means or by chemical neutralization (detoxification) so agents are no longer hazardous.[1] The major objective of decontamination of victims exposed to a hazardous chemical is the prevention of further harm and the optimization of the chance for full clinical recovery.[2] An important secondary objective is to avoid spreading contamination to others and the healthcare facility (HCF). Although accidents from the manufacture, storage, or transportation of chemicals account for most instances of patient contamination, HCFs must now anticipate the intentional use of chemicals (including chemical warfare agents) to potentially contaminate large numbers of victims who may enter the facility individually or en masse with or without prior decontamination. This chapter focuses on the decontamination of patients/victims exposed to chemical warfare agents before entry to an HCF and the issues associated with preventing secondary or cross contamination of healthcare providers and their facilities. Also discussed are the problems associated with treating contaminated patients while wearing personal protective equipment (PPE).

Chemical agents exist in liquid, solid, or vapor form, with inhalation of vapors being the most likely route of exposure. Depending on the chemical's characteristics, physical properties, and exposure pathway, treatment for chemical warfare agent–contaminated patients is similar to other chemical casualties in the HCF environment. Terrorist-induced events are likely to result in psychological as well as physical harm. This is because a chemical attack would likely occur without warning, with an unknown substance, and in a location where large numbers of people are present or likely to pass through. These "outrage" factors elevate the perception of risk and fears for one's safety.[3,4] Other factors—a sense of helplessness and fear of unknown consequences from the exposure to oneself and others—may also result in large numbers of the "walking wounded" converging on an HCF without prior decontamination.

Given the covert measures usually employed by terrorists, healthcare providers should routinely be alert for signs and symptoms of contamination on patients and take immediate steps to protect themselves and their facility from becoming secondary victims. This means that facility managers, especially emergency department directors, should communicate early with first responders about unusual incidents to ensure prompt notification about any potentially contaminated patients. The same personnel should have the authority to lockdown the HCF and reroute response teams and self-presenting victims to appropriate decontamination areas.

Decontamination is generally the task of first responders (e.g., firefighters and hazardous materials [HazMat] teams) trained to use PPE and to process victims through decontamination units at the site of the chemical release. After an accidental release, the chemical's characteristics (including toxicity, persistence, and health effects) are frequently known through information on material safety data sheets or from managers or employees at the release site. In a terrorist event, on the other hand, the chemical substance will likely be unknown, the dose uncertain, and the consequent health effects undetermined. If the victims include children and infants, input from pediatricians and poison specialists will be needed. All victims will require debriefing (even if the chemical agents remain unknown at the time) after decontamination and treatment.

Field decontamination procedures are carried out in both rural and urban settings by full-time first responders or part-time volunteers with or without special equipment or training. Field decontamination of the potentially exposed often occurs as a precautionary measure, especially when health effects are unclear. Working with the hypothesis that removal of clothing reduces the majority of contaminants, most field decontamination efforts involve clothing removal and showering either in a special decontamination unit (e.g., trailer on expedient setup) or by hosing off from firefighting hoses.[5] The objective of field decontamination is to transfer a clean victim to an HCF without contaminating the conveying vehicle or exposing others. Given the large uncertainty of field decontamination effectiveness, most victims undergo another round of decontamination at the HCF to ensure the level of cleanliness needed to protect the facility, an issue that has prompted many complaints from victims. However, it is essential that the

*The submitted manuscript has been authored by a contractor of the U.S. Government under Contract No. DE-AC05-00OR22725. Accordingly, the U.S. Government retains a non-exclusive, royalty-free license to reproduce, distribute, prepare derivative works, and perform or display publicly the published form of this Contribution on behalf of the U.S. Government.

459

HCF be able to lockdown as soon as the potential for contaminated victims arrival is detected to protect critical assets such as healthcare providers, the HCF, and the existing patient population.

The most important element of treatment after exposure to a chemical warfare agent is to immediately remove the agent through decontamination. Decontamination that is delayed or ineffective can escalate the number of casualties when very toxic substances, such as nerve agents, are involved. If injuries are life threatening, victims are sometimes transported with minimal attention to the decontamination unit before arrival at the HCF. This problem can be exacerbated if communications between the field response units and medical facility fail to describe the event so the HCF can take advance precautions, such as suiting up personnel in PPE, performing lockdown, and initiating decontamination setup. In a terrorist event, the number of victims transporting themselves to emergency departments could quickly overwhelm resources, as happened in the Tokyo subway incident.[6]

Treating a chemical warfare agent–contaminated patient is similar to handling patients contaminated by other hazardous chemicals, such as organophosphate pesticides, and requires similar precautions. Over 95% of surface contaminants can be eliminated by removing clothing and showering.[7] Although the process is well known and easy to accomplish with ambulatory victims, injured patients require increased numbers of personnel and resources to perform decontamination.[8]

The three primary types of decontamination important to the healthcare provider are as follows:

- Personal decontamination (i.e., self- or buddy decontamination when one is exposed)
- Casualty decontamination (i.e., decontamination of casualties), and
- Personnel decontamination (generally, decontamination of noncasualties).

Personal decontamination may or may not involve PPE.[9] More often, personal decontamination (i.e., disrobing and bagging clothing, then showering with copious amounts of soap and water) is needed after an unprotected healthcare provider is exposed while caring for a contaminated patient who presents to an emergency department without alerting the admitting staff. If PPE is worn, all equipment including outer garments, gloves, boots, and respiratory apparatus should be decontaminated after removal. This will avoid the unnecessary cost of replacing expensive and individually fitted PPE. Healthcare providers should also be instructed in the proper donning and doffing of PPE to prevent exposing themselves or others to contaminated clothing surfaces.

Decontamination of chemical casualties and other exposed personnel requires a substantial outlay of resources and personnel.[10,11] Not all decontamination efforts will involve healthcare providers directly because HazMat teams are the general providers. However, medically trained personnel should provide overall supervision. The decontamination of each person should be monitored for adequate removal of agents and not left to the subjective evaluation of victims, especially children.[12,13] This process requires sensitivity and tact when handling civilian casualties, especially in the stressed environment of the disaster aftermath.

Decontamination Solutions

Many substances have been evaluated for their ability to remove contaminants from the skin. Compared with washing the skin with copious amounts of soap and water and irrigating the eyes with clean water, most have been found lacking. The most common problems are skin irritation, toxicity, ineffectiveness, and high cost. Although the military has used substances (such as special wipes) to determine whether the contaminant is removed, most healthcare providers must rely on subjective evaluations to assess decontamination effectiveness.

Disposal of contaminated solutions from decontamination of victims should follow the same procedures as disposal of other hazardous materials. If the contaminant is unknown or is suspected as benign at the time of decontamination, precautions such as holding secured drums of solution until a definitive result is obtained from later laboratory analysis can save the considerable expense of sending the wastewater to a HazMat disposal site. The U.S. Environmental Protection Agency (EPA) notes that in special circumstances where the protection of populations is critical, contaminated water from decontamination can be diverted to storm sewer or sanitary disposal.[14] Although this is likely not an option for persistent biologic agents, most chemical agents would likely be dispersed in this way without causing further harm.

It is often assumed that normal decontamination procedures are performed outside the emergency department by trained HazMat personnel. However, during an emergency, those same providers will likely be involved in search and rescue activities, with decontamination of exposed victims a low priority. Many victims will likely self-evacuate to the nearest medical facility without advising emergency department personnel. After the Tokyo subway release of sarin, it is estimated that more than 10,000 victims presented to medical facilities on their own without any form of decontamination before arrival.[6]

Secondary Contamination

Because of the potential for secondary contamination, it is essential that medical personnel understand the need for and undergo training in the actual use of PPE. Surgical masks are not sufficient to protect against hazardous vapors from a contaminated patient's fluids or body parts.[15] This is also a problem if the contaminant was purposely ingested and regurgitated in vomitus. Some persistent chemical warfare agents are not immediately symptomatic or visually evident on patient's skin, hair, or clothing. For example, sulfur mustard is a persistent oily substance producing signs and symptoms that can be delayed for 2 to 24 hours after exposure. It is also important that deceased victims of chemical agent events (even in body bags) be decontaminated prior to release to prevent secondary contamination of unsuspecting forensic or funerary workers.

A serious issue regarding chemical agents is the general absence of criteria to determine the effectiveness of decontamination efforts. Field decontamination performed by

HazMat personnel is generally considered gross decontamination and should not be considered adequate for admitting patients to a medical facility. This is a serious problem if the medical facility has not planned for decontamination of patients being admitted and healthcare providers respond without determining the cleanliness of patients.[16,17] Reports of emergency departments being closed for several hours after healthcare providers were sickened by fumes from patients only field decontaminated suggest this could be a very real problem in large-scale disasters. Not only would the loss of healthcare providers create difficulties, certifying that the HCF was clean enough to reopen could take several hours or, in the worst cases, several days. One HCF found changing out filters in the cleaning process on a Friday required specially ordered filter media, and the supplier did not work weekends. Only after action by the state's health officer did the supplier comply with the request. In a major disaster that disrupts normal infrastructure channels and communications, deliveries could be delayed for several days.

Chemical agents that might be used in a terror event include a wide variety of substances, ranging from chemical warfare agents such as nerve and sulfur mustard agents to riot control and choking agents. (Some consider toxins such as ricin from the caster bean plant a chemical derivative, but most authorities characterize toxins as biologic agents because they are derived from living matter.) The individual chemical's characteristics and mode of release and the victim's own characteristics will determine how decontamination is performed. For example, most victims exposed but not symptomatic can accomplish decontamination on their own. But patients who are injured, wheelchair bound, elderly, or very young will require assistance. Decontaminating victims on litters often requires a team effort to coordinate the lifting required to move the victim from the dirty (hot) to clean (cold) zones.

An issue with most healthcare providers, especially in the emergency theaters, is the lack of training on wearing PPE while treating victims. Although PPE is becoming more available in emergency departments because of the Joint Commission on Accreditation of Healthcare Organizations' requirement to have an emergency response incident management system that is integrated with the community response system, periodic training in the actual use of equipment during patient treatment is still lacking. Having enough equipment for each person and providing the necessary training (8 hours for some PPE) is often restricted by budgets and the common misperception that a mass-chemical-casualty event will not occur in one's hometown. Since respirators must be fitted for individual use to prevent leakage around the face to protect the mouth and eyes, use of individual pieces of respiratory equipment by multiple persons is not acceptable. Each wearer must also be trained in the proper decontamination of the PPE and how to don and doff the equipment effectively. Otherwise, the facility, victims, and other healthcare providers will be placed at risk of secondary contamination.

Communication with patients and with other healthcare providers is difficult when wearing a full face-mask respirator.[18] Handling equipment and providing care is severely hampered when wearing the recommended 7 mL–thick gloves instead of the more common latex ones. Movements are often hindered by cumbersome outerwear, especially if the facility uses a common air line for the supplied air for respirators. Those who don't want to wear PPE and instead rely on common barrier practices should not be allowed into the arena because the threat of secondary contamination from victims is too serious to allow the practice. Appropriate training in PPE can alleviate the feelings of confinement and dread that often affect first-time users. Enacting policies and publicizing them within the facility will help eliminate those problems with noncompliant personnel during an actual event.

Specific stay and rest times while wearing PPE are mandated by the Occupational Safety and Health Administration (OSHA), especially in hot or cold environments. This adds to the total number of healthcare providers needed during the event. PPE and wear-time requirements dictated by state health authorities or OSHA may be more stringent than federal regulations and should be addressed in training sessions. Jurisdictional disputes over appropriate PPE and the training required should be addressed in reviewing yearly plans and in all Memorandums of Understanding (MOUs) and Memorandums of Agreement (MOAs) with other facility managers.

CURRENT PRACTICES

To prevent the spread of contamination, knowing when and how to decontaminate patients is critical. Decontamination usually requires multiple teams to fully decontaminate victims. Factors to be considered in planning for a decontamination facility at HCFs include the number of patients to be processed, the number of personnel in PPE needed, the frequency of rotating those personnel, and the availability of PPE for rotating shifts.[19,20] This section discusses current decontamination practices at an HCF. This includes the physical layout of a decontamination area for handling both ambulatory and nonambulatory patients, mass decontamination techniques, and self/buddy decontamination procedures.

Physical Layout

Figure 69-1 shows one example of a casualty-receiving decontamination station. This can be situated in a field setting in an area safely distant from the accident site or at a hospital. The areas used for a station should be identified during the planning phase. A properly sited station will permit drainage from the decontamination process to be directed into a sump or a holding pond or container that can be emptied later during the recovery phase. The hot zone is the area considered to be contaminated. The cold zone is free from contamination. Plan for the cold zone to be upwind, uphill, and upstream from the hot zone. Walk-in patients and those who cannot be confirmed as receiving decontamination from a certified HazMat unit in the field go to screening and triage stations in the hot zone before proceeding

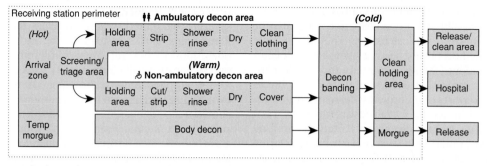

FIGURE 69–1. Layout of a decontamination station outside a healthcare facility. (From Federal Emergency Management Agency. *Don't Be A Victim: Medical Management of Patients Contaminated With Chemical Agents* [training video]. Oak Ridge, Tenn: Oak Ridge National Laboratory; 2003.)

through the decontamination line. Medical personnel should determine whether those decontaminated in the field should be decontaminated again or whether the patient can proceed directly to the triage area.

Site location and layout for decontamination should be predetermined and well known to operators. Maintaining secure perimeter control and clean work areas is important. All staff should be aware of the potential problems of cross or secondary contamination and should know how to process patients through decontamination stations. All of this requires planning and practice through live drills. At a HCF, the decontamination station could be temporarily set up in a parking lot outside the emergency department using a portable unit, or a more permanent decontamination facility could be constructed adjacent to the emergency department. Descriptions of permanent facilities are discussed by Macintyre and colleagues.[8] Common features of most stations include separate lines for ambulatory patients and nonambulatory patients. Each is discussed in more detail below.

Ambulatory Patient Decontamination

The decision about who should proceed through the ambulatory line should be made by medical personnel. The "walking wounded" and others tagged *minimal* can usually be sent to the ambulatory decontamination area, where fewer personnel are needed to supervise the self-decontamination process.

Medical personnel may decide to decontaminate ambulatory victims' wounds and remove bandages before allowing victims to shower. Keep in mind that bandages can readily absorb liquid or aerosols, so passing a victim with bandages across the contamination control line to relatively unprotected personnel could create a secondary hazard. Open wounds should never be decontaminated with a normal soap-and-water solution. First, remove previously applied dressings and foreign bodies from the wound. Then, flush the wound and surrounding areas with water and a tincture of green soap. Carefully decontaminate around the wound by wiping outward, pack the wound, then seal with occlusive dressing before proceeding to full body decontamination.

Ambulatory patients should be instructed to remove all clothing and to bag personal effects. Contaminated clothing should not be removed over the head to avoid

their exposure to the eyes and mucous membranes, but should instead be cut away and discarded. The patient should then shower with copious amounts of soap and water from the head down, leaning the head back to reduce the chance of residue contacting the eyes, nose, or mouth. Encourage careful cleaning of warm, moist areas such as under the armpits and the groin, followed by a thorough overall rinse with clean water.

Once decontaminated, patients should don clean clothing—Tyvek disposables or scrubs work well. Patients then receive a standardized wristband indicating that decontamination has been completed and move to the cold zone staging area for screening and medical treatment. The best assurance a victim is free of contamination is certification of thorough decontamination. Most ambulatory patients will be capable of processing through the ambulatory decontamination lines, but some may need assistance. If possible, separate decontamination lines should be set up for males and females. When only two lines are possible, keep the second line for nonambulatory cases, such as people with wheelchairs or walkers, those on stretchers, or anyone else requiring assistance or supervision.

Patients who were never in the path of a plume or in a contaminated area and who are without signs and symptoms of exposure should not have to be decontaminated. However, if some persons are still concerned about possible contamination, they should be instructed to remove the outer layers of clothing and take a quick 3- to 4-minute shower. Since much of the contamination, whether from liquid or vapor exposure, is completely removed by discarding clothing, that action followed by a rapid shower will likely eliminate 99% to 100% of the contaminant.

Nonambulatory Patient Decontamination

Nonambulatory patients displaying serious signs and symptoms of chemical exposure will be the first ones decontaminated in the nonambulatory area. Rapid decontamination is engaged, involving removal of clothing and a quick, high-volume shower focusing on exposed areas: skin and hair. This should take a maximum of 5 to 10 minutes per patient. Healthcare providers should follow universal precautions when treating these victims, and they may decide to more thoroughly decontaminate a patient if severe signs and symptoms continue. Patients exhibiting moderate signs, or who have a confirmed liquid exposure, will be processed in the normal fashion once the rapid decontamination patients have completed the process. Those with minimal signs and symptoms will follow those with moderate exposures.

Normal decontamination of nonambulatory patients usually takes two to four staff members and 10 to 20 minutes. The casualty's backboard or stretcher should be elevated to limit the amount of runoff exposure to the patient. Each staff member focuses on a quadrant of the victim's body, perhaps using the waistline as a midline. Clothing is cut away or otherwise removed. Starting at the midline, spray or wipe the victim laterally or to the side or back of the victim. The sponge or brush used to decontaminate should be rinsed in the decontamination solution after each wipe. Once the front is finished, roll the victim to the side and proceed to decontaminate the back from the highest to lowest point.

Once the actual wiping process is complete, a liberal amount of solution should be used to rinse the patient, then the patient is dried. The process requires 35 to 50 gallons per patient, and fresh decontamination solution should be used for each patient. Once the patient is cleaned, roll him or her onto a clean stretcher or backboard and transfer across the hotline into the cold area.

Mass Decontamination

Alternatively, victims may be decontaminated in one or more groups; this is called *mass decontamination*. Chemical warfare agents can cause large numbers of casualties if dispersed in a vapor or aerosol, as manifested in the Tokyo subway incident. Such a situation could also occur in a high-profile event at a stadium, concert, or airport. The mass-decontamination process requires cordoning off several areas where a decontamination corridor can be set up with fire department aerials and/or deluge guns in close proximity. The nozzles are set at low volume so as not to inflict damage while maximizing the amount of water to which each victim is exposed. Ambulatory victims progress through the deluge so that they may be grossly decontaminated. In conjunction with removal of clothing, this will likely suffice to decontaminate those victims not exhibiting signs or symptoms of chemical agent exposure.

Another mass-decontamination method is to set up a sprinkler head near the exit point of the hot zone as a rudimentary decontamination shower. In this scenario, water delivered at 500 gallons/minute will produce 8 gallons/second. If the victim remains in the shower for 3 seconds on average, this equals 12 gallons—the amount used in a normal shower. In both scenarios, some clothing is left on, which reduces the effectiveness if vapor has penetrated to the skin.

Potentially contaminated runoff from mass-decontamination stations generally must be disposed of in compliance with local or state environmental regulations. The EPA has also published guidelines on this issue when conditions warrant otherwise.[14] The agency concluded that based on the "good Samaritan" provision in Compre-

hensive Environmental Response, Compensation, and Liability Act, Section 107d, first responders should undertake any necessary emergency action to save lives and protect the public and themselves. Section 107d states that no person will be liable for costs or damages resulting from actions taken or not taken rendering care, assistance, or advice under the National Contingency Plan or at the direction of the on-scene coordinator. This does not preclude liability for damages resulting from negligence. The EPA recommends that once imminent threats to human life are addressed, reasonable attempts should be made to contain wastewater and prevent environmental insult.

Self- and Buddy Decontamination

If resources cannot be mobilized quickly enough to perform systematic and assisted decontamination, it is crucial to have a plan to instruct members of the public potentially exposed to a chemical agent to either perform self-decontamination or assist another to decontaminate ("buddy decontamination"). Instructions should inform people to remove and bag all clothing and personal items such as watches and jewelry and thoroughly wash with copious amounts of soap and water followed by a clean water rinse. People should then don clean clothes and follow official instructions. Eyeglasses can be decontaminated by soaking in household bleach and then rinsing with clean water. Although self- and buddy decontamination will not suffice for entry into the HCF, it will minimize health impacts to the exposed person and help avoid cross contamination.

PITFALLS

Decontamination of victims of a hazardous chemical release is fraught with problems, many of which can be alleviated with appropriate planning. Appropriate PPE is expensive, and maintaining the appropriate level of trained personnel for 24-hour operations will strain budgets and resource allocations.[21] Mass decontamination of victims of a chemical warfare agent release will likely exhaust even the most well-prepared medical facility. If the event is terrorist instigated, there is also the possibility of the perpetrator(s) initiating a secondary hazard or hiding among the casualties. This increases the stress on healthcare providers accustomed to dealing only with a person's medical issues. If the victims include a large number of fatalities, instructions for handling the deceased must be clearly detailed to prevent secondary contamination among medical personnel.

Communications can be problematic. Communications may be difficult between healthcare providers and HazMat responders when the substance is unknown or widespread. Wearing protective respirators complicates communication between patients and healthcare providers. The situation is exacerbated by the potential conflict in agenda between crisis and consequent management teams. Deciding what takes priority—crime investigation or medical care—can be problematic, especially if the event is labeled an act of terrorism. Victims exposed to high levels of chemical warfare agent especially need immediate care to offset immediate and potentially fatal effects, a need that may not be readily apparent to crime scene investigators.

An issue not often considered by healthcare providers is the special decontamination needs of the more vulnerable populations such as elderly persons, children and young adolescents, or immune-compromised persons. Children may compose a significant portion of casualties in a terrorist attack because of their higher breathing rates, thinner skin, larger surface-to-mass ratio, smaller fluid reserves, and lower circulating blood volumes.[21,22] Such groups may also be more vulnerable to negative psychological effects.[23] Likewise, elderly persons may have underlying health problems such as asthma that exacerbate the health effects from a chemical release. Decontamination solutions and areas for disrobing and showering may not be heated. Care should be taken to avoid the necessity of treating victims for exposure (e.g., hypothermia). Having access to personal records of victims may be impossible in mass care situations, and healthcare providers may need to rely on subjective evaluations of stressed victims.

Lack of victim privacy when media personnel are on the scene has also been a problem.[24] Graphic photographs and videos of victims being decontaminated are sought by media outlets but only increase the stressful situation for victims.[25] Securing external perimeters of areas for triage and decontamination of victims while the HCF is in lockdown may prevent such intrusion but may delay essential treatment as well. Innovative news correspondents may pose as victims to gain entry and access to victim's stories. Medical facilities that plan to use expedient items such as large trash bags for patient wear after decontamination should be aware that privacy can and will be a major issue for victims already subjected to unfamiliar decontamination procedures.

Preplanning for chemical agent incidents is still not universal.[26] Although planning for and providing resources for responding to a terrorist event has been advocated by the Joint Commission on Accreditation of Healthcare Organizations (JCAHO) in cooperation with OSHA, studies of healthcare preparedness have found many facilities not in compliance.

The casual openness and use of volunteers at many entries to HCFs present significant vulnerabilities for contamination of the HCF, healthcare providers, and volunteers. A few HCFs provide separate waiting rooms for other reasons than maintaining a space for isolation of contaminated victims. Although this method of receiving patients is not likely to change soon, HCF managers and supervisors should consider reorganizing the environment to more easily adjust to the unexpected influx of contaminated patients after a disaster.

The number of pitfalls that can hinder effective decontamination efforts may seem overwhelming; however, with planning, management support, and appropriate resources and training, such events can be managed with less chaos and confusion. The most important factor is protection of the healthcare provider and the HCF to optimize the care provided to victims.

REFERENCES

1. Office of the Surgeon General, Department of the Army. In: Sidell FR, Takfuji ET, Franz DR, eds. *Textbook of Military Medicine, Part 1: Medical Aspects of Chemical and Biological Warfare*. Washington, DC: Borden Institute, Walter Reed Army Medical Hospital; 1997:352.
2. National Academy Press. *Chemical and Biological Terrorism: Research and Development to Improve Civilian Medical Response*. Washington, DC: National Academy Press; 1999:97.
3. Slovic P, Fischhoff B, Lictenstein S. Facts and Fears: Understanding Perceived Risk. In: Schwing RC, Abers WA, eds. *Societal Risk Assessment: How Safe Is Safe Enough?* New York: Plenum; 1980:181-214.
4. Slovic P. *Perception of Risk*. London: Earthscan Pub; 2002:225-6.
5. Cox RD. Decontamination and management of hazardous materials: exposure victims in emergency departments. *Ann Emerg Med*. 1994;23(4):761-70.
6. Okamura T, Suzuki K, Fukuda A, et al. The Tokyo subway sarin attack: disaster management, part 2—hospital response. *Acad Emerg Med*. 1998;5(6):618-24.
7. Keonig K. Strip and shower: the duck and cover for the 21st century. *Ann Emerg Med*. 2003;42(3):391-4.
8. Macintyre AG, Christopher GW, Eitzen E, et al. Weapons of mass destruction events with contaminated casualties: effective planning for health care facilities. *JAMA* 2000;283(2):242-9.
9. Hick J, Penn P, Hanfling D, et al. Protective equipment for health care facility decontamination personnel: regulations, risks, and recommendations. *Ann Emerg Med*. 2003;42(3):370-80.
10. Burgess JL, Kirk M, Borron SW, et al. Emergency department hazardous materials protocol for contaminated patients. *Ann Emerg Med*. 1999;34(2):205-12.
11. Hick J, Penn P, Hanfling D, et al. Establishing and training health care facility decontamination teams. *Ann Emerg Med*. 2003;42(3):381-90.
12. Rotenberg J, Burklow T, Selanikio J. Weapons of mass destruction: the decontamination of children. *Pediatr Ann*. 2003;32(4):261-7.
13. Wheeler D, Poss W. Mass casualty management in a changing world: an overview of the special needs of the pediatric population during a mass casualty emergency. *Pediatr Ann*. 2003;32(2):98-105.
14. Office of Solid Waste and Emergency Response, Environmental Protection Agency. *First Responder's Environmental Liability Due to Mass Decontamination Runoff. Washington, DC:* Chemical Emergency Preparedness and Prevention Office; 2000.
15. Burgess JL. Hospital evacuation due to hazardous materials incidents. *Am J Emerg Med*. 1999;17(1):50-2.
16. Brennan RJ, Waeckerle JF, Sharp TW, et al. Chemical warfare agents: emergency medical and emergency public health issues. *Ann Emerg Med*. 1999;34(2):91-204.
17. Burgess JL, Blackmon GM, Brodkin CA, et al. Hospital preparedness for hazardous materials incidents and treatment of contaminated patients. *West J Med*. 1997;167(6):387-91.
18. Moles TM. Emergency medical services systems and HAZMAT major incidents. *Resuscitation* 1999;42(2):103-16.
19. Agency for Toxic Substances and Disease Registry. *Hospital Emergency Departments: A Planning Guide for the Management of Contaminated Patients*. Atlanta: U.S. Department of Health and Human Services, Public Health Service ATSDR; 2000. *Managing Hazardous Material Incidents;* vol II.
20. Cone DC, Davidson SJ. Hazardous materials preparedness in the emergency department. *Prehospital Emerg Care*. 1997;1(2):85-90.
21. Burklow T, Yu C, Madsen J. Industrial chemicals: terrorist weapons of opportunity. *Pediatr Ann*. 2003;32(4):230-4.
22. Blaschke G, Palfrey J, Lynch J. Advocating for children during uncertain times. *Pediatr Ann*. 2003;32(4):271-4.
23. Balk SJ, Gitterman BA, Miller MD, et al. Chemical-biological terrorism and its impact on children. *Pediatrics* 2000;105(3):662-70.
24. Vogt B, Sorensen J. *How Clean Is Safe: Lessons Learned From Decontamination Experiences*. Oak Ridge, Tenn: Oak Ridge National Laboratory, ORNL/TM-2002/178; 2002.
25. DiGiovanni C. Domestic terrorism with chemical or biological agents: psychiatric aspects. *Am J Psychiatry* 1999;156(10):1500-5.
26. Treat KN, Williams JM, Furbee PM, et al. Hospital preparedness for weapons of mass destruction incidents: an initial assessment. *Ann Emerg Med*. 2001;35(5):562-5.

chapter 70

Radiation Decontamination*

George A. Alexander

Merriam Webster's Collegiate Dictionary, 10th edition, lists 1936 as the year of the earliest known use of the word *decontaminate* in English.[1] *Decontaminate* is defined as follows:"to rid of contamination (as radioactive material)." To better appreciate the meaning of the word, one should first understand the concept of radiation contamination. Contamination occurs when material containing radioactive particles is deposited on skin, clothing, or any surface area of an inanimate object. A person contaminated with radioactive material will continue to be irradiated until the radioactive material (source of radiation) is eliminated or removed. Interestingly, radiation does not spread in a person; instead, it is the radioactive contamination that can spread. *External contamination* of a person may occur if radioactive material is deposited on external body surfaces or clothing. *Internal contamination* occurs if radioactive material is inhaled, ingested, injected into, or absorbed through wounds. The environment can also become contaminated if radioactive materials are uncontained or spread about.

Comprehensive concepts of radiation decontamination are presented in this chapter. The aim is to provide a framework in which to understand the principles of radiation decontamination and their application in controlling exposures to radioactive contamination. The chapter provides a brief historical perspective of radioactivity, summarizes current practices of radiation decontamination, and highlights obstacles to the execution of an optimal radiation decontamination response plan.

HISTORICAL PERSPECTIVE

Radiation injury to human cells was first recognized within months after Roentgen's discovery of X rays in 1895.[2] In 1896, Becquerel discovered natural radioactivity—the emission of fast electrons from the nuclei of salts of uranium.[3] This mode of radioactive decay was termed *beta decay*. This discovery eventually led to another discovery and isolation of radium by Marie Curie in 1898.[4] In 1899, Rutherford described radioactive decay by the emission of alpha particles (helium nuclei).[5] And, in 1900, Villard was the first to describe electromagnetic radiation release during radioactive decay known as gamma radiation.[3] The three major forms of radioactivity are alpha (α), beta (β), and gamma (γ), named for alpha particles, beta particles, and photon energy, respectively.

After their discovery, X rays and radioactive materials were used with little regard for their biologic effects. The consequences of careless handling and use of radiation sources soon became apparent. Many of the early workers who pioneered the medical applications of ionizing radiation experienced firsthand the deleterious effects of radiation. Curie's discovery of radium led her to receive the Nobel Prize for chemistry in 1911 and brought about the introduction of radium use in medicine and industry.[5] Internal contamination from radium caused injury to many workers of the radium watch dial–painting industry in the 1920s.[6]

In the early twentieth century, the understanding of atomic physics increased rapidly and culminated in the nuclear era. The development of manmade radioactive isotopes during and after World War II was a factor in the establishment of the nuclear industry that had a workforce of several hundred thousand people. Only 97 cases of clinical radiation injury had occurred in this population by 1969.[6] Knowledge of radiation-monitoring procedures was an integral component of the civil defense programs of the 1960s directed against the threat of nuclear weapons use and thermonuclear war. Most of what is known today about radiation decontamination came about after the atomic bomb explosions of World War II and has evolved from three primary areas: therapeutic radiation exposures, radiation accidents, and military preparedness training directed at nuclear weapons-related injuries. The military experience has provided some of the most comprehensive and useful information on radiation decontamination.[7-9]

CURRENT PRACTICE

Basic techniques of radiation decontamination derived from the military can be applied to nonmilitary settings

---

*The views expressed in this chapter are those of the author and do not necessarily represent the official policy or position of the National Cancer Institute, the National Institutes of Health, or the U.S. Department of Health and Human Services.

465

depending on the situation and resources available. Radiation is given off by radioactive particles, most of which appears as dust or debris as in the case of a detonation of a nuclear weapon or radiologic dispersal device. For decontamination purposes, radiation is generally thought of as a solid. Four categories of decontamination are recognized[7]: (1) personal decontamination is decontamination of one's self; (2) casualty decontamination denotes decontamination of patient casualties; (3) personnel decontamination generally means decontamination of workers who are not patients; and (4) mechanical decontamination includes procedures to physically remove radioactive particulates.

Radiation decontamination is not an emergency. Decontamination of casualties is a labor-intensive task. The process demands the dedication of a significant number of personnel and large amounts of time. Appropriate planning and training are a necessity. The demands may require a major contribution of resources.

Monitoring Instruments

A variety of instruments are available for detecting and measuring radiation. Radiation monitoring entails the measurement of radiation fields in the vicinity of a radiation source, measurement of surface contamination, and measurement of airborne radioactivity. Such monitoring methods are also known as radiation surveys. Radiation survey meters are used to evaluate radiation contamination of patients, equipment, or the environment. Old civil defense instruments such as the CD V-700 and CD V-715 survey meters can be used. The CD V-700 meter is used to detect low-intensity gamma and most beta radiation. It can only measure up to 50 mR/hour. The CD V-715 meter is used to measure high-intensity gamma radiation. It can measure up to 500 R/hour; however, it cannot detect beta or alpha radiation. These instruments are also called *Geiger counters* or *Geiger-Mueller meters*.

Newer portable and compact radiation monitor units with digital readouts and alarm systems are commercially available to measure alpha, beta, and/or gamma radiation. Because alpha radiation travels a very short distance in air and is not penetrating, radiation survey instruments cannot detect alpha radiation through even a thin layer of water, blood, dust, paper, or other materials. Most beta emitters can be detected with a survey instrument such as a CD V-700, provided the metal probe cover is opened. Since gamma radiation or X rays frequently accompany the emission of alpha and beta radiation from radioactive isotopes, the latter constitute both an external and internal hazard to humans. Gamma radiation is readily detected with survey instruments.

Radiologic Assessment

In the period immediately after a detonation of, for example, a nuclear or large RDD, there will be considerable uncertainty about the nature and extent of radioactive contamination. It is imperative that radiation measurements be obtained as soon as possible to implement proper protective actions against potential radiologic hazards. On-scene radiologic assessments can be easily and rapidly performed using exposure rate measurements. However, assessments of long-term consequences require knowledge of the specific radioactive isotopes and more specialized skills.[10] An RDD that contains nuclear spent fuel as a radiation source will probably release one or a few radioisotopes on detonation. This simple source is easier to measure and characterize than mixed radiation sources potentially released from nuclear reactors or weapons.

Prehospital Decontamination

State radiation safety or health departments should provide field teams to assist in radiation monitoring at the scene of a nuclear or radiologic incident. The radiologic evaluation of injured patients should be performed by persons with radiation health and safety training under the supervision of on-scene medical personnel.[10] Patient decontamination performed by emergency responders should be brief. The goal should be to remove all gross radioactive dust or debris from body surfaces. If clothing and shoes are contaminated, they should also be removed. These measures may benefit the patient by eliminating sources of radiation exposure and reducing the cumulative absorbed dose the patient would have received. Depending on the severity of injuries and the extent of radiation exposure, these simple decontamination methods may be life-saving while the patient is en route to more definitive care at the nearest hospital emergency department.

Hospital Decontamination

To prevent or minimize the occurrence of radiologic contamination of the hospital facility and hospital staff, a decontamination area should be established outside the hospital, preferably downwind from the clean treatment area or hospital entrance. A patient arrival/triage area should be downwind from the decontamination area. Wind direction is vital since re-suspension of radioactive dust may occur downwind from the contaminated area. Outdoor patient decontamination is always performed upwind from the patient arrival/triage area.[7] Ideally, the decontamination area should be set up to take advantage of the prevailing wind. The setup should be adaptable. Consideration must be given to the security of the decontamination area. An outdoor shower system may also be considered for use of mass decontamination. Portable vacuum units with high-efficiency particulate air filters have reportedly been used to facilitate rapid decontamination outdoors.[11]

An entry control point is necessary to identify and manage movement of clean and contaminated vehicles to the decontamination site. Control of patient and staff movement is critical to ensure that contaminated ambulatory patients and staff do not accidentally contaminate clean areas. A hotline should be established and secured. Any people or equipment leaving a contaminated area must undergo radiologic monitoring to make sure that radioactive contaminants do not enter clean areas. In addition, a radiation emergency area, a location for indoor decontamination, should be part of the radiation emergency plans in the event that patients contaminate the hospital.[11]

Hospitals with nuclear medicine departments have an added resource—a gamma camera. A gamma camera is a perfect device for detecting nuclear fission products from either nuclear detonations or nuclear power plant reactors accidents.

Patient Decontamination

Removal of outer clothing and rapid washing of exposed skin and hair removes 95% of contamination.[7] Standard patient decontamination is normally performed under the supervision of medical personnel.[10] Moist cotton swabs of the nasal mucosa from both sides of the nose should be obtained, labeled, and sealed in separate bags. These swabs can be used as evidence for inhalation of radioactive particles. A 0.5% sodium hypochlorite solution can be used to remove radioactive contamination from intact skin. Radioactive material removed from the patient should be preserved for later analysis to identify the specific radioisotope. Maintain care not to irritate the skin. If skin becomes erythematous, some radioactive isotopes can be absorbed directly through the skin. Surgical irrigating solutions, such as normal saline or lactated Ringer's solution, should be used liberally in wounds, the abdomen, and the chest. These solutions should be removed using suction instead of wiping or sponging. For the eyes, only abundant amounts of water, normal saline, or eye wash solutions are recommended. If feasible, skin wash water should be contained and held for disposal. Contaminated tourniquets are changed with clean ones. Wounds should be covered after adjacent skin is decontaminated to prevent skin contaminants from entering the wound.

Wound Decontamination

During initial decontamination in the receiving/triage area, bandages should be removed and all wounds flushed. If bleeding persists, apply fresh bandages. Highly energetic gamma emitters can present an immediate hazard to contaminated wounds. Particulate matter contaminating a wound should be removed if possible. Alpha and beta emitters left in a wound can cause extensive local injury and may be absorbed into the systemic circulation, where they will be redistributed as internal contaminants; this can cause additional internal organ injury from irradiation. After adequate decontamination of the wound is achieved, it should be copiously irrigated with saline or some other physiologic solution. Aggressive surgery such as amputation is not necessary and should never be used to manage radioactive contamination of a limb. Partial-thickness burns should be extensively irrigated and cleaned with mild solutions to prevent irritation of burned skin. In full-thickness burns, the presence of radioactive contaminants requires specialized surgical treatment.

Mechanical Decontamination

Radiologic contamination may involve one or more radioactive elements. This section addresses the specific decontamination of six common radioactive elements.[8]

The decontamination principles discussed here are also applicable to radiologic contamination by other elements with chemical properties similar to those discussed below.

Cesium

The most common radioisotope of cesium is cesium-137. It emits beta and gamma radiation, decaying to stable barium-137. Cesium-137 is widely used in gamma sources. It occurs in these sources as cesium chloride pellets. Cesium chloride is a soluble salt. The contamination from a sealed-source leak absorbs water, becomes damp, and creeps. Contamination from a sealed cesium source is best decontaminated by wet procedures unless the contamination is on a porous surface, in which case wet procedures should be preceded by vacuuming. Cesium is known to adsorb from a solution onto glass surfaces. Decontaminating a liquid cesium–contaminated surface is best accomplished by wetting the surface, absorbing the solution with a rag or other absorbent material, and rinsing the area several times with water. If the contamination persists, use a detergent solution and scrub with a brush.[8]

Cobalt

The most common radioisotope of cobalt is cobalt-60, a beta and gamma emitter. Metallic cobalt-60 is commonly used in sealed gamma sources. Particles of cobalt dust adhering to small articles are readily removed by ultrasonic cleaners or by dipping the article in a dilute solution of nitric, hydrochloric, or sulfuric acid. Cobalt dust contamination that exists over a large area is best removed by vacuuming. Sealed cobalt sources may leak as a result of electrolytic action between the cobalt and the container. The result is often a soluble cobalt salt, which creeps and spreads. This is best decontaminated with a detergent or an ethylenediamine tetraacetic acid solution, followed by treatment with mineral acids. Contamination from solutions containing cobalt may be treated with water.[8]

Plutonium

The most common isotope in which plutonium may be present as a contaminant is plutonium-239, an alpha emitter. Plutonium contamination may be the result of a nuclear weapons accident, in which case the plutonium will be scattered as a metal or oxide in a dust form. Both forms of plutonium are insoluble. Aging of plutonium-239 contamination is impractical since it has a 24,000-year half-life. Plutonium contamination that covers a small area is best decontaminated by vacuuming. If contamination remains, the area should be washed with a detergent solution. Any contamination that remains can be sealed in a protective coating of paint, varnish, or plastic. Plutonium oxide or metal dust spread over a large area, such as a field, is best decontaminated by removing the top layer of soil and disposing of it as radioactive waste. Personnel should wear respiratory protection when decontaminating or removing the soil.[8]

Strontium

The most common radioisotope of strontium is strontium-90, a beta emitter. The daughter particle of strontium-90 is yttrium-90, which is also a beta emitter. Strontium-90-yttrium-90 is commonly used in sealed beta sources. Generally, it is present as a chlorine or carbonate. The chlorine is hygroscopic; it absorbs water and creeps out of the container. This contamination is best decontaminated by vacuuming, followed by a treatment with water, a complexing agent solution (i.e., substance capable of forming a complex compound with another material in solution), and a mineral acid, in that order. Contamination resulting from a strontium-containing solution is best decontaminated by absorbing the solution with rags or other absorbing materials and washing the area with a detergent solution. If strontium contamination persists, the top layer of the surface should be removed by abrasives or other removal procedures and a sealing coat should be placed over the surface.[8]

Tritium

Tritium is the radioisotope of hydrogen and is a weak beta emitter. If it is released to an area as a gas, the best decontamination method is to flush the area with air. Since inhalation tritium can present an internal hazard, personnel entering an area containing tritium gas should wear an appropriate self-contained type of breathing apparatus. Objects in an area exposed to tritium for any great length of time may absorb the gas and should be disposed of, if possible. They may be degassed, under a vacuum, by flushing with helium or hydrogen. A surface that is monitored as clean may become contaminated again in a matter of hours by percolation. There is no practical way of removing tritium oxide (T_2O) from water due to its similarity to natural water.[8]

Uranium

The most probable source of uranium contamination is a nuclear weapon accident in which the fissionable uranium is spread as a metal or oxide dust. The common isotopes of uranium contamination are uranium-235 and uranium-238. This metal or oxide is insoluble and is best removed from a contaminated surface by brushing or vacuuming, followed by a treatment with mineral acids or oxidizing acids, and then the area should be sealed. Large-area uranium contamination is best decontaminated by removing the top layer of the surface or by sealing it.[8]

Equipment and Building Decontamination

In most instances of equipment and building contamination, a mixture of normal household cleaning practices will remove the radioactive material. Vacuum cleaners that can handle wet material and have high-efficiency particulate air filters are suggested.

Personal Protective Equipment

Members of on-scene field radiologic decontamination teams and hospital-based teams should have appropriate protective equipment to meet all requirements for radiation decontamination. Emergency medical services and hospital personnel responsible for patient decontamination should also be appropriately equipped to protect themselves from the hazards of radioactive contamination.

Respiratory Protective Devices

There are two types of respiratory protective devices: air-purified respirators, which remove contaminants from breathing air by filtering or chemical absorption, and air-supplied respirators, which provide clean air from an outside source or from a tank. Most air-purified respirators (i.e., protective masks) afford excellent protection from inhalation of radioactive material. Radioisotopes such as radon and tritium gas will pass through these filters. However, short exposures to these gases are not considered medically significant. The device providing the greatest factor of safety for a particular radiation incident should be used.

In nuclear weapons accidents or terrorist incidents, most nuclear weapons will contain high explosives in varying amounts—even as much as hundreds of pounds. Detonation of high explosives in nuclear weapons will cause a major radiologic threat—the release of plutonium-239.[12] When associated with a fire, metallic plutonium may burn, producing radioactive plutonium oxide particles and serious inhalation and wound deposition hazards. In these situations, use of self-contained breathing apparatuses should be considered.

In RDD incidents in which radioactive contamination is associated with fire and dangerous chemical fumes from burning metals and plastics, use of self-contained breathing apparatuses should be considered. Such devices enable radiation response/decontamination workers to enter a contaminated or oxygen-deficient environment, up to the limits of the respirator. They should be used when it is necessary to enter a highly contaminated environment to rescue persons, for example, from RDD incidents or nuclear power plant accidents.

Protective Clothing

Anticontamination suits are commercially available for use in nuclear and radiologic disasters. Chemical-protective clothing provides excellent protection against radioactive contamination while also offering protection from chemical and biologic agents or hazards. A wide variety of chemical-protective clothing is available to protect the body, including gloves, boots, coveralls, and total-encapsulation protective suits. Standard hospital barrier clothing that is used in universal precautions is adequate for protection of hospital personnel who provide emergency evaluation and treatment to limited numbers of radiologically contaminated patients. In these instances, hospital personnel should be decontaminated after the patients' emergency treatment and decontamination.

Radiation Dosimeters

There are a variety of detectors used to measure a person's level of radiation exposure.[13] Film badges, thermoluminescent dosimeters (TLDs), pocket dosimeters, or other devices should be used by radiation decontamination personnel, emergency responders, and hospital medical providers who are involved in any nuclear accident or terrorist incident.

Film badges are the most common dosimeter in use. They are worn on the outer clothing and are used to measure gamma, X-ray, and high-energy beta radiation. A badge consists of a small piece of photographic film wrapped in an opaque cover and held in a metal frame. It can be worn as a ring or pinned to clothing. Radiation interacts with the atoms in the film to expose the film. At periodic intervals, the film is removed and is developed to determine the amount of radiation exposure. A film badge provides a permanent record of radiation exposure.

TLDs are used for measuring gamma, X-ray, and beta radiation exposures. They can be worn as rings or body badges. They contain small chips of lithium fluoride that absorb ionizing radiation energy and displace electrons from their ground state. The electrons then become trapped in a metastable state but can be restored to their original ground state by heating. When heated, the electrons return to their ground state and light is emitted. A TLD readout instrument is used to heat the chips and measure the emitted light. The amount of light emitted is related to the dose of radiation absorbed by the TLD and to the radiation exposure dose of the individual. TLDs are beginning to replace film badges.

A pocket dosimeter is a direct-reading portable unit shaped like a fountain pen with a pocket clip. It is worn on the trunk of the body and is generally used to measure X-ray and gamma radiation. It should be used in conjunction with a TLD rather than in place of TLD use.

The pocket dosimeter consists of a quartz fiber, a scale, a lens to observe movement of the fiber across the scale, and an ionization chamber. The quartz fiber is charged electrostatically until it reaches zero on the scale. When the dosimeter is exposed to radiation, some of the atoms of air in the chamber become ionized. This causes the static electricity charge to leak from the quartz fiber in direct response to the amount of radiation present. As the charge is lost, the fiber moves to some new position on the scale that indicates the amount of radiation exposure.

The main advantage of the pocket dosimeter is that it can be read immediately by the wearer, even while working in a radiation-contaminated environment, instead of waiting for processing of a film badge or TLD. However, since pocket dosimeters lose their electrical charge over time, they may give a false indication of radiation exposure. When practicable, use of two dosimeters can prevent false interpretation of a person's exposure. One should assume that the lower reading is the actual exposure.

Basic Radiation Safety

During a nuclear or radiologic disaster, it is vital that emergency medical responders, decontamination team personnel, and hospital healthcare providers adhere to the basic principles of radiation safety. These actions will help to prevent or minimize the risk of these persons becoming radiation casualties due to exposure to radioactive contaminants. The three basic principles of radiation protection are time, distance, and shielding.

Time

The longer the exposure to radioactive contaminants, the greater is the possibility of radiation injury. There is a direct relationship between the exposure dose received and the duration of exposure. Reducing exposure time in a contaminated area will reduce the radiation exposure. The maximum acceptable exposure time can be calculated based on the exposure dose rate measured using radiation survey meters at a given incident scene and the maximum dose that is needed to accomplish radiation decontamination or other task. In practice, the dose received in completing a task may be spread over several workers so that no one person's exposure exceeds guide levels.

Distance

The inverse square law states that the dose from a radiation point source decreases with the square of the distance from the source. For example, doubling the distance from the source of radiation, the exposure would be decreased to $(\frac{1}{2})^2$, or one fourth, of the original amount. In nuclear or radiologic incidents, the radiation source may not be equivalent to a point source and so the inverse square law can be used as an approximation. In most instances, the approximation should be adequate. Maintaining a safe distance is especially critical. The larger the distance from a radiation source, the lower the dose.

There are certain emergency response operations that cannot be performed without some exposure of workers. In these situations, all unnecessary exposure to radiation should be avoided, even if it means barring workers from entering contaminated areas. These hazardous areas should be barricaded or roped off to form a restricted area that cannot be entered by non–radiation workers or bystanders.

Shielding

Shielding is generally used to safeguard against radiation from radioactive sources. The more mass placed between a source and a person, the less radiation the person will receive. This should be the guiding principle. Proper shielding from a source requires knowledge of the type of radiation hazard.[13] Different types of shielding are required for alpha, beta, and gamma radiation. Light clothing will provide protection and prevent contamination of the body from alpha radiation. Light metals such as aluminum are preferred for shielding from beta emissions. A sheet of aluminum can stop most beta radiation. Plexiglas is another shielding material that is effective against beta particles. Since gamma radiation is more penetrating than alpha and beta particles, higher-density materials such as lead, tungsten, steel, and concrete are ideal for shielding gamma rays. As the thickness of these materials increases, the intensity of the gamma radiation will decrease.

PITFALLS

Obstacles preventing the delivery of proper radiation decontamination procedures in response to a radiation catastrophe include the following:

- Lack of adequate radiation decontamination planning by emergency medical and hospital responders for possible nuclear or radiologic accidents and/or terrorist incidents;
- Lack of commitment of resources for radiation decontamination preparedness by emergency and hospital disaster planners;
- Lack of consultation and involvement of medical or health physicists in planning radiation decontamination plans and protocols;
- Lack of coordination with local and state radiologic health and safety agencies;
- Lack of understanding by medical providers and assigned decontamination team personnel of the basic science of radioactive isotopes and principles of radiation injury;
- Lack of adequate training in radiation decontamination techniques;
- Lack of recognition of the importance of radiation safety by emergency medical response personnel;
- Lack of proper radiation safety equipment and monitoring devices and instruments.

REFERENCES

1. *Merriam-Webster's Collegiate Dictionary*. 10th ed. Springfield, Mass: Merriam-Webster; 1997.
2. Zajtchuk R, Jenkins DP, Bellamy RF, et al, eds. *Medical Consequences of Nuclear Warfare*. Vol 2. Falls Church, Va: TMM Publications, Office of the Surgeon General; 1989.
3. Hendee WR. *Medical Radiation Physics*. Chicago: Year Book Medical Publishers; 1970.
4. Wilson W. *A Hundred Years of Physics*. London: Gerald Duckworth; 1950.
5. Weber RL. *Pioneers of Science: Nobel Prize Winners in Physics*. London: The Institute of Physics; 1980.
6. Wald N. Radiation injury. In: Cassel C, McCally M, Abraham H, eds. *Nuclear Weapons and Nuclear War: A Source Book for Health Professionals*. New York: Praeger; 1984:121-38.
7. Jarrett D, ed. *Medical Management of Radiological Casualties: Handbook*. Bethesda, Md: Armed Forces Radiobiology Research Institute; 1999. AFRRI special publication 99-2.
8. U.S. Department of the Army and the Commandant, Marine Corps. *NBC Decontamination. Army Field Manual 3-5; Marine Corps Warfighting Publication 3-37.3*. Washington DC: July 28, 2000.
9. U.S. Army Center for Health Promotion and Preventive Medicine. Washington DC: *The Medical NBC Battlebook. USACHPPM Tech Guide 244*. 2000.
10. National Council of Radiation Protection and Measurement. *Management of Terrorist Events Involving Radioactive Material: Report No. 138*. Bethesda, Md: National Council on Radiation Protection and Measurement; 2001.
11. Fong FH Jr. Nuclear detonations: evaluation and response. In: Hogan DE, Burstein JL, eds. *Disaster Medicine*. Philadelphia: Lippincott Williams & Wilkins; 2002:317-39.
12. Berger M, Byrd B, West CM, et al. *Transport of Radioactive Materials: Q&A About Incident Response*. Oak Ridge, Tenn: Oak Ridge Associated Universities; 1992.
13. Martin JE. *Physics for Radiation Protection*. New York: John Wiley & Sons; 2000.

PART II

Management of Specific Event Types

chapter 71

Introduction to Natural Disasters

Debra D. Schnelle

This text is designed as a comprehensive study of disaster medicine that also includes ready-made resources for the practitioner of disaster medicine. Part I, Overview of Disaster Management, serves as a definitive informational text for the professional working in the field of disaster management. The goal of Part II is to provide a quick reference for an exhaustive list of possible disaster scenarios. This introductory chapter provides an analytical framework common to all disasters, so that each scenario can be understood within a common frame of reference. The analytical framework offers definitions and provides a structure for the study of natural disasters in general.

This framework is the result of more than seven years of work conducted by the Steering Committee of the Task Force on Quality Control of Disaster Management, which is under the oversight of the World Association for Disaster and Emergency Medicine (WADEM) and the Nordic Society for Disaster Medicine. These organizations recently published their work, *Health Disaster Management Guidelines for Evaluation and Research in the Utstein Style,*[1] which provides much more detail concerning the concepts summarized here.

Natural disasters are a part of the human experience, and as the size of human societies increases, it appears that the *impact* of natural disasters on human society is growing, for the following four reasons[1]:

- Disasters are continuing to increase in frequency
- Disasters are affecting more citizens of the world community
- The economic costs associated with disasters are increasing at an alarming rate
- More people are moving to areas subject to natural hazards, for example, along hurricane-vulnerable coasts (many living in vulnerable mobile homes) and areas near earthquake faults or in flood plains

Unfortunately, the uncertainties of a natural disaster—how and when it will occur, what "type" of disaster will occur, and the ability of the affected population to withstand the effects of the disaster—all combine to create a "threat" not easily understood by any single professional perspective, specialty, or discipline. After each disaster, expert sources release a plethora of "reports" that recount personal experiences or consensus agreements from the experts on the lessons learned from the disas-ter. Unfortunately, few of these reports or evaluations appear to lead to sustained improvements in the response to natural disasters.

Important information is lost, errors and inefficiencies are perpetuated, and, in many settings, vulnerability continues to increase. Often, the impact of an intervention is assessed by *quantifying the output and not the outcome.* It is clear that some relief and assistance efforts not only are ineffective in meeting defined needs, but also actually are counter-productive and impair potentially beneficial responses and measures. More than 50% of the medical supplies sent to Bosnia during the recent conflicts not only were inappropriate or useless, but also cost the Bosnian government 34 million dollars to dispose of them.[1]

Examples such as this indicate the need for common definitions and a common conceptual framework for understanding natural disasters and systematically improving the quality of interventions designed to mitigate the natural disaster's impact on society.

The analytical framework outlined in the following is an adaptation of the conceptual model developed by WADEM; it is presented in detail in *Concepts of Operation of Health Service Support in an NBC Environment.*[2] Although the analytical framework in this textbook focuses on the chemical, biologic, radiologic, and nuclear (CBRN) threat, the adaptation remains broadly consistent with the WADEM conceptual model, due to the scope encompassed by the WADEM efforts and its rigorous development of definitions.

To begin, the word *disaster* has almost as many definitions as there are disasters—or the number of disciplines involved in disaster management. However, both the World Health Organization (WHO) and the United Nations (UN) present the following definition[1]: a natural disaster is "the result of a vast ecological breakdown in the relationships between man and his environment, a serious and sudden (or slow, as in drought) disruption on such a scale that the stricken community needs extraordinary efforts to cope with it, often with outside help or international aid." This definition is particularly useful because it differentiates between the *event* that caused the disaster and the *damage* associated with the disaster. From this definition, an understanding emerges that "all disasters are related to a specific hazard...."[1]

473

Hazards are classified by type in three classes: natural (e.g., seismic, climactic); manmade (e.g., a result of technology, such as the release of CBR substances; explosions; or fire); and mixed (a combination of natural and manmade). Section Seven of this textbook focuses on natural disasters, but the framework and definitions apply to all of the sections in Part II.

Events, then, are the realization or delivery of a hazard and can be characterized by onset, intensity, duration, scale, and magnitude.[1] *Damage* is defined as harm or injury that impairs the value or usefulness of something, or the health or normal function of persons. *Impact* is defined as the actual process of contact between an event and a society or a society's immediate perimeter.[1] These definitions can be understood separately or as different phases of the disaster (Fig. 71-1). A society exists in a state that can be characterized by its major functional components (medical, public health, sanitation, shelter, food, energy supplies, etc.).[1] Hazards may exist or be common in this environment, such as hurricanes, earthquakes, tornadoes, or floods.

When these hazards are realized, the event occurs, producing damage of varying degrees and types. The impact resulting from the infliction of the damage on a society is "dependent upon the vulnerability and preparedness of the environment and the society for that event."[1] This definition of a disaster as a progression from situation, to hazard, to event, to damage, and then to impact leads to the understanding that effective disaster response consists of intervening between these states to minimize the impact of the event to the greatest extent possible (see Fig. 71-1).

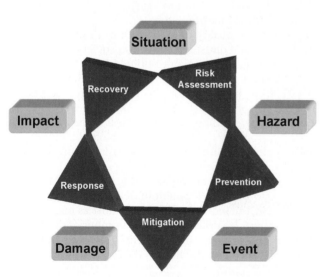

FIGURE 71–1. Phases of natural disasters and appropriate interventions. (From North Atlantic Treaty Organization, Nuclear, Biological, Chemical/Medical Working Group. Concepts of Health Service Support in an NBC Environment. Oct 2003.)

The first intervention is risk assessment—a comprehensive analysis of all possible hazards. WADEM defines hazard assessment as "identification and scaling of latent conditions that represent a threat."[1] The second intervention—planning and preparedness—is the most effective means of "prevention" to a natural disaster.[1] *Planning* is defined as[1]:

The process used to develop contingencies in preparation for an event that is likely to occur at some time. Planning includes warning systems, evacuation, relocation of dwellings (e.g., for floods), stores of food and water, temporary shelter, energy, management strategies, disaster drills and exercises, etc.

Preparedness is defined as "the aggregate of all measures and policies taken by humans before the event."[1]

The third intervention is mitigation and in this context refers to the mitigation of the damage *after* an event.[2] The fourth intervention is *response*, defined as "an answer to a defined need or request."[1] Finally, the fifth intervention is recovery, or "the restoration or replacement for all of the damage of an event."[1]

All of these interventions serve one or more of the following objectives[1]:

- Reduce the likelihood of damage that results from an event
- Minimize the damage
- Improve the resilience and capacity of the society and thus reduce the impact of the event
- Direct the recovery from the damage

Each of the following chapters in this section focuses on a particular type of natural hazard and describes the most common events associated with that hazard. Practical considerations for the hazard assessment and planning/preparation interventions are presented as preincident actions, and the mitigation, response, and recovery interventions are presented as postincident actions.

Finally, unique considerations, pitfalls, and case presentations are offered to place each of these natural disasters within the common framework presented in this chapter.

REFERENCES

1. Task Force on Quality Control of Disaster Management, the World Association for Disaster and Emergency Medicine, the Nordic Society for Disaster Medicine. Health Disaster Management: Guidelines for Evaluation and Research in the Utstein Style. Volume I. Conceptual Framework of Disasters. *Prehospital Disaster Med.* 2003;17(Suppl 3):1-177.
2. North Atlantic Treaty Organization, Nuclear, Biological, Chemical/Medical Working Group. Concepts of Health Service Support in an NBC Environment. Oct 2003.

chapter 72

Hurricanes, Cyclones, and Typhoons

Eric Sergienko

 ## DESCRIPTION OF EVENT

Cyclonic weather throughout the tropics has caused hundreds of thousands of deaths and billions of dollars of property damage in the last 100 years. Cyclones can occur in the Atlantic, Western or Eastern Pacific, or Indian Oceans. They can occur at any time of the year.

Tropical cyclones start as waves of warm air. In the Atlantic, these typically start as waves coming off of the Sahara. A tropical cyclone forms over the ocean, and then increases in strength and size, depending on the moisture and heat that it derives. As it moves over the ocean, it draws energy from the warm water, pulling it up into an organized weather system. Water must be at least 26.5°C (80°F). Rapid cooling of the atmosphere, enough to create thunderstorms, liberates the heat from the ocean and allows a cyclone to develop. There must be adequate moisture at about 5 km above sea level for the thunderstorms to continue. And this must occur far enough away from the equator (about 500 km) for the Coriolos effect to occur, resulting in the rotation of the storm. Finally, there must be a near-surface disturbance to create a vortex. If vertical wind shear between the surface and the upper troposphere occurs, this can prevent a cyclone from occurring or can significantly weaken an existing storm.

As the wave becomes organized, it may be classified as a tropical disturbance. These appear to have an organized convection (e.g., squall lines or multiple cell thunderstorms) and a discrete identity for at least 24 hours. They may not have increased winds, and they do not have a closed circulation or eye formation.

Tropical depressions generate sustained surface wind speeds of less than 17 m/s (34 knots, or 39 mph). Depressions are poorly organized, but they do have closed circulation. They do not have the classic "eye" formation that is seen with more organized storms.

Tropical storms generate winds that range from 17 m/s (34 knots, or 39 mph) to 32 m/s (63 knots, or 73 mph). At this intensity there is a distinct organization to the storm with rain bands forming outward from the center. On achieving this level, the storm is assigned a name. Names can be retired if they are associated with a devastating storm. Of the 60 or so tropical waves coming off of Africa in a year, 10 will become named storms.

Tropical cyclones that generate sustained surface winds greater than 32 m/s have titles associated with the location from where they originate: hurricanes (From the Carib language, meaning "eye of the god") form in the mid-Atlantic, Caribbean, or Northeast Pacific oceans. Typhoons form in the Western Pacific. Cyclones form in the Indian Ocean.

The typical season for Atlantic and Eastern Pacific hurricanes is from June to November. Although typhoons can develop any time of the year, they are more common from May until December.

Tropical cyclones are classified by the strength of their sustained winds. The Saffir-Simpson scale rates cyclones on a scale from 1 to 5 (Table 72-1). In addition, super-typhoons are typhoons that maintain wind speeds greater than 140 knots.

Movement of a cyclone is generally east to west as the storm forms in the tropics. It is kept in the tropics by a subtropical ridge. The storm gradually moves away from the tropics and becomes extratropical, finally dissipating in the regions outside the 45th parallel. The weaker the subtropical ridge, the earlier it turns away from the equator and dissipates.

Although the intensity of the winds is predictive of damage, equally important is how rapidly a storm moves through an area. A slow-moving storm will allow for a greater degree of damage than a fast-moving storm. Also one has to consider the amount of rainfall associated with the cyclone, which can lead to significant flooding and landslides. In addition, a storm surge associated with tropical storms causes further flooding and damage to coastal areas. Finally, a tropical storm can spawn tornadoes and waterspouts that can cause additional damage.[1,2]

The worst natural disaster in the United States occurred in 1900 in Galveston, Texas, when a storm surge of 15.7 feet flooded the island, which has a maximum elevation of 8.7 feet. Eight thousand people, one-fifth of the population, died. The most deadly natural disaster in the western hemisphere was Hurricane Mitch in 1998, which resulted in approximately 12,000 deaths in Central America, predominantly from flooding and mudslides. Similarly, more than 500,000 deaths occurred when a cyclone coming off the Bay of Bengal in 1970 caused flooding in Bangladesh and India[3]. Economically, Hurricane Andrew caused more than $20 billion worth of damage.[4,5] In 2005, Hurricane katrina devastated the gulf coast of the United States and

TABLE 72-1 SAFFIR-SIMPSON HURRICANE SCALE

CATEGORY	SUSTAINED WINDS (MPH)	DESCRIPTION	DAMAGE	EXAMPLE
Tropical storm	39–73			
1	74–95	Minimal	No real damage to buildings; damage to unanchored mobile homes	Allison, 1995
2	96–110	Moderate	Damage to building roofs, doors, and windows; considerable damage to mobile homes; flooding damage; trees down	Bonnie, 1998
3	111–130	Extensive	Some damage to small residences and utility buildings; mobile homes destroyed; coastal flooding, causing destruction of smaller buildings and damage to larger ones; flooding inland	Opal, 1995
4	131–155	Extreme	Complete roof failure on small buildings; major erosion; flooding well inland	Hugo, 1989
5	156 and up	Catastrophic	Roof failure on residences and industrial buildings; complete building failures possible; major flooding on shoreline structures	Andrew, 1992

Adapted from National Weather Service National Hurricane Center. The Saffir-Simpson Hurricane Scale Available at: www.nhc.noaa.gov/aboutsshs.shtml.

resulted in the evacuation of New Orleans. As of this writing, the full extent of the destruction in terms of loss of property and life is not fully known, but clearly Katrina was one of the worst hurricanes in U.S. history.

 PREINCIDENT ACTIONS

Planning for a tropical storm involves preparations for all of the threats associated with the storm: high winds, flooding, landslides, and storm surge.

Preparations for tropical weather should be an ongoing activity starting at the onset of the tropical storm season. Whereas some preparations should be made at the start of the season, others can wait until storm activity is anticipated. Typical hospital emergency management plans are organized based on a timeline that starts at the beginning of the storm season and continues through the arrival of storm-force winds to the post-storm recovery efforts.

Some planning should start with the construction or remodeling of the hospital. Hospitals in areas where storms occur should be constructed to withstand high winds and flooding. Storm shutters should be used to protect all exterior openings. Redundant power sources should be considered, with a final backup being small portable generators capable of powering essential equipment in an individual unit. Redundant communications systems with civil defense and emergency medical services are essential because multiple system failures can occur.

Another consideration for medical facilities, regardless of size, is the evacuation of patients and staff farther inland and away from the predicted storm track.

Therefore, the facility's evacuation annex should include relocation of patients to a distant facility.

At the start of the storm season, sandbags should be available to barricade low-lying doors susceptible to flooding. Damage control equipment should be available. Plywood sheeting for blown-out windows, 2 × 4 boards for reinforcing doors and other structures that may be stressed by prolonged winds, and vacuums that can handle water (wet/dry vacuum) are essential. Facility engineers and damage control parties must be designated as essential personnel and receive training on mitigation of storm damage. Generators should be fully fueled and maintained.

Before a storm, employees should be alerted to bring in personal items that may be required for a prolonged stay in the medical treatment facility. This should include food, bedding, and medications. Employees who are in the facility during the storm should ensure that their families and residences are prepared before the storm.

Enough durable and expendable medical equipment and pharmaceuticals should be stocked to allow for unsupported operations for up to 72 hours. Disposable equipment (e.g., suture sets) should be considered if sterilization systems should fail. Alternative means of cleaning, such as alcohol-based hand sanitizers, should be obtained. Food and water must be stocked to feed and hydrate staff, patients, and family of patients. The fuel tanks of vehicles, both personal and hospital-associated, should be filled. Waste systems may be damaged, so alternative means of disposing liquid and solid waste, including biohazardous material, must be considered.

Traditionally, pregnant women, who are either at least 36 weeks' gestation or are in the third trimester and expecting complications with delivery, have been advised to report to the hospital before the storm's arrival. Precipitous labor may occur due to decreased barometric pressure, although this has never been validated.

During the Storm

Generally, damage control predominates during the passage of a tropical cyclone over a medical facility. In an intense storm, there will be minimal movement outdoors, so new patients will not be arriving in large numbers.

If emergency medical services are required to perform a rescue during high winds, it is advisable to use military vehicles (such as Hummers) or at least heavy four-wheel drive vehicles rather than a standard ambulance. Because of its high profile and relative low weight, a traditional ambulance is at risk of being blown over or flooded away. Further, it is beneficial to send two vehicles in a convoy rather than sending a vehicle by itself.

Communications will deteriorate during the storm. Cellular systems will go down as repeater cells are destroyed. The same is true for handheld radios beyond line of sight as their repeaters are damaged. Landline analog phones seem to be the most rugged, and amateur radio operators can serve as a backup.

Deaths during the storm will occur due to multiple causes. The largest cause of death in flat areas is flooding. Oftentimes, these deaths involve the drowning of persons trapped in vehicles. In areas with hills, landslides may be the most prominent cause of death. Drownings from swimming, boating, or surfing in storm waters do occur despite warnings to the contrary. Deaths that can occur post-storm may be indirectly due to power outages as people are electrocuted when power lines are re-energized and from the use of candles, which can lead to house fires. Equally frustrating are deaths related to carbon monoxide caused by the use of generators or charcoal stoves/grills without proper ventilation.[6,7]

 ## POSTINCIDENT ACTIONS

A rapid needs assessment for the hospital and the community should be performed. Repairs required for maintaining hospital operations should be done. Durable and expendable medical equipment destroyed or damaged during the storm should be noted, and replacement equipment should be ordered. Typically, power will be out, so consideration should be made for patients with medications that require refrigeration. "Social" admissions may be needed to maintain patients' health status. Post-storm morbidity in the community is associated with disruption in the infrastructure and attempts to restore normal function. Those with chronic medical problems or patients who require regular routine medical procedures such as dialysis experience an exacerbation due to the stresses of the uncontrolled environment and/or loss or medications and durable medical equipment. Injuries occur during cleanup of storm damage and may include lacerations, concussions, and plantar puncture wounds. Illnesses are associated with lack of safe water sources or proper food handling and the inability to dispose of waste. In developing countries, cholera and other diarrheal diseases often occur. Finally, anxiety and posttraumatic stress can occur among survivors.[8,9]

 ## MEDICAL TREATMENT OF CASUALTIES

There may be a greater likelihood to admit patients who are unable to take care of themselves at home until the community's infrastructure has been re-established.

There also is a tendency to use antibiotic wound prophylaxis and to administer early updates of tetanus post-storm due to the increased concern over wound contamination and the inability to properly clean the wound. It may be more appropriate to use delayed primary closure.[10]

It may be difficult to obtain ancillary or laboratory studies in a hospital that is stressed by a surge in patients or damaged radiology or laboratory spaces. Consideration for prioritizing studies may be necessary in these situations.

Foodborne and waterborne diseases are possible, even in developed countries. Most of these are spread through fecal-oral contamination. Public health actions may prevent an outbreak. Notices to boil or chlorinate water should be posted. Both depression and posttraumatic stress disorder (PTSD) are common after large storms. In one survey after Hurricane Andrew, the incidences of depression and PTSD among survivors were 36% and 30%, respectively. Although there is significant debate over what methods are most effective in minimizing the psychological sequelae of a disaster, cognitive therapy and supportive psychotherapy may be useful, along with short-term use of antianxiety and sleep medications. Recognition that healthcare providers could be part of the disaster and may need intervention is also important in maintaining a functional disaster response.[11,12]

 ## UNIQUE CONSIDERATIONS

The hospital in the midst of a tropical cyclone is just as prone to being damaged or rendered unusable as any other building in the area. Consideration must be given in the pre-storm period to evacuate all patients who are able to be transported. Essential staffing should be maintained during the storm, including keeping providers in house. The bulk of hospital staff should be available after the storm since that is the time the majority of new patients will arrive.

 ## PITFALLS

1. Failing to plan for catastrophic weather when located in a zone that experiences such hazards: Storm preparation and planning, including tabletop exercises, should be done yearly to ensure that the hospital is adequately equipped and trained for cyclonic weather.

2. Failure to evacuate, when possible: Smaller community hospitals should consider this as part of their routine for larger tropical storms. Moving critically ill patients will free up beds for incoming casualties and minimize the number of staff needed in-hospital during the storm. Larger hospitals in coastal or flood prone areas should also consider this option.[13]

3. Failure to have redundant systems: Both power and communications systems tend to fail during cyclonic weather.

4. Thinking that the worst is over when the storm has passed: The post-storm period is just as likely to produce injuries, illness, and fatalities.

 CASE PRESENTATION

Supertyphoon Ponsonga struck the island of Guam in the Western Pacific on Dec. 11, 2002. Ponsonga started as a tropical disturbance to the east of Chuuk. As it progressed across the Pacific, it became increasingly more organized and powerful. The majority of computer models initially predicted the storm would pass south of Guam. An outlier model predicted a direct hit. Both the military and government of Guam issued statements for higher conditions of readiness. As the storm continued to track toward Guam, aircraft and ships moved out of its path. The eye of the storm made landfall over the north end of the island. Although the official wind gauge was destroyed by the typhoon, the wind gusts were estimated to be greater than 200 mph, with sustained winds of 150 mph. In addition, the storm track went over the island at a speed of approximately 6 knots. This sustained wind over an unusually long period led to significant structural damage. Most nonreinforced structures were destroyed. The pediatric intensive care unit of the island's civilian hospital, Guam Memorial Hospital, was destroyed, and the adult intensive care unit was significantly damaged. Naval Hospital Guam experienced significant water damage, and the emergency department's equipment storage room was destroyed. The emergency medical services system lost several ambulances, which were blown over by the storm.

In addition, during the storm, several people trapped in buildings were rescued, and thunderstorms caused a fuel depot to ignite. Three deaths were attributed to Ponsonga. In the post-storm environment, the emergency departments of both hospitals were overrun with patients with minor traumatic injuries that had occurred during the storm. Resource sharing, including personnel, was used to maintain critical care. Critically ill patients were transferred to the naval hospital. Within 72 hours, an expeditionary medical squadron that was deployed from an air base in Japan had co-located with Guam Memorial Hospital. Two additional disaster medical assistance teams deployed to the island from the U.S. mainland. Initially, acute injuries were treated, but largely these teams were involved in the care of routine medical problems.

REFERENCES

1. Atlantic Oceanographic and Meteorological Laboratory. Hurricane Research Division. Frequently asked questions. Available at: http://www.aoml.noaa.gov/hrd/tcfaq/tcfaqHED.html.

2. National Weather Service National Hurricane Center. Available at: http://www.nhc.noaa.gov.

3. Century's Top Weather, Water and Climate Events. Available at: http://www.noaanews.noaa.gov/stories/s334.htm.

4. Jarrell JD, Mayfield M, Rappaport E. NOAA Technical Memorandum NWS TPC-1: The Deadliest, Costliest, and Most Intense Hurricanes from 1900 to 2000. Available at: http://www.aoml.noaa.gov/hrd/Landsea/deadly/.

5. Anonymous. The devastating path of Hurricane Mitch in Central America. *Disasters: Preparedness and Mitigation in the Americas.* 1999;75:S1-4.

6. George-McDowell N, Landron F, Glenn J, et al. Deaths associated with Hurricanes Marilyn and Opal—United States, September-October 1995. *MMWR.* 1996;45(2):32-4.

7. Carmichael C, Neasman A, Rivera L, Wurm G, et al. Morbidity and mortality associated with Hurricane Floyd—North Carolina, September-October 1999. *MMWR.* 2000;49(17):369-72.

8. Hopkins RS. Comprehensive assessment of health needs 2 months after Hurricane Andrew—Dade County. *MMWR.* 1993;42(22):434-5.

9. Waring SC, desVignes-Kendrick M, Arafat RR, et al. Tropical Storm Allison rapid needs assessment—Houston, Texas, June 2001. *MMWR.* 2002;51(17):366-9.

10. Capellan O, Hollander JE. Management of lacerations in the emergency department. *Emerg Med Clinic North Am.* 2003;21(1):205-31.

11. Garakani A. General disaster psychiatry. *Psychiatr Clin North Am.* 2004;27(3):391.

12. Raphael B. Debriefing: its evolution and current status. *Psychiatr Clin North Am.* 2004;27(3):407.

13. Nates JL. Combined external and internal hospital disaster: impact and response in a Houston trauma intensive care unit. *Crit Care Med.* 2004;32(3):686-90.

chapter 73

Earthquake

Bruce M. Becker

 ## DESCRIPTION OF EVENT

At 11:40 AM on Dec. 7, 1988, a massive earthquake struck northwestern Armenia. The epicenter was between the cities of Spitak and Stepanavan. Leninakan, a larger and more populous city, located 35 miles south of Spitak, was also severely affected. The earthquake registered 6.9 on the Richter scale and was followed by multiple aftershocks that lasted for days. Because the earthquake occurred in the late morning of a weekday, in the winter, and in a mountainous region of Armenia, most adults were at work or home and most children were inside at school. The majority of buildings in the affected cities and towns were destroyed. Water, sewage, and gas lines running under the city streets were ripped apart. Natural gas leaking from broken pipelines caught fire, and soon much of Leninakan was a burning conflagration. Many people were trapped inside the collapsed buildings and suffered from smoke inhalation. In other sites, broken water mains flooded buildings and streets. In Leninakan, a large clock tower still stands, partially destroyed in the town square, with its iron hands frozen at 11:41 AM. The clock has not been fixed but remains as a memorial to the earthquake. Roads were destroyed, blocking access to these cities and the towns between them. People who survived the initial quake, escaping from collapsing buildings, returned again and again to try to rescue their friends and relatives from the rubble. By the night of Dec. 7, 1988, almost 500,000 people were homeless in the earthquake region, squatting by fires in the streets and fields and trying to arrange temporary shelter. At the time of the earthquake, Mikhail Gorbachev was preparing to visit the United States. International news media attention was focused on the former Soviet Union. When Gorbachev interrupted his visit to attend to the disaster area, the news media quickly focused on the Armenian earthquake, providing tremendous coverage. This coverage initiated one of the largest international acute disaster relief efforts ever mounted.

To this day, the number of casualties is unknown. The region had recently been the site of a large immigration of Armenians from other republics of the former Soviet Union and from Nagorno Karabakh, an Armenian terri-tory that had been annexed by Azerbaijan, a hostile neighbor. (Soon after the quake, Nagorno Karabakh became the site of a civil war and uprising.) Estimates of casualties from the earthquake and its aftermath ranged from 30,000 to 75,000 people dead and hundreds of thousands injured. Because roadways were the only means of transportation into Spitak and Leninakan, and because these roadways were compromised by the earthquake, there was a significant lag time between the disaster's impact and the arrival of local response. Medical infrastructure in the city was completely destroyed or rendered inoperable, and many of the healthcare workers, including physicians and nurses, were killed or injured. Relief workers were forced to rely on air transportation. The Leninakan airport was small and inadequate, and very soon its runway became so congested that relief planes could not land. Within 48 hours of the quake, the weather had worsened, with rain and snow falling, putting the now homeless residents of these destroyed cities at risk for hypothermia.

The destruction of infrastructure was almost unimaginable. Almost 400 schools and universities were destroyed along with 85 hospitals and clinics. Fifty-eight villages, 90 collective farms, and 200 large state farms were destroyed. The psychological effects were even more far reaching. The average survivor lost between 10 to 15 relatives, their homes, jobs, and all of their possessions. The country's nuclear reactor, a Chernobyl-style facility, had been built on the same fault line that caused the earthquake. Amazingly, it was not affected; however, the government immediately shut it down, thus cutting electricity to most of the country. It did not resume operating for years. Soviet and international relief efforts were extensive. Almost 5000 tons of drugs and consumable medical supplies were delivered to Armenia. Thousands of Soviet physicians and other medical relief workers and hundreds of international workers poured into the country to provide aid. Most remained for about 2 weeks. Five years later the cities of Leninakan (renamed Gyumri after the fall of the Soviet Union and the extirpations of Lenin and Stalin from all city names) and Spitak remained in rubble, with few hospitals and clinics rebuilt or restored to providing functional medical services.

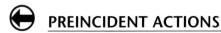

PREINCIDENT ACTIONS

Preincident actions in earthquake-prone regions fall into two categories. The first focuses on structural preparations and engineering and design issues intended to strengthen and improve buildings to decrease the likelihood of massive destruction in the face of an earthquake event. These engineering decisions may also focus on the positioning, strengthening, and layout of utility pipes, roadways, and power plants and the relative proximity of potentially dangerous structures, such as factories producing or storing toxic materials and fuel storage facilities, to fault lines and potential earthquake epicenters. The fault system in northwest Armenia had been well defined in the past; nevertheless, very few appropriate engineering and structural preparations had been put into place. The older buildings in Armenia, especially in the northwest, were made from huge blocks of a native Armenian stone called *tufa*, which is volcanic but strong. In fact, one of the last standing buildings in Gyumri was the great Armenian apostolic church, which was made completely of huge blocks of tufa. Most of the housing constructed in the decades before the earthquake, however, was much shoddier. This was the result of two forces acting in concert: an unprecedented demand for housing triggered by the large-scale immigration to the region from other parts of the Soviet Union, as previously described, and the deep and inherent corruption of the Soviet system itself. It was well known that collective farms and industries paid almost no wages to workers, especially during the last years of the regime, as it began to fall apart economically and politically. Those who were successful either initiated private business enterprise or became involved in corrupt practices, such as acquisitioning sturdy building materials from the government for construction of large apartments and then selling the materials on their own while using cheaper-grade concrete or concrete thinned with sand with few reinforcement bars to construct dwellings. The result of these building practices was the construction of edifices with little capacity to resist earthquakes. When the temblor struck Dec. 7, 1988, most of the newly constructed and tall apartment buildings in Gyumri and Spitak crumbled to the earth like so many sand castles washed away by an incoming tide.

The second set of preincident actions for a country or region with populous regions and cities in the area of large earthquake faults is the development and implementation of a disaster response plan that should include training medical providers and stockpiling equipment to facilitate rapid action in the event of an earthquake. The former Soviet Union's medical structure was reactive, rather than proactive, and slow to accept conceptual changes from the West. There was no emergency medicine in Armenia before the earthquake and only a very primitive prehospital care system. Search and rescue teams and earth-moving equipment, which are vital for appropriate search and rescue operations after an earthquake, were not readily available. The medical system was so economically devastated in the years before the fall of the Soviet Union that even some of the most basic equipment for medical procedures was not available in medium to large cities in republics across the former Soviet Union. Therefore, when the earthquake struck, there were virtually no resources available to provide disaster response to Gyumri, Spitak, or the villages in between. The few surviving local health workers organized the small amount of undamaged medical equipment available and were able to mount a small immediate local response. Many healthcare workers responded from Yerevan, the capital city; however, as previously noted, transportation was very difficult—there is only one road into the earthquake region from the south, and much of it was destroyed by the earthquake. Search and rescue teams and equipment came first from the former Soviet Union and then from other countries; personnel, machinery, and supplies had to be flown into the airport in Yerevan and then trucked to the earthquake zone. This delay proved deadly for people trapped in the rubble of falling buildings, many of whom perished.

POSTINCIDENT ACTIONS

One of the most important concepts in disaster response today is that of command and control. There has to be a central authority that oversees the disaster response and controls the communications; logistics; requests for and distribution of resources; distribution of information; allocation of search and rescue teams and equipment, medical equipment, surgical equipment, primary care and subspecialty healthcare physicians, and allied healthcare workers; and construction of temporary healthcare facilities. This central authority is also responsible for the control, preparation, and distribution of other vital public health elements of the relief efforts, including sanitation, water, shelter, food, clothing, and psychosocial support. Large-scale international disaster responses, such as those mounted in Armenia after the earthquake, are well intentioned and successful in providing lifesaving interventions; nevertheless, they are inefficient and resource intensive. One problem that responders sometimes encounter is that many of the teams from different countries do not share a common language or common system in their approach to the response. They may have different equipment and drugs that cannot be shared across systems and are often unknown to healthcare practitioners in the host country. This lack of coordination can lead to extensive duplication of some services and the lack of other services completely. Some of this was magnified in Armenia because of the latent tensions between Armenia and Russia, in the wake of the dissolution of the former Soviet Union. There was a lack of trust of intentions on both sides that impeded the pace and efficiency of the response effort. Disaster responders from different countries are often reluctant to submit to a central command and control or Incident Command System that is being directed by administration and personnel from a country other than their own.

The tremendous amount of media attention that was focused on Armenia immediately after the earthquake was both a blessing and a curse. It engendered a tremendous amount of international response, bringing healthcare workers, allied health personnel, search and rescue teams, fire rescue personnel, structural engineers, psychologists, and others from all over the world to Armenia with a huge amount of relief supplies. On the other hand, of the almost 5000 tons of drugs and medical supplies eventually delivered, less than 30% were usable by healthcare workers in Armenia. More than 10% of the drugs delivered were expired or about to expire, and an equal percentage of the medical equipment sent was outdated, broken, or not functional. Twenty percent of all materials delivered as foreign aid had to be destroyed by the Armenians by the end of 1989 at considerable cost.[1]

In the ideal postimpact phase of an earthquake, the fire chief or fire rescue commander (of Spitak, Gyumri, Yerevan, or Armenia) would have initiated a command center and set up an Incident Command System. All other healthcare workers, search and rescue workers, structural engineers, and others involved in the rescue effort would have been dispatched through and monitored by the command center. All supplies, drugs, and other equipment would have been inventoried, sorted, and distributed through the command center, which also would have controlled the apportioning of casualties and would have maintained a database of all persons uncovered, discovered, or otherwise affected in the earthquake area. Such an orderly response is rarely seen in the postdisaster phase, especially in countries already suffering from economic, political, and social upheaval. Certainly this was the case in Armenia in 1988.

 ## MEDICAL TREATMENT OF CASUALTIES

Medical casualties in the impact and postimpact phases of an earthquake disaster fall into three categories: acute, subacute, and chronic. Acute injuries from the impact of an earthquake, as clearly witnessed in the cities of Armenia, are caused by collapsing buildings, falling rubble, fire, and dust inhalation. Most people caught in collapsing buildings, especially structures greater than two stories, are killed instantly or trapped in pockets. Some of those trapped have body parts pinned under extremely heavy loads, timbers, or stone. Even when rescued, they will often have crush syndrome and acute renal failure. Others are caught up in the flash fires that accompany the rupture of natural gas pipes and suffer extensive body burns or smoke inhalation, leading to severe morbidity and mortality. A third group of patients suffers acute and chronic respiratory disease from the inhalation of the large amount of particulate matter that is aerosolized by the collapse of concrete and stone buildings and mixed with smoke from the generalized fires throughout a region. Depending on climatic conditions, hypothermia can also be a consideration.

The cities affected by the earthquake in Armenia were located in a mountainous, snowy region; the earthquake occurred in winter. Five hundred thousand people were homeless, and of those, many had minor to moderate orthopedic and soft tissue injuries. One of the unique acute medical problems associated with earthquakes is crush syndrome. In some ways, the timing of the Armenian earthquake was quite fortuitous, considering the large incidence of crush syndrome and secondary renal failure. The American Society of Nephrology was having its annual meeting Dec. 11, 1988. The official Soviet request for dialysis was made to the nephrologists at that meeting and the international nephrology community responded.[2] Hospitals in Yerevan had 10 antiquated dialysis machines. The system was overwhelmed by the almost 400 patients with acute renal failure from crush syndrome who were extricated from the rubble of the earthquake. About 150 of these patients were flown to Moscow for dialysis treatment. Many others were treated by machinery sent by the international nephrology community rendering humanitarian assistance in response to the earthquake.[3] This acute response also had positive long-term outcomes for Armenia in that an extensive sustainable dialysis program was set up in the postearthquake days and continues.[4,5]

Subacute injuries and medical illnesses after the impact of an earthquake often include those that patients sustain while attempting to rescue other victims trapped in the rubble. These injuries are quite common since many of the buildings in a zone devastated by an earthquake are rendered structurally unstable and are subject to further collapse if people attempt to enter them to perform hand excavation and rescue; aftershocks are common. There are also many new hazards created by the collapse of building structures and the rupture of underground utility pipes and underground or above-ground electric wires. These secondary injuries are less severe than those sustained during the earthquake; nevertheless, they require appropriate intervention if patients are to heal properly without infection and long-term disability. Illness in the subacute phase includes exacerbation of chronic medical problems no longer being treated with appropriate medications or equipment destroyed during the disaster. These illnesses may include diabetes, hypertension, coronary artery disease, and pulmonary disease. Asthma and chronic obstructive pulmonary disease often flare in response to deteriorating air quality and the rapid spread of acute respiratory illness through a population weakened by compromised nutrition; sleep deprivation; and lack of clothing, housing, and food; and stress. Smoke from fires caused directly by the disaster as well as smoke from open fires uses for cooking and keeping warm exacerbate these problems. Other infectious disease entities of concern include gastroenteritis from the consumption of spoiled food when refrigeration is not available and contaminated water from ruptured water mains and surface water contaminated by toxins and fecal run-off.

Chronic medical problems are seen in the weeks and months of the postimpact phase of an earthquake and include the ramifications of chronic disease entities untreated or partially treated during that time and the infectious complications of a population displaced into temporary and congested housing lacking proper food, clothing, and shelter. In addition, disruption of the social milieu may lead to psychiatric illness, including posttraumatic stress disorder (PTSD) and depression. PTSD and depression may persist for months to years after the impact.[6,7] In fact, treatment for these problems both in children and adults has been ongoing for years after the Armenian earthquake.[8-10]

 UNIQUE CONSIDERATIONS

There are several considerations that are unique to the disaster medical response to an earthquake.

1. A small but salvageable number of persons is often trapped by falling building debris in an earthquake. Rapid deployment of appropriately trained search and rescue teams with dogs and high-tech listening devices is necessary to locate and save these people. Search and rescue equipment was very limited initially in response to the Armenian earthquake. It was on-scene after considerable delay during the rescue effort. Consequently, most people trapped in the rubble in Gyumri and Spitak died.

2. The most common injuries in an earthquake are traumatic injuries to the head and body, including closed head injury and orthopedic injuries. Disaster medical response teams must be prepared to handle these neurosurgical, orthopedic, and soft tissue injuries to provide appropriate medical treatment to casualties. Crush syndrome is more common in earthquakes than in any other disaster. The response team should have appropriate intravenous solutions and the equipment and skills to evaluate tissue compartment syndromes, perform fasciectomies, and treat crush syndrome. Laboratory capacity is necessary to monitor renal function and provide dialysis if necessary.

3. Other injuries commonly seen in earthquakes, especially in urban areas, are burns; inhalation injuries from smoke; and exacerbation of chronic or subacute respiratory illness, including asthma from the inhalation of dust, smoke, and debris. Disaster medical response teams must be prepared to treat patients with these problems.

4. Earthquakes massively destroy infrastructure, rendering hospitals and medical clinics inoperable and unusable. Basic utilities are also usually devastated, including gas lines, water mains, sewage facilities, and electrical power plants. The disaster response team must be prepared to provide these basic services, including water, shelter, and energy as well as temporary equipped medical facilities. Even if hospitals and clinics remain standing after an earthquake, they may be structurally unusable and extremely dangerous to enter.

5. The earthquake site is quite dangerous for rescue workers. Building debris, loose wires, and leaking gas, water, and sewage are common. Rescue workers entering buildings to perform search and rescue operations or to unearth buried casualties are often putting themselves at risk if the buildings are structurally unstable. Aftershocks are common after the initial impact of an earthquake and can trigger the collapse of structures that remain standing.

 PITFALLS

1. Not implementing search and rescue operations early. Search and rescue personnel with heavy earth moving equipment can be very effective if mobilized in a timely fashion and are available proximate to the impact of the earthquake. These operations have discovered and unearthed survivors trapped in the rubble; however, this part of the disaster response is very cost-intensive and, generally, the number of victims saved is small relative to the total number of casualties that requires intensive short- and long-term medical care.

2. Identification and treatment of crush syndrome. Crush syndrome is common in patients pinned under small or large amounts of debris and trapped for extensive periods, leading to necrosis of the pinned extremities. Rescue workers should be fully educated and carry protocols on how to respond properly to patients who potentially have crush syndrome and incipient renal failure. The response team needs to have access to dialysis and nephrology consultation.

3. Even though major orthopedic injuries, crush syndrome, hemodialysis, and other major medical subspecialty interventions are interesting and often grab media attention, the most important part of the medical response to earthquakes is couched within public health and primary healthcare. The major issue facing most survivors of an earthquake is the restoration of infrastructure, including water, shelter, food, sanitation, and basic medical facilities with primary healthcare services. Any relief effort that ignores these issues will only have a short and expensive impact for a small number of patients without any sustained impact on the short-, medium-, or long-term health of the affected population.

4. Early attention to anxiety and psychological stress imposed by the disaster can ameliorate the long-term disability and impaired functional capacity associated with PTSD, chronic anxiety, and depression on the population. Disaster medical response teams must engage psychologists and psychiatrists to participate actively from the very beginning of the response.

5. Although human nature calls for an immediate active *intervention*, the best disaster medical response to an earthquake demands a rapid and immediate *assessment* with communication of information back to planning entities removed from the disaster site so that appropriate allocations of equipment, medicines, medical personnel, search and rescue teams, and other resources can be made.

6. Disaster systems concepts such as an Incident Command System and Command and Control must be imposed on any disaster response to avoid ineffective and inefficient interventions resulting in duplication, waste, miscommunication, and unnecessary further loss of life.

REFERENCES

1. Autier P, Ferir MC, Hairapetien A, et al. Drug supply in the aftermath of the 1988 Armenian earthquake. *Lancet.* 1998;335 (8702):1388-90.
2. Eknoyan G. The Armenian earthquake of 1988: a milestone in the evolution of nephrology advances in renal replacement and therapy. *Adv Ren Replace Ther.* 2003;10(2):87-92.
3. Tattersall JE, Richards NT, McCann M, et al. Acute hemodialysis during the Armenian earthquake disaster. *Injury.* 1990;21(1):25-8.
4. Eknoyan G. Acute renal failure in the Armenian earthquake. *Renal Failure.* 1992;14(3):241-4.
5. Leumann E, Bernhardt JP, Babloyian A, et al. From dialysis to basic paediatric nephrology: an unorthodox project applied in Yerevan Armenia. *Pediatr Nephrol.* 1994;8(2):252-5.
6. Goenjian AK, Karayan I, Pynoos RS, et al. Outcome of psychotherapy among early adolescents after trauma. *Am J Psychiatry.* 1997;154(4):536-42.
7. Goenjian AK, Yehuda R, Steinberg AM, et al. Basal cortisol, dexamethasone, suppression of cortisol, and MHPG in adolescents after the 1988 earthquake. *Am J Psychiatry.* 1996;153(7):929-34.
8. Goenjian AK, Pynoos RS, Steinberg AM, et al. Psychiatric comorbidities in children after the 1988 earthquake in Armenia. *J Am Acad Child Adolesc Psychiatry.* 1995;34(9):1174-84.
9. Goenjian AK. A mental health relief programme in Armenia after the 1988 earthquake: implementation and clinical observations. *Br J Psychiatry.* 1993;163: 230-9.
10. Goenjian AK, Najarian LM, Pynoos RS, et al. Post-traumatic stress reactions after single and double trauma. *Acta Psychiatr Scand.* 1994;90(3):214-21.

chapter 74

Tornado

Michael D. Jones and James Pfaff

 DESCRIPTION OF EVENT

Tornadoes are one of nature's most violent storms. In an average year, about 800 tornadoes are reported across the United States, resulting in 80 deaths and over 1500 injuries.[1] A tornado is a violently rotating column of air extending from swelling cumulonimbus clouds to the ground. The most violent tornadoes are capable of tremendous destruction with wind speeds of 250 mph or more. Damage paths can be in excess of 1 mile wide and 50 miles long.[2]

Tornado severity is graded using the Fujita-Pearson Tornado Scale (Table 74-1). This scale ranges from designations of F0 to F5. Originally designed as a measurement of structural damage caused by a tornado, the scale is now often used to describe the wind speeds associated with a tornado. Measurements of actual tornado wind speeds are not usually available, and the assignment of a Fujita designation may vary for any one tornado, even among experts. Still, this scale is the preferred method for rating the severity of these storms. The great majority of tornadoes are rated F0-F1 with wind speeds under 113 mph, causing only mild structural damage and rarely leading to significant injuries or death. Only 1%-2% of tornadoes each year are designated as F4-F5 (wind speeds greater than 206 mph), but these rare monstrous storms cause over 50% of the tornado-related fatalities in the United States each year.[3]

Tornadoes occur with equal frequency in all countries of the world that have land mass in the middle latitudes, but the unique landscape and weather patterns of the United States cause it to have the most intense tornadoes of any country. Between 1950 and 2003, over 4663 deaths and 80,376 injuries were reported as directly related to tornadic storms in the United States. In addition to the loss of life and the frequent injuries, tornadoes were responsible for over $20 trillion in property and crop damage between 1950 and 2003.[4] Tornadoes come in all shapes and sizes and can occur anywhere in the United States at any time of the year. In the southern states, peak tornado season is March through May, whereas peak months in the northern states are during the summer.[2] Because of the consistent high frequency of tornadoes seen in the region including northern Texas, Oklahoma, Kansas, and Nebraska, this area has become known as "Tornado Alley."[5] The probability that any one particular city in North America will be struck by a tornado has been calculated as once every 250 years.[6] This probability is much higher for communities in Tornado Alley. For example, Oklahoma City has been struck by significant tornadoes 26 times in the past 100 years.[7]

Tornadoes strike with little or no warning. Because of investments in research and observation systems such as the NEXRAD Doppler radar, interactive computer systems, and other forecasting technology, the lead time for tornadoes has nearly doubled from a national average of 5 minutes in the early 1990s to nearly 11 minutes today. Major storms are often picked up or spotted and warnings made more than 20 minutes before the tornado touches down.[1] In the United States, all severe weather watches and warnings are issued by the Storm Prediction Center (SPC) in Norman, Oklahoma. The SPC is a division of the National Weather Service (NWS). The SPC issues a *tornado watch* when their forecasting systems indicate there is a region where tornadoes and other kinds of severe weather are possible in the next several hours. This is the time to turn on the TV or radio to the local weather channel and quickly review tornado disaster plans. The SPC issues a *tornado warning* only when a tornado has been spotted or when Doppler radar has detected a thunderstorm circulation that can spawn

TABLE 74-1   FUJITA-PEARSON TORNADO SCALE

CATEGORY	WIND SPEED (MPH)	TYPES OF DAMAGE INFLICTED
F0	40–72	Small trees uprooted, broken tree limbs
F1	73–112	Roofs damaged, mobile homes uprooted
F2	113–157	Roofs removed, mobile homes demolished
F3	158–206	Roofs and walls torn down, all trees uprooted
F4	207–260	Homes leveled, foundations moved
F5	261–318	Buildings destroyed, cars thrown >100 meters

a tornado at any moment.[8] When a tornado warning is issued, immediate action to ensure safety during a tornado should be undertaken. Despite the improved surveillance and severe weather warning systems, communities that hope to prevent unnecessary death and injury from tornado disasters must prepare long before the warning sirens are sounding.

Pre-Incident Actions

The most important preincident action is to develop a tornado disaster plan and to rehearse that plan regularly. Such rehearsals should be especially frequent in communities within Tornado Alley. The Federal Emergency Management Agency (FEMA) has published a *State and Local Guide for All-Hazard Emergency Operations Planning* (SLG 101), which can be downloaded from their Web site.[9] The SLG 101 has an appendix addressing specific issues for tornado planning.

Communication

Command/Control

Designate a clear command and control structure involving police, fire, EMS, and local hospital emergency rooms with capability for these entities to communicate on radio devices that do not depend on the local power grid for functionality.

Warning Systems

Make certain all public buildings, trailer home parks, nursing homes, and all hospitals have 24/7 access to local weather reports and a method for receiving severe weather watch and warning information from the SPC. Active warning systems (weather alert sirens, weather alert radios, and loudspeakers) are more effective than passive warning systems (conventional radio and TV).[10]

Injury Prevention

Warning/Shelter

Timely warning of an approaching tornado and appropriate sheltering have proved to be the most important factors in preventing injury and death in the face of tornadic storms.[11-13]

Focused Education

Public health education regarding tornado warning systems and safe sheltering during tornados should be provided to the populations most at risk. These include:

1. People in mobile homes
2. The elderly, very young, and physically or mentally impaired.
3. People who may not understand the warnings because of a language barrier.[1,9]

Sheltering Guidelines

FEMA, the Centers for Disease Control and Prevention (CDC), and the NWS have published guidelines detailing the safest sheltering actions to take in case of a tornado warning. These are summarized in Table 74-2.

Emergency Medical Response

Hospital Power/Water Supply

Medical facilities are not immune from tornado damage.[14] Electrical power and clean, running water are essential to medical care following a tornado. All hospitals should have plans for short-term back-up power and water supply should the main power and water lines be damaged.

Trauma System Triage/Transport

An organized trauma system with a centralized communication system has been shown to be highly effective and efficient in ensuring that the sickest patients go to the highest level care facilities following a tornado disaster.[15] Even with such a system in place, a significant minority of patients will require transfer from community hospitals to higher-level trauma centers. Agreements for such transfers should be worked out before a mass casualty incident occurs. Aeromedical transport has been shown to be of great benefit when they come to rural hospitals, or when the normal urban roadways are damaged or closed because of the disaster.[16]

Traffic Control at Hospitals

Traffic control has consistently been reported as a problem in and around emergency departments following a tornado disaster. Disaster plans should include

---

TABLE 74-2 SHELTERING GUIDELINES IN CASE OF TORNADO WARNING

In General:

1. Stay away from windows.
2. When a warning is issued, move to the safest area immediately.
3. If possible, put on a helmet.
4. Get under a sturdy piece of furniture and cover yourself with a blanket, pillows, or mattress.

IF YOU ARE:	YOU SHOULD:
Outside	Get inside a building. If stuck outside, stay away from cars and trees. Lie down in a ditch or culvert and cover your head and neck with your hands.
In a mobile home	Leave the mobile home. Go to a community shelter. If no shelter is available, see "Outside" above.
In a car	Move the car off the road. Leave the vehicle. Do not seek shelter under an overpass. If stuck outside, see above.
At work or school	Go to the designated interior room or hallway away from windows, and get under a sturdy piece of furniture.
In a house	Go to the basement. If there is no basement, go to an interior room or hallway away from windows, get under a sturdy piece of furniture, and cover yourself with a blanket.

directions for hospital security or local police to secure the access and egress routes from local hospitals. These agencies should understand where to direct the walking wounded, privately owned vehicles, and EMS vehicles for appropriate triage and evaluation.[17]

Healthcare Provider Training

The majority of patients arriving at hospitals following a tornado disaster will arrive by private vehicles. Some of these patients may have severe injuries. Healthcare personnel should be trained in proper spinal immobilization and vehicle extraction techniques in order to avoid further injury to these patients who have not benefited from prehospital medical care.[8,17]

Postincident Actions

Search/Rescue

Reports of tornado disasters—including the 1970 tornado in Lubbock, Texas and the 1996 tornado in Topeka, Kansas—support the intuitive idea that the most severely injured victims and the majority of those killed will be found in the core area of the tornado strike.[8] Severely injured victims are likely to be thrown by the tornado, struck by flying debris, or found in buildings with the greatest structural damage. An aerial survey using fire, EMS, or police helicopters can greatly assist rescue efforts by defining the regions of greatest damage and guiding search teams to locations where the most injured patients are likely to be found. Such surveys may be hindered by severe weather still lingering in the region. Search-and-rescue teams and first responders should protect themselves from hazards such as downed power-lines, gas leaks, and potentially unstable building structures. This is especially important since most tornado fatalities are not prevented by rapid EMS transport. Most patients that die in tornado disasters do so at the scene prior to EMS arrival.[8] Multiple reports of tornado disasters confirm that very few patients that arrive at the hospital alive die during hospitalization.[8,15,18,19]

EMS Triage

EMS units should be deployed carefully along the area of the tornado strike. Early responding units will likely become overwhelmed with casualties and must be supported by other units or aeromedical transport systems that can move the severely injured patients to the area hospitals and resupply the units in the field. Casualty collection points should be set up using mobile EMS vehicles or public buildings such as schools or churches. These collection points should be carefully selected to avoid radio blackout zones so that the medical command/control personnel can stay in close contact with the providers in the field to coordinate evacuation resources. If aeromedical transport is to be used, personnel must be trained in selecting and marking safe landing zones for the helicopters.

Hospital Triage

As in any mass casualty situation, it is imperative that open and precise communication channels are in place to allow triage personnel, emergency department physicians, and operating room personnel and surgeons to communicate as casualties arrive. Casualties following a tornado usually arrive in a bimodal fashion, with the least severely injured arriving first, usually within 5 to 30 minutes after the disaster. The severely wounded will arrive by EMS transport and by privately owned vehicles usually 1-4 hours after the tornado strike.[17,20] Plans should be designed to allocate appropriate resources to the least injured without overwhelming personnel and space that will be needed by critically injured patients.

Monitor Ongoing Weather Alerts

It is not uncommon for multiple tornadoes to touch down in a region over a period of several hours. The emergency response teams and emergency departments should have access to NOAA weather alert radios and should constantly monitor the storm. Heavy flooding and/or hail may alter the medical response as well.

Medical Treatment of Casualties

Types of Injuries

The majority of injuries from tornado disasters are complex, contaminated soft-tissue wounds. Fractures are the second most common injury and the most common cause for hospitalization.[8,10-12,15,19-20] Many fractures are open and require surgical wash-outs and reductions.[21] Head injuries are the most common fatal injuries following tornado disasters.[20,22] Nearly 50% of patients seen in emergency departments following tornado disasters will have soft tissue wounds as their chief complaint. Many of these wounds will be severely contaminated with mud and debris.[8,9,22] Wound infections caused by gram-negative bacteria such as *Escherichia coli, Klebsiella, Serratia, Proteus,* and *Pseudomonas* are common in wounds sustained during tornadoes.[23-25]

A clean water supply, good lighting, large numbers of suture repair kits, and ample wound care materials are essential resources for emergency departments in a tornado response. In the case of water line damage, emergency departments must have access to a short-term emergency water supply. Some have suggested that without clean water, emergency departments should not even attempt to treat patients following a tornado but instead act as triage or command/control headquarters.[8,26] An emergency supply of high-powered flashlights should be kept in all emergency departments and the batteries checked regularly. Car headlights have been used as a temporary lighting mode in tornado disasters that caused loss of power to hospital centers.

At 6 PM on May 15, you are working in a community hospital on the outskirts of Kansas City and your triage nurse comes running into the emergency department (ED) screaming "A huge tornado has been spotted just 5 miles from here. The news says it's headed right into the metropolitan area!!!" Because of the frequency of tornadoes in the region, your head nurse knows the drill and immediately activates the hospital tornado response plan. Suddenly the power goes out in the hospital. Thanks to the backup generator, the lights, monitors, and computers are back up within minutes.

One of the new techs is assigned to watch three local news stations on the TVs in the waiting room and keep the head nurse posted on any new weather advisories or other public emergency announcements. This tech is also provided with a battery-powered weather alert (NOAA) radio that is kept in the emergency department for use during weather-related disasters. The operating room (OR) is notified of the possibility of mass-casualty incoming traumas, and the in-hospital radio system is tested to ensure adequate communications between the ED and the OR. All on-call physicians are alerted of the impending mass casualty and asked to respond ASAP. A call is made to the local police asking for assistance in organizing a controlled traffic pattern into and away from the ED. The hospital public affairs director is alerted via beeper and asked to organize a press-briefing area away from the ED.

Over the next 5 hours your hospital receives some 200 tornado-related patients. Almost 70% of these patients arrive by private vehicle and must be triaged by ED and hospital staff. Thanks to recent training, all victims of blunt trauma or other high-risk injuries are carefully immobilized and c-collars are placed by the triage personnel.

Again, thanks to the well-rehearsed hospital and regional disaster plan, you are able to provide appropriate care for all of these patients. During your shift, you and your colleagues treat 70 patients with soft tissue injuries, including

30 lacerations, 2 corneal abrasions, and 38 contusions. Halfway through the shift the city water is shut off because of tornado damage to several of the main lines. Luckily the hospital has an emergency hot and cold water supply that allows for continued appropriate cleansing of your patients wounds, most of which are highly contaminated with soil and other debris.

Almost 50 of the 200 patients are not physically injured but just don't know where to go and need direction to the emergency shelters in the area being set up by the Red Cross and other relief agencies. Twenty-six patients present with head injuries ranging from mild concussions to skull fractures and ICH. Three of these patients require emergent transfer to the regional tertiary care facility for neurosurgical intervention. The local fire and EMS system provides two air ambulances, which make these transfers possible despite extensive damage and congestion on the local highways between your facility and the receiving hospital. During the shift you and your colleagues manage 18 patients with fractures and dislocations, 14 patients with blunt trauma to the chest and abdomen (one of whom has a pneumothorax requiring tube thoracotomy and 6 of whom are sent to the OR for emergent operative procedures), 18 sprains/strains, and one patient with a penetrating injury to the neck resulting in spinal cord injury. (This patient is also transferred via air ambulance to the regional tertiary care facility.) In all, you admit 35 patients with tornado-related injuries. Four of these go to the regional trauma center, four go to your ICU, six go to the OR, and 21 go to ward beds.

Driving home after your shift you contemplate the magnitude of the disaster you have just witnessed. You realize how grateful you are for all those "mandatory" disaster response drills the city has required you to reluctantly participate in over the past several years. You shudder to think what might have happened had you, the hospital, and your staff been totally unprepared for the events of the past 12 hours.

Unique Considerations

Most tornado-related deaths occur prior to arrival at the hospital. Rapid EMS transport may not affect mortality from tornadoes.

Soft tissue wounds from tornadoes should be considered highly contaminated, and delayed primary closure may be a prudent approach to wound management.

PITFALLS

Up to 50% of soft tissue wounds and contusions from tornado disasters are sustained during search-and-rescue efforts.

REFERENCES

1. National Oceanic and Atmospheric Administration. Available at: http://www.noaa.gov/.
2. National Severe Storms Laboratory. Available at: http://www.nssl.noaa.gov/.
3. Lillibridge S. Tornadoes. In: Noji E, ed. *The Public Health Consequences of Disasters*. New York: Oxford University Press; 1997, pp 228-44.
4. National Climatic Data Center. Available at: http://www.ncdc.noaa.gov/oa/ncdc.html.
5. Concannon P, Brooks H, Doswell C. Climatological Risk of Strong and Violent Tornadoes in the United States. Second Conference on Environmental Applications of the American Meteorological Society. 2000. Available at http://www.nssl.noaa.gov/users/brooks/public_html/concannon/.
6. Saunderson L. Tornadoes. In: Gregg M, ed. *The Public Health Consequences of Disaster, 1989*. Atlanta, GA: Centers for Disease Control; 1989;127:39-49.
7. Galway J. Ten famous tornado outbreaks. *Weatherwise* 1981; 34:100-9.
8. Bohonos J, Hogan D. The medical impact of tornadoes in North America. *J Emerg Med*. 1999;17:67-73.
9. Federal Emergency Management Agency. Available at: http://www.fema.gov/fema/first_res.shtm.
10. Liu S, Wuenemoen L, Malilay J, et al. Assessment of a severe-weather system and disaster preparedness, Calhoun county, Alabama, 1994. *Am J Pub Health*. 1996;86:87-9.
11. Duclos P, Ing R. Injuries and risk factors for injuries from the 29 May 1982 tornado, Marion, Illinois. *Int J Epidemiol*. 1989;18:213-9.
12. Brenner S, Noji E. Tornado injuries related to housing in the Plainfield tornado. *Int J Epidemiol*. 1995;24:144-9.
13. Glass R, Craven R, Bregman D, et al. Injuries from the Wichita Falls tornado: implications for prevention. *Science* 1980;207:734-8.

14. Anonymous. Salt Lake hospital survives close brush with twister, power outage. *Profiles in Healthcare Marketing*. 1999;15(6):48-9.

15. May A, McGwin G, Lancaster L, et al. The April 8, 1998 Tornado: Assessment of the trauma system response and the resulting injuries. *J Trauma*. 2000;48:666-72.

16. Hogan D, Askins D, Osburn A. The May 3, 1999, tornado in Oklahoma City. *Ann Emerg Med*. 1999;34:225-6.

17. Hogan D. Tornadoes. In: Hogan D, Burstein DE, eds: *Disaster Medicine*. Philadelphia: Lippincott-Williams and Wilkins; 2002, pp 171-8.

18. May B, Hogan D, Feighner K. Impact of a tornado on a community hospital. *JAOA* 2002;102:225-8.

19. Millie M, Senkowski C, Stuart L, et al. Tornado disaster in rural Georgia: Triage response, injury patterns, lessons learned. *Am Surgeon*. 2000;66:223-8.

20. Mandelbaum I, Noahrwold D, Boyer D. Management of tornado casualties. *J Trauma*. 1966;6:353-61.

21. Rosenfield L, McQueen D, Lucas G. Orthopedic injuries from the Andover, Kansas tornado. *J Trauma*. 1994;36:676-9.

22. Brenner S, Noji E. Head and neck injuries from 1990 Illinois tornado. *Am J Pub Health*. 1992;82: 1296-7.

23. Brenner S, Noji E. Wound infections after tornadoes. *J Trauma*. 1992;33:643.

24. Ivy J. Infections encountered in tornado and automobile accident victims. *J Indiana State Med Assoc*. 1968;61:1657-61.

25. Gilbert D, Sanford J, Kutscher E, et al. Microbiologic study of wound infections in tornado casualties. *Arch Environ Health*. 1973;26:125-30.

26. Johnson J. Tornado as teacher: lessons learned in caring for tornado victims lead to revision of one hospital's disaster plan. *Hospitals JAHA*. 1970;44:40-2.

chapter 75

Flood

Sylvia H. Kim

DESCRIPTION OF EVENT

Floods are the most common natural disasters. They cause greater mortality than any other natural disaster.[1] Worldwide, floods account for approximately 40% of natural disasters. In the United States, approximately 146 deaths are caused by floods each year, the majority associated with flash floods.[2] Floods cost the nation $3.8 billion each year.[3]

Floods continue to be the No. 1 natural disaster in the United States in terms of lives lost and property damage. In 1889, more than 2200 deaths were due to flash flooding from a dam break in Johnstown, Penn. In 1976, a 19 foot wall of water near the Big Thompson River near Denver, Colo., killed 140 people camping nearby.[4] More recently, in 2001, Tropical Storm Allison resulted in 41 deaths, $2 billion in property damage, and decades of research lost by scientists at the Texas Medical Center.[5]

Floods may be caused by an abundance of rainfall; melting snow; or the expanding development of wetlands, which reduces absorption of rainfall. Flash floods occur within 6 hours of a rain event, after a dam or levee fails, or after the sudden release of water from an ice or debris jam. Flash floods are the No. 1 cause of natural disaster–related death.[3]

Most communities in the United States can experience flooding. In fact, flash floods occur in all 50 states.[6] Communities at greatest risk are those in low-lying areas, near water, and located downstream from a dam.[4] In October 1998, flooding in Central Texas resulted in 31 deaths. Of the 16 incidents of vehicles being driven across flood waters, 11 (69%) occurred in areas with a prior history of flooding.[7]

PREINCIDENT ACTIONS

Hospitals should determine whether they are located in a flood-prone area. The National Weather Service issues flood watches and warnings, which are organized by state, and publishes these listings at *www.nws.noaa.gov*. These projections are based on precipitation and lake and river levels.[8] Flood watches are posted 12 to 36 hours before possible flooding events. Flood watches indicate a hazardous event is occurring or will occur within 30 minutes.[3] A flood watch should be used for early evacuation planning.

Evacuation routes should be planned and practiced. For planning purposes, flood hazard maps are available from the Federal Emergency Management Agency at *www.fema.gov/mit/tsd*. The usual routes of access to and from the hospital may be flooded, therefore alternative routes should be planned in advance. As with any natural disaster, transport times will likely increase, and hospital personnel should expect ambulance arrival without prior dispatch. There will be greater reliance on alternative means of transport, including aeromedical and marine units.[8] In one extreme case, flood waters isolated a community in Grand Forks, N.D. A temporary shelter for medical care that was capable of laboratory tests, radiology and other ancillary services was established.[9]

An emergency communications system should be available. Communication lines among hospitals, prehospital staff, and patients may be affected by floods. Telephone lines, 911 dispatch lines, and emergency medical service communication with hospitals may be impaired. Create a plan for redundant communications capabilities, including two-way radios and dedicated channels, cell phones, and Internet connectivity.[10] An emergency communications system plan should be in place to request further staffing, services, or evacuation assistance.

Floods are long-term events and may last days to weeks, or longer.[6] Therefore, disaster supplies should be available and include a portable battery-operated radio, flashlights, batteries, first aid kits, nonperishable food, and water.[4]

POSTINCIDENT ACTIONS

During a flood, battery-operated radios or televisions should be used. The National Oceanic and Atmospheric Administration (NOAA) Weather Radio broadcasts warnings from the National Weather Service 24 hours a day. Hospitals not equipped with the special radio receiver to pick up the signal can obtain timely information at *iwin.nws.noaa.gov/iwin/nationalwarnings.html* or from television and radio.

Hospital staff and patients should immediately be evacuated according to a pre-established disaster plan. If no plan is in place, seek shelter at higher ground. Avoid walking or driving through flood water. The force from 6 inches of flood water can cause one to fall. Cars can easily be swept away by just 2 feet of flood water.[4] Research from the Georgia flood in 1994 showed that 71% of flood deaths were associated with submersion in vehicles.[2]

 ## MEDICAL TREATMENT OF CASUALTIES

Approximately 0.2% to 2% of flood survivors will require urgent medical care.[1] The main cause of death during floods is drowning, with victims typically found some time after the flood recedes. Because it is often difficult to reach victims during the acute phase of a flood, it is relatively uncommon for near-drowning victims to present to emergency departments..[11] Fast-flowing flood waters carry cars, trees, and other large debris that can result in trauma, including orthopedic injuries and lacerations.[1,11] In addition, there have been reports of flood waters displacing snakes and other animals, resulting in increased animal bites.[12,13] Also, the preponderance of water during the event and still water postevent results in an increase in insect bites and vectorborne illnesses. Flood waters also may contaminate the local water supply and sewage system.[1,13]

The Centers for Disease Control and Prevention[13] analyzed data from emergency departments in 20 hospitals during Hurricane Floyd in North Carolina during September and October 1999. The medical examiner found that 52 deaths were directly related to the storm. Four causes of injury/illness accounted for 63% of all emergency room visits during this period: orthopedic and soft tissue injury (28%), respiratory illness (15%), gastrointestinal illness (11%), and cardiovascular disease (9%). The majority (24/52, or 67%) of deaths was due to drowning, primarily associated with vehicles. There were 19 cases of hypothermia and 10 cases of carbon monoxide poisoning. There was also an increase in suicide attempts, violence, dog bites, and arthropod bites compared with the same period the prior year. Finally, five deaths occurred among prehospital personnel.[13]

Not surprisingly, drowning is the primary cause of death during floods. Patients who are submerged in cold water for 40 minutes have been successfully resuscitated to attain complete neurologic recovery secondary to the neuroprotective effects of hypothermia.[1] Therefore, cardiopulmonary resuscitation should be performed as soon as possible after securing the scene. Cervical spine injuries should be suspected, and immobilization should be maintained.[14] The patient should be rewarmed using external and internal rewarming techniques, as indicated. Resuscitation efforts should be continued until the patient's temperature is 32° to 35°C (90° to 95°F); at that point, decisions regarding the utility of continuing resuscitation are made.[15]

Flood waters carry a large amount of debris, such as cars and tree limbs, and result in traumatic injuries. Orthopedic injuries should be reduced, splinted, and managed accordingly. Most injuries during floods that require urgent medical attention include lacerations,

rashes, and ulcers. These wounds are contaminated and should be conservatively managed by irrigation and healing by secondary intention. Among those lacerations that are closed primarily, the majority require reopening secondary to infection.[1]

Floods cause water contamination and an increase in vectorborne illnesses. Water contamination often results from damage to the water purification and sewage systems. Contaminated water sources result in waterborne disease transmission, including *Escherichia coli*, *Shigella*, *Salmonella*, and hepatitis A virus. The large areas of stagnant water that typically remain days or weeks after the initial flood event create a breeding medium for vector-borne illnesses..

Flood waters may also result in the spread of chemicals stored above ground. In addition, temporary shelters to house those displaced by flooding may result in crowded and unsanitary living conditions, increasing the incidence of gastrointestinal illness among other infectious illnesses.[1]

The force from flood waters may also down power lines, flood electrical circuits, and submerge electrical equipment, increasing the risk of fires and electrical hazards.[4,8]

Finally, victims of floods, as well as other natural disasters, are at an increased risk of mental illness and substance abuse. In one study, there was an increase in suicide rates of 13.8% compared with predisaster rates.[16] As of this writing we are beginning to see evidence of this in the flood regions resulting from Hurricane Katrina that struck the Gulf Coast of the United States in 2005.

 ## UNIQUE CONSIDERATIONS

Floods are the most common natural disasters and affect all 50 states. Flood waters can remain for days, weeks, or longer. As a result, flood-related injuries and illnesses may continue to present over a long period of time. Drowning is the No. 1 cause of death and is often related to vehicles attempting to cross flood waters. Deaths also occur among healthcare providers, but increased natural disaster training may decrease this occurrence. In addition to drowning, flood victims are at an increased risk for hypothermia, contaminated wounds, and waterborne infections. Water and sewage treatment facilities may be damaged by flood waters and result in water contamination.

Most communities in the United States can experience flooding. Flash floods occur in all 50 states and most countries. Areas at greatest risk are low-lying, near water, and located downstream from a dam.[4] For planning purposes, flood hazard maps should be obtained in advance and evacuation routes planned accordingly. In the event of flood warnings, evacuate early because a vehicle can be swept away with the force from as little as 2 feet of water.

 ## PITFALLS

- Failure to plan flood evacuation routes before a flood event
- Delayed evacuation by those in a flood watch area

- Failure to know who is in command of disaster operations in the local area
- Closing contaminated lacerations
- Failure to continue resuscitation of a patient who is hypothermic
- Notify the unified command/management structure and obtain directions
- Listen to a radio or television for local flood information
- Obtain your emergency kit and emergency communication (including battery-operated radio)
- Be prepared to evacuate patients and staff and know the evacuation route
- Communicate with other facilities to determine who has the capacity to accept your patients

REFERENCES

1. Noji E. Natural Disaster Management. In: Auerbach P, ed. *Wilderness Medicine: Management of Wilderness and Environmental Emergencies.* 3rd ed. St. Louis: Mosby; 1995:644-63.
2. Centers for Disease Control and Prevention. Flood-related mortality—Georgia, July 4-14, 1994. *MMWR.* 1994;43(29):526-30.
3. National Disaster Education Coalition. Flood and Flash Flood. Available at: http://www.disastercenter.com/guide/flood.html.
4. Federal Emergency Management Agency. Fact Sheet: Floods and Flash Floods. Available at: http://www.fema.gov/library/prepand-prev.shtm#floods.
5. Sirbaugh P, Bradley R, Macias C, et al. The Houston flood of 2001: the Texas Medical Center and lessons learned. *Clin Pediatr Emerg Med.* 2002;3:275-83.
6. US Department of Commerce, National Oceanic and Atmospheric Administration, National Weather Service. Floods: The Awesome Power. Available at: http://www.nws.noaa.gov/om/brochures/Floodsbrochure_9_04_low.pdf.
7. Centers for Disease Control and Prevention. Storm-related mortality—Central Texas, October 17-31, 1998. *MMWR.* 2000;49(7):133-5.
8. Floyd K. Floods. In: Hogan D, Burstein J, eds. *Disaster Medicine.* Philadelphia: Lippincott Williams & Wilkins; 2002:187-93.
9. Stensrud K. Floodwaters bring docs to the front. *Minnesota Med.* 1997;80(8):14-19.
10. Joint Commission on Accreditation of Healthcare Organizations. Health Care at the Crossroads: Strategies for Creating and Sustaining Community-wide Emergency Preparedness Systems. Available at: http://www.jcaho.org/about+us/public +policy+initiatives/ emergency_preparedness.pdf.
11. Pan American Health Organization. Emergency Health Management after Natural Disaster. Scientific Publication 407. Washington DC: Pan American Health Organization; 1981.
12. Ussher J. Philippine flood disaster. *J R Nav Med Serv.* 1973; 59(2):81.
13. Centers for Disease Control and Prevention. Morbidity and mortality associated with Hurricane Floyd—North Carolina, September-October 1999. *MMWR.* 2000;49(23):518.
14. Braun R, Kristel S. Environmental emergencies. *Emerg Med Clin North Am.* 1997;15:451.
15. Jolly B, Ghezzi K. Accidental hypothermia. *Emerg Med Clin North Am.* 1992;10:311.
16. Axelrod C, Killam PP, Gaston MH, Stinson N. Primary health care and the Midwest flood disaster. *Public Health Rep.* 1994: 109(5):601-5.

chapter 76

Tsunami

Prasanthi Ramanujam and Thea James

DESCRIPTION OF EVENT

Tsunami is a series of waves formed by displaced water due to disturbance of the sea floor that enters the coastal areas, causing serious damage. *Tsunami* (pronounced tsoo-nah-mee) is a Japanese word that literally means "harbor wave." Tsunamis are appropriately named so because they are silent and unseen in the ocean waters, but are fierce on the shallow coastal waters. They are commonly referred to as tidal waves or seismic sea waves. This is entirely misleading because neither of these terms fully characterizes tsunamis. Tidal waves are caused by the gravitational pull of the moon, sun, or planets, whereas seismic sea waves are the result of earthquakes. Tsunamis can also be caused by nonseismic activity and usually occur due to the following three major geologic movements:

1. **A fault movement on the sea floor occurring during an earthquake:** When tectonic earthquakes (those associated with the crustal deformation of earth) occur in the ocean floor, the harmony of the ocean is disturbed. This results in the displacement of the water mass, creating a wave. When a large area of the sea floor is involved, tsunami waves are created. Tsunamis can occur in any oceanic region of the world but are more common in the Pacific coast. The zone of Earth where tsunamis terrorize the Pacific Island coast is called the "Ring of Fire." This zone of extreme seismic activity circles the Pacific Ocean from south of Chile to the coast of North America and westward along the Aleutian Islands arc, extending south to Japan and the Philippines, westward to Malaysia and Indonesia, and eastward through New Guinea, the Southern Pacific Island groups, and New Zealand.[1]
2. **A landslide:** This begins above the sea, plunges into the water, or occurs under water and creates a violent disturbance in the waterfront as the landslide disseminates into the ocean floor, generating a tsunami.
3. **A sub-marine explosion:** This is the result of a volcanic eruption, creating a mechanical force that lifts the water column, which generates a tsunami. Landslides and cosmic-body impacts thrust the water from above, as the energy and force from falling debris are transferred to the water, stirring up a tsunami wave.[2]

Categories of Tsunamis

There are three categories of tsunami. Depending on the area affected, they are categorized as local, regional, or Pacific. Local tsunamis are confined to small areas and are commonly caused by coastal or sub-marine landslides and volcanic explosions. Regional tsunamis are the most common and are undersized because of deficient energy or lack of a favorable geographic location. Pacific-wide tsunamis are less common but have the potential for causing major damage.[1]

Characteristics of a Tsunami

Once tsunamis are generated, the energy propagates a horizontal wave through the ocean, similar to ripples formed by tossing a rock into a pond. A series of waves, called a *tsunami wave train,* spreads outward in all directions from the source of activity. The waves follow each other in 5- to 90-minute intervals.[2] The original tsunami then divides into two types: one goes to the nearest coast (a local tsunami) and the other one travels into the deep ocean (a distant tsunami).[1] The speed at which the waves travel varies depending on the ocean depth, which implies that the local tsunami travels at slower speeds than the deep ocean wave. Tsunamis in deep water may travel as fast as 500 mph, compared with the normal wave speed of around 60 mph. Despite traveling at such great speeds on the open ocean, at that depth, they only reach one or two feet, producing a small uprise of the sea surface, often going unnoticed by sea travelers. However, as a tsunami comes closer to the coast, the wave height increases due to a decrease in ocean depth. People who have survived tsunamis describe them as giant "walls of water." On shore, the initial sign of a tsunami depends on what part of the wave first reaches the land: a wave crest causes a rise in water level, but a wave trough causes a recession.[2] The terminology used to measure the height of water above the referenced sea level is called *run up.*[3] Tsunamis may reach a maximum run up on shore of 10, 20, and even 30 meters. Unlike many descriptions of tsunami-like monster waves, the waves come onto the shore more like uncontrollable fast tides, and much of the damage inflicted is caused by their strong currents and debris.

The small number of tsunamis that form vertical walls of turbulent water near the shore line are called *bores.*[1] Once a tsunami hits the shore, some of its energy reverts into the ocean. In some cases, a tsunami can generate a particular type of wave called an *edge wave,* which swings back and forth along a coastal shore, resulting in successive multiple waves.[3]

 ## PREINCIDENT ACTIONS

Once tsunamis are formed, they cannot be stopped; hence, strategies to lessen their effects are crucial. Salient features of a preparedness program include improving awareness and mitigation of the hazards. The foremost step is to increase knowledge among decision-making authorities, emergency personnel, and the public. Mitigation involves steps to decrease the impact of the event at the time of occurrence. The features recommended by the 1995 National Oceanic and Atmospheric Administration's (NOAA) Tsunami Hazard Mitigation plan[4] are as follows:

1. **Identifying an approaching tsunami and attempting to reduce false alarms:** The Pacific Tsunami Warning Center (PTWC) is an operational center for the Tsunami Warning System in the Pacific coast (TWSP). It has been the international warning center since 1965, when a formal arrangement was made. PTWC is able to locate seismic activities that are potentially tsunami-generating in the Pacific coast or surrounding areas by continuously obtaining seismographic data from more than 150 stations around the Pacific and other international agencies running such stations and networks.[5][6] This method is not foolproof; false alarm rates are extremely high. To improve the accuracy of reporting, Japan and NOAA have planted multiple bottom-pressure sensors that detect a tsunami traveling overhead. This information is communicated to the shore via satellite links using a buoy in the ocean. If the extent of destruction is determined to be wide, entire Pacific coastal areas are given a warning. Regional warning centers exist, which are responsible for the issuing warnings to specific countries and their coastal areas. For example, the Japan Meteorological Agency provides tsunami warnings to Japan and also to Korea and Russia for events occurring in the Sea of Japan or East Sea. The Center Polynesien de Prevention des Tsunamis provides warnings to French Polynesia and Chile. In the United States, West Coast/Alaska Tsunami Warning Center (WC/ATWC) provides tsunami warnings to the U.S. West Coast and Canada, and PTWC provides tsunami warnings to Hawaii and all other U.S. interests in the Pacific.[6]
2. **Utilization of resources for communication and evacuation:** Local preparedness planning consists of determining safe evacuation pathways, setting up shelters, critical facilities, and strengthening structures that cannot be relocated and are in the path of inundation of a tsunami. As preparations are being undertaken, alerting systems are used to spread the information

and to communicate effectively about the evacuation measures. Local tsunamis pose major challenges. They are associated with earthquakes that cause damage to the infrastructure, leading to difficult evacuation plans. This is further complicated by a tsunami arriving minutes after events like earthquakes leaving less time for emergency response. Planning committees have made recommendations for this setting. They include disseminating an inundation map obtained using computer-generated simulations to plan mapping of the critical zones and to predict the areas prone to devastation. Other strategies are improvising warning systems and notifying the public immediately after earthquakes of the likelihood that a tsunami will result.[4]

3. **Support for state and local agencies' long-term tsunami mitigation program:** Multistate projects have been proposed, along with individual state programs, to raise the public's level of awareness and preparation for an event. Apart from federal and state actions, various organizations exist to help coordinate federal, state, and local emergency management agencies; the public; and the NWS (National Weather Service) tsunami warning system. This helps maintain the safety of the public by increasing awareness. The various guidelines at the community level include:

- Establish minimum community standards, which depend on the size of the community. Create a 24-hour operations system, with the ability to receive, disseminate, and activate warning systems in the community. There also should be communicative abilities between other emergency centers and tsunami warning centers.[7]
- Disseminate information to the public using means such as NWS (NOAA weather radio), television, and a statewide telecommunications network located at public buildings.[7]
- Improve awareness and preplanning among the community by conducting awareness programs in schools, hospitals, and community meetings. Define the areas in the community for shelter, provide hazard zones and evacuation maps, and conduct practice evacuation drills in schools.[7]

 ## POSTINCIDENT ACTIONS

Preventing a disaster from happening is paramount, but when it is impossible to avert the natural disaster, timely applications of management strategies gain importance. The postincident action phase is composed of emergency response activities that transition into rehabilitation phase activities that culminate in the reconstruction phase. Emergency response efforts actually evolve from the final stages of the preincident phase and have many overlapping features. Examples include (a) evacuation of people to safe places, which in the case of a tsunami can be inland or to a higher altitude, and (b) provisions for emergency shelter and temporary lodging to people who are displaced after the event. The next stage begins with the dispatch of search and rescue teams to look for injured people who need medical assistance. Because damage to water pipes in the affected areas is likely, provision of short-term food and water is essential for the displaced population. Water disinfection and purification become important after the disaster to prevent epidemics from water contamination. Public announcements regarding safety standards for water storage and disinfection, even after flooding, should be made as a preventive health measure. Epidemiologic surveillance in areas affected by flooding is important because overcrowding among the displaced population and overflow of industrial, agricultural, and sewage systems can pose serious health hazards. Subsequent management steps consist of reestablishing communication with remote areas, restoring infrastructure by re-opening roads, clearing debris, and repairing damaged housing and public buildings. The final phase consists of providing employment by creating opportunities, offering technical assistance to industries and for agricultural recovery, and encouraging activities that help rebuild the area.[8,9]

 ## MEDICAL TREATMENT OF CASUALTIES

Mass casualties can exceed system capabilities during disasters. This becomes a burden on the local system until outside help arrives. Steps to hasten the delivery of treatment to the injured include triage, on-site stabilization, and transportation to the local hospital. The goal of triage is to prioritize injured patients by identifying those whose injuries are critical and in need of prompt medical attention and arranging for either on-site treatment or quick transfer. Patients who have minimal likelihood of survival from major injuries despite optimal care are provided only comfort measures. There are two different systems of triage for mass casualties, and they are qualitative and quantitative. The former system is based on the patient's injury relative to others who are injured and to available care and requires timely reassessment. The latter is based on a clinical score for the patient at time of initial presentation to predict outcome. Triage begins with arrival of the emergency medical personnel on-scene. This is followed by relative assessment of the demand on available supplies. If the numbers overwhelm available help, the need for additional services is rapidly communicated to the emergency dispatch center. Triage set up begins with designating the most qualified medical person to be the provisional triage officer. With the arrival of more help from outside, this role should be taken by the most knowledgeable person with triage experience. Various adjuncts to triage help with the identification of which triage category the patient is placed in and with enforcing the use of a classification system, such as immediate, delayed, minor, and expectant, depending on the injury severity and prognosis. Priority one triage, based on the initial clinical picture, includes patients with impending airway issues, such as asphyxia, respiratory obstruction, sucking chest wounds, tension pneumothorax, maxillofacial wounds with impending air-

way compromise, shock, and major medical problems. Delayed triage, or priority two, includes patients with visceral, vascular, facial, spinal cord, and genitourinary injuries; thoracic injuries without asphyxia; and victims with less chance of survival. Once patients are triaged, a decision must be made as to whether to transport them to a nearby hospital or provide on-site care by setting up the necessary facilities. This decision is based on the number of available qualified transport personnel. If the system is overwhelmed by the number of patients awaiting rapid transportation, advanced-field medical treatment may be necessary. If rescue personnel or patients are in an unsafe environment, rapid transport becomes a necessity. Emergency communications should be used to alert local hospitals about the mass casualty situation and the need for resources to handle multiple-trauma patients. Hospitals, in turn should, report to the disaster operations center the current status on bed availability, the number of casualties they have received, and the availability of supplies to manage the crisis.[9]

 ## UNIQUE CONSIDERATIONS

- Tsunami is rightfully called the harbor wave because its effects are devastating on coastal areas.
- Tsunamis are not one single wave but consist of a wave train and travel at great speeds in the ocean.
- Unlike other tides, tsunamis are caused mostly by seismic activity, which adds to the damage caused by a tsunami.
- Tsunamis are unique in that their propagation involves the entire depth from the ocean surface to the bottom, accounting for their tremendous energy.[1]
- The issuance of a tsunami warning means that evidence exists for a potentially destructive tsunami and evacuation is strongly advised. On the other hand, a watch status means that a tsunami may have been generated, the wave travel time is more than 3 hours, and evacuation is needed if the watch is upgraded to a warning.[1]
- For tsunamis of distant origin, the danger areas are 50 feet above sea level and within 1 mile of the coast.
- For tsunamis of local origin, potential danger areas are those less than 100 feet above sea level and within 1 mile of the coast.[8]

 ## PITFALLS

- Tidal wave is a misnomer for tsunami because the latter can be extremely dangerous with devastating effects.
- Tsunami run up (height of the water above sea level) varies with the geography of the land, leading to different degrees of damage along the coastline.
- Local tsunamis can follow a seismic activity very quickly, leaving less time for incident preparation.
- False alarms during the preincident phase can pose a major drain on available resources.
- Early return of people to their settlements without anticipating the wave train or to witness the tsunami can result in significant morbidity and mortality.

Papua New Guinea is a group of islands including the eastern half of the island of New Guinea between the Coral Sea and the South Pacific Ocean, east of Indonesia. On July 17, 1998, at 6:49 PM local time, these islands experienced an earthquake with a magnitude of 7.1 near the northwest coast. This was soon followed by three dreadful tsunamis that killed about 2182 people and left more than 10,000 people in the villages of Sissano, Warupu, and Arop homeless. The tsunamis affected a 40-km coastline of a narrow strip of land, largely a swamp area between the ocean and a lagoon that was home to 15,000 tribal people who subsisted on farming and fishing. About 20 minutes after the first earthquake, the trough of the first tsunami arrived with a 7- to 10-meter crest that destroyed the village and swept the debris into the lagoon 500 meters inland from the coast. The destruction was enormous and included three schools, a heath center, mission buildings, churches, bridges, and the government administration center. Common injuries included multiple bony and soft tissue injuries, development of gangrene, near-drownings, and loss of lives from impalement onto tree stumps.[10]

The tsunami of southeast Asia on Dec. 26, 2004, deserves mention for the death and devastation it caused in the region. An undersea earthquake with a magnitude of 9.0 on the Richter scale in the Indian Ocean originated off the western coast of Northern Sumatra. This fourth-largest earthquake since 1900 resulted in the generation of a tsunami, which affected the coastal regions of Indonesia, Thailand, Sri Lanka, and South India. Waves were as tall as 50 feet and traveled more than 1 mile inward in some areas. Damage also was recorded in South Africa, about 5000 miles from the epicenter. The estimated number of deaths in the affected region was about 300,000 and the displaced population about 1.5 million. The waves also inflicted major environmental damage on the regions. There was infiltration of fresh water supplies, spread of solid and liquid wastes, damage to ecosystems, and much more. The economic damages are unquantifiable and included loss of industrial infrastructure on the coastline, destruction of fishing fleet, and a breakdown of the tourism industry. The devastation has created a lot of awareness in the region about tsunamis and has created a need for establishing warning systems in the Indian Ocean.[11]

Multiple case reports from different parts of the world have resulted in improvements to existing disaster mitigation plans. Lessons learned from historic events include the following:

- Establish a global communication network that recognizes and warns the population in high-risk areas about possible tsunamis
- Quickly sense an approaching tsunami after ground-shaking and loud oceanic noises.[10]
- Identify areas of land between a lagoon and the ocean as high-risk areas for inundation, thereby avoiding rebuilding after a tsunami[10]
- Train the local population to handle the immediate disaster needs in case of a tsunami strike until further support systems can be deployed
- Recognize that mangroves are a source of floating debris that can cause more physical damage and that lagoon areas are less of an impediment for tsunamis, exposing more inland to destruction[10]

REFERENCES

1. British Columbia Ministry of Public Safety & Solicitor General. British Columbia Tsunami Warning and Alerting Plan 2000. Available at: http://www.pep.bc.ca/hazard_plans/tsunami 2001/Tsunami_Warning_and_Alerting_Plan-2001.pdf.
2. Reed SB. Natural and human-made hazards: mitigation and management issues. In: Auerbach, PS ed. *Wilderness Medicine*. 4th ed. St. Louis: Mosby; 2001.
3. U.S. Geological Survey. Tsunamis and Earthquakes: Tsunami Research at the USGS. Available at: http://walrus.wr.usgs.gov/tsunami/.
4. National Oceanic and Atmospheric Administration. National Tsunami Hazard Mitigation Program. Available at: http://www.pmel.noaa.gov/tsunami-hazard
5. The University of Washington Earth and Space Sciences. The Tsunami Warning System. Available at: http://www.ess.washington.edu/ tsunami/general/warning/warning.html
6. National Weather Service. Tsunami Warning Centers. Available at: http://www.prh.noaa.gov/itic/library/pubs/great_waves
7. State of Alaska Division of Homeland Security and Emergency Management. Tsunami Mitigation. Available at: http://www.ak-prepared.com/plans/mitigation/tsunami.htm.
8. University of Wisconsin Disaster Management Center. Natural Hazards: Causes and Effects. Lesson 3: Tsunamis. Available at: http://dmc.engr.wisc.edu/courses/hazards/BB02-03.html
9. Noji EK. Natural disaster management. In: Auerbach PS, ed. *Wilderness Medicine*. 4th ed. St. Louis: Mosby; 2001.
10. James F, Lander LS, Whiteside PA, Lockridge PA. Two decades of global tsunamis 1982-2002. *Science of Tsunami Hazards*. 2003; 21(1):3.
11. Wikipedia. 2004/Indian Ocean Earthquake. Available at: http://en.wikipedia.org/wiki/ 2004/Indian_Ocean_Earthquake.

chapter 77

Heat Wave

Alison Sisitsky

 ## DESCRIPTION OF EVENT

A heat wave is a prolonged period of heat and humidity. The duration of heat plays an important role in how people are affected. Illness tends to occur within 2 days of excessive heat. However, there are certain populations who are at increased risk, and may exhibit symptoms earlier. The elderly, very young, those with preexisting diseases, those taking various drugs/medications, and urban dwellers are more susceptible to heat-related illness.

Each year, hundreds of people die from heat-related illnesses. The Centers for Disease Control and Prevention estimated that from 1979 to 1997 there were 7000 U.S. deaths attributable to extreme heat. There were 600 deaths during the Chicago heat wave of July 1995. The next summer, during the 1996 Summer Olympics in Atlanta, Ga., 1059 people were treated for heat-related illness. Of those who died, 89% were either spectators or volunteers.[1]

There are four mechanisms by which the human body is able to dissipate heat. Radiation is the passive transfer of heat by electromagnetic waves. This accounts for 65% of heat transfer. Evaporation is the transition of liquid into gas. This only occurs when the outside temperature reaches 95°F, and it accounts for 30% of heat transfer. Convection is heat loss to air and water vapor molecules that surround the body. It only accounts for 10% of heat transfer. Finally, conduction is heat transfer via direct physical contact. It is only responsible for 2% of heat transfer.[2]

Heat waves are among the most common emergencies and are the leading environmental cause of death in the United States, followed by cold-related deaths during winter months (Fig. 77-1).

 ## PREINCIDENT ACTIONS

The most important action in preventing illness during a heat wave is public education before the heat wave begins. The National Weather Service issues alerts when a potential heat wave is near. The heat index (HI) is the temperature the body feels when heat and humidity are combined. For example, if the air temperature is 90°F and the relative humidity is 60%, the HI is 99°F.[1]

Educating the public allows people to protect themselves from excessive heat exposure. If the following recommendations are adhered to, the risk of heat-related illnesses could be reduced. Reduce strenuous activity or reschedule outdoor activities until the coolest time of day. Dress with lightweight clothing and light colors. Avoid restrictive hats that will block sweating and evaporation of heat. Drink large amounts of water or other nonalcoholic beverages. Avoid alcohol intake. Spend as much time as possible in air-conditioning and avoid direct sun exposure.[3]

 ## POSTINCIDENT ACTIONS

In the prehospital setting, remove the patient from the heat. Disrobe the patient and apply ice packs to the neck, axilla, and groin. In addition, placing a wet sheet over the body will encourage heat loss from the body to the environment. Intravenous fluid should be started. If the patient has an altered mental status, consider administering glucose, thiamine, and naloxone.

Always assess vital functions, and obtain an accurate core temperature with a rectal probe. Laboratory evaluation should include a complete blood count to assess for leukocytosis as well as electrolyte levels and a urinalysis. Hypernatremia can exist with severe dehydration. Acute renal failure and myoglobinuria may be present with rhabdomyolysis. If heat stroke is suspected, liver function tests and coagulation studies are needed to assess for hepatic necrosis or disseminated intravascular coagulation.

Further diagnostic tests should include an electrocardiogram in an elderly patient or anyone with cardiac risk factors, head computed tomography for patients with an altered mental status, and a chest x-ray for evidence of respiratory distress.[4,5]

 ## MEDICAL TREATMENT OF CASUALTIES

Immediate cooling should include spraying the disrobed patient with cool mist; fanning mist with bedside fans; and applying ice packs to the neck, axilla, and groin.

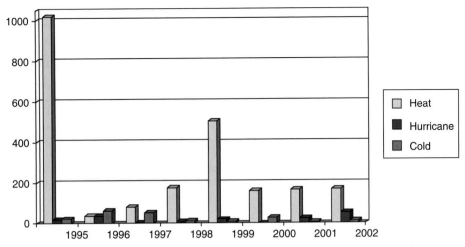

FIGURE 77–1. Heat fatalities. Between 1995 and 2002 in the United States heat-related deaths outnumbered both hurricane- and cold-related deaths. (Graph adapted from data collected at http://www.disastercenter.com.)

Immersion in cold water is effective if the patient's condition is stable, but it is difficult to manage patients who have any evidence of cardiovascular compromise.

For patients whose hyperthermia (temperature >104°F) persists, iced peritoneal lavage and cardiopulmonary bypass should be considered.

While active cooling is taking place, hydration should be started with 0.5 to 1 L of normal saline. Pediatric patients should receive a 20-mL/kg bolus.

Medications to consider include analgesics for muscle cramps; benzodiazepines for seizures or severe shivering; and glucose, thiamine, and naloxone for altered mental status.

Patients with evidence of heat stroke (hyperthermia, anhidrosis, and altered mental status) should be admitted to an intensive care unit. Patients with heat exhaustion (hyperthermia [temperature >104°F], central nervous system dysfunction, dehydration, nausea/vomiting, and diaphoresis) or the elderly should be admitted for electrolyte abnormalities and evidence of rhabdomyolysis.[4,5]

 UNIQUE CONSIDERATIONS

Patients at extremes of age are at increased risk of heat-related illnesses. Children have an increased body surface area to mass ratio, which increases their risk. Hydration of pediatric patients consists of a 20-mL/kg bolus of intravenous fluid. If hypoglycemia is present, give 2 mL/kg of D25W over 1 minute intravenously.

Elderly patients are at increased risk secondary to underlying medical conditions and medications that worsen heat illness. Taking a thorough history and a physical examination will help guide therapy.

Risk factors for serious heat injury are outlined in Table 77-1.[2,4,5]

 PITFALLS

Consider other causes of hyperthermia in patients with altered mental status. The differential diagnosis includes

TABLE 77-1 RISK FACTORS FOR SERIOUS HEAT INJURY

Dehydration
Obesity
Heavy clothing
Poor physical fitness
Cardiovascular disease
Skin diseases (burns, eczema, scleroderma, psoriasis)
Febrile illnesses
Hyperthyroidism
Alcoholism
Drug use (cocaine, amphetamines, opiates, LSD, PCP)
Poor socioeconomic conditions
Medications (antipsychotics, anticholinergics, calcium-channel blockers, beta blockers, diuretics, alpha agonists, sympathomimetics)

CASE PRESENTATION

Today is the local marathon. There are 2000 runners participating in the event. The local temperature is predicted to reach 99°F. The race started 2 hours ago and medical control is calling with questions. Not only do they have runners with symptoms of heat-related illness, many of the spectators are symptomatic. Currently, they would like to bring three patients. Patient 1 is a 40-year-old male with vomiting and severe abdominal pain who was unable to finish the race. Patient 2 is a 4-year-old female spectator who had a syncopal episode while waiting for her mom to finish the race. Patient 3 is an 85-year-old female who was providing water for the participants, but became diaphoretic and short of breath and is now unresponsive. While you are online with medical control, the triage nurse is handing you a note with five expected patients that were called in. How can you prepare to treat these people, and what care do they need?

alcohol withdrawal, neuroleptic malignant syndrome, malignant hyperthermia, toxicities (anticholinergics, salicylates, PCP, cocaine, amphetamine), infectious sources (tetanus, sepsis, encephalitis, meningitis, brain abscess, typhoid fever, malaria), endocrine abnormalities (thyroid storm, diabetic ketoacidosis), status epilepticus, and cerebral hemorrhage.

For patients with hyperthermia, do not forget to consider an acute cardiac event or a severe electrolyte abnormality.

Consider other causes of altered mental status, including hypoglycemia, thiamine deficiency, or opiate overdose.[6]

REFERENCES

1. Wetterhall SF, et al. Medical care delivery at the 1996 Summer Games. *JAMA* 1998:279, 1463-1468.
2. Moran DS, Gaffin SL. Clinical management of heat-related illnesses. In: Aurebach PS, ed. *Wilderness Medicine*. 4th ed. St. Louis: Mosby; 2001:290-317.
3. The Disaster Center. Available at: http://www.disastercenter.com
4. Walker JS, Barnes SB. Heat emergencies. In: Tintinalli JE, ed. *Emergency Medicine: A Comprehensive Study Guide*. 5th ed. New York: McGraw-Hill; 2000:1237-42.
5. Doucette M. Hyperthermia. In: Schaider J, et al, eds. *Rosen and Barkin's 5-Minute Emergency Medicine Consult*. 2nd ed. Philadelphia: Lippincott Williams & Wilkins; 2003:562-3.
6. Schmidt E, Nichols C. Heat- and sun-related illnesses. In: Harwood-Nuss A, Wolfson AB, Linden CH, Shepherd SM, Stenklyft PH, eds. *The Clinical Practice of Emergency Medicine*. 3rd ed. Philadelphia: Lippincott Williams & Wilkins; 2001:1667-70.

chapter 78

Winter Storm

Alison Sisitsky

 DESCRIPTION OF EVENT

Heavy snow, high winds, and freezing rain can combine to create winter storms. The National Weather Service provides public information related to the severity of the storm expected. The various types of winter storm are blizzard, heavy snow, sleet, and ice storm. A blizzard is a combination of low temperatures, snow, and wind speeds up to 35 miles per hour resulting in less than a quarter mile of visibility. Heavy snow is 6 or more inches of falling snow in less than 12 hours. Sleet is frozen raindrops that bounce when hitting the ground. Finally, ice storms occur when rain hits the ground and freezes. The ice can accumulate on roads and power lines, causing damage and creating dangerous electrical hazards.[1]

The incidence of winter storms is approximately 105 per year in the continental United States. Causes of death related to winter storms include traffic accidents, overexertion, and exposure.[2] Of these deaths, 70% occur in automobiles, and 25% occur out in the storm.[1]

 PREINCIDENT ACTIONS

Before a winter storm hits, the most important action is to prepare the public. This includes educating the public about when to expect a storm, how to find out if one is coming, and how to handle the possible dangers associated with it.

The National Weather Service will issue alerts on the radio and television within 24 hours of a possible storm. The alerts are graded from watch to advisory to warning. When dangerous weather is predicted, a watch is issued. During the storm, an advisory is issued that alerts the public to dangerous winter weather. When a warning is issued, the weather is very dangerous and could be life-threatening.[1]

The public should have a winter storm plan as well as various supplies. Every home should have extra blankets and warm clothing, including coats, gloves, hats, and water-resistant boots. A disaster kit should be assembled. The American Red Cross recommends a first aid kit, a battery-powered weather radio, extra batteries, canned food, can opener, bottled water (1 gallon per person per day for 3 days), and extra warm clothing. In addition, cars should be winterized in the late fall, including placing a disaster kit inside the car.[1]

When a winter storm warning is issued, the public should follow these general rules: stay indoors but if one must go outside, wear several light layers of clothing, a hat, and gloves; protect the skin from wind chill; walk carefully on snow and ice; and avoid overexertion when removing snow.

If one gets stuck in a car, it is advised to stay inside the car after placing a bright cloth on the antenna. To stay warm, start the car and use the heater for 10 minutes every hour. Continue to move the arms and legs while sitting in the car to keep the body warm.[1]

Prehospital treatment consists of keeping the patient warm with minimal movement if the patient is hypothermic. Assess vital functions, remove cold or wet clothing, and apply dry blankets. Refer to hypothermia treatment described later in the chapter. It is not recommended to begin cardiopulmonary resuscitation if a pulse is palpable and transport time is brief.

 POSTINCIDENT ACTIONS

Remove the patient from the cold environment as soon as possible. Remove all wet and cold clothes to prevent further heat loss.[3]

The medical conditions to consider in a patient caught in a winter storm are hypothermia (mild, moderate, and severe), frostbite, carbon monoxide poisoning, and overexertion injuries.[3]

It is important to keep roads clear of snow and ice as soon as possible. Driveways and sidewalks around the hospital also must be clear to keep patients safe upon arrival.

 MEDICAL TREATMENT OF CASUALTIES

Assess vital functions, and determine core temperature. Blood should be evaluated for possible complications, including lactic acidosis, rhabdomyolysis, and bleeding diatheses. A toxicology screen is recommended as well. An electrocardiogram should be obtained to evaluate for prolongation of the intervals, elevation of the J point (Osborne wave) (Fig. 78-1), and dysrhythmias.[3]

Mild hypothermia is when the core temperature is between 32° and 35°C. Patients with mild hypothermia may experience tachypnea, tachycardia, shivering, or mild altered mental status. Passive external rewarming should be initiated after removing wet clothing. Blankets or any other insulation should be adequate to assist endogenous thermogenesis. Moderate hypothermia is when the core temperature is between 28° and 32°C. These patients may have decreased heart rate and cardiac output and generalized central nervous system depression. They are at risk for renal failure, atrial fibrillation, and bradycardia. Paradoxical undressing may be witnessed. Immediate passive and active external rewarming should be initiated. Warm blankets, heating pads, and warm air should be applied to the patient to decrease further heat loss. The heat should be applied to the patient's torso to prevent core temperature afterdrop. The goal is to prevent extensive peripheral vasodilation that occurs naturally after the patient is removed from the cold and is rewarmed. Cold blood is shunted to the core, causing decrease in body temperature as well as hypotension, poor cardiac perfusion, and risk of ventricular fibrillation.[4-6]

Severe hypothermia is when the core body temperature is below 28°C. Patients with severe hypothermia are at risk for hypotension, bradycardia, ventricular fibrillation, pulmonary edema, and coma. Move these patients carefully to avoid inducing ventricular fibrillation. Active internal rewarming is necessary in these patients and can be done with the external techniques previously described. Humidified oxygen and warm intravenous fluids are minimally invasive ways to warm the severely hypothermic patient. The peritoneal cavity, pleural spaces, and bladder can be irrigated with 45°C fluid.

Pleural irrigation should be reserved for those without a cardiac rhythm to avoid inducing ventricular fibrillation with chest tube placement. Blood warming by hemodialysis and cardiopulmonary bypass are acceptable means to raise the core body temperature. Protocols for aggressive and invasive rewarming procedures should be developed in cooperation with other departments involved in these processes prior to an incident requiring such measures.[4-6]

Arrhythmias related to hypothermia were formerly treated with bretylium, but this medication is no longer available. Arrhythmias should be treated according to advanced cardiac life support (ACLS) guidelines and may be refractory until the patient is normothermic.[5]

Cold-induced tissue injuries are common during winter storms. Risk factors include altered mental status, advanced age, malnutrition, and peripheral vascular disease. Tissue injuries range from mild (frostnip) to severe (frostbite). Frostbite is local injury from contact with temperatures below 2°C. The first phase of frostbite is the initial freeze injury when cell damage occurs. The second phase is the reperfusion injury that occurs while rewarming. The full extent of the injury may not be obvious on initial presentation. Do not rub or manipulate the frozen part. Treatment should consist of rapid rewarming in a water bath kept between 40° and 42°C. The affected extremity should be immersed for 15 to 30 minutes. Blisters should be left intact, and a sterile dressing with antibiotic ointment should cover any that have burst. Other remedies include aloe vera and ibuprofen. Tetanus status needs to be updated. Patients should be advised to avoid smoking as well.[3,7,8]

Carbon monoxide poisoning should be considered in patients with headache, dizziness, nausea, vomiting, confusion, seizures, or coma. Apply 100% oxygen, and consider hyperbaric oxygen therapy if the patient's condition is stable and a chamber is easily accessible.

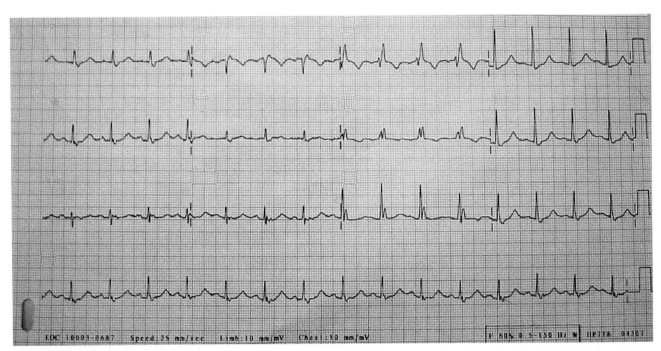

FIGURE 78–1. Electrocardiogram of a hypothermic patient with characteristic J waves after the QRS complexes.

Arterial blood gas and carboxyhemoglobin levels will help guide therapy.[9]

Epidemics of carbon monoxide toxicity may be encountered when heat and electricity are cut off for prolonged periods due to storms. The indoor use of heat generation utilizing fossil fuels contributes to cases (as was seen in the 1999 ice storms in upstate New York).

 ## UNIQUE CONSIDERATIONS

Extremes of age are risk factors for cold-induced illnesses. As one ages, the shivering mechanism may not be adequate, and therefore there is an increased risk of hypothermia. Infants have a large body surface to mass ratio and can lose heat quickly. The elderly and children may be unable to carry out actions to warm themselves.

Medications such as barbiturates, benzodiazepines, chlorpromazine, and tricyclic antidepressants can increase the risk of hypothermia.

 ## PITFALLS

- Always assess the entire patient.
- Think of other causes of altered mental status and consider giving naloxone, thiamine, and glucose.

CASE PRESENTATION

Yesterday, the National Weather Service issued a winter storm warning. A blizzard is expected to hit this morning. Snow began falling late last night, and local schools are closed. Emergency medical services have just arrived with a homeless man found unresponsive under a bridge. He is naked, feels frozen, and has a thready pulse. They have intubated him in the field and started intravenous fluid, but they cannot get a blood pressure reading. What else can be done to save this patient?

- Do not forget to evaluate for hypothermia in the patient who presents with frostbite.
- For patients with frostbite, do not rub the affected part. Monitor the rewarming bath temperature to avoid extremity refreezing. Obtain surgical consult for severe frostbite that involves structures below the subcutaneous tissues. Warn patients about the dangers of reexposing the area to cold temperatures.
- For patients with hypothermia, always obtain an accurate rectal temperature. Remember that arrhythmias are best treated with rewarming. Do not handle the patient roughly because it may induce arrhythmias. Continue to resuscitate patients until the core temperature is at least 32°C. Continue fluid resuscitation, and watch for core temperature afterdrop.[3,5]

REFERENCES

1. Thousands Without Power After Southeast Ice Storm, 2000, CNN.com. Available at: http://edition.cnn.com/2000/WEATHER/01/24/ice.storm.02/
2. Spitalnic SJ, Jagminas L, Cox J. An association between snowfall and ED presentation of cardiac arrest. *Am J Emerg Med.* 1996; 14(6):572-3.
3. Schaider J. Hypothermia. In: Schaider J, et al, eds. *Rosen and Barkin's 5-Minute Emergency Medicine Consult.* 2nd ed. Philadelphia: Lippincott Williams & Wilkins; 2003:584-5.
4. UpToDate. Available at: http://www.uptodate.com.
5. Currier J. Hypothermia. In: Harwood-Nuss A, Wolfson AB, Linden CH, Shepherd SM, Stenklyft PH, eds. *The Clinical Practice of Emergency Medicine.* 3rd ed. Philadelphia: Lippincott Williams & Wilkins; 2001:1664-7.
6. Danzl D. Accidental hypothermia. In: Aurebach PS, ed. *Wilderness Medicine.* 4th ed. St. Louis: Mosby; 2001:135-77.
7. Gonzalez F, Leong K. Cold-induced tissue injuries. In: Harwood-Nuss A, Wolfson AB, Linden CH, Shepherd SM, Stenklyft PH, eds. *The Clinical Practice of Emergency Medicine.* 3rd ed. Philadelphia: Lippincott Williams & Wilkins; 2001:1661-4.
8. Arnold P. Frostbite. In: Schaider J, et al, eds. *Rosen and Barkin's 5-Minute Emergency Medicine Consult.* 2nd ed. Philadelphia: Lippincott Williams & Wilkins, 2003:436-7.
9. Chang A, Hamilton R. Direct relationship between unintentional workplace carbon monoxide deaths and average U.S. monthly temperature. Academic Emergency Medicine *AEMJ* 2002;9:531.

chapter 79

Volcanic Eruption

Gregory Jay

DESCRIPTION OF EVENT

Volcanic eruptions have the potential to produce significant loss of life and far-reaching medical and socioeconomic disruption. More than 270,000 volcano-related fatalities have been recorded since 1700, with the number of fatal eruptions averaging two to four events per year.[1-3] Eighty percent of the world's active volcanoes are located around the Pacific Basin where continental and seafloor plate subduction occurs.[1,4] In 1990 approximately 10% of the world's population lived within 100 km of an active volcano.[1] With the continued growth in world population and urbanization, the risk of trauma and death from volcanic eruptions will only increase.

The violence or force of a volcanic eruption determines the characteristic of injuries produced. A volcanic eruption is the ejection of gases and solid material from a vent or hole in the Earth's surface. Outgassing, or release of volatiles dissolved in magma, provides the motive force for an eruption. While magma rises to the Earth's surface, the decreasing pressure on molten rock allows volatiles and gases in the melt to be released.[5] The higher the silica content of the melt, the more viscous and polymerized it remains, stabilizing volatiles and gases.[1] When pressure is suddenly released on magma with a high dissolved volatile concentration, rapid and explosive outgassing may occur. This produces the typical violent or explosive eruption during which lava bombs and plumes of ash are ejected. When magma has a low silica content, outgassing occurs more gradually, and a more gentle, or effusive, eruption ensues.[6] The volcanoes located along plate subduction zones tend to produce more violent eruptions because of the high silica and dissolved volatile concentration in their magma.[1]

A variety of physical and chemical hazards are associated with volcanic eruptions. Lava is responsible for very few fatalities. The flow is often slow and can be easily avoided. Pyroclastic flows are responsible for the most deaths.[2] A pyroclastic flow is a mass of hot volcanic ash, lava fragments, and gases that erupts from a volcano and moves rapidly down its slope at speeds of up to a few hundred miles per hour.[6-8] Rocks and debris within the flow may be hurled at great speed, causing severe secondary blast injury. Pyroclastic flows are extremely destructive and fatal to nearly all life in the area through which they travel. The temperatures in a pyroclastic flow may be as high as 600° to 900°C, causing severe, if not fatal, burns.[6]

Pyroclastic flows may extend a great distance from the site of an eruption. Flows commonly travel up to 15 km from a vent; during the Mount St. Helens eruption in 1980, flows reached 17 miles.[7] Pyroclastic flows often occur multiple times during an eruption and have also been reported in the absence of violent eruption.[9,10]

Another common cause of volcanic eruption–related fatalities is tephra. Tephra includes all of the solid fragments of magma and volcanic rock ejected from a volcano during an eruption.[6,8] Ejecta can cause severe head injury, burns, and blunt trauma.[11] Tephra fragments less than 2 mm are termed *ash,* 2- to 64-mm fragments are called *lapilli,* and fragments larger than 64 mm are often called *lava bombs* or *blocks.* Lava blocks and bombs generally follow a more ballistic trajectory after ejection, landing a few meters to several kilometers away from the site of eruption. The path and final point of impact is dependent on the initial "muzzle velocity" of the fragment.[6] Ballistic fragments are a serious hazard near a vent, but become a more minor hazard as distance increases from the site of eruption. Air resistance also prevents ballistic fragments less than a few centimeters in diameter from being hurled more than a few hundred meters from a vent.[6]

Ash clouds pose a potential health hazard. Small particles of tephra rise on convection currents within a hot eruption cloud and may drift for hundreds of kilometers downwind from the active volcano.[6] Tephra deposits tend to become finer grained farther downwind because the coarser particles of ash and lapilli fall nearer the volcano.[6] In very large eruptions, tephra accumulations may reach several meters in depth, and the associated lapilli and ashfall may be heavy enough to induce darkness at midday.[6] Although the mean diameter of tephra grains decreases with distance from a vent, the percentage of respirable ash, particles less than 10 μm in diameter, does not necessarily increase.[6]

Currently very little research is available regarding the respiratory effects of volcanic ash. There was concern about the development of acute silicosis from exposure to ash with high silica and cristobalite content.[12,13] However, no cases of acute silicosis were reported in studies of eruptions at Soufriere Volcano in Montserrat and of the Mount St. Helens eruption in 1980, where high concentrations of cristobalite and silica were recorded in ash samples.[12,13] These studies did note a slight increase in bronchial reactivity and wheeze in children during the Montserrat eruptions and a doubling of asthma- and bronchitis-related emergency department (ED) visits, compared with the previous year, during the Mount St. Helens eruption.[13,14] It is believed that no cases of acute silicosis were reported because people were not exposed to high enough concentrations of silica-laden ash for a long enough duration to develop the condition.[13] The risk of silicosis from prolonged ash exposure may be more substantial, but it is difficult to quantify.[13]

During ashfalls, the amount of total suspended particles (TSP) in the air is a useful predictor of ED visits for some respiratory conditions. The number of ED visits for respiratory complaints during the Mount St. Helens eruption was highest when the TSP concentration was greater than 30,000 μg/m³.[14] The number of ED visits did decline with decreasing TSP levels, but it did not return to normal levels until 3 weeks after peak TSP levels were recorded.[14] The increase in ED visits during high TSP levels was greatest for asthmatics.[14] (An important factor to remember is that rain significantly reduces TSP levels.[14])

Volcanic gases also pose a potential health threat. To determine the hazards from volcanic gas, the composition of the volcanic gas emissions and the prevailing weather conditions should be assessed.[6,15,16] Water vapor is the most abundant volcanic gas released, followed by carbon dioxide and sulfur dioxide.[5,6] Volcanic emissions may also include smaller amounts of hydrogen sulfide, hydrogen, carbon monoxide, hydrogen chloride, hydrogen fluoride, helium, and trace amounts of other gases.[5]

The volcanic gases that pose the greatest threat to people, animals, and agriculture are sulfur dioxide, carbon dioxide, and hydrogen fluoride.[5] Sulfur dioxide may produce an irritant effect in the upper and lower airways, on mucosal surfaces, in the eyes, and on the skin.[5,17] Few studies have been performed to assess the health risk of volcanic gas emissions. One study, performed in Hawaii, of volcanic sulfur dioxide emissions was inconclusive in respect to its effect on reactive airway disease.[18] Sulfur dioxide does produce acid rain, which may react with zinc in galvanizing on sheet metal roofs and release heavy metals into drinking water and catchments.[16]

Hydrogen fluoride also induces an irritant response in the upper and lower respiratory tracts, but it is of greatest risk to livestock secondary to ingestion. Ash becomes impregnated with hydrogen fluoride, and upon ingestion, the fluoride produces fluorosis and death of the animal.[5] Fluorosis is a theoretical risk to a human population posteruption, but it can be avoided by cleaning ash off of food before ingestion and checking the fluoride levels of local drinking water.

Carbon dioxide is the second most common gas released during volcanic activity. Carbon dioxide is odorless, colorless, and heavier than air, thus it will collect in low-lying areas. Breathing air with a carbon dioxide concentration greater than 20% to 30% can rapidly induce unconsciousness and death through asphyxiation.[5] If a substantial release of carbon dioxide has occurred or is sus-

pected, venturing into depressions or cellars in the area should be avoided. The carbon dioxide and air boundary can be sharply demarcated, with one step placing a person within a lethal concentration of carbon dioxide.[5]

The other gases tend to be released in much smaller quantities during an eruption. An important consideration is hydrogen sulfide. It is a highly toxic gas that is relatively dense and may collect in depressions and low-lying areas.[6] Hydrogen sulfide gives off a "rotten egg" odor and can cause eye and upper respiratory tract irritation, pulmonary edema with prolonged exposure, and death through cellular asphyxiation.[5,17] It is important to determine the emissions spectrum of a volcano to ensure that larger concentrations of dangerous trace gases are not present.

Volcanic debris flows, termed *lahars,* and mudslides can be very destructive. Loose fragments of rock mixed with water from rainfall, melted snowpack, or another source forms a thick slurry that travels down the mountain side or valley at speeds that may be greater than 50 km per hour.[6,19] The high sediment concentration of the flow destroys buildings, bridges, and other structures, which would usually survive a flood.[6] People caught in the flows almost universally perish.[6]

Lahars also occur when a volcano is quiescent. Both the heavy rainfall from hurricanes and the disruption of volcanic debris and sediment by earthquakes have produced lahars and mudslides.[20,21] Lahars may also be formed by lake breakouts. This happens weeks to months after an eruption when a river blocked by a mudslide or other volcanic deposit overflows the newly formed dam. Erosion of the blockage and the walls of the river channel downstream from the initial surge of water allows tremendous volumes of sediment to be incorporated into the flow.[22] This is termed a *cold lahar;* in comparison, the lahar formed by hot volcanic debris may remain hot far downstream.[6]

Volcanoes pose a unique threat in regard to gas release in the absence of visible eruption. In 1984 at Lake Monoun in Cameroon, 73 people were killed by carbon dioxide released by lake water turnover.[23] A similar event occurred in 1986 at Lake Nyos in Cameroon, a crater lake. Approximately 1700 people in low-lying areas were killed by a massive release of carbon dioxide.[23] Carbon dioxide is believed to have gradually accumulated in the deep waters of the lake. Rain or a landslide may have been responsible for the lake water turnover and gas release at Lake Nyos.

Other risks associated with volcanic eruptions are lightning, tsunamis, and earthquakes. Lightning discharges and lightning strikes from ash clouds occur during eruptions and have caused electrocution injuries.[24] Please see the chapters on tsunamis (Chapter 76) and earthquakes (Chapter 73) for further information about these forms of disaster.

 ## PREINCIDENT ACTIONS

The following are important preincident questions to ask:

- Is there a volcano in close proximity to your medical facility that may be at risk of eruption? To determine this, contact the U.S. Geological Survey or an equivalent authoritative source.

- Does your facility have a mass casualty plan in case of an eruption? Refer to the section on the basics of disaster management (Part 1 of the book) for assistance in developing an organized strategy for dealing with mass casualties.
- Does your medical facility need to be evacuated in the event of an eruption? Medical facilities were evacuated during the eruption of the Rabaul Volcano in Papua New Guinea in 1994 because it was in the fallout zone.[24] If your facility is in a valley or plain with a history of lahars or mudslides, it may need to be evacuated.
- Is a disaster plan prepared, and has it been practiced to allow the timely notification and evacuation of your hospital and the populations at risk? Preparation is crucial, considering that the majority of the deaths during an eruption occur within the first 24 hours.[2] Please refer to the basics of disaster management of this book (Chapter 1) for assistance in creating a disaster plan appropriate for your facility.
- If your facility may require evacuation during an eruption, is there an evacuation plan prepared and coordinated with the appropriate nearest medical facilities outside of the potential fallout zone?
- Does your facility have appropriate supplies and personal protective equipment? Your facility may benefit from having detectors for sulfur dioxide, hydrogen sulfide, carbon dioxide, and carbon monoxide available in case of gas release.[15] Special masks may be needed for protection from gases and dust. Particulate masks do not provide adequate protection. Based on experience from the World Trade Center disaster, the New York Committee for Occupational Safety and Health has recommended the use of National Institute for Occupational Safety and Health (NIOSH)–approved air-purifying respirators of N-100 or N-95 grade.[25] Other useful protective equipment would include hard hats or helmets and heat-resistant clothing.[11]
- Does your facility have adequate internal resources for continued short-term operation if isolated by disruption of local infrastructure? If not, do you have a plan for communication and procurement of needed assistance?

 POSTINCIDENT ACTIONS

1. Activation of disaster plan with appropriate allocation of resources.
2. Distribution and use of appropriate personal protective equipment.
3. Situational awareness. Avoid low-lying areas where lahars or pyroclastic flows have occurred because of the risk of repeat episodes. Avoid basements or depressions where toxic gases may have accumulated unless air quality has been tested.
4. Be alert for repeat eruptions. The volcano may erupt multiple times.
5. Monitor ash and tephra accumulation on buildings in the medical facility. Tephra causes the most injuries

through building collapse. If ash clearing is undertaken, make sure that appropriate personal protective equipment is worn and that the conditions are safe enough to allow removal of the ash. If there is any concern about the risk of building collapse, consider evacuating the facility or building.

6. Monitor air quality and provide appropriate public health warnings. Those at risk for chronic obstructive pulmonary disease and asthma exacerbations may benefit from staying indoors, if it is safe to do so, while TSP concentrations are high.

 MEDICAL TREATMENT OF CASUALTIES

Casualties during a volcanic eruption can be complex and require sophisticated and intensive multisystem trauma care. Detailing of all the medical treatments potentially required is beyond the scope of this chapter. The important factor to consider is the mechanism of volcanic-related injury in anticipating patient care needs. The broad categories of injuries seen are burns, crush injuries, head trauma, inhalation injuries, toxic exposure to gases, blunt force trauma, and amputations. For further information and recommendations please refer to the basics of disaster management of this book (Part 1), the accidental disaster section (chapter 57), and the following chapters: accidental versus intentional event (Chapter 57) building and bridge collapse (Chapters 169 and 170), landslide (Chapter 81) and building fires (Chapter 156).

 UNIQUE CONSIDERATIONS

1. Gas release from lake water turnover in the absence of visible volcanic activity.
2. Dormant or suspected dormant volcano reactivation.

 PITFALLS

1. Failure to assess whether your medical facility is at risk from volcanic eruption and failure to incorporate this eventuality into the hospital disaster plan.
2. Lack of consideration for a volcano's historic eruptive pattern when preparing a disaster plan.
3. Failure of your medical facility to procure adequate and appropriate supplies to deal with a volcanic eruption. Personal protective equipment should include heat-resistant coveralls, hard hats, and NIOSH-recommended respirators.
4. Failure to appreciate the risk for volcanic-related injuries in the absence of visible volcanic activity. Examples include mudslides, lahars, and volcanic gas release.
5. Failure to consider the need to evacuate a hospital posteruption and to determine whether the receiving facility is in a safe zone that will not be endangered by future or repeated eruptions.

CASE PRESENTATION

The eruption of the Galeras Volcano in Colombia in 1993 provides a better understanding of the need for adequate personal protective equipment and a more clear understanding of the injury spectrum that may be suffered during a volcanic eruption. Six volcanologists and three tourists were killed when the volcano erupted without warning. Autopsies showed that individuals closest to the eruption site within the caldera were torn apart by the force of the eruption. Those farther away from the eruption suffered burns from ejecta, fractures, concussions, and other head injuries from bombardment with ejecta. Analysis of the tragedy suggested that hard hats would provide some protection from head injuries during escape. Heat-resistant and water-repellent coveralls could limit the risk of burns and clothing ignition.[11]

REFERENCES

1. Small C, Naumann T. The global distribution of human population and recent volcanism. *Environmental Hazards*. 2001;3:93-109.
2. Simkin T, Siebert L, Blong R. Disasters: volcanic fatalities—lessons from the historical record. *Science*. 2001;5502:255.
3. US Geological Survey. Types and Effects of Volcanic Hazards. Available at: http://volcanoes.usgs.gov/Hazards/What/hazards.html.
4. Bernstein RS, Baxter PJ, Buist AS. Introduction to the epidemiological aspects of explosive volcanism. *Am J Public Health*. 1986;76(3 Suppl):3-9.
5. US Geological Survey. Volcanic Gases and Their Effects. Available at: http://volcanoes.usgs.gov/Hazards/What/VolGas/volgas. html.
6. Newhall CG, Fruchter JS. Volcanic activity: a review for health professionals. *Am J Public Health*. 1986;76(3 Suppl):10-24.
7. US Geological Survey. Effects of Pyroclastic Surge at Mount St Helens, Washington, May 18, 1980. Available at: http://volcanoes.usgs.gov/Hazards/Effects/MSHsurge_effects. html.
8. Decker RW, Decker BB. *Mountains of Fire: The Nature of Volcanoes*. New York: Cambridge University Press; 1991:1-40.
9. US Geological Survey. Dome Collapses Generate Pyroclastic Flows at Unzen volcano, Japan. Available at: http://volcanoes.usgs. gov/Hazards/What/PF/PFUnzen. html.
10. US Geological Survey. Effects of Pyroclastic Flows and Surges at Soufriere Hills Volcano, Montserrat. Available at: http://volcanoes. usgs.gov/Hazards/Effects/Soufrie reHills_PFeffects.html.
11. Baxter PJ, Gresham A. Deaths and injuries in eruption of Galeras Volcano, Colombia, 14 January 1993. *J Volcanology Geothermal Research*. 1997;77:325-38.
12. Martin TR, Covert D, Butler J. Inhaling volcanic ash. *Chest*. 1981;80(1 Suppl):85-8.
13. Searl A, Nicholl A, Baxter PJ. Assessment of the exposure of islanders to ash from the Soufriere Hills volcano, Montserrat, British West Indies. *Occup Environ Med*. 2002;59:523-31.
14. Baxter PJ, Ing R, Falk H, Plikaytis B. Mount St. Helens eruptions: the acute respiratory effects of volcanic ash in a North American community. *Arch Environ Health*. 1983;38(3):138-43.
15. Baxter PJ, Berstein MD, Buist AS. Preventative health measures in volcanic eruptions. *Am J Public Health*. 1986;76(3 Suppl):84-90.
16. US Geological Survey. Long-lasting Eruption of Kilauea Volcano, Hawai`i Leads to Volcanic-Air Pollution. Available at: http://volcanoes.usgs.gov/Hazards/What/Vol Gas/VolGasPollution.html.
17. Olson KR, et al. Poisoning and drug overdose. 3rd ed. Stamford, Conn: Appleton & Lange; 1999:181-8.
18. Mannino DM, Ruben S, et al. Emergency department visits and hospitalizations for respiratory disease on the island of Hawaii, 1981 to 1991. *Hawaii Med J*. 1996;55:48-54
19. US Geological Survey. "What's That Cloud Upriver?" An Eyewitness Account of a Lahar by USGS Geologist Jeff Marso. Available at: http://volcanoes.usgs.gov/Hazards/What/Lahars/ Santiaguito_89. html.
20. US Geological Survey. Intense Rainfall During Hurricane Mitch Triggers Deadly Landslide and Lahar at Casita Volcano, Nicaragua, on October 30, 1998. Available at: http://volcanoes.usgs.gov/ Hazards/What/Lahars/Cas itaLahar.html.
21. US Geological Survey. Earthquake on June 6, 1994, Triggers Landslides and Catastrophic Lahar Near Nevado del Huila Volcano, Colombia. Available at: http://volcanoes.usgs.gov/Hazards/What/ Lahar s/HuilaLahar.html.
22. US Geological Survey. Lahars Caused by Lake Breakouts. Available at: http://volcanoes.usgs.gov/Hazards/What/Lahars/LakeLahar.html.
23. Baxter PJ, Kapila M, Mfonfu D. Lake Nyos disaster, Cameroon, 1986: the medical effects of large scale emission of carbon dioxide? *BMJ*. 1989;298:1437-41.
24. Dent AW, Davies G, Barrett P, de Saint Ours PJ. The 1994 eruption of the Rabaul volcano, Papua New Guinea: injuries sustained and medical response. *Med J Aust*. 1995;163:536-9.
25. New York Committee for Occupational Safety and Health. NYCOSH WTC Factsheet 4: Cleaning Up Indoor Dust and Debris in the World Trade Center Area. Available at: http://www.nycosh.org/ environment_wtc/wtc-dust-factsheet.html.

chapter 80

Famine

Laura Macnow and Hilarie Cranmer

 DESCRIPTION OF EVENT

Famine is the most extreme form of lack of access to enough food and is often the result of natural or man-made disasters. Famine has been defined as "a condition of populations in which a substantial increase in deaths is associated with inadequate food consumption."[1] Natural disasters such as drought, floods, crop infestations, and livestock diseases that limit a population's food production are often popularly thought of as the events precipitating famine; however, insufficient access to food is now more commonly the result of war, civil strife, and economic collapse. Famine is usually caused by an exacerbation of preexisting conditions of poverty, debt, underemployment, and high malnutrition prevalence in a population, so that when added burdens arise, widespread starvation can occur rapidly.[2]

Famine is a complex emergency often involving massive population displacements between and within countries, and as such, complicates the ability of agencies to coordinate relief efforts and provide ongoing surveillance of the emergency.

The usual consequences of mass starvation during famine are increased malnutrition and mortality.[3] Manifestations of starvation depend on the individual's previous nutritional status, age, and severity of food deprivation.[4] Malnutrition is the objective physical or laboratory findings of physical deterioration as a result of inadequate nutrient intake and encompasses a range of conditions, including acute malnutrition (characterized by wasting), chronic malnutrition (characterized by stunting or nutritional edema), and micronutrient deficiencies.[5]

To assess the prevalence of moderate-to-severe malnutrition in a population, it is a commonly accepted practice to do anthropometric surveys in a random sample of children younger than 5 years using the weight-for-height (WFH) index[2,5]; these data are a reliable indicator of malnutrition in the wider population. Because weight is more sensitive to sudden changes in food availability,[2] the WFH index is used instead of height-for-age (which measures stunting). Mean upper arm circumference (MUAC) can also be measured to screen for acute malnutrition. The presence of edema, however, may confound these indices, and clinical judg-ment must be used in their evaluation. Additionally, anthropometric data may be skewed by concurrent mortality rates. Anthropometric data are commonly interpreted using z scores (or standard deviation [SD] scores) where:

$$\frac{z \text{ score}}{(\text{or SD score})} = \frac{\text{Observed Value} - \text{Median Value of the Reference Population}}{\text{Standard Deviation Value of Reference Population}}$$

The WHO Global Database on Child Growth and Malnutrition[6] uses a z-score cut-off point of less than -2 SD to classify low weight-for-age, low height-for-age, and low weight-for-height as moderate and severe undernutrition, and less than -3 SD to define severe undernutrition.[6] If more than 8% of the children samples have a z score of less than -2, a nutritional emergency exists. An excess of even 1% of children with z scores of less than -3 indicates a need for immediate action.[2]

Famines are often assessed and reported in terms of cases, rates, or degrees of malnutrition, or the number of deaths from malnutrition and its complications. Crude mortality rates (CMRs) can be useful for evaluating the severity of a disaster, using 1 death/10,000 population/day as the cut-off for an emergency.[2]

Although the most direct and obvious results of famine are severe malnutrition and death, the immediate cause of death in affected individuals is usually a communicable disease, most commonly measles, diarrheal illness, acute respiratory infections (ARIs), and malaria. Displaced populations and refugees almost always experience higher CMRs compared with nondisplaced populations, and this is likely due to increased risk of communicable disease associated with crowded, often unsanitary camps. Malnutrition predisposes individuals to certain micronutrient deficiencies, notably vitamin A deficiency; communicable diseases such as measles and diarrhea further deplete vitamin A stores and can cause worsening immune compromise and xerophthalmia, corneal xerosis, and ulceration and scarring, and can eventually lead to blindness.[2] Other important micronutrient deficiencies include vitamin C, niacin, iron, iodine, and thiamine deficiency.

PREINCIDENT ACTIONS

- Advance detection and monitoring of economic, social, and environmental factors that influence the development of food shortages and famine. Early warning systems may rely on community involvement. Local people can collect data on what they see as signs of growing food insecurity; for example, an increase in the number of animals sold in local markets may indicate that families need cash to buy food because their crops have failed.[7] This information is used in conjunction with satellite imaging and meteorologic data to create the whole picture of drought and its effects.
- Support of socially responsible community development, including education about preserving the huge local ranges of hardy crop types and encouraging food production of a wide variety of crops, bred to be hardy and grown together in a robust mixed-crop pattern. This will help communities recover quickly in the event of natural disasters.[7] Mono-cropping can increase vulnerability in times of natural or economic disasters, as can deforestation, desertification, and poor agricultural practices.[2]
- Coordination of relief agencies.
- Development of standard case management protocols.
- Establishment of reserves of essential supplies (medical and nutritional).
- Development of environmental management plans.

 POSTINCIDENT ACTIONS

- Media and worldwide notification.
- Perform field assessment: determine total refugee or displaced population, determine age-sex breakdown and average family/household size, identify at-risk groups (children <5 years old, pregnant and lactating women, elderly, disabled/wounded persons). This information is needed to estimate quantities of relief supplies and for effective surveillance of mortality/morbidity rates.
- Initiate health and nutrition surveillance systems.
- Assess prior health/nutritional status, and determine prevalence of acute malnutrition and micronutrient deficiencies in children younger than 5 years old (this serves as a proxy for malnutrition in the general population).
- Calculate crude, age-, sex-, and cause-specific mortality rates and morbidity rates of diseases.
- Assess local community resources, and determine important health beliefs and traditions.
- Evaluate environmental conditions, such as water sources, sanitation arrangements, local disease vectors and epidemiology, and availability of materials for shelter and fuel.
- Evaluate resources such as food supplies and distribution systems, and assess logistics for food transport and storage.
- Ensure ongoing surveillance of communities' health and nutritional status and evaluate the effectiveness of the intervention and quality of care delivered.[2]

 MEDICAL TREATMENT OF CASUALTIES

Medical treatment of victims of famine must include preventive as well as curative measures. Regardless of immunization status, all children up to age 16 should be immunized against measles. If vaccine supplies are limited, higher-risk children (up to age 5) should be immunized preferentially. One should never withhold immunization because of fever, ARI, diarrhea, HIV, or malnutrition. Vitamin A treatment should be instituted concomitantly. All children with clinical measles should receive 200,000 IU oral vitamin A (half-dose for children <12 months); children with complicated measles should receive a second dose on day 2. Individuals with eye symptoms of vitamin A deficiency should receive 200,000 IU oral vitamin A on day 1, day 2, and then again 1 to 4 weeks later (half-dose for children <12 months).

Diarrheal illness in malnourished populations is generally caused by the same pathogens that cause diarrhea in developing countries: *Escherichia coli, Shigella,* and *Salmonella.* Oral rehydration therapy (ORT) is a mainstay in the treatment of diarrhea, and chemotherapy should not be used for routine treatment of uncomplicated, watery diarrhea unless cholera, *Shigella, Giardia,* or amoebic dysentery is suspected. Preventive measures are of extreme importance in control of diarrheal illness and include providing adequate quantities of clean water, good sanitation, personal hygiene education, and promotion of breast-feeding of infants.[2,5]

Nutritional interventions can be categorized as general ration distribution to the affected population, blanket supplementary feeding to all members of an identified risk group, targeted dry (take-home) supplementary feeding centers for the moderately malnourished, and therapeutic feeding centers for the severely malnourished. General rations must supply at least 2100 kcal/person/day, of which 17% of calories are in the form of fats and 12% of calories are derived from protein.[5] Food should ideally be distributed in a community setting (avoiding risk of communicable disease associated with mass feeding centers), and adequate fuel and cooking utensils should be available. Supplemental feeding programs should be provided to acutely undernourished children younger than 5 years old, pregnant and lactating women, elderly individuals, and chronically ill individuals. The disadvantage of dry (take-home) supplemental feedings is that sharing of the ration among family members is likely. Therapeutic feeding programs (TFPs) are reserved for severely malnourished children (z score of less than −3, clinical edema); feedings are provided in on-site, resource-intensive centers. Children should receive 150 kcal and 3 g of protein for each kilogram of body weight in four to six feedings per day.[2] Nasogastric feedings may be needed. Close monitoring is essential, and weight gain should be targeted to 10 g/1 kg of body weight/day. TFPs have serious limitations, and there have been suggestions that community-based therapeutic care is likely to be more successful. TFPs are resource-intensive and require skilled staff and imported therapeutic products; international standards require one care provider for every 10 patients, with a maximum of 100 patients per center.[8] Criticisms of TFPs include that they take months to become operational, have low coverage, are extremely expensive, undermine local health infrastructure, disempower communities, and promote the congregation of people around them, increasing risk of communicable diseases.[8] Admitted children usually depend on the presence of their mothers to care for them around the clock, taking the mothers away from their community and decreasing their ability to look after their other children. Community-based therapeutic care, on the other hand, may be as successful overall as TFPs at decreasing overall mortality, while being more cost-effective and less disruptive to communities and families. A ready-to-use therapeutic food (RUTF) made from peanuts, dried skimmed milk, sugar, and a specially formulated mineral/vitamin mix can be distributed in a paste form, which keeps it from spoiling for several months, and is equally nutritious as TFP feedings. Proponents of community-based therapeutic care suggest that, when used to complement TFPs, overall death rates from starvation can be reduced while providing socio-economic and educational benefits for the families of the malnourished.[8]

 ## UNIQUE CONSIDERATIONS

The demographic groups that are most at risk during famine are young children and women, and it is important that establishment of Maternal and Child Health (MCH) care be given high priority to provide care for pregnant and lactating women and children younger than 2 years of age. Services should include health

 CASE PRESENTATION

You have volunteered to work in a refugee camp in Rwanda. Your first patient is a 5-year-old with a cough and a rash. Physical examination reveals a severely malnourished child with a nonproductive cough. The rash is diffuse and has been present for at least 3 days. The child also has a fever and diarrhea.

education as well as routine monitoring, immunization, nutritional rehabilitation, micronutrient supplementation, and curative care. Breast-feeding should be encouraged for children, minimally up to age 6 months, and preferably up to 2 years. Local female health workers should be trained to provide culturally appropriate education and care. Ideally, one MCH clinic per 5000 population should be set up.[2]

 ## PITFALLS

- Failure to recognize early warning signs of famine
- Failure to mobilize resources and coordinate relief agencies
- Neglect of preventive programs (e.g., immunizations, ORT, hygiene education), and failure to prevent communicable diseases
- Failure to preferentially target vulnerable populations
- Lack of variety in basic relief rations (risk of micronutrient deficiencies)
- Failure to recognize importance of cultural practices, beliefs, and taboos, and failure to involve the refugee community and its leaders in relief work

REFERENCES

1. Toole MJ, Foster S. Famines. In: Gregg MB, ed. *The Public Health Consequences of Disasters*. Atlanta: US Department of Health and Human Services, Public Health Service, Centers for Disease Control and Prevention; 1989:79-89.
2. Centers for Disease Control and Prevention. Famine-affected, refugee, and displaced populations: recommendations for public health issues. *MMWR* 1992;41(RR-13):1-76.
3. Noji EK. *The Public Health Consequences of Disaster*. New York: Oxford University Press; 1997.
4. Graham G. Starvation in the modern world. *New Engl J Med*. 1993;328:1058-61.
5. The Sphere Project. Minimum standards in food security, nutrition and food aid. In: Sphere Handbook, 2004 Revised Edition. Available at: http://www.sphereproject.org/handbook/hdbkpdf/hdbk_c3.pdf.
6. World Health Organization. WHO Global Database on Child Growth and Malnutrition. Available at: http://www.who.int/nutgrowthdb.
7. International Federation of Red Cross and Red Crescent Societies. *World Disasters Report: Focus on Reducing Risk*. Geneva: International Federation of Red Cross; 2002.
8. Collins S. Changing the way we address severe malnutrition during famine. *Lancet* 2001;358:498-501.

chapter 81

Landslides*

Mark E. Keim

 DESCRIPTION OF EVENT

The term *landslide* includes a wide range of ground movement, such as rock falls, deep failure of slopes, and shallow debris flows. This chapter uses landslide terminology as presented by Varnes[1] and Cruden and Varnes.[2] As used, the term *landslide* will include all types of gravity-induced mass movements, ranging from rock falls through slides/slumps, avalanches, and flows, and it includes both subaerial and submarine mass movements triggered mainly by precipitation (including snowmelt), seismic activity, and volcanic eruptions. For simplification, the term *debris flow* will include mud flows, debris torrents, and lahars (volcanic debris flows).

Debris flows are fast-moving landslides that occur in a wide range of environments. A debris flow is a rapidly moving mass of water and material that is mainly composed of sand, gravel, and cobbles, but typically includes trees, cars, small buildings, and other anthropogenic material. A debris flow typically has the consistency of wet concrete and moves at speeds in excess of 16 meters per second (35 miles per hour).[3]

Although gravity acting on an over-steepened slope is the primary reason for a landslide, there are other contributing factors[4]:

- Erosion by rivers, glaciers, or ocean waves creates over-steepened slopes
- Rock and soil slopes are weakened through saturation by snowmelt or heavy rains
- Earthquakes create stresses that make weak slopes fail
- Earthquakes of magnitude 4.0 and greater have been known to trigger landslides
- Volcanic eruptions produce loose ash deposits, heavy rain, and debris flows
- Excess weight from accumulation of rain or snow, stockpiling of rock or ore, waste piles, or manmade structures may stress weak slopes to failure and other structures

*The material in this chapter reflects solely the views of the author. It does not necessarily reflect the policies or recommendations of the Centers for Disease Control and Prevention or the U.S. Department of Health and Human Services.

The world's largest landslides are prehistoric. Their remains are displayed as significant morphologic features on the Earth's surface. Most very large landslides have been triggered by earthquakes or volcanic eruptions.[5]

The world's largest historic landslide is the 1980 Mount St. Helens rock slide–debris avalanche in the Cascade Range of southwestern Washington State, which was triggered by a catastrophic volcanic eruption.[6] This 24-km–long, 2.8-km³ landslide buried about 60 km² of the valley of the North Fork Toutle River under a cover of hummocky-surfaced, poorly sorted debris, ranging in size from clay to blocks of volcanic rocks with individual volumes as large as several thousand cubic meters.[5]

Landslides occur in every state and U.S. territory. The Appalachian Mountains, the Rocky Mountains, and the Pacific Coastal Ranges as well as some parts of Alaska and Hawaii have severe landslide problems. Landslides cost an estimated $1 billion to $3 billion per year in the United States alone. During 1990-1999, landslides were second only to hurricanes as the leading cause of death resulting from environmental disasters in the hazard-prone Pacific basin (4 times more than earthquakes and 30 times more than volcanoes).[7]

Landslides and debris flows triggered by earthquakes accounted for most of the fatalities and serious injuries in several recent earthquakes, including those in Peru (1970), Tajikistan (1989), the Philippines (1990), and Colombia (1994).[8] In 1985, a lahar from Nevada del Ruiz volcano traveled over 30 miles and killed at least 23,000 people.[9] In 1999, rainstorms induced thousands of landslides along the coast of northern Venezuela and resulted in a death toll estimated at 19,000 to 30,000 people and total damage estimated at $1.9 billion[3,10] (Fig. 81-1).

Landslides impact public health by causing injuries and severe property destruction. Landslide mortality is largely related to trauma and asphyxiation. Landslide morbidity is largely associated with traumatic injuries and a disruption of water, sanitation, shelter, and the locally grown food supply of the affected population[11] (Fig. 81-2).

Landslides triggered during the 1994 Northridge earthquake resulted in an outbreak of 203 cases of coccidioidomycosis when arthrospores were spread in dust clouds.[12] Debris flows associated with massive

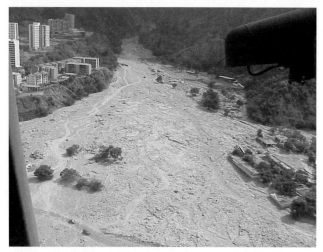
FIGURE 81–1. Large debris flow channel caused during 1999 Venezuela landslides.

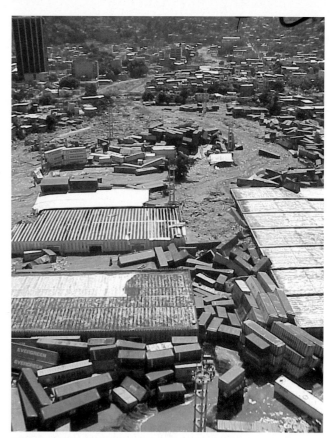
FIGURE 81–3. Venezuelan port warehouses storing hazardous materials were inundated by debris flow in 1999.

floods in northern Venezuela on Dec. 16 and 17, 1999 destroyed part of the port facilities in LaGuaira. The port facilities contained customs warehouses known to store hazardous materials, including corrosives, organic solvents, oxidants, compressed gases, heavy metals, and explosives. These chemicals were inundated by the debris flow, which came dangerously close to causing an explosion and toxic exposure with the potential to affect 80,000 nearby residents as well as closing that nation's largest airport and second largest seaport[13,14] (Fig. 81-3).

Pre-Incident Actions

Landslides usually strike without warning. Therefore, pre-incident actions in prevention, preparedness, and mitigation are by far the most effective means of protecting life and property. Although the physical cause of many landslides cannot be removed, geologic investiga-

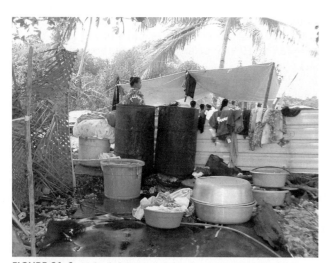
FIGURE 81–2. Makeshift living conditions of homeless family after 2002 landslides in Chuuk, Micronesia.

tions, good engineering practices, and effective enforcement of land-use management regulations can reduce landslide hazards.[4] Two mitigation strategies can be implemented to protect property: (1) large structural flood control measures and (2) avoidance of the affected area. Land-use regulations can be used to reduce hazards by limiting the type or amount of development in high risk areas. In high-risk zones where development and reconstruction are inevitable, steps such as orienting buildings and streets parallel to the down-slope direction of debris flow will minimize the width of the building exposed and allow streets to serve as overflow channels.[3] Monitoring, warning, and evacuation are nonstructural approaches to hazard mitigation that reduce potential loss of life. Early warning systems based on weather forecasts and rainfall information can substantially improve emergency managers' responses to warn and evacuate threatened communities. Areas such as Hong Kong, San Francisco, and Denver use warning systems such as sirens and radio bulletins to alert residents of potentially threatening conditions.[3] The public, first responders, emergency managers, and decision-makers should be educated regarding hazard awareness, as well as emergency preparedness, mitigation, and response measures.[15] Box 81-1 list areas that are generally more prone to landslide hazards:[3,16] Box 81-2 lists what to do if a home is suspected as being at risk for landslide danger.[16] Box 81-3 lists features that may be noticed prior to major landsliding.[16]

Post-Incident Actions

Landslides are associated with high rates of traumatic injury and mortality. If there is an imminent risk of landslides, individuals should stay alert and awake. Many debris-flow fatalities occur when people are sleeping. They should also listen to an NOAA Weather Radio or portable, battery-powered radio or television for warnings of intense rainfall. They should be especially alert when driving. Embankments along roadsides are particularly susceptible to landslides.[17] During a landslide, persons at risk should take immediate steps to get out of the down-slope path of the flow or, if unable to evacuate, to protect themselves inside of a building. If escape is not possible, individuals should attempt to curl up into a ball and protect their head.[17] Box 81-4 lists recommendations for actions to be considered after a landslide has occurred. [17]

Whenever possible, search-and-rescue operations should be performed by properly trained and adequately equipped professional rescuers. First-arriving incident commanders need to establish safety zones immediately. Soil engineers should be called and an emergency warning system, such as a siren blowing steadily for 30 seconds, immediately established. In the safety briefing of the Incident Action Plan, the incident commander should stress that evacuation and "all-clear" signals are not for discussion and must be obeyed immediately.

The organized literature for such rescues is minimal. In the absence of an engineer assessment, general guidelines for safety zones have been recommended as follows[15]:

Cold Zone

1. 100 feet from the outside edge of each side of the debris flow in situations involving stream order 1 situations ("stream order" is the geological classification of drainages; the number increases as the size and number of drainages increase)
2. 1000 feet from the sides and base of debris flows that are occurring on slopes that are 26 degrees or greater and involve areas with stream orders 2–4; and
3. 500 feet from the sides and base of flows in stream order 5 and above, which occur at the mouth of large canyons and have largely ceased flowing. All of these recommendations are based on weather reports of diminishing or ceasing rainfall. If rain continues, all distances should be increased.

Warm Zone

The warm zone is the area inside the distances mentioned for the cold zone, up to the edge of the flow. Safety gear should be worn by all personnel in that zone.

Hot Zone

The hot zone is the area on the debris field. All personnel on the field should have complete safety gear. All personnel in the warm and hot zones should be logged in and out of the areas.

With respect to personal safety equipment for rescuers, foot and leg protection is mandatory. Personal flotation devices should be worn if there is danger of further flows. Helmets and harnesses should be worn on steep slopes. A harness—at least a tubular webbing "hasty" harness—must be worn, even on reasonably flat terrain, in the event the rescuer becomes trapped. Additional equipment might include: work gloves; a small backpack or load-bearing rig for water bottles, or a "camel-back" irrigation system; small folding shovels; face masks; and goggles. All rescuers should be tethered from dry ground, if possible.

Small inflatable rafts assist rescuers in crossing soft mud and serve as a stable work platform. An air-filled hose—either laced back and forth through a roof ladder and then filled with air to make a field-expedient raft, or simply pulled out onto the mud as a handhold—is extremely useful. Helpful technical and USAR-type gear includes: ropes, "A" frames and confined-space tripods, plywood and shoring materials, and rescue "hardware," such as carabiners and pulleys.

Chances of survival in a debris flow or mudslide are best on the edges and decrease toward the center. Most survivors are found in a zone that makes up about a quarter of the flow width, immediately along its edges. As a result, most rescues can be conducted using simple techniques from dry ground.

If a victim is mired higher than his or her waist, shore-based thrown lines are likely not going to work because there is simply too much suction on the victim. The rescuers will need to go out and extricate the victim by breaking the suction. The two best techniques involve air and water. A 1-inch fire hose with a metal "root wand"

affixed to the end can be shoved along the edge of the victim's body. When the water is turned on, it creates a "slurry" next to the victim and releases the suction. Air has also been suggested, which involves using an SCBA bottle and a rigid hose that can be shoved down in the mud. Air charged into the mud creates large air bubbles that also help break the suction. It may become necessary to build an "island" around the victim so that a vertical pull can be attempted, using either a ladder "A" frame or a tripod. Combined with air and water, such techniques may free victims trapped all the way to their necks. Rescuers should also remain vigilant of the possibility of exposure to hazardous materials and should plan appropriately for response to hazardous materials exposures including decontamination of rescuers at the scene.

Medical Treatment of Casualties

The treatment of landslide casualties is the same as that for other causes of traumatic injury. In the case of mass casualties, an incident management system should be established and a system for triage of casualty care should be in place. After extended entrapments, extricated victims may have medical complications ranging from hypothermia, impaired airway, and compartment syndrome.

UNIQUE CONSIDERATIONS AND PITFALLS

The single most important issue regarding landslides is the priority of pre-incident prevention and mitigation efforts. Landslide morbidity and mortality is high and many of these deaths and injuries are preventable given the appropriate level of pre-incident intervention. In

CASE PRESENTATION

A desperate search for survivors is under way on a remote Pacific island after a typhoon triggered landslides that wiped out entire families. A typhoon struck the small Pacific nation 4 days ago. An official from the national Disaster Office told news agencies that there were 31 confirmed deaths. About 100 people are reported to have been injured and over 2000 are now homeless. Many of the deaths known were on one island. "Whole families are just left with one or two people," he said. "It is a very bad time. There is a lot of suffering and a lot of pain." But he said there could be worse to come. "We are still searching," he said. "We are expecting many more. We have not been able to reach the outer islands yet." Survivors are in dire need of food, water, and medical supplies. No outside help has reached them. Many of the seriously injured are unable to receive the medical treatment they need. The U.S. Joint Typhoon Warning Center says seas of about 18 feet with winds gusting to 90 mph are expected to continue through tomorrow. Rescuers are unable to transport heavy equipment to the affected islands. There are no local urban search-and-rescue teams in existence.

most cases, emergency response is often much too little and much too late to make a significant impact. The major pitfall of emergency management related to landslides is an over-reliance upon response compared with the overwhelming cost-effectiveness of prevention and mitigation. Another pitfall is to underestimate the public health needs of those populations displaced by the disaster.[11] In addition to an obvious lack of food security, shelter, and adequate sanitations, these populations are more prone to incur additional injuries, disease, and lingering mental illness (see Fig. 81-2).

REFERENCES

1. Varnes DJ. Slope movement types and processes. In: Schuster RL, Krizek RJ, eds. *Landslides: Analysis and Control*. Washington DC: National Research Council; *Transp Res Bd Spec Rept* 176, 1978, pp 11-33.
2. Cruden DM, Varnes DJ. Landslide types and processes. In Turner AK, Schuster RL, eds. *Landslides: Investigation and Mitigation*. Washington DC: National Research Council; Transp. Res. Bd. Spec. Rept. 247, 1996, pp 36-75.
3. Larsen M, Wieczorek G, Eaton L, et al. Natural Hazards on Alluvial Fans: The Venezuela debris flow and flash flood disaster. Washington DC: U.S. Department of the Interior; U.S. Geological Survey Fact Sheet 103-01. Available at: http://pubs.usgs.gov/fs/fs-0103-01/fs-0103-01.pdf.
4. Anonymous. Landslide hazard fact sheet. U.S. Geological Survey. Available at: http://landslides.usgs.gov/ html_files/nlic/page5.html.
5. Schuster RL. Engineering geologic effects of the 1980 eruptions of Mount St. Helens. In: Galster R, ed. *Engineering Geology in Washington*. Olympia, Wash: Washington Division of Geological Bulletin, 1989;78(2):1203-28.
6. Voight RB, Janda RJ, Glicken H, Douglass PM. Nature and mechanisms of the Mount St. Helens rock-slide avalanche of 18 May 1980. *Geotechnique* 1983;33(3):243-73.
7. Anonymous. *World Disasters Report*. Geneva, Switzerland: International Federation of Red Cross and Red Crescent Societies; 2000.
8. Noji E. Earthquakes. In: Noji, E, ed. *Public Health Consequences of Disasters*. New York, NY: Oxford University Press; 1997.
9. Voight B. The 1985 Nevada del Ruiz volcano catastrophe: anatomy and retrospection. *J Volcanolog Geotherm Res*. 1990;44:349-86.
10. Sancio R. Disaster in Venezuela: The floods and landslides of December 1999. *Natural Hazards Observer*. March 24;4:2002.
11. UN Office for the Coordination of Humanitarian Affairs (OCHA). Tropical Storm Chata'an, Federated States of Micronesia. *OCHA Situation Report No. 2*. July 16, 2004. Available at: http://landslides.usgs.gov/html_files/News/2002/Micronesia_Tropical_Storm_Chataan-Jul%202002%20Micronesia_Report_2.htm.
12. Centers for Disease Control and Prevention. Coccidioidomycosis following the Northridge earthquake—California, 1994. *MMWR* 1994;43:194-5.
13. Keim M, Humphrey A, Dreyfus A, et al. Situation assessment report involving the hazardous material disaster site at LaGuaira Port, Venezuela. *CDC Report to Office of Foreign Disaster Assistance*. U.S. Agency for International Development, Jan. 10, 2000.
14. Anonymous. Venezuela seeks contractors for hazardous cleanup. *Hazardous Substances Spill Report*. Jan. 27, 2000; 3:2,.
15. Segerstrom J. A dirty job: Rescuers face the growing problem of debris flows, mudslides and estuary rescues. *Adv Rescue Technol*. Feb/Mar;2004;41-7.
16. Anonymous. Features that may indicate catastrophic landslide movement. U.S. Geological Survey. Available at: http://landslides.usgs.gov/html_files/nlic/page3.html.
17. Anonymous. Informing the public about hazards: landslides and debris flow. Federal Emergency Management Agency. Available at: http://www.fema.gov/hazards/landslides/.

chapter 82

Avalanche

Jason A. Tracy

DESCRIPTION OF EVENT

Deaths caused by avalanches are on the rise as more recreationalists are undertaking "extreme" outdoor sporting activities. Climbers, backcountry skiers, out-of-bounds skiers, and snowmobilers comprise a majority of these fatalities.[1] As many as 80% of these casualties are due to asphyxiation after snow burial[2-4]; time to extrication is the critical factor to survival. There is a 92% chance of survival in open areas if victims are found within 15 minutes; however, these odds decrease to 30% after 35 minutes.[3,5] This statistic differs dramatically among building-confined avalanche victims, for whom there is only a 31% chance of survival if extricated within 190 minutes.[5] Although rare, avalanches triggered by topographic or meteorologic conditions can be devastating to ill-prepared building inhabitants or to those traveling on exposed roadways.[6]

Professional rescue teams, compared with recreationalists, can improve survival of these victims, since time to extrication can be dramatically improved to within the "golden 15 minutes." Depth of burial is also a critical survival factor; approximately 50% of individuals who are completely buried (head and chest under snow) will likely die, whereas only 4% of those who are partially buried will succumb to death.[6] No avalanche victim buried to depths greater than 7 feet has ever survived in the United States.[4]

Asphyxiation from burial or from sudden burial-site airway obstruction causes the majority of avalanche deaths. However, it is clear from autopsy studies that blunt trauma also plays a significant role, not only as a cause of death, but as a critical consideration during rescue efforts.[4,7] Injuries most commonly sustained by avalanche victims include craniofacial trauma with a high likelihood of closed head injuries,[7] and chest and abdominal trauma.[8] Trauma is reportedly the cause of death in up to 13% of all avalanche disaster cases.[9]

Creating an air space in the entombment site has been postulated as the reason that 7% of all victims survive for as long as 130 minutes postburial.[5] As long as icing of the air space ("ice lensing") does not occur, carbon dioxide diffusion can commence and delay asphyxiation.[4,10] Appropriate survival training and readily available rescue equipment can reduce the time to rescue and prolong the oxygen supply.

Although hypothermia may prevent hypoxic damage,[6] it can also cause vascular instability and death when core body temperatures fall below the 32°C hypothermic threshold.[11] In hypothermic-inducing conditions, body temperatures will fall predictably by approximately 3°C per hour. Complete burial limits the time up to which hypothermia avoidance is possible—90 minutes. Beyond the 90-minute cut-off, significant hypothermia in these conditions will occur.[6]

PREINCIDENT ACTIONS

Avalanche avoidance through appropriate training is the mainstay of prevention. Local weather conditions should be verified before any backcountry traveling. Training for at-risk individuals includes condition analysis as well as proper safety and rescue equipment usage. Individuals in an avalanche area should carry a snow shovel, which is used not only for rescue purposes, but also for building "snow pits" to analyze conditions. Long probes (ranging from 10 to 12 feet in length when extended) and/or personal avalanche beacons, both of which are useful for finding buried victims, are also requisite recreationalist trekking gear. Personal avalanche beacons have become the most widely used personal rescue devices worldwide. When buried, these devices emit a signal that can be received by active rescuers.[12] Newer survival equipment includes the artificial air pocket device (AvaLung), the ABS-Avalanche Airbag System, and the Avalanche Ball. Each of these devices provides a unique way of preventing death.[4] As previously discussed, professional rescue teams improve avalanche victim survival through their ability to rapidly locate and extricate a buried victim. Regardless of extrication team training, it is critical that potential burial-site air pockets are preserved during extrication because any loss of this space will lead to rapid death.

POSTINCIDENT ACTIONS

Rapid location and extrication of buried victims are the key to survival. The last known location of a victim should be marked before launching the search and rescue effort. Subsequent topologic scanning for body parts or debris and probing or rescue-beacon searching should immediately ensue. If a limited number of rescuers are in an isolated location, all immediate efforts should be focused on victim location. If they are close to a phone or if there is rescuer surplus, then a makeshift contact team can be organized and sent quickly to notify a professional rescue team. Once victims are extricated, medical treatment should occur immediately.[12]

 ## MEDICAL TREATMENT OF CASUALTIES

Initial management of all avalanche victims should focus on the ABCs (airway, breathing, and circulation) of resuscitation. Immediate interment-site airway protection is critical; airway obstruction or respiratory arrest must be managed immediately using standard advanced cardiac life support (ACLS) guidelines. Due to potential cardiac instability, gentle handling of all hypothermic patients is mandatory.[13] Core temperature and electrocardiogram monitoring should commence as soon as qualified personnel are available. Core temperature monitoring is best achieved via esophageal or rectal measurement, although the less-reliable epitympanic method is an acceptable alternative.[13,14]

Prehospital assessment and treatment of hypothermia will likely be required for victims with prolonged burial (greater than 35 minutes). Assessment of hypothermia using the Swiss Society of Mountain Medicine guidelines can be performed by those with limited medical training and is based on the patient's mental status and presence or absence of shivering. In a patient who is alert and shivering, the core temperature is presumably between 32° to 35°C. Drowsiness and the absence of shivering are causes for concern, since this combination is symptomatic of a very low core body temperature (potentially as low as 28°C). If the temperature is less than this, the patient is likely to be unconscious and/or not breathing.[6,14,15]

Rapid triage of multiple victims is determined on-scene, with cessation of resuscitative efforts applied to appropriate patients. Death determination on-scene limits futile use of resources and limits risk to rescue teams during patient extrication. Burial time, presence or absence of a burial-site air pocket, and core body temperature are all used as death determination factors. All patients with a burial time of less than 35 minutes and/or a core body temperature greater than 32°C should undergo ACLS treatment with rapid hospital transfer. Death pronouncement can occur in asystolic patients with no evidence of an air pocket or presence of obvious airway obstruction, with a burial time greater than 35 minutes, and/or with a body temperature of less than 32°C. If there is any evidence of an air pocket, hospital transport should occur regardless of burial time. The receiving facility should have cardiopulmonary bypass capabilities, since this method of active internal rewarming has had the best success.[6,14,15]

Treatment of hypothermia should commence as soon as extrication occurs; the type of treatment will depend on available equipment and training level of on-site rescuers. Passive rewarming occurs through the removal of wet clothes; shielding from the wind; and application of blankets, aluminum foils, or bivouac bags. Initial warming procedures should be performed on all hypothermic patients and is commonly the only treatment required for patients who can shiver.[13] Active external rewarming occurs with heat packs applied to the trunk. Warm, sweet drinks should be provided to those who are conscious.[6,14,15] ACLS recommendations limit active external warming applications to the trunk area only, for fear of "afterdrop" hypothermia. Afterdrop hypothermia, caused by warming of the extremities, can lead to recirculation of cold peripheral blood to the central circulation system, culminating in a substantial decline in core body temperature.[13] Active internal rewarming in the field is best achieved through the use of warm, humidified oxygen. This can be achieved through either application of a mask or through endotracheal intubation.[6,14,15] Hospital treatment of severe hypothermia victims (less than 30°C by ACLS guidelines) should be more aggressive and includes warm intravenous fluids and warm lavage of the peritoneum, pleural cavity, and gastric mucosa with cardiopulmonary bypass being the ultimate goal. Internal rewarming should continue until the core temperature reaches 35°C or there is return of spontaneous circulation.[13]

Severely hypothermic patients with confirmed ventricular fibrillation should not receive any intravenous medications but should receive a maximum of three attempts at defibrillation. Intravenous medications and defibrillation are ineffective at this temperature. Once the core temperature reaches 30°C, normal ACLS protocols should be followed.[13] Serum potassium levels should be carefully monitored after avalanche burial because hyperkalemia is expected.[13] All resuscitation efforts should cease for patients with substantially prolonged burial times (greater than 35 minutes) and high serum potassium levels (greater than 12 mmol/L).

Although hypoxia and hypothermia usually prevail as initial treatment priorities, attention to other life threats should not be overlooked. Traumatic injuries should be assessed as previously discussed. In victims with obvious traumatic injuries, transport to a trauma center should occur per local protocols. In-hospital evaluation of these patients includes complete trauma and medical requirement assessments.

 ## UNIQUE CONSIDERATIONS

Hypothermic patients with prolonged burial in an oxygen-available tomb are potentially salvageable with active internal rewarming. Otherwise, resuscitative efforts among severely hypothermic patients or among patients with airway obstructions and burial times of greater than 35 minutes should cease.

 ## PITFALLS

- Inadequate avalanche training of backcountry explorers
- Improper rescue techniques
- Failure to preserve a victim's air pocket

Fourteen high school students, two mountain guides, and one parent were backcountry skiing in British Columbia's Glacier National Park during the winter of 2003. The skiing conditions were perfect with 2 feet of fresh powder on the 550-yard-wide trail.

The leaders, both avalanche-certified instructors, confirmed conditions for the day as being "moderate—natural avalanches are unlikely, but human triggers are possible." However, the area above their route was deemed to be at "considerable" avalanche risk.

While traveling, the group used the skills taught in their avalanche awareness and rescue courses—all paired skiers traveled 30 to 50 feet apart, and they routinely recited their rescue procedures. Each skier carried a shovel and a probe and wore an avalanche beacon.

At 11:45 AM, an 850-yard-wide avalanche came from above and buried most of the skiers. One of the freed members called for help on his satellite phone, and within 40 minutes, 10 rescuers were on-scene. Within 120 minutes, all members of the group were recovered, but seven of the students ultimately died.[16]

- Inappropriate triage of avalanche victims
- Inappropriate treatment of hypothermic patients

REFERENCES

1. Page CE, Atkins D, Shockley LW, Yaron M. Avalanche deaths in the United States: a 45-year analysis. *Wilderness Environ Med.* 1999;10(3):146-51.
2. Ammann WJ. Epidemiological trends in avalanche accidents [abstract]. *Wilderness Environ Med.* 2001;12(2):139.
3. Falk M, Brugger H, Adler-Kastner L. Avalanche survival chances. *Nature.* 1994;368(6466):21.
4. Radwin MI, Grissom CK. Technological advances in avalanche survival. *Wilderness Environ Med.* 2002;13(2):143-52.
5. Falk M, Brugger H, Adler-Kastner L. Calculation of survival as a function of avalanche burial [abstract]. *Wilderness Environ Med.* 2001;12(2):140-1.
6. Brugger H, Durrer B, Adler-Kastner L, Falk M, Tschirky F. Field management of avalanche victims. *Resuscitation.* 2001;51(1):7-15.
7. Grossman MD, Saffle JR, Thomas F, Tremper B. Avalanche trauma. *J Trauma.* 1989;29(12):1705-9.
8. Johnson SM, Johnson AC, Barton RG. Avalanche trauma and closed head injury: adding insult to injury. *Wilderness Environ Med.* 2001;12(4):244-7.
9. Stalsberg H, Albretsen C, Gilbert M, et al. Mechanism of death in avalanche victims. *Virchows Arch A Pathol Anat Histopathol.* 1989;414(5):415-22.
10. Radwin MI, Grissom CK, Scholand MB, Harmston CH. Normal oxygenation and ventilation during snow burial by the exclusion of exhaled carbon dioxide. *Wilderness Environ Med.* 2001;12(4):256-62.
11. Danzl DF, Pozos RS. Accidental hypothermia. *New Engl J Med.* 1994;331(26):1756-60.
12. Williams K, Armstrong BR, Armstrong BL. Avalanches. In: Auerbach PS, ed. *Disaster Medicine.* 4th ed. St Louis: Mosby; 2001:44-73.
13. American Heart Association. Part 8: advanced challenges in resuscitation. Section 3: special challenges in ECC 3A: hypothermia. *Resuscitation.* 2000;46(1-3):267-71.
14. Brugger H, Durrer B, International Commission for Mountain Emergency Medicine. On-site treatment of avalanche victims ICAR-MEDCOM-recommendation. *High Alt Med Biol.* 2002;3(4):421-5.
15. Brugger H, Durrer B, Adler-Kastner L. On-site triage of avalanche victims with asystole by the emergency doctor. *Resuscitation.* 1996;31(1):11-16.
16. Dohrmann G. A deadly avalanche. *SI Adventure*; February 17, 2003.

chapter 8 3

Introduction to Nuclear/Radiologic Disasters

Dale M. Molé

A familiarity with the medical aspects of nuclear or radiologic incidents is essential for any clinician in the 21st century. In addition to an increase in the number of nuclear power reactors around the world, the once unthinkable use of nuclear or radiologic devices against innocent noncombatants by terrorist groups or rogue nations may become reality in our lifetime. Underscoring this concern is the rampant proliferation of nuclear weapons technology within the Third World, the likelihood of stolen or black market tactical nuclear weapons from the former Soviet Union,[1] and the diversion of ubiquitous industrial and medical radioactive sources for nefarious uses.[2]

In the age of global terrorism, few things generate as much fear in the general public as radiation and its potential to produce painful death, malignant disease, or genetic mutations. Since radiation is undetectable by our normal senses, when used, its psychologic effectiveness to achieve sinister goals is enhanced. Public perceptions, or in most cases misperceptions, regarding the risk of even low-dose radiation exposure makes the use of radioactive materials a very effective terror weapon.

Few in the general public realize that we live in a world surrounded by natural radiation sources. Cosmic rays from outer space; radioactive minerals on Earth; and some radioactivity in food, water, and air provide the majority of radiation exposure we receive. Additional exposure may be the result of medical procedures (e.g., radiographs, nuclear medicine studies). Even the human body contains natural radioactive materials, such as carbon-14, potassium-40, and polonium-210.[3] With the exception of radon, found in excessive amounts in poorly ventilated dwellings in some parts of the United States, this low level of radiation has not been demonstrated to have any adverse clinical effects.

Radiation Physics

Radiation consists of either particles or electromagnetic waves, both of which deposit energy when interacting with matter. Radiation of sufficient energy to displace electrons from atoms, creating an ion and a free electron, is called *ionizing radiation. Particulate ionizing radiation* is made up of any atomic or subatomic particles, but the ones of clinical interest are alpha particles, beta particles, and neutrons. X-rays and gamma rays are types of *electromagnetic radiation* energetic enough to produce ionization. Less energetic forms of electromagnetic radiation (radiant heat, light, lasers, radio, microwaves) expend energy mainly in the form of heat when interacting with matter, but they do not produce ions; hence, these are classified as *nonionizing radiation*.

Matter consists of atoms. All atoms have a small central nucleus composed of protons (positive charge) and neutrons (no charge) that are surrounded by orbiting clouds of electrons (negative charge). The atomic number, unique for each element and descriptive of its particular physical and chemical characteristics, is equivalent to the number of protons in the nucleus (e.g., since hydrogen has one proton, its atomic number is 1). The atomic mass is essentially equivalent to the number of protons plus the number of neutrons (e.g., ordinary carbon has six protons [atomic number 6], but it has an atomic mass number of 12 (six protons plus six neutrons.) Since ordinary carbon-12 is electrically neutral, it has six orbital electrons. Atoms of the same element (the same number of protons) having different atomic mass (different numbers of neutrons) are called isotopes. The isotopes of hydrogen include hydrogen-2, or deuterium, with one proton and one neutron and hydrogen-3, or tritium, with one proton and two neutrons.

The forces between various components of the nucleus determine the stability of an atom. Neutrons appear to play an important role in binding protons together, with the ratio of protons to neutrons determining the stability of an atom. Too many or too few neutrons in the nucleus cause the atom to be unstable, which then decays or emits particles and/or energy to become more stable.

Alpha radiation consists of a helium nucleus (two protons and two neutrons). This relatively massive particle is only able to travel a short distance in air (1-2 cm) and is stopped by a sheet of paper or the top layer of skin. However, if inhaled or ingested, it can produce large exposures to internal organs.

Beta radiation is an electron emitted from an unstable nucleus. Beta particles penetrate deeper into tissue than alpha particles, but usually not beyond the few top layers of skin. They are completely absorbed by thin layers of glass, plastic, cloth, or metal foils. Beta particles of high energy can cause skin burns and are hazardous if ingested or inhaled.

Neutron radiation is produced when a neutron is emitted from the unstable nucleus of an atom, usually during nuclear fission in an atomic bomb or nuclear reactor. Being electrically neutral, neutrons are very penetrating and cause secondary beta and gamma radiation to be emitted when interacting with matter.

Gamma rays and *x-rays* are ionizing forms of electromagnetic radiation. Both are very penetrating and capable of delivering significant radiation doses to internal organs without ingestion or inhalation. Identical except for place of origin, gamma rays are emitted from an unstable nucleus, whereas x-rays originate from the outer electron shells of the atom.

The amount of ionizing radiation deposited in tissue or matter is called the *absorbed dose,* conventionally expressed in units of *radiation absorbed dose (rad).* The International System of Units for absorbed radiation is the gray (Gy). One gray is equal to 1 joule per kilogram and is equivalent to 100 rads.

The biologic effect produced by each type of ionizing radiation depends on the mass, electrical charge, and energy of the radiation. Hence, the same absorbed dose of one type of ionizing radiation can result in more or less biologic damage than the same absorbed dose of another type. This is because the *linear energy transfer,* or LET—the amount of energy deposited in a unit of track length—is different for different types of radiation. One gray of alpha radiation will result in more damage to cells than 1 gray of beta radiation. To standardize the tissue damage produced by the different types of radiation, we use a measure of equivalent biologic effects produced or equivalent dose. The absorbed dose multiplied by a quality factor produces an equivalent dose. The quality factor for most x-rays, gamma rays, and beta particles is 1, so the absorbed dose and equivalent dose are essentially equal. Alpha particles have a quality factor of 20, and neutrons have quality factors between 5 and 20, depending on their individual energies. Expressed in conventional units, rads multiplied by the quality factor for that particular type of radiation equals *radiation equivalent, man,* or *rem.* The international unit is the sievert (Sv). Since gamma radiation has a quality factor of one, 1 Gy (100 rad) of gamma radiation equals 1 Sv (100 rem).

Important factors in reducing radiation exposure are time, distance, and shielding. The absorbed dose is directly proportional to the length of time an individual is exposed and inversely proportional to the square of the distance from the radioactive source. Doubling the distance decreases the absorbed dose by a factor of four. The use of lead, concrete, or other shielding material significantly reduces or eliminates exposure.

Radioactivity decreases or decays with time. The *half-life* of a particular radioisotope is the length of time required for one-half of the radioactive material to decay or in most cases become nonradioactive. Some radioisotopes have half-lives of hours or days; others have half-lives of years or centuries. The decay rate can have an

important effect on medical management decisions regarding decontamination and/or treatment.

Biologic Effects

Ionizing radiation interacts with living cells by producing charged water molecules (i.e., free hydroxyl radicals) or by direct ionization of deoxyribonucleic acid. Clinical symptoms (acute radiation syndrome) occur if enough cells are damaged and die, or if the killed cells are essential for human survival. Rapidly dividing cells, such as bone marrow cells or the intestinal mucosa, are the most sensitive to radiation, whereas slowly dividing cells (e.g., central nervous system) are the most radio-resistant. Nonlethal radiation doses may cause some cells to undergo malignant transformation, leading to radiation-induced cancers years or decades after exposure.[4]

Nuclear or Radiologic Scenarios

History is replete with accidents involving radioactive materials. Fortunately, most involved exposure to only a few people. An exception was the Chernobyl incident in 1986 when reactor unit number four exploded, exposing the reactor core and dispersing radioactive material over a wide area. One hundred thirty-four people developed acute radiation syndrome, with 28 deaths directly related to radiation exposure. A dramatic increase in thyroid cancers among those who were either very young or in utero at the time of exposure has been noted.[5]

Occasionally, individuals without criminal intent can create radiologic hazards for themselves and the community. Such was the case of David Hahn, the "radioactive Boy Scout," who attempted to build a breeder reactor in his backyard shed and ended up causing an expensive Environmental Protection Agency cleanup as well as terrifying his neighbors.

Terrorist groups such as Aum Shinri Kyo and Al-Qaeda, as well as state sponsors of terrorism, have tried to acquire radiologic/nuclear material and technology. The father of the Pakistani atomic bomb, A.Q. Khan, peddled nuclear weapon expertise to many rogue nations and terror organizations.[7]

In addition to Third World countries or terror groups trying to develop a nuclear weapons program beginning with uranium ore,[8] an expensive and technologically intensive undertaking, there are other more likely nuclear or radiologic scenarios:

- Using radioactive materials to fabricate a radiation emission device (RED), or the detonation of a radiologic dispersion device (RDD) (i.e., "dirty bomb")[9]
- Sabotage of nuclear facilities (e.g., nuclear power plants) with the subsequent release of large amounts of radioactivity[10]
- The detonation of an improvised nuclear device made from fissile material acquired by theft or purchased[11]
- The detonation of an intact nuclear weapon acquired by theft or on the black market[12]

An RED irradiates passersby with high levels of radiation. Such a device is highly radioactive and poses a significant threat to those who place it. It therefore requires some degree of sophistication to safely construct and deploy. A device using "induced criticality" could expose those nearby to lethal doses of neutron radiation and gamma rays in just moments.[13]

RDDs are often referred to as weapons of mass *disruption* since their psychologic and economic effects far outweigh the physical damage to life or property.[14] The so-called dirty bomb consists of radioactive material surrounding or mixed in a conventional explosive. Those injured by blast effects from the explosion are contaminated by the radioactive material, as are the rescue workers.

The accidental contamination of the village of Goiânia, Brazil, in 1987 from an orphaned cancer radiotherapy source provides an insight to the consequences of an RDD. Junkyard workers broke open the lead shielding surrounding a medical radioactive source and exposed the 20-g cesium-137 chloride capsule. Soon afterward, 13 people became ill and sought medical care. Four people died. By the time authorities discovered what had happened, 249 people were affected by radiation and thousands more rushed to emergency departments fearing contamination. Economic damage as a result of clean-up ran into the millions of dollars—6000 tons of clothing, furniture, soil, and other materials had to be packed into steel drums and buried in an abandoned quarry.[15]

A nuclear reactor accident (e.g., Chernobyl) or sabotage remains an ongoing concern. In August 2003, 19 individuals were arrested for plotting to destroy a nuclear power plant on the shore of Lake Ontario, Canada. The method of attack used on Sept. 11, 2001, raised concerns that terrorists could use a commercial airliner as a guided missile against a nuclear power plant. A study produced for the Nuclear Energy Institute using the Boeing 767-400 as the attacking aircraft suggests that the reactor containment building, as well as irradiated fuel storage facilities, would survive a direct impact.[16]

A nuclear weapon detonation is the ultimate terrorist nightmare. The destructive effects from a nuclear explosion include widespread blast effects, burns from the initial flash and burning debris, and ionizing radiation from the fission process initially, followed by radioactive fallout. It has been estimated that a 10-kiloton weapon detonated at Grand Central Station in Manhattan would kill 500,000 people immediately, injure hundreds of thousands more, force the evacuation of all of Manhattan, and result in direct economic damage of well over $1 trillion.

Terrorists may achieve a nuclear detonation by obtaining highly enriched uranium (HEU) and constructing a crude atomic bomb (improvised nuclear device [IND]). Many experts believe that a technologically sophisticated terrorist group could construct a nuclear weapon from HEU without state support. A plutonium bomb is much more difficult to construct and probably exceeds the abilities of substate organizations. Given the cost and complexity of a nuclear materials enrichment program, making a bomb from uranium ore is not currently feasible for a substate organization. Of concern, however, is the 130 research nuclear reactors around the world using HEU in the reactor core, many with minimal security and vulnerable to theft.

Nuclear fission is the process underlying the explosive power of an atomic bomb. When atoms of a fissile material (e.g., uranium-235 [U-235] or plutonium-239 [Pu-239]) absorb a neutron, they split or fission into two atoms of roughly equal mass, producing enormous amounts of energy, as well as additional neutrons that cause other atoms to fission. If enough fissile material is present (i.e., *critical mass*), a *chain reaction* will progress at a geometric rate, resulting in the liberation of tremendous quantities of energy in the form of heat, light, and radiation. The critical mass required for a self-sustaining chain reaction is a function of the shape, density, and type of fissile material. By surrounding the bomb core with a neutron reflector or tamper, the amount of material required to reach critical mass is significantly reduced. The critical mass for a bare sphere of U-235 is 56 kg, but with a thick tamper, this is reduced to about 15 kg. For Pu-239, critical mass is 11 kg and 5 kg, respectively.

Since the critical mass of a particular fissile material decreases as the density increases by an inverse square relationship, an implosion device requires much less material than one using a gun-assembly method.

Fission weapons require the "assembly" of a supercritical mass from a subcritical mass to occur in a very short period; otherwise, the weapon is blown apart before significant amounts of material have undergone fission, significantly lowering the yield. There are two classical assembly methods—gun and implosion (Fig. 83-1). Gun assembly is useful only for U-235 and involves firing a subcritical projectile of U-235 into a subcritical target of U-235 to create a supercritical mass. This is the easiest type of atomic bomb to make and did not even require testing before operational use over Hiroshima, Japan.[17]

An implosion device uses high explosives to create an inwardly directed shock wave that compresses a sphere of fissile material, increasing density to supercritical levels. Although very efficient, it requires much more sophisticated technology since the explosive "lenses" must detonate at exactly the same instant to produce a nuclear explosion. Also, a neutron generator emits a burst of neutrons to initiate the chain reaction at the point of maximum compression.[18]

Russia has many tactical nuclear weapons that are more widely dispersed and not as well guarded as strategic weapons. With the dissolution of the Soviet Union, there is uncertainty regarding the whereabouts of every weapon. It is not known whether any were sold on the black market, and if so, whether they remain fully functional.

HISTORICAL PERSPECTIVE

X-rays were first discovered in 1895 by Wilhelm Roentgen while experimenting with cathode ray tubes and were used in medical diagnosis only a few months later. The following year, Henri Becquerel, while conducting some experiments with uranium salts, discovered radioactivity.[19] The danger of this mysterious new force was not fully appreciated. Initially, radiation was viewed as healthy, perhaps because of the small

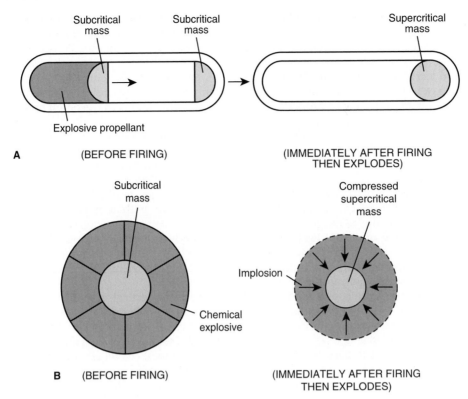

FIGURE 83–1. Principles of gun-assembly **(A)** and implosion-type **(B)** nuclear devices.

amounts of radium and radon detected in waters in the health spas of Europe. Despite some evidence of the harmful effects of excessive radiation, such as the deep skin burns to those scientific pioneers who handled unsealed radioactive sources, radioactive material was added to everything from toothpaste to drinking water in an effort to provide a healthful, stimulating effect. Shoe salesmen used portable x-ray machines to check shoe fit. Radium was painted on tonsils and adenoids to reduce the size of lymphoid tissue. Radium was also used together with surgery to provide the "Curie therapy" for cancer patients before the development of effective chemotherapy.

With the discovery of nuclear fission by Otto Hahn, Lise Meitner, and O.R. Frisch in 1939 came the realization that this process could be used to make a bomb.[20] On Dec. 2, 1942, Enrico Fermi succeeded in creating the world's first self-sustaining nuclear chain reaction under the squash courts at the University of Chicago. During the World War II, both Germany[21] and Japan[22] pursued atomic bomb development. The world changed forever on July 16, 1945, with the detonation of the atomic bomb in the New Mexico desert.[23]

The following month, World War II ended with the use of atomic weapons on Hiroshima and Nagasaki, Japan. The pictures of the devastation in Japan helped shape public perception regarding the dangers of radiation. This was further enhanced by decades of science fiction movies and anti-nuclear literature. Movie images, from giant ants and humans to reactor cores melting through the Earth or melting flesh from bones, convinced many in the general public that any amount of radiation is an immediate threat to life.

CURRENT PRACTICE

External irradiation is the exposure of the entire body or just a part of it to an external source of penetrating radiation. Unless exposed to high-intensity neutron radiation, a patient is not radioactive from external irradiation and no special protective measures are required of medical personnel.

Acute radiation syndrome (ARS) is the primary threat to life after exposure to major doses of radiation.[24] The diagnosis of ARS is based on a history of exposure and clinical findings (Table 83-1). ARS occurs when the entire body is exposed to a large dose of penetrating external radiation over a short period. There are three classic acute radiation syndromes.

Bone marrow, or hematopoietic, syndrome usually occurs with doses higher than 2 Sv (200 rem), depending on the premorbid state of health. Destruction or depression of the bone marrow produces a pancytopenia, resulting in increased susceptibility to infection and clotting abnormalities. As long as the bone marrow is not completely destroyed, granulocyte stimulating factors may enhance regeneration.

Gastrointestinal syndrome occurs with doses greater than 6 Sv (600 rem). Cell death and sloughing of the intestinal mucosa result initially in nausea, vomiting, and diarrhea. Since gastrointestinal symptoms coincide with

TABLE 83-1 ACUTE RADIATION SYNDROME

1 Gray (Gy) = 100 rads   1 centiGray (cGy) = 1 rad

WHOLE BODY RADIATION FROM EXTERNAL RADIATION OR INTERNAL ABSORPTION

Phase of syndrome	Feature	Subclinical range		Sublethal range		Lethal range	
		0 – 100 rad or cGy	100-200 rad 1-2 Gy	200-600 rad 2-6 Gy	600-800 rad 6-8 Gy	800-3000 rad 8-30 Gy	>3000 rad >30 Gy
Prodromal phase	Nausea, vomiting	None	5%-50%	50%-100%	75%-100%	90%-100%	100%
	Time of onset		3-6 hr	2-4 hr	1-2 hr	<1 hr	Minutes
	Duration		<24 hr	<24 hr	<48 hr	<48 hr	N/A
	Lymphocyte count	Unaffected	Minimally decreased	<1000 at 24 hr	<500 at 24 hr	Decreases within hours	Decreases within hours
	CNS function	No impairment	No impairment	Cognitive impairment for 6-20 hr	Cognitive impairment for >24 hr	Rapid incapacitation, often after a lucid period of up to several hours	
Latent phase (subclinical)	Absence of symptoms	>2 wks	7-15 days	0-7 days	0-2 days	None	
Acute radiation illness or "manifest illness" phase	Signs and symptoms	None	Moderate leukopenia	Severe leukopenia, purpura, hemorrhage Pneumonia Hair loss after 300 rad/3 Gy	Diarrhea, fever, electrolyte disturbance	Diarrhea, fever, electrolyte disturbance	Convulsions, ataxia, tremor, lethargy
	Time of onset	None		2 days to 2 wks		1-3 days	
	Critical period	None	>2 wks	4-6 wks: Most potential for effective medical intervention		2-14 days	1-48 hr
	Organ system	None		Hematopoietic and respiratory (mucosal) systems		GI tract Mucosal systems	CNS
Hospitalization	% Duration	0	<5%	90%	100%	100%	100%
			45-60 days	60-90 days	90+ days	Weeks to months	Days to weeks
Mortality		None	Minimal	Low with aggressive therapy	High	Very high, significant neurologic symptoms indicate lethal dose	

From Armed Forces Radiobiology Research Institute. Available at: http://www.afrri.usuhs.mil/www/outreach/pdf/pcktcard.pdf.

hematologic abnormalities, dehydration, electrolyte imbalances, and sepsis are part of the natural disease course. Severe bloody diarrhea is an ominous sign.

Cardiovascular (CV)/central nervous system (CNS) syndrome occurs with doses exceeding 20 Sv (2000 rem). The almost immediate nausea, vomiting, ataxia, and convulsions are the result of diffuse microvascular leaks in the central nervous system, causing edema and increased intracranial pressure. Cardiovascular collapse from a transient post-irradiation vasodilation has been observed.[25]

ARS progresses through the following four clinical phases:

- *The prodromal phase* occurs within hours of exposure and may last for up to 2 days. Symptoms are a function of the total radiation absorbed dose and include anorexia, nausea, vomiting, diarrhea, fatigue, fever, respiratory distress, and agitation. Treatment should be symptomatic.
- *The latent phase* is a transitional period in which the patient is asymptomatic. This may last as long as 3 weeks, but is much shorter with higher radiation exposures.
- *The illness phase* produces overt clinical manifestations, including infection as a result of leukopenia, bleeding from thrombocytopenia, diarrhea, electrolyte imbalances, altered mental status, and shock.
- *The death or recovery phase* often occurs over weeks or months.

The clinical phases of ARS are related to cell reproduction, with the fastest-dividing cells affected earliest. The time of onset after exposure of general signs and symptoms related to the hematopoietic and gastrointestinal systems are good markers for prognosis. After exposure, a shorter time until symptom onset is associated with a poorer prognosis.

A more specific indicator is the absolute lymphocyte count (ALC). A 50% drop in lymphocytes at 24 hours postexposure is indicative of significant radiation injury.[26] At 48 hours postexposure, if the ALC is greater than 1200, the patient likely received a nonlethal dose. An ALC between 300 and 1200 indicates significant exposure and the need for hospitalization. If the ALC is less than 300, the patient is critically ill and should be considered for colony-stimulating factors. The ALC may be an unreliable indicator in a patient with combined injuries.

Cutaneous radiation syndrome (CRS) is the constellation of symptoms resulting from acute exposure to beta radiation or x-rays. This can occur when radioactive isotopes contaminate the patient's clothes or skin. Although similar in appearance to thermal burns, radiation burns may take several days to appear. Dermal changes can help estimate the dose of radiation received, so it is important to observe for signs of erythema, pain, blister formation, and necrosis. Sequelae from CRS include vascular insufficiency developing months or years after exposure and causing necrosis or ulceration of previously healed tissue, and sometimes requiring hyperbaric oxygen therapy, plastic surgery, or amputation. Because of radiation's effect on dividing cells, if a radiation patient requires emergency surgery, it

should be done within the first 24 to 48 hours after the radiation injury; otherwise, the surgery should be delayed for 3 months.

Radioactive contamination occurs if radioactive materials are deposited internally, externally, or both. Patients can be radioactive and require decontamination when radioisotopes are inhaled, ingested, or deposited in wounds. *Incorporation* occurs if radioactive materials are taken up by cells and incorporated into tissues or organs.

Effective treatment of internal contamination requires knowledge of the type and chemical form of the radioisotope. The goal is to hasten elimination and prevent incorporation. This is accomplished by reducing absorption (with Prussian blue in the case of cesium), by using dilution techniques (forcing fluids with tritium), chelation (plutonium), or through the use of blocking agents (potassium iodide for radioactive iodine).

External contamination is not usually a medical emergency. Simply removing clothing will eliminate 90% of the contamination. Water and detergent effectively remove skin contamination. Uncontaminated wounds should be covered before decontamination. Contaminated wounds should be treated conventionally with pressurized normal saline irrigation. Residual radioactivity often comes off with dressing changes, in exudates, or with the eschar. If the wound remains contaminated with long-lived radioisotopes, wound excision should be considered. All contaminated clothing and materials should be placed in labeled plastic bags for proper disposal.

Successfully treating radioactive-contaminated injured people requires teamwork and practice. In addition to the usual emergency medicine personnel, the hospital health physicist or radiation safety officer is essential, both for assistance in conducting surveys of the patient with radiation detection equipment and in providing additional advice regarding decontamination. Emergency department patient decontamination and treatment exercises should occur at least annually to ensure proper decontamination technique, reinforce appropriate treatment priorities, and provide familiarity with radiation detection equipment and personal dosimeters.

It is likely that patients will present with mixed injuries (i.e., trauma combined with significant radiation exposure or contamination). Evaluate, resuscitate, and stabilize the patient before completing decontamination.

Triage decisions based on radiation exposure can be difficult when there are large numbers of casualties since the individual exposure is unknown. Early onset of ARS symptoms portends a poor outcome. The Armed Forces Radiobiology Research Institute has a Biodosimetry Assessment Tool (BAT) available for download at its Web site.

Surgeons operating on irradiated patients should consider them to be immunocompromised. Impaired wound healing, as well as fluid balance, electrolyte, and clotting abnormalities, should be expected. The earlier the patient is operated on after exposure, the better. If operations are performed early, surgical wounds should be in the healing phase when the immune system is at its nadir. Because of the high potential for sepsis, wound debridement must be meticulous.[27] Prophylactic antibiotics should be considered for any patient with combined injuries of radiation exposure, burns, and classical trauma, and should be continued until the absolute neutrophil count rises above 500 and the patient is afebrile for at least 24 hours. The use of hematopoietic growth factors shortens the duration of neutropenia and should be started as soon as significant radiation exposure is identified.

 PITFALLS

- Failure to treat life-threatening injuries or stabilize a patient because of concern regarding radioactive contamination on clothing or skin
- Failure to plan, train, and exercise the emergency management of radiologic events
- Lack of personal dosimetry equipment for medical workers
- Poor decontamination skills
- Failure to set and monitor radiation boundaries to prevent the spread of contamination throughout the hospital
- Failure to provide timely and appropriate risk communication regarding the hazards of radiation exposure

RESOURCES

Armed Forces Radiobiology Research Institute (AFRRI). Available at: http://www.afrri.usuhs.mil.

Radiation Emergency Assistance Center/Training Site (REAC/TS). Available at: http://www.orau.gov/reacts.

Centers for Disease Control and Prevention. Available at: http://www.bt.cdc.gov.

REFERENCES

1. Sokov N, Potter W. *"Suitcase Nukes": A Reassessment*. Monterey, Calif: Monterey Center for Nonproliferation Studies; 2004.
2. Wald M. Uranium reactors on campus raise security concerns. *New York Times*. August 15, 2004. http://ucnuclearfree.org/articles/2004/08/15_wald_uranium-reactors-campus.htm
3. Ford J. *Radiation, People and the Environment*. Vienna: International Atomic Energy Agency; 2004.
4. Mettler F, Upton A. *Medical Effects of Ionizing Radiation*. Philadelphia: WB Saunders; 1995.

5. Gusev I, Guskova A, Mettler F. *Medical Management of Radiation Accidents*. Boca Raton, Fla: CRC Press; 2001.
6. Silverstein K. *The Radioactive Boy Scout*. New York: Random House; 2004.
7. Ferguson C, Potter W. *The Four Faces of Nuclear Terrorism*. Monterey, Calif: Monterey Center for Nonproliferation Studies; 2004.
8. Bhatia S, McGrory D. *Brighter Than the Baghdad Sun*. Washington, DC: Regnery Publishing; 2000.
9. Edwards R. Risk of radioactive "dirty bomb" growing. *New Scientist*. June 2004. Available at: http://www.newscientist.com/article.ns?id=dn5061.
10. Brown D. Canada arrests 19 as security threats. *Washington Post*. August 23, 2003, page A20.
11. Mark JC, Taylor T, Eyster E, Maraman W, Wechsler J. Can terrorists build nuclear weapons? In: Leventhal P, Alexander Y, eds. *Preventing Nuclear Terrorism*. Lexington, Mass: Lexington Books; 1987.
12. Alexander B, Millar A. *Tactical Nuclear Weapons*. Washington: Brassey's; 2003.
13. Mettler F, Voelz G, et al. Criticality accidents. In: Gusev I, Guskova A, Mettler FA, eds. *Medical Management of Radiation Accidents*. Boca Raton, Fla: CRC Press; 2001
14. Levi M, Kelly H. Weapons of mass disruption. *Scientific American*. November 2002. pages 77-81, http://www.fas.org/resource/03212005140554.pdf
15. O'Neill K. *The Nuclear Terrorist Threat*. Washington, DC: Institute for Science and International Security; 1997.
16. Hardy G, Arros J, Merz K. *Aircraft Crash Impact Analyses Demonstrate Nuclear Power Plant's Structural Strength*. San Diego: ABS Consulting/ANATECH; 2002.
17. Henriksen P, Westfall C. Critical Assemblies and Nuclear Physics. In: Hoddeson L, Henriksen PW, Meade RA, Westfall CL, eds. *Critical Assembly: A Technical History of Los Alamos During the Oppenheimer Years, 1943-1945*. New York: Cambridge University Press; 1993.
18. Serber V. *The Los Alamos Primer: The First Lectures on How to Build an Atom Bomb*. Berkeley: University of California Press; 1992.
19. Sacks O. *Uncle Tungsten*. New York: Alfred A. Knopf; 2001.
20. Hahn O. From the natural transmutations of uranium to its artificial fission. Nobel Lecture. December 13, 1946; Stockholm. Available at: http://nobelprize.org/chemistry/laureates/1944/hahn-lecture.pdf.
21. Irving D. *The German Atomic Bomb*. New York: Da Capo Press; 1967.
22. Wilcox R. *Japan's Secret War*. New York: William Morrow & Company; 1985.
23. Rhodes R. *The Making of the Atomic Bomb*. New York: Simon and Schuster; 1986.
24. Mettler F, Voelz G. Major radiation exposure—what to expect and how to respond. *New Engl J Med*. 2002;346(20):1554-61.
25. Hawkins R, Cockerham L. Postirradiation cardiovascular dysfunction. In: Conklin J, Walker R, eds. *Military Radiobiology*. San Diego: Academic Press; 1987.
26. Jarrett D. *Medical Management of Radiological Casualties*. Bethesda, Md: Armed Forces Radiobiology Research Institute; 1999.
27. Eiseman B, Bond V. Surgical care of nuclear casualties. *Surg Gynecol Obstet*. 1978;146:877-83.

chapter 84

Ionizing Radiation Incident

Carrie Barton

DESCRIPTION OF EVENT

Exposure to significant levels of radiation is a rare occurrence but an everyday possibility. It can occur through occupational exposure at a medical facility or among persons processing nuclear materials or waste. Other sources include a nuclear power plant reactor core accident, a nuclear weapon detonation, a dirty bomb, or radioactive material placed accidentally or intentionally in an area exposing the public. It is important to understand the different types of radiation to understand the ways it affects the body.

Ionizing radiation includes alpha and beta particles, x-rays and gamma rays, and neutrons. Alpha particles are composed of two protons and two neutrons, are relatively large, and are easily stopped; colliding with matter causes them to lose their energy. A single piece of paper has enough density to stop them, as does the epidermis of the skin. Because they give up their energy over a very short distance, they have the most potential to cause damage, but because they are stopped easily before reaching the dermis, they are not a significant source of injury unless exposure is through broken skin, inhalation, or ingestion.[1,2] Examples of alpha emitters are uranium, plutonium, americium (found in smoke detectors), and radon (a naturally occurring gas and the major source of natural radiation exposure).[3]

Beta radiation is composed of electron-like particles. They are much smaller, will travel about 1 meter through air, and can penetrate 1 to 2 cm into human tissue. They are stopped by higher-density material, such as a few millimeters of aluminum.[1,2] Beta particles can cause severe local damage to the dermal tissue as well as areas of bony prominence, such as the wrist and hands; these particles also can cause bone necrosis. Morbidity from beta radiation skin injury is proportional to the body surface area affected, similar to thermal burns. Examples of beta emitters are nuclear fallout, tritium (used in emergency lighting, gauges, and nuclear weapons), and radiostrontium (produced in nuclear reactors).[4]

X-rays and gamma rays are, like sunlight, a form of electromagnetic radiation composed of photons, which have no mass or electrical charge. They are generated during a fission reaction but are primarily encountered in medical use.

Both gamma radiation and x-rays travel several meters and are not stopped by human tissue. They require 5 cm of lead to be stopped.[5] They result in whole body irradiation and are associated with acute radiation syndrome. Sources of gamma radiation include radiocesium, which is a by-product in nuclear fuel and is often used as a radiation source for medical treatments. Radiocesium is considered likely to be used in a "dirty bomb" due to its abundant use as a source.[2]

Neutrons are released during nuclear fission, such as in a criticality device, a nuclear reactor, or a nuclear detonation. They are very penetrating and pass through the body, where they collide with other atomic nuclei, causing them to become unstable and therefore radioactive, giving off alpha and beta particles and gamma rays. Although gamma irradiation alone does not render a person or object radioactive, a survivor of a neutron exposure would be rendered only minimally radioactive and would not present a great enough threat to prevent appropriate healthcare intervention.[6]

PREINCIDENT ACTIONS

Local hazardous materials (HazMat) teams should have the ability to detect radiation. Hospitals should also have access to real-time detection equipment, such as Geiger counters, in the event patients present with a reported exposure. Remember that most detectors do not detect alpha radiation. If the equipment is not kept in the emergency department, arrangements should be made beforehand to have 24-hour access to devices used elsewhere in the hospital. The hospital's radiation safety officer should be on call in a hospital's disaster plan for any known radiation exposure or for any intentional explosion until a "dirty bomb" scenario is ruled out. Planning to be able to decontaminate mass numbers of patients is similar to chemical decontamination; however, emergency intervention should be done before decontamination when indicated.[6]

POSTINCIDENT ACTIONS

There are four types of radiation exposure: (1) irradiation, (2) external contamination, (3) internal contamination, and (4) incorporation. In the event of a "dirty bomb" or detonation, patients may have both trauma injuries and radiation exposure; don't forget to use standard trauma assessment and intervention.[7] Radiologic injury is always of secondary importance to traumatic injury.

Irradiated patients pose no hazard to healthcare workers or other patients. Patients suspected of any type of contamination should be treated with contact and respiratory precautions and examined with radiation detection equipment. This should ideally be managed by the radiation safety officer. For patients with a stable condition who are awaiting decontamination of particulate matter (e.g., from a "dirty bomb" or possible fallout exposure), it is advised to take swabs of the ears and nares before decontamination for later testing to help confirm the exposure.

Healthcare providers should take respiratory precautions when treating a person externally contaminated with radioactive dust. Patients should avoid making airborne any particulate dust to prevent inhalation. This is especially important during removal of clothing. There must be no eating or drinking in the contamination area, and all patients and healthcare workers must be decontaminated and screened with detection equipment before entering the clean area. If necessary, the emergency room can be divided into a clean area and a dirty area. If so, plastic and/or sheets should be taped in place on the floor and on frequently used door handles etc. to prevent long-term contamination of the facility.

Clothing should be removed and saved for further testing to determine presence, type, and quantity of exposure and for evidence, if indicated. Patients should be washed with soap and water before entry into the hospital when possible. Plastic bags for clothing and temporary garments for patients (e.g., paper scrubs, sheets) should be available. Runoff water from decontamination must be collected with the same priority used with chemical contaminants.[4]

Healthcare providers should only use instruments to remove radioactive shrapnel because touching the material could result in severe local damage to their hands. All material removed during contamination should be saved and stored behind shielding or away from persons. If a patient has radioactive shrapnel that cannot be immediately removed and he or she requires immediate care for another life-threatening illness, lead shields may be placed over the affected area and patient care initiated before full decontamination.

Internal contamination occurs after swallowing or inhaling radioactive material and allows radiation to contact the gastrointestinal endothelial lining and respiratory parenchyma. Although alpha radiation is relatively benign when shielded by the epidermis, because it gives up its energy over a very short distance, when unshielded, alpha particles cause severe damage. Radioactive shrapnel can cause deep tissue radiation damage and prolonged exposure to radiation. The decision to remove radioactive shrapnel must balance long-term risk against aggressive surgical morbidity.

Radioactive material may be incorporated into the body after internal contamination from inhaled or swallowed radioactive particulate matter. If ingested or inhaled, it has the potential to be absorbed and deposited in vital organs, or absorbed into macrophages and deposited in lymph nodes. This incorporated radioactive material can damage organ tissue over time. If this is not accompanied by more serious injuries, it is usually concerning as a cause of increased long-term cancer rates and not acute illness. Many sources of radiation are more concerning for their heavy metal components and toxicity than for their radiation effects.

Radiation causes two clinical syndromes: cutaneous radiation syndrome (caused by local tissue damage, usually due to alpha or, more likely, beta radiation) and acute radiation syndrome (ARS) (caused by whole body radiation, usually due to gamma radiation). Both of these have delayed presentations and are characterized by four stages: the prodrome, a latent asymptomatic stage, the manifest illness stage, and finally death or a period of recovery. The rapidity of progression through these stages is directly related to the severity of the exposure. The presence of burns without a known thermal or chemical exposure or the presence of immune suppression without a cause (especially associated with acute onset of general alopecia) should prompt consideration of an occult radiation exposure.

Cutaneous radiation syndrome is caused by localized damage to the basilar layer of the dermis, which leads to blistering. The vascular tissue is often destroyed, causing delayed necrosis. During the prodrome, which occurs hours after the exposure,[2] persons may notice redness or itching of the affected area. During the latent phase, there are no symptoms, and the affected skin appears normal. This phase may last minutes to weeks, depending on the severity of the exposure.[2] The manifest illness phase is characterized by local hair loss, blistering, and necrosis as the dermal tissue dies without adequate vascular supply. There may be underlying bone necrosis as well. Hair loss is expected to occur about 17 to 21 days after exposure.[2] There may be dry desquamation (peeling of the skin) or wet desquamation (blisters and bullae). Desquamation may occur within hours or up to 2 to 4 weeks after exposure. Necrosis can develop in days to months.

ARS is caused by whole body radiation and affects stem cells with high mitotic rates first (particularly the hematopoietic cells of the bone marrow, the endothelial microvilli of the small intestine, spermatogenesis, and hair follicles), leading to many of the clinical features.[3] Lymphocytes are the most radiosensitive cell in the body and are used to estimate the dose of radiation received.[1,7] Both the acute and cutaneous radiation syndromes may simultaneously be manifest.

The prodromal phase is characterized by gastrointestinal symptoms—nausea, vomiting, and diarrhea. Onset of ARS can be minutes to weeks after exposure, can last for minutes to days, and can be episodic. Onset within 2 hours indicates a life-threatening exposure, although other causes of nausea and vomiting should be considered. Persons may appear healthy during the latent period, which may last 2 to 3 weeks, but after extremely high radiation doses, this phase may be minimal. The manifest illness includes up to three syndromes and lasts days to months. Fatal infectious complications usually occur during the initial 2 to 3 months. Full recovery will require weeks and potentially up to 2 years.

The three types of manifest illness in ARS are (1) bone marrow, (2) gastrointestinal, and (3) cardiovascular/central nervous syndrome. The signs and symptoms are based on the amount of damage done, with different organ systems being variably sensitive. Bone marrow is the most sensitive, and medically significant doses will cause marrow suppression only. Higher doses will cause damage to the gastrointestinal lining as well, and very high doses result in all three constellations of signs and symptoms. Bone marrow symptoms are caused by the pancytopenia that follows irradiation and is marked by severe anemia and immunosuppression. Neutrophil counts drop after 2 to 4 days, but thrombocytopenia can take 2 to 4 weeks to be seen.[8] There may be a misleading transient initial period of thrombocytosis after exposure. If fatal, death usually occurs within a few months and usually due to infection and hemorrhage.[1]

Radiation exposures severe enough to cause gastrointestinal damage are usually fatal, and death may occur within 2 weeks. Damage to the intestinal villi leads to endothelial sloughing, diarrhea, hemorrhage, malabsorption, and opportunistic infections as bacteria transit the intestinal lining concomitant with immune suppression. Death is due to dehydration, infection, and/or electrolyte imbalances. Very severe exposures can cause nervousness, confusion, severe nausea and vomiting, convulsions, and coma. Death due to cardiovascular/central nervous system damage occurs within 3 days.

MEDICAL TREATMENT OF CASUALTIES

Decontaminate patients if indicated. Remember that irradiated patients are not radioactive and do not require decontamination. Decontamination can be postponed in patients with trauma or burn injuries or medical disorders requiring emergent intervention. Collect swabs from patients with a stable condition before decontamination. In a mass casualty situation, remember to transfer patients with a stable condition early so that resources will remain for new patients and those whose condition is not stable for transfer. Mortality increases dramatically when surgeries are performed more than 48 hours after whole body irradiation injury. It is important that all surgeries be performed during this window, or delayed up to 3 months. For patients with internal contamination and incorporation, bodily fluids may contain traces of radioactive isotopes.

In a mass casualty scenario, analgesia and antiemetics may be the only appropriate treatment for patients with fatal exposures or major trauma. Patients with absolute lymphocyte counts less than 1000/mm^3 12 to 24 hours after exposure will eventually require reverse isolation

and will likely not survive. For patients whose radiation exposure is amenable to treatment, several interventions are appropriate. Trauma injuries should be addressed rapidly, and radiation skin injury may initially be treated similar to thermal burns. Prophylactic antibiotics are controversial but should be considered. Bone marrow stimulation may be helpful. Pulmonary contamination may require pulmonary lavage, but this should be discussed with an expert in treatment of radiation injuries before implementation and is not an emergency. Shrapnel and other foreign bodies may require debridement, but destructive surgery for removal is not indicated. Depleted uranium fragments have been left in numerous persons who have had close monitoring without complications.[9]

Patients whose condition is stable and who are without symptoms should have baseline laboratory samples drawn, including blood, urea, nitrogen; creatinine; complete blood count; and urinalysis. They may then be discharged home with arrangements made to have their 24- to 48-hour postexposure lymphocyte count checked and are to be instructed to seek immediate care for any symptoms of acute radiation sickness or cutaneous radiation syndrome.

Although patients presenting with radiation pose little risk to healthcare workers, pregnant healthcare workers should not participate in their treatment, and other healthcare workers should rotate out often to minimize the exposure to any contaminated individual. Ideally, providers will receive dosimeters from their radiation safety officer to ensure no provider gets an exposure above occupational safety guidelines. Because radiation exposure is such a rare occurrence, management should include prompt consult of the Radiation Emergency Assistance Center/Training Site (REAC/TS).[10]

 ## PITFALLS

- Make sure the radiation detection equipment has working batteries!
- Any noise from the detection equipment will alarm patients; do not turn the equipment's sound on unless headphones are used.
- Make sure a baseline radiation level is checked remote from those potentially contaminated to prevent a false elevation determination.
- Scanning too quickly will fail to detect radiation, so go slow.
- Geiger counters do not detect alpha radiation.

REFERENCES

1. Tucci M, Camporesi E. Risks and effects of radiation terrorism. *Semin Anesth Perioperative Med Pain.* 2003;22(4).
2. Leikin J, McFee R, Walter F, Edsall K. A primer for nuclear terrorism. *Disease-A-Month.* 2003;49(8).
3. Upton A. Radiation injury. In: Goldman L, Bennett JC, eds. *Cecil Textbook of Medicine.* 21st ed. Philadelphia: WB Saunders; 2000:62-8.
4. Smith J, Spano M, et al. *Interim Guidelines for Hospital Response to Mass Casualties from a Radiological Incident.* Atlanta: Centers for Disease Control and Prevention, Department of Health and Human Services; 2003.

5. Rutherford M, Seward J. Radiation injuries and illnesses in pediatric emergency medicine. *Clin Pediatr Emerg Med.* 2001;2(3).

6. Reeves G. Radiation injuries. *Crit Care Clin.* 1999;15(2):457-73.

7. Markovchick V. Radiation injuries. In: Marx J, Hockberger R, Walls R, eds. *Rosen's Emergency Medicine: Concepts and Clinical Practice.* 5th ed. St. Louis: Mosby; 2002:2055-63.

8. Dainiak N. Hematologic consequences of exposure to ionizing radiation. *Exp Hematol.* 2002;30(6):513-28.

9. Lee H, Gabriel R, Bolton P. Depleted uranium—is it really a health issue? *Lancet Oncol.* 2001;2(4):197.

10. Radiation Emergency Assistance Center/Training Site. Available at: http://www.orau.gov/reacts.

Nuclear Detonation*

William E. Dickerson

 DESCRIPTION OF EVENT

The detonation of a nuclear device is, perhaps, the most ominous of terrorist scenarios. Although unlikely, the consequence of such an event must be considered as part of a robust disaster preparedness program. If a terrorist organization detonates a nuclear device equivalent to 10 kilotons (KT) of trinitrotoluene (TNT) in a truck parked in a large city, one can expect a series of catastrophic events. There would be immediate casualties due to the blast, heat, and radiation from the bomb. Because this would most likely be a surface burst, radioactive fallout would also be produced, which would travel for several miles, depending on the size of the particles and weather conditions.[1] The Hiroshima nuclear detonation in August 1945 was equivalent to approximately 15 KT of TNT and was an air burst, which produced minimal fallout. Approximately 100,000 people died within 4 months in the city with a population of about 310,000. The result of such a blast today would cause enormous casualties and structural destruction and result in an area of contamination that may require a prolonged quarantine.

 PREINCIDENT ACTIONS

If there is warning of a potential nuclear detonation, the population can be instructed to evacuate or find shelter, but forewarning is unlikely. Every medical center should include in its emergency preparedness program a radiation disaster plan, which identifies personnel assignments and duties for a radiation decontamination and management team. Since teamwork is essential, training and exercises are necessary. Every team must have a medical or health physicist familiar with the detection and management of radiation hazards, and subject matter experts should be identified who can guide the treatment of radiation casualties. Reference materials such as those in the References section of this chapter should be available.

 POSTINCIDENT ACTIONS

After a radiologic disaster, local responders and facilities will be overwhelmed. The infrastructure will be damaged, and there will be chaos. Most likely, the city mayor will request assistance from the state, and the state governor will request federal aid. A federal emergency will be declared, and the National Response Plan and/or Federal Radiation Emergency Response Plan will be activated. However, as in all disasters, the local communities will have to rely on their own resources for the first several hours. (See Chapter 61, Nuclear Disaster Management.)

Initially, it may not be apparent that the blast or bomb was a nuclear device. However, the extensive area of complete destruction stretching within approximately a 1-km radius from ground zero; the blast winds, which would be felt kilometers away from ground zero; and the probable appearance of a mushroom cloud will indicate that there was a nuclear detonation. The distribution of energy from a nuclear detonation is approximately 50% blast, 35% thermal radiation, 4% initial ionizing radiation (first minute), 10% residual nuclear radiation (fallout), and 1% electromagnetic pulse (EMP).[2] The percentage of casualties from each modality is not clear. Nuclear weapons with a yield of 10 KT or less have a higher percentage of radiation casualties than do nuclear weapons with a yield of more than 10 KT. Thermal radiation is the primary cause of injury from weapons larger than 10 KT because the thermal envelope extends well beyond the radiation contours.[2] The approximate range for casualties from a 10-KT weapon is as follows[3]:

- 590 meters for 50% mortality from blast effects
- 1800 meters for 50% mortality from thermal burns
- 790 meters for 4-Gy initial nuclear radiation (approximately 50% lethality)
- 9600 meters for 4-Gy fallout in first hour after the blast

Any combination of blast, burn, and radiation injury will cause synergistic effects worse than only one type of injury.

First responders will need to evaluate the areas near victims for high levels of radioactivity. It is recommended that first responders use a radiation dose of 0.1 Sv per hour as a "turn-around" dose. However, for lifesaving purposes, a dose of 0.5 Sv or more may be received if the situation warrants it and the responder is aware of the potential health effects.[3]

---

*All material in this chapter is in the public domain, with the exception of any borrowed figures or tables.

State response will include National Guard and Civil Support Team involvement. Federal response will include early actions by the Department of Energy to identify the extent of surface and atmospheric radiation and actions by the Department of Defense, the National Disaster Medical System, the Strategic National Stockpile, and other federal agencies to provide emergency and long-term assistance. (See Section Two, Governmental Resources.)

Radiation Protection Guidance

1. **Time, distance, and shielding.**
   - Time: Limit the time exposed to radioactive material.
   - Distance: The radiation dose received from a source decreases as the inverse square of the distance from the source increases.
   - Shielding: The more material (especially earth, water, concrete, or metal) between a radiation source and a victim, the less dose to a victim. Therefore, one of the best places to take shelter from initial radiation and fallout is in an underground basement away from any windows.
2. **Do not look at a nuclear fireball, even from a distance:** Flash-blindness and retinal burns may occur up to 20 km from the source during the daytime and up to 50 km at night.[2]
3. **The 7/10 rule:** For every sevenfold increase in time after a nuclear detonation, the dose rate of early fallout decreases by a factor of approximately 10.[4] For example, if the radiation dose 1 hour after a detonation is taken as a reference, then the radiation dose at 7 hours would be 0.1 of the dose rate at 1 hour. The radiation dose at 49 hours would be $0.1 \times 0.1 = 0.01$, and the radiation dose rate at 343 hours ($7 \times 7 \times 7$, or about 14 days after a detonation) would be $0.1 \times 0.1 \times 0.1$ or 1/1000th of the radiation level at 1 hour. Therefore, maintaining shelter for 14 days would significantly reduce the radiation exposure from fallout.
4. **Take shelter or evacuate:** Due to radioactive fallout, the government may initially advise people to take shelter if they are within a specific radial distance, such as 30 miles, from the hypocenter. Later, after radiation plume data are available, the government may direct some population areas to take shelter and others to evacuate based on the predicted downwind path of the plume.
5. **Should potassium iodide be taken to block the uptake of radioactive iodine?** In general, the answer is no. The fission products that make up fallout include more than 300 different isotopes of 36 elements. Radioactive iodine is no more of a problem than other radioactive isotopes unless the radioactive iodine is inhaled or ingested. In this case, it will concentrate in the thyroid gland.[4] The best measure to take is to avoid inhaling radioactive fallout or ingesting crops or milk contaminated with radioactive iodine. The food supply should be monitored for radioactive contamination. In a situation such as a nuclear reactor accident where large amounts of radioactive iodine might have been released, potassium iodide would more likely be beneficial.

MEDICAL TREATMENT OF CASUALTIES

The area in the vicinity of ground zero will be completely devastated with no survivors. Continuing out in a radius from ground zero, the percentage of immediate survivors will increase. First responders will be overloaded, and most ambulatory victims will need to walk to the nearest medical facility. Medical facilities closest to ground zero may not be functional, and local medical facilities that are functional will be overloaded beyond their surge capacity. (See Chapter 28, Surge Capacity.) Victims with blast and thermal injuries may initially outnumber victims with only radiation injury due to the latent nature of manifest radiation injury. (See Chapter 83, Introduction to Nuclear/Radiologic Disasters.)

Local medical facilities should:

- Activate their disaster plan.
- Secure their medical center to control patient flow and avoid having contaminated patients contaminate the facility.

The following radiation safety precautions should be taken:

- Follow the guidance of the facility's radiation safety officer.
- Wear personal protective equipment (PPE), such as surgical face masks, caps, gowns, double gloves, and shoe covers, with dosimeters if performing triage or decontamination procedures. (See Chapter 36, Personal Protective Equipment.)
- Perform triage and decontamination outside the medical facility if possible.

First triage and treat life-threatening injuries, then decontaminate. Be aware that the risk of radiation injury to care providers treating those exposed is exceedingly low. In fact, there are no known instances in which nurses, physicians, or other medical professionals have become ill due to their involvement in caring for someone injured in a radiation accident. (See Chapter 43, Triage, and Chapter 70, Radiation Decontamination.)

Blast Injury

Important differences exist between the blast effects from a nuclear weapon and the effects due to a conventional high-explosive bomb. With a nuclear weapon, the combination of high peak overpressure, high wind (or dynamic) pressure, and longer duration of the positive (compression) phase of the blast wave results in "mass distortion" of buildings similar to that produced by earthquakes and hurricanes. An ordinary explosion will usually damage only part of a large structure, but the blast from a nuclear weapon can surround and destroy whole buildings.[4] (See Chapter 141, Introduction to Explosions and Blasts.)

Burn Injury

Thermal injury may initially be difficult to differentiate from skin injury due to radiation. One difference is that thermal injury occurs early, and radiation skin injury may not appear for several days. The combination of thermal burns and irradiation significantly increases mortality.[5] Thermal injury may also cause eye injury. Two types of eye injury are temporary blindness, which occurs if a person indirectly sees the flash of a nuclear fireball, and permanent blindness, which occurs from looking directly at a fireball and results in retinal damage.[6] (See Chapter 155, Introduction to Fires and Burns.)

Acute Radiation Injury

Radiation injury may occur alone or in combination with blast and/or thermal burn injuries. Combined injuries result in a significantly worse prognosis than radiation injury alone. For the diagnosis and treatment of acute radiation injury, the following principles should be used (see Chapter 84, Ionizing Radiation Incident):

- Treat life-threatening injuries (e.g., airway, breathing, circulation) first.
- Decontaminate. The removal of clothes may remove up to 90% of external contamination.
- Anticipate combined injuries (e.g., radiation plus blast and/or thermal).
- Close open wounds within 48 hours of the event for best results.
- Base early dose estimates on symptoms and changes in lymphocyte counts. The Biodosimetry Assessment Tool (BAT) is a computer program that assists with dose estimates and is available free at the Armed Forces Radiobiology Research Institute (AFRRI) Web site (*www.afrri.usubs.mil*).[7]

Acute Radiation Syndrome

Acute radiation syndrome (ARS) may require early use of hematopoietic colony stimulating factors such as filgrastim (Table 85-1). ARS may occur miles from an incident due to radioactive fallout (Fig. 85-1). There will probably be no major role for the use of potassium iodide, Prussian blue, or diethylenetriamine pentaacetic acid (DTPA) after a nuclear detonation. See chapters 83 and 84 for a more thorough discussion of ARS.

Delayed Radiation Effects (2 to 4 Weeks After Event)

Due to the delayed onset of the hematopoietic subsyndrome of ARS, some patients may do well for 2 to 4 weeks before developing manifest symptoms with neutropenia and infections. If these patients could be identified the first few days after the event, they could be assigned to distant, even out-of-state, facilities for treatment of their impending symptoms.

Psychologic Injury

Long-term follow-up care will be necessary to identify late effects from radiation injury and trauma and to assist with posttraumatic stress symptoms. (See Chapter 8, Psychological Impact of Disaster.)

 UNIQUE CONSIDERATIONS

The following should be considered when treating patients as a result of a radiologic event:

- Hospital surge capacity for all services will be exceeded. It will be best for many victims with minimal injury to go home, shower, change clothes, and take shelter.
- For acute radiation injuries, first check airway, breathing, and circulation, and then perform radiation decontamination.
- Decontaminate and triage outside a medical facility if possible to avoid contaminating the medical facility.
- Mass deaths will exceed immediate storage and burial capacity.

TABLE 85-1 TREATMENT GUIDELINES FOR RADIATION EXPOSURE*

NATURE OF INCIDENT	PROPOSED RADIATION DOSE FOR CYTOKINES: FILGRASTIM (G-CSF) OR SARGRAMOSTIM (GM-CSF)	PROPOSED RADIATION DOSE FOR ANTIBIOTICS†	PROPOSED RADIATION DOSE FOR STEM CELL TRANSPLANTATION
<100 casualties, healthy, no other injuries	3-10 Gy	2-10 Gy	7-10 Gy for allogeneic 4-10 Gy if autograft stored or syngeneic donor available
<100 casualties, but multiple injuries or burns	2-6 Gy	2-6 Gy	Not applicable
Mass casualties, >100 casualties, healthy, no other injuries	3-7 Gy	2-7 Gy	7-10 Gy for allogeneic 4-10 Gy if autograft stored or syngeneic donor available
Mass casualties, >100 casualties, multiple injuries or burns	2-6 Gy	2-6 Gy	Not applicable

*This table summarizes the consensus guidelines of the Strategic National Stockpile Radiation Working Group. (Adapted from Waselenko J, MacVittie TJ, Blakely WF, et al. Medical management of the acute radiation syndrome: recommendations of the Strategic National Stockpile Radiation Working Group. *Ann Intern Med.* 2004;140[12]:1037-51, W-64-W-67.)
†Prophylactic antibiotics should be administered to neutropenic patients who have received the whole-body or significant partial-body dose listed in the table. Prophylactic antibiotics in general include a fluoroquinolone, acyclovir (if the patient is seropositive for herpes simplex virus or has a medical history of this virus), and fluconazole.

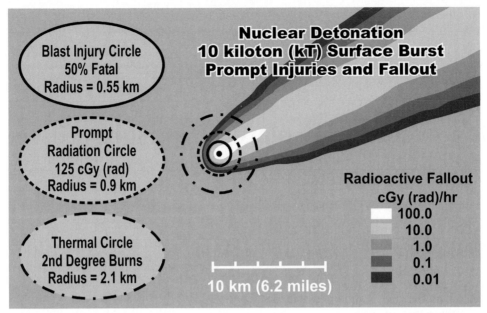

FIGURE 85–1. A 10-KT nuclear detonation, surface burst, hazard prediction assessment capability (HPAC) plot[8] with wind 10 mph from the southeast. The plot shows both prompt effects and fallout 4 hours after detonation. Prompt effects include blast injury fatal in 50% of victims out to a radius of 0.55 km, radiation injury of 125 cGy (rad) out to a 0.9-km radius, and second-degree burns out to a 2.1-km radius. Fallout shows a 100 cGy/hour area out to about 5 km downwind and much larger distance coverages for 10 cGy/hour and less.[8]

 PITFALLS

In the event of a nuclear detonation, there will be damage to the community infrastructure with limited communications and limited services. Failure to secure the medical center will result in radiation contamination throughout the facility. Health professionals may fail to anticipate the manifest illness phase of pure radiation casualties.

Management

In a mass casualty situation, this patient is expectant. He received a dose, which by itself would be lethal to about 50% of the population. His second-degree burns will have a synergistic effect on his morbidity. Survival

might be possible if all medical resources are available (e.g., the patient might require several weeks of care in an intensive care unit). In a mass casualty situation, triage may require that his treatment include only comfort measures. In that case, the patient would develop progressive symptoms of ARS and succumb within a few days.

REFERENCES

1. Radiation Effects Research Foundation. Frequently Asked Questions about the Atomic-bomb Survivor Research Program. Available at: http://www.rerf.or.jp/top/qae.htm.
2. *The Medical NBC Battlebook*. Tech Guide 244. Aberdeen Proving Ground, Md: US Army Center for Health Promotion and Preventive Medicine; 2002:2-23.
3. *Management of Terrorist Events Involving Radioactive Material. NCRP Report No. 138.* Bethesda, Md: National Council on Radiation Protection and Measurements; 2001:23, 95-98.
4. Glasstone S, Dolan PJ. *The Effects of Nuclear Weapons.* 3rd ed. Washington, DC: US Department of Defense and US Energy Research and Development Administration, 1977.
5. Armed Forces Radiobiology Research Institute. *Medical Management of Radiological Casualties Handbook.* 2nd ed. Bethesda, Md: Armed Forces Radiobiology Research Institute; 2003:39. Available at: http://www.afrri.usuhs.mil.
6. Walker RI, Cerveny TJ, eds. *Textbook of Military Medicine: Medical Consequences of Nuclear Warfare.* Falls Church, Va: TMM Publications, Office of the Surgeon General, Department of the Army, United States of America; 1989:6, 7. Available at: http://www.afrri.usuhs.mil.
7. Armed Forces Radiobiology Research Institute. Biodosimetry Assessment Tool (BAT). Available at: http://www.afrri.usuhs.mil.
8. Hazard Prediction Assessment Capability (HPAC) plot performed by the Armed Forces Radiobiology Research Institute. Bethesda, Md. Available at: http://www.dtra.mil/Toolbox/Directorates/td/programs/acec/hpac.cfm.

 CASE PRESENTATION

A 40-year-old white male is seen in the emergency department several hours after a nuclear detonation by a terrorist organization. The patient was working approximately three-fourths of a mile from a nuclear blast. He started vomiting 3 hours after the event. His lymphocyte count dropped from a level of 1000/mm³ 12 hours after the event to a level of 500/mm³ 24 hours after the event. According to the Biodosimetry Assessment Tool (BAT), he was exposed to approximately 4 Gy of radiation. The patient also has second-degree thermal burns over 60% of his body.

Radiation Accident—Isolated Exposure

Jeanette A. Linder and Lawrence S. Linder

DESCRIPTION OF EVENT

Intentional radiation exposure is an integral part of medical care, industrial monitoring, calibration, signage, nuclear reactors, sterilization of agricultural products, and x-ray screening of luggage and cargo. Accidental exposure from radioactive sources and x-ray–producing machines can easily occur with minor variations in practice, loss of custody of radioactive sources, or equipment malfunction. Although accidents are infrequent, rapid recognition of an exposure and intervention can prevent significant, and sometimes fatal, outcomes. Conversely, the risk to the healthcare worker is minimal, provided that simple precautions are taken.

Ionizing radiation is capable of creating ions. These ions then cause cell damage to varying degrees, depending on the total dose, the portion and proportion of body exposed, the duration of exposure, and comorbidities.

Radiation exposure is commonly divided into two broad categories: external irradiation and contamination. Exposures from an external source are described in this chapter. Both internal and external contamination are described in Chapter 87. This chapter focuses on the simplest form of radiation accident: isolated external exposures to a single person over a finite period.

Sealed radioactive sources and radiation generators (diagnostic and therapeutic x-ray machines) can cause external radiation without contamination. X-ray machines do not deposit lasting radioactivity in a person. Radioactive sources, on the other hand, are sometimes implanted into patients, permanently or temporarily. High-activity sources are also used in industry for imaging. Sources can be sealed within metal or unsealed in liquid or powder form. Unsealed or damaged sources can transfer radioactivity (i.e., contaminate) and are discussed in Chapter 87.

The most commonly encountered forms of radiation are:

- *Al*pha: Topic*al*, absorbed/shielded by clothing or paper
- *B*eta: *B*arely penetrate only a few millimeters
- *G*amma: *G*o all the way through, deeply penetrate
- *N*eutrons: *N*astiest and *n*uclear, deeply penetrate and cause more damage than gamma

Sealed sources containing iridium-192, cesium-137, and cobalt-60 are commonly used in industry and medicine. These beta and gamma emitters are the primary cause of isolated exposure without contamination.[1] Alpha and neutron emissions usually occur in nuclear reactions, such as nuclear power plant accidents and nuclear detonations and are discussed in Chapters 85 and 88.

PREINCIDENT ACTIONS

Preparation for a rare event involves ensuring rapid access to infrequently used references and an early warning system. Any facility using radioactive materials or x-ray equipment must have a detailed plan to minimize exposure and respond to unintentional exposure. Exposure limits are defined by Occupational Safety and Health Administration guidelines, which vary for the general public, radiation workers, and disaster recovery workers.[2,3] Incorporating the radiation safety plans of nearby industrial facilities, including mines, nuclear facilities, municipal landfills, metal works, and radiation therapy accelerators, may help prepare for the most likely accidents.

Basic precautions, such as shielding, minimal handling, and maintaining exposure at a maximal distance and minimal time, provide primary prevention of radiation accidents. An orphan source is one not under the custody of an authorized radiation safety officer (RSO). To help prevent orphan sources, all radioactive sources, sealed and unsealed, should be registered, clearly labeled, inventoried, and stored in a locked facility that is clearly marked as radioactive storage with access limited to authorized personnel. Orphan sources are addressed in Chapter 87.

Hospitals must post radiation detectors at strategic locations around diagnostic and therapeutic radiation use areas.[2] They must clearly signal removal of a source or failure to turn off a radiation generator. Hospitals may also consider placing detectors at hospital entrances. Alarm levels are suggested in the National Council on Radiation Protection and Measurements (NCRP) *Report No. 138—Management of Terrorist Events Involving*

Radioactive Material.[3] The benefits and consequences of immediate detection and possible disproportionate emotional reactions should be considered when choosing a threshold for alarms or whether to post monitors at all. Be sure to discuss alarm levels with an RSO and a method of rapidly communicating the alarm (audible versus electronic message to a remote authority, on-site or off-site).

Simple forms are available for documentation of signs, symptoms, and details of exposure (isotope or beam generator, direct contact or exposure to a beam, time of exposure, distance, whole versus partial body, single incident, intermittent exposure, or ongoing exposure with contamination). These forms are available online and in multiple texts.[4,5]

A communication plan for radiation accidents should describe reporting to your RSO and a radiation specialist. If your hospital does not have specialists who can treat radiation injury, you can call the Radiation Emergency Assistance Center/Training Site in Oak Ridge, Tenn. (REAC/TS at [865] 576-1005) or the Medical Radiobiology Advisory Team (MRAT at [301] 295-0316 daytime; [301] 295-0530 after hours) at the Armed Forces Radiobiology Research Institute (AFRRI) for advice. Local and federal authorities may also need to be notified. If there is a significant exposure, either large dose or multiple victims, REAC/TS (for civilian incidents) and/or MRAT (for military incidents) should be notified.

References on basic care of radiation accidents, both hard copies and electronic, are available. Computers can have clearly labeled Web site shortcuts in a separate corner of the desktop for rapid access. The Biodosimetry Assessment Tool (BAT) is detailed later in this chapter and is one of the most useful resources. Other resources include: AFRRI: www.afrri.usuhs.mil, accessed October 11, 2005. A PDF file of Medical Management of Radiological Casualties: Handbook, 2nd edition, can be downloaded at: www.afrri.usuhs.mil/www/outreach/pdf/2e dmmrchandbook.pdf.

- U.S. Centers for Disease Control and Prevention (CDC): www.bt.cdc.gov/radiation.
- U.S. Food and Drug Administration (FDA): www.fda.gov/cder/drugprepare/default.htm#Radiation.
- REAC/TS: www.orau.gov/reacts.
- American College of Radiology (ACR): http://www.acr.org/s_acr/sec.asp?CID=3127&DID=18846. This site contains preapproved patient education handouts and the ACR's disaster preparedness publication, *Disaster Preparedness for Radiology Professionals.*

Basic medical fact sheets and patient handouts are available on the CDC Web site. Patient education should address the following:

1. Short- and long-term health risks of radiation exposure: physical and psychologic
2. Signs and symptoms requiring medical intervention, especially subacute to chronic
3. References to Web sites and other literature for further support

4. Ways to prevent further exposure
5. Referral to a radiation specialist

Basic equipment for detection and management of radiation accidents includes a variety of radiation detectors. Preparedness plans should be reviewed and tested periodically, and supplies should be inventoried.

 ## POSTINCIDENT ACTIONS

The most common accidental single exposures occur with previously identified sources and beam generators.[1,6] Most medical and nuclear reactor facilities can immediately identify the radioactive source(s) (usually iridium-192, cobalt-60, cesium-137) or a generated beam and an approximate dose. Details about the isotope and form of exposure (topical, inhaled, ingested, or absorbed through skin) will focus medical care on the critical organ for that particular isotope and exposed body site. Irradiation by a completely removed isotope, such as a sealed source, or a machine-generated beam over a finite period is much simpler and is the focus of this chapter.

Recognition of a radiation accident may be elusive. The signs and symptoms of radiation sickness are similar to many common syndromes, including thermal burns, gastroenteritis, vague malaise, nausea, and vomiting.[1] Burns without previous thermal or solar exposure, nausea, vomiting, epilation, and/or bone marrow suppression, especially in clusters of patients, may be due to unidentified radiation exposure. The history and physical should address therapeutic, diagnostic, and occupational sources of radiation, particularly in close proximity to nuclear reactors, scientific laboratories, particle accelerators, or other facilities with high radiation exposure.

Unrecognized exposure to radiation is uncommon, but can be deduced from signs and symptoms over time.[6] Whole-body radiation exposure causes predictable and proportional declines in blood counts, increasing constitutional symptoms, and other factors.[7] Once a radiation accident has been confirmed, you should follow your emergency department's (ED's) communication protocol and notify at least the RSO and a radiation specialist.

 ## MEDICAL TREATMENT OF CASUALTIES

Initial emergency care is the same for both the nonradiation and radiation casualty. Airway, breathing, and circulation are always the first priority.[3] Radiologic exposure does not cause immediate loss of consciousness; you should assess other toxic exposures or trauma in the immediately unconscious patient. Once the patient's condition is stabilized, the most important distinction for initial medical management is contamination versus irradiation. Irradiated patients have no detectable radioactivity and pose no risk to providers.[6]

The history and accompanying documentation usually quickly identify the source, machine or isotope; form of isotope (sealed or unsealed); body distance and position from the source; and approximate dose. One must determine whether the exposure was whole body, local, or both. Small portions of the body can tolerate much larger exposures than the whole body. Sequelae of whole-body irradiation can quickly escalate without immediate intervention, whereas partial-body exposures can often be observed and treated days to weeks after the exposure, when local symptoms occur, if necessary.[1,8,9]

Localized Exposure

Acute treatment of uncontaminated local exposures is similar to that of thermal burns or other trauma.[9,10] Trauma of the irradiated area must be avoided. The time course to development of erythema, epilation (hair loss), desquamation, and blistering requires days to weeks. These signs usually result in predictable cutaneous changes, which vary depending on the dose and distribution of exposure. Consequences of exposure and the time delay until those consequences become clinically apparent will vary with the volume of tissue exposed and the dose absorbed.[8] Epilation occurs in 2 to 3 weeks at doses greater than approximately 3 Gy.[9] The threshold for erythema being visible on day 1 is 10 Gy; the erythema rapidly dissipates at relatively low doses, then recurs days to weeks later. Twenty Gy local irradiation causes moist desquamation and possibly ulceration in about 2 weeks. Delayed or lack of healing of ulceration is caused by 25 Gy and greater. Higher doses shorten the time in which these changes develop. Local radiation tissue injury can be treated in a manner similar to thermal burns, but manipulation of erythematous tissue should only be undertaken with severe trepidation. Ulcerated areas will gradually expand to include surrounding erythematous regions as the tissue injury is expressed over time. Follow-up care should be transferred to a radiation specialist.[8,10,11]

Patients with signs of local exposure may also have lesser degrees of whole-body exposure. Other injuries will hinder recovery from whole-body exposure. All patients should be monitored for acute radiation sickness or some other phase of radiation exposure, as noted later in the chapter. In patients with concomitant total body exposure, closure of wounds should be done either within 36 to 48 hours before bone marrow suppression or several weeks to months later once the marrow has recovered.[10-12]

Whole-Body or Large Partial-Body Exposure

Radiation exposure of ~1 Gy or more to large portions of the body causes predictable syndromes. The time to emesis (first vomiting after exposure [TE]), lymphocyte depletion kinetics, and chromosome aberrations are dose-dependent over time.[7,9,11] A sophisticated but user-friendly software program, BAT, is a free download from the AFRRI Web site (www.afrri.usuhs.mil) and is based on these indicators.[11,13] Signs and symptoms and validated data can be systematically recorded in the program at varying intervals. The program will calculate estimated doses based on input data and physical parameters.

Initial symptoms of acute radiation sickness can occur within minutes to days after whole-body exposure. Affected systems increase with increasing dose in the following order: hematopoietic, gastrointestinal, cardiovascular, then central nervous system.[7,9,10] Each syndrome has four phases: (1) prodromal, (2) latent, (3) manifest illness, and (4) recovery or death. The prodromal phase is predictive of the severity of subsequent phases. Prodromal symptoms include nausea, vomiting, diarrhea, fatigue, weakness, headache, parotid pain, and erythema. The time between exposure and the first episode of emesis (time to emesis, or TE) often correlates with general ranges of total body dose. A TE of less than 4 hours may indicate a significant whole-body dose of 3.5 Gy or more. Without appropriate medical treatment, a whole-body dose of approximately 3.5 Gy is generally considered lethal to 50% of patients within 60 days ($LD_{50/60}$). The $LD_{50/60}$ may nearly double to 6 to 7 Gy with aggressive intervention.[10,11] Without medical care, this 6- to 7-Gy dose would allow few survivors. A TE of less than 1 hour possibly indicates a lethal exposure even with intensive medical care; palliative care is recommended if the supralethal dosage is confirmed by clinical evaluation. Healthy adults with a TE of more than 4 hours, which implies a dose of less than 1 to 2 Gy whole body, will probably survive without medical care, unless additional medical factors complicate the issue. If there are mass casualties, patients without concomitant injuries who have a TE of more than 4 hours can be triaged to delayed evaluation in 24 to 72 hours, but reevaluation is mandatory.[14]

The speed at which lymphocyte counts decrease is directly proportional to the whole-body dose. An absolute lymphocyte count (ALC) decline of 50% or more within 24 hours indicates at least a moderate whole-body dose. If the victim has other injuries, then ALC is a less reliable predictor.[7,10,13]

Physical Examination

Initial physical examination should focus on vital signs (fever, hypotension, orthostasis), skin manifestations (erythema, blistering, onycholysis, edema, desquamation, petechiae), central nervous system deficits (motor, sensory, ataxia, mental status, cognition), and abdominal signs (pain or tenderness).[10]

Laboratory Studies

A complete blood count with differential and platelet count should be drawn immediately and at least three times per day for several days in anyone with prodromal symptoms. Blood samples for cytogenetic studies should be drawn around 24 hours after exposure. Verify in which tube to collect blood (currently 10 mL in a lithium-heparin collection tube), proper labeling, and storage temperature with MRAT or your RSO.[11]

Treatment

Treatment is stratified by the estimated total body dose in addition to treatment of known injuries or infections.

Estimated dose, probability of survival, and treatment are based on signs, symptoms, and approximate blood counts in Table 86-1 or by the results of serial data input into the BAT program.[1,13,15]

The Strategic National Stockpile Radiation Working Group (SNS) has consolidated the seminal literature on radiation injury. It recommends treatment of neutropenic or anticipated neutropenic patients with: (1) broad-spectrum prophylaxis using a fluoroquinolone with streptococcal coverage or augmented with penicillin or amoxicillin; (2) acyclovir; and (3) fluconazole. Known sites of infection should be managed according to established guidelines. Underlying foci of current or new infection are likely to be due to loss of integrity of the integument or gastrointestinal tract. Add anaerobic coverage when there is known bowel injury.[10]

The SNS recommends supportive care with cytokines (G-CSF, Peg-G-CSF, GM-CSF), prophylactic and therapeutic antibiotics, leukoreduced/irradiated transfusions, antiemetics, antidiarrheals, opiates, parenteral fluids, and nutrition.[10] In patients with concomitant total-body exposure, closure of wounds should be done either within 36 to 48 hours before bone marrow suppression or months later when the marrow has recovered.[10-12] Treatment should be transferred to a radiation specialist or should continue under the guidance of REAC/TS, MRAT, or other response teams. Long-term care should be transferred to a specialist in radiation injury. When chronic, nonhealing wounds are present as late effects of exposure to radiation, consideration of hyperbaric oxygen therapy should be made before and after attempts at flaps or skin grafts, and consultation from a specialist in hyperbaric medicine should be sought as part of a multispecialty approach to wound healing.[16,17]

 UNIQUE CONSIDERATIONS

All radiation accident victims carry some risk of an induced malignancy.[3] This is usually far less than

TABLE 86-1   RESPONSE CATEGORIES

RESPONSE CATEGORY	WBE	PROBABILITY OF SURVIVAL*	CLINICAL SIGNS†	ALC‡	ANC§	TREATMENT
1	~0.4 to 1.4 Sv	~100% without treatment	None or minimal	0.5-2	>2	Follow-up as outpatient
2	~1.3 to 5.5 Sv	>60 days with treatment	Mild N, V, D, F	0.3-0.8	Initial ↑ days 10-20, ↓ days 25-30	Antibiotics Transfuse platelets (prn) Follow-up for infections Antiemetics ‖
3	~4.4 to 8.0 Sv	Survival with intense treatment	N, V, F, Er, D, Ep	0.2-0.5	Initial ↑, then ↓ days 15-25	Reverse isolation Replacement/ transfusions Growth factors Fluids Gut bacterial decontamination Antiemetics ‖
4	~9 to 11 Sv	10-15 days 100% mortality without transplant	N, V, D, early Er and edema, CNS	0-0.1 in 3 days	Early ↑, then ↓ in 6 days	Reverse isolation Gnotobiotic treatment Fluids and electrolytes Stem cell transplant Antibiotics, antifungals, and antivirals Transfusions Cytokines Antiemetics ‖
5	>11 Sv	<7-12 days	CNS, shock, edema, N, V	0-0.1 within hours	Initial ↑, then ↓ by day 5	Palliative only

(Data from Turai I, Veress K. Radiation accidents: occurrence, types, consequences, medical management, and the lessons to be learned. *Central Eur J Occup Environ Med.* 2001;7:3-14; Blakely W, Prasanna P, Miller A. Update on current and new developments in biological dose-assessment techniques. In: Ricks R, Berger M, O'Hara F, eds. *The Medical Basis for Radiation-accident Preparedness: The Clinical Care of Victims.* Proceedings of the Fourth International REAC/TS Conference on The Medical Basis for Radiation-Accident Preparedness. New York: Parthenon Publishing Group; 2002:23-32; and Mettler F, Guskova A. Treatment of acute radiation sickness. In: Gusev I, Guskova A, Mettler F, eds. *Medical Management of Radiation Accidents.* 2nd ed. Boca Raton, Fla: CRC Press; 2001: 53-67.)
WBE, Whole-body exposure in sieverts, which include a radiobiologic quality factor (equivalent to Gy for most radiation exposure); ↓, nadir
Survival may be reduced with concomitant injuries and comorbidities.
†*Clinical signs* are N = nausea, V = vomiting, D = diarrhea, F = fatigue, Er = erythema, Ep = epilation, CNS = central nervous system perturbations.
‡*ALC,* Absolute lymphocyte count in units of 10⁹/L.
§*ANC,* Absolute neutrophil count in units of 10⁹/L.
‖Nausea and vomiting can be quite severe after large doses to the abdomen or moderate whole body doses.[12] The most effective antiemetics are 5HT-3 antagonists.[15]

anticipated and only slightly greater than the preincident risk, since radiation is a relatively weak carcinogen.[3] Risk is related to quality and dose of radiation, affected organs, age at the time of exposure, and other risk factors.[3] Education about the usual small increase in risk may diminish stress significantly. General educational materials can initially allay fears, and subsequent consultation with a radiation specialist can better define risks and proper surveillance.

Loss of fertility is common with irradiation of the gonads. This may be temporary or permanent, depending on dose, depth of penetration, age, and maturation of the patient.[3] Doses to the testes of 0.15 Gy are likely to cause temporary sterility, but 3.5 Gy or more will cause permanent sterility. Ovarian doses for permanent sterility range from 2.5 to 6 Gy.[3] There has been some recovery of fertility even in major radiation accidents, such as Chernobyl recovery workers.[18]

Fetal doses should be estimated separately from whole-body and local doses to a pregnant woman. In some cases, the fetus receives a lower whole-body dose than the mother due to natural shielding of the baby by surrounding structures. Very low doses of only 0.1 to 1 Gy can be very harmful to the fetus depending on the stage of gestation. Exposure to ionizing radiation before implantation usually results in undetectable death of the fetus or failure to implant. Exposure during organogenesis (weeks ~3 to 7) may cause malformations. Later exposure during weeks 8 to 25 causes decreasing IQ with increasing dose. There is a small increased risk of childhood cancers and leukemias.[3]

Patients, family members, co-workers, recovery workers, and even healthcare providers often require some psychologic intervention. The emotional trauma and possible stigma of radiation exposure can be intense and outlast the physical manifestations. Acute stress reactions of insomnia, impaired concentration, and social withdrawal should be anticipated. If the radiation accident is associated with an act of terrorism, then psychologic effects will increase. Patients should be followed-up long term for signs of posttraumatic stress disorder. Groups at particularly high risk are children, mothers of young children, pregnant women, emergency personnel, recovery and cleanup workers, and those with a history of mental illness. Education and early intervention can prevent much of this psychologic stress.[9,19]

 PITFALLS

Failure to prepare a response plan and learn basic radiation medicine can lead to excessive morbidity and mortality or failure to recognize an accidental or intentional radiation incident by terrorists. There are multiple educational resources and a sample emergency plan on the Web sites listed in this chapter.[20] REAC/TS and AFRRI provide physician training online and at various courses, remote and on-site, at varying levels of intensity for first responders, ED personnel, and radiation specialists. Detailed references are provided by multiple government agencies and other organizations, including the CDC, AFRRI, and ACR. If communications systems are not

operational, several resources, such as the latest edition of the *Medical Management of Radiological Casualties: Handbook* and the Biodosimetry Assessment Tool (BAT), can be stored on a portable memory device. Basic facts sheets on medical management and documentation of radiation emergencies are on the CDC Web site (www.bt.cdc.gov/radiation). The latest drug recommendations and approvals will be noted on the U.S. Food and Drug Administration Web site (www.fda.gov/cder/drugprepare/default.htm#Radiation).

REFERENCES

1. Turai I, Veress K. Radiation accidents: occurrence, types, consequences, medical management, and the lessons to be learned. *Central Eur J Occup Environ Med.* 2001;7:3-14.
2. *OSHA Occupational Radiation Safety Manual and CD.* Los Angeles, Calif: University Of HealthCare; 2003.
3. National Council on Radiation Protection and Measurements. *Report No. 138—Management of Terrorist Events Involving Radioactive Material.* Bethesda, Md: National Council on Radiation Protection and Measurements; 2001.

4. National Council on Radiation Protection and Measurements. *Report No. 65—Management of Persons Accidentally Contaminated with Radionuclides*. Bethesda, Md: National Council on Radiation Protection and Measurements; 1980.

5. US Centers for Disease Control and Prevention. Radiation Emergencies. Available at: http://www.bt.cdc.gov/radiation. Accessed October 10, 2005.

6. Mettler F, Kelsey C. Fundamentals of radiation accidents. In: Gusev I, Guskova A, Mettler F, eds. *Medical Management of Radiation Accidents*. 2nd ed. Boca Raton, Fla: CRC Press; 2001:1-13.

7. Guskova A, Baranov A, Gusev I. Acute radiation sickness: underlying principles and assessment. In: Gusev I, Guskova A, Mettler F, eds. *Medical Management of Radiation Accidents*. 2nd ed. Boca Raton, Fla: CRC Press; 2001:33-51.

8. Guskova A. Radiation sickness classification. In: Gusev I, Guskova A, Mettler F, eds. *Medical Management of Radiation Accidents*. 2nd ed. Boca Raton, Fla: CRC Press; 2001:15-22.

9. Mettler F, Voelz G. Major radiation exposure—what to expect and how to respond. *New Engl J Med*. 2002;346:1554-61.

10. Waselenko J, MacVittie T, Blakely W, et al. Medical management of the acute radiation syndrome: recommendations of the Strategic National Stockpile Radiation Working Group. *Ann Intern Med*. 2004;140:1037-51.

11. Jarrett D, ed. *Medical Management of Radiological Casualties: Handbook*. 2nd ed. AFRRI Special Publication 03-1. Bethesda, Md:Armed Forces Radiobiology Research Institute; 2003. Available at: http://www.afrri.usuhs.mil. Accessed October 10, 2005.

12. Barabanova A. Local radiation injury. In: Gusev I, Guskova A, Mettler F, eds. *Medical Management of Radiation Accidents*. 2nd ed. Boca Raton, Fla: CRC Press; 2001:223-240.

13. Blakely W, Prasanna P, Miller A. Update on current and new developments in biological dose-assessment techniques. In: Ricks R, Berger M, O'Hara F, eds. *The Medical Basis for Radiation-accident Preparedness: The Clinical Care of Victims*. Proceedings of the Fourth International REAC/TS Conference on The Medical Basis for Radiation-Accident Preparedness. New York: Parthenon Publishing Group; 2002:23-32.

14. US Department of Homeland Security Working Group on Radiological Dispersal Device (RDD) Preparedness. Medical Preparedness and Response Sub-Group. Available at: http://www1.va.gov/emshg/docs/Radiologic_Medical_Counter measures_051403.pdf. Accessed October 10, 2005.

15. Mettler F, Guskova A. Treatment of acute radiation sickness. In: Gusev I, Guskova A, Mettler F, eds. *Medical Management of Radiation Accidents*. 2nd ed. Boca Raton, Fla: CRC Press; 2001: 53-67.

16. Marx RA. Radiation injury to tissue. In: Kindwall EP, Whelan HT, eds. *Hyperbaric Medicine Practice*. 2nd ed. Flagstaff, Ariz: Best Publishing Co; 1999:665-723.

17. Feldmeier JJ, Matos LA. Delayed radiation injuries (soft tissue and bony necrosis). In: Feldmeier JJ, ed. *Hyperbaric Oxygen 2003— Indications and Results: The Hyperbaric Oxygen Therapy Committee Report*. Kensington, Md: Undersea and Hyperbaric Medical Society; 2003:87-100.

18. Guskova A, Gusev I. Medical aspects of the accident at Chernobyl. In: Gusev I, Guskova A, Mettler F, eds. *Medical Management of Radiation Accidents*. 2nd ed. Boca Raton, Fla: CRC Press; 2001: 195-210.

19. Berger M, Sadoff R. Psychological support of radiation accident patients, families, and staff. In: Gusev I, Guskova A, Mettler F, eds. *Medical Management of Radiation Accidents*. 2nd ed. Boca Raton, Fla: CRC Press; 2001:191-200.

20. Appendix 1: Sample radiation emergency plan for a medical facility. In: Gusev I, Guskova A, Mettler F, eds. *Medical Management of Radiation Accidents*. 2nd ed. Boca Raton, Fla: CRC Press; 2001: 557-570.

chapter 87

Radiation Accident—Dispersed Exposure

Jeanette A. Linder and Lawrence S. Linder

 ## DESCRIPTION OF EVENT

Dispersed ionizing radiation accidents are caused by unsealed or damaged radiation sources. Contamination can be external or internal (by injection, ingestion, inhalation, or absorption through intact skin or wounds). The most common dispersed exposures have been medical and industrial accidents.[1] Less commonly, orphan sources, those no longer in the custody of a radiation safety officer (RSO), were knowingly or unwittingly transported and/or altered by unauthorized persons. Coupling an orphan source with a conventional explosive will create a dirty bomb. Fortunately, the small amounts of radioactivity dispersed by a dirty bomb or from spraying radioactive powders or liquid would be unlikely to cause significant illness beyond psychological terror.[2] Radiation dispersal devices and other intentional dispersion are addressed in Chapter 87. The most dangerous and feared dispersed exposure is due to nuclear explosion, and this is addressed in Chapter 85.

Beta, gamma, and minimal neutron exposure are most prevalent in industry and medicine, whereas alpha and neutron emitters usually occur in nuclear reactions, such as those in nuclear power plants or nuclear detonations. Medical or industrial sources are the ones most likely to be dispersed, either accidentally or intentionally, in a dirty bomb.[1] These sources are usually sealed in metal. In decreasing frequency, accidents can involve iridium-192, cobalt-60, and cesium-137, which emit penetrating gamma and minimal beta radiation.[1] Iodine-125 and palladium-103 seeds are weak gamma and beta emitters. They are commonly used in radiation oncology for permanent implantation of the prostate gland and other organs and usually pose little to no risk. Many unsealed sources are used in scientific laboratories and nuclear medicine testing and treatment, including tritium-3, iodine-131, iodine-125, strontium-90, and technetium-99m. The chemical and radiation characteristics of each isotope will determine which organs are affected. The effective time of exposure without intervention depends on the body's incorporation and/or excretion of that substance or the vehicle on which the isotope is carried. Incorporation of an isotope into tissues may be temporary or permanent and depends on the chemical nature,

size of the particles, phase state (liquid versus solid), and route of entry. For example, radium can be permanently incorporated into bone matrix, whereas iodine is taken up into the thyroid. Others may eventually be excreted in the urine or feces without intervention. Table 87-1 provides basic facts for the most commonly encountered isotopes in accidents.[3-6] The RSO and agencies such as the Radiation Emergency Assistance Center/Training Site (REAC/TS) in Oak Ridge, TN (865-576-1005), will provide detailed information on detection, dose estimation, decontamination, and consequence prevention and management.

 ## PREINCIDENT ACTIONS

As in Chapter 86, reparation for a rare event involves ensuring rapid access to infrequently used references and an early warning system. In the case of contamination with dispersed radioactive materials, patients may know they were contaminated during medical or industrial accidents. For the rare case of accidental or intentional contamination that has yet to be identified, mounted radiation monitors at strategic entrances to the hospital may detect undeclared or unrecognized radioactivity. Alarm levels are suggested in the National Council on Radiation Protection and Measurements (NCRP) report number 138.[7] The benefits of immediate detection and consequences of possible disproportionate emotional reactions should be considered when choosing a threshold for alarming or deciding whether to post monitors at all. This will require a well-thought-out floor plan, response, and notification of appropriate authorities, including the local RSO and radiation specialists. Sample emergency plans are available on various Web sites and in radiation texts.[8] Hospital and clinic emergency preparedness exercises should include a radiation-exposed patient or scenario to ensure familiarity with and provide practice of the radiation response, containment, and treatment procedures by the emergency department and other hospital staff members.

First responders to any detonation should always survey for radioactivity on arrival.[7] First responders at the accident site may receive significant doses; however,

TABLE 87-1   DECONTAMINATION OF COMMON ELEMENTS IN INDUSTRIAL AND MEDICAL ACCIDENTS*

ELEMENT	EMISSIONS	CRITICAL ORGAN	EFFECTIVE T$_{1/2}$†	DECONTAMINATION
Cesium-137	Beta, gamma	Total body	70 days	Prussian blue (Radiogardase) 3 g po 3 times per day (adults and adolescents); 1 g po 3 times/day (2-12 years old); consider lavage and purgatives
Cobalt-60	Beta, gamma	Total body	10 days	Lavage, purgatives, penicillamine
Iodine-125, iodine-131	Beta, gamma	Thyroid	Iodine-125, 42 days; iodine-131, 8 days	Potassium iodide: 0-1 month, 16 mg/day; >1 month to 3 years, 32 mg/day; >3 to 12 years and < 70 kg, 65 mg/day; adults or ≥70 kg, 130 mg/day; consider lavage
Iridium-192	Beta, gamma	Lung	74 days	Lavage for large quantities
Technetium-99m	Gamma	Total body	5 hours	Potassium perchlorate to reduce thyroid dose
Tritium-3	Beta	Total body	12 days	Forced fluids
Uranium-235 and uranium-238	Alpha	Kidney,‡ bone, liver, lung	Can be permanent if in bone	Bicarbonate to alkalinize the urine

(Data from U.S. Food and Drug Administration. Prussian blue, Radiogardase, package insert. Available at: http://www.fda.gov/cder/drug/infopage/prussian_blue/default. htm, accessed October 11, 2005; U.S. Food and Drug Administration. Guidance: Potassium iodide as a thyroid blocking agent in radiation emergencies. Available at: http://www.fda.gov/cder/guidance/4825fnl.htm, accessed October 11, 2005; *Management of Persons Accidentally Contaminated with Radionuclides.* NCRP report no. 65. Bethesda, Md: National Council on Radiation Protection and Measurements; 1980; and Jarrett D, ed. *Medical Management of Radiation Casualties: Handbook.* 2nd ed. AFRRI special publication 03-1. Bethesda, Md: Armed Forces Radiobiology Research Institute; 2003. Available at: http://www.afrri.usuhs.mil, accessed October 11, 2005.
*See Chapter 86 for a description of possible elements and types of radioactivity.
†Effective t$_{1/2}$ combines radioactive and chemical properties and rates of elimination without decontamination efforts.
‡The kidney is most vulnerable to large amounts of uranium due to the chemical properties of this heavy metal. Uranium can ultimately be deposited in bone.
po, Per os; qd, once per day.

with proper real-time monitoring, limited time, and maximal distance, exposures can be acceptable. When following simple procedures, providers receive very little exposure even while caring for large numbers of contaminated victims. It is reassuring that no U.S. healthcare worker who has adhered to simple precautions has become contaminated from handling a contaminated patient.[9] Habitual use of gowns, double gloves, masks, and hair and shoe covers and remaining within the contaminated zone until cleared for exit by the RSO will keep exposures well within limits in nearly all scenarios.[10] Any site the patient has visited prior to decontamination must be considered radioactive and, therefore, a hot zone. An adjacent transitional or warm zone is for step-off as protective clothing and gear are removed. Radioactive materials deposited on clothing and skin can be quickly decontaminated up to 90% simply by removing clothing and washing gently with soap and water. Personnel are then monitored to ensure minimal to no residual activity before they step into the cold zone.[5,6]

A floor plan should be detailed in an accident-preparedness plan. Only essential equipment and necessary furniture should be in the hot zone. Supplies and personnel are brought in only as needed. A defined pathway from the entry point/ambulance reception to the treatment area should be covered in plastic and roped off with radioactive warning signs. Traffic through the emergency department must be tightly monitored to minimize spread of contamination. A detailed security plan restricting admittance to authorized personnel and patients should be clearly defined before any incident occurs.[11] If the radioactive contaminant may be airborne, air handlers and ventilation should be isolated, if possible.

Background radiation levels for various hospital locations should be documented well in advance of an accident.[12] Plans must map the locations and use of beta-gamma detectors and alpha detectors. Plans should also address personal dosimeters of varying types (defined by the RSO), a large supply of sealable plastic containers, various sizes of plastic bags, radiation warning signs, ropes, plastic for covering the floor, gowns, gloves, tape, and current references on management of contaminated patients.[7,11] The Web sites, agencies, and literature mentioned in Chapter 86 are essential.

Protective clothing and gear in the hospital setting is nearly the same as for universal precautions. The exception is double gloving. If time allows, tape the first pair of gloves to gown sleeves so they are not removed when the top pair is frequently removed. All other seams and transitions, pants legs and shoe covers, can be taped. Detailed instructions on donning and removing protective clothing and gear are available from the Centers for Disease Control and Prevention (CDC).[13] Lead aprons are not recommended. The weight of the aprons may cause overheating, accelerate fatigue, and slow down providers, with little to no benefit.

Details of whom to notify, education of providers and patients, and other details of the disaster plan are summarized in Chapter 86 and detailed in multiple other references.[5-9,11]

 ## POSTINCIDENT ACTIONS

Initial emergency care is the same for both nonradiation and radiation casualties. Airway, breathing, and circulation are always the first priorities. In other words, patients with life-threatening conditions are treated first and decontaminated second. Stable patients can be decontaminated first.[6] Radiologic exposure does not cause immediate loss of consciousness; assess other toxic exposures or trauma in the immediately unconscious patient. One exception is that there may be transient incapacitation after extremely high doses to the head or whole body.[14] Once stabilized, the most important distinction for initial medical management is contamination (radioactive material present on or within the body) versus irradiation (previous exposure without any radioactive material deposited on or within the body).

The history and accompanying documentation usually quickly identify the source, machine or isotope, form of isotope (sealed or unsealed), body distance and position from the source, and approximate dose. One must determine whether the exposure was whole body or local. Sequelae of whole body irradiation can quickly escalate without immediate intervention, whereas partial body exposures can often be observed and treated days to weeks later when or if signs and symptoms develop.[1,11,15]

First responders should complete an identification tag specifying the usual triage information plus radiation-specific details. Information for internal contamination should include the radionuclide, route of contamination, nasal counts, wound counts, whole body counts, bioassay samples already collected, and treatment initiated. Data for external exposure to penetrating radiation should include the location and position of patient with respect to the source, exact time and duration of exposure, whether a dosimeter was used and where it was located, who has the dosimeter and its current location, type of symptoms, time to onset of symptoms, and treatment at the site of the accident/assessment/facility.[5]

Ambulatory patients should be decontaminated, if possible, before transport to the hospital, especially at a facility with its own decontamination process. A radiation dispersal device may contaminate as many as 1000 victims,[2] most of whom will be ambulatory. The few who are not ambulatory most likely have significant blast injuries. Ambulatory patients should remove clothing in a manner that minimizes further contamination, taking care not to contact undergarments and skin with the external surfaces of the garments being removed. Removing clothing and washing gently with soap and water will remove significant amounts of surface contamination. Splashing into eyes, mouth, nose, and open wounds must be avoided to minimize internal contamination. Cover all wounds to prevent further contamination and limit contamination of clean areas by the wound. Washing should be repeated until the radioactivity is less than twice that of the background activity, until it is unwise to continue due to medical conditions or impending skin abrasion, or until further measures fail to decrease activity significantly. Wastewater and any shiny or metallic particles should be retained and identified as radioactive contaminate. Abrasions and shaving should be avoided. Hair can be clipped, if necessary. All clothing and hair should be sealed in a labeled bag for assessment by the RSO.[5,6] When decontamination efforts fail to reduce any radioactivity, suspect internal contamination with a gamma-emitter.[5]

Patients requiring transport by stretcher, if stable, should have clothing cut off.[6] The patient should then be wrapped in cloth sheets, not plastic, to minimize the spread of radioactive material and minimize hyperthermia.[6,13] First responders should notify the hospital before arrival that a contaminated patient is on the way. They should also provide additional medical information including the following:

1. Other injuries and medical conditions besides radioactive exposure/contamination;
2. Whether toxic or corrosive chemicals are involved in addition to the radionuclides;
3. Whether the compounds are soluble or insoluble and the size of the particles;
4. Measurements from the site of the accident that will help determine dose;
5. What decontamination efforts have already been attempted, and whether they were successful;
6. Verification that clothing removed at the site has been saved to allow identification of isotope and dose estimation;
7. Which excreta, swipes, and samples have been collected, time of collection, current location, when analyses will be completed and by whom; and
8. Any previous radiation therapy or accidental exposure.[5,6,7,9]

Co-morbidities may affect the clearance, absorption, or tolerance of decontamination measures (e.g., renal disease may affect the tolerance of chelators).[5] Once stable, either first responders or hospital providers should swab nasal cavities and collect multiple samples of excreta and blood. All metal fragments should be removed with forceps and monitored. If these are contaminated debris or particles from a damaged source, your RSO will direct you to seal high-activity sources in lead containers or at least 6 feet from personnel.[2]

 ## MEDICAL TREATMENT OF CASUALTIES

As stated above, initial emergency care is the same for both the nonradiation and the radiation casualty. Once airway, breathing, and circulation are stable, radiation surveys and decontamination can be considered. First, one must identify that a radiation accident has occurred. Occupational and therapeutic exposures may be easily identified after a brief history is taken or a discussion with supervisors or treating physicians is undertaken. More elusive to diagnosis are accidental exposures to unsealed or damaged orphan sources in the community at landfills or construction sites or in malfunctioning equipment. One should include radiation exposure in the differential diagnosis of unexplained bone marrow suppression; skin burns or desquamation with no history of thermal injury; and clusters of people with unexplained nausea, vomiting, and decreasing blood counts currently or several days to weeks earlier.[1] Radiation detectors mounted at hospital entries might identify significant contamination.

External or internal contamination will determine the initial intervention. There also may be a combination of external penetrating radiation with concomitant contamination. Prodromal symptoms and serial peripheral blood counts should predict the overall total body dose, including external components not necessarily identified at the time of presentation.

Once the patient is stable, surface surveys and nasal swabs with a moist cotton-tipped applicator or filter paper swab can be obtained by gently rotating the swabs over accessible surfaces. This should not be done by the patient, who might contaminate the swab with material already on hands and clothing.[5] Nasal swab counts represent approximately 5% of lung activity.[2]

Medical intervention should be orderly and should include the following:

1. Triage and medical stabilization;
2. External decontamination: remove clothing, wash skin, irrigate wounds (collect bandages and attempt to collect drainage), clip and collect hair if stubborn to shampooing;
3. Documentation of prodromal symptoms or whole body exposure: nausea, time to emesis, diarrhea, transient incapacitation, hypotension (the presence of all indicates very high dose), parotid pain, erythema;
4. Documentation of signs and symptoms of local exposure (erythema, dry and moist desquamation);
5. Initial complete blood count with differential and platelet count immediately and every 4 to 6 hours for at least 24 to 48 hours;
6. Collection of all excreta for at least 48 hours;
7. Collection of blood at 24 hours for cytogenetics;
8. Nasal swabs; and
9. Internal decontamination (see Table 87-1).

LOCALIZED EXTERNAL CONTAMINATION

Removing clothing and gently washing with soap and water will remove significant amounts of external contamination. When the skin is unbroken and levels fall below twice background levels, decontamination can stop. Even with broken skin and other injuries, there are no immediate consequences of localized exposure.

Patients with localized external contamination may have also had significant external radiation and may manifest acute radiation syndrome (ARS). Only those casualties who were in intimate contact with the source before its dissemination are likely to exhibit this level of injury. Evaluation and treatment of ARS are the same as described in Chapter 86. Radiation specialists and agencies (REAC/TS for civilian events and/or the Medical Radiobiology Advisory Team, MRAT, for military events) should be contacted upon confirmation of a dispersed exposure.

INTERNAL CONTAMINATION

Initial evaluation and treatment are the same as for the externally irradiated patient with respect to ARS. Once a patient's condition is stabilized, measures to reduce internal contamination and incorporation (binding radioactive material into tissues or bone) can proceed. The route of entry and particular isotope will determine decontamination methods. Currently recommended interventions and drugs for each isotope can be found on numerous Web sites, such as those maintained by the CDC and the U.S. Food and Drug Administration (FDA). The four main mechanisms of internal decontamination are as follows: (1) reducing uptake; (2) isotopic dilution or use of blocking agents; (3) mobilizing agents; and (4) chelation.[5] See Table 87-1 for specific interventions.

Reducing Uptake

Nasopharyngeal, bronchoalveolar, and gastric lavage (within 1 to 2 hours of ingestion), emetics, purgatives, and enemas may significantly reduce contamination.[2,5-7] Prussian blue, recently approved by the FDA as Radiogardase, prevents absorption of cesium-134 and cesium-137 and promotes excretion in stool.[3]

Blocking Agents

Blocking uptake of the radioactive material, also called *isotopic dilution,* can decrease uptake into stable metabolic pools, such as bone, where uptake becomes permanent. For instance, potassium iodide will block radioactive iodine if given before or within 4 to 6 hours of exposure. Potassium iodide will not block any other isotopes, although patients and families may request it.[4,5,16] It has no medical value except for the emergency treatment of radioiodine exposure. See Table 87-1 for doses of potassium iodide.

Mobilizing Agents

Mobilizing agents accelerate excretion in feces or urine. Forced fluids will reduce uptake and increase the excretion of tritium-3 in the urine. Alkalinizing the urine with bicarbonate can increase excretion of uranium.[5,7]

Chelation

Americium-241, plutonium-238-239, and curium can be chelated with pentetate calcium trisodium and pentetate zinc trisodium; these older agents were recently approved by the FDA for this use. Care must be exerted because these agents also bind endogenous metals in the body, (i.e., zinc, magnesium, and manganese), and plasma levels should be monitored. Depletion of these trace metals can interfere with necessary cellular mitotic processes. Mineral and vitamin supplements may be indicated. In animal studies, chelates with uranium and neptunium were less stable than chelates of americium, plutonium, and curium, in vivo, resulting in deposition of uranium and neptunium in tissues including bone, and thus they are *not* expected to be effective for uranium or neptunium.[17-21] Ethylenediamine tetraacetic acid can also be used, on the recommendation of REAC/TS or a radiation specialist. Chelated salts are then excreted by glomerular filtration in the urine.[5,7]

Collect blood, urine, feces, wound exudates, and dressings at least three times per day for at least 48 hours. Initial excreta may underestimate exposure before transit through the intestines. Any initial orifices with activity above background should be swiped periodically. Be careful not to cause abrasions, which could cause further internal contamination. Collect blood for cytogenetics at around 24 hours. Your RSO and radiation specialists will help identify those patients who require subsequent surveys. Patients who are not hospitalized must be given containers and instructed to collect all excreta. Each sample must be labeled with the time and date for proper dosimetry assessment. All contaminated instruments, specimens, clothing, and equipment should be saved in separate containers and labeled with patient name, time, and date. These samples will contribute to identifying isotopes and approximate dose. Radioactive tissue should NOT be removed as a means of decontamination unless under the guidance of a trained radiologic physician. Extreme measures, such as amputation, are rarely indicated except for unremovable embedded highly radioactive particulate contamination with long-lived sources. Destructive surgeries should only be performed after complete evaluation by, and on recommendation of, a radiation medicine specialist.[5,7]

CASE PRESENTATION

A salvage worker finds an "EXIT" sign among the rubble of an office building. It is crushed and no longer glowing. During the 2-hour drive back to the landfill, the exit sign rests on the front seat of his truck, approximately 14 inches from his right hip. Upon arrival at the landfill, he notices the radioactive warning label on the back of the sign indicating that it contains tritium,[3] H. The worker abandons the sign and rushes to the emergency department in a panic.

This worker is relieved to hear that tritium is a rapidly dispersed gas that was probably not even present at the time that he found the broken exit sign. He has no signs or symptoms of radiation exposure (i.e., no erythema of the closest body part, the right hip, and no prodromal symptoms or signs). Local HazMat authorities are dispatched to recover the sign, and after examination, they determine that it no longer contains radioactive material. Your RSO has verified only background levels of beta radiation on the patient. Urine specimens taken at the time of arrival and 1 hour later are negative for beta activity above background. The patient is reassured that even if there were tritium present in his urine, and therefore throughout his body, tritium is a pure beta emitter that is exhaled, and, if metabolized, excreted in the urine. It would be unlikely to cause any signs or symptoms.

You reassure the patient that he is fine. A full analysis by authorities to better define his exposure and risk of consequences is not indicated in this case because there was no true exposure. This worker is referred to his primary care physician for follow-up and psychological assessment. If a true radiologic exposure had been validated, then the RSO would have reported the incident to REAC/TS, and both local and perhaps federal authorities could have performed a full analysis and recommended treatment and follow-up of this patient. Regardless of the absence of radiation injury, this patient has likely suffered some emotional injury and needs psychological follow-up. This can be done with his primary care physician or with a radiation medicine specialist a day or so later for reassurance.

UNIQUE CONSIDERATIONS

The number of casualties involved in a radiation accident may range from one patient to thousands contaminated by a dirty bomb. The number of patients with significant exposure will usually be quite small. The only people exposed to very high activity contamination due to a dirty bomb are usually those involved in its production or delivery, i.e., the terrorists themselves. Triage may differ depending on the number of casualties and total whole body doses. The Strategic National Stockpile Radiation Working Group (SNS) has published guidelines for triage of fewer than or more than 100 casualties.[9]

Accidents involving pregnant women or young children are unique. Internal contamination of the pregnant woman can increase or decrease the relative fetal dose, depending on the element, route of exposure, and age of gestation. Internal contamination with elements excreted in the urine may increase the fetal dose because of the proximity to the bladder. Developing organs in the fetus or young child may have greatly increased uptake of particular elements, especially iodine. The threshold dose for giving potassium iodide is much lower for them ($\geq$0.05 Gy expected dose) compared with adults 18 to 40 years old ($\geq$0.1 Gy expected dose) and adults older than 40 years (5 Gy).[4]

All radiation accident victims carry some increased lifetime risk of an induced malignancy.[7] This is usually far less than anticipated and only slightly above the preincident risk because radiation is a relatively weak carcinogen.[7] Risk is related to quality and dose of radiation, affected organs, age at the time of exposure, and other risk factors.[7] Education about the usual small increase in risk may diminish stress significantly. General educational materials can initially allay fears, and subsequent consultation with a radiation specialist can better define risks and proper surveillance.

Mortuary procedures and burial of contaminated corpses must be coordinated with an RSO. The NCRP and the Disaster Mortuary Operational Response Team provide guidelines (see http://www.dmort.org) for handling deceased patients with radioactivity significantly above background levels.[2,7] Most decedents can be decontaminated for conventional burial; however, cremation may be restricted. All corpses must be stored in the hot zone until decontaminated and released by an RSO.[7]

Finally, psychological stress can be intense and long-lasting in victims, relatives, coworkers, first responders, and providers.[7,16] Counseling and educational handouts can allay many fears. The stigma of radiation exposure and posttraumatic stress disorder may require long-term psychological follow-up.[5,16] Preparation of general and specific educational handouts in advance can provide quick reassurance. The CDC Web site has several excellent handouts on these topics. Local electronic storage is appropriate, as authoritative Internet sites will likely be overloaded during an incident. Your facility should prepare specific instructions in advance relative to the known industrial and medical radiologic hazards in your region.

 ## PITFALLS

Rapid assessment and limited contamination will only be possible by providers who promptly recognize radiation accidents and appropriately institute a predetermined response plan. Failure to have detection equipment available and accessible can lead to delays in initial interventions. Failure to consider radiation scenarios in disaster exercises can lead to inadequate responses in the event of a true radiologic emergency.

REFERENCES

1. Turai I, Veress K. Radiation accidents: occurrence, types, consequences, medical management, and the lessons to be learned. *CEJOEM* 2001;7:3-14.
2. Department of Homeland Security Working Group on Radiological Dispersal Device (RDD) Preparedness, Medical Preparedness and Response Sub-Group. 5/1/03 Version. Available at: http://www1.va.gov/emshg/docs/Radiologic_Medical_Countermeasures_051403.pdf.
3. U.S. Food and Drug Administration. Prussian blue, Radiogardase, package insert. Available at: http://www.fda.gov/cder/drug/infopage/prussian_blue/default.ht Accessed October 11, 2005.
4. U.S. Food and Drug Administration. Guidance: Potassium iodide as a thyroid blocking agent in radiation emergencies. Available at: http://www.fda.gov/cder/guidance/4825fnl.htm. Accessed October 11, 2005.
5. *Management of Persons Accidentally Contaminated with Radionuclides*. NCRP report no. 65. Bethesda, Md: National Council on Radiation Protection and Measurements; 1980.
6. Jarrett D, ed. *Medical Management of Radiological Casualties: Handbook*. 2nd ed. AFRRI special publication 03-1. Bethesda, Md:Armed Forces Radiobiology Research Institute; 2003. Available at: http://www.afrri.usuhs.mil. Accessed October 11, 2005.
7. *Management of Terrorist Events Involving Radioactive Material*. NCRP report no. 138. Bethesda, Md: National Council on Radiation Protection and Measurements; 2001.
8. Appendix 1: Sample radiation emergency plan for a medical facility. In: Gusev, I, Guskova, A, Mettler, F, eds. *Medical Management of Radiation Accidents*. 2nd ed. Boca Raton, Fla: CRC Press; 2001:557-570.
9. Waselenko J, MacVittie T, Blakely W, et al. Medical management of the acute radiation syndrome: recommendations of the Strategic National Stockpile Radiation Working Group. *Ann Intern Med*. 2004;140:1037-51.
10. Mettler F, Kelsey C. Fundamentals of radiation accidents. In: Gusev I, Guskova A, Mettler, F, eds. *Medical Management of Radiation Accidents*. 2nd ed. Boca Raton, Fla: CRC Press; 2001:1-13.
11. Mettler F, Voelz G. Major radiation exposure—what to expect and how to respond. *N Engl J Med*. 2002;346:1554-61.
12. Farb D. OSHA Occupational Radiation Safety Manual and CD. Los Angeles: University of Health Care; 2003.
13. Centers for Disease Control and Prevention. Emergency preparedness and response: radiation emergencies. Available at: http://www.bt.cdc.gov/radiation. Accessed October 11, 2005.
14. Guskova A, Baranov A, Gusev I. Acute radiation sickness: underlying principles and assessment. In: Gusev I, Guskova A, Mettler, F, eds. *Medical Management of Radiation Accidents*. 2nd ed. Boca Raton, Fla: CRC Press; 2001:33-51.
15. Guskova A. Radiation sickness classification. In: Gusev I, Guskova A, Mettler, F, eds. *Medical Management of Radiation Accidents*. 2nd ed. Boca Raton, Fla: CRC Press; 2001:15-22.
16. Berger M, Sadoff R. Psychological support of radiation accident patients, families, and staff. In: Gusev I, Guskova A, Mettler, F, eds. *Medical Management of Radiation Accidents*. 2nd ed. Boca Raton, Fla: CRC Press;2001:191-200.
17. Package insert: NDA 21-749 Pentetate calcium trisodium injection. Hameln, Germany: Hameln Pharmaceuticals gmbh; 2004.
18. Package insert: NDA 21-751 Pentetate zinc trisodium injection. Hameln, Germany: Hameln Pharmaceuticals gmbh; 2004.
19. Centers for Disease Control and Prevention. CDC fact sheet on DTPA. Available at: http://www.bt.cdc.gov/radiation/dtpa.asp. Accessed October 11, 2005.
20. Fasano A. Pathophysiology and management of radiation injury of the gastrointestinal tract. In: Ricks R, Berger M, O'Hara F, eds. *The Medical Basis for Radiation-Accident Preparedness: The Clinical Care of Victims*. Proceedings of the Fourth International REAC/TS Conference on the Medical Basis for Radiation-Accident Preparedness. New York:The Parthenon; 2002:149-60.
21. Voelz G. Assessment and treatment of internal contamination: general principles. In: Gusev I, Guskova A, Mettler, F, eds. *Medical Management of Radiation Accidents*. 2nd ed. Boca Raton, Fla: CRC Press; 2001:319-36.

chapter 88

Nuclear Power Plant Meltdown

William Porcaro

 DESCRIPTION OF EVENT

Nuclear power plants that provide safe, clean energy to many areas of the globe have the potential to cause massive disasters, both through accidents and terrorist events. About 17% of the world's energy is generated by nuclear fission. Whereas only about 15% of U.S. power is nuclear generated, the French create about 75% of their energy by the nuclear route.[1] Figure 88-1 shows a schematic of a typical nuclear power plant. A catastrophic meltdown would pose many threats, ranging from various flavors of radiation escaping into the atmosphere to more conventional dangers such as steam and fire. Commercial U.S. nuclear reactors have been cited numerous times in the media as potential targets for terrorist attacks.

Risk for radiation leak and exposure may occur at many points. In the most drastic situation, a fire, coolant failure, control rod failure, or sabotage may allow a reactor to overheat and melt itself. As the reactor self-destructs, radioactive solids and gases may be released into the environment. Volatile radioactive isotopes may also be elaborated from the core, including those of iodine and the noble gases. Over 100 radioactive elements were elaborated into the atmosphere during the core fire caused by exploding gases in the number four reactor at Chernobyl. The vast majority of these isotopes decayed quite quickly. The most dangerous and longest-lasting isotopes are of iodine, strontium, and cesium, which possess half-lives of 8 days, 29 years, and 30 years respectively. Internalized strontium may lead to leukemia. Cesium, which traveled the farthest, may be linked with liver and spleen pathology.[2] Experience from nuclear incidents and nuclear medicine accidents has proved the long-term implications of such a release, most notably the increase in childhood thyroid cancer attributed to radioactive iodine.[3]

In addition to the health hazards posed by radioactive materials, nuclear power plants harbor many other potential hazards. The steam and high pressures that exist in the reactor coolant systems and heat exchangers in pressurized water reactors may cause severe thermal burns because either simple steam or radioactive steam may be evolved. Over the past 50 years, there have been several instances of nuclear power plant disasters and near disasters. In 1952, the Chalk River nuclear reactor near Ottawa, Ontario, sustained a partial meltdown of the uranium fuel core after four control rods were accidentally removed. Millions of gallons of radioactive water accumulated inside the reactor, but no injuries occurred. In 1957, fire in a graphite-cooled reactor north of Liverpool, England, spewed radiation over the countryside. In 1976, near Greifswald, East Germany, the radioactive core of a reactor nearly melted down due to the failure of safety systems during a fire. At Three Mile Island, near Harrisburg, Pa, coolant loss allowed overheating and partial meltdown of the uranium core in one of two reactors, and some radioactive water and gases were released.

On April 26, 1986, the worst nuclear accident in history occurred at the Chernobyl power plant in Kiev, U.S.S.R. (now Ukraine). During a shutdown for routine maintenance, a test was performed to see whether enough energy could be maintained to operate emergency equipment and cooling pumps. As workers tried to compensate, they accidentally caused a power surge estimated at 100 times nominal power output. This surge caused part of the fuel rods to rupture and react with water, creating a steam and hydrogen gas explosion and a subsequent graphite fire that destroyed the core. The lack of a containment facility and thermal loft resulted in the release of tremendous amounts of radioactive material into the atmosphere. The failure of officials to acknowledge the incident to the general public resulted in the ingestion of contaminated foodstuffs during the days immediately after the meltdown. The estimated death toll was 31, but the total number of casualties is unknown.

In addition to nuclear power plants, many TRIGA nuclear reactors (a brand name that stands for Training Research Isotopes, General Atomics, the builder) used for research exist primarily in universities throughout the world. They are often located in densely populated urban areas with relatively minimal security. TRIGA reactors are considered "inherently safe." Their safety profile is based on the construction of their fuel rods, which force overheating fuel to limit the fission process and stop the nuclear reaction. Even when all of the control rods are simultaneously removed by

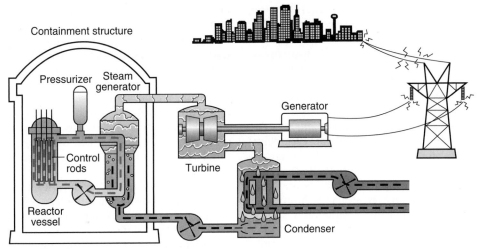

FIGURE 88–1. Anatomy of a pressurized water reactor. (From the U.S. Nuclear Regulatory Commission Web site. Available at: http://www.nrc.gov/reading-rm/basic-ref/students/reactors.html.)

accident or deliberate intent, the reactor cannot generate enough heat to cause a problem; it simply shuts down.[4]

 PREINCIDENT ACTIONS:

Hospitals that may receive victims after a nuclear power plant incident should have the capability to detect radioactivity, primarily through the use of Geiger counters. Large institutions should have a Radiologic Emergency Response Team that can be activated when needed. This group may be composed of emergency department providers, security personnel, radiation safety officers, maintenance personnel, and laboratory support. Staff should be fitted with appropriate anti-contamination clothing, including double gloving so that the outer pair can be removed when contaminated. Personnel should also be issued dosimeters to track their exposure. A radiation decontamination area should be prepared with plastic lining and plastic waste containers. Flooring should be covered and cordoned off. Special ventilation to isolate the area is desirable but not necessary because there is very low likelihood that radioactive material will become aerosolized.[5]

Evacuation plans are paramount to preparation for a nuclear power plant meltdown. All Nuclear Regulatory Commission–regulated power plants have community contingency plans as a requirement for licensure. In addition to local and state authorities, the Federal Emergency Management Agency (FEMA) plays a role in orchestrating these strategies. One of the special concerns surrounding nuclear power plant meltdowns involves radioactive iodine and exposure to the thyroid gland. Appropriate plans must be in place for the prophylaxis or treatment of persons who live in close proximity to nuclear power plants to decrease their risk of thyroid cancer if a release occurs, by providing prompt potassium iodide to compete with released radioactive iodine for binding sites in the thyroid. Preparedness should be practiced through exercises involving power plants and area hospitals.

 POSTINCIDENT ACTIONS

After a nuclear power plant incident has occurred, containment of radioactive contaminants in and around the facility continues to be a priority. The Chernobyl Exclusion Zone served as an evacuation area and continues to use natural and manmade boundaries to prevent migration of radionuclides and to control the illegal harvesting of contaminated foodstuffs. Evacuation of the at-risk population will lead to the need for sheltering and medical care of large numbers of evacuees and screening for necessary prophylaxis.

Numerous other details must be considered after a meltdown, including radioactive and hazardous waste removal, economic sustainability in the surrounding areas, and food supply/agriculture. Contaminated soil leads to contamination of plants and animals and their products, such as milk and beef.[6]

 MEDICAL TREATMENT OF CASUALTIES

Victims from a nuclear power plant meltdown or persons potentially exposed from the surrounding area must be evaluated for possible contamination. However, immediate medical attention must be paid to serious or life-threatening problems. At triage, a brief radiologic survey should be performed to determine exposure. Non-acutely ill victims should have clothing removed and sealed in plastic bags by staff wearing proper protective equipment. Wounds that may be contaminated should be cleansed, after thorough draping to avoid spread of radioactive material. Cleansing of intact skin must be performed in a manner that limits mechanical or chemical irritation to avoid deeper spread of the radioactive material.

Contaminated orifices may require special attention; for example, decontaminating the mouth may require aggressive brushing with toothpaste or gargling with 3% hydrogen peroxide.[5] Irrigation solutions used to clean open contaminated wounds must be carefully retained and surveyed, so they can be disposed of properly.

Victims who are believed to have suffered radioactive contamination should have several basic laboratory studies. All specimens must be sealed in plastic and sent in properly labeled containers that specify name, date, time of sampling, area of samples, and size of sample areas. Complete blood count with stat differentials must be obtained to follow absolute lymphocyte counts, and this should be repeated approximately every 6 hours for 2 days to monitor for bone marrow suppression in any patient suspected to have suffered whole body irradiation. Urinalysis should also be performed on all victims of radiologic injury to ensure proper renal function, which is necessary to clear possible internal contamination. Externally contaminated patients should have swabs from wounds and all body orifices sent to be monitored for radioactivity. In cases where internal contamination is suspected (i.e., inhalation, ingestion, or absorption), 4 days of 24-hour urine and feces should be sampled for detection of radionuclides excreted from the body.

Acute radiation syndrome may be seen in victims who were in close proximity to the reactor meltdown such as plant workers, first responder firemen and law enforcement officers, or EMS officials who were unable to use appropriate precautions. Signs and symptoms arise secondary to cellular deficiencies and the reactions of various cells, tissues, and organ systems to ionizing radiation.

In addition to radiologic injuries, traditional emergencies may present during a nuclear power plant incident. Steam is a real and present danger in all power plants. From a nuclear standpoint, radioactive steam may serve as a medium to rapidly spread nuclear fallout and allow it to penetrate the body through burns and inspiration. However, the dangers of injuries inflicted by nonradioactive steam should not be underestimated. Severe thermal skin burns as well as inhalational burns to the distal airway causing stridor and respiratory distress and failure should be anticipated. In August 2004, nonradioactive steam leaked from a nuclear power plant in Mihama, Japan, killing four workers and severely burning seven others.

As discussed in the unique considerations section, patients from areas of radioactive iodine fallout should be treated with potassium iodide within 4 hours of exposure.

UNIQUE CONSIDERATIONS

Like all nuclear/radiologic events, the factors of time, distance, and shielding are crucial at determining human exposure and ultimately disease and outcome of a nuclear power plant meltdown. Simple actions such as rapid and orderly evacuation from contaminated areas, rapid and effective decontamination, and containment of hazardous waste can greatly reduce risk. As alluded to above, any time there is a leak of radioactive material into the environment, concerns about soil and plant/animal food sources come into play. Therefore, an adequate, noncontaminated food and water supply must be ensured.

The increased risk of thyroid cancer in children must be anticipated. Strong consideration must be given to the treatment of children and infants with potassium iodide when there is risk for inhalation of contaminated air or ingestion of contaminated food. Administered before or within 4 hours after intake of radioactive iodine, potassium iodide can block or reduce the accumulation of radioactive iodine in the thyroid, thereby reducing the risk of cancer.[7]

If a genuine nuclear power plant meltdown has occurred, concerns about public response during and after the incident will almost certainly arise. The public is often quite eager to obtain as much information as possible regarding the incident. When instructions are given, they must be clear and repeated, and the rationale for the warnings and instructions must be provided.[8]

CASE PRESENTATION

It's 6 PM on a Friday during a hectic emergency department shift. The medical control radio alarms, and you learn that there has been an incident at a nuclear power plant reactor in a neighboring state. Authorities have learned that an international terrorist group has had operatives in the plant for the past several years. This afternoon, these radicals were able to defeat the control rod safety features and plant cooling system to initiate a core meltdown. Simultaneously, others detonated a huge truck bomb to form a breach in the plant's concrete-containment system. It is now believed that a radioactive plume has escaped from the plant and is traveling toward the city.

The area surrounding the plant is currently being evacuated. Rescue efforts are under way at the plant and numerous victims are being airlifted to your facility. The department triage nurse also tells you that there are a number of people calling and presenting to the hospital concerned that they are contaminated with radiation.

You immediately initiate a disaster code within the hospital and begin looking for your hospital's plans on how to manage a mass radiologic disaster. You take the following initial steps: You notify the hospital's radiation safety officer on call, considering it is after hours and they have likely already left the facility. You meet with the nurses in your emergency department and start to discharge all stable walk-in patients in your waiting room after explaining what has happened, keeping only those patients who truly appear ill. You also ensure that the emergency department is being prepared to receive radiologically exposed and possibly contaminated patients. You check the batteries in the radiation-detection device kept in the emergency department, in case you need it before the radiation safety officer arrives. The remainder of this chapter discusses some of the unique considerations and possible pitfalls that may be associated with the simulated preceding case.

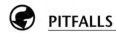 **PITFALLS**

Well-crafted and rehearsed strategies are the key to success during the genuine incident. Failure to appropriately set up decontamination areas and unsuccessful decontamination may lead to dispersing contaminated patients throughout the hospital, further exposing these patients as well as contaminating the staff caring for them. Studies suggest that evacuation time estimates are crucial for proper emergency response planning. Evacuation time estimates must consider many factors, ranging from traffic management to uncontrollable events such as weather, when projecting for an event.[8] "Shelter in place" should always be considered.

Although treatment or prophylaxis with potassium iodide is relatively safe for children, there are some risks, including gastrointestinal effects or even hypersensitivity reactions. Additionally, thyroidal adverse effects may result from stable iodine administration, especially in iodine-deficient patients or in connection with thyroid disorders, such as autoimmune thyroiditis or Graves' disease.[7]

REFERENCES

1. Brain M. How nuclear power works. Available at: http://science.howstuffworks.com/nuclear-power.htm.
2. Chernobyl + 15, Frequently asked questions. Available at: http://www.iaea.org/NewsCenter/Features/Chernobyl-15/index.shtml.
3. Mettler FA Jr, Voelz GL. Major radiation exposure: what to expect and how to respond. *N Engl J Med.* 2002;346(20):1554-61.
4. TRIGA nuclear reactors, General Atomics Cooperation Web site. Available at: http://triga.ga.com.
5. Oak Ridge Institute for Science and Education. Radiation Emergency Assistance Center/Training Site (REAC/TS). Available at: http://www.orau.gov/reacts.
6. International Conference, 15 Years After the Chernobyl Accident. *Lessons Learned: Executive Summary.* Kyiv, Ukraine: April 18-20, 2001. http://www.iaea.org/NewsCenter/Features/Chernobyl-15/execsum_eng.pdf.
7. *Guidelines for Iodine Prophylaxis Following Nuclear Accidents, Update 1999.* Geneva: World Health Organization; 1999.
8. Mileti DS, Peek L. The social psychology of public response to warnings of a nuclear power plant accident. *J Hazardous Mater.* 2000;75:181-94.

SUGGESTED READINGS

British Energy Web site. Available at: http://www.british-energy.com.

International Atomic Energy Agency. Promoting safety in nuclear installations. Available at: http://www.iaea.org/Publications/ Factsheets/English/safetynuclinstall.pdf

International Atomic Energy Agency. The International Nuclear Event Scale for prompt communication of safety significance. Available at: http://www.iaea.org/Publications/ Factsheets/English/ines-e.pdf

International Nuclear Safety Center at Argonne National Laboratory, U.S. Department of Energy Nuclear Energy Institute Source Book on Soviet-Designed Nuclear Power Plants. Available at: http://www.insc.anl.gov/sov_des/sov_des.php

Nuclear and Chemical Accidents, 2005. Family Education Network; Boston, MA 2005. Available at: http://www.infoplease.com/ipa/A0001457.html.

Tintinalli JE, et al. *Emergency Medicine: A Comprehensive Study Guide.* 5th ed. American College of Emergency Physicians; 2000:1303-17.

Urbanik T. Evacuation time estimates for nuclear power plants. *J Hazardous Mater.* 2000;75:165-80.

U.S. Department of Homeland Security, Federal Emergency Management Agency. Nuclear Power Plant Emergency Fact Sheet. Available at: http://www.fema.gov/pdf/hazards/nuclear.pdf

chapter 89

Introduction to Chemical Disasters

David Marcozzi

This chapter serves as an overview and a broad outline toward managing victims of chemical releases, both accidental and intentional, including those related to terrorism. Although the specific agents that may be released vary immensely, the clinical approach to response is fairly uniform. When a chemical release occurs, rapid and effective response is dependent on thorough pre-event planning, appropriate medical treatment, and subsequent post-event analysis to allow for refinements in future response operations. These steps help to ensure rapid deployment of resources, accurate identification and treatment of victims, and protection of medical providers, the environment, and the scene for law enforcement.

Chemical exposures may come from environmental, industrial, warfare, or terrorism sources. Historically in the United States, the overwhelming majority of chemical-release incidents have been the result of industrial accidents, the effects of which may be in sharp contrast to those of intentional releases.

In the present world climate, the potential for chemical warfare and terrorism, the intent of which are to produce casualties, continues to change our planning, response, and overall perspective. *Chemical warfare* refers to the utilization of weapons using the toxic properties of certain chemicals to produce debilitating physiologic, psychological, and economic effects on their targets. Chemical terrorism is the use of chemical agents to further political or social objectives by intimidating or coercing any segment of a government or of a civilian population. The exact number of states and stateless groups that possess chemical agents is difficult to assess, but industrial chemicals are widely available throughout the world. This has been pointed out by the U.S. Central Intelligence Agency to Congress and its committees:

> Although U.S. intelligence is increasing its emphasis and resources on many of these issues, there is continued and growing risk of surprise. We focus much of our intelligence collection and analysis on some ten states, but even concerning those states, there are important gaps in our knowledge. . . . Moreover, we have identified well over 50 states that are of concern as suppliers, conduits, or potential proliferants.[1]

The threat of terrorists using chemical, biological, radiological, and nuclear (CBRN) materials appears to be rising—particularly since the 11 September attacks. Several of the 30 designated foreign terrorist organizations and other non-state actors worldwide have expressed interest in CBRN.[2]

A response to any hazardous material (HazMat) release, whether as a result of deployment from these new threats or from an accidental industrial release, must be well coordinated among HazMat teams, hospitals, fire, emergency medical services (EMS), Emergency Management and law enforcement personnel. Paramount to chemical releases is the mandate for quick and efficient deployment of resources to extricate, decontaminate, and treat the largest number of victims ensuring the greatest benefit to the greatest number of casualties. Simultaneously, there are fundamental principles to which any chemical exposure response must adhere to ensure the protection of healthcare workers, the environment, and the potential crime scene.

HISTORICAL PERSPECTIVE

No significant intentional mass-casualty chemical disaster has yet occurred on U.S. soil. The sad reality is that an event of that nature, related to an act of war, terrorism, or a major industrial sabotage, will likely occur in the future with the potential to affect hundreds or thousands of people. The distress caused by the use of such an agent or the accidental release of a toxic chemical would be psychologically traumatic for many more.

The first employment of chemical weapons in modern times was in World War I by the Germans at Ypres, Belgium, on April 15, 1915 (Box 89-1). That afternoon, German units released an estimated 150 tons of chlorine gas against Allied troops. Its use was followed on Dec. 19, 1915, by the use of phosgene, which like chlorine was denser than air but which had a greater predilection than did chlorine to produce death from pulmonary edema (see Chapter 93). Still later in the war, sulfur mustard (a liquid at ambient temperatures) was introduced. As a persistent agent, sulfur mustard remained in the environment for weeks and could act as a barrier to troop movements. Mustard was subsequently used extensively and with decisive results by Italy in Abyssinia (now Ethiopia) in 1935 (see Chapter 92). Nerve agents are organophosphorus anticholinesterases and are the most potent chemical warfare agents. These agents were first developed in the 1930s by the German scientist Gerhard Schrader in conjunction with his research on insecticides. Nerve agents include the nonpersistent G-series agents and the V agents, which are environmentally persistent (see Chapter 91).

Chemical agents were not extensively used during World War II due to the fear of retaliation and because chemical weapons are of limited use in a mobile front in which their use would slow the advance of one's own troops. In addition, chemical warfare requires supply from railroads, which were available in the fixed fronts of World War I but which were not well suited to supply to the often rapidly mobile fronts of World War II. However, the fear that the German military might use such weapons led to the production of mustard agent bombs by the United States, to be used only if the Axis forces used chemical weapons first. Such weapons were shipped to Europe on a U.S. Liberty ship, the John Harvey, in 1943. Before the unloading of the vessel in Bari Harbor, Italy, it was struck by a direct hit during a Luftwaffe air raid and exploded, killing the entire crew and spreading its toxic mustard agent throughout the port and into the air, affecting hundreds of servicemen and civilians.[3] The incident was kept secret for decades. Dozens of shiploads of such toxic chemicals, many of them captured German weapons, were scuttled in waters off shore in the Norwegian Trench and the Baltic Sea, and many agents were brought back to the United States and scuttled in the Gulf of Mexico. The environmental impact has been poorly studied, but many instances of fishermen injured by such weapons in Europe have been reported.[3] In 1974, the United States signed the Geneva Protocol of 1925, which bans the use of poisonous substances in war. At that time, the United States reserved the right to retaliate in kind if an enemy were to use any chemical agent against it; the power to order such retaliation resided with the president. On April 4, 1984, President Ronald Reagan called for an international ban on chemical weapons, and the United States currently has a no-use policy for any official chemical agents (the official U.S. military definition of chemical agents excludes riot-control agents, herbicides, and smoke-and-flame material from consideration as chemical agents; this distinction is not universally accepted internationally) and is in the process of dismantling its chemical-agent stockpiles. The United States has additionally renounced the use of herbicides and riot-control agents in war, except in retaliation.

In June 1994, a team of cultists from Aum Shinri Kyo sprayed vaporized sarin for 10 minutes at residential quarters in Matsumoto, Japan. Three judges staying at the residence were about to rule on a civil case over a

BOX 89-1 A HISTORY OF CHEMICAL WEAPONS

1899
An international peace conference held in The Hague leads to an agreement prohibiting the use of projectiles filled with poison gas.
1915
First large-scale use of chemical agents on the World War I battlefields near Ypres (Ieper), Belgium.
1918
By the end of World War I, the use of over 100,000 tons of toxic chemicals during the war had resulted in the deaths of 90,000 soldiers and had caused more than a million casualties.
1925
The Geneva Protocol is concluded. This treaty bans the use of both bacteriologic and chemical weapons but is not enough to stop countries from producing, stockpiling, or using chemical weapons thereafter.
1972
The countries of the world conclude the Biological and Toxin Weapons Convention in Geneva and commit themselves to continue negotiations on a treaty to ban chemical weapons as well.
1984-1989
Iraq uses chemical weapons against Iran and (in 1988) against its own Kurdish citizens in the town of Halabja.
1992
The negotiators in Geneva agree on the text of the Convention on the Prohibition of Development, Production, Stockpiling, and Use of Chemical Weapons and on Their Destruction (Chemical Weapons Convention).
1993
The Chemical Weapons Convention (CWC) is opened for signature at a January signing ceremony in Paris; 130 countries show support for the CWC and for international disarmament by signing the convention. In February 1993, a Preparatory Commission is set up in The Hague to prepare for the entry into force of the convention.
1995
In Japan, the Aum Shinri Kyo cult releases the chemical agent sarin in a terrorist attack on the Tokyo subway.
1997
The CWC enters into force for 87 original member countries. The organization created by the Convention to carry out the terms of the Convention, the Organisation for the Prohibition of Chemical Weapons (OPCW), opens its headquarters in The Hague.
2003
The CWC has grown into an international regime with 152 member countries (as of May 6, 2003), covering 90% of the world's population, 92% of the world's landmass, and 98% of its chemical industry. The OPCW has overseen the destruction of nearly 10% of the stockpiles of chemical weapons declared to it.

fraudulent land deal involving the cult. In this attack, 7 people were killed and 144 injured, many of them seriously.[4]

On March 20, 1995, in a more well-known incident, members of the Aum Shinri Kyo cult released the G-series nerve agent sarin in the Tokyo subway system during rush hour, killing 11 and injuring more than 5500 people.[5,6] Secondary contamination occurred in more than 20% of healthcare workers at St. Luke's International Hospital, a facility near the release site. Eighty percent of patients arrived via means not involving their EMS system. This release served as the modern-day landmark event with regard to chemical warfare on civilians. The response to this incident has been extensively reviewed. In addition to the physical effects of the release that required immediate treatment, 60% of victims suffered from posttraumatic stress disorder, persisting in several cases for more than 6 months.

Chemical exposures on U.S. soil are predominantly industrially related accidental releases. HazMat transportation incidents are reported to the U.S. Department of Transportation. For the last 10 years, of the almost 156,500 incidents that occurred, 3218 injuries and 226 deaths were reported.[7]

In another data set, a total of 13,808 emergency events relating to hazardous substances were reported in 1999 and 2000 to the Hazardous Substances Emergency Events Surveillance System (HSEES), which collects information from approximately 15 states.[8] These data deserve review and can help focus efforts with regard to pre-event planning for HazMat releases. Approximately 70% of the reported events occurred at fixed facilities, with 96% of all events involving only one substance. The nature of the agent was balanced, with a spill occurring in 54.0% of the releases, followed by 41.7% for air releases, 6.8% for fires, and 1.2% for explosions. Ammonia, sulfur dioxide, and sulfuric acid were the most frequently released substances. Fortunately, only 9.1% of all events resulted in victims. Of the events that did involve victims, 73.2% involved only one or two casualties. It should be noted that the HSEES reports do not cover hazardous materials events occurring due to petroleum products. Interpretation of the data from the HSEES and the Department of Transportation, whose morbidity and mortality are low, demonstrates a marked contrast to the potential results of a terrorism or warfare chemical release, where the intent is aimed at producing casualties—both physical and psychological.

CURRENT PRACTICE

Any chemical release has the potential to produce mass casualties. The safe and effective management of the scene, patients, and environment depends on prioritizing scene safety and staff protection for emergency responders and hospital personnel.

Pre-event planning and training are critical to maximize resources and to ensure that those most in need receive aid while preventing rescue and hospital workers from becoming patients themselves. Unfortunately, HazMat preparedness has largely been reactive instead of

preemptive. Although no community can prepare for every chemical emergency, the potential for mass casualties and secondary contamination can be mitigated with the help of a Hazard Vulnerability Analysis. Before an event, many issues need to be addressed (Box 89-2), all of which are important for a sufficient response to chemical disasters. These topics are addressed in this text and should be referred to accordingly. In attending to these various issues, a local emergency planning committee, hospital, private organization, or government agency should systematically address each concern in the local area and cover additional ones specific to its scope of practice, environment, level of risk, and capabilities.

Depending on the chemical or chemicals released, the mode of dissemination, the properties of each agent, various physical effects, and various degrees of symptoms and signs will result. Many key terms, acronyms, and principles relating to chemical properties are important to understand (Box 89-3).

Unlike bioterrorist incidents, an event of this nature is unlikely to be covert. Due to the presence of a foreign chemical in the environment, effects will likely be seen immediately—within minutes or hours. Within 90 minutes of an event, 50% to 80% of the acute casualties will likely arrive at the closest medical facilities (Figure 89-1).[9]

Depending on the type of chemical release, different interventions, antidotes, and treatments will be needed for the casualties. Decontamination of victims remains a primary medical response. The maneuvers of removal of clothing or the application of soap and water (or simply copious amounts of water) limit further absorption of a toxicant by the victim and serve to protect medical providers from secondary contamination. Decontamination by means of chemical compounds such as alkaline bleach solutions may cause more tissue damage, leading to further penetration of agent, and physical or mechanical decontamination should be preferred over decontamination using chemicals. Immediate medical care may need to be provided before full-body decontamination, but removal of all agent visible on body surfaces should never be delayed. Immediate local, or spot, decontamination of skin and wounds can make the difference between life and death, since many chemicals are absorbed quickly and since chemicals already in transit through the skin are no longer amenable to surface contamination. Spot decontamination should always

BOX 89-2 PRE-EVENT CONSIDERATIONS

Hazard vulnerability analysis
Personal protective equipment
Decontamination capabilities
HazMat training
Public education
Press cooperation
Patient-surge capacity
Additional mobilizable resources and personnel
Coordinated response between all agencies
Communications plan
Evacuation and shelter-in-place plans

BOX 89-3 HAZMAT DEFINITIONS

- **Flash point**: The temperature at which a liquid will give off enough flammable vapor to burn. Because there are several flash-point test methods, and because flash points may vary for the same material depending on the method used, the test method must be indicated when the flash point is given.
- **Immediately dangerous to life and health (IDLH)**: Any condition that may result in damage to health that cannot be repaired. IDLH situations include explosive and oxygen-deficient environments and the presence of class A poisons or substances that can be absorbed through the skin.
- **Lower explosive limit (LEL)**: The lowest concentration (i.e., lowest percentage of the substance in air) that will produce a flash of fire when an ignition source (e.g., heat, arc, flame) is present.
- **Manifest form**: The form required by the EPA to track hazardous wastes.
- **Material safety data sheet (MSDS)**: An informational sheet that is sent with hazardous materials. It lists chemical properties, emergency response procedures, reactivity data, control measures, safe handling procedures, and the manufacturer.
- **Permissible exposure limit (PEL)**: The highest level of a substance to which a person can be exposed. This limit is set by the Occupational Safety and Health Administration (OSHA).
- **Short-term exposure limit (STEL)**: An exposure limit that sets the maximum concentration that a worker can be exposed to during a 15-minute period.
- **Threshold limit value (TLV)**: The airborne concentration of a material to which nearly all persons can be exposed day after day without adverse effects. The American Conference of Industrial Hygienists expresses TLVs in three ways:
  - **TLV-TWA**: The allowable time-weighted average concentration for a normal 8-hour workday.
  - **TLV-STEL**: The short-term exposure limit, or maximum concentration for a continuous 15-minute exposure period (maximum of four such periods a day, with at least 60 minutes between exposure periods and provided that the daily TLV-TWA is not exceeded).
  - **TLV-C**: The ceiling exposure limit or "the concentration that should not be exceeded during any part of the working exposure ... a 15-minute period except for those substances which may cause immediate irritation ..."
- **Time-weighted average (TWA)**: A measurement to determine the average exposure of a worker to a substance over a typical 8-hour work shift. The actual exposure is then compared to OSHA standards or other professional guidelines.
- **Upper explosive limit (UEL)** or **upper flammable limit (UFL)** (pertaining to a vapor or gas): The highest concentration (i.e., highest percentage of the substance in air) that will produce a flash of fire when an ignition source (e.g., heat, arc, or flame) is present. At higher concentrations, the mixture is too "rich" to burn. See also lower explosive limit.
- **Vapor density**: The weight of a vapor or gas compared with the weight of an equal volume of air; an expression of the density of the vapor or gas. Materials lighter than air have vapor densities less than 1.0. Materials heavier than air have vapor densities greater than 1.0.
- **Vapor pressure**: The pressure (usually, a partial pressure acting as one component of the total pressure of the atmosphere) exerted by the vapor arising from a solid or liquid.
- **Volatility**: The tendency of a substance to evaporate (this property is directly correlated with speed of evaporation).

receive the same high priority as airway, breathing, circulation, and specific antidotal therapy and should therefore be included as one of the "ABCDDs" (airway, breathing, circulation, decontamination [spot], and drugs [specific antidotes]) of the immediate medical response

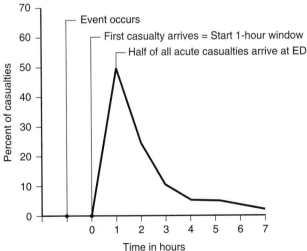

FIGURE 89–1. Predicted emergency department casualties.

to a chemical casualty (J.M. Madsen, personal communication, November 1, 2004). Casualties who are triaged as low priority may be escorted to a waiting area after decontamination to allow for appropriate treatment of those requiring emergent attention. Continued reevaluation of the victims is of the utmost importance because effects and routes of exposure may differ from patient to patient, thus affecting the time of onset of symptoms and signs. Initial recognition and a careful step-by-step approach to victims exposed to a chemical agent are paramount; this approach should use a logical progression from agent through agent in the environment to agent on and in the host and then follow through with an appreciation of toxicologic principles such as toxicokinetics (i.e., absorption, distribution, biotransformation, and elimination), toxicodynamics (i.e., mechanism of action), the continuum of exposure (from external dose through internal dose and biologic effective dose to early biologic effects, altered structure and function, and clinical intoxication), and clinical pearls such as the inverse relationship between the dose of most agents and their latent (clinically asymptomatic) periods.

This toxicologic approach is often not stressed in the education and training of healthcare providers but provides a vital framework for the clinical evaluation of casualties exposed to chemicals. It can be summarized by means of one or more acronyms suitable for posting in ambulances and emergency departments and for memorization (see Table 89-1) and Table 89-2 [J.M. Madsen, personal communication, November 1, 2004]). Knowledge of specific symptoms and signs of each agent is of great importance, as this will determine further efforts and treatment. Accurate triage systems incorporating immediate, delayed, minimal, and expectant categories are required to allow the medical resources to effectively reach those in greatest need. Depending on their level of training, specialized teams may be inserted into the warm and hot zones to provide triage and medical stabilization before decontamination. After full-body decontamination, secondary triage may occur and subsequent medical management may be instituted.

As stated, based on patient presentations, specific treatments and antidotes may be instituted for each agent once confirmation or suspected agent recognition occurs. It is unlikely that toxicant identification will occur prior to casualties presenting to a healthcare provider or institution. Therefore, the ability of prehospital and hospital providers to recognize toxidromes associated with chemical agents is essential. This initial recognition can be lifesaving for the patients, their providers, and even for patients in an institution not involved in the event.

The U.S. Centers for Disease Control and Prevention divide chemical agents into 13 categories (Box 89-4). These categories are based either on chemical properties of the agent or on specific physiologic or psychological effects the agents induce in victims. Toxicologic effects will vary depending on the agent, means of dissemination, amount and concentration of the agent, length of time of exposure, environmental conditions, and the location or locations of release.

TABLE 89-1 *ASBESTOS*: ACRONYM FOR THE SYSTEMATIC APPROACH TO THE EVALUATION OF CHEMICAL CASUALTIES

Agent(s)	Type(s) and estimated dose
State(s)	Solid? Liquid? Gas? Vapor? Aerosol? Combinations?
Body site(s)	Where exposed/route(s) of entry? *[exposure/absorption]*
Effects	Local? Systemic? *[distribution]*
Severity	Mild? Moderate? Severe? *[(a) of effects; (b) of exposure]*
Time course	Onset? Latent period? Getting better/worse? Prognosis?
Other diagnoses	Instead of? *[differential diagnoses]* In addition to?
Synergism	Combined effects of multiple exposures or insults?

(From Madsen JM. Toxins as weapons of mass destruction: a comparison and contrast with biological-warfare and chemical-warfare agents. *Clin Lab Med.* 2001;21(3):593-605.)

After triage and treatment of casualties, issues must be addressed relating to environmental contamination, law enforcement, and critical-incident stress debriefing. The release of a toxic agent into the environment and subsequent rapid decontamination of victims may well result in the substance permeating the nearby infrastructure, soil, water table, or sewer systems. The U.S. Environmental Protection Agency (EPA), specialized private and federal teams, HazMat environmental response teams, and local and state public works must be involved in the clean-up of such an event. In a terrorism event, the location is also a crime scene. Although preservation of life is the primary concern, it should be understood by all parties that any and all debris, patients, and clothing are

TABLE 89-2 ALTERNATIVE ACRONYMS TO *ASBESTOS* FOR THE SYSTEMATIC APPROACH TO THE EVALUATION OF CHEMICAL CASUALTIES

TOXICANT

*T*oxicant/toxidrome	Agent: does it fit with a specific toxidrome?
*O*utside the body	Solid? Liquid? Gas? Vapor? Aerosol? Combinations?
*X*ing into the body	Where did agent cross into the body? *[exposure/absorption]*
*I*nside the body	Where did agent go inside the body? *[distribution]*
*C*hronology	*Past:* Duration of exposure? Onset? Latent period?
	Present: Getting better or worse?
	Future: Prognosis?
*A*dditional diagnoses	Possible coexisting diagnoses?
*N*et effect of diagnoses	Interaction among all diagnoses; patient as a whole
*T*riage	Priority for treatment, decontamination, evacuation

POISON

*P*oison(s)	Type(s) and estimated dose
*O*utside the body	Solid? Liquid? Gas? Vapor? Aerosol? Combinations?
*I*nto/inside the body	Where did it get into the body? *[exposure, absorption]*
	Where did it go inside the body? *[distribution]*
*S*equence of events	Time course *[past, present, future]*
	Onset? Latent period? Getting better or worse? Prognosis?
*O*ther diagnoses	Instead of? *[differential diagnoses]* In addition to?
*N*et effect of diagnoses	Interaction among all diagnoses; patient as a whole

potential evidence and should be treated as carefully as possible to preserve maximum authenticity and validity. Finally, after the event, it is important to plan for involved parties to undergo stress debriefing. After an event of such magnitude, psychologists, psychiatrists, social workers, and licensed professional counselors should be consulted to provide support to all involved personnel.

Whatever the type of chemical release—intentional or accidental—effective pre-event planning and preparation are paramount to ensuring that an optimal response will be delivered to the injured persons, that preservation of the crime scene will be maintained, and that protection of the environment will be considered.

 PITFALLS

Chemical disasters pose unique issues to patients, healthcare providers, and the environment. The involvement of a chemical toxicant adds another element to an already complicated paradigm. Mass-casualty incidents involving biologic or radiologic agents often lead to delayed effects in casualties; moreover, biologic and radiologic agents in contact with the skin usually do not pose a high risk of percutaneous absorption. In contrast, many chemical agents (especially, although not exclusively, as liquids) can begin penetrating the skin within seconds of contact and can relatively quickly build up to a lethal internal dose.

CASE PRESENTATION

At noon on any given Sunday, your professional football team takes the field. The crowds are out in force to support their favorite team. The security checks have not hampered the enthusiasm of the crowd, and as the game kicks off anticipation for a win is high. Near the end of the first half of the game, large explosions occur outside the stadium, outside the inner security perimeter. They are audible to all inside the stadium and are seemingly very close. In panic, the crowds begin to move away from the explosions. Their fairly orderly evacuation is met with terror as a previously staged secondary device explodes. With its detonation, a strong odor, which some compare to that of geraniums, becomes apparent. As the plume spreads, fans near the detonation who were not immediately killed begin to complain of chest pain and to cough severely. In addition to their respiratory complaints, the victims begin to complain of burning of their skin and intense eye pain.

The number of dead and of severely and partially injured patients totals, at best initial estimates, close to 1000. The scene at the stadium is described as chaotic, with evacuation degenerating into a mass exodus and with many trampled. Crowd control, decontamination, security, and triage are difficult to establish in the initial minutes; news crews, EMS personnel, police, and firemen continue to rush to the scene. As the news breaks minutes later, you realize your hospital is closest to the stadium, and you are the only physician on duty in the emergency department. You immediately do the following:

- Activate your facility's Multicasualty Incident (MCI) Emergency Preparedness Plan and notify your hospital administrator and Incident Command Center (ICC)[DM11] director.
- Notify personnel in your emergency department to start alerting people in the waiting room that if they have minor medical problems, to leave and see their own physician, but if they are there for severe chest pain, shortness of breath, high fevers, or abdominal pain, they should stay and wait to be seen.
- Make contact with the trauma service and make sure they know of the impending surge of hospital patients.
- Notify your emergency department backup personnel to come in, as they will likely be needed.
- Activate your hospital HazMat response plan, and have your decontamination tent(s) brought out, erected, and prepared to receive contaminated patients responding on their own who did not wait for Fire/EMS to activate decontamination at the site.
- Make contact with your Hospital Incident Commander under Hospital Emergency Incident Command System (HEICS) to make sure the HEICS management system has been activated and is up and running.
- Prepare to receive patients for triage either to decontamination site or to the usual areas of your hospital uses during an MCI. Review triage procedures with the other members of the triage team from your emergency department.
- Consider a phone call to the local or regional Poison Control Center, advise them of what you have heard about the events at the stadium, and review what their recommendations are for the suspected agent(s).
- Meet with on-call security and make sure they understand the nature of the events and their need to have at least one or two members suit up in personal protective equipment to manage the potential of unruly contaminated patients.

The first patients begin to arrive.

Depending on the chemicals and their forms in the environment, clinical effects may be of short onset or may be delayed even though tissue damage may begin within seconds or minutes of exposure. Thus, lifesaving interventions for victims of biologic and radiologic agents are often those administered at the hospital level, whereas the lives of chemical casualties, even those who may not yet have developed clinical signs or symptoms, may be saved or lost well before transport to a hospital and in many cases even before the arrival of emergency medical responders. This critical difference between chemical agents in general and biologic or radiologic agents has crucial implications for preparation (including education and training) and response.

Because immediate intervention may be lifesaving, the general public should be educated about the importance of prompt removal (by physical or mechanical means such as adsorption followed by brushing, plucking, picking, or flushing with field-expedient materials) of the agent and about the importance of basic life-support measures (i.e., the ABCDDs). For example, it is possible that many victims of the October 2002 storming of the Moscow theater occupied by Chechnyan terrorists might have survived exposure to an opioid or anesthetic agent (see Chapters 97 and 100) had attention been given at the scene to basic airway management.

Emergency medical responders need to emphasize these urgently required interventions, and both emergency responders and hospital personnel need to see the overall picture by means of the use of an easily posted or memorized mnemonic device such as ASBESTOS, TOXICANT, or POISON (see Tables 89-4 and 89-5). Those involved in hospital stockpiling of antidotes need to realize that although administration of vaccines or antibiotics after biologic agent exposure may in many cases be delayed until patients arrive at a hospital, chemical agent antidotes need to be prepositioned for immediate use by emergency responders, who will not have time to wait for antidotes shipped from national stockpiles.

As stressed repeatedly throughout this chapter, chemical disasters, in contrast to other disasters, require advance planning for prompt local (spot) decontamination, for subsequent thorough (full-body) decontamination, for the capability to set up and perform mass decontamination in an efficient manner, and for a quick, logical, and systematic toxicologic review of the situation and the patient. A coordinated, preplanned strategy for immediate deployment of resources to accomplish these goals is mandatory. This approach may at times conflict with the prehospital tenet of "scene safety," since it is certainly possible that victims will present to healthcare providers and to police and fire personnel prior to agent decontamination and identification. A remedy to this dilemma is additional advanced training—including the maintenance of a high index of suspicion for potential chemical exposures—for all public service and hospital personnel with regard to HazMat incidents. The current level of mass casualty weapon preparedness in the United States may not be acceptable for realistic, immediate hot and warm zone operations.

The philosophy of preparing "specialized teams" to respond may simply not be practical in chemical-release incidents, since the event and patients will not wait for deployment of these groups. Instead, casualties will walk, drive, or be driven to a healthcare facility, diverting the hazard from the prehospital providers to the hospital and increasing the potential for contamination at the hospital. The likelihood in a chemical scenario is that the responding teams will be treating those casualties who are the most critical (including immediate casualties) or who are expectant. Therefore, increased training and equipment (including ventilatory support and specific antidotes) is mandatory for emergency response personnel.

One problem with chemical response is that it occurs infrequently and disrupts the routine of daily patient care involving trauma and medical illness. A high index of suspicion, early recognition, the ability to assess the situation toxicologically and systematically, and agent-specific treatment are all essential and can make the difference between life and death for a casualty. This is perhaps our greatest vulnerability. Our comfort with everyday cases far surpasses our ability to care for, recognize, and treat victims from chemical exposures. This is a natural behavioral phenomenon but one that can no longer be tolerated. Additional education and training is necessary so that competence and confidence with HazMat agents increases (see Box 89-4).

Another concern is the ability to handle the surge of patients presenting to the medical system. Prehospital and fixed-facility plans should be implemented and regularly drilled so that a large influx of patients can be accommodated and cared for. These plans should include consideration of alternative care sites, appropriate diversion of patients to nonlocal hospitals that are already absorbing the majority of patients, and the ability to "treat and street" the worried well.

Any disaster scenario is fraught with difficulties. In almost all cases, communication will be one area of complication. Some of the issues that need to be addressed include the following: number and type of radios, frequency coordination, redundancy of equipment, backup power, the ability of a communication system to adapt to the additional resources entering the theater of operations, and the availability of specialized devices so that teams within the hot zone are able to communicate.

The approach to chemical exposures and disasters must be proactive rather than reactive. Comfort and confidence with everyday practices must include preparedness for all hazards. The great potential for healthcare workers to be injured and the necessity of rapid patient identification and treatment need to be recognized. Victims of chemical disasters depend on the ability of emergency responders and hospital personnel to think of the possibility of chemical exposure, to recognize and manage toxidromes and injuries, and to assess the overall scenario just as competently and confidently as they would manage cases of acute pharyngitis, for example. This degree of preparedness, competence, and confidence must remain the goal of planning, training, education, and response to the accidental or intentional release of chemicals in a mass-casualty setting.

REFERENCES

1. Statement by Director of Central Intelligence, George J. Tenet, Before the Senate Foreign Relations Committee on The Worldwide Threat in 2000: Global Realities of Our National Security "as prepared for delivery"; March 21, 2000. Available at: http://www.cia.gov/cia/public_affairs/speeches/2000/dci_speech_032100.html.
2. Director of Central Intelligence Unclassified Report to Congress on the Acquisition of Technology Relating to Weapons of Mass Destruction and Advanced Conventional Munitions, January 1 through June 30, 2001. Available at: http://www.cia.gov/cia/reports/721_reports/jan_jun2003.htm.
3. Reminick G. *Nightmare in Bari: The World War II Liberty Ship Poison Gas Disaster and Cover-up.* Palo Alto, Calif: The Glencannon Press; 2001.
4. Kaplan D. Aum Shinrikyo (1995). In: Tucker JB, ed. *Toxic Terror: Assessing Terrorist Use of Chemical and Biological Weapons.* Cambridge, Mass: MIT Press; 2000:207-26.
5. Ohbu S, Yamashina A, et al. Sarin poisoning on Tokyo subway. *South Med J.* 1997;90(6):587-93.
6. Suzuki T, Morita H, et al. Sarin poisoning in Tokyo subway. *Lancet* 1995;345(8955):980.
7. Hazardous Materials Information System, U.S. Department of Transportation. Data as of June 13, 2005. Available at: http://hazmat.dot.gov/pubs/inc/data/tentr.pdf.
8. Agency for Toxic Substances and Disease Registry. *Hazardous Substances Emergency Events Surveillance Annual Report, 2000.* Atlanta: US Department of Health and Human Services; 1994.
9. U.S. Centers for Disease Control and Prevention. Mass Trauma Preparedness and Response. CDC Injury Center Web site, June 2004. Available at: http://www.cdc.gov/masstrauma/preparedness/predictor.htm.

chapter 90

Industrial Chemical Disasters*

Mark E. Keim

 DESCRIPTION OF EVENT

Definition

An *industrial chemical disaster* is defined as the release or spill of a toxic chemical that results in an abrupt and serious disruption of the functioning of a society, causing widespread human, material, or environmental losses that exceed the ability of the affected society to cope using only its own resources.

The chemical release itself may be acute or chronic in duration. It can be overt or insidious in its onset. Although less dramatic than a major explosion, environmental contamination from the toxic residue of industrialization has resulted in health and environmental problems of immense proportions.[1]

Industrial chemical disasters may occur as the result of fire, explosion,[2] and chemical releases or spills.[3] Between 1993 and 2001, most major chemical releases or spills in the United States involved a single substance at fixed facilities.[4,5] The substance was most frequently a volatile hydrocarbon compound followed by ammonia, sulfur dioxide, carbon monoxide, and nitric oxide, in that order.[4] Employees were the most commonly reported victims.[4] Toxic chemicals are more strongly associated with worker injury, whereas flammables are more strongly associated with property damage.[6]

Scope of the Problem

Incidents involving either slow or explosive release of chemicals are common and on the increase.[7] Between 1988 and 1992, more than 34,000 chemical release events were reported in the United States alone.[8] During 2001, a total of 8978 events were reported.[4] A 1989 study showed that, on average, 1.6 hazardous substance emergency events occur per day in the United States, resulting in death, injury, or evacuation.[9]

Chemical Release Events in Developing Countries

In many rapidly industrializing countries, less elaborate measurers for the protection of the environment, human health, and safety have been an important item in economic negotiations, and these have often led to unfair international division of risks.[1,10-12] This "comparative powerlessness of certain societies to control risk" has been described as sociopolitical amplification of risk.[10]

Between 1945 and 1991, India, Brazil, Mexico, and China led the world in the number of chemical releases resulting in greater than five fatalities.[12] The largest industrial chemical disaster in world history occurred in Bhopal, India, in 1984. The Bhopal disaster killed over 2500 persons and affected an additional 200,000 to 300,000.[13]

Poverty and Vulnerability to Chemical Disasters

In general, poverty is the single most important risk factor for vulnerability to disasters.[14] In one study of over 15,000 industrial facilities located in some 2333 counties in the United States between 1994 and 2000, larger and more chemically intensive facilities tended to be located in counties with larger African American populations, and higher-risk facilities were more likely to be found in counties with sizable poor and/or minority populations that disproportionately bear the collateral environmental, property, and health risks.[15]

 PREINCIDENT ACTIONS

Risk Management Strategies

Recently, the overall approach to emergencies and disasters has shifted from ad hoc postdisaster activities to a more systematic and comprehensive process of risk management that also emphasizes the importance of predisaster activities including prevention, mitigation, and preparedness.[14] *Risk management* is the process of selecting and implementing prevention and control measures to achieve an acceptable level of that risk at an acceptable cost. In general, risk management is composed of four main elements: risk assessment,

---

*The material in this chapter solely reflects the views of the author. It does not necessarily reflect the policies or recommendations of the Centers for Disease Control and Prevention or the U.S. Department of Health and Human Services.

countermeasure determination, cost-benefit analysis, and risk communication.

Emergency Preparedness

Elements of emergency preparedness typically include emergency planning, training and education, warning systems, specialized communication systems, surveillance activities, information databases and resource management systems, resource stocks, emergency exercises, population protection measures, and incident management systems.

Emergency Planning

During an emergency, time constraints place a premium on available plans, data, and record-keeping systems. Planning and preparedness are essential and carefully crafted procedures, and checklists can help; at the same time, prior training in how to respond during emergency situations will aid in handling the difficult circumstances involved.[16] Disaster plans should also be developed for all special facilities, such as schools, hospitals, and nursing homes, which may be at risk for industrial chemical disasters.[16-18]

Information Databases and Resource Management Systems

There are several widely available software and Internet-based tools that have been widely used to rapidly access information regarding hazardous materials. Examples of these software programs include the following:

- TOMES Plus (CD-ROM database), Micromedex, Inc.
- Chemical Hazards Response Information System, U.S. Coast Guard
- TOXNET, National Library of Medicine, Special Information Services

A list of related information available on the Internet can also be found on the U.S. Centers for Disease Control and Prevention (CDC) Web site at http://www.cdc.gov/exposurereport.

Table 90-1 includes a list of other resources that planners and responders can use in the event of industrial chemical disasters.

TABLE 90-1 RESOURCES FOR INFORMATION RELATED TO INDUSTRIAL CHEMICAL RELEASES

INFORMATION RESOURCE	APPLICATION
Major Hazard Incident Data Service (MHIDAS)	A database of incidents involving hazardous materials that had an off-site impact or had the potential to have an off-site impact. MHIDAS features searchable codified and textual information on more than 11,000 incidents involving the transportation, storage, and processing of hazardous materials over the past 20 years.
Environmental Protection Agency (EPA) Toxic Release Inventory (TRI)	A publicly available EPA database that contains information on toxic chemical releases and other waste management activities reported annually by certain covered industry groups as well as federal facilities.
Chemical Transportation Emergency Center (CHEMTREC)	Provides its preregistered customers with a 24-hour emergency telephone number for shipments of hazardous materials or dangerous goods assistance in identifying the hazardous substance and precautionary measures. There is an annual fee for this service.
National Library of Medicine	Offers many electronic databases such as MEDLINE and TOXLINE, which provide literature references, and CHEMLINE and TOXLIT, which provide information from books and journals and information on other hazardous-materials databases.
National Institute of Occupational Safety and Health (NIOSH) Pocket Guide to Chemical Hazards	Offers key information and data on 198 chemicals or substance groupings that are commonly found in the workplace
2000 Emergency Response Guidebook (ERG2000)	Developed jointly by Transport Canada, the U.S. Department of Transportation, and the Secretariat of Transport and Communications for use by first responders at the scene of a transportation incident involving dangerous goods. It is primarily meant to guide first responders in quickly identifying specific hazards and in protecting themselves and the general public.
National Response Center (NRC)	Provides 24-hour assistance and hazardous-materials information to people responding to major industrial accidents.
Agency for Toxic Substances and Disease Registry (ATSDR)	Provides 24-hour assistance to emergency responders who require assistance in managing hazardous-materials emergencies. Such assistance includes information on treatment protocols, laboratory support, and emergency consultation related to assessment and decontamination.
Hazardous Substances Emergency Events Surveillance (HSEES)	Established by ATSDR to collect and analyze information about releases of hazardous substances that need to be cleaned up or neutralized according to federal, state, or local law, as well as threatened releases that result in a public health action such as an evacuation.
National Pesticide Telecommunications Network (NPTN)	Provides information for dealing with pesticide exposures to medical personnel and emergency responders.
CDC	The Second National Report on Human Exposure to Environmental Chemicals provides an ongoing assessment of the exposure of the U.S. population to environmental chemicals using biomonitoring.
Toxic Exposure Surveillance System (TESS)	A comprehensive poisoning surveillance database compiled by the American Association of Poison Control Centers (AAPCC). The cumulative AAPCC database now contains 33.8 million human poison exposure cases. These data are used to identify hazards early, to focus prevention education, to guide clinical research, and to direct training.

Specialized Communication Systems

Coordination of activities of an on-site facility with those located off-site is essential in an emergency.[19] National, regional, and local public health departments must be linked in a network of real-time communication with the medical response community, public safety, regional poison control centers, and regional laboratory capacities for integration of information management, passive and active surveillance systems, and epidemiologic investigation.[20-23]

Resource Stocks

A lack of hospital preparedness for chemical casualty care has been well documented in regions throughout the United States.[24-29] In 1999, Congress charged the Department of Health and Human Services (HHS) and the CDC with establishing the National Pharmaceutical Stockpile (NPS). In March 2003, the NPS became the Strategic National Stockpile (SNS), managed jointly by the Department of Homeland Security (DHS) and HHS. The SNS is a national repository of antibiotics, chemical antidotes, antitoxins, life-support medications, intravenous-administration supplies, airway maintenance supplies, and medical/surgical items. The SNS supplements and resupplies state and local public health agencies within 12 hours of federal deployment. Local communities should therefore be prepared to operate on their own during the critical first 12 hours of a chemical disaster without assistance from the SNS. In addition, local communities should be prepared to receive, protect, and store the SNS, and develop distribution plans for ensuring its use in a timely fashion.

Training and Education

Caregivers should be familiar with basic principles of toxicology, trauma, burn care, mass-casualty management, occupational safety and health, and hazardous materials decontamination as well as incident management systems. Public health officials should also be aware of population protection measures, information resources, environmental health, environmental law, public warning systems, and risk communication.

Warning Systems

To mount a safe and timely evacuation in the event of an industrial chemical disaster, there must first be an effective system in place for warning the population at risk.[1,16,17,22] The system must use redundant methods of communication, including direct contact. It must also address the needs of special populations such as persons with disabilities and extremes of age as well as those with language differences. Recent advances in the telecommunications arena allow for reverse 911 systems to be used as a new method of communicating hazards to local residents.

Exercises

Exercises are a common way of monitoring and evaluating parts of emergency preparedness programs. The purpose of an exercise, and the aspect of emergency preparedness to be tested, must be carefully decided and fairly specific. Adequate predrill instruction and training are vital for success. Special attention should be given to the training of personnel to wear personal protective equipment at the decontamination and initial triage sites.[18]

 POSTINCIDENT ACTIONS

Detection and Management of the Consequences of Industrial Chemical Disasters

The primary functions that must be performed at any toxic release remain fairly consistent. Box 90-1 contains a listing of these actions[16,19,30]:

Assessment and Surveillance for Industrial Chemical Disasters

The primary role of rapid assessment after an industrial chemical disaster is to gain timely and accurate information suitable for directing efficacious action to minimize health impacts. Activities of a rapid assessment should focus on information objectives that can be undertaken consecutively and/or concurrently. Box 90-2 lists examples of such objectives.[1,16,31]

Triage for Chemical Exposures

The clinical condition of exposure victims may be triaged according to four main categories as follows:

BOX 90-1 PRIMARY FUNCTIONS THAT MUST BE PERFORMED AT ANY TOXIC RELEASE

- Rapid assessment
- Scene control and establishment of a perimeter
- Product identification and information gathering
- Pre-entry examination and characterization of site
- Selection and donning of appropriate personal protective clothing and equipment
- Establishment of a decontamination area
- Entry planning and preparation of equipment and supplies
- Victim rescue from release area
- Containment of spill
- Neutralization of spill/release
- Decontamination of victims and responders
- Triage of injured
- Consultation with toxicologist/emergency department/Poison Control Center
- Medical care, including antidotes
- Transport of patients
- Post-entry evaluation of rescuers and equipment
- Delegation of final clean-up to responsible party
- Record-keeping and after-action reporting

- Determine the types, size, and distribution of the release
- Identify the specific type(s) of chemicals and their by-products
- Characterize the hazardous release site
- Identify human exposure pathways
- Define the populations at risk
- Conduct a toxicologic evaluation and assessment
- Describe morbidity and mortality
- Identify appropriate treatment regimens
- Evaluate emergency medical care and health service capabilities
- Ensure provision of appropriate medical care
- Identify and evaluate environmental control strategies
- Evaluate evacuation and mass care strategies
- Develop criteria for defining comprehensive databases

(1) nonambulatory injured; (2) ambulatory injured; (3) ambulatory noninjured; and (4) dead or expectant.

Historically, nonambulatory injured victims of chemical exposures have made up a small percentage of event survivors. Although some of these victims may be transported to the hospital via bystanders, most will be treated and transported by first responders. These casualties should be decontaminated and transported immediately.

Ambulatory injured and ambulatory noninjured victims comprise the largest group (80% to 90% in most series).[32] They will self-evacuate from the area of release and thus mitigate their exposure. Many will be transported to the closest hospital without decontamination via bystanders. Ambulatory injured casualties should be decontaminated immediately and then transported to the hospital. If these patients present to the hospital outside of the emergency medical system, they should be decontaminated immediately upon arrival to the hospital. Ambulatory noninjured victims should be triaged to a secondary location by non-ambulance transportation for registry, interview, and a secondary medical assessment by emergency medical personnel.

Decontamination

Decontamination is a process of removing or reducing the concentration of harmful substances. It should be performed whenever there is a likelihood of contamination or risk of secondary exposure.[19] The most important factor in effective decontamination is the speed of removal of the agent.[33] Copious skin lavage with water or gentle cleansing with soap and water has proved to be beneficial for both liquid and solid substances. It may be difficult to determine whether a victim has been exposed to a chemical; responders and hospital personnel should assume that these victims are contaminated, since it takes too long to prove otherwise.

Population Protection Measures

Proper evacuation can save lives and decrease disruption of social networks.[5,17] However, since mass evacuation may result in disrupted health or other critical services, it may by itself cause a disaster and therefore should not be entered into lightly in the absence of accurate predictive models for population exposure. Many modeling tools are available to assist in creating a database of industrial chemicals present at a local industrial site, rapidly estimating plume-dispersion patterns, and predicting the consequences of a technologic or natural hazard using real-time weather models. Examples of these tools include Computer-Aided Management of Emergency Operations (CAMEO)[34] and The Consequence Assessment Tools Set (CATS).[35] Once modeling has been completed for potential areas at risk, the decision can be made regarding the need for evacuation or shelter-in-place contingencies.[17]

Population protection measures may include population evacuation, sheltering in place, and individual protection measures. Sheltering in place may be necessary when sufficient time for evacuation is not available. Generally, providing individual protection measures in the way of protective gear is impractical and potentially dangerous to the general population.[36]

The effectiveness of shelter-in-place strategies is time dependent and is not always applicable. Shelter-in-place strategies are employed when it is safer for a population to remain indoors as opposed to an outdoor evacuation. Indoor shelters may initially provide protection from atmospheric releases as compared to the outdoor environment during the early timing after a chemical release. However, 30 to 60 minutes after the plume dispersion has ceased, chemical levels indoors may actually then exceed outdoor concentrations. Recommendations for population protection measures should therefore be based on an accurate exposure modeling system and should not remain static over time. Box 90-3 is a list of recommendations for implementing effective population evacuations.[3,5]

Risk Communication

The public will have obvious concerns about their exposure to fire, smoke, and hazardous materials.[37] Public health and medical personnel should anticipate this need for information and develop public advisories and risk communication strategies for early implementation during such an event. A well-executed risk communication response effort will increase an organization's credibility.[38]

MEDICAL TREATMENT OF CASUALTIES

In spite of the enormous challenge presented in the identification of chemical hazards, there are certain generalizations that can be made to simplify disaster medical response. Toxic chemicals can be categorized by their known health effects. For ease of case and incident management, a broad variety of hazardous chemicals can be divided into 13 basic categories (see Box 90-4).

Aside from an extremely limited number of antidote therapies, medical management of nearly all toxic chemical exposures involves mostly supportive therapy.[22] Even if there may be an antidote available for a specific exposure, many times the clinician may not be able to identify the offending agent in enough time to guide effective therapy.

Thus, the acute health effects of a broad variety of hazardous chemicals, as categorized in Box 90-4, may actually be expected to invoke demands for medical resources that address a very narrow range of medical conditions. Table 90-2 represents four main basic medical conditions that can be expected to occur as major short-term sequelae following severe exposures to any of these chemical hazards. It then also identifies a mere

TABLE 90-2 EMERGENCY MEDICAL CONDITIONS AND NEEDS ASSOCIATED WITH CHEMICAL EXPOSURES

SYNDROME AND CAUSATIVE AGENTS	MEDICAL THERAPEUTIC NEEDS
Burns and Trauma	
Corrosives, vesicants, explosives, oxidants, incendiaries, radiologics	Intravenous fluid and supplies Pain medications Pulmonary products Splints and bandages
Respiratory Failure	
Corrosives, military agents, explosives, oxidants, incendiaries, asphyxiants, irritants, pharmaceuticals, metals	Pulmonary products Ventilators and supplies Antidotes (when available) Tranquilizing medications
Cardiovascular Shock	
Pesticides, asphyxiants, pharmaceuticals	Intravenous fluids and supplies Cardiovascular products Antidotes (when available)
Neurologic Toxicity	
Pesticides, pharmaceuticals, radiologics	Antidotes (when available)

eight categories of emergency medical therapeutics that would become necessary to treat these four syndrome complexes.[22]

CASE PRESENTATION

At 1:00 AM, a tank containing methyl isocyanate (MIC) located at a pesticide plant ruptures and releases its entire contents. The public siren is sounded only for a few minutes. The toxic plume extends as far as 5 miles from the plant and covers an area of 25 square miles. A thermal inversion traps the plume over the most highly populated areas of a nearby impoverished community of 800,000 people.

By 3:00 AM, all 40 tons of the lung-damaging MIC is released, leaving thousands of local residents dead and hundreds of thousands exposed. Over 80% of the deaths occur before people enter the medical care system. Most deaths occur due to anoxia and cardiac arrest as a result of pulmonary edema caused by the effects on lung tissue. Emergency response is ad hoc, chaotic, and limited by the lack of lighting and of street identification within the poor community.

Fifteen years later, the national Supreme Court directs the company operating the plant to pay a total of $470 million in full settlement of all claims arising from the tragedy. Twenty years after the incident, the Supreme Court orders the national government to distribute the balance of compensation remaining from the chemical company settlement among the 566,876 survivors whose claims have been successfully settled. The average payout amount is equal to $570 per person.

UNIQUE CONSIDERATIONS

Industrial chemical disasters are also unique in the degree of complexity that an event entails. In this case, the very nature of response changes as assessments become less certain and older forms of intelligence gathering become obsolete. Decision-making becomes less centralized and more interdependent and may be influenced by local and distant theaters of operation. Responders are forced to act in a collective and integrated fashion within an unconventional network of personnel also unfamiliar with this catastrophic breakdown phenomenon.[22,39]

In addition, the public tends to judge all technologic hazards more harshly than natural hazards of a similar magnitude and to attach to them much more of a public concern and perception of risk.[5,7,39-41] There are also special problems in chemical emergencies with respect to exactly how to handle the overwhelming numbers of mass media representatives.[7] For this reason, risk communication and public information become critical components of the response to these incidents.

 PITFALLS

Lack of Knowledge

One major pitfall involving industrial chemical disasters is the relative lack of knowledge regarding the adverse health effects of many of the chemicals that are currently on the market. More than 600 new chemical substances enter the marketplace each month.[42] Researchers estimate that only 7% of all known chemical substances have been fully investigated.[13] Measuring human exposure to chemical substances through laboratory sampling also has its limitations.[1] In some cases, consequences can be revealed only by means of formal, sometimes complex, and often long-term investigations.[5]

Lack of Familiarity

Another pitfall of industrial chemical disasters is a fundamental lack of familiarity among the medical community, including emergency care providers. Baxter[43] observes that health professionals are more used to planning for trauma than for mass chemical exposure. The direct effects of the disaster can be compounded by ineffective management or leadership, legal difficulties, economic or political limitations, and psychological stress.[16]

Lack of Community Preparedness

There is also a fundamental and endemic lack of preparedness among communities at risk for industrial chemical disasters.[1,24-29] An additional impediment to local planning efforts is the fact that the most relevant resources rest in the hands of extra-community groups (i.e., state and federal assets) rather than with the community organizations that invariably are confronted with the immediate postincident response.[7] Local Emergency Planning Councils, mandated by the Superfund Amendment, often lack regular input by the healthcare community.

High Occupational Health Risk Posed to Responders

Workers and first responders are often the first and most frequently injured populations in the case of industrial chemical release events.[1,37,42,44] Most injuries of this group of emergency personnel occur in the first few minutes of responding, with firefighters and police being the most frequent victims.[44] Injuries from hazardous substances emergency events are also becoming increasingly more common among hospital personnel as a result of secondary contamination.[45]

REFERENCES

1. Lillibridge S. Industrial disasters. In: Noji ER, ed. *The Public Health Consequences of Disasters*. New York: Oxford University Press; 1997:354-72.
2. Hull D, Grindlinger G, Hirsch E. The clinical consequences of an industrial plant explosion. *J Trauma*. 1985;25(4):303-7.
3. Duclos P, Sanderson L, Thompson F, et al. Community evacuation following a chlorine release, Mississippi. *Disasters* 1987;11(4):286-9.
4. Agency for Toxic Substances and Disease Registry. *2001 HSEES Annual Report*. Hazardous Substances Emergency Events Surveillance (HSEES). Atlanta: U.S Department of Health and Human Services; 2002.
5. Bertazzi P. Industrial disasters and epidemiology. *Scan J Work Environ Health*. 1989;15:85-100.
6. Elliott M, Lowe R. The role of hazardousness and regulatory practice in the accidental release of chemicals at U.S. industrial facilities. *Risk Anal*. 2003;23(5):883-96.
7. Quarantelli E, Gray J. Research findings on community and organizational preparations for and responses to acute chemical emergencies. *Public Management*. 1986;68:11-13.
8. National Environmental Law Center and the US Public Research Interest Group. *Chemical Releases Statistics*. Washington, DC: Associated Press International; 1994.
9. Binder S. Deaths, injuries and evacuations from acute hazardous materials releases. *Am J Public Health*. 1989;79:1042-4.
10. Firpo de Souza Porto M, Machado de Freitas C. Major chemical accidents and industrializing countries: the socio-political amplification of risk. *Risk Anal*. 1996;16:(1)19-29.
11. Brown H, Himelberger J, White A. Development of environment interactions in the export of hazardous technologies. *Technol Forecast Soc Change*. 1993;43:125-55.
12. Glickman T, Golding D, Terry K. *Fatal Hazardous Materials Accidents in Industry: Domestic and Foreign Experience from 1945 to 1991*. Washington, DC: Center for Risk Management; 1993.
13. Mehta PS, Mehta AS, Mehta SJ, et al. Bhopal tragedy's health effects. *JAMA* 1990;264(21):2781-7.
14. Clack Z, Keim M, MacIntyre A, Yeskey K. Emergency health and risk management in sub-Saharan Africa: a lesson from the embassy bombings in Tanzania and Kenya. *Prehospital Disaster Med*. 2002;17(2):59-66.
15. Elliott M, Wang Y, Lowe R, et al. Environmental justice: frequency and severity of US chemical industry accidents and the socio-economic status of surrounding communities. *J Epidemiol Community Health*. 2004;58:24-30.
16. Falk H. Industrial/chemical disasters: medical care, public health and epidemiology in the acute phase. In: Bourdeau P, Green G. eds. *Methods for Assessing and Reducing Injury from Chemical Accidents*. New York: John Wiley and Sons; 1989:105-14.
17. Rogers G, Sorensen J, Long J, et al. Emergency planning for chemical agent releases. *Environmental Professional*. 1989;11:396-408.
18. Tur-Kaspa I, Lev E, Hendler I, et al. Preparing hospitals for toxicological mass casualty events. *Crit Care Med*. 1999;27(5):1004-08.

19. McCunney R. Emergency response to environmental toxic incidents: the role of the occupational physician. *Occup Med.* 1996;46(5):397-401.

20. Keim M, Kaufmann A, Rodgers G. *Recommendations for Office of Emergency Preparedness/CDC Surveillance, Laboratory and Informational Support Initiative.* Atlanta: Centers for Disease Control and Prevention, National Center for Environmental Health; 1998.

21. Brennan RJ, Waeckerle JL, Sharp TW, Lillibridge SR. Chemical warfare agents: emergency medical and emergency public health issues. *Ann Emerg Med.* 1999;34:(2)191-204.

22. Keim M. Intentional chemical disasters. In: Hogan D, Burstein J, eds. *Disaster Medicine.* Philadelphia: Lippincott, Williams & Wilkins; 2002:340-8.

23. Delgado R, Gonzalez P, Alvarez T, et al. Preparation for response to an industrial disaster in Spain. *Public Health.* 2003;117:260-1.

24. Ghilarducci DP, Pirrallo RG, Hegmann KT. Hazardous materials readiness of United States Level 1 trauma centers. *J Occup Environ Med.* 2000;42(7):683-92.

25. Wetter DC, Daniell WE, Treser CD. Hospital preparedness for victims of chemical or biological terrorism. *Am J Pub Health.* 2001;91:710-6.

26. Chyka, PA, Conner HG. Availability of antidotes in rural and urban hospitals in Tennessee. *Am J Hosp Pharm.* 1994;51:1346-8.

27. Dart RC, Stark Y, Fulton B. Insufficient stocking of poisoning antidotes in hospital pharmacies. *JAMA* 1996;276:1508-10.

28. Woolf AD, Chrisanthus K. On-site availability of selected antidotes: results of a survey of Massachusetts hospitals. *Am J Emerg Med.* 1997;15:62-6.

29. Keim M, Pesik N, Twum-Danso N. Lack of hospital preparedness for chemical terrorism in a major US city: 1996-2000. *Prehospital Disaster Med.* 2003;18(3):193-9.

30. Staten C. Emergency response to chemical/biological terrorist incidents. *Emergency Response & Research Institute.* 1997. Available at: http://www.emergency.com/cbwlesn1.htm.

31. Sanderson L. Toxicologic disasters: natural and technologic. In: Sullivan JB, Krieger GR, eds. *Hazardous Materials Toxicology: Clinical Principles of Environmental Health.* Baltimore: Williams & Wilkins; 1992.

32. Levitin H, Siegelson H, Dickinson S, et al. Decontamination of mass casualties: evaluating existing dogma. *Prehospital Disaster Med.* 2003;18(3):200-7.

33. Curreri P, Morris M, Pruitt B. The treatment of chemical burns: specialized diagnostic, therapeutic, and prognostic considerations. *J Trauma.* 1970;10:634-42.

34. U.S. Environmental Protection Agency. Computer-Aided Management of Emergency Operations (CAMEO) Web site. Available at: http://epa.gov/ceppo/cameo/.

35. Kirkpatrick J, Howard J, Reed D. Assessing homeland chemical hazards outside the military gates: industrial hazard threat assessments for department of defense installations. *Science Total Environ.* 2002;288:111-7.

36. Golan E, Shemer J, Arad M, et al. Medical limitations of gas masks for civilian populations: the 1991 experience. *Mil Med.* 1992;157:444-6.

37. Hsu E, Grabowski J, Chotani R, et al. Effects on local emergency departments of large scale urban chemical fire with hazardous material spill. *Prehospital Disaster Med.* 2002;17(4):196-201.

38. Fernandez L, Merzer M. *Janes Crisis Communications Handbook.* Surrey, England: Janes Information Group; 2003.

39. Lagadec P. Accidents, crises, breakdowns. Paper presented at the Society of Chemical Industry, London. January 9, 1998.

40. Slovic P. Perception of risk. *Science* 1987;236:280-5.

41. Glickman TS, Golding D, Silverman ED. *Acts of God and Acts of Man: Major Trends in Natural Disasters and Major Industrial Accidents [discussion paper].* Washington, DC: Center for Risk Management, Resources for the Future; 1991

42. Doyle C, Upfal M, Little N. Disaster management of possible toxic exposure. In: Haddad L, ed. *Clinical Management of Poisoning and Drug Overdose.* Philadelphia: WB Saunders; 1990;483-500.

43. Baxter P. 1991 Major chemical disasters: Britain's health services are poorly prepared. *BMJ* 1991;302:61-2.

44. Zeitz P, Berkowitz Z, Orr M, et al. Frequency and type of injuries in responders of hazardous substances emergency events, 1996 to 1998. *J Occup Environ Med.* 2000;42:1115-20.

45. Cox R. Decontamination and management of hazardous materials exposure victims in the emergency department. *Ann Emerg Med.* 1994;23:761-70.

chapter 91

Nerve Agent Attack

David Davis and David Marcozzi

 ## DESCRIPTION OF EVENT

The prospect of nerve agent exposure during wartime and a terrorist event is a very real and well-documented concern.[1,2] Still, the potential for nerve agent intoxication is not limited to intentional exposures. The well-described nerve agents tabun, sarin, soman, and VX were developed in the early part of the twentieth century as derivatives of pesticides with their initial intended uses as such. However, their prospect as chemical warfare agents was soon realized, and development to this end was undertaken. Currently, the commercial agricultural industry continues to use analogs of these precursor pesticides. Given current agricultural practices, the manufacturing, distribution, and application of these pesticides may also represent a significant potential for mass exposure to nerve agents.[3]

Nerve agents are anticholinesterases, which can be divided into three distinct categories: quaternary ammonium alcohols, carbamates, and organophosphates. Each of these classes has its distinctive characteristics, but all anticholinesterases achieve their toxic effects through inhibition of the enzyme acetylcholinesterase. Acetylcholine is an important neurotransmitter in the human nervous system. Under normal physiologic conditions, acetylcholine is hydrolyzed by acetylcholinesterase into acetate and choline. Anticholinesterases disrupt this reaction by forming stable complexes with acetylcholinesterase, resulting in preservation of the neurotransmitter.[4] Consequently, widespread hyperactivity (with subsequent fatigue and failure) of cholinergic end organs ensues secondary to the accumulation of acetylcholine. Toxicity is related to hyperstimulation of nicotinic and muscarinic receptors in neurons, muscle, and exocrine glands. Nicotinic effects result from extensive sympathetic and parasympathetic ganglionic outflow as well as somatic neuromuscular junction hyperactivity in skeletal muscle. Muscarinic effects are the product of increased postganglionic parasympathetic stimulation of smooth muscles, exocrine glands, and neurons in the central nervous system (CNS).

Quaternary ammonium compounds inhibit cholinesterase activity through a fleeting ionic interaction that lasts only milliseconds, limiting the toxicity of these agents. Carbamates are common components of many household insecticides. Carbamates inhibit acetylcholinesterase through the covalent bonding of the chemicals carbaryl group to the enzymes active site.[5] Unlike the acetylated form of the enzyme, the carbamylated form is much more resistant to hydrolysis. However, the reaction is reversible because reactivation of acetylcholinesterase occurs spontaneously when the carbamate is hydrolyzed.[6] Hydrolysis takes an average of 2 to 6 hours and is in part responsible for the limited toxicity of carbamates. The inability of carbamates to cross the blood-brain barrier also explains their lack of CNS effects.[7] Exposure to these compounds usually occurs either through intentional ingestion, cutaneous absorption, or inhalation of droplets.

The organophosphates, which are technically organophosphorus esters, comprise the last and largest group of acetylcholinesterase inhibitors. A complete list of these agents is beyond the scope of this chapter, but they include pesticides such as diazinon, malathion, parathion, dichlorvos, and chlorpyrifos as well as the G-series and V-series nerve agents used as chemical warfare agents. The common denominator of this group of agents is their phosphoric acid backbone. A phosphorylated acetylcholinesterase is a remarkably stable complex and the reaction in effect irreversible, as normal physiologic chemistry does not allow for spontaneous hydrolysis. Furthermore, the enzyme will undergo "aging" if not reactivated.[8] *Aging* refers to a conformational change of the phosphorylated acetylcholinesterase, rendering the enzyme permanently disabled.

Organophosphates may exist as powders, epoxies, and resins but are most commonly encountered as odorless, colorless liquids. They are also highly lipophilic substances. As such, transcutaneous absorption is the most frequently seen exposure for organophosphate pesticides. Evaporation of organophosphates can occur, however, and inhalation may lead to rapid development of systemic toxicity. In particular, the classically described G-agent nerve "gases" sarin (GB), soman (GD), and tabun (GA) possess sufficiently high enough vapor pressures to produce lethal vapor concentrations at room temperature.[8,9] (These agents never actually boil at usual environmental temperatures but rather evaporate; *nerve gas* is therefore a misnomer.) Vapor pressure represents the pressure at which the vapor and liquid phases of a substance will equilibrate in a closed system, or more simply, the point at which a liquid will cease spontaneous vaporization. In most cases, these agents will completely vaporize because their release is unlikely to occur in a closed area. Additionally, sarin, soman, and tabun are relatively volatile compared with other organophosphates. *Volatility* refers to the ease with which a substance will evaporate[10] and correlates directly with speed of evaporation.

Another organophosphate nerve agent, VX, is the most potent chemical warfare agent; a single droplet of VX on the skin can be fatal. VX exists solely as a liquid with a low vapor pressure and volatility, making spontaneous evaporation highly unlikely.[11] However, it is well absorbed through the skin.

Organophosphates may be aerosolized with mechanical sprayers, during crop dusting, or from the combustion of an explosive device. As these agents persist in the environment, secondary vaporization or "off gassing" may occur.[12] This is an important fact to remember because although protective clothing will minimize dermal exposure, the agent may still evaporate and be inhaled.

 PREINCIDENT CONSIDERATIONS

Hospital, community, and military preparedness for any massive chemical exposure is imperative. Decontamination strategies must be incorporated into disaster protocols. A more comprehensive outline of decontamination tactics can be found in Chapter 70. There are several caveats when preparing protocols to handle nerve-agent disasters.[13]

During nerve agent exposure, systemic absorption is continuous as long as the agent is in contact with epithelial surfaces or in transit through the skin. Respiratory exposure can be terminated either by masking the victim or by removing the victim from the incident site. Percutaneous absorption will continue as long as the agent is in contact with skin; moreover, agent already in transit through the skin is not removed by decontamination of skin surfaces. For this reason, skin decontamination is imperative and must begin as soon as possible. This is achieved by immediate removal (by adsorption, flushing, or both) at the incident site of any agent seen on the skin—local, or so-called "spot" decontamination, which may mean the difference between life and death for nerve agent casualties. Skin irrigation is accompanied or followed by prompt removal of all clothing. Irrigation of exposed skin and hair may be performed with saline or soapy water, although in mass-casualty situations, water will be the most well-tolerated, abundant, and readily available decontaminating solution. Sodium hypochlorite (i.e., household bleach) is no longer recommended as a dermal cleansing solution but is still the solution of choice for decontaminating equipment because it effectively neutralizes organophosphates. Eyes should be irrigated with water only. General recommendations are to spend 10 to 15 minutes irrigating the skin and eyes. However, in the event of a disaster related to nerve agents, practical decisions about length of irrigation will have to be made and

tailored to individual situations based on the severity of incident, the number of casualties, and the availability of resources.

Ideally, in cases of ingestion of organophosphate pesticides, gastrointestinal decontamination would also begin at the scene but will most likely be delayed until the patient reaches a healthcare facility. When available and indicated, activated charcoal (1 g/kg) should be administered orally or via nasogastric tube.

Emergency crews need to ensure adequate self-protection during the extrication, decontamination, and transport of casualties. Butyl or nitrile rubber gloves, boots, suits, and masks provide protection from nerve agent absorption; conventional latex and vinyl gloves do not.[14] The importance of appropriate protective equipment and thorough decontamination should not be underemphasized. Attention to these details not only prevents rescue workers from becoming intoxicated through dermal contact with nerve agents but also prevents those healthcare workers downstream who will be providing definitive care for the patient from contacting the nerve agent and subsequently becoming casualties.

Military healthcare providers are faced with several unique challenges and options in preparing for nerve agent attack. First, soldiers must be trained to recognize a chemical attack and to don appropriate personal protective equipment properly and swiftly.[12] Second, if military intelligence suggests a high probability of attack with the nerve agent soman, soldiers may be pretreated with pyridostigmine bromide. Pyridostigmine is a carbamate that when administered before exposure to soman will functionally "protect" some of the acetylcholinesterase by reversibly binding to it. Subsequent spontaneous hydrolysis of the carbamate releases the enzyme for return to normal activity.[15,16] Pyridostigmine is well tolerated with few side effects and is dispensed in a blister pack containing 30-mg tablets; one tablet is taken every 8 hours for a usual maximum of 14 days. Lastly, the U.S. military issues the MARK I autoinjector kit. Each kit contains one 0.5-mL preloaded autoinjectable syringe containing 2 mg of atropine and a 2-mL syringe containing 600 mg of the oxime 2-pralidoxime chloride. A combination autoinjector syringe, the Antidote Treatment Nerve Agent Autoinjector, which contains both atropine and 2-pralidoxime chloride, is in development. Soldiers should be familiar with indications for and administration of these kits.

 POSTINCIDENT CONSIDERATIONS

Prompt recognition of the cholinergic crisis associated with nerve agent exposure is critical in directing treatment. Nicotinic effects include weakness, hypertension, hyperglycemia, local or generalized muscle fasciculations, tachycardia, and mydriasis, although mydriasis is almost inevitably overridden by miosis induced by hyperstimulation of muscarinic receptors. Muscarinic effects include diaphoresis, urinary incontinence, miosis, bronchorrhea, bronchospasm, emesis, lacrimation, loose stools, and salivation (remembered with the acronym DUMBBELLS).[8,17] (Bradycardia is also a muscarinic effect but in humans is usually overridden by tachycardia from nicotinic stimulation in sympathetic ganglia.) Since the end-organ response to excessive cholinergic stimulation is first hyperactivity and then fatigue and failure, another way of organizing these effects is to list effects from organ-system hyperactivity and then effects from subsequent organ-system failure. For example, overactivity of neurons in the brain causes seizures (manifested in an as-yet-unparalyzed patient as convulsions); subsequent fatigue and failure of the respiratory center in the medulla leads to central apnea. Similarly, increased stimulation of skeletal muscle produced twitching and fasciculations eventually followed by weakness and paralysis (usually flaccid paralysis). An important consideration is that any constellation of these symptoms may initially be present depending on the route of exposure and the dose of agent. Inhalation immediately leads to bronchorrhea and respiratory difficulty, whereas dermal contamination may manifest as local muscle fasciculations and diaphoresis before the onset of systemic symptoms. However, sudden collapse with apnea and convulsions may occur after high doses either from inhalation or percutaneous exposure; the difference is that, for a fatal dose, effects from skin exposure will be delayed for 20 to 30 minutes because of passage of the agent through the epidermis to the dermal vasculature. The mechanism of death from nerve agent exposure is primarily respiratory in nature as progressive bronchorrhea, bronchospasm, direct paralysis of the diaphragm, and especially central apnea. Confusion, seizures, apnea, and coma are ominous CNS symptoms indicative of severe intoxication.[9]

After recognition of the cholinergic toxidrome, post-exposure triage can aid in managing mass casualties and in directing initial medical treatment. Exposed victims should be triaged as mild, moderate, or severe based on their clinical presentation, which will depend in part on the type and route of exposure and the dose of agent (Table 91-1). Emphasis should be on recognizing the syndrome and broadly grouping casualties to facilitate rapid medical treatment. Initial treatment will be based on triaging casualties into one of these categories.[9,17,18]

Laboratory values are of little clinical utility in the immediate management of nerve agent poisonings. Erythrocyte-cholinesterase levels may be drawn and do correlate with serum cholinesterase levels after acute exposures, but this is not a readily available test and has much intersubject variability, making it most useful in occupational settings where an individual baseline can be determined for each worker. Plasma-cholinesterase levels measure butyrylcholinesterase, also called *pseudocholinesterase*, and may be used to monitor the return of serum cholinesterase activity during recovery. Initial medical treatment should always be clinically dictated. Initial electrocardiography may show either sinus tachycardia or bradycardia, although tachycardia is actually somewhat more common in patients with nerve agent injuries. Also, those patients with severe or chronic exposures to organophosphate pesticides may develop a delayed-onset polyneuropathy or chronic organophosphorus-induced delayed neurotoxicity with a stocking/glove distribution. This neuropathy may be permanent[9,11] but appears to occur seldom if ever with nerve agents.

 ## MEDICAL MANAGEMENT OF CASUALTIES

After primary decontamination, medical management of organophosphate exposure is directed at blocking cholinergic-receptor stimulation and reactivating acetylcholinesterase. Management of known quaternary ammonium or carbamate intoxication does not usually require specific medical therapy but rather general supportive measures, although atropine by itself has been used in cases of carbamate poisonings.[19]

Supportive care should always start with the ABCs (i.e., airway, breathing, and circulation) and appropriate

---

TABLE 91-1 NERVE AGENT SIGNS AND SYMPTOMS BASED ON SEVERITY AND ROUTE OF EXPOSURE*

SYMPTOM SEVERITY AND TRIAGE LEVELS	TYPE OF EXPOSURE	
	Liquid	**Vapor**
Mild	Localized fasciculations and diaphoresis; no miosis	Miosis; dim vision; rhinorrhea
Moderate	Mild symptoms and: gastrointestinal cramping; nausea/vomiting; generalized weakness and fasciculations	Mild symptoms and: salivation/lacrimation; wheezing; dyspnea; bronchorrhea; bronchoconstriction
Severe	Mild/moderate symptoms and: apnea; convulsions/seizures; confusion/coma; flaccid paralysis; bowel/bladder incontinence	Mild/moderate symptoms and: apnea; convulsions/seizures; confusion/coma; flaccid paralysis; bowel/bladder incontinence

*Note: The signs and symptoms of severe exposure may occur after progression through mild and moderate effects or may occur suddenly, depending on the dose. Effects from inhalation will be immediate; a latent period of 20 minutes to 18 hours is seen after liquid exposure; the length of this latent period is inversely correlated with dose.

advanced life support protocols. Aggressive airway management is often needed. Usually supplemental oxygen and suctioning of airway secretions is sufficient in cases of organophosphate-pesticide poisoning, although high doses of nerve agents will likely require endotracheal intubation and ventilatory support. Paralytic agents are rarely needed, but if necessary a short-acting competitive neuromuscular blocker such as vecuronium or rocuronium should be used. Avoid use of succinylcholine, which may have prolonged effects.[4,8,9]

Atropine is a competitive cholinergic blocking agent and when administered will aid in alleviating muscarinic symptoms[8,20] but will not control nicotinic symptoms such as muscle fasciculations, weakness, or flaccid paralysis. Initial dosing is based on symptoms and triaged categories of victims (Table 91-2). Atropine has a short half-life and can be given every 5 to 10 minutes at a dose of 2 mg in adults and 0.05 to 0.1 mg/kg in children. The maximal single dose for children should not exceed 1 mg. Administration of atropine should continue until airway resistance is minimized, respiratory secretions dried, and dyspnea resolved. Total doses of up to 1 to 2 g have been required in cases of intoxication with organophosphorus pesticides, but nerve agent poisoning should seldom require more than a total of about 20 to 30 mg of atropine, as long as oximes are also administered.

With organophosphate intoxication, definitive treatment is aimed at reactivating acetylcholinesterase. Reactivation is achieved through the administration of an oxime-containing compound. Oximes reactivate acetylcholinesterase by displacing the phosphate moiety from the enzyme. However, reactivation is not possible after aging. Although nerve agents begin aging almost immediately, the half-lives of aging are hours to days for most of the agents. The exception is soman, which has an aging half-life of approximately 2 minutes. Thus, oxime administration to a soman-poisoned patient after five half-lives (about 10 minutes) is unlikely to have any effect.[17,20] Currently, pralidoxime chloride (2-PAM chloride) is the only oxime approved by the Food and Drug Administration (FDA) for use in the United States. Again, initial dosing is based on symptom severity. However, because of potential adverse effects from overdosage, repeat intramuscular administration of oximes after the initial 1800- to 2000-mg dose given to severely intoxicated adults should be delayed for an additional hour.

CASE PRESENTATION

You are called to the scene of an explosion that has rocked a crowded downtown park. Initial reports are vague and indicate several blast injuries. Additionally, there is speculation that a chemical agent was released during the explosion.

The first casualty that you see is a 35-year-old previously healthy businessman who walks into the triage area. He is complaining of a headache and blurry vision. His vital signs are stable, but you do notice that his pupils seem markedly constricted. Next, medics bring over an 8-year-old girl. She is actively seizing on arrival. Her vital signs include a pulse of 110, blood pressure of 95/60, and oxygen saturation of 85%. This patient has some minor superficial abrasions, is incontinent of bowel and bladder, is extremely diaphoretic, and is salivating profusely. As you order a benzodiazepine to treat the seizure, the medic who assisted with transporting the young girl collapses. He loses consciousness only transiently and on awakening seems confused. He is also complaining of difficulty breathing and feeling weak. In the interim, the police have identified debris from the explosion; this debris includes the remains of a duffel bag, an explosive device, and a canister of some sort.

Benzodiazepines are the treatment of choice for organophosphate-induced seizures. Prophylactic administration of benzodiazepines is recommended in all cases of severe organophosphate exposure to minimize the risk of subsequent seizures. Remember, although benzodiazepines do control convulsions, increased neuronal activity still consumes a significant amount of oxygen, and adequate oxygenation is imperative to preserve CNS function in severely exposed patients. Most experience is with diazepam, but other benzodiazepines including midazolam would also be appropriate. See Table 91-2 for recommended dosing.

Other medical therapies include inhaled nebulized ipratropium bromide, a synthetic analog of atropine. Ipratropium will be helpful in relieving bronchoconstriction and reducing airway secretions. There have been a few case reports of hemodialysis followed by hemoperfusion for direct removal of organophosphate compounds.[8,15]

TABLE 91-2 RECOMMENDED INITIAL DOSING OF ANTIDOTES

	INFANTS (0-2 YEARS)	CHILDREN (<10 YEARS)	ADOLESCENTS	ADULTS	ELDERLY
Mild/Moderate Symptoms	Atropine, 0.05 mg/kg; pralidoxime, 15 mg/kg	Atropine, 1 mg; pralidoxime, 15 mg/kg	Atropine, 2 mg; pralidoxime 15 mg/kg	Atropine, 2-4 mg; pralidoxime, 600 mg	Atropine, 1 mg; pralidoxime, 10 mg/kg
Severe Symptoms	Atropine, 0.1 mg/kg; pralidoxime, 25 mg/kg; diazepam, 0.2-0.5 mg/kg	Atropine, 1 mg; pralidoxime, 25 mg/kg; diazepam, 0.2-0.5 mg/kg	Atropine, 4 mg; pralidoxime, 25 mg/kg; diazepam, 0.2-0.5 mg/kg	Atropine, 6 mg; pralidoxime, 1800 mg; diazepam, 10 mg	Atropine, 2-4 mg; pralidoxime, 25 mg/kg; diazepam, 0.5 mg/kg

Atropine and diazepam may be given intramuscularly (IM) or intravenously (IV). Pralidoxime may be given IM as a single dose or infused IV over 30 minutes.[8,9,21]

For military exposures, soldiers will have to administer the Mark I kits to themselves or to severely exposed colleagues. Each kit contains one 0.5-mL autoinjectable syringe filled with 2 mg of atropine and a 2-mL autoinjector containing 600 mg of pralidoxime. Those incurring mild exposures receive one kit, moderate exposures two kits, and severe exposures three kits as well as 10 mg of diazepam.[12]

 ## UNIQUE CONSIDERATIONS

A civilian nerve agent attack will invariably affect a diverse group of people. What cannot be predicted is how coexisting injuries and comorbidities will affect treatment and outcomes of those persons exposed to nerve agents, except that synergism is known to occur between nerve agents and other agents, including other chemicals, biologic agents, radiation, conventional wounds, and preexisting medical conditions.

While treating children, keep in mind that they posses several distinct physiologic characteristics that make them particularly susceptible to nerve agent poisoning. Children have lower basal levels of acetylcholinesterase, more permeable skin, and higher minute ventilation than do adults.[22,23]

With regard to pregnancy, several studies and case reports have shown atropine to be safe during pregnancy. Currently, there is no evidence of atropine having increased teratogenic potential.[24] Atropine is an FDA pregnancy category C drug.[25] Experience with the oximes is much more limited. Only case reports on the use of pralidoxime during pregnancy exist. Thus far, there have been no reported instances of increased or unexpected teratogenesis related to pralidoxime use. Pralidoxime is also an FDA pregnancy category C drug.[25] Benzodiazepines have been studied more extensively and have been shown to increase the risk of teratogenesis.[26,27] Consequently, benzodiazepines are FDA pregnancy category D drugs.[25]

In the treatment of pregnant women, the potential benefits to the patient must always be weighed against the potential risks to the fetus. If the pregnant patient is known to have exposure to a carbamate, atropine may be the only pharmacologic therapy needed and will be safe. However, in the case of severe organophosphate exposure, none of the previously mentioned therapeutic interventions should be withheld. In mild to moderate organophosphate exposure, benzodiazepines are not indicated, although atropine and pralidoxime should still be used.

 ## PITFALLS

Several potential pitfalls in response to a nerve agent attack exist. These include the following:

- Failure to immediately notify local, state, and federal authorities, including the Federal Bureau of Investigation and the Centers for Disease Control and Prevention, in the event of a suspected nerve agent attack.

- Failure to initiate decontamination immediately. Do not delay spot decontamination in favor of later full-body decontamination. Physical or mechanical removal of agent takes priority over the use of chemical decontaminants such as bleach. If soap is not immediately available, begin irrigation with copious amounts of water.

- Failure to use appropriate clinical end points for atropine administration. Administration of atropine should continue until respiratory secretions are clear and airway compromise has resolved. Inappropriate end points for atropine administration include miosis (which may persist for up to 2 months), heart rate, and nicotinic effects such as twitching or weakness.

- Failure to consider nerve agents as a possible etiology for respiratory distress or generalized weakness in the case of exposure to an unknown chemical agent.

REFERENCES

1. Okumura T, Takasu N, Ishimatsu S, et al. Report on 640 victims of the Tokyo subway sarin attack. *Ann Emerg Med.* 1996;28:129-35.
2. Blanc P. The legacy of war gas. *Am J Med.* 1999;106(6):689-90.
3. Watson WA, Litovitz TL, Rodgers GC Jr, et al. 2002 annual report of the American Association of Poison Control Centers Toxic Exposure Surveillance System. *Am J Emerg Med.* 2003;21:353-421.
4. Miller R. Drugs and the autonomic nervous system. In: *Anesthesia.* 5th ed. Philadelphia: Churchill Livingstone; 2000:550-66.
5. Tafuri J, Roberts J. Organophosphate poisoning. *Ann Emerg Med.* 1987;16:193.
6. Saadeh AM. Metabolic complications of organophosphate and carbamate poisoning. *Trop Doct.* 2001;31:149-52.
7. Mycek M, Harvey RA, Champe PC. Cholinergic agonist and cholinergic antagonist. In: *Pharmacology.* 2nd ed. Lippincott's Illustrated Reviews. Philadelphia: Lippincott; 2000:40-7.
8. Leiken JB, Thomas RG, Walter FG, et al. A review of nerve agent exposure for the critical care physician. *Crit Care Med.* 2002;30:2346-54.
9. Takala J, de Jong R. Nerve gas terrorism: a grim challenge to anesthesiologists. *Anesth Analg.* 2003;96:819-25.
10. Macintosh R, Mushin WW, Epstein HG. Vapor pressure. In: *Physics for the Anesthetist.* 3rd ed. Oxford, England: Blackwell Scientific Publications; 1963:68.
11. Marrs TC, Maynard RL, Sidell FR. Organophosphate nerve agents. In: *Chemical Warfare Agents: Toxicology and Treatment.* New York: Wiley; 1999:83-100.
12. McKee CB, Collins L. *The Medical NBC Battlebook: USACHPPM Tech Guide 244.* U.S. Army Center for Health and Preventive Medicine (USACHPPM); 2000.
13. Jones J, Terndrup T, Franz D, Eitzen E. Future challenges in preparing for and responding to bioterrorism events. *Emerg Med Clin North Am.* 2002;20:501-24.
14. King JM, Frelin AJ. Impact of the chemical protective ensemble on the performance of basic medical tasks. *Military Med.* 1984;149:496-501.
15. Keller JR, Hurst CG, Dunn MA. Pyridostigmine used as nerve agent pretreatment under wartime conditions. *JAMA* 1994;266:693-5.
16. Lallement G, Foquin A, Dorandeu F, et al. Subchronic administration of various pretreatments of nerve agent poisoning: I. protection of blood and central cholinesterase's innocuousness towards blood-brain barrier permeability. *Drug Chem Toxicol.* 2001;24:151-64.
17. Abraham R. Practical guidelines for acute care of victims of bioterrorism: conventional injuries and concomitant nerve agent intoxication. *Anesthesiology.* 2002;97:989-1004.
18. U.S. Army Medical Research Institute of Chemical Defense (USAMRICD). *Medical Management of Chemical Casualties Handbook.* 3rd ed. U.S. Army; 1999.
19. Simpson JR, William M. Recognition and management of acute pesticide poisoning. *Am Fam Phys.* 2002;65:1599-604.
20. Mokhlesi B, Corbridge T. Toxicology in the critically ill patient. *Clin Chest Med.* 2003;24:689-711.

21. U.S. Centers for Disease Control and Prevention, Agency for Toxic Substances and Disease Registry. Medical Management Guidelines: Nerve agents. January 2004. Available at: http://www.bt.cdc. gov/agent/sarin/index.asp.

22. Henretig F, Cielsak T, et al. Environmental emergencies, bioterrorism and pediatric emergencies. *Clin Pediatr Emerg Med.* 2001;2:211-21.

23. Reigart J, Roberts J. Pesticides in children. *Pediatr Clin North Am.* 2001;48:1185-98.

24. Bailey B. Are there teratogenic risks associated with antidotes used in the acute management of poisoned pregnant women? *Birth Defects Res A Clin Mol Teratol.* 2003;67:122-40.

25. Hick J. Protective equipment for health care facility decontamination personnel: regulations, risks, and recommendations. *Ann Emerg Med.* 2003;42:370-80.

26. Weinstock L, Cohen LS, Bailey JW, et al. Obstetrical and neonatal outcome following clonazepam use during pregnancy: a case series. *Psychother Psychosom.* 2001;70:158-62.

27. Fleming T. *PDR Pharmacopoeia Pocket Dosing Guide.* New Jersey: Thompson PDR; 2004:173, 251.

chapter 92

Vesicant Agent Attack

Lara K. Kulchycki

 DESCRIPTION OF EVENT

Vesicants are chemical warfare agents named for their ability to cause skin blisters, or *vesicles*. These chemicals produce severe damage to the eyes, lungs, and skin through direct contact or inhalation of vapor.[1] Multiple nations maintain vesicant stores because these agents are simple to manufacture and can incapacitate large numbers of people with a single deployment. The prototypical vesicant is mustard. Two types of mustard agents exist: the nitrogen mustards (HN-1, HN-2, and HN-3), known for their medicinal uses as chemotherapy drugs, and the sulfur mustards (H, HD, HT), which are known only for their combat applications. Subsequent discussion of *mustard* refers only to the sulfur compounds. Other variants of these agents are tabulated elsewhere.[2]

Mustard is a yellowish-brown, oily liquid with an odor comparable to that of mustard, garlic, or onion. It does not boil until 217°C (423°F) and thus is not mustard "gas," but it freezes at 14°C (58°F); mustard-lewisite mixtures remain liquid at lower temperatures. It was heavily used in World War I and was outlawed by the Geneva Gas Protocols of 1925, but the United States was not a signatory to that agreement. Rumors of possible use of mustard by the German and Italian armies in World War II led to the secret production of mustard bombs by the United States to be used only if the Axis forces used them first. Although never intentionally used, a disastrous attack on a U.S. Liberty ship loaded with a secret cargo of mustard bombs occurred as part of an air attack on the Italian port of Bari in 1943, exposing many hundreds of Allied soldiers and sailors to this agent.[3] It was used again in the Iran-Iraq war in the 1980s. It causes ocular, respiratory, and dermatologic symptoms that develop 1 or more hours after exposure. Eye effects range from tearing and conjunctival irritation to ocular pain, photophobia, corneal ulceration, and blindness. Mustard respiratory signs and symptoms include rhinorrhea, dysphonia, productive cough, hemoptysis, and dyspnea. Mustard burns are more likely to appear on warm, moist areas of the body such as the neck, axillae, and groin. Patients first notice skin erythema, burning pain, and intense pruritus, followed several hours later by vesication. Other mustard effects may include nausea, vomiting, tremor, ataxia, and convulsions. Symptom onset is usually delayed for 2 to 12 hours after initial contact.

Since mustards are alkylating agents that interfere with nucleic acid synthesis, leukopenia can be a clinically significant problem. Drops in neutrophil counts usually appear by days 3 to 5 and can be precipitous, predisposing injured skin and airways to superinfection. Deaths, although uncommon, usually occur days after exposure from bronchopneumonia or sepsis. The case fatality rate from World War I was surprisingly low, approximately 3%. This preantibiotic statistic underscores that vesicants are maiming agents, intended to disable rather than kill and generating large numbers of casualties requiring extended medical care.

Lewisite (L) is an arsenical vesicant sometimes combined with mustard (HL). Lewisite is a colorless oily liquid, but with impurities it is amber and smells like geraniums. It causes symptoms very similar to those of mustard but is distinguished from mustard by its quick onset of discomfort, within seconds to a minute or two. Casualties may be less likely to receive blinding injuries from vapor since early-onset blepharospasm can limit exposure. Large exposures are notable for causing "lewisite shock" from increased capillary permeability, renal failure, and hepatic necrosis.

Phosgene oxime (CX) is not a true vesicant because it does not cause the blistering seen with mustard and lewisite. It is more precisely classified as an *urticant,* or nettle agent, and causes wheals and blanching comparable to nettle stings. It is not to be confused with phosgene (CG), a pulmonary irritant that smells like hay. Phosgene oxime is a colorless solid or yellowish-brown liquid with immediate corrosive effects. Patients experience instantaneous skin blanching and burning, eye pain, and respiratory distress. It is notable for causing pulmonary edema and pulmonary-vessel thromboses. There are no documented battlefield uses of this chemical, and consequently few data exist on the clinical course and optimal treatment regimens.

 PREINCIDENT ACTIONS

Every community and each hospital should have a documented disaster plan for mass-casualty incidents and release of toxic chemicals. Emergency personnel should be provided with, and trained in the use of, personal protective equipment and the implementation of the disaster response protocol.

 POSTINCIDENT ACTIONS

Medical personnel coordinating a disaster response must notify appropriate local and regional healthcare providers as well as law enforcement and public health officials. If possible, a hotline should be established to disseminate information to the public.

First responders at the scene of a suspected chemical attack will need to create rapid scene control to prevent the spread of contamination and minimize the number of injuries. Any rescuer working in the hot zone will require personal protective equipment as well as a pressure-demand, self-contained breathing apparatus (SCBA) to guard against exposure to liquid and vaporized agents.

Vesicant absorption is both rapid and irreversible. Decontamination occurring after the first few minutes of exposure may be too late to prevent the eventual development of skin lesions (although lesion appearance is delayed, the damage from mustard begins within a few minutes) but may prevent systemic absorption of a lethal dose from liquid still in contact with the skin. Late decontamination can also prevent the incapacitation of first responders by liquid agent or off-gassing vapor from chemical attack victims.

Chemical casualties should be removed from the scene and brought to the designated decontamination zone. Patients' eyes should be flushed with water for 5 to 10 minutes. No ocular patches or occlusive dressings should be applied. All contaminated clothing must be removed and double-bagged, and the skin should be washed with either soap and water or dilute 0.5% sodium hypochlorite solution. If water is unavailable, absorbent materials such as flour or fuller's earth can be applied to soak up liquid agent on the skin; these substances should then be washed off after several seconds of contact. Contaminated equipment can also be cleaned with dilute sodium hypochlorite. After decontamination, patients can be transferred to the designated medical treatment facility, where they can be retriaged.

 MEDICAL TREATMENT OF CASUALTIES

Initial medical treatment and stabilization may need to occur in the hot zone, especially for patients with other significant injuries, large chemical exposures, or preexisting airway disease. As always, a quick assessment of the ABCs (i.e., airway, breathing, and circulation) is the initial step.

Constructing a timeline of symptom onset can be crucial in determining the agent used in a chemical attack. Immediate onset of lacrimation, blepharospasm, and burning skin pain argues for the use of lewisite or phosgene oxime. A latent period of 2 to 12 hours is more consistent with the use of mustard. Despite active investigation, there are currently no sensitive, specific, and readily available laboratory tests to confirm exposure to a particular vesicant,[4] although urinary analysis for thiodiglycol, a metabolite of sulfur mustard, is available at military reference-laboratory facilities. Providers must keep in mind that the deployed weapon may have contained multiple chemicals, including nerve agents, each of which may require a different treatment algorithm.

Specific medical management guidelines for exposure to vesicant agents have been compiled by the Agency for Toxic Substances and Disease Registry, a division of the U.S. Department of Health and Human Services designated to assist with emergency medical response to release of toxic substances. Links to these clinical guidelines can be found on the Web site for the Centers for Disease Control and Prevention.[5-7]

Eye injuries require ophthalmic antibiotic ointments to prevent lid adhesion and infection, and mydriatic agents for analgesia if there is underlying iritis. Corticosteroid ointments are sometimes recommended to decrease inflammation, but these should be administered only after consultation with an ophthalmologist. Short-term visual incapacitation is common after vesicant eye injury, but most patients recover full function.[8] Hence, reassurance for all but the most severely injured is both appropriate and humane.

Respiratory injuries are treated with supportive measures including oxygen, bronchodilators, and ventilatory support, as needed. Pulse oximetry and chest radiographs can aid in clinical assessment. Patients with preexisting reactive airway disease may have more severe reactions to inhalation injury and require careful monitoring. Antibiotics are best withheld until sputum cultures or other clinical evidence confirms infection with a specific organism. Productive cough is a common symptom of chemical bronchitis and by itself does not warrant the use of antibiotics. In severe respiratory injury, the airway can become plugged with necrotic debris and urgent bronchoscopy with deep suctioning may be needed.

Treatment of chemical burns is similar to that required for thermal injuries, including wound care, debridement, topical antibiotics, intravenous fluid replacement, and systemic analgesics. Vesicant skin burns are usually only partial thickness but take nearly twice the time to heal as comparable thermal injuries.[9,10] Maintenance of strict wound hygiene and avoidance of secondary infection is crucial in patients incurring injury from mustard, since leukopenia is a delayed effect of exposure to higher doses. The use of systemic antibiotics should be avoided unless there is specific evidence of infection. Involvement of burn specialists would be appropriate for ongoing management of such patients.

Data from the Iran-Iraq war suggest that fluid losses occurring in conjunction with vesicant burns are less extreme than those encountered in the case of thermal burns of equivalent body surface area. Care providers must be cautious because overzealous fluid replacement can lead to pulmonary edema, further compromising respiratory function in patients with vesicant airway injury.[1,11]

In case of vesicant ingestion, care providers should neither induce emesis nor attempt decontamination with activated charcoal. Symptoms of nausea and vomiting can be treated with standard antiemetic agents.

A set of routine laboratory tests, including a complete blood count (CBC) and serum electrolytes as well as kidney and liver function tests, is warranted for patients who will be admitted. The CBC is a baseline by which to measure the subsequent leukopenia of patients with mustard injury or the hemolytic anemia of lewisite patients. Kidney and liver function tests are particularly important in lewisite exposure since it is known to cause multi-organ failure.

Of the vesicants, only Lewisite has a specific antidote. The chelating agent British anti-lewisite (BAL), also known as dimercaprol, enhances urinary excretion of arsenic and improves clinical outcome in exposed patients.[12] The lewisite protocol suggests a dose of 2.5 to 5 mg/kg delivered intramuscularly (IM) every 4 hours for four doses. Dose frequency can be increased to every 2 hours in cases of severe poisoning. The drug is dissolved in peanut oil and is thus contraindicated in patients with peanut allergy. Water-soluble BAL analogs exist but are still experimental; they are unlikely to be readily available in the instance of a chemical disaster.[13] Side effects to IM administration are both common and dose-related, leading many experts to recommend BAL be given only to patients with shock or significant pulmonary injury. Side effects include injection site reactions, hypertension, tachycardia, headache, nausea, vomiting, perioral and extremity paresthesias, anxiety, chest pain, and fever.[14]

Patients with mild symptoms should be observed for a period of about 24 hours. If symptoms have not progressed, the patients can be discharged with instructions to return if new manifestations appear.

CASE PRESENTATION

Your hospital's emergency department is put on alert for a report of a mass-casualty incident. An explosion occurred during a local sporting event. According to emergency medical services and firefighter personnel at the scene, victims reported a cloud of smoke with a strange garlic smell that permeated the stands after the blast. Victims closest to the explosion were found with a yellow, oily residue on their skin and clothing. The first of the injured will be arriving in your trauma bay within 5 minutes. No immediate identification of the attack agent is available.

UNIQUE CONSIDERATIONS

Patients may not show any initial signs of chemical injury. A variable delay in symptom onset can occur with different agents, variations in the amount and route of exposure, and various weather conditions. This latent period can cloud initial clinical evaluation and delay the onset of decontamination procedures. Even if first responders are vigilant and well trained, contaminated patients or equipment may gain entrance to hospitals and cause additional casualties. For sulfur mustard, knowledge of the latent period is useful in estimating absorbed dose because the

length of the latent period is inversely correlated with dose. For example, the appearance of respiratory signs and symptoms within 4 hours of inhalational exposure portends a poor outcome.

Proper management of a vesicant attack will require significant medical and financial resources, including facilities equipped for the prolonged hospitalization of casualties and consultation services with specialists in toxicology, burn surgery, ophthalmology, and pulmonary medicine. In addition, the psychological burdens to patients, families, and caregivers cannot be ignored. Crisis counseling for victims and debriefing for staff is a key component of the disaster response. Chronic medical sequelae, although beyond the scope of this chapter, will add to the toll of a chemical attack.

 ## PITFALLS

Several potential pitfalls in response to a vesicant agent attack exist. These include the following:

- Failure to suspect chemical injury and initiate prompt decontamination because casualties do not yet exhibit the symptoms of vesicant injury.
- Failure to notify appropriate public health, local government, and law enforcement officials as soon as chemical attack is suspected.
- Failure to treat urgent injuries and respiratory compromise during decontamination.
- Failure to maintain a strict hot zone.
- Failure to recognize and treat concomitant exposures to other chemical weapons, such as nerve agents.
- Failure to appreciate the severity of vesicant burns on initial presentation.
- Failure to prevent overhydration in patients with chemical burns.
- Failure to withhold systemic antibiotics until there is specific evidence of skin or respiratory-tract bacterial infection.
- Failure to involve the appropriate specialty consultants, including toxicologists, burn surgeons, ophthalmologists, and pulmonologists.
- Failure to provide counseling and emotional support to victims and medical personnel in the event of a chemical attack.[15]

REFERENCES

1. Zajtchuk R, Bellamy RF, eds. *Textbook of Military Medicine*. Washington, DC: Office of The Surgeon General; 1997:197-228.
2. Noort D, Benschop HP, Black RM. Biomonitoring of exposure to chemical warfare agents: a review. *Toxicol Appl Pharmacol*. 2002;184:116-26.
3. U.S. Centers for Disease Control and Prevention, Agency for Toxic Substances and Disease Registry. Sulfur mustard medical management guidelines. Available at: http://www.bt.cdc.gov/agent/sulfur-mustard/index.asp.
4. U.S. Centers for Disease Control and Prevention, Agency for Toxic Substances and Disease Registry. Lewisite medical management guidelines. Available at: http://www.bt.cdc.gov/agent/lewisite/index.asp.
5. U.S. Centers for Disease Control and Prevention, Agency for Toxic Substances and Disease Registry. Phosgene oxime medical man-

agement guidelines. Available at: http://www.bt.cdc.gov/agent/phosgene-oxime/index.asp.

6. Safarinejad MR, Moosavi SA, Montazeri B. Ocular injuries caused by mustard gas: diagnosis, treatment, and medical defense. *Mil Med.* 2001;166:67-70.

7. Mellor SG, Rice P, Cooper GJ. Vesicant burns. *Br J Plast Surg.* 1991;44:434-7.

8. Momeni A-Z, Enshaeih S, Meghdadi M, et al. Skin manifestation of mustard gas: a clinical study of 535 patients exposed to mustard gas. *Arch Dermatol.* 1992;128:775-81.

9. Willems J. Clinical management of mustard gas casualties. *Ann Med Militaris (Belgicae)* 1989;3(Suppl):1-60.

10. Vilensky JA, Redman K. British anti-Lewisite (dimercaprol): an amazing history. *Ann Emerg Med.* 2003;41:378-83.

11. Munro NB, Watson AP, Ambrose KR, et al. Treating exposure to chemical warfare agents: implications for health care providers and community emergency planning. *Environ Health Perspect.* 1990;89:205-15.

12. *Goldfrank's Toxicologic Emergencies.* 6th ed. Stamford, Conn: Appleton & Lange, 1274-6.

13. Reminick G. *Nightmare in Bari: The World War II Liberty Ship Poison Gas Disaster and Cover-up.* Palo Alto, Calif: Glencannon Press; 2001:266.

14. Ellison DH. *Handbook of Chemical and Biological Warfare Agents.* Boca Raton, Fla: CRC Press; 2000:133-8.

15. Romano Jr JA, King JM. Psychological factors in chemical warfare and terrorism [Chapter 13]. In: Somani SM, Romano Jr JA, eds. *Chemical Warfare Agents: Toxicity at Low Levels.* Boca Raton, Fla: CRC Press; 2001:393-408.

chapter 93

Respiratory Agent Attack (Toxic Inhalational Injury)

Stephen J. Traub

 DESCRIPTION OF EVENT

Many chemical and biologic agents are capable of causing respiratory symptoms. Ricin (see Chapter 136) and the trichothecene mycotoxins (see Chapter 135) may cause pulmonary syndromes ranging from cough to acute pulmonary edema; *Bacillus anthracis* (see Chapter 102), the causative agent of anthrax, may cause a lethal pneumonitis; vesicant agents (see Chapter 92) may cause acute lung injury in addition to ocular and dermal toxicity; and the organophosphorous nerve agents (see Chapter 91) may produce suffocating pulmonary secretions. This chapter, however, is limited to a discussion of three agents that are gases under environmental conditions and whose main target organ is the lung. Phosgene (military chemical weapon designation, CG) and diphosgene (DP) have similar toxicities and are considered together; chlorine (no military chemical weapon designation) is considered separately. These toxicants cause a dose-dependent pulmonary syndrome that may range from a mild cough through reactive airways disease to acute lung injury and the adult respiratory distress syndrome.

Phosgene, also known as carbonyl chloride (COCl2), is the reactive species formed by the decomposition of diphosgene. Both phosgene and diphosgene have relatively low water solubility and so are capable of diffusing deeply into the lungs, to the level of the alveoli, before reacting. The exact mechanism of toxicity of phosgene is incompletely understood but is thought to involve some combination or reaction with the amino or thiol groups of alveolar proteins or the phosphate groups of surfactant, reaction with water to form hydrochloric acid, or free-radical formation that then initiates further cellular toxicity.

The aqueous solubility of chlorine gas (Cl_2) is intermediate between the low values for the phosgenes and the high solubilities of strong mineral acids and bases. Not only can chlorine diffuse into the alveoli (like phosgenes) before exerting toxicity, but it can also irritate and damage the larger airways. Soldiers gassed with chlorine in World War I exhibited an almost equal distribution of large-airway and small-airway damage. The reaction of

chlorine gas with alveolar water generates several toxic species, such as hypochlorous acid, hydrochloric acid, molecular oxygen, and free-radical oxygen species. It is the oxygen species that are thought to mediate much of the alveolar pulmonary damage, whereas the acid species mediate the upper respiratory symptoms that may be seen in massive exposures (see below).

A respiratory agent attack could occur in almost any setting. Closed ventilation areas, such as a theater or a government building, intuitively seem particularly vulnerable to such attacks. These gases, however, may also be devastatingly effective in open areas, as occurred on the battlefields of World War I. They might also be used at large gatherings (such as sporting events) or on crowded city streets. All of these gases are denser than air and would thus stay at the level of the victims rather than quickly dissipating into the atmosphere.

Both phosgene and chlorine are used for industrial purposes and could easily be diverted for a large-scale terrorist attack.[1] Chlorine gas can also be produced by mixing household cleaning agents and is thus an inexpensive and easily produced chemical weapon that could inflict terror (if not mass casualties) in any crowed area such as a movie theater or subway.

Respiratory agent attack should be suspected when more than one person begins complaining of unexpected pulmonary symptoms. Tissue damage from these agents begins almost immediately. Depending on the dose to which the victims are exposed, however, effects may develop within minutes or be delayed for several hours. Upper-airway irritation and noise (i.e., coughing, sneezing, inspiratory stridor, and wheezing) are usually of short onset, whereas the dyspnea that heralds incipient pulmonary edema from alveolar damage is usually delayed for hours; the length of this latent period is inversely correlated with dose. Onset of dyspnea within 4 hours of exposure to phosgenes indicates a very high dose and portends a grave outcome. The odor or appearance of the air may also help to identify the event and causative agent. Phosgene is colorless but has the odor of freshly mown hay; chlorine gas is yellow and pungent and has a characteristic odor of bleach. The toxic effects of phosgene can occur at environmental levels of 1.5 to 2 ppm, whereas the aroma is detectable at 2 to 3 ppm; hence, toxicity can occur without subject awareness.[2]

 PREINCIDENT ACTIONS

Every hospital in the United States should have a plan in place to treat victims of a chemical agent attack. Such a plan should include, at the very least, a means to identify victims of a chemical agent attack, a procedure to triage them to appropriate areas, a decontamination plan, and a treatment strategy. The establishment of a pulmonary care team with respiratory therapists may be beneficial in the hospital response plan to assist in monitoring a surge of patients with respiratory complaints. In the event of a true attack, hospital response should include notification of local, state, and federal authorities.

There are no antidotes to poisoning from the phosgenes or chlorine and thus no specific stockpiles that must be kept on hand, although ample supplies of standard bronchodilators should be ensured. Treatment is supportive (see below).

 POSTINCIDENT ACTIONS

Clinicians who suspect respiratory agent poisoning, or any chemical weapons attack, should immediately contact local, state, and federal authorities. Law enforcement, firefighters/hazardous materials and emergency medical services officials will coordinate scene control, triage, evacuation, and containment, which are crucial steps in the management of any chemical weapons attack. Because the site will likely be a crime scene, Federal Bureau of Investigation/law enforcement officials will control evidence gathering and chain of evidence.

The hospital chemical-exposure plan should be activated because more potential victims should be expected. The regional poison control center should also be contacted; the center may be aware of other cases at nearby hospitals and thus serve as a clearinghouse for epidemiologic information.[3] It is also an indispensable resource for questions regarding diagnosis and management. In the United States, callers can be automatically connected to the closest regional poison control center by dialing 1-800-222-1222.

 MEDICAL TREATMENT OF CASUALTIES

The initial approach to the victim of a respiratory agent attack begins with assessing and securing the patient's airway, breathing, and circulation.

- **Airway.** A victim with a massive exposure may present in obvious respiratory failure and need immediate intubation. All patients should be monitored for decompensation throughout treatment because progressive deterioration may necessitate intubation in a patient who initially appeared stable. Sudden stridorous airway sounds should generate immediate concern for acute laryngospasm from newly generated hydrochloric acid from phosgene hydrolysis, and emergent airway management may be necessary.[4]
- **Breathing.** All patients should be placed on high-flow oxygen; this may be discontinued if the oxygen saturation is subsequently found to be normal by transcutaneous pulse oximetry or arterial-blood-gas analysis. Wheezing may be present even in patients with no history of reactive airway disease and should be treated with beta$_2$-selective agonists such as albuterol. Acute lung injury and the acute respiratory distress syndrome may occur after a respiratory agent attack and should be managed with low (6 ml/kg) tidal volumes in accordance with currently accepted standards.[5,6]
- **Circulation.** Two large-bore intravenous lines (18 gauge or larger) should be placed to volume resuscitate the patient if necessary.

Once the airway, breathing, and circulation are secured, other treatment strategies may be considered depending on the agent involved.

- **Phosgenes.** Nonsteroidal anti-inflammatory drugs (NSAIDs)[7] and corticosteroids[8] are relatively benign interventions that may have a role in the treatment of poisoning by the phosgenes. Reasonable dosing regimens for NSAIDs are ibuprofen, 400 mg taken by mouth every 6 hours, or ketorolac, 30 mg given intravenously (IV) every 6 hours. A reasonable dosing regimen for corticosteroids is methylprednisolone, 1 mg/kg IV every 8 hours until pulmonary toxicity resolves, followed by an appropriate taper. IV isoproterenol[9] and aminophylline[10] have shown benefits in animal models, as has inhaled N-acetylcysteine.[11] These treatments, however, carry a significant risk of iatrogenic toxicity, lack any human data to support them, and cannot be recommended at this time.
- **Chlorine gas.** Corticosteroids, either inhaled[12] or IV,[13] may help speed lung recovery in chlorine-gas poisoning. They should be given as soon as possible because the beneficial effects appear to decrease with time.[14] A reasonable dosing regimen is methylprednisolone, 1 mg/kg IV every 8 hours until pulmonary toxicity resolves, followed by an appropriate taper. Nebulized sodium bicarbonate has been advocated as a means to neutralize the acidic species generated in the alveoli,[15] but there are no data to support its use in patients with any more than trivial toxicity, and its routine use cannot be recommended.

 UNIQUE CONSIDERATIONS

Liquids, such as nerve agents (see Chapter 91) or vesicant agents (see Chapter 92), are most lethal when allowed to evaporate or when aerosolized; as such, they require some form of dispersal mechanism (e.g., a small explosion or a machine to generate a spray) to achieve their maximum effect. True gases, such as the phosgenes and chlorine, require no such dispersal mechanism; they require only that the container be opened to the atmosphere or that they be synthesized in an open-air reaction (e.g., the mixing of cleaning supplies in a bucket).

A disheveled subway rider with several bags of belongings is observed to be cleaning the interior of one of the subway cars during the afternoon commute. Although he clearly does not work for the subway, his actions seem harmless and he is not approached by the other riders. As he exits at one stop, no one notices that he has left behind several containers and a bucket under one of the benches.

Shortly after the subway pulls from the station, a rider notices a yellow gas with a pungent odor coming from the bucket. Panic quickly engulfs the car, as three passengers begin coughing and screaming that they "cannot breathe." Another passenger activates the emergency brake, stopping the train. The passengers chaotically exit the car, and the resulting stampede is later determined to have caused more injuries than the gas attack.

Several persons are taken to the nearest emergency department complaining of coughing and burning of the eyes and mouth. Their symptoms, coupled with the history of a yellow gas and the unmistakable smell of bleach, lead the emergency department workers to conclude that the subway riders were victims of an attack with chlorine gas. The riders are decontaminated in accordance with the hospital chemical-exposure protocol. The emergency department notifies the local authorities, who state that they will contact the appropriate state and federal authorities.

The riders with pulmonary complaints are all observed for several hours and discharged. Examination of the crime scene reveals a bottle of drain opener (active ingredient: sulfuric acid) and chlorine bleach, both purchased from a local drugstore. When mixed together, the two liquids generated chlorine gas.

The phosgenes and chlorine are also somewhat unique in that their toxicity is primarily pulmonary (although chlorine gas may also cause significant ocular and mucous-membrane irritation). Other chemical agents may have pulmonary toxicity, but this is a secondary effect. The toxicity of vesicant agents is primarily dermal, and the toxicity of nerve agents is primarily related to the peripheral and central nervous systems.

 PITFALLS

Several potential pitfalls in response to a respiratory agent attack exist. These include the following:

- Failing to consider the phosgenes and chlorine as potential agents of attack.
- Failing to obtain important historical information, such as the presence of an odor of freshly mown hay (phosgene) or bleach (chlorine) or the presence of a yellow-colored gas (chlorine).
- Assuming that respiratory complaints in patients from a mass-casualty incident are due to smoke inhalation.

- Failing to notify local, state, and federal authorities when a respiratory agent attack is suspected.
- Failing to observe victims of respiratory agent attack closely to monitor for deterioration of their conditions.
- Failing to recognize that patients without signs, symptoms, or laboratory evidence of pulmonary damage may nevertheless have been exposed to a pulmonary agent such as the phosgenes or chlorine. Such patients should be observed carefully (ideally, for at least 8 to 24 hours) for the development of dyspnea and pulmonary edema.
- Failure to prospectively account for all active and spare ventilators in the hospital, and failure to have a source of backup ventilators on short notice, in the event of a surge of patients with respiratory failure from a respiratory agent attack.

REFERENCES

1. Burklow TR, Yu CE, Madsen JM. Industrial chemicals: terrorist weapons of opportunity. *Pediatr Ann*. 2003;32(4):230-4.
2. Ware LB, Matthay MA. The acute respiratory distress syndrome. *N Engl J Med*. 2000;342(18):1334-49.
3. Sciuto AM, Stotts RR, Hurt HH. Efficacy of ibuprofen and pentoxifylline in the treatment of phosgene-induced acute lung injury. *J Appl Toxicol*. 1996;16(5):381-4.
4. Borak J, Diller WF. Phosgene exposure: mechanisms of injury and treatment strategies. *J Occup Environ Med*. 2001;43(2):110-9.
5. Sciuto AM, Strickland PT, Gurtner GH. Post-exposure treatment with isoproterenol attenuates pulmonary edema in phosgene-exposed rabbits. *J Appl Toxicol*. 1998;18(5):321-9.
6. Sciuto AM, Strickland PT, Kennedy TP, et al. Postexposure treatment with aminophylline protects against phosgene-induced acute lung injury. *Exp Lung Res*. 1997;23(4):317-32.
7. Sciuto AM, Strickland PT, Kennedy TP, et al. Protective effects of N-acetylcysteine treatment after phosgene exposure in rabbits. *Am J Respir Crit Care Med*. 1995;151(3 Pt 1):768-72.
8. Gunnarsson M, Walther SM, Seidal T, et al. Effects of inhalation of corticosteroids immediately after experimental chlorine gas lung injury. *J Trauma*. 2000;48(1):101-7.
9. Demnati R, Fraser R, Martin JG, et al. Effects of dexamethasone on functional and pathological changes in rat bronchi caused by high acute exposure to chlorine. *Toxicol Sci*. 1998;45(2):242-6.
10. Wang J, Zhang L, Walther SM. Inhaled budesonide in experimental chlorine gas lung injury: influence of time interval between injury and treatment. *Intensive Care Med*. 2002;28(3):352-7.
11. Bosse GM. Nebulized sodium bicarbonate in the treatment of chlorine gas inhalation. *J Toxicol Clin Toxicol*. 1994;32(3):233-41.
12. Moore DH, Alexander SM. Emergency response to a chemical warfare agent incident: domestic preparedness, first response, and public health considerations [Chapter 14]. In: Somani SM, Romano Jr JA, eds. *Chemical Warfare Agents: Toxicity at Low Levels*. Boca Raton, Fla: CRC Press; 2001:417.
13. Urbanetti JS. Toxic inhalational injury [Chapter 9]. In: Sidell FR, Takafuji ET, Franz DR, eds. *Textbook of Military Medicine, Part 1: Warfare, Weaponry and the Casualty—Medical Aspects of Chemical and Biological Warfare*. Washington, DC: Office of the Surgeon General at TMM Publications; 1997:257-8.
14. Piantadosi CA, Schwartz DA. The acute respiratory distress syndrome. *Ann Internal Med*. 2004;141:460-70.
15. Vilke GM, Jacoby I, Manoguerra AS, et al. Disaster preparedness of poison control centers in the United States. *J Toxicol Clin Toxicol*. 1996;34:53-8.

chapter 94

Cyanide Attack*

Mark E. Keim

 ## DESCRIPTION OF EVENT

Cyanide—much of it in the form of salts, such as sodium, potassium, and calcium cyanide—is widely used in industry. Hundreds of thousands of tons of cyanide are manufactured annually in the United States alone. The cyanides of military (and possibly terrorist) interest are the volatile liquids hydrogen cyanide (North Atlantic Treaty Organisation designation, AC) and cyanogen chloride (CK).[1]

A covert cyanide attack involving food or water contamination with ingestion as a route of exposure would likely initially present in a manner similar to that of a covert biologic attack. In this sense, the first indications of attack may be an unusual cluster of cases or a more diffuse increase in the number of patients presenting with an initially unknown illness. In this covert scenario, forensic and/or epidemiologic investigation may be necessary to confirm the cause of the event. Obviously, an abruptly high incidence, a close temporal relationship, or a more focal cluster of cases will increase the suspicion of a common causative agent.

Cyanide released as a liquid or an aerosol can pose a liquid hazard via penetration through even intact skin, but the greater risk in a terrorist attack is the inhalation of aerosol, vapor, or gas. A cyanide attack involving inhalational exposure is more likely to present in a manner similar to that of other hazardous-material (HazMat) release events, with a well-localized incident scene and an associated cluster of attack victims. In this scenario, an accurate and timely history of the event will be important in guiding response decision-making and clinical diagnosis. Lethal concentrations of cyanide vapor or gas typically kill rapidly, dissipate quickly, and leave no toxic residue. It must not be forgotten that smoke-inhalation casualties from any terrorist scenario, even one using only conventional weapons, may also exhibit cyanide toxicity.[2,3]

 ## PREINCIDENT ACTIONS

The Importance of Local Preparedness

Preparation for the 1996 Olympic Games in Atlanta demonstrated an ability to stockpile and mobilize resources (including chemical antidotes) given sufficient advance notice.[4] Since then, the development of specialized chemical and biologic incident-response teams within the National Disaster Medical System as well as the pharmaceutical reserve and delivery systems of the Strategic National Stockpile have augmented regional and national capacity.

However, with chemical releases (and especially cyanide), lethal effects can occur within minutes after exposure. The characteristically rapid onset of cyanide toxicity offers only a very narrow window of opportunity for clinical intervention, thus limiting the potential effectiveness of resources other than those that are immediately available at the community first-responder level. The inclusion of cyanide antidote in prehospital formularies is nearly nonexistent in the United States due to the inherent toxicity and narrow therapeutic range of currently available medications.[5] Unfortunately, hospital preparedness for many chemical emergencies and disasters is also reportedly inadequate.[6-10] One particular study noted a decrease in hospital-based availability of cyanide antidotes in a major U.S. city between 1996 and 2000.[10]

The character of HazMat risk has also changed in the wake of recent acts of terror. Emergency responders, including both law enforcement and emergency medical services care providers, are not only potential victims but potential targets.[11,12] Several publications have recently agreed that, "At the community level, planning for chemical-biologic catastrophes begins with development of local health resources."[13-15] Boxes 94-1 and 94-2 list recommendations for preincident actions that can be undertaken to mitigate the potential impact of a terrorist attack involving cyanide.

 ## POSTINCIDENT ACTIONS

Scene Safety

The first step in the response to any HazMat release incident is to limit any further exposure to the victims, as well

---

*The material in this chapter solely reflects the views of the author. It does not necessarily reflect the policies or recommendations of the Centers for Disease Control and Prevention or the U.S. Department of Health and Human Services.

as to others, including first responders. Despite an increased awareness of chemical terrorism among first responders, in one simulated chemical weapons release in New York City, first responders entered the site without adequate personal protective gear.[21] Despite an extensive pre-staging of national assets in preparation for potential terrorist use of mass-casualty weapons at the 1996 Atlanta Olympics, many medical and investigational responders entered Olympic Centennial Park immediately after the bomb explosion and before any chemical hazard characterization. A thorough assessment of scene safety is paramount to any subsequent rescue activities. Rescuers should also keep in mind the possibility of secondary devices meant to injure the first responders.[22]

Termination of Exposure and Decontamination

Once the scene has been declared safe for entry or the proper personal protective equipment is employed, the next step is to remove the victims from the area of any potential further exposure. No decontamination is necessary if it is known that the cyanide exposure was in the form of vapor or gas. The health risk from vapor released from clothing contaminated by cyanide gas, vapor, or fine aerosol is not significant. Simple removal of outer clothing will provide an added precaution against any such potential for exposure but should not delay the initiation of emergency medical therapy.

In the case of direct dermal exposures to liquid or dry cyanide compounds, contaminated clothing should be removed immediately and the skin should be decontaminated using copious amounts of water or soap and water. There may also be instances when cyanide contamination is combined with conventional wound injuries. In these cases, bandages are removed in the decontamination area and the wounds are flushed. Dressings and tourniquets are replaced with new ones. Splints are thoroughly decontaminated (but removed only by a physician).[1] The new dressings are removed in the operating room and submerged in 5% sodium hypochlorite or placed into a plastic bag and sealed. Cyanide is quite volatile, so it is extremely unlikely that liquid cyanide will remain in a wound. The risk from vapor off-gassing from chemically contaminated fragments and cloth in wounds is very low and not significant. A chemical protective mask is not required for surgical personnel.[1]

The 1978 mass suicide in Jonestown, Guyana, dramatically illustrates the potential for mass casualties due to cyanide ingestion. In the case of cyanide ingestion, gastrointestinal decontamination should include gastric lavage, cathartics, and activated charcoal. Responders should also take personal protective precautions to avoid dermal exposures to cyanide-contaminated emesis or gastric contents.

 ## MEDICAL TREATMENT OF CASUALTIES

Mechanism of Toxicity

The cyanide ion can rapidly bind with certain metallic complexes, particularly those containing cobalt and trivalent iron. Cyanide can combine with the ferric iron in the cytochrome-oxidase complex in mitochondria, thus preventing intracellular use of oxygen. The cell must then switch to anaerobic metabolism, creating lactic acid and metabolic acidosis and leading to progressive tissue hypoxia to the point of cell death. The organs most sensitive to this hypoxia are the central nervous system and the heart.

Therapy

The primary goal of therapy is to remove cyanide from the cytochrome-oxidase complex. Methemoglobin has a high affinity for cyanide, and cyanide will preferentially, although only temporarily, bind to methemoglobin instead of cytochrome oxidase. Amyl nitrite and sodium nitrite are used to induce methemoglobinemia.[1] However, induction of methemoglobinemia can result in serious side effects, especially in children.[23] Methemoglobin levels should be monitored and not be allowed to exceed 35% to 40%.[24]

A secondary goal is to bind cyanide irreversibly so that it cannot reenter mitochondria. This detoxification is produced by administration of sodium thiosulfate, which binds to cyanide irreversibly in a one-way reaction that is catalyzed by the enzyme rhodanese and that produces thiocyanate, which is rapidly excreted by the kidneys.

Amyl nitrite, sodium nitrite, and sodium thiosulfate are commercially available in the form of a cyanide antidote kit (CAK). The CAK itself is not without its own inherent toxicity and adverse effects. Sodium nitrite can cause severe hypotension.[25] High thiocyanate levels (>10 mg/dL) have been associated with vomiting, psychosis, arthralgias, and myalgia. Anaphylaxis is a rare event. The most serious potential adverse effect from the use of CAK is the production of toxic levels of methemoglobin, although concentrations greater than 40% are identifiable by the appearance of cyanosis and can be treated by the administration of methylene blue. The methemoglobin-induced decrease in the oxygen-carrying capacity of the blood has led to recommendations of caution when the CAK is used to treat smoke-inhalation victims,[26] but risks of nitrite use in this situation may be overstated.[27] Moreover, waiting for laboratory confirmation of cyanide exposure before beginning to administer the CAK may represent a potentially fatal delay in life-saving intervention. Nevertheless, fatal methemoglobinemia from an iatrogenic overdose of sodium nitrite has claimed the life of at least one child who consumed a sublethal dose of cyanide.[23]

Hydroxocobalamin has been recognized as an antidote for cyanide toxicity for over 40 years.[28-30] It is in active use in France as an antidote for cyanide intoxication, and excellent data about its efficacy, safety, and adverse reactions are available. Hydroxocobalamin reacts stoichiometrically with cyanide to form cyanocobalamin (vitamin B_{12}). Hydroxocobalamin is rarely used in the United States as a cyanide antidote,[31] but after the publication of articles advocating its use for cyanide disasters,[5] several pharmaceutical companies are investigating the feasibility of formulation for such use in the United States.

Supportive care for cyanide toxicity is also an important goal during the resuscitative phase of therapy and usually involves oxygenation and sodium bicarbonate for correction of the metabolic acidosis.[32] Anticonvulsants such as benzodiazepines are used to control seizures.[33]

Table 94-1 provides a list of recommendations for detection, decontamination, and therapy for cyanide toxicity.

Triage of Cyanide Mass Casualties

Mass-casualty events may necessitate the triage of casualties. In most cases, given the rapidity of the effect of cyanide, by the time the responder arrives on the scene of an aerosol or vapor release, the casualties will be asymptomatic, exhibiting acute effects, recovering from acute effects, or dead. Table 94-2 lists a triage scheme that may be applied to these four categories.[34]

An evening memorial service was held in a church hall. The meeting was attended by 60 men, women, and children. Everyone was seated in the middle of the hall. During the service, most of those present began to experience dizziness, lightheadedness, nausea, and weakness. Within minutes, a 54-year-old man seated near the back of the hall lost consciousness and fell off his chair. An ambulance was called. Within the next few minutes, many of those in the hall also became unconscious, starting with those seated immediately surrounding the 54-year-old casualty. On entering the hall, one emergency medical technician (EMT) complained of feeling dizzy and stumbled to the ground. His partner, who had not yet entered the hall, noted the mass casualties inside and immediately called for backup before entering to rescue his fallen comrade.

Thereafter, a fleet of ambulances was dispatched to the scene. After they had arrived, police and ambulance services established that a large number of people, including both of the previously dispatched EMTs, were affected. A major incident was declared, and the local HazMat response team was dispatched while police established and maintained a perimeter around the scene.

After the arrival of the HazMat response team, an entry was made into the open doors of the building and all 62 patients were found to be inside. Twelve patients, including one of the EMTs, were conscious and breathing but weak. Twenty-eight patients, including one EMT, were apneic and convulsing, although all still had a pulse. Ten patients were unconscious but breathing. Twelve patients were apneic and asystolic. The HazMat response team opened all doors and windows to the room and immediately removed everyone but the 12 asystolic patients.

Fifty patients were transferred to a warm zone for removal of outer clothing before evacuation. Thirty-eight patients were triaged for immediate transport to the hospital. While en route, oxygen therapy was initiated for all 38 patients, several of whom also required assisted ventilation. At the hospital, 28 patients were found to be dead on arrival, eight patients remained unconscious but breathing, and two had regained consciousness. The hospital had enough CAKs on hand to care for one patient. Antidotal therapy was initiated for one patient, and the rest were treated with 100% high-flow oxygen. All eight recovered. The entire community was shocked and deeply saddened by this event. The surviving EMT expressed profound remorse for not having saved his partner.

UNIQUE CONSIDERATIONS

During World War I, both AC and CK were used as chemical warfare agents. Neither form of cyanide was highly successful as a weapon, partly because of the incomplete filling of projectiles and partly because of the use of bursting charges that set most of the hydrogen cyanide on fire.

AC is formed when a cyanide salt is mixed with an acid. Hydrogen cyanide is a liquid that boils at 25.6°C (78.1°F) but evaporates rapidly at usual temperatures. The vapor and gas are lighter than air and persist for only a few minutes in the open atmosphere. These factors made AC difficult to disperse in a lethal concentration using relatively small payloads on the open battlefield.

CK is similarly released when a saturated solution of potassium cyanide salt is mixed with chlorine. Cyanogen chloride boils at 13.8°C (56.8°F), and its vapor and gas are heavier and less volatile than AC. The toxicity of CK is similar to that of AC, but CK had the additional mucosal-irritant and pulmonary effects of its chlorine component.

During World War II, the Nazis used AC absorbed onto Zyklon B, a dispersible pharmaceutical base, as a means for prisoner extermination within the confined space of death-camp gas chambers. During the 1980s, Iraq is reported to have used cyanide-like agents in incidents involving Syria,[35] Iraqi Kurds,[36] and possibly Iran.[37] The largest industrial chemical disaster in world history occurred in Bhopal, India, in 1984. The Bhopal disaster killed over 2500 persons and affected an additional 200,000 to 300,000.[38] Although methyl isocyanate contains a cyanide moiety, methyl isocyanate itself is primarily a pulmonary agent that causes pulmonary edema at moderate doses and has additional irritative effects on larger (central) airways at higher doses.[38,39]

AC is still used in modern gas chambers for capital punishment in a process involving the reaction of cyanide salts with acid. Precursors of AC were also found in several Tokyo subway restrooms in the weeks after the 1995 sarin nerve agent attack in that city.[1] Cyanide has been implicated in the covert poisoning of commercial foodstuffs[1] and drug products,[40] and terrorists are reported to have expressed an ongoing interest in the use of cyanide compounds—including chemicals from industrial sources—as weapons.[41,42]

Inhalation and ingestion are the most likely routes of exposure in mass casualties during a terrorist event. Dermal toxicity can occur with cyanide but is less likely to affect large numbers compared with inhalation or ingestion. Dispersing a respirable aerosol in the open atmosphere requires a high-energy–generating system to produce the small particle size, appropriate weather conditions to ensure that the aerosol cloud stays near the ground, and adequate concentrations of the agent to produce the toxic effect.[1] The release of cyanide vapor or gas within an enclosed public space or building would likely maximize its potential toxicity and minimize the difficulty of its deployment for inhalational exposure. However, a large amount of liquid is required to produce vapor sufficient to cause mass casualties.[1] Introduction of cyanide, probably as cyanide salts, into the food and water supply may be another feasible scenario that could seek to exploit the physical and toxicologic characteristics of cyanide. Inhalational exposure to lethal concentrations of cyanide gas usually kills within minutes. Odor thresholds for AC are highly variable, and 40% to 60% of adults cannot detect its characteristic smell of bitter almonds.[43,44] CK may be more readily detectable by the victim because of its chlorine-like irritation of the eyes, lungs, and mucous membranes. After exposure to lower concentrations, or exposure to lethal amounts via ingestion, the effects are slower to develop.

TABLE 94-1 OVERVIEW OF RECOMMENDATIONS FOR DETECTION, DECONTAMINATION, AND THERAPY OF CYANIDE EXPOSURES

Likely method of dissemination	1. Liquid, aerosol, vapor, or gas
	2. In water or food
Odor	Bitter almonds (although description is variable)
Vapor heavier than air	AC: No
	CK: Yes
Persistency in soil >24 hours	Nonpersistent
Detection equipment	**Military:**
	AC vapor or gas: M256A1 kit, ICAD
	CK vapor or gas: M256A1 kit
	Commercial:
	Draeger CDS kit
Skin decontamination solution[28]	Wet decontamination is usually not necessary for vapor exposure.
	For liquid or solids: water with or without soap (preferred); 0.5% sodium hypochlorite solution (bleach water) (usually not necessary).
Onset of symptoms	Immediate
Mild effects	Dizziness, nausea, feeling of weakness
Severe effects	Gasping, syncope, seizures, apnea, asystole
Adult therapy[29]	**Amyl nitrite:**
	1 amp (0.2 mL) for 30 to 60 seconds along with 100% oxygen until IV access is obtained
	Sodium nitrite:
	300 mg (10 mL 3% sol) IV over 5 to 20 minutes; slow infusion if patient develops hypotension
	Sodium thiosulfate:
	12.5 g (50 mL) IV delivered over 10 minutes; repeat at half initial dose in 1 hour if symptoms persist
	Lorazepam:
	4 mg IV/IM over 2 to 5 minutes and repeated as needed
Pediatric therapy[29]	**Amyl nitrite:**
	Pediatric dose not established
	Sodium nitrite:
	0.33 mL/kg of 10% solution IV over 5 to 20 minutes, not to exceed 300 mg
	Sodium thiosulfate:
	1.65 mL/kg of 25% solution over 10 minutes, not to exceed 12.5 g; repeat in 1 hour at half initial dose if symptoms persist
	Lorazepam:
	4 mg IV/IM over 2 to 5 minutes; repeat as needed
Supportive therapy	Assisted ventilation

TABLE 94-2 TRIAGE RECOMMENDATIONS FOR CYANIDE MASS CASUALTIES[30]

TRIAGE CATEGORY	CLINICAL SIGNS	RECOMMENDED INTERVENTION
Minimal	Conscious and breathing	No antidotes, no oxygen
Immediate	Convulsions and apnea	Antidotes and oxygen
Delayed	Unconscious but breathing	Antidotes and oxygen
Expectant	No cardiac activity	No care unless resources are available for resuscitation

Ingestion of a lethal dose of cyanide may allow for a 15- to 60-minute window of survival time during which antidote may be administered, although loss of consciousness has been reported in as little as 1 minute following ingestion of a high dose of liquid cyanide or cyanide in solution.

 PITFALLS

There are several factors that may complicate a timely and accurate diagnosis in the event of a cyanide attack. These include the following:

1. Cyanide toxicity is not a common patient presentation and clinicians may have little or no experience in diagnosis. Sublethal symptoms are often nonspecific, and lethal exposures may present as nonspecific cardiorespiratory arrest.
2. Measurements of blood cyanide levels are almost never available during the treatment phase, although laboratory determination of a decreased arteriovenous oxygen gradient can usually be performed relatively quickly and can serve as a valuable indicator of exposure.
3. Cyanide levels tend to fall in stored samples because of the short half-life of the compound.

Signs and symptoms of cyanide toxicity are often relatively nonspecific and may offer little indication of the causation in absence of other historical data. Early signs and symptoms may include transient hyperpnea, headache, diaphoresis, flushing, weakness, vertigo, dyspnea, and findings of central nervous system excitement progressing to seizures. With high inhalational doses, gasping may be nearly immediate and may progress to collapse, apnea, and convulsions within 30 to 60 seconds, with death ensuing within 6 to 8 minutes. In the case of CK exposure, victims may also complain of irritation of the eyes and mucous membranes. Cyanide casualties are classically described as having flushed skin rather than cyanosis, but many patients are nevertheless cyanotic.[43] The telltale odor of bitter almonds may not be always be appreciated because 40% to 60% of the population lacks the gene that enables detection of this odor.[44,45] Late-appearing indications of central nervous system depression, such as coma and dilated pupils, are prominent but nonspecific signs of cyanide intoxication.

REFERENCES

1. Baskin SI, Brewer TG. Cyanide poisoning. In: Zajtchuk R, Bellamy R, eds. *Textbook of Military Medicine*. Volume 1: Sidell FR, Takafuji ET, Franz DR, eds. Medical Aspects of Chemical and Biological Warfare. Washington, DC: Office of the Surgeon General, Department of the Army; 1997.

2. Koschel MJ. Where there's smoke, there may be cyanide. *Am J Nurs*. 2002;102:39-42.

3. Alcorta R. Smoke inhalation and acute cyanide poisoning: hydrogen cyanide poisoning proves increasingly common in smoke-inhalation victims. *JEMS* 2004; 29(8):Suppl 6-15; quiz suppl 16-17.

4. Sharp TW, Brennan RJ, Keim M, et al. Medical preparedness for a terrorist event involving biological or chemical agents during the 1996 Atlanta Olympic games. *Ann Emerg Med*. 1998;32:214-23.

5. Sauer SW, Keim ME. Hydroxocobalamin: improved public health readiness for cyanide disasters. *Ann Emerg Med*. 2001;37:631-41.

6. Cone DC, Davidson SJ. Hazardous materials preparedness in the emergency department. *Prehospital Emerg Care*. 1997;1:85-90.

7. Burgess JL, Blackmun GM, Bodkin CA. Hospital preparedness for hazardous materials incidents and treatment of contaminated patients. *West J Med*. 1997;167:387-91.

8 Ghilarducci DP, Pirrallo RG, Hegmann KT. Hazardous materials readiness of United States level 1 trauma centers. *J Occup Environ Med*. 2000;42:683-92.

9. Wetter DC, Daniell WE, Treser CD. Hospital preparedness for victims of chemical or biological terrorism. *Am J Public Health*. 2001;91:710-6.

10. Keim ME, Pesik N, Twum-Danso N. Lack of hospital preparedness for chemical terrorism in a major US city 1996-2000. *Prehospital Disaster Med*. 2003;18(3):193-9.

11. Eckstein M. The medical response to modern terrorism: why the "rules of engagement" have changed. *Ann Emerg Med*. 1999; 34(2):219-21.

12. Nakajama T, Sato S, Morita H, et al. Sarin poisoning of a rescue team in the Matsumoto sarin incident in Japan. *Occup Environ Med*. 1997;54:697-701.

13. Nozaki H, Hori S, Shinosawa Y, et al. Secondary exposure of medical staff to sarin vapor in the emergency room. *Intensive Care Med*. 1995;21:1032-5.

14. American Academy of Pediatrics. Chemical-biological terrorism and its impact on children: a subject review. *Pediatrics* 2000; 3:662-70.

15. Brennan RJ, Waeckerle JF, Sharp TW, et al. Chemical warfare agents: emergency medical and emergency public health issues. *Ann Emerg Med*. 1999;34(2):191-204.

16. Keim ME, Kaufmann AF. Principles of emergency response to bioterrorism. *Ann Emerg Med*. 1999;34:177-82.

17. Keim ME, Kaufmann AF, Rodgers GC. *Recommendations for OEP/CDC Surveillance, Laboratory and Informational Support Initiative*. Atlanta: U.S. Centers for Disease Control and Prevention, National Center for Environmental Health; 1998.

18. Joint Commission on Accreditation of Healthcare Organizations. *2000 Comprehensive Accreditation Manual for Hospitals*. Oakbrook Terrace, Ill: JCAHO; 2000.

19. 29 Code of Federal Regulations Part 1910.120. Occupational Safety and Health Standards. Washington, DC: U.S. Government Printing Office; 1995.

20. Adler J. The protection and sheltering policy in hospitals. *Prehospital Disaster Med*. 1990;5:265-7.

21. American Hospital Association. *Hospital Preparedness for Mass Casualties: Summary of an Invitational Forum, Final Report*. Washington, DC: American Hospital Association; 2000.

22. Tucker JB. National Health and Medical Services response to incidents of chemical and biological terrorism. *JAMA* 1997;278:396-8.

23. Berlin CM Jr. The treatment of cyanide poisoning in children. *Pediatrics* 1970;46:793-6.

24. Bunn HF. Disorders of hemoglobin. In Braunwald E, Wilson JD, Martin JB, et al. *Harrison's Principles of Internal Medicine*. 11th ed. New York: McGraw-Hill; 1987:1518-27.

25. Bowden CA, Krenzelok EP. Clinical applications of commonly used contemporary antidotes: a US perspective. *Drug Saf*. 1997;16:9-47.

26. Hall AH, Kulig KW, Rumack BH. Suspected cyanide poisoning in smoke inhalation: complications of sodium nitrite therapy. *J Toxicol Clin Exp*. 1989;9:3-9.

27. Kirk MA, Gerace R, Kulig KW. Cyanide and methemoglobin kinetics in smoke inhalation victims treated with the cyanide antidote kit. *Ann Emerg Med*. 1993;22:1413-8.

28. Mushett C, Kelley KL, Boxer GE, et al. Antidotal efficacy of vitamin B12a (hydroxo-cobalamin) in experimental cyanide poisoning. *Proc Soc Exp Biol Med*. 1952;81:234-7.

29. Lovatt E. Cobalt compounds as antidote for hydrocyanic acid. *Br J Pharmacol* 1964;23:455-75.

30. Yacoub M, Faure J, Morena H, et al. Acute hydrocyanic acid intoxication: current data on the metabolism of cyanide and treatment by hydroxocobalamin [French]. *Eur J Toxicol Environ Hyg*. 1974;7:22-9.

31. Litovitz TL, Klein-Schwartz W, Caravati EM, et al. 1998 annual report of the American Association of Poison Control Centers Toxic Exposure Surveillance System. *Am J Emerg Med*. 1999;17:435-87.

32. Anonymous. Cyanide. In: *Medical Management of Chemical Casualties*. Aberdeen Proving Ground, Md: Chemical Casualty Care Office, U.S. Army Medical Research Institute of Chemical Defense; 1995.

33. Pennardt A. CBRNE: cyanides, hydrogen. Available at: http://www.emedicine.com/emerg/topic909.htm.

34. Anonymous. Cyanide. In: Sidell FR, Patrick WC, Dashiell TR, eds. *Janes Chem-Bio Handbook*. Alexandria, Va: Janes Information Group; 1998.

35. Lang JS, Mullin D, Fenyvesi C, et al. Is 'the protector of lions' losing his touch? *US News and World Report*. November 1986;10:29.

36. Heylin M, ed. US decries apparent chemical arms attack. *Chem Eng News*. 1988;66:23.

37. Anonymous. Medical expert reports the use of chemical weapons in Iran-Iraq War. *UN Chronicle*. 1985;22:24-6.

38. Mehta PS, Mehta AS, Mehta SJ, et al. Bhopal tragedy's health effects. *JAMA* 1990;264:2781-7.

39. Anderson N. Disaster epidemiology: lessons from Bhopal. In: Murray V, ed. *Major Chemical Disasters: Medical Aspects of Management*. London: Royal Society of Medicine Services Limited; 1990:183-95.

40. Wolnick KA, Fricke FL, Bonnin E, et al. The Tylenol tampering incident: tracing the source. *Anal Chem*. 1984;56:466A-70A, 474A.

41. Anonymous. Averted New Year's attack included use of poison gas bombs. *Newsweek* February 7, 2000. Available at: http://www.prnewswire.com/cgi-bin/stories.pl?ACCT=104&STORY=/www/story/01-30-2000/0001127257&EDATE=.

42. Associated Press. Minnesota Protesters Left Poison. *Washington Post*. July 25, 2000. Available at: pdm.medicine.wisc.edu/18-3pdfs/193keim.pdf.

43. van Heijst AN, Douze JM, van Kesteren RG, et al. Therapeutic problems in cyanide poisoning. *J Toxicol Clin Toxicol*. 1987;25:383-98.

44. Gonzalez ER. Cyanide evades some noses, overpowers others [letter]. *JAMA* 1982;248:2211.

45. Dhames MS. Acute cyanide poisoning [letter]. *Anaesthesia* 1983;38:168.

chapter 95

Antimuscarinic Agent Attack

Fermin Barrueto, Jr. and Lewis S. Nelson

 ## DESCRIPTION OF EVENT

There are five recognized muscarinic receptor subtypes (M1 through M5) located primarily within the parasympathetic nervous system and the brain. Peripherally, they are located postsynaptically on secretory organs and glands; and within the CNS, they are concentrated in various areas such as the striatum, the cerebral cortex, and the hippocampus. Muscarinic antagonists such as atropine, scopolamine, hyoscyamine, and 3-quinuclidinyl benzilate cause a constellation of signs and symptoms known as the *antimuscarinic,* or *anticholinergic,* toxidrome, because cholinergic activation of end organs is partially blocked. The clinical presentation is in general the opposite of that seen in the cholinergic crisis induced by nerve agents. The peripheral antimuscarinic effects are well described and include mydriasis, loss of visual accommodation leading to blurred vision, drying of mucous membranes, urinary retention, anhidrosis, hyperthermia, tachycardia, and hypertension. The central anticholinergic effects include confusion, delirium, memory loss, paresthesias, speech difficulty, characteristic hallucinations (e.g., concrete, describable, and Lilliputian—that is, decreasing in size over time), disrobing, picking and plucking (so-called phantom behaviors, or "woolgathering"), and, with very high doses, seizures.[1]

It is precisely these central effects for which antimuscarinic chemical warfare agents were developed. The anticholinergic toxidrome is sometimes summarized as being exemplified by patients who are "blind as a bat" (from mydriasis and paralysis of accommodation), "dry as a bone," "hot as a hare," "red as a beet," and "mad as a hatter"—the first four representing peripheral effects and the final description referring to effects in the central nervous system (CNS). These agents are classified as *incapacitating*; that is, they are neurotoxic but not typically lethal. The intent of dispersing these agents is to prevent a military force from performing its duties efficiently or to disrupt a military or civilian infrastructure. A similar syndrome can be seen after the ingestion of jimson weed due to natural scopolamine-like agents found in the seeds; this plant could theoretically be used as a source for antimuscarinic agent.

Although atropine is the prototypical antimuscarinic agent, 3-quinuclidinyl benzilate, or QNB (North Atlantic

Treaty Organisation [NATO] code, BZ), is the prototype for use as an incapacitating agent because of its physicochemical properties (which allow it to be dispersed easily and which make it resistant to heat and persistent in the environment for weeks), its potency, and its high safety ratio.[1] BZ was produced in the United States in the early 1960s and received its NATO code either because it was a benzilate or because of the "buzz" associated with its use (it was also known as "Agent Buzz").[1,2] Destruction of U.S. stockpiles of BZ began in the 1980s when it was realized that this agent was unpredictable and had little practical utility.[2] BZ is now primarily used as a research marker in Alzheimer's disease.[3,4]

BZ is an odorless crystalline solid that can be absorbed by many routes (e.g., intramuscular, intravenous, inhalation, oral, transdermal), but a chemical attack would likely involve inhalation of aerosol or ingestion of contaminated food or water.[2] This agent is a more potent competitive antagonist of muscarinic acetylcholine receptors than is atropine. The onset of peripheral antimuscarinic signs and symptoms after inhalation of an aerosol is usually between 20 minutes and 4 hours after exposure but can be delayed if delivery occurs by other routes.[2] Hallucinations appear approximately 6 hours after exposure and may persist for up to 3 to 4 days. BZ is very potent but has a wide safety profile, with an ICt_{50} (the concentration-time product at which half of an exposed group will become incapacitated) of only 112 mgzmin/m^3 but an LCt_{50} (the concentration-time product at which 50% of those exposed will die) of 200,000 mgzmin/m^3—a safety factor of nearly 2000[2]; its intraperitoneal LD_{50} (the dose at which 50% of those exposed will die) in mice is 18 to 25 mg/kg.[5]

It has been alleged that Bosnian Serbs used BZ in July 1995 against 15,000 Bosniak civilians fleeing from Srebrenica to Tuzla.[6] Although survivors experienced hallucinations and believed that they were victims of a chemical attack, some believe that stress, starvation, and exhaustion were more likely causes.[6]

 ## PREINCIDENT ACTIONS

The temporally related presentation of a group of patients with the combination of peripheral and CNS

signs and symptoms of the antimuscarinic toxidrome should raise the suspicion of a chemical attack with an antimuscarinic agent. Such an event should prompt notification of local and state health departments. The local hospital disaster plan should be implemented immediately so that proper measures can be taken for decontamination, prevention of secondary exposures, and efficient management of a mass-casualty event. The availability of the antidote, physostigmine, should be checked, and the number of patients who could be treated in the event of a mass exposure should be ascertained.

 ## POSTINCIDENT ACTIONS

Physical examination, history, and epidemiology are the primary tools to assist with diagnosis. Hospital-based laboratory confirmation of BZ is not readily available, and no standard laboratory tests will assist with the diagnosis. A gas chromatography/mass spectrometry confirmatory urine test is available through health authorities,[7] although the results will not be available in a clinically relevant fashion. Clinical response to the administration of physostigmine can be a practical diagnostic aid.

 ## MEDICAL TREATMENT OF CASUALTIES

Initial treatment involves removing patients from the exposure. The removal of clothes and decontamination of skin with water is indicated if the exposure occurred through ambient aerosol exposure or from transdermal exposure but is not indicated if contaminated food was the source. Standard precautions with the addition of eye protection and neoprene or butyl rubber gloves should be used by healthcare providers to prevent secondary exposure.[2] Assessment of the patient's hemodynamic status and airway are necessary; however, the most challenging issue may be controlling the patient's agitated delirium. Behavioral control should be easily accomplished by titrating a benzodiazepine, such as diazepam, lorazepam, or midazolam, to sedation along with judicious use of soft physical restraints. It should be remembered that use of physical restraints can exacerbate body heat retention from excess muscular activity, if a patient is attempting to resist restraint, and may contribute to hyperthermia. Benzodiazepines should be in plentiful supply for most hospitals and can be as practically efficacious as the antidotal use of physostigmine.[8] Antipsychotic sedatives such as haloperidol are probably best avoided or used only in combination with benzodiazepines. Patients can die from too high a dose of BZ, from self-injury related to hallucinations or illusions, or from heat stress caused by anhidrosis. Careful attention to body temperature should always be a component of supportive care of patients who have been exposed to BZ.

The antidote to poisoning by an antimuscarinic agent is physostigmine, an acetylcholinesterase inhibitor. Physostigmine, a nonpolar tertiary-amine carbamate, crosses the blood-brain barrier, reversibly binds with tissue acetylcholinesterase in postsynaptic membranes, and

temporarily increases the concentration of acetylcholine in the synapse. This extra acetylcholine competes with BZ for occupancy of postsynaptic muscarinic receptors and helps to overcome the cholinergic blockade induced by BZ.[8] Although physostigmine is clinically beneficial, its reversible binding mandates multiple repeat intramuscular dosing every 30 to 60 minutes (or careful calibration of an intravenous drip) and makes its use labor-intensive and practical only with a few patients at a time. For example, a patient given 6.4 mg of BZ intramuscularly required 200 mg of physostigmine over 72 hours to maintain normal functional competence.[9] Although safe when used in small titrated amounts and with frequent clinical reassessment, physostigmine can cause cholinergic effects such as dyspnea, apnea, bradycardia, and seizures if administered too rapidly. In a mass-casualty incident, physostigmine and the personnel to administer it and to monitor its use would be in short supply. In these situations, benzodiazepines would be best for safe, rapid, and effective management.

Vomiting should not be induced if the agent has been ingested. The use of orally activated charcoal in this situation, although likely safe in an alert patient, has not been evaluated. Clinical laboratory investigation, including cerebrospinal fluid analysis, should be performed as indicated, at least until the diagnosis is clear. This will allow

 ### CASE PRESENTATION

Over a period of 48 hours, 12 patients who are known to abuse heroin presented to a single hospital emergency department with agitated delirium. Their vital signs revealed mild hypertension, tachycardia, and temperature elevation to 38.3°C (101°F) in several patients and to 40°C (104°F) in a few. Their physical examinations showed markedly dry skin and mucous membranes along with a mumbling incoherent speech and random movements on the stretcher. Their pupils were in most cases large (6 mm), a finding that was particularly atypical for heroin users, who generally have notably small pupils. Several patients were unconscious, and after receiving naloxone, developed an agitated delirium similar to that described in this chapter. Patients were restrained, sedated with benzodiazepines, cooled as needed, and given fluids intravenously.

An outbreak of encephalitis was initially considered, and several patients had lumbar punctures to obtain cerebrospinal fluid for analysis, which always yielded normal results. When the possibility of an anticholinergic agent was being considered, one patient was evaluated for possible contraindications to physostigmine administration and was then given 2 mg of physostigmine intravenously over 5 minutes. This patient, who initially was delirious and hallucinating, became alert, oriented, and able to give a history of insufflating what he had believed to be heroin. A sample of this heroin was obtained and analyzed by public health authorities, revealing synthetic scopolamine. (This case was adapted from an epidemic in the United States 1995-1996.[10])

3-Quinuclidinyl benzilate   Benzilic acid   3-Quinuclidinol

FIGURE 95–1. Hydrolysis of 3-quinuclidinyl benzilate (BZ) will occur at pH > 11.

the clinician to exclude other diagnoses, including infectious etiologies, because these patients will often present with temperature elevation (due to psychomotor agitation and anhidrosis) and an altered mental status.

 ## UNIQUE CONSIDERATIONS

Complications resulting from exposure to BZ include acute-angle closure glaucoma secondary to the mydriasis, rhabdomyolysis due to psychomotor agitation, ileus, urinary retention requiring Foley catheterization, pneumonia or hypoxia due to prolonged stupor or aspiration, and heat damage from heat retention secondary to anhidrosis.

3-Quinuclidinyl benzilate is a bicyclic ester that will hydrolyze in an alkaline solution of pH > 11 to benzylic acid and 3-quinuclidinol within minutes; both of these hydrolysis products are much less toxic than the parent compound (Figure 95-1).[5,11] This may be relevant in decontamination of surfaces and medical equipment.

 ## PITFALLS

Several potential pitfalls in response to a nerve agent attack exist. These include the following:

- Disorganization of hospital and local emergency medical services, should they become overwhelmed by many patients with agitated delirium
- Failure to recognize that numerous patients requiring attention (including restraint in many cases) will mandate efficient allocation of hospital resources and personnel to avoid resource depletion and staff exhaustion
- Inadequate decontamination of patients exposed externally, resulting in secondary exposure to healthcare workers, particularly rescue workers and paramedics
- Failure to be diligent in identifying other injuries when confronted with multiple patients
- Failure to suspect the diagnosis of an antimuscarinic agent, resulting in the administration of medications with antimuscarinic effects (e.g., haloperidol) that may worsen the patient's condition

- Failure to restrain potentially disruptive patients who have been exposed to BZ
- Failure to recognize the potential for heat stress in anhidrotic patients who have been exposed to BZ

REFERENCES

1. Ketchum JS. The Human Assessment of BZ. Edgewood Arsenal, Md: Chemical Research and Development Laboratory; 1963. Technical Memorandum 20-29. Cited in: Ketchum JS, Sidell FR. Incapacitating agents. In: Sidell FR, Takafuji TE, Franz DR, eds. *Textbook of Military Medicine: Medical Aspects of Chemical and Biological Warfare*. Falls Church, Va: Office of the Surgeon General, U.S. Army; 1997:287-305.
2. U.S. Army Center for Health Promotion and Preventive Medicine: Psychedelic agent 3: quinuclidinyl benzilate (BZ). The Deputy for Technical Services' Publication: Detailed Chemical Facts Sheets; 1998. Available at: http://chppm-www.apgea.army.mil/dts/dtchemfs.htm.
3. Wyper DJ, Brown D, Patterson J, et al. Deficits in iodine-labelled 3-quinuclidinyl benzilate binding in relation to cerebral blood flow in patients with Alzheimer's disease. *Eur J Nucl Med*. 1993; 20:379-86.
4. Hiramatsu Y, Eckelman WC, Baum BJ. Interaction of iodinated quinuclidinyl benzilate enantiomers with M3 muscarinic receptors. *Life Sci*. 1994;54:1777-83.
5. Guidelines for 3-quinuclidinyl benzilate. In: Subcommittee on Guidelines for Military Field Drinking-Water Quality, Committee on Toxicology, Board on Environmental Studies and Toxicology, National Research Council. *Guidelines for Chemical Warfare Agents in Military Field Drinking Water*. The National Academies Press; 1995:15-8.
6. Hay A. Surviving the impossible: the long march from Srebrenica. An investigation of the possible use of chemical warfare agents. *Med Confl Surviv*. 1998;14:120-55.
7. Byrd GD, Paule RC, Sander LC, et al. Determination of 3-quinuclidinyl benzilate (QNB) and its major metabolites in urine by isotope dilution gas chromatography/mass spectrometry. *J Anal Toxicol*. 1992;16:182-7.
8. Burns MJ, Linden CH, Graudins A, et al. A comparison of physostigmine and benzodiazepines for the treatment of anticholinergic poisoning. *Ann Emerg Med*. 2000;35:374-81.
9. Ketchum JS. *The Human Assessment of BZ*. Technical Memorandum 20-29. Edgewood Arsenal, Md: Chemical Research and Development Laboratory; 1963.
10. U.S. Centers for Disease Control and Prevention. Scopolamine poisoning among heroin users—New York City, Newark, Philadelphia, and Baltimore, 1995 and 1996. *JAMA* 1996;276:92-3.
11. Hull LA, Rosenblatt DH, Epstein J. 3-Quinuclidinyl benzilate hydrolysis in dilute aqueous solution. *J Pharm Sci*. 1979;68:856-9.

chapter 96

LSD, Other Indoles, and Phenylethylamine Derivative Attack

Fiona E. Gallahue

 DESCRIPTION OF EVENT

d-Lysergic acid diethylamide (LSD), an indole alkylamine, also known as LSD-25, was discovered by Albert Hofmann in 1938 while he was working for Sandoz Company. In 1943, Hofmann became intoxicated by LSD through accidental exposure, and 3 days later he intentionally took LSD. His experience with LSD paved the way for neuropsychiatric studies using LSD and later, in 1951, for U.S. Central Intelligence Agency (CIA) experimentation with human subjects using LSD and similar mind-altering drugs. The results of most of these CIA experiments are still classified, but some documents that have been made available describe how the American government intended for LSD to be used as a weapon. Psilocin and psilocybin, indole alkylamines derived from hallucinogenic mushrooms, were also considered and allegedly tested. Mescaline, a phenylethylamine derivative derived from the peyote cactus, was also reportedly selected for testing on human subjects. Because these substances have cross-tolerance and similar side effects and treatment, and because they were once considered by the American government as potential chemical weapons, we will narrow our focus to these hallucinogens rather than including the entire spectrum of phenylethylamine derivatives (e.g., 3,4-methylenedioxyamphetamine [MDA] and related amphetamines) or the other indole alkylamines (e.g., bufotenine, ibogaine).[1,2]

LSD, mescaline, peyote, psilocin, and psilocybin have all been classified as Schedule I drugs since the passage in 1970 of the Controlled Substance Act. These agents have somewhat similar (although not identical) effects but differ in potency: 1000 mcg of mescaline is equivalent to 1.0 mcg of LSD or 100 mcg of psilocybin.[3]

LSD, the most potent of these drugs, is generally taken orally at doses between 1 and 16 mcg/kg. There is a proportional relationship between the dose and the psychophysiologic effect of LSD, with 50 to 100 mcg constituting a mild dose, 100 to 250 mcg representing a moderate dose, and 250 to 500 mcg considered to be a strong dose.[4,5] LSD is odorless and tasteless and is usually ingested orally, although it can be smoked, snorted, or injected. It has a plasma half-life of 100 minutes but can

be detected in plasma or urine for up to 3 days, and it is metabolized in the liver, with urinary excretion of metabolites.[6] The clinical effects begin within 30 to 60 minutes and peak at 2 to 4 hours; the majority of the symptoms resolve within 12 hours.[5,7,8] Studies conducted in simulated military settings demonstrated that even well-trained units become totally disorganized after ingesting total oral doses of less than 200 mcg.[9] Affected persons usually cannot carry out a series of instructions or concentrate on a complex task, but they might be capable of isolated impulsive actions. Behavior is said to unpredictable although well coordinated.[9]

Although LSD has an LD_{50} (the amount needed to kill 50% of an exposed group) of 14,000 mcg (nearly 30 times the 500-mcg strong dose), LSD is not considered a safe drug.[10] Acute psychotic reactions have been reported. Trauma resulting from accidents or self-destructive behavior, suicide, or homicide can occur; deaths from LSD are more likely from these effects than from the direct toxicity of the compound.[1,7,11]

LSD resembles serotonin chemically and acts on serotonin and dopamine receptors. Sympathomimetic effects commonly seen with LSD intoxication include dilated pupils, tachycardia, hypertension, and hyperreflexia.[5,6] The mind-altering properties of LSD can cause euphoria, anxiety, and paranoia with intense visual and auditory hallucinations that tend to be abstract, colorful, expansive, and often ineffable (in contrast to the concrete, lilliputian, and easily describable hallucinations from anticholinergic compounds). Synesthesia (sensory crossover) is frequently present, although tactile hallucinations are uncommon.[6,7] Abnormalities of serotonin-induced platelet aggregation may result in abnormal clotting and poor clot retraction. Although cardiovascular complications are infrequent, reports exist of supraventricular tachycardia and myocardial infarction.[6] Severe manifestations of toxicity include hyperthermia, seizures, and rhabdomyolysis.[8]

Mescaline is a hallucinogenic alkaloid derived from the North American peyote cactus and that also occurs in several species of the genus *Trichocereus* of South American cacti. Mescaline, or 3,4,5-trimethoxyphenylamine, can be taken directly from the peyote cactus or derived synthetically. The ritual use of mescaline-containing cacti is documented from the sixteenth century; mescaline itself was first isolated from peyote in 1896 and was first synthesized in 1918. Peyote is commonly ingested in the form of brown discoid "mescal buttons," which are the sun-dried crowns of the cactus. Each button may contain 45 to 100 mg of mescaline. The hallucinogenic dose is 5 mg/kg. Taken orally, mescaline is rapidly absorbed from the gastrointestinal tract and has an unpleasantly bitter taste. It can also be taken intravenously with similar side effects and with a similar duration of effects. (The popular Mexican liquor called *mescal* does not come from peyote and does not contain mescaline.)

The effects of mescaline begin within 30 minutes to 2 hours of ingestion and peak at about 4 hours, with a total duration of 8 to 14 hours. Like LSD, mescaline is metabolized in the liver and excreted in the urine. Clinically, the effects are similar to those of LSD but with the additional initial symptoms of nausea, vomiting, sweating, generalized discomfort, dizziness, and headache, all of which generally occur during the first hour after ingestion and shortly before the onset of hallucinogenic effects. Large doses can produce hypotension, bradycardia, and respiratory depression.[5,7]

Psilocybin (4-phosphoryloxy-*N,N*-dimethyltryptamine) and psilocin (4-hydroxyl-*N,N*-dimethyltryptamine) are members of the indole alkylamine hallucinogens derived from tryptophan. These drugs were first isolated in 1958 from hallucinogenic mushrooms used by Mexican Indians for centuries. Psilocybin is more resistant to oxidation than psilocin and retains its activity in dried mushrooms. Psilocin is approximately 1.5 times as potent as psilocybin, but otherwise these two drugs are pharmacologically similar; in fact, psilocin is the active metabolite of psilocybin in the body. A 100-mcg dose of psilocybin is equivalent to 1 mcg of LSD and 1000 mcg of mescaline. The LD_{50} of intravenous psilocybin has been reported to be 280 mg/kg.[3]

Peyote mushrooms can be ingested raw, dried, as a brew, or stewed. The dose to produce hallucinogenic effects in nontolerant adults is approximately 6 to 12 mg. Little correlation has been found between clinical effects and the number of mushrooms ingested. Approximately 50% of the hallucinogenic compounds are absorbed via the gastrointestinal tract, and distribution occurs to most tissues, including the brain; most excretion is renal. Signs and symptoms develop within 30 to 60 minutes, with the psychedelic effects peaking between 30 minutes and 2 hours and lasting from 3 to 15 hours.[3,5,10] Both compounds primarily affect serotonergic neurotransmission. Clinical effects of the drug are mostly sympathomimetic and include pupillary dilation, piloerection, tachycardia, and hyperreflexia. The hallucinations are usually visual but may be auditory or tactile. Both dysphoria and euphoria are commonly reported mood alterations. Nausea, cramping, abdominal pain, and a sensation of swelling of parts of the body are potential adverse responses. Deaths from psilocin and psilocybin are rare but have been reported from ingestion by a 6-year-old child who experienced hyperthermia and status epilepticus.[5]

All of these drugs have cross-tolerance to each other; the tolerance develops rapidly (within days) without the development of physical dependence and also regresses rapidly, within 3 to 4 days of withdrawal.

Flashbacks, or recurrences of hallucinogenic imagery days to years after the initial experience, have been described often with LSD but also with mescaline. Their etiology is unknown, but these flashbacks do decrease in their intensity with time and can be treated adequately with benzodiazepines in significantly affected patients. Flashbacks can be precipitated by triggers such as stress, exercise, and illness.[5]

LSD chemically resembles serotonin and interacts with the 5-hydroxytryptamine, or 5-HT, receptor. As might be expected, there is evidence (from a small retrospective cohort study by Bonson and Murphy[12]) of cross-reactivity between LSD and various antidepressants. In this study, patients taking selective serotonin-reuptake inhibitors (SSRI agents) and monoamine oxidase inhibitors reported decreased responses to LSD, whereas those taking tricyclic antidepressants and lithium experienced increased responses. Psilocybin also chemically resembles serotonin, and similar interactions might be expected between psilocybin and these antidepressants.

Since LSD is the most potent of these agents, the most difficult to detect (being odorless and tasteless), and the compound that was reportedly most tested by governmental agencies in the 1960s, this agent may be the most likely of the indoles and phenylethylamine derivatives to be used in an attack.[13]

Difficulties in covert distribution of LSD limit its utility as a chemical weapon. The compound could be released into water, but impossibly high quantities would be needed to contaminate a large water source such as a reservoir. Moreover, chlorine in concentrations found in water-treatment plants can deactivate LSD by oxidation. Delivery distal to such treatment facilities is possible but also impractical (because of dilution) even for someone intent on targeting a single building.[1] LSD could also be delivered in an aerial drop so that a bomb filled with LSD would explode at ground level or several feet above the ground. The local population would become intoxicated through inhalation.[1] LSD could potentially be aerosolized, but it would have to be dispersed relatively close to the intended targets, a mode of delivery that might be acceptable to some but perhaps not all terrorists, depending on the situation. With a particle size of approximately 5 microns, the ID_{50} (the dose that incapacitates 50% of the exposed population) was estimated to be 5.6 mcg/kg, approximately twice the ID_{50} of the parenteral route.[9]

If an immediate effect in a particular location is desired, the fact that LSD has a latent period of 30 minutes or longer might be a disadvantage, since exposed victims might well have moved to different areas by the time that they begin hallucinating. However, this delay in action might be advantageous in a covert release of agent. Another potential problem is the fact that SSRI antidepressants are used commonly in the American populace and might have protective effects in these patients. Nevertheless, biologic variability is likely to ensure that a significant proportion of intended victims will still be affected.

PREINCIDENT ACTIONS

Hospitals and emergency personnel should be well trained for the event of a potential chemical weapons attack. Protocols for these events should include removal of the victims from the contaminating source and the use of protective equipment to avoid inhalation, ingestion, or transdermal exposure to the toxicant. Although person-to-person transmission of LSD from a terrorist attack would not be expected, aerosolized LSD could theoretically remain on skin, clothing, or environmental surfaces; whether secondary aerosolization would be significant for this compound would depend on a multitude of as-yet-uninvestigated variables. If settling of aerosolized product on skin or clothing is of concern, washing of the skin with water (with or without soap) and washing of clothes would likely suffice. Since LSD detection equipment is not readily available, the detection of small amounts covertly released into the environment could be difficult.

POSTINCIDENT ACTIONS

LSD and similar hallucinogenic agents in a mass-casualty event should be relatively easy for most clinicians to detect clinically, given the onset of action of approximately 30 to 60 minutes, the sympathomimetic effects, and the types of hallucinations induced. LSD intoxication would be difficult to distinguish from poisoning by the other psychedelic indoles and by phenylethylamine derivatives, but management of all these types of cases is similar. The differential diagnosis also includes acute panic reactions, schizophrenia, and exposure to phencyclidine (PCP), amphetamines, and anticholinergic compounds.[14] The appropriate authorities should be contacted to identify and eliminate the contaminating source.

MEDICAL TREATMENT OF CASUALTIES

Treatment is usually supportive, and patients can often be managed adequately without medications if they can be reassured and treated in a calm, quiet area.[15] Some patients with more severe agitation may require medication. In this situation, a moderately long-acting benzodiazepine such as lorazepam 2 mg or diazepam 5 mg administered intravenously would be the best choice. Although haloperidol 5 mg given intramuscularly/intravenously or 10 mg given orally can also be used effectively for LSD-induced agitation not responding adequately to benzodiazepines, it should not be used routinely for drug-induced hallucinations. Haloperidol and the phenothiazines are contraindicated for patients with anticholinergic poisoning, which could be mistaken for LSD psychosis without a careful examination.

UNIQUE CONSIDERATIONS

Because LSD can be oxidized by large amounts of chlorine, contaminated water sources could potentially be appropriately treated and used safely.

Because LSD, mescaline, and psilocybin are rapidly metabolized and are excreted primarily in the urine, these drugs can be most easily detected in the urine through an immunologic method such as the enzyme multiplied immunoassay technique (EMIT) for confirmatory testing.[16]

Some studies have suggested that SSRI agents may decrease the severity of the effects of LSD and psilocybin. In certain situations, it may be useful to consider using SSRIs as protective medications for personnel at high risk for being exposed to LSD. However, more testing needs to be done before a definitive recommendation can be made.

PITFALLS

Several potential pitfalls exist in responding to an attack. These include the following:

- Failure to notify the appropriate agencies to find the source of the contaminating drug
- Failure to use proper protective equipment in removal of patients, causing additional victims

- Failure to remove hallucinating patients to a quiet, controlled area
- Failure to consider amphetamines, anticholinergic agents, schizophrenia, and acute panic reactions in the differential diagnosis
- Use of haloperidol for hallucinations without being certain of the cause

ACKNOWLEDGMENTS

I would like to especially thank Dr. Lewis Nelson, Dr. Robert Hoffman, and Mary Ann Howland, PharmD, from the New York Poison Control Center for their help and support.

REFERENCES

1. Buckman J. Brainwashing, LSD, and CIA: historical and ethical perspective. *Int J Soc Psychiatry*. 1977;23:8-19.
2. Lee MA, Schlain B. *Acid Dreams: The Complete Social History of LSD: The CIA, the Sixties and Beyond*. Grove Press; 1985.
3. Passie T, Seifert J, Schneider U, et al. The pharmacology of psilocybin. *Addict Biol*. 2002;7:357-64.
4. Lycaeum Web site. Available at: http://www.lycaeum.org.
5. Leikin JB, Krantz AJ, Zell-Kanter M, et al. Clinical features and management of intoxication due to hallucinogenic drugs. *Med Toxicol Adverse Drug Exp*. 1989;4:324-50.
6. Ghuran A, Nolan J. Recreational drug misuse: issues for the cardiologist. *Heart* 2000;83:627-33.
7. Williams LC, Keyes C. Psychoactive drugs. In: Ford MD, Delaney KA, Ling LJ, et al, eds. *Ford: Clinical Toxicology*. Philadelphia: WB Saunders; 2001:640-9.
8. Lemke T, Wang R. Emergency department observation for toxicologic exposures. *Emerg Med Clin North Am*. 2001;19:155-67, viii.
9. Ketchum JS, Sidell FR. Incapacitating agents [Chapter 11]. In: Zajtchuk R, ed. *Textbook of Military Medicine, Part I: Warfare, Weaponry, and the Casualty: Medical Aspects of Chemical and Biological Warfare*. Washington, DC: Office of the Surgeon General, U.S. Army, TMM Publications, Border Institute; 1997:293.
10. Clark RF, Williams SR. Hallucinogens. In: Marx JA, ed. *Rosen's Emergency Medicine: Concepts and Clinical Practice*. St Louis: Mosby; 2002:2137-50.
11. Sotiropoulos A. Injury to the bladder: unusual complication of lysergic acid diethylamide. *Urology* 1974;3:755-8.
12. Bonson KR, Murphy DL. Alterations in responses to LSD in humans associated with chronic administration of tricyclic antidepressants, monoamine oxidase inhibitors or lithium. *Behav Brain Res*. 1996;73:229-33.
13. Yensen R. LSD and psychotherapy. *J Psychoactive Drugs*. 1985;17:267-77.
14. Perry P. LSD psychosis. In: Clinical Psychology Seminar, Virtual Hospital. Available at http://www.vh.org/adult/provider/psychiatry/CPS/28.html.
15. Schlicht J, Mitcheson M, Henry M. Medical aspects of large outdoor festivals. *Lancet* 1972;1(7757):948-52.
16. Bodin K, Svensson JO. Determination of LSD in urine with high-performance liquid chromatography—mass spectrometry. *Ther Drug Monit*. 2001;23:389-93.

chapter 97

Opioid Agent Attack

Rick G. Kulkarni

 DESCRIPTION OF EVENT

In cultivation since circa 300 BCE, pure opium is a mixture of alkaloids extracted from the sap of unripened seedpods of *Papaver somniferous* (the Asian, or opium, poppy). Opiates, such as heroin, codeine, and morphine, are natural derivatives of these alkaloids. Synthetic opium-like narcotic compounds, such as oxycodone, meperidine, and fentanyl and its derivatives (e.g., carfentanil and sufentanil) are also available. Originally, *opioid* meant a synthetic narcotic not derived from opium, but the term is increasingly applied to opiates as well as to synthetic narcotics; *opiate* is still reserved for the naturally occurring alkaloids with a morphine or thebaine backbone.[1,2]

The postsynaptic binding of opioids to receptors in the central nervous system (CNS) and in the gastrointestinal tract leads to hyperpolarization of neuronal cell membranes, inhibition of neurotransmission, and, depending on the affected cell population, either depression or excitation of end organs. The physiologic effects of opioids are mediated principally through three major kinds of opioid receptors: OP1 (δ), OP2 (κ), and OP3 (μ). All three types of receptors can mediate analgesia and respiratory depression, but OP1 (δ) receptors are responsible primarily for spinal analgesia, OP2 (κ) receptors are more selective for sedation (although they also mediate miosis, analgesia, and respiratory depression), and OP3 (μ) receptors are the most important for respiratory depression, miosis, constipation, and euphoria (with subsequent dependence in chronic users).[3] The opioid antagonists (e.g., naloxone, nalmefene, naltrexone) have greater affinity for OP3 (μ) receptors than for OP1 or OP2 receptors and are all effective in reversing the respiratory depression associated with acute opioid overdoses. Naltrexone, however, is usually reserved for the treatment of opioid addiction.[1,2]

CLINICAL PRESENTATION

Opioid toxicity characteristically presents with a depressed level of consciousness and should be suspected when the clinical triad of CNS depression, respiratory depression, and pupillary miosis are present. The differential diagnosis of miosis also includes clonidine, cholinergic crisis (from cholinergic agents, organophosphorous pesticides, or nerve agents), phenothiazines, phencyclidine, and sedative-hypnotic drugs as well as pontine and subarachnoid hemorrhage. However, pupillary dilatation can be seen in hypoxic opioid patients as well as in persons exposed to mixtures containing both an opioid and an anticholinergic agent such as atropine or scopolamine. Drowsiness, euphoria, ventricular arrhythmias, and acute mental status changes are frequently seen. Often, intoxication leads to respiratory impairment with bradypnea and hypopnea. In moderate-to-severe opioid intoxication, the respiratory rate can be as low as four breaths per minute; and frank respiratory arrest can occur. Generalized seizures are infrequent and occur mostly in infants and children because of initial excitation of the CNS. Nystagmus is also infrequent but has been reported.[1,2]

LIKELY AGENTS IN AN ATTACK

Oral ingestion and respiratory exposure are the two most likely routes of absorption in an opioid agent attack. Both routes provide easy absorption for most opioids. Peak effects are reached by 90 minutes after ingestion and within 10 minutes of inhalation.[4] The synthetic opioid fentanyl and its derivatives as a group are the most likely agents to be used in a terrorist attack (Table 97-1).[5] Their high potency (approximately 10 to 10,000 times that of morphine) and the fact that they can be aerosolized to induce unconsciousness and long-lasting respiratory depression in animals make them ideal agents in this regard.[6-8]

 PREINCIDENT ACTIONS

Preparedness is the single most important action that can be taken to prevent mass casualties from an opioid attack. The critical factors in minimizing the number of casualties in such an attack are as follows: (1) reaching casualties as soon as possible; (2) securing the airway. (3) implementing assisted ventilation either noninvasively or invasively; and (4) rapid treatment with the

TABLE 97-1 CHARACTERISTICS OF OPIOIDS, INCLUDING FENTANYL DERIVATIVES

AGENT	OPIOID POTENCY (COMPARED WITH MORPHINE)	THERAPEUTIC INDEX*
Morphine	1	70
Meperidine	0.5	5
Fentanyl	300	300
Sufentanil	4500	25,000
Alfentanil	75	1100
Remifentanil	220	33,000
Carfentanil	10,000	10,600

*Therapeutic index = median lethal dose (LD_{50})/lowest median effective dose (ED_{50}).

specific opioid antagonist naloxone. Recognition of the use of opioid agents as the primary contributing factor to the state of the victims is paramount, and in view of the relatively high profile given to chemical warfare agents such as nerve agents, a number of unconscious victims with respiratory depression (or apnea) and miosis who are not responsive to nerve agent antidotes should initiate the suspicion of other causes, including opioid agent attack. Communities at high risk for such an attack must familiarize their first responders, including firefighters, police personnel, and emergency medical technicians/paramedics, with the typical presentation and the differential diagnosis of a person exposed to such agents. In addition, consideration should be given to equip such personnel not only with devices to assist ventilation but also with naloxone.

Training and equipping of healthcare facilities in high-risk metropolitan areas for the treatment of a large number of patients exposed to an opioid agent is also an important link in the chain of adequate preparedness. Although there are no official position statements from government agencies or professional organizations addressing this specific possibility at this time, hospital disaster committees should include this topic in their general emergency preparedness plan. At a minimum, high-risk areas should be able to provide on-scene emergency medical services (including fast rescue and supportive care during transport), noninvasive and invasive artificial ventilation to affected persons, and sufficient doses of naloxone.[1,2]

 POSTINCIDENT ACTIONS

Once an opioid agent attack is identified, a preformulated action plan must be activated immediately. An attack with an opioid agent will likely take place in an enclosed area containing hundreds of people. Implementation of the facility evacuation plan is the first step to isolate persons not already under the effects of the agent and to remove them from the affected area.

For those persons who are affected, rescue personnel wearing personal protective equipment should implement rapid control measures even before the arrival of medical personnel. These measures are fundamental for three important reasons:

1. Proper positioning of the patient in the left-lateral-decubitus position can prevent aspiration of gastric contents and can minimize the risk of the tongue falling back to occlude the airway.
2. The ability of the medical rescue team to deliver artificial ventilation and naloxone can be severely limited if the victims cannot be accessed easily (for example, victims sitting in the middle seats of rows in a theater may be difficult to reach where they are).
3. Without intervention, the ensuing confusion can create a situation in which persons are not properly categorized or treated.

Because local supplies of antidotes can be rapidly depleted in a mass-casualty situation, additional stocks of naloxone should be requested early from adjoining communities.[1,2]

Appropriate local, state, and federal public-health and law-enforcement authorities should be notified.

 MEDICAL TREATMENT OF CASUALTIES

Treatment should be tailored to the clinical presentation of victims. For those who are awake and not disoriented, the only intervention necessary may be to escort the victims into an open area outside the zone of contamination. Those who are sleepy or just lethargic but who are easily arousable should also be escorted to an open area and kept under observation for progression of symptoms. Patients who are unconscious but still breathing should also be moved to an open area and administered adequate intramuscular doses of naloxone in 2.0-mg increments (0.1 mg/kg for pediatric patients) to awaken them. The onset of antidotal effects after intramuscular naloxone administration is 1 to 3 minutes, with maximal effects observed within 5 minutes. Repeat doses are indicated for partial response and can be repeated as often as needed. Because the clinical half-life of naloxone is between 20 and 60 minutes, assigned medical staff should observe patients for a period of no less than 1 hour to ensure that opioid effects do not recur. Nalmefene, if available, could be used in intramuscular doses of 0.5 to 1.0 mg, with a maximal efficacy seen at a total dose of 1.5 mg.

Finally, those patients who are unconscious with significantly depressed respirations or who are frankly apneic should receive immediate artificial ventilation, preferably with noninvasive techniques such as a bag-valve-mask device connected to 100% oxygen. They should also be given naloxone until they are awake and breathing spontaneously. These persons should be triaged and transported to local hospitals for continued administration of naloxone as needed and for further monitoring for at least 12 to 24 hours.

All affected victims should be examined and assessed for blunt trauma from possible falls resulting from opioid-induced unconsciousness. If there is concern regarding neck injury or head injury, the patient should be placed on a backboard and into a cervical collar and should be transported to a local hospital for further evaluation and treatment.

Although opioids have not been used directly by terrorists in large-scale attacks, the potential of these agents to create mass casualties is illustrated by their use in October 2002 by Spetsnaz commando units of the Russian Federal Security Service (FSB) against Chechen terrorists who had taken control of a theater in Moscow.[9,10] Minister of Health Yuri Shevchenko later identified the agent used as a fentanyl derivative, and it has been speculated that this opioid compound had been aerosolized either alone or in combination with an anesthetic agent. Approximately 120 hostages died. Shevchenko asserted that over a thousand doses of "antidote" were available and were used, but many casualties appear to have been removed from the theater and placed into positions, either on the ground or in buses, in which their airways were not secured.[9,10] This incident demonstrates that use of an opioid agent on a large group of people can represent a major medical disaster and that proper evacuation of casualties and careful attention to airway and ventilation can be matters of life and death quite apart from the issue of antidotes. An attack can quickly overwhelm limited medical resources available in the affected area. Proper preparation and planning can help save lives in a catastrophic event.[11-13]

 # UNIQUE CONSIDERATIONS

An opioid agent attack will likely take place in a closed space filled with hundreds of people because this combination presents an ideal opportunity for causing mass casualties. Because respiratory depression is the usual mechanism of death from opioid intoxication, absolutely crucial elements of response will include speed in reaching victims, evaluation of airway and breathing, and maintenance of airway and ventilation during and after evacuation from the scene. Naloxone should be administered as soon as is practical but is not so important in the immediate response as securing and maintaining an open airway and ensuring adequate ventilation. Naloxone stocks may become quickly depleted during an outbreak, and early consideration should be given to ordering more antidote.

Awareness for blunt trauma from falls sustained due to unconsciousness induced by the opioid agent and from potential mass hysteria during exit from an enclosed space should be considered.

Recognition by first responders, hazardous-materials teams, and other rescue personnel of the clinical picture of opioid exposure in humans and of the essentials of speedy rescue, appropriate evacuation, and the primacy of airway support and ventilation can make the difference between a relatively good outcome and a catastrophe involving hundreds of casualties. Although there have been no reported incidents of a terrorist attack

 ## CASE PRESENTATION

The grand opening of a new concert hall in Los Angeles is today. The auditorium has a maximum capacity of 800 patrons and accommodates an additional 200 performers and support staff. During the first intermission, several patrons in the back of the concert hall report hearing a hissing sound. Two security-staff personnel are called to the scene of the noise and locate three large canisters hidden behind the curtains and vigorously discharging an odorless substance into the hallway. Before they can remove the canisters, they succumb to the unknown gas and fall unconscious to the floor. Moments later, several of the patrons in the vicinity of the reported noise begin to slump into their seats or to sit down in the hallways. Others complain of nausea and begin to vomit. In a few minutes, more patrons begin to experience similar symptoms in a progressive fashion toward the front of the stage. Approximately 5 minutes after the first group of people have begun to experience symptoms, the majority of the persons in the theater are unconscious. The performers and those at the front of the stage have panicked and are rushing for two clearly marked exits at the front of the concert hall.

Hazardous materials staff arrive at the scene, which was cordoned off by the police within 10 minutes of the first report. Entering the concert hall in personal protective equipment, they find hundreds of unconscious victims.

Many of the victims are not breathing. When the unit commander notes pinpoint pupils in every victim he examines, he immediately suspects a nerve agent attack and radios the operational commander to have nerve agent antidotes brought to the scene. Rescue team members inside the hall pull victims from their seats, move them to the aisles, and then remove them from the concert hall. Outside, the victims are placed on their sides to prevent aspiration of gastric contents, and their airways are secured. Two of the apneic patients are successfully intubated by paramedics, and artificial ventilation by bag-valve-mask is begun with no significant airway resistance noted. The lack of airway resistance and the failure of victims to respond to nerve agent antidotes leads to a consideration of the differential diagnosis of pinpoint pupils and to the possibility of an opioid agent attack. Naloxone from arriving ambulances is administered via intramuscular injection first to the apneic but not intubated patients, and when spontaneous respiration resumes within 2 or 3 minutes of injection in two of these patients, this finding is reported to the hospital and additional naloxone is requested. Most of the unconscious persons wake up and resume adequate respirations, but approximately 80 persons are declared dead at the scene despite receiving large amounts of naloxone. An additional five persons are declared dead at local hospitals. None of the rescuers are affected or succumb to the agent.

involving an opioid agent, the possibility of such an attack cannot be excluded. Increased vigilance among enclosed venues capable of holding hundreds of people is indicated.

 PITFALLS

Several potential pitfalls in response to an opioid agent attack exist. These include the following:

- Failure to create a plan for mass treatment in the event of an attack
- Failure to staff and supply a high-risk area with adequate stocks of naloxone
- Failure to recognize or report an attack from an opioid agent
- Misdiagnosis of a victim of an opioid agent attack as one of nerve agent attack
- Delay in reaching casualties with respiratory depression or apnea
- Failure to position victims properly and to attend to airway and ventilation issues
- Failure to recognize the clinical presentation of opioid toxicity and to institute specific antidotal treatment with naloxone

REFERENCES

1. Wax PM, Becker CE, Curry SC. Unexpected "gas" casualties in Moscow: a medical toxicology perspective. *Ann Emerg Med*. 2003;41:700-5.
2. Toxicity, Narcotics. eMedicine.com. Available at: http://www.emedicine.com.
3. Worsley MH, Macleod AD, Brodie MJ, et al. Inhaled fentanyl as a method of analgesia. *Anesthesia* 1990;45:449-51.
4. Mather LE, Woodhouse A, Ward ME, et al. Pulmonary administration of aerosolized fentanyl: pharmacokinetic analysis of systemic delivery. *Br J Clin Pharmacol*. 1998;46:37-43.
5. Van Bever WF, Niemegeers CJ, Schellekens KH, et al. N-4-Substituted 1-(2-arylethyl)-4-piperidinyl-N-phenylpropanamides, a novel series of extremely potent analgesics with unusually high safety margin. *Arzneimittel-Forschung*. 1976;26:1548-51.
6. Jaffe AB, Sharpe LG, Jaffe JH. Rats self-administer sufentanil in aerosol form. *Psychopharmacology* 1989;99:289-93.
7. Kreeger TJ, Seal US. Immobilization of gray wolves (*Canis lupus*) with sufentanil citrate. *J Wildlife Dis*. 1990;26:561-3.
8. Baker JR, Gatesman TJ. Use of carfentanil and a ketamine-xylazine mixture to immobilise wild grey seals (*Halichoerus grypus*). *Vet Rec*. 1985;116:208-10.
9. Lethal Moscow gas an opiate? CBS News Web site. October 29, 2002. Available at: http://www.cbsnews.com/stories/2002/10/29/world/main527298.shtml.
10. Ruppe D. CWC: Experts differ on whether Russian hostage rescue violated treaty. *Global Security Newswire*. October 30, 2002. Available at: http://www.nti.org/d_newswire/issues/thisweek/2002_11_1_chmw.html.
11. Lakoski JM, Murray WB, Kenny JM. The advantages and limitations of calmatives for use as a non-lethal technique. The Sunshine Project Web site. Available at: http://www.sunshine-project.org.
12. Glenski JA, Friesen RH, Lane GA. Low-dose sufentanil as a supplement to halothane/N$_2$O anaesthesia in infants and children. *Can J Anaesth*. 1988;35:379-84.
13. Committee for an Assessment of Non-Lethal Weapons Science and Technology, National Research Council. *An Assessment of Non-Lethal Weapons Science and Technology*. Washington, DC: National Academies Press; 2003.

chapter 98

Riot-Control Agent Attack

Sam Shen

 ## DESCRIPTION OF EVENT

Riot-control agents are commonly known as "tear gas," irritants, harassing agents, and lacrimators. These agents are used by the military for training purposes and by law enforcement officers for riot control. The North Atlantic Treaty Organization (NATO) has assigned these compounds two-letter codes. The agents include 1-chloroacetophenone (NATO code, CN), o-chlorobenzylidene malononitrile (CS), bromobenzylcyanide (CA), and dibenz (b,f)-1:4-oxazepine (CR). Oleoresin capsicum (OC), an oily extract of the capsaicin found in pepper plants, is also used by law enforcement officers and, often mixed with CN, in products for personal protection. Because of their long chemical names, they are generally referred to by their NATO codes except for OC, which is often called *pepper spray*. These compounds are similar in the following respects[1]:

- Production of sensory irritation causing severe discomfort
- Quick onset of action
- Short duration of effects after exposure
- High safety profile (ratio of lethal to effective dose)

Diphenylaminearsine, or adamsite (DM), is an agent that causes vomiting and is also used for riot control, but it differs in several aspects[1]:

- Its onset of action is delayed for several minutes after exposure.
- It produces nausea, vomiting, diarrhea, abdominal cramping, and other systemic effects (including headache and depression) in addition to the mucosal irritation characteristic of the other riot-control agents.
- It produces less severe effects on the skin.

When properly used, these agents can cause extreme discomfort and temporarily disable the victim.[2] Due to the high safety profile of these compounds, riot-control agents are an attractive option for incapacitation by military and law enforcement personnel. They are sometimes called *nonlethal,* or *less-lethal,* agents because their intent is to incapacitate rather than to produce serious injury or death and because of their high safety ratios; however, it should be kept in mind that a sufficiently high dose can prove fatal.

The first widely used agent was CN, which was developed in 1871; in about 1912, ethylbromoacetate was used to control riots in Paris.[1] As Mace, CN was also subsequently marketed for personal protection. Subsequent agents were developed that produced similar results but possessed better safety profiles, higher potencies, or both.[3] CS is more potent and less toxic.[3] It is the agent most commonly used today and was introduced for common civil use in 1967.[4,5] CA was developed toward the end of World War I but is rarely used today. CR is the newest compound in this class and is the most potent, with a high safety profile and such low volatility that its effects deep in the lungs are minimal.[1] DM is primarily a vomiting agent but will be discussed as a riot-control agent because of its similar effects and management steps.

Riot-control agents are liquids or solids ("tear gas" is a misnomer) and can be dispersed as fine droplets or particles or in solution. They may be combined with an explosive substance in grenades or released as a smoke of particles from handheld devices.[6,7] Consequently, the effects are from direct contact with skin, eyes, or mucous membranes and from inhalation.

EFFECTS OF RIOT-CONTROL AGENTS

Riot-control agents are nonlethal when used properly. Reports of death are infrequent and are usually due to toxic pulmonary damage leading to pulmonary edema.[2] Symptoms usually occur within 1 minute of exposure and last approximately 30 minutes.[6] These agents have minimal long-term effects.[5] The predominant systems affected are the eyes, nose, lungs, and skin.[3]

Eyes

The eye is extremely sensitive to irritants. Exposure to an agent will produce an intense burning sensation leading to tearing, blepharospasm, photophobia, and conjunctival injection.[6,8] The victim will subsequently close his or her eyes reflexively. Although the vision of the victim will be near normal, the blepharospasm will hinder the ability of the victim to see. Most of these effects disappear in 20 minutes, although conjunctivitis may persist for 24 hours.[3]

In addition to the sensory effects, the ejection of the agent particles can cause blunt trauma to the cornea, and small particles can be embedded in the tissue of the eye.

Nose

If riot-control agents make contact with the mucous membranes of the nose, they will produce rhinorrhea, sneezing, and burning.[3,8]

Lung

One of the more serious effects of riot-control agents involves the airways. In addition to a burning sensation, irritation of the bronchial lining can produce bronchoconstriction, coughing, and dyspnea. Effects from higher doses include pulmonary edema and chemical pneumonitis.[2] The agents can also worsen underlying lung disease such as asthma or chronic obstructive pulmonary disease.[2]

Due to numerous reported deaths in custody patients who had been exposed to OC, many of whom had been restrained, pulmonary function testing was studied in normal subjects given OC or placebo to inhale. OC does not result in abnormal spirometry, hypoxemia, or hypoventilation in either the sitting, or prone–maximal restraint position.[9]

Skin

If riot-control agents make contact with the skin, they will produce erythema and a burning or tingling sensation.[2] Prolonged exposure can produce vesicles and burns similar to thermal burns. These symptoms are exacerbated in hot or humid weather.[2]

Metabolic System

Some studies have suggested that CS can be metabolized to cyanide in peripheral tissues.[2,10] However, the risk of cyanide toxicity from inhalational exposure to CS appears to be minimal.[1]

Gastrointestinal System

Exposure can produce nausea, vomiting, and diarrhea.[2] DM is the riot control agent responsible for predominantly gastrointestinal symptoms in addition to mucosal irritation.

Pregnancy

One animal study showed no significant effects from CS on pregnancy.[2,8]

 ## PREINCIDENT ACTION

The effects of riot-control agents are usually self-limiting. Therefore, victims often will not seek medical care initially. Victims may seek assistance if symptoms persist or if complications develop. Emergency medicine physicians should wear impermeable gloves and goggles to avoid exposure to the agents before treating casualties.[3,6] Facilities should be prepared for the disrobing and showering of patients before they enter the emergency department.[8]

 ## POSTINCIDENT ACTION

Since the agents are released into the air, evacuation is important to eliminate further exposure. Therefore, victims must be advised to do the following[11]:

- Immediately leave the scene where riot control agents were released.
- Move to an area where fresh air is available.
- Move to higher ground, since riot-control agents can linger as dense, low-lying clouds.

 ## MEDICAL TREATMENT OF CASUALTIES

There is no antidote for riot-control agents. Their effects are self-limiting and usually last no more than 15 to 30 minutes, although erythema of the skin may persist longer.[1] Medical management consists primarily of supportive care for each affected system. Initially, it is important to decrease any possible further contact with the agents through the following decontamination methods[11]:

- Remove clothing that may have agent particles on it. Do not pull clothing over the victim's head. Instead, clothing should be cut off to minimize potential further contact.
- The victim should be washed with copious amounts of soap and water even though wetting of the skin may temporarily increase the severity of the burning sensation from the agent.

The specific management steps are directed to each system affected.

Eye

The first step involves blowing dry air into the eyes to help the dissolved agents vaporize.[6] This should be followed by irrigation of the eyes with cold water or saline. If irrigation is performed before drying the eyes, one can prolong the burning sensation in the eyes. Although 5% sodium bisulfite was once recommended for treatment of exposure, its use is no longer advised.[12] A careful slit-lamp examination should be performed to evaluate for corneal impaction injuries secondary to the blast of the agent particles. If a corneal injury is present, any visible foreign bodies should be removed and topical antibiotics should be prescribed.

Lungs

The most serious complications occur in the lungs. Initially, humidified oxygen can provide relief. Inhaled beta-2 agonists may be given for dyspnea and bronchospasm.[6] Because the clinical onset of pulmonary injury, especially pulmonary edema, can be delayed, patients should be admitted for observation. Victims should also be admitted if they have respiratory complaints or underlying lung disease.[2]

Skin

Any solid powder or smoke particles should be gently brushed from the skin. After copious irrigation with soap and water (a measure that may be briefly painful), burns should be treated the same as any other types of burns. If dermatitis or erythema persists, topical steroids or antipruritic agents may be applied.[2,6]

CASE PRESENTATION

There has been an ongoing strike by workers at a local factory. The local news has reported that many protesters have become disruptive and violent. In fact, law enforcement officers were called to the site of the factory strike to restore order. Unfortunately, there were too many demonstrators to control safely. As the crowd of angry factory workers became more agitated, they began throwing objects at the police. Consequently, the officers had to use riot-control agents to contain the situation.

In the emergency department, emergency medical services personnel start to bring you patients complaining of shortness of breath, tearing, and burning sensation in their eyes, nose, and skin.

UNIQUE CONSIDERATIONS

Riot-control agents are fast-acting compounds that cause significant discomfort but are nonlethal when used properly. Whereas other chemical agents may cause worsening of symptoms over time, symptoms of riot-control agents often recede with time. Death is rare and, when it occurs, usually ensues from pulmonary complications. Symptoms will improve over time without long-term sequelae, so supportive care is the main treatment.

PITFALLS

Several potential pitfalls exist in treating injuries involving riot-control agents. These include the following:

- Failure to evacuate victims from area of exposure
- Failure to remove clothing or any materials that may have come in contact with the agents from the victims

- Failure to blow dry eyes before irrigating them with water or saline after exposure
- Failure to brush affected skin before washing with soap and water to eliminate further exposure
- Use of bleach for skin decontamination[13]
- Failure to admit patients with respiratory symptoms or underlying lung disease
- Failure to decontaminate any patient with riot-control agent contamination before loading onto a medical helicopter; the spread of such agents around the cockpit during flight could immobilize the pilot and endanger the lives of the patient and crew

REFERENCES

1. Sidell F. Riot control agents. In: *Medical Aspects of Chemical and Biological Warfare*. Borden Institute, Walter Reed Army Medical Center Office of the Surgeon General, U.S. Army U.S. Army Medical Dept. Center and School, U.S. Army Medical Research and Material Command Uniformed Services University of the Health Sciences; 1997:307-24.
2. Hu H, Fine J, Epstein P, et al. Tear gas: harassing agent or toxic chemical weapon? *JAMA* 1989;262:660-3.
3. Beswick FW. Chemical agents used in riot control and warfare. *Hum Toxicol*. 1983;2:247-56.
4. Kalman SM. Riot control agents. Introduction. Fed Proc. 1971 Jan-Feb; 30(1):84-5.
5. Karagama YG, Newton JR, Newbegin CJ. Short-term and long-term physical effects of exposure to CS spray. *J R Soc Med*. 2003;96:172-4.
6. Yih J-P. CS gas injury to the eye. *BMJ* 1995;311:276.
7. Smith J. The use of chemical incapacitant sprays: a review. *J Trauma*. 2002;52:595-600.
8. Sanford JP. Medical aspects of riot control (harassing) agents. *Ann Rev Med*. 1976;27:421-9.
9. Cucunell SA, Swentzel KC, Biskup R, et al. Biochemical interactions and metabolic fate of riot control agents. *Fed Proc*. 1971;30:86-91.
10. U.S. Army Medical Research Institute of Chemical Defense. Riot control agents. In: *Medical Management of Chemical Casualties Handbook*. 2nd ed. Md: 1995.
11. Lee BH, Knopp R, Richardson ML. Treatment of exposure to chemical personal protection agents. *Ann Emerg Med*. 1984;13:487-8.
12. Harrison JM, Inch TD. A novel rearrangement of the adduct from CS-epoxide and dioxin-2-hydroperoxide. *Tetrahedron Lett*. 1981;22:679-82.
13. Chan TC, Vilke GM, Clausen J, et al. The effect of oleoresin capsicum "pepper spray" inhalation on respiratory function. *J Forensic Sci*. 2002;47:299-304.

chapter 99

Nicotinic Agent Attack

Sage W. Wiener and Lewis S. Nelson

DESCRIPTION OF EVENT

Nicotine has long been recognized as a toxin in humans by reason of its action as a direct agonist at the nicotinic family of acetylcholine receptors (a family in fact defined by the affinity for nicotine). These receptors are present at the neuromuscular junction (NMJ), in both sympathetic and parasympathetic ganglia, and in the central nervous system (CNS).[1]

More recently recognized nicotinic acetylcholine receptor agonists include epibatidine and anatoxin-a, among others.[1-3] Epibatidine is derived from the skin of the *Epibatobades* frog (a species of "poison dart" frogs) and has been studied as an analgesic that acts through incompletely understood central nicotinic cholinergic pathways.[4] Anatoxin-a is found in species from several genera of cyanobacteria (formerly known as blue-green algae).[3] It should not be confused with *amatoxin*, a cyclopeptide RNA polymerase inhibitor found in several hepatotoxic mushrooms, or with *anatoxin-a(s)*, a cyanobacterial toxin that acts purely as a cholinesterase inhibitor without accompanying nicotinic agonist activity (the *s* refers to the *salivation* caused from excess acetylcholine at muscarinic receptors).

Anatoxin-a and epibatidine differ from nicotine primarily in potency. The LD_{50} (the dose required to kill 50% of those exposed) of anatoxin-a is 200 to 250 µg/kg body weight (mouse, ip),[3] and the LD_{50} of epibatidine (rat, iv) is less than 125 nmol/kg.[5] By comparison, a lethal dose of nicotine is estimated to be between 0.5 and 1.0 mg/kg in humans.[6] Epibatidine is also more specific than nicotine at the ganglionic and CNS subtypes of nicotinic receptor and does not act at the NMJ.[1] Another difference between these agents is that in vitro, epibatidine appears to have some agonist action at muscarinic acetylcholine receptors as well.[7] It is unclear, however, whether muscarinic effects would be seen clinically after human exposure.

Although nicotine has never been known to be developed as a chemical weapon by any government, it has been weaponized more than once by domestic criminals. In 1997, Thomas Leahy was found to possess ricin and botulinum toxins as well as a spray bottle filled with nicotine sulfate dissolved in dimethyl sulfoxide (an organic solvent also known as DMSO). Because his intent with the other agents was difficult to prove, he was initially only charged and convicted for the weaponization of the nicotine sulfate, although he subsequently pled guilty to the other charges.[8] Another incident of domestic terrorism involving nicotine is discussed in the case at the end of this chapter. Neither epibatidine nor anatoxin-a is known to have been developed for state, terrorist-group, or individual use.

The potential for the use of nicotine in a chemical attack is enhanced by its many possible means of delivery and routes of absorption. Nicotine freebase is an oily liquid but is relatively unstable in air. Nicotine salts, however, are solids that are readily dissolved in water or organic solvents. Therefore, these salts could potentially be dispersed as an aerosol of liquid or powder. Nicotine can be absorbed transdermally, as evidenced by "green tobacco sickness." In this illness, acute nicotine toxicity occurs in those who harvest wet tobacco without protection for their skin.[9] Nicotine patches for smoking cessation take advantage of this principle. Clearly, if nicotine were suspended in a solvent with good dermal penetration (DMSO would be an option) and then aerosolized, the potential for systemic toxicity from dermal exposure would be great. Nicotine is also stable to pyrolysis and may be absorbed through inhalation, as in tobacco smoking. Nicotine is orally bioavailable, and numerous case series exist of children with nicotine toxicity from ingestion of tobacco products.[10-18] Much less is known about the absorption and bioavailability of epibatidine and anatoxin-a through different routes. Epibatidine is available as an off-white powder and is soluble in organic solvents including alcohol. Anatoxin-a is a light brown solid that is soluble in water. Anatoxin-a appears to cause illness through ingestion in animal models.[19] Few data exist regarding the oral bioavailability of epibatidine or the inhalational absorption of either toxin. One feature of anatoxin-a that might make it ill-suited to chemical terrorism is that it is susceptible to photolysis, rapidly breaking down in the presence of sunlight.[20] Thus, while an incident involving contamination of food is possible, an incident involving outdoor dispersion of an aerosol seems extremely unlikely.

The clinical effects of nicotinic poisoning depend in part on the route of absorption. Most data have been gathered in the context of exposure through ingestion, in which significant nausea and vomiting are early features. In one review of 143 children with symptoms after ingestion of cigarettes or cigarette butts, 99% (138 children) vomited; 74% (104 children) did so within 20 minutes.[10] These features are also seen in toxicity from dermal absorption, but they may not be the first sign of exposure. Other early findings include dizziness and dyspnea. In one reported case of dermal exposure, dizziness, dyspnea, "unsteadiness," and nausea occurred within 30 minutes.[21] Flushing and pallor of the skin have both been reported after nicotine exposure, and diaphoresis may be present as well.[11,12,14] Cardiac effects include both hypertension and hypotension as well as palpitations and dysrhythmias ranging from sinus bradycardia and sinus tachycardia to sinoatrial block, atrial fibrillation, and asystole.[10,12-14,16,17] These seemingly contradictory effects are better understood when one considers that the effects of nicotine on the autonomic nervous system are mediated through its action at both sympathetic and parasympathetic ganglia. Which effects predominate in any individual patient can be difficult to predict. Nicotine also acts as a depolarizing neuromuscular blocker at the NMJ.[1] Thus, early muscle spasms and fasciculations may occur, followed by weakness, hypotonia, and even flaccid paralysis.[10,12,13] Nicotinic cholinergic agonism in the CNS leads to seizures and altered mental status. In children, both lethargy and irritability have been reported after tobacco ingestion.[10-14,16] Patients with less severe poisoning may present with headache or dizziness.[10,11,15] Seizures are uncommon in typical cases of cigarette ingestion and when present suggest a more severe exposure.[10] Severe exposures can lead to permanent neurologic devastation.[22]

Little is known about clinical findings in humans after poisoning with epibatidine or anatoxin-a; there are no reported cases. Presumably, because of the greater potency of these agents, patients would clinically resemble those with severe nicotine toxicity. If epibatidine were used, it is possible that muscarinic findings would be present as well, which would make the distinction from nerve agent poisoning even more challenging; however, the absence of neuromuscular signs and symptoms might actually clarify the diagnosis.

 ## PREINCIDENT ACTIONS

Disaster planning and education are the most important preincident actions that can be taken in preparation of an attack involving cholinergic agents. Coordination between the U.S. Department of Agriculture, the Food and Drug Administration, and law enforcement and counterterrorism agencies is likely to facilitate early detection of incidents involving food and water contamination. Syndromic surveillance of emergency department triage complaints may also play a role because food and water contamination may initially appear as gastrointestinal (GI) illness. Although atropine is already stockpiled in many hospitals because of preparations for nerve agent attack, this measure is unlikely to be helpful because muscarinic effects will be inconsequential in most patients. Other than basic preparedness for chemical terrorism such as personal protective equipment and

decontamination facilities, no specific physical infrastructure or supplies are required in the hospital for preparation for a nicotinic agonist attack.

Technology originally developed for workplace monitoring exists for detection of small amounts of nicotine in the air.[23] It is also possible to test water supplies for cyanobacteria,[3] and anatoxin-a can be detected by gas chromatography with an electron-capture detector.[24] In the future, it may be possible to deploy chemical detectors in strategic sampling locations to provide early warning of a chemical attack.

 ## POSTINCIDENT ACTIONS

The most important actions after a nicotinic agent attack (besides rescue and care of exposed patients) are prompt notification of the appropriate authorities and decontamination of affected areas. This differs little from the response to other types of chemical attack. If anatoxin is known to have been the agent involved, maximizing exposure of the involved area to sunlight will help to rapidly destroy the toxin; anatoxin-a spontaneously degrades in direct sunlight, with a half-life of about 1 hour.[20]

 ## MEDICAL TREATMENT OF CASUALTIES

Although nicotinic cholinergic antagonists exist, there are no clinical data on their use in human poisoning with nicotinic agents. In addition, of the ganglionic blockers, hexamethonium and trimethaphan are not available for clinical use, and mecamylamine is available in tablet form only, making it unsuitable for use in an emergency. Furthermore, nicotinic cholinergic antagonists at the NMJ are not useful to treat paralysis, as they are themselves paralytic agents. There is thus no useful antidote to nicotine or nicotinic-agonist exposure, and supportive care is the mainstay of therapy.

As in most chemical-attack scenarios, rapid removal of just that clothing that has been soaked and of agent visible on the skin (local, or "spot," decontamination) is crucial to prevent continued absorption and should be accomplished in concert with attention to airway, breathing, and circulation. Patients without a secure airway or who need ventilatory support need these interventions at approximately the same time that local decontamination is being done and before full-body disrobing and decontamination. Mouth-to-mouth ventilation should never be performed because it can pose risks to the rescuer, particularly after a GI exposure.[25] For full-body decontamination, removal of the patient's clothes, shoes, belt, watch, and jewelry should be followed by irrigation of the skin with copious amounts of water with or without soap (soap may be useful for oily substances such as nicotine freebase or any of these agents dissolved in an organic solvent).

Hemodynamic support should include intravenous fluid boluses followed by vasoconstrictor agents such as norepinephrine as needed to treat hypotension.

Therapy for hypertension should be approached with caution, because hemodynamic collapse may be precipitous.[26] In the absence of end-organ effects of severe hypertension, pharmacologic intervention should probably be avoided. Dysrhythmias should be managed according to the usual practice. Seizures should be treated with benzodiazepines or barbiturates. Other anticonvulsants are unlikely to be helpful and are not indicated. Vomiting should be managed with antiemetics, and oral activated charcoal should be administered, particularly after GI exposures.[27] Because nicotine exhibits a certain degree of enteroenteric circulation, oral activated charcoal even after dermal or inhalational exposure could theoretically be of benefit.[26]

Suspected cases should be reported to the regional poison control center. Poison control centers can recognize developing epidemics, assist with patient management, and help contact other health and law enforcement authorities in the event of an attack. Because symptoms occur early after exposure, minimal observation is required for patients who present with no clinical abnormalities.

Poisoning by a nicotinic agonist may be difficult to distinguish from nerve agent poisoning, and it is possible that patients exposed to these agents might conceivably be treated in the field with Mark I kits containing atropine and pralidoxime. If possible, this should be avoided. Although there may be some role for atropine in patients with bradydysrhythmias, bronchorrhea, or other severe muscarinic symptoms, there is no role for pralidoxime, an oxime cholinesterase reactivator. In fact, aggressive oxime therapy may do more harm than good because pralidoxime is itself a weak cholinesterase inhibitor with the potential to cause cholinergic excess.

 ## UNIQUE CONSIDERATIONS

The most notable feature of nicotinic-agonist poisoning is its similarity to poisoning by cholinesterase inhibitors such as organophosphate pesticides and nerve agents. Enhanced parasympathetic outflow (with resulting muscarinic effects) due to ganglionic stimulation may further confuse the clinical findings and mimic organophosphate poisoning. Without identification of the product at the scene, it is unlikely that this distinction will be possible in the event of a chemical attack. Failure to respond to atropine and oximes (or worsening of symptoms with oxime therapy) may be the only clue. Fortunately, as there is no specific therapy for nicotinic-agonist poisoning, chemical attacks with these agents are otherwise managed as are any generic chemical exposure; good decontamination and supportive care is the only therapy needed.

 ## PITFALLS

Several potential pitfalls exist in responding to an cholinergic agent attack. These include the following:

- During disaster planning and provider education, failure to consider the possibility of nicotinic agonists as mass-casualty chemical agents
- Failure to consider a chemical attack with a nicotinic agonist after an epidemic of a GI illness
- Misdiagnosis of nicotinic-agonist poisoning as poisoning by organophosphate pesticides or nerve agents
- Administration of atropine therapy to patients with nicotinic-agonist poisoning and with no significant muscarinic signs or symptoms
- Administration of oxime therapy to patients with nicotinic-agonist poisoning
- Failure to involve public health and law enforcement authorities when a chemical attack is suspected
- Failure to call the regional poison control center to report cases and to get assistance with management

 ### CASE PRESENTATION

In 2003, a total of 18 patients from four different families developed nausea, vomiting, dizziness, and burning of the mouth after eating ground beef. One of the patients required evaluation in the emergency department for atrial fibrillation. The pattern of illness suggested contamination at a single store rather than at a meat-processing plant. A recall was issued for approximately 1,700 pounds of ground beef with sell-by dates including the 3 days potentially involved. Samples of the ground beef were sent for analysis. Although testing for food-borne pathogens was negative, it was quickly determined that the samples contained nicotine at a concentration of 300 mg/kg of ground beef. Since a lethal dose of nicotine is about 50 mg, about one-third pound of beef would have represented a life-threatening ingestion. Investigators thus became suspicious of contamination with a nicotine-containing pesticide because these were widely available in the community. However, none of these pesticides was used or sold in the store where the contamination occurred. Several weeks later, a man formerly employed as a meat cutter in the supermarket was arrested and charged with poisoning the meat with Black Leaf 40, a pesticide containing 40% nicotine. A public health notice was issued, and 148 people were interviewed after reporting illness; 92 were ultimately determined to have suffered illness consistent with nicotine poisoning.[6]

REFERENCES

1. Hoffman BB, Taylor P. Neurotransmission. In: Hardman JG, Limbird LE, Gilman AG, eds. *Goodman & Gilman's The Pharmacological Basis of Therapeutics.* 10th ed. New York: McGraw-Hill Medical Publishing Division; 2001:115-53.
2. Rupniak NM, Patel S, Marwood R, et al. Antinociceptive and toxic effects of (+) epibatidine oxalate attributable to nicotinic agonist activity. *Br J Pharmacol.* 1994;113:1487-93.
3. Hitzfeld BC, Höger SJ, Dietrich DR. Cyanobacterial toxins: removal during drinking water treatment, and human risk assessment. *Environmental Health Perspectives.* 2000;108:113-22.
4. Dukat M, Glennon RA. Epibatidine: impact on nicotinic receptor research. *Cellular and Molecular Neurobiology.* 2003;23:365-78.
5. Kassiou M, Bottlaender M, Loc'h C, et al. Pharmacological evaluation of a Br-76 analog of epibatidine: a potent ligand for studying brain nicotinic acetylcholine receptors. *Synapse* 2002;45:95-104.

6. Boulton M, Stanbury M, Wade D, et al. Nicotine poisoning after ingestion of contaminated ground beef. *MMWR* 2003;52:413-6.

7. Kommalage M, Hoglund AU. (+/−) Epibatidine increases acetylcholine release partly through an action on muscarinic receptors. *Pharmacol Toxicol.* 2004;94:238-44.

8. Threat of Bioterrorism in America. Statement for the Record of Robert M. Burnham, Chief, Domestic Terrorism Section before the United States House of Representatives Subcommittee on Oversight and Investigations, May 20, 1999. Available at: http://www.fas.org/irp/congress/1999_hr/990520-bioleg3.htm.

9. Ballard T, Ehlers J, Freund E, et al. Green tobacco sickness: occupational nicotine poisoning in tobacco workers. *Arch Environ Health.* 1995;50:384-9.

10. McGee D, Brabson T, McCarthy J, et al. Four-year review of cigarette ingestions in children. *Pediatr Emerg Care.* 1995;11:13-6.

11. Lewander W, Wine H, Carnevale R, et al. Ingestion of cigarettes and cigarette butts by children—Rhode Island, January 1994-July 1996. *MMWR* 1997;46:125-8.

12. Smolinske SC, Spoerke DG, Spiller SK, et al. Cigarette and nicotine chewing gum toxicity in children. *Human Toxicol.* 1988;7:27-31.

13. Oberst BB, McIntyre RA. Acute nicotine poisoning. *Pediatrics* 1953;11:338-40.

14. Mensch AR, Holden M. Nicotine overdose after a single piece of nicotine gum. *Chest* 1984;86:801-2.

15. Haruda F. "Hip-pocket" sign in the diagnosis of nicotine poisoning. *Pediatrics* 1989;84:196.

16. Malizia E, Andreucci G, Alfani F, et al. Acute intoxication with nicotine alkaloids and cannabinoids in children from ingestion of cigarettes. *Human Toxicol.* 1983;2:315-6.

17. Petridou E, Polychronopoulou A, Kouri N, et al. Childhood poisoning from ingestion of cigarettes. *Lancet* 1995;346:1296-7.

18. Sisselman SG, Mofenson HC, Caraccio TR. Childhood poisoning from ingestion of cigarettes. *Lancet* 1996;347:200-1.

19. Stevens DK, Krieger RI. Effect of route of exposure and repeated doses on the acute toxicity in mice of the cyanobacterial nicotinic alkaloid anatoxin-a. *Toxicon.* 1991;29:134-8.

20. Stevens DK, Krieger RI. Stability studies on the cyanobacterial nicotinic alkaloid anatoxin-a. *Toxicol.* 1991;29:134-8.

21. Davies P, Levy S, Pahari A, et al. Acute nicotine poisoning associated with a traditional remedy for eczema. *Arch Dis Childhood.* 2001;85:500-2.

22. Rogers AJ, Denk LD, Wax PM. Catastrophic brain injury after nicotine insecticide ingestion. *J Emerg Med.* 2004;26:169-72.

23. Pendergrass SM, Krake AM, Jaycox LB. Development of a versatile method for the detection of nicotine in air. *AIHAJ.* 2000;61:469-72.

24. Stevens DK, Krieger RI. Analysis of anatoxin-a by GC/ECD. *J Anal Toxicol.* 1988;12:126-31.

25. Koksal N, Buyukbese MA, Guven A, et al. Organophosphate intoxication as a consequence of mouth-to-mouth breathing from an affected case. *Chest* 2002;122:740-1.

26. Salomon ME. Nicotine and tobacco preparations. In: Goldfrank LR, Flomenbaum NE, Lewin NA, et al. *Goldfrank's Toxicologic Emergencies.* 7th ed. New York: McGraw-Hill Medical Publishing Division; 2002:1075-84.

27. Geller RJ, Singleton KL, Tarantino ML, et al. Nosocomial poisoning associated with emergency department treatment of organophosphate toxicity—Georgia, 2000. *J Toxicol Clin Toxicol.* 2001;39:109-11.

chapter 100

Anesthetic-Agent Attack

Kinjal N. Sethuraman and K. Sophia Dyer

 ## DESCRIPTION OF EVENT

In the 1830s, ether, the earliest anesthetic agent, began to be used for sedation and pain control in the United States.[1] Today, however, ether and various other anesthetics such as chloroform and cyclopropane are no longer in use because of the danger of explosion and the potential for fatal consequences from their use. Initially, they were replaced by nonflammable agents such as halothane and nitrous oxide; however, halothane itself, because of its hepatotoxicity and cardiotoxicity, has now been largely superseded by halogenated ethers such as isoflurane and enflurane. These drugs are typically delivered via inhalation after intravenous sedation. A major advantage of inhaled anesthetics for anesthesiologists is that the level of sedation can be rapidly modified to remain within the therapeutic window and to achieve desired analgesia, amnesia, muscle relaxation, and paralysis.[2]

Anesthetic agents are not known to have been used on the battlefield or by terrorists, but recently an event in Russia brought the issue of the topic of anesthetic agents as potential mass-casualty weapons into sharp focus.[3-5] In 2002, a "knockout gas," bluish-gray in color and with a sweet taste, was used by the Russian Army to incapacitate Chechnyan hostage-takers while elite Spetsnaz forces of the Russian army attempted to rescue 800 hostages in a Moscow theater.[6] It has been speculated that the gas contained halothane or another anesthetic agent mixed with an opioid compound (see Chapter 97).[7,8] One hundred twenty-seven hostages, including several children, died from the gas. It was reported that the gas was released for over 20 minutes at an unknown concentration. The preincident health of some of the victims may have led to the high mortality rate, but some hostages had virtually no response to the agents.[7] Hospitals that received victims of the attack were allegedly not informed of the gases used and thus had to experiment with reversal agents.[8,9] As television footage shows, many affected hostages removed from the theater were placed onto the ground or onto buses in positions that risked airway compromise and underscored the necessity of attention to airway and breathing in these casualties quite apart from considerations of specific antidotal treatment.[7]

Although newer anesthetic gases are relatively safe, older agents have several properties that could make them appealing for criminal purposes:

- Ease of availability
- Portability
- Volatility
- Mass dissemination
- Rapid onset of action
- Low warning properties
- Potential to incapacitate or kill
- Possible use of remote trigger
- Novel to first responder
- Can also be used as explosives in high concentrations

In this chapter, we will focus on some of the more common agents.

If a terrorist attack occurs with any agent, first responders need to be well prepared. The response team needs to act quickly to triage, evacuate, and attend to airway and breathing in affected casualties and to determine which agent or agents were used, the agent concentration, and the method of distribution. The odor, taste, color, signs, and symptoms will vary by agent. Therefore, interviewing victims can be helpful in identifying the gas or gases used. Since these agents share significant inhalational hazards with a quick onset of action, they could pose a hazard both to original victims and also first responders.

CHARACTERISTIC PROPERTIES OF POTENTIAL TERROR AGENTS

The following agents are described as examples of the range of physicochemical properties and effects of the many compounds that have been used as inhalational anesthetics. Clinicians should always be aware of potential interactions from combinations of agents, as in the Moscow theater incident. Attention to presenting symptoms, descriptions by victims, and information from hazardous materials specialists can aid in clarification of the chemical used.

Victims of inhaled anesthetic agents will experience confusion, relaxation, dizziness, drowsiness, and various respiratory symptoms that can include choking, a burning sensation in the mouth or nose, and respiratory distress. Less water-soluble agents such as nitrous oxide will stealthily cause effects in the smaller, peripheral airways but less pronounced skin, mucous-membrane, or central-airway damage.[10]

The mean alveolar concentration (MAC) is used as a measure of the strength of an anesthetic. It represents the *minimum* concentration necessary to cause unresponsiveness in 50% of the general population.[11] Simply put, the higher the MAC, the less potent the gas. The MAC is influenced by many factors including age of victim, the victim's comorbidities and metabolism, combination with another anesthetic or analgesic agent, and preexposure vital signs.[2] The solubility of an anesthetic in blood is described by the blood-gas partition coefficient (BGPC), which expresses, in liters, the amount of an agent that will dissolve in 1 liter of blood exposed to air containing the anesthetic. The lower the BGPC, the faster the onset of an anesthetic and the faster it will wear off.

Diethyl Ether

Diethyl ether ($C_4H_{10}O$) is a flammable, volatile, colorless liquid with a sweet taste and ethereal odor.[12] It is soluble in alcohol, acetone, benzene, and chloroform. Its boiling point is only 94°F (34.5°C). When exposed to fire or heat, ether releases carbon monoxide; exposure to light causes ether to break down into flammable peroxides.[12] Ether, with a BGPC of 12, is more soluble in blood than either halothane or nitrous oxide. The MAC of ether is 2.0%. Because of the explosive nature of ether, the National Fire Protection Association has given ether a flammability rating of 4, corresponding to an extreme fire hazard.[13] Although ether works well as an anesthetic, its propensity to explode prompted anesthetists to find alternative inhaled agents such as chloroform, cyclopropane, and halothane.

Anesthesia induction occurs at a concentration of 100,000 to 150,000 ppm and is maintained with 50,000 ppm.[13] Very small doses to eyes or skin can cause corneal injury and burns.[14] Toxic exposures to ethers (as with other anesthetics) can occur through inhalation, eye or skin contact, and ingestion. The effect of ether is dose dependent. Symptoms consist of skin, eye, and mucosal irritation leading to an increase in bronchial secretions. Dizziness, drowsiness, bradycardia, hypothermia, or acute excitement may also occur. Laryngospasm, loss of consciousness, and death may result. The after-effects of emergence from ether-induced anesthesia include nausea, vomiting, and headache.[15]

Newer ethers are halogenated and include enflurane, desflurane, and sevoflurane. They are not flammable, have fewer side effects, are efficient as anesthetic agents, and cause less end-organ damage.[1] They may be potentially used by terrorists as incapacitating agents.

Nitrous Oxide

Nitrous oxide (N_2O)[16] is a weak anesthetic (MAC of 105) often combined with other agents to produce adequate analgesia and anesthesia. Induction and maintenance of anesthesia require very high concentrations of nitrous oxide, and hypoxia may result if high concentrations of oxygen are not coadministered. During minor procedures, lower concentrations are used for sedation. Nitrous oxide is found commonly in aerosol sprays, and its abuse potential is accordingly high. Prolonged use can cause peripheral nerve damage, psychosis, perceptual impairment, and hyperpyrexia.[17]

Nitrous oxide administered in high doses has been found to cause arrhythmias, malignant hyperthermia, seizures, pneumomediastinum, and subcutaneous emphysema. Nausea and vomiting are early signs of nitrous oxide toxicity.[18]

Chloroform

Chloroform ($CHCl_3$)[18] is a colorless, volatile chlorinated hydrocarbon that is often mixed with ethanol. It has a sweet, burning taste and a pungent odor. As a byproduct of chlorination, chloroform is present in low concentrations in chlorinated water[19] but exposure to these low concentrations is insufficient to cause anesthesia. It is also produced from the reduction of carbon tetrachloride (CCl_4) with moist iron.

Although no longer used as an anesthetic,[1] chloroform is still used an intermediate in chemical syntheses. One of the Freon refrigerants is an example of the current use of chloroform. Moreover, chloroform has been widely popularized as a knockout agent to induce consciousness when poured onto a handkerchief or other cloth and held over the mouth and nose. And its well-known use for this purpose may make it a more likely choice for terrorists for either small-scale or mass-casualty use.

The toxic dose of chloroform is 7 to 25 mg/dL (0.59 to 2.1 mmol/L).[20] At inhaled concentrations of less than 1500 ppm, physical effects of dizziness, tiredness, and headache are reported; and anesthesia occurs at a range of 1500 to 30,000 ppm. Chloroform causes irritation to the respiratory tract. It will cause dry mouth, sedation, confusion, and loss of consciousness within 5 to 10 minutes, and unconsciousness may last up to 30 minutes after removal from exposure. Fatalities occur after 5 to 10 minutes at doses of 25,000 ppm or greater by inhalation.[20]

Death can occur from cardiac arrest and hepatic toxicity with peak elevation of hepatic enzymes 3 to 4 days after exposure and a subsequent return of liver-function tests to normal in survivors.[20] Pulmonary toxicity from intravenous injection of chloroform peaks after 3 days. Renal and hepatic toxicity may also occur from phosgene ($COCl_2$), a byproduct that results from exposure of chloroform to sunlight and air (see Chapter 95).[21] Other byproducts include hydrochloric acid (HCl), carbon monoxide (CO), inorganic chloride, and formaldehyde.[21] Pulmonary exposure to HCl and phosgene can result in pulmonary edema, bronchial pneumonia, and subsequent lung abscesses.

Victims exposed to chloroform need supportive care, including cardiac and pulmonary monitoring in an intensive care unit as clinically indicated. While there is no antidote for chloroform, liver toxicity in animals may be prevented by using N-acetylcysteine (NAC) after exposure, since chloroform and its byproducts deplete glutathione stores.[20,22] However, no studies have evaluated the use of NAC for this purpose in humans.[23]

Cyclopropane

Cyclopropane (C_3H_6) is a hydrocarbon ring that was discovered in 1882; it began to be used as an anesthetic in 1933.[1] It is extremely flammable and is thus no longer used clinically. Cyclopropane, a gas at room temperature, is caustic to eyes but not to the skin. At concentrations greater than 40%, cyclopropane causes irritation to the eyes and respiratory tract. Its density is greater than air, and if released into the environment, it will hug the ground.[14] At higher concentrations, it causes nausea, disorientation, dizziness, and incoordination. If released in a closed area, cyclopropane, as is the case with all hydrocarbons, will displace oxygen and cause asphyxiation.[24]

Autopsy results from accidental death after cyclopropane ingestion showed hemorrhagic edema of the lungs.[14] Cardiac output, stroke volume, and heart rate are all affected by high concentrations of cyclopropane, but these parameters return to normal a few minutes after the agent is removed.[25] Cyclopropane causes decreases in renal blood flow and glomerular filtration rate.[26] Malignant hyperthermia from cyclopropane has been reported; it can be resolved with cooling and perhaps by the administration of dantrolene.[27] Cyclopropane has also been shown to alter cognitive function, especially the ability to learn, for up to a week after exposure.[28]

Halothane

Halothane ($C_2HBrClF_3$) continues to be used occasionally as an anesthetic, analgesic, and amnesic. Halothane is a colorless, volatile, nonflammable liquid unique for its sweet taste and odor. It is the most potent inhaled anesthetic, with a MAC of 0.77.[2] The MAC is commonly reduced by administering a coagent. The MAC for patients who are older, hypothermic, hypotensive, or hypoxic will be lower.[29] Halothane is highly soluble in both blood and fat; this behavior accounts for its prolonged emergence from anesthesia.[2] When exposed to light, heat, flames, and acids, halothane will decompose into other toxic fumes or metabolites (e.g., bromide, chlorine, and fluorine). The dose used for anesthesia ranges between 5000 to 30,000 ppm,[30] or 0.5% to 3% concentration in oxygen.[31,32] Even if victims are exposed to less than 5000 ppm, they will show impaired manual dexterity and word-finding difficulties.

Acute exposure to this agent causes severe irritation to all exposed areas. Hypotension, dizziness, somnolence, lethargy, and changes in mental status are all potential symptoms. Exposure to halothane may lead to hepatic failure, cardiac arrhythmias, and malignant hyperthermia.[31,33,34] Liver failure from other halogenated anesthetics is less common. Long-term, chronic exposure to halothane can increase the risk of some cancers and can increase rates of spontaneous abortions and of congenital abnormalities in newborns of exposed mothers.[35]

Diagnosis of halothane toxicity is based mainly on history, physical examination, and basic laboratory analyses. Attributing hepatic failure to halothane is difficult, since the clinical presentation is identical to other causes of hepatitis. An assay for halothane-related antibodies is available for experimental use but is not practical in emergency or disaster settings. Halothane metabolites can be detected in the urine up to 1 week after exposure.[31]

 ## PREINCIDENT ACTIONS

Because terrorist attacks are for the most part unpredictable, it is important for emergency medical services, law enforcement, and local, state, and national agencies to be prepared for any type of attack at any given time. For attacks using anesthetic agents, the focus should be on rapid access to casualties, prompt evacuation, careful attention to airway and ventilation (especially during transport and positioning), general supportive care, identification of agent, and ample supply of reversal agents. In Moscow, although the Russian military had an "antidote" (probably naloxone) to the agents used, claims were made that there were not enough medical personnel to administer the drug.[7] There are no antidotes to ether, chloroform, cyclopropane, or halothane, and the importance of attention to airway, breathing, and circulation cannot be overemphasized.

The first gas masks were developed as a response to the use of inhaled gases at Ypres during World War I.[3] In any given situation, appropriate respiratory protection should be worn by emergency medical services personnel, healthcare workers, and law enforcement personnel until the area in question has been cleared of inhalation risk. Many first-responding agencies may not have the available detection equipment to identify exactly the type of anesthetic gas used or even the general class of anesthetic gases used, thus making it even more important to use proper equipment. The typical canister respirator either with a full face piece or partial face piece, which is very portable and varying in comfort, will not offer protection in an atmosphere of depleted oxygen. If oxygen displacement has occurred, a supplied air respirator (either through a tank or air line) is the only appropriate respiratory protection. Many portable sensors are available for measuring ambient oxygen concentrations, either as individual items or components in other detection equipment. Several companies market canister respirators for application in event of the use of weapons of mass destruction. In general, these products are not specifically tested against many of the anesthetic agents discussed in this chapter, as of the time of this writing. An organic vapor canister might trap some of these agents, with the obvious exception of the inorganic nitrous oxide. However, this will depend on concentration values within the acceptable range. In addition, the canister testing information should be evaluated to see whether it has been tested against the known agent. Given that this might be difficult to accomplish in a critical time period, a self-contained breathing apparatus will offer the best protection for an unknown environment.

 ## POSTINCIDENT ACTIONS

As with any potential exposure to an inhalational toxin, protection of the victims from further exposure and guarding against exposure in responders is vital. If in doubt as to the type of chemical, the highest level of respiratory protection is recommended—in many cases, this is a supplied air respirator. Because some of these products are volatile, precautions against direct flame and any equipment that could potentially generate a spark are prudent. The most important immediate actions to take are to reach victims (who may already be apneic) as soon as possible, to ensure a patent and protected airway, to increase ventilation, to decrease exposure, and to provide oxygen to victims.

MEDICAL TREATMENT OF CASUALTIES

It is important to interview survivors and gather as many data as possible to determine the agent used. The volatility of anesthetic agents may decrease the utility of air samples, but such samples can help to identify other agents that may have been used in combination with the agents. It is important to consider the potential of a mixture of agents even after the identification of a specific agent. Once victims are at a hospital, laboratory studies that can be obtained relatively quickly can be helpful in the management of exposed patients. These studies include arterial-blood-gas and carboxy-hemoglobin determinations, liver-function tests, a complete blood count, and a comprehensive metabolic panel. A chest radiograph is also useful in the setting of suspected chemical pneumonitis or pulmonary edema, although dyspnea is usually the first indicator of incipient pulmonary edema.

CASE PRESENTATION

It is a hot and humid summer day on a holiday weekend in Baltimore. Air conditioners are working overtime. The threat of rain forever looms overhead, as it always seems to do in the mid-Atlantic region of the United States. As shopping continues to be a national pastime, several hundred shoppers have packed into a local mall. Security is nonexistent due to budget cuts and the economic slump.

Nearly 20 men holding machine guns, wearing masks, and carrying cylinders that could be mistaken for helium tanks easily enter the mall. They strategically release the gas in the cylinders into the air-conditioning system.

After a few minutes, people with asthma start feeling their chests tighten. Others start to choke, as their eyes burn. Still more involuntarily fall asleep. Those near the doors try to run outside for fresh air, but the electrically controlled doors are locked shut.

The masked men make their presence known to the few who are fighting off the weight of their eyelids. They have taken the mall over for two purposes: to steal, and to make it known to the Westerners that they are not safe.

PITFALLS

Several potential pitfalls exist in response to an anesthetic opioid nerve agent attack. These include the following:

- Failure to recognize that an attack has taken place
- Failure to reach potentially apneic patients as soon as possible
- Failure to attend adequately to airway, breathing, and circulation in casualties before, during, and after transport to medical treatment facilities
- Failure to notify proper local, state, national, and international agencies
- Failure to identify the agent or agents used
- Failure to follow the identification of a specific chemical agent by consideration of the possibility of simultaneous use of an anesthetic agent
- Failure to remove igniting factors or flammable objects from scene
- Failure to use gloves and appropriate respiratory protection
- Failure to evacuate or ventilate area
- Failure to notify hospitals
- Failure to have enough personnel available

REFERENCES

1. Vandam L. History of anesthetic practice. In: Miller RD, ed. *Anesthesia*. Vol V. Philadelphia: Churchill Livingston; 2000.
2. Schwinn DA, Shafer SL. Basic principles of pharmacology related to anesthesia. In: Miller RD ed. *Anesthesia*. Vol V. Philadelphia: Churchill Livingston; 2000.
3. Gas killed hostages in raid. CNN Web site. October 27, 2002. Available at: http://www.cnn.com/2002/WORLD/europe/10/27/moscow.putin/index.html.
4. Moscow doctor: gas killed 116 hostages. CBS News Web site. October 27, 2002. Available at: http://www.cbsnews.com/stories/2002/10/28/world/main527107.shtml.
5. Bismuth C, Borron S, Baud FJ, et al. Chemical weapons: documented use and compounds on the horizon. *Toxicol Lett*. 2004;149:11-8.
6. Reed D. Terror in Moscow. HBO Documentaries; June 2004.
7. Wax PM, Becker CE, Curry SC. Unexpected "gas" casualties in Moscow: a medical toxicology perspective. *Ann Emerg Med*. 2003; 41:700-5.
8. Lethal Moscow gas an opiate? CBS News Web site. October 29, 2002. Available at: http://www.cbsnews.com/stories/2002/10/29/world/main527298.shtml.
9. Anger grows over gas tactics. CNN Web site. October 28, 2002. Available at: http://archives.cnn.com/2002/WORLD/europe/10/28/moscow.gas/.
10. Greenfield RA, Brown BR, Hutchins JB, et al. Microbiological, biological, and chemical weapons of warfare and terrorism. *Am J Med Sci*. 2002;323:326-40.
11. Marshall BE, Longenecker DE. General anesthetics. In: Hardman JG, Limbird LE, Molinoff PB, et al, eds. *Goodman and Gilman's The Pharmacological Basis of Therapeutics*. Vol IX. New York: McGraw-Hill; 1996.
12. Occupational Health and Safety Administration, US Department of Labor. Ethyl ether: material data safety sheet. April 27, 1999. Available at: http://www.osha.gov/SLTC/healthguidelines/ethylether/.
13. Hathaway GJ, Proctor NH, Hughes JP, et al. *Proctor and Hughes' Chemical Hazards of the Workplace*. Vol III. New York: Van Nostrand Reinhold; 1991.
14. Grant WM. *Toxicology of the Eye*. Springfield, Ill: Charles C Thomas; 1962.
15. Clayton G, Clayton F. *Patty's Industrial Hygiene and Toxicology*. 3rd ed. New York: John Wiley & Sons; 1981.
16. OSHA Health Guidelines. Occupational Safety and Health Guideline for nitrous oxide. Available at: http://www.osha.gov/SLTC/healthguidelines/nitrousoxide/recognition.html.
17. Murray MJ, Murray WJ. Nitrous oxide availability. *J Clin Pharmacol*. 1980;20:202-5.
18. Haddad K, Pearson C. Chlorinated hydrocarbons. In: Ellenhorn MJ, Barceloux DG, eds. *Medical Toxicology: Diagnosis and Treatment of Human Poisonings*. Philadelphia: WB Saunders; 1998.

19. Rook JJ. Formation of haloforms during chlorination of natural waters. *Water Treatment Exam*. 1974;23:234-43.

20. Maynard SM. Appendix D: drugs and toxins: therapeutic and toxic levels. In Ford MD, ed. *Clinical Toxicology*. Vol 1. Philadelphia: WB Saunders; 2001.

21. Van Dyke RA. On the fate of chloroform. *Anesthesiology* 1969; 30:264-72.

22. el-Shenawy NS, Abdel-Rahman MS. The mechanism of chloroform toxicity in isolated rat hepatocytes. *Toxicol Lett*. 1993;69:77-85.

23. Flanagan RJ, Meredith TJ. Use of N-acetylcysteine in clinical toxicology. *Am J Med*. 1991;91:131S-9S.

24. Barasch ST, Booth S, Modell JH. Hypercapnia during cyclopropane anesthesia: a case report. *Anesth Analg*. 1976;55:439-41.

25. Cullen DJ, Eger EI, Gregory GA. The cardiovascular effects of cyclopropane in man. *Anesthesiology* 1969;31:398-406.

26. Deutsch S, Pierce EC, Vandam LD. Cyclopropane effects on renal function in man. *Anesthesiology* 1967;28:547-58.

27. Lips FJ, Newland M, Dutton G. Malignant hyperthermia triggered by cyclopropane during cesarean section. *Anesthesiology* 1928;56: 144-6.

28. James FM. The effect of cyclopropane anesthesia without surgical operation on mental function of normal man. *Anesthesiology* 1969;30:264-72.

29. Dale O, Brown BR. Clinical pharmacokinetics of the inhalational anesthetics. *Clin Pharmacokinet*. 1987;145-67.

30. OSHA Health Guidelines. Occupational Safety and Health Guidelines for Halothane. Available at: http://www.osha.gov/SLTC/healthguidelines/halothane/recognition.html.

31. Halothane: Drugdex Drug Evaluations. DRUGDEX® System. Greenwood Village, Colo: Thomson MICROMEDEX.

32. *Product Information: Fluothane®, Halothane (Liquid for Vaporization)*. Philadelphia: Wyeth-Ayerst Laboratories; 1998.

33. Viitanen H, Baer G, et al. The hemodynamic and Holter-electrocardiogram changes during halothane and sevoflurane anesthesia for adenoidectomy in children aged one to three years. *Anesth Analg*. 1999;87:1423-5.

34. Humphrey DM. *Technical Info Fluothane®, Halothane*. Philadelphia: Wyeth-Ayerst Laboratories; 2002.

35. *Material Safety Data Sheet 2-Bromo-2-chloro-1,1,1-trifluoroethane*. Milwaukee, Wisc: Aldrich Chemical Co; May 1992.

chapter 101

Introduction to Biologic Agents

Andrew S. Nugent and Eric W. Dickson

On Aug. 6, 1945, at 8:16 AM, the detonation of "Little Boy" over the city of Hiroshima, Japan, ushered in the age of nuclear weapons and warfare. The first known use of the second element of NBC (nuclear, biologic, and chemical) weapons of mass destruction is not as dramatic nor as well documented but likely took place in 6th century BC, when the Assyrians used rye ergot to poison the wells of their adversaries.[1] Knowing a good idea when they saw it, Scythian, Roman, Greek, and Persian archers tipped their arrows with manure and other biologic agents circa 400 to 300 BC. Many other uses of human sickness to wage war followed; perhaps the most destructive occurred when the Tartars used trebuchets to hurl plague-infected corpses into the city of Caffa in the year 1346. Sailors fleeing the ensuing epidemic may have inadvertently initiated the Great Plague by spreading the illness to Genoa, Italy (although this has been recently questioned).[2-4] Biologic warfare was not limited to the "Old World." Pizzaro, the British, and the Americans used smallpox-infected blankets to produce mass casualties among their adversaries.[5]

U.S. research into offensive biologic weapons continued until 1969, when President Richard Nixon renounced the use of biologic weapons as killing or incapacitating agents. Although most nations signed the Biological Weapons Convention in 1975, many experts believe that biologic weapons programs still exist in Russia, North Korea, and until recently, Iraq. It is estimated that 10 countries have stockpiled biologic weapons either now or in the recent past.[6] Since the early 1980s, the risk of the use of biologic weapons has increased dramatically with the rise of modern terrorism because these agents are relatively easy and inexpensive to make and weaponize and have the potential to kill large numbers of individuals, while sowing terror into millions of survivors.

The organisms and toxins that can be used as biologic weapons have been categorized by the U.S. Centers for Disease Control and Prevention (CDC) into three categories (A, B, and C [Table 101-1]). Agents classified as Category A by the CDC are of the highest priority because of the risk of their imminent use. Each of the Category A agents is easily disseminated, may result in much mortality, and has the ability to cause public panic, outcomes that are perceived to be among the main goals of a terrorist attack. All other significant bacteria that could possibly be used as bioweapons fall into the CDC's Category B; these are moderately easy to disseminate and have much less potential for severe mortality, although morbidity may be high. Category C is reserved for emerging infectious illnesses that may be bioengineered in the future as weapons.

Beyond the psychologic impact of a biologic weapon attack, several conditions must be met in order for a biologic agent to be useful as a weapon; lethality and infectivity of an organism alone are not sufficient. For example, Ebola is highly transmissible unless proper precautions are used and has a high mortality rate. However, Ebola does not persist in the environment and kills too quickly to allow for widespread exposure to infected individuals. This limits dissemination (e.g., formation of an epidemic) in the population. Thus, Ebola is unlikely to make an ideal weapon unless weaponized in a form that rapidly infects a large segment of the population.

With that in mind, several criteria must be met for an organism or toxin to be an effective biologic weapon, including the following: (1) the organism or toxin must be easily obtainable, culturable, and stable in the environment; (2) the organism or toxin must have the ability to be weaponized with a delivery system that allows widespread dissemination and/or be highly transmissible (by human, insect, or animal vector) while also allowing time for individuals to infect others in society; (3) the organism or toxin must be able to incapacitate or kill a large segment of the population (e.g., there is no innate resistance or easy treatment).

The first barrier to weaponization is delivery. Biologic agents can be delivered by several routes: inhalation of an aerosol, such as with anthrax; ingestion, such as with enterohemorrhagic *Escherichia coli*; or transcutaneously (e.g., the use of plague-infected fleas in Manchuria during World War II). Delivering and disseminating biologic agents effectively is not easy. Distribution via explosive device can reduce the efficiency of the delivered organisms to as low as 5%. However, it is not only delivery to a location that is important. Aerosolized particles that are too large will settle out of the atmosphere, and particles that are too small will not be trapped effectively in the lung, reducing infectivity. For this reason, aerosolized particles must be between 1 and 10 μm, and an efficient delivery system must be used; aerosolization using compressed gas can achieve 70% efficiency.[7] Weather and

TABLE 101-1 CDC CATEGORIES OF BIOLOGIC WEAPON AGENTS

CATEGORY	DEFINITION	AGENTS
A	Organisms that pose a high risk to national security because they are easily disseminated or transferred from person to person, they can result in high mortality rate and have the potential for major public health impact, may cause public panic and social disruption, and require special action for public health preparedness.	*Bacillus anthracis* (anthrax) *Yersinia pestis* (plague) *Francisella tularensis* (tularemia) Botulinum toxin Variola (smallpox) Viral hemorrhagic fevers (Marburg, Ebola, etc.)
B	Organisms that are moderately easy to disseminate, result in moderate morbidity and low mortality rates, and require the CDC's diagnostic capacity and enhanced disease surveillance.	*Brucella* (brucellosis) *Coxiella brunetti* (Q fever) *Rickettsia rickettsii* (Rocky Mountain spotted fever) *Vibrio cholerae* (cholera) *Shigella dysenteriae* (shigellosis) *Salmonella* species (salmonellosis) *Salmonella typhi* (typhoid fever) *Burkholderia mallei* (glanders) *Burkholderia pseudomallei* (melioidosis) *Chlamydia psittaci* (psittacosis) *Escherichia coli* 0157:H7 and others(enterohemorrhagic *E. coli*) Hantavirus, flavivirus, and others
C	Emerging pathogens capable of being engineered for mass dissemination in the future due to availability, ease of production and dissemination, and potential for high morbidity and mortality resulting in a major health impact.	

electrical charge are other barriers to the effective dispersion of a biologic agent. For example, rain will remove particles from the atmosphere, and high wind speed can disperse an agent away from the intended target, whereas low wind speed will allow the aerosol to settle too rapidly. Electrical forces affect distribution as well. There is a natural electrostatic attraction between particles and surfaces. Unless compensated for, this electrostatic charge limits aerosolization. The problem of electrostatic charges can be overcome but is difficult and requires expertise.[8] Alternatively, electrostatic charge can be used as an advantage when designing environmental filtering systems.[9,10] Because of the variability of outdoor conditions, an indoor release of a biologic agent may be more desirable for terrorists since it requires a smaller amount of the agent and can be targeted to a specific population of interest (as was accomplished with anthrax in the Hart Office building in 2001). Conversely, an indoor release is not as likely to cause mass casualties unless the organism is highly infective during an asymptomatic incubation period and can be disseminated person to person.

A second route of delivery is by oral ingestion. There are barriers to the effective transmission of biologic agents in the water system, primarily the use of water purification in the United States. For this reason, the release of a biologic agent in the water supply may be less effective than contaminating the food supply.

The archetype for biologic weapons is anthrax. Anthrax is easily obtainable, easily weaponized, stable when released (spores can persist in the environment for up to 40 years), and highly lethal. One hundred kilograms of aerosolized anthrax spores have the potential to kill up to 3 million people. Because of efficient delivery, the lack of person-to-person infectivity and limited secondary aerosolization are not barriers to its effective use as a biologic weapon. Thus, even though it is unlikely that infection will persist or spread much beyond the initial casualties, anthrax still makes an ideal weapon.

SURVEILLANCE

The role of surveillance is a subject of much debate. Surveillance depends on the recognition of occurrences of diseases/organisms/symptoms beyond that which would be expected as a background rate or outside of a disease's natural range. One of the major weaknesses in surveillance systems is the lack of sensitivity and specificity. Even though it is critical to detect the presence of a pathogen, it is also important to avoid mobilizing a response to false-positive tests. A second weakness is that by the time symptom or organism surveillance is able to pick up a pattern of illness in a community, the illness may already be well established. Environmental monitoring, on the other hand, has the potential to identify pathogens before they become ensconced in the community. Environmental monitoring includes the routine monitoring of food and water supplies as well as the general environment. Autonomous monitoring devices are available (August 2004) that perform testing (e.g., on air) at a predefined interval for infectious, chemical, and radiologic agents.[11] More information on surveillance is available at the CDC Web site (www.cdc.gov) and in *Morbidity and Mortality Weekly Report*.[12] Readers with an interest in worldwide surveillance may wish to subscribe to ProMed-mail (www.promedmail.org), which is a free mailing list that reports symptomatic outbreaks of known diseases and unidentified symptom complexes worldwide.

Each of the chapters in Section 10 will review the likely scenario and consequences of an attack with a specific biologic agent. Much of the information provided is based on our understanding of the agent's pathogenicity in nature. In many cases, how a given agent will behave when delivered as a weapon is extrapolated from these data. Early recognition and isolation minimize morbidity and mortality of the primarily exposed and reduce secondary infection. For the clinician, this is implemented by early identification of a cluster of patients with similar symptoms or the occurrence of a

TABLE 101-2 DIFFERENTIAL DIAGNOSIS OF SYNDROMES POSSIBLY CAUSED BY BIOLOGIC WARFARE AGENTS

SYNDROME	CATEGORY A BIOTERRORISM DISEASES	CATEGORY B BIOTERRORISM DISEASES	CATEGORY C BIOTERRORISM DISEASES	NATURALLY OCCURRING DISEASES
Respiratory tract infection with fever	Inhalational anthrax Tularemia Pneumonic plague	Inhalational glanders Inhalational ricin Melioidosis Q fever Typhus	Legionellosis SARS, Hantavirus (2nd stage)	Diphtheria *E. coli* Histoplasmosis Influenza Malaria Measles Respiratory syncytial virus
Gastroenteritis	Anthrax Tularemia Ebola Plague Marburg	Acute brucellosis Cholera Giardia *Cryptosporidium* Q fever Ricin/abrin toxins Paralytic shellfish toxins	Hantavirus Norovirus Legionellosis	Cestodes *Clostridium difficile* *Helicobacter pylori* Hepatitis A & E Leishmaniasis-Visceral Rocky Mt. spotted fever
Rash with fever	Ebola Marburg Pneumonic plague Smallpox	Glanders typhus	Lyme disease Dengue fever	Typhoid fever Chickenpox Measles Monkeypox Mumps Rubella Rocky Mt. spotted fever
Influenza-like illness	Plague Smallpox Anthrax Tularemia Ebola	Q fever Typhus Brucellosis Glanders	Hantavirus Nipah virus Legionellosis Lyme disease SARS	Diphtheria Influenza Malaria Measles Mononucleosis Rift Valley fever Respiratory syncytial virus Yellow fever
Sepsis, nontraumatic shock	Ebola Lassa fever Marburg	*E. coli*	Hantavirus	Cytomegalovirus *Enterococcus faecium* *Histoplasmosis* Listeriosis *Staphylococcus epidermidis* *Streptococcus pneumonia* Toxic shock syndrome *Yersinia entercolitica*
Meningitis, encephalitis-like syndrome	Anthrax Ebola Lassa fever	Eastern equine Encephalitis Venezuelan equine encephalitis Q fever	St. Louis encephalitis West Nile virus Lyme disease Japanese encephalitis Nipah virus	Chickenpox Dengue Epstein-Barr virus *Haemophilus influenza* Influenza A & B Malaria Measles Viral meningitis Rift Valley fever Rocky Mt. spotted fever
Botulism-like illness	Botulism			Diphtheria Listeriosis

(Table reproduced with permission Kristin Uhde, PhD, and Center for Biological Defense, College of Public Health, University of Southern Florida.)

disease outside of its normal range. Table 101-2 provides a summary of the symptoms and a differential diagnosis that are observed during a possible bioterrorism attack.[13]

REFERENCES

1. Kortepeter M, Christopher G, Cieslak T, Culpepper R, Darling R, Pavlin J, eds. *Medical Management of Biological Casualties Handbook*. Fort Detrick, Frederick, Md: US Army Medical Research Institute of Infectious Diseases; 2001:1-12.
2. Derbes VJ. De Mussis and the great plague of 1348: a forgotten episode of bacteriological warfare. *JAMA*. 1966;196(1):179-82.
3. Christopher GW, Cieslak TJ, Pavlin JA, Eitzen EM. Biological warfare: a historical perspective. *JAMA*. 1997;278(5):412-17.
4. Wheelis M. Biological warfare at the 1346 siege of Caffa. *Emerg Infect Dis*. 2002;8(9):971-5. Available at: http://www.cdc.gov/ncidod/EID/vol8no9/01-0536.htm.
5. Noah DL, Huebner KD, Darling RG, Waeckerle JF. The history and threat of biological warfare and terrorism. *Emerg Med Clin North Am*. 2002;20(2):255-71.
6. Jakobs MK. The history of biologic warfare and terrorism. *Dermatol Clin*. 2004;22:231-46.
7. Federation of American Scientists. Militarily Critical Technologies List. (MCTL) Part II: Weapons of Mass Destruction Technologies. Section III: Biological Weapons Technology. Available at: http://www.fas.org/irp/threat/mctl98-2/.
8. Gomez A. The Electrospray and its application to targeted drug inhalation. *Respir Care*. 2002;47:1419-31.
9. Utrup LJ, Frey AH. Fate of bioterrorism-relevant viruses and bacteria, including spores, aerosolized into an indoor air environment. *Exp Biol Med*. 2004;229:345-50.
10. Weber RW. Meteorologic variables in aerobiology. *Immunol Allergy Clin North Am*. 2003;23:411-22.
11. Bravata MD, McDonald KM, Smith WM, et al. Systematic review: surveillance systems for early detection of bioterrorism-related diseases. *Ann Intern Med*. 2004;140:910-22.
12. Syndromic surveillance. Reports from a national conference, 2003. *Morb Mortal Wkly Rep*. 2004;53(Suppl):1-264.
13. Center for Biological Defense, College of Public Health, University of Southern Florida. Syndromic Surveillance. Available at: http://www.bt.usf.edu/files/SurveillancePacket%20Draft.pdf.

chapter 102

Bacillus Anthracis (Anthrax) Attack

Christo C. Courban

 ## DESCRIPTION OF EVENT

Anthrax, a category A bioterrorism agent, is a zoonotic disease caused by *Bacillus anthracis*, an aerobic, nonmotile, spore-forming, gram-positive bacillus that is ubiquitous in soil. Anthrax is primarily a disease of herbivores, including sheep; cattle; goats; horses; and, less commonly, pigs.

The first known description of anthrax (approximately 1400 BC) is in the Old Testament where it represented the fifth plague on Egypt, the killing of the Egyptian cattle. The "Black Bane" outbreak (named after the black eschars caused by cutaneous anthrax) took place in Europe in the 1600s and killed 60,000 people and many more cattle. In 1881, Robert Koch definitively identified *B. anthracis* as the cause of cutaneous anthrax, making it the first disease for which a microbial cause was identified. Soon thereafter, Pasteur developed an effective vaccine. Despite all efforts, anthrax remains a sporadic problem in Africa, the Middle East, some parts of South America, and Asia.

B. anthracis makes an almost perfect biologic weapon—it is easily weaponized; can be aerosolized; has a high mortality rate; and the spores are highly resistant to drying, heat, gamma radiation, ultraviolet light, and many disinfectants. Additionally, the spores can remain dormant in the environment for up to 40 years. Several countries have developed weaponized anthrax, which was used during WWII by the Japanese in Manchuria. It is estimated that the release of 100 kg of anthrax spores in a major city could lead to up to 3 million deaths, making anthrax potentially as lethal as a hydrogen bomb. For comparison, it is estimated that Iraq had 8500 L of concentrated *B. anthracis* in 1991, all of which was subsequently destroyed. Concern about the use of anthrax spores as a biologic weapon was heightened dramatically in 1979 when an epidemic of inhalation anthrax occurred downwind of a weapons research facility in Sverdlovsk, Russia, with cases occurring up to 50 km away and almost 6 weeks after the release. Indeed, anthrax was used as a biologic weapon in 2001 when anthrax spores were disseminated via the U.S. Postal Service along the Eastern Seaboard of the United States. Twenty-two cases of anthrax were identified, half of which were inhalation type anthrax and half cutaneous, resulting in five fatalities among those with inhalation anthrax.

Transmission

Anthrax infection occurs by three methods: contact with broken skin, inhalation of spores, and ingestion. Naturally occurring infections are due mainly to contact with infected animals or animal products, such as hides or poorly cooked meats. Historically, the number of inhaled spores required to cause infection in 50% of individuals was thought to be approximately 10,000. More recent data suggest that as few as 1 to 3 spores may be sufficient to cause disease, depending on particle size. This estimate is tempered somewhat by the observation that many hide and wool workers are exposed to high concentrations of aerosolized spores on an ongoing basis with subsequent infection occurring only in a minority of individuals. There is no person-to-person transmission of anthrax, with the exception of the cutaneous form, which can be spread by skin contact.

Virulence

The virulence of anthrax is dependent on its ability to produce three distinct proteins: lethal *factor* (LF), protective antigen (PA), and edema *factor* (EF). Edema *toxin,* formed when edema *factor* and protective antigen bind, interferes with water homeostasis, causing severe, localized edema seen in cutaneous anthrax. Edema *toxin* also inhibits neutrophil function, impairing the host's ability to defend itself against infection. Lethal *toxin* is also composed by the binding of two subunits: the lethal *factor* and protective antigen. Lethal toxin is responsible for, among other things, the release of TNF-alpha and interleukin B-1, which are responsible for the systemic reaction leading rapidly to death. One area of investigation has been the search for an inhibitor that can block the binding of protective antigen with lethal factor and edema factor, thus preventing the formation of lethal toxin and edema toxin.

Inhaled Anthrax

Inhaled anthrax is the most serious form likely to occur after a bioterrorism event. Inhalational anthrax victims typically present 1 to 5 days after exposure, with a median incubation time of 4 days.[1] However, cases have occurred up to 6 weeks after exposure to anthrax spores (thus the suggestion for prolonged prophylaxis). Inhaled anthrax does not cause a true pneumonia. Rather, the lungs act only as a portal for infection. After the inhalation of anthrax spores into the alveoli, the spores are picked up by macrophages that transport them to the mediastinal and peribronchial lymph nodes. Activated spores divide rapidly, causing hemorrhagic mediastinitis and subsequent dissemination to the rest of the body via the blood, causing toxemia and sepsis.[2]

Presenting complaints are that of a nonspecific flulike illness, often including occasional nonproductive cough, fevers, chills, sweats, malaise, myalgia, and chest discomfort. Rhinorrhea is notably absent. If untreated, this prodrome can last for 48 to 72 hours, after which the patient's condition may improve before a severe and precipitous decline. Within 24 to 48 hours of the onset of respiratory disease, patients develop bacteremia, with disease progression to hemorrhagic mediastinitis, pleural effusions, and septic shock. Patients often become dyspneic and cyanotic, with increasing chest and/or abdominal pain and diaphoresis. Stridor may also be present because of obstruction of the trachea by enlarged lymph nodes. Up to 50% of patients with pulmonary anthrax develop meningitis with associated subarachnoid hemorrhages. The detection of hemorrhagic cerebrospinal fluid with gram-positive bacilli and polymorphonuclear pleocytosis can aid in making the diagnosis.[3]

Chest radiographs characteristically show a widened mediastinum with pleural effusions and relative sparing of the lung parenchyma. Computed tomography (CT) of the chest should be considered if inhalation anthrax is suspected and the diagnosis is in doubt. CT scan is more sensitive and specific for detecting mediastinal lymphadenopathy, in which there is a normal white cell count or a mild leukocytosis with a left shift.[4]

The differential diagnosis of inhalational anthrax is wide and includes mycoplasma, influenza, legionella, tularemia, and psittacosis. *Characteristics that differentiate anthrax from influenza and other influenza-like illnesses include the following:* wide mediastinum on radiograph (70%), pleural effusion (80%), absence of rhinorrhea (only 10% of patients with anthrax infection will have rhinorrhea), absence of sore throat (found in only 20%), dyspnea (80%), and nausea and/or vomiting (80%). Before September 2001, inhalation anthrax was estimated to have a mortality rate of up to 95%. With modern antibiotics and aggressive supportive care, the mortality rate has been reduced to 50%. This reduction in mortality is attributed to prompt recognition of the disease, aggressive concomitant antimicrobial therapy, and improvements in supportive care techniques. However, in the face of a major attack, medical services will likely be overwhelmed and it will not be possible to provide intensive care for all cases. Thus, the mortality of cases may be higher than 50% and possibly approach 95%.

Cutaneous Anthrax

As seen during 2001, cutaneous anthrax is likely to occur regardless of the mode of attack. Cutaneous anthrax represents 95% of background cases of anthrax in the United States. Cutaneous anthrax presents as a painless pruritic papule generally appearing 1 to 7, but up to 12, days after exposure in an area of compromised skin integrity. Within 48 hours, vesicles containing a serosanguineous fluid surround the papule, with extensive associated edema. The vesicles rupture, necrose, and enlarge, forming the characteristic painless, black (hence "anthrax" from the Greek "anthracis," or coal), ulcerated lesion. Debridement of such lesions should be avoided because this may facilitate bacteremia. However, with concurrent administration of antibiotics, this prohibition does not extend to diagnostic skin biopsies, which is part of the recommended evaluation for cutaneous anthrax.[5] The eschar dries and falls off in 1 to 2 weeks, leaving little or no scar. Lymphangitis and painful lymphadenopathy associated with systemic symptoms occur in some patients. Mortality is due to systemic invasion and may be as high as 20% of those with cutaneous anthrax without treatment. Even though antibiotics do not affect the course of the local eschar, they can prevent systemic infection. The differential diagnosis of cutaneous anthrax includes ecthyma gangrenosum, brown recluse spider bite, orf, and glanders among others. *The presence of purulence suggests an etiology other than anthrax unless there is a secondary infection.*

Gastrointestinal Anthrax

Gastrointestinal anthrax occurs 2 to 5 days after ingestion of poorly cooked, contaminated meat or poisoned food sources. Patients generally develop ulcers in the mouth, esophagus, terminal ileum, or cecum. Symptoms initially include nausea, vomiting, fever, and abdominal discomfort that progress rapidly to bloody diarrhea and signs suggestive of peritonitis. Gastric ulcers with associated hematemesis, hemorrhagic mesenteric lymphadenitis, and massive ascites may also occur.[6] Gastrointestinal anthrax can mimic an acute abdomen, ascites with peritonitis, and a perforated viscus. The mortality rate of gastrointestinal anthrax approaches 100%. It has been suggested that early aggressive therapy may reduce the mortality rate. However, the diagnosis is often overlooked until the patient's condition is already terminal.

Specimen Collection and Organism Identification

Anthrax is so prolific that the organism may be seen on a Gram stain of blood. Cultures of blood, pleural fluid, and cerebrospinal fluid may be used to identify the organism in suspected cases. Surveillance cultures in exposed individuals (e.g., nasal swabs) are used as an epidemiologic tool and should not be routinely obtained. If possible, cultures should be obtained prior to the initiation of antibiotic therapy, since blood can be sterilized after only one or two doses of antibiotics. The organism can be easily cultured on 5% sheep blood agar or MacConkey's agar; growth can be expected in 6 to 24 hours. *Treatment should be initiated on clinical grounds. Withholding treatment while waiting for culture results will lead to increased mortality.* Although initial identification of the organism can be done in a local laboratory, specialized testing must be done in one of the laboratories certified to do so. More information about these laboratories is available at *www.bt.cdc.gov/labissues*.

Identification of anthrax spores at the site of an attack is problematic. Handheld identification devices generally require 10,000 or more spores. Additionally, there is a cross-reactivity between *B. cereus* and other bacillus species. Several rapid identification techniques have been developed since 2001, including a nucleic acid-based test that can identify as few as 10 spores within 4 hours, a polymerase chain reaction (PCR) based test, and others.

Autonomous detection systems (ADS) that perform a PCR or immunoassay test at a defined interval (e.g., 1.5 hours) have been developed for anthrax and are being deployed in 300 high-speed mail handling facilities. Further details about ADS, including necessary criteria for deployment, can be found at the Centers for Disease Control and Prevention Web site (*www.cdc. gov/mmwr/preview/mmwrhtml/rr53e430-2a1.htm*).

Isolation

There are no data suggesting that person-to-person transmission of inhalational anthrax occurs; hence, patients with suspected anthrax may be hospitalized in a standard hospital room with standard universal precautions. Contact precautions should be used with patients who have cutaneous lesions because direct exposure to vesicle secretions of such lesions may result in secondary cutaneous infection.[7]

 ## MEDICAL TREATMENT OF CASUALTIES

Guidelines for therapy are subject to change and may vary at the time of an anthrax attack. This is because weaponized *B. anthracis* may be engineered to be resistant to multiple antibiotics. A summary of current treatment suggestions is found in Tables 102-1 and 102-2.

TABLE 102-1 INHALATIONAL ANTHRAX TREATMENT PROTOCOL[*,†] FOR CASES ASSOCIATED WITH BIOTERRORISM ATTACK

CATEGORY	INITIAL THERAPY (INTRAVENOUS)[‡§]	DURATION

Adults	Ciprofloxacin 400 mg every 12 hrs[*]
	
	 or
	 Doxycycline 100 mg every 12 hrs[¶]
	 and
	 One or two additional antimicrobials[§]
		IV treatment initially.[‖] Switch to oral antimicrobial therapy when clinically appropriate:
		     Ciprofloxacin 500 mg po BID
		     or
		     Doxycycline 100 mg po BID
		 Continue for 60 days (IV and po combined)[#]

Children	Ciprofloxacin 10-15 mg/kg every 12 hrs[**,††] or Doxycycline:[¶,‡‡] >8 yrs and >45 kg: 100 mg every 12 hrs >8 yrs and <45 kg: 2.2 mg/kg every 12 hrs <8 yrs: 2.2 mg/kg every 12 hrs and One or two additional antimicrobials[§]	IV treatment initially.[‖] Switch to oral antimicrobial therapy when clinically appropriate: Ciprofloxacin 10-15 mg/kg po every 12 hrs[‡‡] or Doxycycline:[†††] >8 yrs and >45 kg: 100 mg po BID >8 yrs and <45 kg: 2.2 mg/kg po BID <8 yrs: 2.2 mg/kg po BID Continue for 60 days (IV and po combined)[§§]
Pregnant women[§§]	Same for nonpregnant adults (the high death rate from the infection outweighs the risk posed by the antimicrobial agent)	IV treatment initially. Switch to oral antimicrobial therapy when clinically appropriate.[†] Oral therapy regimens same for nonpregnant adults.
Immunocompromised persons	Same for nonimmunocompromised persons and children	Same for nonimmunocompromised persons and children.

(From Centres for Disease Control and Prevention: Update: investigation of bioterrorism-related anthrax and interim guidelines for exposure management and antimicrobial therapy. *Morb Mortal Wkly Rep.* 2001;50:909-19.)

[*]For gastrointestinal and oropharyngeal anthrax, use regimens recommended for inhalational anthrax.

[†]Ciprofloxacin or doxycycline should be considered an essential part of first-line therapy for inhalational anthrax.

[‡]Steroids may be considered as an adjunct therapy for patients with severe edema and for meningitis based on experience with bacterial meningitis of other etiologies.

[§]Other agents with in vitro activity include rifampin, vancomycin, penicillin, ampicillin, chloramphenicol, imipenem, clindamycin, and clarithromycin. Because of concerns of constitutive and inducible beta-lactamases in *Bacillus anthracis*, penicillin and ampicillin should not be used alone. Consultation with an infectious disease specialist is advised.

[‖]Initial therapy may be altered based on clinical course of the patient; one or two antimicrobial agents (e.g., ciprofloxacin or doxycycline) may be adequate as the patient improves.

[¶]If meningitis is suspected, doxycycline may be less optimal because of poor central nervous system penetration.

[#]Because of the potential persistence of spores after an aerosol exposure, antimicrobial therapy should be continued for 60 days.

[**]If intravenous ciprofloxacin is not available, oral ciprofloxacin may be acceptable because it is rapidly and well absorbed from the gastrointestinal tract with no substantial loss by first-pass metabolism. Maximum serum concentrations are attained 1-2 hours after oral dosing but may not be achieved if vomiting or ileus is present.

[††]In children, ciprofloxacin dosage should not exceed 1 g/day.

[‡‡]The American Academy of Pediatrics recommends treatment of young children with tetracyclines for serious infections (e.g., Rocky Mountain spotted fever).

[§§]Although tetracyclines are not recommended during pregnancy, their use may be indicated for life-threatening illness. Adverse effects on developing teeth and bones are dose related; therefore, doxycycline might be used for a short time (7-14 days) before 6 months of gestation.

TABLE 102-2 CUTANEOUS ANTHRAX TREATMENT PROTOCOL* FOR CASES ASSOCIATED WITH BIOTERRORISM ATTACK

CATEGORY	INITIAL THERAPY (ORAL)†	DURATION
Adults*	Ciprofloxacin 500 mg BID or Doxycycline 100 mg BID	60 days‡
Children*	Ciprofloxacin 10-15 mg/kg every 12 hrs (not to exceed 1 g/day)† or Doxycycline:§ >8 yrs and >45 kg: 100 mg every 12 hrs >8 yrs and <45 kg: 2.2 mg/kg every 12 hrs <8 yrs: 2.2 mg/kg every 12 hrs	60 days‡
Pregnant women*,‖	Ciprofloxacin 500 mg BID or Doxycycline 100 mg BID	60 days‡
Immunocompromised persons*	Same for nonimmunocompromised persons and children	60 days‡

(From Centres for Disease Control and Prevention: Update: investigation of bioterrorism-related anthrax and interim guidelines for exposure management and antimicrobial therapy. *Morb Mortal Wkly Rep.* 2001;50:909-19.)

*Cutaneous anthrax with signs of systemic involvement, extensive edema, or lesions on the head or neck requires intravenous therapy, and a multidrug approach is recommended (see Table 102-1).

†Ciprofloxacin or doxycycline should be considered first-line therapy. Amoxicillin 500 mg po TID for adults or 80 mg/kg/day divided every 8 hours for children is an option for completion of therapy after clinical improvement. Oral amoxicillin dose is based on the need to achieve appropriate minimum inhibitory concentration levels.

‡Previous guidelines have suggested treating cutaneous anthrax for 7-10 days, but 60 days is recommended in the setting of this attack, given the likelihood of exposure to aerosolized *B. anthracis.*[6]

§The American Academy of Pediatrics recommends treatment of young children with tetracyclines for serious infections (e.g., Rocky Mountain spotted fever).

‖Although tetracyclines or ciprofloxacin are not recommended during pregnancy, their use may be indicated for life-threatening illness. Adverse effects on developing teeth and bones are dose related; therefore, doxycycline might be used for a short time (7-14 days) before 6 months of gestation.

Because of the lack of adequate central nervous system penetration by doxycycline, ciprofloxacin should be the drug of choice for central nervous system anthrax.[3,8] This recommendation may be extended to all patients with inhalational anthrax, given the high rate of associated meningitis. Penicillin, cephalosporins, and trimethoprim-sulfamethoxazole should not be used *for treatment* because of resistance. Chest tube drainage of the recurrent, often hemorrhagic, pleural effusions has been shown to lead to quite dramatic clinical improvement and should be strongly considered.

Treatment of Exposed Individuals

Treatment is not advocated for asymptomatic persons unless public, health, or law-enforcement authorities have ascertained that there is a risk of exposure. Ciprofloxacin 500 mg orally twice daily for 60 days is recommended (Table 102-3). In addition to antibiotics, some authorities have recommended 3 doses of vaccine at diagnosis and at 2 weeks and 4 weeks after exposure.[9] Boosters should be given at 6, 12, and 18 months and yearly thereafter. Vaccination of exposed individuals may be prudent and may be recommended in the event of an attack. It is likely that amoxicillin can be used in children and pregnant women as a *prophylactic* drug since many strains of anthrax are sensitive to penicillin. Again, these recommendations[10] are subject to change based on recommendations made at the time of an incident.

The majority of patients who receive prophylaxis cannot tolerate the therapy. At 30 days, as few as 40% of individuals were noted to be taking prophylactic medications (this was 70% of high-risk exposures). Common side effects at 14 days include "severe" gastrointestinal

symptoms (13%-19%); fainting, dizziness, and lightheadedness (7%-13%); and heartburn and gastroesophageal reflux disease (8%).[9,10]

 PREINCIDENT ACTIONS

Personal protective equipment should be available. Stockpiling of antibiotics in local or national stores and rapid distribution systems can prevent delays in postexposure antibiotic prophylaxis. Prophylactic vaccination is indicated only in individuals who will be repeatedly exposed to anthrax spores, such as those in Bioterrorism Level B laboratories, those working with imported raw hides, and wool and cleaning crews.

 POSTINCIDENT ACTION

Reaerosolization of *B. anthracis* spores is uncommon. Cleansing of the skin, potentially contaminated clothing, and the environment may reduce the risk of acquiring cutaneous and gastrointestinal forms of disease.[11]

For decontamination, sporicidal solutions, such as commercially available bleach or 0.5% hypochlorite solution (a 1:10 dilution of household bleach), should be used. These substances may be corrosive to some surfaces. Dressings from cutaneous lesions are considered a biohazard.

It is the responsibility of the treating physician to report all suspected or confirmed cases of anthrax to the local and state public health departments and laboratories as well as the local police department. Updated information regarding these requirements can be found

TABLE 102-3 INTERIM RECOMMENDATIONS FOR POSTEXPOSURE PROPHY-LAXIS FOR PREVENTION OF INHALATIONAL ANTHRAX AFTER INTENTIONAL EXPOSURE TO *BACILLUS ANTHRACIS*

CATEGORY	INITIAL THERAPY	DURATION
Adults (including pregnant women and immunocompromised persons)	Ciprofloxacin 500 mg po BID or Doxycycline 100 mg po BID	60 days
Children	Ciprofloxacin 10-15 mg/kg po Q 12 hrs* or Doxycycline:>8 yrs and >45 kg: 100 mg po BID >8 yrs and ≤45 kg: 2.2 mg/kg po BID ≤8 yrs: 2.2 mg/kg po BID	60 days

*Ciprofloxacin dose should not exceed 1 g per day in children.
(From *Morb Mortal Wkly Rep. 2001*; 50:909-19.)

on the Centers for Disease Control and Prevention's Web site at www.bt.cdc.gov.

 UNIQUE CONSIDERATIONS

Isolation of the source of infection may be valuable for public health and law enforcement officials. If, for example, an envelope is the source of infection, the source

CASE PRESENTATION

An envelope containing anthrax is sent to a member of Congress. There are several infected individuals. Other sources of anthrax are found in the mail throughout the country. Because of concern about anthrax, every person who finds a white powder presents to the emergency department convinced he or she needs antibiotic prophylaxis for anthrax or at least cultures, as do close relatives and co-workers and everyone who was in the mall last Saturday when someone scattered baking soda. The emergency department is overwhelmed by the walking well. What are some of the steps necessary to manage this event?

should be placed in a plastic bag. If a plastic bag is not available, the source should be covered with a sheet or other barrier. All windows in the infected building should be closed, the ventilation system should be turned off, and exposed individuals should be instructed to remove possibly contaminated clothing and shower before presenting to the emergency department.

 PITFALLS

- Failure to remain vigilant.
- Failure to treat for an adequate length of time and with multidrug regimens.
- Failure to consider inhalation anthrax as the cause of flulike symptoms.
- Failure to notify appropriate authorities in suspected or confirmed cases of anthrax.

REFERENCES

1. Dixon TC, Meselson M, Guillemin J, Hanna PC. Anthrax. *New Engl J Med.* 1999;341:815-26.
2. Inglesby TV, Henderson DA, Bartlett JG, et al. Anthrax as a biological weapon: medical and public health management [Erratum appears in *JAMA.* 2000;283:1963]. *JAMA.* 1999;281:1735-45.
3. Friedlander AM. Anthrax: clinical features, pathogenesis, and potential biological warfare threat. In: Remington JS, Swartz MN, eds. *Current Clinical Topics in Infectious Disease.* Vol. 20. Malden, Mass:Blackwell Science; 200:335-49.
4. Jernigan DB, Raghunathan PL, Bell BP, et al. Investigation of bioterrorism-related anthrax, United States, 2001: epidemiologic findings. *Emerg Infect Dis.* 2002;8:1019-28.
5. Update: investigation of bioterrorism-related anthrax and interim guidelines for clinical evaluation of persons with possible anthrax. *Morb Mortal Wkly Rep.* 2001;50:941-8.
6. Swartz MN. Recognition and management of anthrax—an update. *New Engl J Med.* 2001;345:1621-6.
7. Anonymous. Bioterrorism alleging use of anthrax and interim guidelines for management—United States, 1998. *Morb Mortal Wkly Rep.* 1999;48:69-74.
8. Bell DM, Kosarsky PE, Stephens DS. Conference summary: clinical issues in the prophylaxis, diagnosis and treatment of anthrax. *Emerg Infect Dis.* 2002;8:222-5.
9. Centers for Disease Control and Prevention. Use of anthrax vaccine in response to terrorism: supplemental recommendations of the Advisory Committee on Immunization Practices. *MMWR Morb Mortal Wkly Rep.* 2002;51(45):1024-6.
10. Centers for Disease Control and Prevention. Update: investigation of anthrax associated with intentional exposure and interim public health guidelines, October 2001. *MMWR Morb Mortal Wkly Rep* 2001;50:889-97.
11. APIC Bioterrorism Task Force, Centers for Disease Control and Prevention Hospital Infections Program Bioterrorism Working Group. Bioterrorism Readiness Plan: A Template for Health care Facilities. Available at: http://www.cdc.gov/ncidod/hip/Bio/13apr99APIC-CDCBioterrorism.PDF.

chapter 103

Yersinia Pestis (Plague) Attack

Jeremiah D. Schuur and Jonathan Harris Valente

 ## DESCRIPTION OF EVENT

A bioterrorism event leading to multiple cases of the plague would likely result from airborne dispersal of a weaponized form of *Yersinia pestis* and would cause a pulmonary variant of the plague called *pneumonic plague*.[1] During World War II, in two separate incidents, the Japanese dropped clay pots filled with *Y. pestis*–contaminated rice and fleas over the Chinese cities of Shusien in Chekiang province and Changteh in Hunan province. This tactic led to outbreaks of bubonic plague.[2,3] However, this would not be the optimal way for terrorists to spread the plague because bubonic plague requires a bite from a flea. In addition, bubonic plague is not spread directly from person to person like the pneumonic form.

Pneumonic plague may occur as a secondary pneumonia due to hematogenous spread from bubonic plague. This is the most common form of naturally occurring pneumonic plague. Primary pneumonic plague occurs after inhalation of aerosolized *Y. pestis* bacilli, either from person-to-person transmission or via an intentional attack. Pneumonic plague is rapidly progressive and can spread from person to person via aerosolized droplets. The incubation period for pneumonic plague (1 to 6 days) is shorter than that of the bubonic form (2 to 8 days).[4,5] Control of the disease would be complex because affected people without knowledge of the exposure could spread disease by travel to other regions.[6-8]

Pneumonic plague presents clinically as a rapidly progressive respiratory syndrome that is often associated with fever, cough, shortness of breath, chest pain, hemoptysis, malaise, myalgia, nausea and vomiting, sputum or blood cultures with gram-negative rods, and radiographic findings of pneumonia. Chest roentgenograms of patients with pneumonic plague usually show patchy bronchopneumonic infiltrates as well as segmental or lobar consolidation with or without confluence. They may show cavitary lesions or bilateral diffuse infiltrates characteristic of acute respiratory distress syndrome.[9]

It has been estimated that if 50 kg of weaponized *Y. pestis* were released as an aerosol over a city of 5 million people, pneumonic plague could occur in as many as 150,000 persons, 36,000 of whom would be expected to die.[10]

 ## PREINCIDENT ACTIONS

An intentional plague outbreak should be considered one of the most likely bioterrorism scenarios for which emergency providers need to prepare. Pneumonic plague would most likely occur naturally as a complication of bubonic plague in the setting of a major bubonic plague outbreak.[11] *Y. pestis* is not stable in the environment, and it is readily destroyed by drying and sunlight exposure. If *Y. pestis* were released into the air in a bioterrorism attack, it would likely survive for less than an hour. Due to these factors, preparation for environmental decontamination is less important than in other similar attacks, such as with anthrax.[7,8,10]

No vaccine is currently available. The U.S. manufactured vaccine (Greer) was discontinued in 1999 and was not protective for the pneumonic form of the plague. Research is under way, and a new vaccine protective against pneumonic plague is in advanced development.[6,8] There are no early warning systems for the detection of *Y. pestis* if an aerosolized form were dispersed. In addition, there are no rapid diagnostic tests to detect *Y. pestis* in suspected patients.[8,12]

 ## POSTINCIDENT ACTIONS

All cases of pneumonic plague should be considered terrorism-related until proven otherwise. Hospital infection control officers and local and state, national health, and law enforcement officials should be notified immediately of any suspected cases of the plague.

The risk for reaerosolization of *Y. pestis* from the contaminated clothing of exposed persons is low. Under ideal conditions, *Y. pestis* can survive in the environment for about 1 hour, and since patients will present with symptoms after 24 hours, there is no need for routine decontamination. In situations where there may have been recent, gross exposure to *Y. pestis*, decontamination of skin and potentially contaminated fomites (e.g., clothing or environmental surfaces) may be considered to reduce the risk of cutaneous or bubonic forms of the disease.

The plan for decontaminating patients may include several steps. Patients should be instructed to remove contaminated clothing. Clothing should be stored in labeled, plastic bags and gently handled to avoid dispersal of *Y. pestis*. Patients should be instructed to shower thoroughly with soap and water. Environmental surface decontamination may be performed using an Environmental Protection Agency–registered, facility-approved sporicidal/germicidal agent or a 0.5% hypochlorite solution (one part household bleach added to nine parts water).[1,13,14]

In its natural form, pneumonic plague is transmitted person to person via large droplets (not via fine-particle aerosol) and requires close personal contact (2 meters or less) for effective transmission.[4,15,16] Patients with symptoms suggestive of pneumonic plague should be isolated using droplet precautions in addition to standard precautions. Patients with suspected pneumonic plague should be placed in a private room when possible. It is appropriate to cohort symptomatic patients with similar symptoms and the same presumptive diagnosis (i.e., pneumonic plague) when private rooms are not available. Maintain spatial separation of at least 3 feet between infected patients and others when cohorting is not possible. Avoid placement of patients requiring droplet precautions in the same room with an immunocompromised patient. Special air handling is not necessary, and doors may remain open. Patient transport should be limited to essential medical purposes. When transport is necessary, minimize dispersal of droplets by placing a surgical-type mask on the patient. Isolation precautions should be continued for 2 days after initiation of antibiotics and until some clinical improvement occurs in patients with pneumonic plague.[8]

 ## MEDICAL TREATMENT OF CASUALTIES

Specific antibiotic treatment must be initiated within 24 hours after symptom onset, otherwise pneumonic plague is nearly uniformly fatal.[6,8] Table 103-1 shows the Working Group on Civilian Biodefense's antibiotic recommendations for pneumonic plague.[8] These consensus-based recommendations cover contained exposures, mass casualty exposures, and postexposure prophylaxis. They are based on the best available evidence. However, it should be noted that there is a lack of published trials in treating plague in humans and a limited number of studies in animals. A number of possible therapeutic regimens for treating plague have not been prospectively studied or approved by the Food and Drug Administration.

In a contained casualty setting, parenteral antibiotics are recommended for all symptomatic patients. In a mass casualty incident, local resources must be evaluated and if sufficient supplies of parenteral antibiotics are not available, oral antibiotics may be used. Oral antibiotics should also be given for 7 days as postexposure prophylaxis. Individuals refusing postexposure antibiotics should be observed for fever or cough for 1 week, although isolation is not recommended.[6,8] Several antibiotics that should not be used for pneumonic plague include rifampin, aztreonam, ceftazidime, cefotetan, and cefazolin.[20]

Laboratory testing is needed to confirm pneumonic plague. A sputum Gram stain should be used emergently because it may reveal bipolar staining gram-negative bacilli or coccobacilli. *Y. pestis* is described as having a bipolar (also termed "safety pin") staining best seen with Giemsa or Wayson stains.[21] The only gram-negative bacilli to cause rapidly progressing pulmonary symptoms are *Y. pestis* and *Bacillus anthracis*. Blood or sputum cultures should demonstrate growth within 24 to 48 hours, although some laboratory systems may misidentify *Y. pestis*.[22] Laboratory personnel should be notified when *Y. pestis* is suspected to decrease the chance of laboratory exposure and to increase the diagnostic yield. Biosafety Level 2 conditions are acceptable for routine laboratory procedures.[8] Serologic tests are useful for bubonic plague, but since patients do not seroconvert until between 5 and 20 days postexposure, they would be of little use in a pneumonic plague outbreak.[4]

Due to the severity of pneumonic plague, patients may require advanced supportive measures including mechanical ventilation, pressors, and invasive monitoring. Clinical deterioration despite appropriate antimicrobial treatment should raise the possibility of an antimicrobial-resistant strain of *Y. pestis*. This has been reported to occur naturally as well as via genetic engineering by Soviet scientists.[23]

 ## UNIQUE CONSIDERATIONS

Y. pestis must be considered one of the most likely bacteria to be used as a bioterrorism agent. *Y. pestis* has been used as a biowarfare agent throughout history, it is readily available worldwide in nature and biologic laboratories, and mass production is relatively simple. Although aerosolized *Y. pestis* is not known to have ever been used, it has been successfully weaponized by the former Soviet Union and could be effectively dispersed as an aerosol.[8,23] Under proper conditions, such a release could lead to widespread epidemic pneumonic plague with continued human-to-human transmission. Cases would not present for at least 24 hours after exposure. Pneumonic plague is highly contagious and virulent, and antimicrobial treatment must be initiated within 24 hours to improve survival. Without appropriate antibiotic treatment and supportive care, numerous casualties would result.

 ## PITFALLS

- Failure to notify appropriate public health and law enforcement agencies when an outbreak of pneumonic plague is suspected or confirmed
- Failure to consider pneumonic plague as the etiologic agent in major pneumonia endemics or pandemics
- Failure to use droplet precautions and standard precautions in potential cases of pneumonic plague
- Failure to initiate specific antibiotic therapy within 24 hours of symptom onset
- Failure to provide postexposure antibiotic prophylaxis

TABLE 103-1 RECOMMENDATIONS FOR ANTIMICROBIAL TREATMENT OF PNEUMONIC PLAGUE*

PATIENT CATEGORY	RECOMMENDED THERAPY
Contained Casualty Setting	
Adults	Preferred choices
	Streptomycin, 1 g IM twice daily
	Gentamicin, 5 mg/kg IM or IV once daily or 2 mg/kg loading dose followed by 1.7 mg/kg IM or IV 3 times daily[†]
	Alternative choices
	Doxycycline, 100 mg IV twice daily or 200 mg IV once daily
	Ciprofloxacin, 400 mg IV twice daily[‡]
	Chloramphenicol, 25 mg/kg IV 4 times daily[§]
Children[‖]	Preferred choices
	Streptomycin, 15 mg/kg IM twice daily (maximum daily dose, 2 g)
	Gentamicin, 2.5 mg/kg IM or IV 3 times daily[†]
	Alternative choices
	Doxycycline,
	If >45 kg, give adult dosage
	If <45 kg, give 2.2 mg/kg IV twice daily (maximum, 200 mg/d)
	Ciprofloxacin, 15 mg/kg IV twice daily[‡]
	Chloramphenicol, 25 mg/kg IV 4 times daily[§]
Pregnant women[¶]	Preferred choice
	Gentamicin, 5 mg/kg IM or IV once daily or 2 mg/kg loading dose followed by 1.7 mg/kg IM or IV 3 times daily[†]
	Alternative choices
	Doxycycline, 100 mg IV twice daily or 200 mg IV once daily
	Ciprofloxacin, 400 mg IV twice daily[‡]
Mass Casualty Setting and Postexposure Prophylaxis[#]	
Adults	Preferred choices
	Doxycycline, 100 mg orally twice daily[††]
	Ciprofloxacin, 500 mg orally twice daily[‡]
	Alternative choice
	Chloramphenicol, 25 mg/kg orally 4 times daily[§,**]
Children[‖]	Preferred choice
	Doxycycline,[††]
	If <45 kg, give adult dosage
	If >45 kg, then give 2.2 mg/kg orally twice daily
	Ciprofloxacin, 20 mg/kg orally twice daily
	Alternative choices
	Chloramphenicol, 25 mg/kg orally 4 times daily[§,**]
Pregnant women[¶]	Preferred choices
	Doxycycline, 100 mg orally twice daily[††]
	Ciprofloxacin, 500 mg orally twice daily
	Alternative choices
	Chloramphenicol, 25 mg/kg orally 4 times daily[§,**]

(From Inglesby TV, et al. Consensus Statement: Plague as a Biological Weapon: Medical & Public Health Management. *JAMA*. 2000;283[17]:2281-90.)

*These are consensus recommendations of the Working Group on Civilian Biodefense and are not necessarily approved by the Food and Drug Administration. One antimicrobial agent should be selected. Therapy should be continued for 10 days. Oral therapy should be substituted when patient's condition improves. IM indicates intramuscularly; IV, intravenously.

[†]Aminoglycosides must be adjusted according to renal function. Evidence suggests that gentamicin, 5 mg/kg IM or IV once daily, would be efficacious in children, although this is not yet widely accepted in clinical practice. Neonates up to 1 week of age and premature infants should receive gentamicin, 2.5 mg/kg IV twice daily.

[‡]Other fluoroquinolones can be substituted at doses appropriate for age. Ciprofloxacin dosage should not exceed 1 g/d in children.

[§]Concentration should be maintained between 5 and 20 µg/mL. Concentrations greater than 25 µg/mL can cause reversible bone marrow suppression.[17,18]

[‖]Refer to "Management of Special Groups" for details. In children, ciprofloxacin dose should not exceed 1 g/d, chloramphenicol should not exceed 4 g/d. Children younger than 2 years should not receive chloramphenicol.

[¶]In neonates, gentamicin loading dose of 4 mg/kg should be given initially.[19]

[#]Duration of treatment of plague in mass casualty setting is 10 days. Duration of postexposure prophylaxis to prevent plague infection is 7 days.

[**]Children younger than 2 years should not receive chloramphenicol. Oral formulation available only outside the United States.

[††]Tetracycline could be substituted for doxycycline.

CASE PRESENTATION

It is a Tuesday afternoon in August in your emergency department, and you have just encountered your third patient with a history of high fever, cough, shortness of breath, nausea, vomiting, and chest pain. The first patient was a 24-year-old healthy male diagnosed with pneumonia. He was admitted for intravenous antibiotics and fluids secondary to persistent hypoxia, tachypnea, and dehydration. The second patient was a 40-year-old female with a similar story; however, she needed intubation and admission to the intensive care unit for respiratory distress and hypoxia. You see a few more patients in what appears to be a typical work day. As you read the next chart, you recall that the last name of the woman whom you admitted to the intensive care unit earlier in the morning is the same as this patient's last name; it is her husband. He is an ill-appearing 42-year-old male wearing a T-shirt from the air show that occurred over the weekend. You remember that he had been sweating and coughing while in the emergency department with his wife earlier in the morning. During your interview, he states that he and his wife had been at the air show. "It was a great show. I especially liked the stunt planes that were spraying the smoke!" You finish your evaluation and determine that he also has pneumonia. It is near the end of your shift and one of your colleagues arrives to relieve you. He states, "I'm here for work, but I don't feel that well. I think I may need to call the back-up person in to work. I have been getting this really bad cold, and this morning I had a fever. The kids are all sick, too, with the same thing." It crosses your mind that he was the medical director at the air show.

REFERENCES

1. APIC Bioterrorism Task Force, CDC Hospital Infections Program Bioterrorism Working Group. Bioterrorism Readiness Plan: A Template for Healthcare Facilities. Available at: http://www.cdc.gov/ncidod/hip/Bio/13apr99APIC-CDCBioterrorism.PDF.
2. Noah DL, Huebner KD, Darling RG, et al. The history and threat of biological warfare and terrorism. *Emerg Med Clin North Am.* 2002;20(2):255-71.
3. Williams P, Wallace D. Unit 731: Japan's Secret Biological Warfare in World War II. New York: The Free Press; 1989.
4. Dennis DT, Gage KL, Gratz N, et al. Plague Manual: Epidemiology, Distribution, Surveillance and Control. Available at: http://www.who.int/csr/resources/publications/plague/whocdscsredc992a.pdf.
5. Gani R, Leach S. Epidemiologic determinants for modeling pneumonic plague outbreaks. *Emerg Infectious Dis.* 2004;10(4):608-14.
6. Miller JM. Agents of bioterrorism: preparing for bioterrorism at the community health care level. *Infect Dis Clin North Am.* 2001;15(4):1127-56.
7. US Centers for Disease Control and Prevention. Frequently asked questions (FAQ) about plague. Available at: http://www.bt.cdc.gov/agent/plague/faq.asp.
8. Inglesby TV, Dennis DT, Henderson DA, et al. Plague as a biological weapon: medical and public health management. *JAMA.* 2000;283(17):2281-90.
9. Mettler FA, Mann JM. Radiographic manifestations of plague in New Mexico, 1975-1980. A review of 42 proved cases. *Radiology.* 1981;139:561-5.
10. Health Aspects of Chemical and Biological Weapons. Geneva, Switzerland: World Health Organization; 1970:98-109.
11. Cunha BA. Anthrax, tularemia, plague, ebola, or smallpox as agents of bioterrorism: recognition in the emergency room. *Clin Microbiol Infect.* 2002;8: 489-503.
12. Center for Biosecurity at University of Pittsburgh Medical Center. Plague. Available at: http://www.upmc-biosecurity.org/pages/agents/plague.html.
13. US Centers for Disease Control and Prevention, the Hospital Infection Control Practices Advisory Committee (HICPAC). Recommendations for isolation precautions in hospitals. *Am J Infect Control.* 1996;24:24-52.
14. American Public Health Association. Control of communicable diseases in man. Washington, DC: American Public Health Association; 1995.
15. Meyer K. Pneumonic plague. *Bacteriol Rev.* 1961;25:249-61.
16. Doll JM, Zeitz PS, Ettestad P, Bucholtz AL, Davis T, Gage K. Cat-transmitted fatal pneumonic plague in a person who traveled from Colorado to Arizona. *Am J Trop Med Hyg.* 1994;51:109-14.
17. American Hospital Formulary Service. AHFS Drug Information. Bethesda, Md: American Society of Health System Pharmacists; 2000.
18. Scott JL, Finegold SM, Belkin GA, et al. A controlled double blind study of the hematologic toxicity of chloramphenicol. *New Engl J Med.* 1965;272:113-42.
19. Watterberg KL, Kelly HW, Angelus P, Backstrom C. The need for a loading dose of gentamicin in neonates. *Ther Drug Monit.* 1989;11:16-20.
20. Byrne WR, Welkos SL, Pitt ML, et al. Antibiotic treatment of experimental pneumonic plague in mice. *Antimicrob Agents Chemother.* 1998;42:675-81.
21. McGovern TW, Friedlander AM. Plague. In: Sidell FR, Takafuji ET, Franz DR. Medical Aspects of Chemical and Biological Warfare. Washington, DC: Office of The Surgeon General; 1997:479-502. Available at: http://www.nbc-med.org/SiteContent/HomePage/WhatsNew/MedAspects/Ch-23Rprntblscx699.pdf.
22. Wilmoth BA, Chu MC, Quan TC. Identification of Yersinia pestis by BBL Crystal Enteric/Nonfermenter Identification System. *J Clin Microbiol.* 1996;34:2829-30.
23. Alibek K, Handelman S. Biohazard. New York: Random House; 1999.

chapter 104

Francisella Tularensis (Tularemia) Attack

Irving Jacoby

 ## DESCRIPTION OF EVENT

Tularemia, known also as rabbit fever, hare fever, deerfly fever, or lemming fever, is a zoonotic bacterial illness caused by a small, gram-negative coccobacillus, *Francisella tularensis,* that infects more than 150 animal species, can be transmitted to humans, and is associated with a wide variety of clinical presentations. Reservoirs for this disease include terrestrial and aquatic mammals, such as rabbits, hares, ground squirrels, voles, muskrats, water and other rats, and skunks. Most recently, it has been identified in prairie dogs.[1] Additionally, *F. tularensis* survives in amoebae, which may explain the association of this bacterium with swamps and waterways.[2] The primary vectors are ticks, mosquitoes, and biting flies, such as the deerfly.

Four subspecies are currently recognized by microbiologists, with somewhat different geographic distributions. *F. tularensis* subspecies *tularensis,* also known as Type A, is found almost exclusively in North America and is considered a more virulent strain in humans, whereas the *F. tularensis* subspecies *holarctica* (Type B) is found throughout the northern hemisphere, predominantly in Europe, and is associated with a milder disease state. *F. tularensis* subspecies *novicida* is also found in North America, and subspecies *mediasiatica* is found in Kazakhstan and Uzbekistan.[2] Transmission to humans occurs in a number of ways, including the handling of infected animal tissues or fluids; bites from infected arthropods, particularly ticks and mosquitoes that have fed on infected animals; direct contact or ingestion of contaminated water or food; and via the inhalation of infective aerosols. Examining an open culture plate has resulted in human infection in laboratory workers, and Biosafety Level 3 facilities must be used for work with the organism. Historic origins related to human infection have been presented elsewhere.[3] No human-to-human transmission has ever been documented; hence, isolation is not required. Most naturally occurring cases in the United States are seen from May to August, although infection can occur at any time.

Tularemia is high on the list of dangerous weaponizable biologic agents due to its extreme infectivity once aerosolized, ease of dissemination, and substantial capacity to cause morbidity and mortality. One of the most infectious pathogens known, as few as 10 to 50 inhaled organisms have been shown to be capable of producing disease.[4,5] Tularemia has historically been a part of biologic weapons programs in the last century. It was one of the agents studied at Japanese germ warfare research units operating in Manchuria between 1932 and 1945. Ken Alibek suggests that the tularemia outbreak that infected thousands of Soviet and German soldiers before the Battle of Stalingrad in 1942 was related to weaponized tularemia developed by the Soviets, which spread out of control by wind changes,[6] although this remains controversial.[7] *F. tularensis* weapons were produced and stockpiled at the biologic warfare production facility of the U.S. Army at the Pine Bluff Arsenal, Ark., by 1954 to 1955, but were destroyed by 1973.[8] Vaccine-immune and antibiotic-resistant strains of tularemia were prepared by Biopreparat, the covert Soviet biologic weapons effort, in the 1980s.[6]

Clinical manifestations of disease in humans are varied and often depend on the mode of transmission, site of infection, and the virulence and dose of the infecting organism. Presenting syndromes are glandular, ulceroglandular, oculoglandular, oropharyngeal, pneumonic, typhoidal, and septic.

The most common forms of naturally acquired disease are ulceroglandular and glandular. A cutaneous papule forms at the site of the bite or cutaneous inoculation from an infected animal hide or carcass, and involvement of regional lymph nodes occurs. The pustule suppurates and ulcerates within a few days. Lymph nodes can swell to a large size and resemble the buboes of bubonic plague or the adenopathy of cat scratch disease. An eschar may form and resemble anthrax. Symptoms include fever, chills, headache, and myalgia. Glandular tularemia is present when there is adenopathy without ulceration.

Oculoglandular disease occurs when inoculation takes place directly into the eye, often by a finger that has viable organisms on it, and ulceration of the conjunctiva may be seen. Pronounced chemosis and pre-auricular node enlargement are manifest.

Oropharyngeal tularemia occurs after ingestion of contaminated water or food. Stomatitis, exudative tonsillitis, or pharyngitis may occur with or without ulceration. Lymphadenopathy of cervical or retropharyngeal nodes can be marked.

Tularemia pneumonia follows either inhalation of contaminated aerosols or is secondary to bacterial spread from a local site and is a much more serious form of tularemia. Mortality rates of 30% are reported for this form. The pneumonia is accompanied by hilar adenopathy, dry cough, shortness of breath, and chest pain, either substernal or pleuritic. The term "lawnmower tularemia" was first used when two cases of pneumonic tularemia were reported to have occurred in adolescent males who mowed over a dead rabbit with presumptive aerosolization and inhalation of contaminated fomites. Both were treated with streptomycin and recovered.[9] A larger outbreak was reported with patients who had mowed lawns and cut brush on Martha's Vineyard in 2001.[10] Adult respiratory distress syndrome has been reported in association with tularemic pneumonia.[11]

Typhoidal tularemia refers to illness characterized by systemic infectious manifestations of fever and chills, but without cutaneous, ocular, lymphatic, or pulmonary findings. Diarrhea and abdominal pain may predominate.

Tularemic sepsis is severe and often fatal. The patient is toxic-appearing, confused, and may become comatose. Systemic inflammatory response syndrome (SIRS) may occur with shock and disseminated intravascular coagulation.[11]

Standard blood, wound, and body fluid cultures should be sent for detection of *F. tularensis*. Because the organism may grow on conventional culture media, it is important to notify laboratory personnel of your suspicion for this organism because growth on a plate represents a significant contagion risk to the laboratory worker.[12] Notification in advance may also increase the likelihood of detecting the organism because use of special media can enhance growth and recovery. If organisms suggestive of *Francisella* are grown by a standard hospital laboratory, further steps in identification may need to be halted, with referral of the isolate to a Centers for Disease Control and Prevention (CDC) reference or national laboratory for definitive identification and sensitivity testing. Such laboratories would be part of the CDC's Laboratory Response Network (LRN) where standardized, unpublished protocols are followed when dealing with such suspected agents of bioterrorism.

Other clinical tests for general use can be ordered, such as commercially available serologic tests for *F. tularensis* antibody, antigen capture enzyme-linked immunosorbent assay (cELISA), and polymerase chain reaction/TaqMan assays, for detecting antigen in inactivated clinical samples. If present, pleural fluid should be tapped and sent for staining, culture, and direct fluorescent antibody (DFA) testing.

 PREINCIDENT ACTIONS

Tularemia is typically a rural disease, and, although urban and suburban exposures may occur, occurrence in the latter situations may signal the possibility of a terrorist attack, even when a link to an animal vector can be made, since known contaminated hides or fomites could be circulated as a terrorist act. Given the greater severity of Type A disease and the inhalational route, and the known weaponization of *F. tularensis*, a terrorist attack is most likely to be perpetrated via the aerosolized route. However, identification of an index case is key in defending against a tularemic terrorist attack. An index case may represent autoinoculation by the perpetrator. Detecting an uncommon disease can be enhanced by ongoing public health communications of isolated occurrences or outbreaks in a real-time continuum.[13] The similarity of many of the clinical manifestations of tularemia to other more common syndromic presentations would make it difficult to come up with tularemia as an immediate diagnosis because it is unlikely to be a leading cause of community-acquired pneumonia or conjunctivitis. The careful history of live or dead animal exposures would be an important source of clues to suggest the need for a diagnostic workup for tularemia. Familiarization with the different syndromic presentations of tularemia remains the most important tool in your armamentarium.

Vaccination before exposure is a way of preparing for an attack. The former Soviet Union used a live-attenuated vaccine strain (LVS) for decades, starting in the 1930s, to immunize millions of people living in endemic areas. In the United States, an investigational new drug is approved for clinical trials. A retrospective study of laboratory workers working with *F. tularensis* at a U.S. Army research facility found a decrease in risk of infection from 5.70 cases of typhoidal tularemia per 1000 person-years of risk with a killed vaccine to 0.27 cases per 1000 person-years of risk after introduction of an LVS vaccine.[14] However, the incidence of ulceroglandular tularemia was unchanged, albeit cases were moderated. LVS vaccine is currently the only effective vaccine under investigation, but it is not available for clinical use at this time, since data required for licensing were not adequately documented during the manufacture of current lots, and the older method of growth using shaker culture no longer meets current good manufacturing processes. A new process for production must be devised to obtain licensure.[15] Improved vaccines are needed since the LVS vaccine requires scarification, is cumbersome, and difficult to standardize. Current vaccine efforts are reviewed elsewhere.[15,16]

 POSTINCIDENT ACTIONS

The local or state health department should be alerted if tularemia is highly suspected, particularly if multiple patients present with a compatible illness.

If prompt recognition of an attack with a tularemia bioweapon occurs during the early incubation period, exposed persons should be treated prophylactically, with either doxycycline 100 mg p.o. twice daily or ciprofloxacin 500 mg p.o. bid for 14 days.

If an attack has been identified only after cases are occurring, it has been recommended by the Working Group on Civilian Biodefense that persons potentially exposed should begin a fever watch. Persons who develop an otherwise unexplained fever or flulike illness within 14 days should begin treatment as noted later in the chapter.[17]

If a laboratory worker has had a potentially high-risk infective exposure to *F. tularensis*, such as via a spill, centrifuge accident, needlestick exposure, or exposure to an open culture plate, oral postexposure prophylaxis should be given. With low-risk events, the laboratory worker can be placed on a fever watch and treated if any symptoms develop within 14 days of exposure.

Laboratory spills of infectious *F. tularensis* broth or suspension should be decontaminated with 10% bleach solution; after 10 minutes, it is recommended that 70% solution of alcohol be used to further clean the area and reduce the corrosive effects of the bleach.[17]

Isolation is not recommended for infected patients, given lack of human-to-human transmission. Close contacts of patients with diagnosed disease thus do not require prophylaxis.

If the LVS vaccine were available, immunity would take 2 weeks to develop and hence has no role in protecting against inhalational exposure after the fact.

 ## MEDICAL TREATMENT OF CASUALTIES

Treatment of tularemia is antibiotic-based. The preferred first-line choice of antibiotics for adults is streptomycin 1 g intramuscularly twice daily or gentamicin 5 mg/kg intramuscularly or intravenously once daily for 10 days.[18]

For patients allergic to aminoglycosides, alternatives are doxycycline 100 mg intravenously twice daily; chloramphenicol 15 mg/kg intravenously four times daily for 14 to 21 days. Ciprofloxacin 400 mg intravenously twice daily for 10 days; other fluoroquinolones have also been used.[19]

In pregnant women, preferred choices are gentamicin or streptomycin; alternative choices are ciprofloxacin or doxycycline.

Bioterrorist attacks using resistant strains are a possibility. Culturing to obtain isolates for sensitivity testing is essential. This should be suspected if patients fail to respond to first-line therapy.

Supportive care is critical for fluid management and the detection and treatment of the complications of sepsis, including shock, acute respiratory distress syndrome, disseminated intravascular coagulation, rhabdomyolysis, and organ failure.

 ## UNIQUE CONSIDERATIONS

It would be expected that tularemia would have a slower progression of illness and a lower case fatality rate than inhalational anthrax or pneumonic plague. Presumptive laboratory diagnosis of anthrax or plague would likely be made more rapidly than tularemia, due to the need for referral to reference laboratories.

Outbreaks of tularemia in patients from an urban setting should trigger suspicion of a bioterrorist attack. A World Health Organization expert committee in 1970 gave an estimate that aerosol dispersal of 50 kg of virulent *F. tularensis* over a metropolitan area with 5 million inhabitants would result in 250,000 incapacitating casualties, including 19,000 deaths.[20]

Painful pre-auricular lymphadenopathy is a hallmark of oculoglandular tularemia and distinguishes it from cat scratch disease, tuberculosis, sporotrichosis, and syphilis.

Epidemiologic workup may be needed to determine the reservoir in a given outbreak. The occurrence of an outbreak of tularemia in a war-torn area, although suggestive of possible bioterrorism, can be related to factors such as environmental disruption, as was recently shown in Kosovo.[21]

 ## PITFALLS

Although intuitively one might think that only pneumonic tularemia would occur from an airborne attack with viable organisms, airborne transmission can result in an initial clinical illness without prominent respiratory symptoms.

Mild inhalational disease in a rural setting can be indistinguishable from Q fever.

Due to the many varied presentations of classical tularemia, the differential diagnosis is very broad. Add to

 ### CASE PRESENTATION

You are on duty at an academic medical center emergency department. A 41-year-old male presents for fever, cough, and pleuritic chest pain. The patient reports he has been ill for 3 days. No one else is ill at home. His social history includes the following: No travel, no hunting, and the patient lives in a suburban area of a Midwestern metropolitan area. The review of his systems is positive for diffuse myalgia and shortness of breath. On examination, he is mildly ill-appearing. His pulse is 112; respiratory rate, 20 with splinting respirations; temperature, 103.0; and blood pressure, 114/68 mm Hg. His oxygen saturation is 94% on room air. The patient's skin examination is normal, and no insect or tick bites are found. The HEENT (head, ears, eyes, nose, throat) examination is normal, but some submandibular lymph nodes feel prominent. Lung sounds are decreased in the left base posteriorly, and a pleural friction rub is heard. Chest radiograph shows a widened mediastinum, with a left pleural effusion, but no obvious pulmonary infiltrates are seen. Your differential diagnosis includes viral pleurisy, bacterial empyema, and mediastinitis with its attendant differential. You start the workup by ordering blood and sputum cultures, a complete blood count, differential, electrolytes, liver function tests, and coagulation tests. You mention the case to your double-coverage colleague, who replies that he admitted a similar patient last night from the same suburban neighborhood and had heard about another case during the prior shift. You return to the patient and ask about any unusual occurrences over the past week involving animals or hides, and he reports that he was outdoors 5 days ago in a suburban shopping mall when a spray plane had passed overhead spraying what he had assumed was insecticide for mosquitoes. He wondered whether he might have gotten sprayed with insecticide, which he thought may have caused the illness. You had not heard of such spraying taking place. You call the local health department now, despite no definitive diagnosis, and relay your suspicions of a possible terrorist attack. You then contemplate the differential, adding bioterrorism-type agents; plan further workup and initial treatment; and call the hospitalist to admit the patient for a pleural tap and intravenous antibiotics.

that the unusual manifestations of tularemia, including pericarditis, lymphocytic meningitis, hepatitis, endocarditis, osteomyelitis, sepsis and septic shock, and rhabdomyolysis, and it is apparent that tularemia could be missed easily in the urban setting, until laboratory confirmation is made.

REFERENCES

1. Avashia SB, Petersen JM, Lindley CM, et al. First reported prairie dog-to-human tularemia transmission, Texas, 2002. *Emerging Infect Dis.* 2004;10:483-86.
2. Titball RW, Sjøstedt A. Francisella tularensis: an overview. *Am Soc Microbiol (ASM) News.* 2003;69(11):558-63.
3. Weinberg AN. Commentary: Wherry WB, Lamb BH. Infection of man with Bacterium tularense. *J Infect Dis.* 2004;189:1317-31.
4. Saslaw S, Eigelsbach HT, Prior JA, et al. Tularemia vaccine study. II. Respiratory challenge. *Arch Int Med.* 1961;107:702-14.
5. McCrumb FR. Aerosol infection of man with Pasteurella tularensis. *Bacteriol Rev.* 1961;25:262-7.
6. Alibek K. Biohazard. New York: Dell Publishing; 1999: 15-28, 29-38.
7. Croddy E, Krcalova S. Editorial: tularemia, biological warfare and the battle for Stalingrad (1942-43). *Milit Med.* 2001;166(10):837-8.
8. Franz DR, Parrott CD, Takafuji ET. The U.S. biological warfare and biological defense programs. In: Sidell FR, Takafuji ET, Franz DR, eds. Textbook of Military Medicine, Part I: Warfare, Weaponry and the Casualty: Medical Aspects of Chemical and Biological Warfare. Washington, DC: Office of the Surgeon General, Department of the Army; 1997:425-36.
9. McCarthy VP, Murphy MD. Lawnmower tularemia. *Pediatr Infect Dis J.* 1990;9:298-9.
10. Feldman KA, Enscore RE, Lathrop SL, et al. An outbreak of primary pneumonic tularemia on Martha's Vineyard. *New Engl J Med.* 2001;345:1601-6.
11. Sunderrajan EV, Hutton J, Marienfeld D. Adult respiratory distress syndrome secondary to tularemia pneumonia. *Arch Int Med.* 1985;145:1435-7.
12. Shapiro DS, Schwartz DR. Exposure of laboratory workers to Francisella tularensis despite a bioterrorism procedure. *J Clin Microbiol.* 2002;40(6):2778-81.
13. Dembeck ZF, Buckman RL, Fowler SK, et al. Missed sentinel case of naturally occurring pneumonic tularemia outbreak: lessons for detection of bioterrorism. *J Am Board Fam Pract.* 2003;16: 339-42.
14. Burke DS. Immunization against tularemia: analysis of the effectiveness of live Francisella tularensis vaccine in prevention of laboratory-acquired tularemia. *J Infect Dis.* 1977;135:55-60.
15. Nierengarten MB, Lutwick LI. Biowarfare vaccines: developing new tularemia vaccines. Medscape Infectious Diseases 2004; Available at: http://www.medscape.com/viewarticle/431539.6.
16. Ellis J, Oyston PC, Green M, et al. Tularemia. *Clin Microbiol Rev.* 2002;15(4):631-46.
17. Dennis DT, Inglesby TV, Henderson DA, et al. Tularemia as a biological weapon: medical and public health management. *JAMA.* 2001;285(21):2763-73.
18. Enderlin G, Morales L, Jacobs RF, et al. Streptomycin and alternative agents for the treatment of tularemia: review of the literature. *Clin Infect Dis.* 1994;19(1):42-7.
19. Johansson A, Berglund L, Gothefors L, et al. Ciprofloxacin for treatment of tularemia in children. *Pediatr Infect Dis.* 2000;19(5):449-53.
20. Health Aspects of Chemical and Biological Weapons. Geneva, Switzerland: World Health Organization; 1970:105-7.
21. Reintjes R, Dedushaj I, Gjini A, et al. Tularemia outbreak investigation in Kosovo: case control and environmental studies. *Emerg Infect Dis.* 2002;8(1):1-8.

chapter 105

Brucella Species (Brucellosis) Attack

Teriggi J. Ciccone

DESCRIPTION OF EVENT

Brucellosis, also known as Mediterranean fever, undulant fever, and Malta fever, is a protean clinical syndrome caused by a number of species within the genus *Brucella*. *Brucellae* are small, gram-negative aerobic coccobacilli. Clinical cases of brucellosis are rare in North America, occurring almost exclusively in workers exposed to livestock; however, the syndrome is endemic throughout agrarian areas with poor food and sanitation standards, such as in the Middle East, India, and Latin America. Domesticated animals such as cattle, swine, sheep, and dogs comprise *Brucellae's* natural reservoir.

One of the first biologic agents to be weaponized by the United States,[1] *Brucella* is classified as a category B agent by the Centers for Disease Control and Prevention (CDC).[2] Several characteristics of *Brucellae* make them ideal candidates for production into biologic weapons. *Brucellae* can be manipulated in the laboratory and manufactured into particles measuring 1 to 5 μm in diameter. Particles of this size are ideally suited to enter into and remain in the alveolar spaces of the lung where they initiate the disease process described later in the chapter. Such weaponized particles are highly virulent, with only 10 to 100 organisms required to cause infection.[3] Additionally, *Brucellae* species are very hardy organisms and can survive for prolonged periods in storage and under hostile conditions. In soil or water, these organisms may survive for up to 10 weeks.[4] However, unlike the CDC category A agents (*Bacillus anthracis*, *Francisella tularensis*), the *Brucellae* have very low mortality among immunocompetent hosts, with only about a 2% mortality rate.[5,6] Additionally, a prolonged incubation period on the scale of months between exposure and clinical illness limits the terrorist's ability to cause a large number of casualties in a short time period.

Due to the low mortality and prolonged incubation period, medical and public health officials may not recognize a *Brucella* attack for quite some time. The most likely scenario would involve a large number of otherwise healthy individuals presenting over weeks to months with vague, multisystem complaints. An attack would most likely occur in an urban area where airborne particles could be spread over a heavily populated area. Once a few cases of brucellosis are confirmed in an urban area among persons without exposure to domesticated animals, the possibility of a bioattack should be highly considered.

In affected individuals, after respiratory, gastrointestinal, or mucous membrane inoculation, the bacteria spread hematogenously to various organ systems. Weeks to months later, clinical manifestations begin to arise. Patients experience intermittent and irregular fevers over weeks and possibly months. Other constitutional symptoms such as chills, fatigue, malaise, sweats, and headache may occur. Pulmonary manifestations are generally rare, even after inhalation.[6] Patients may complain of cough in addition to constitutional symptoms. Interstitial pneumonitis, hilar lymphadenopathy, pleural effusions, and empyema may be found on chest x-ray. Gastrointestinal manifestations are more common, and involve nausea, vomiting, anorexia, diarrhea, and abdominal pain. Rarer gastrointestinal manifestations include hepatitis, pancreatitis, cholangitis, or hepatic and splenic abscesses. Musculoskeletal manifestations, such as arthralgias of the axial skeleton and larger joints, occur in up to 60% of patients[4] and may offer the most specific clue to the diagnosis of brucellosis. Sacroiliitis is most commonly found, and may proceed to osteomyelitis. Central nervous system manifestations occur rarely and may range from depression to meningoencephalitis.[7] Acute orchitis and epididymitis have been reported.[8] Although rare, endocarditis is the most common cause of death from *Brucellae* infections.[9]

Laboratory data are generally low yield and nonspecific; however, anemia with thrombocytopenia may be found on complete blood count. Serum white blood cell count may reveal lymphocytic pleocytosis. Elevated liver transaminases may occur in cases of hepatic involvement. *Brucellae* species grow quite slow in culture media, and cultures should be maintained for 4 to 6 weeks if the diagnosis is suspected. Bone marrow cultures have been shown to provide a higher yield than blood cultures.[6]

PREINCIDENT ACTIONS

Hospital, emergency department, and outpatient facilities should all have general disaster plans in place in the event

621

of a bioterrorist attack. Mass casualty events require coordination of local, state, and federal public safety resources. Both emergency medical service and hospital-based triage systems may need to be altered in the event of a large number of patients seeking medical care within a brief time period. Isolation procedures should be in place in the event of an attack with known person-to-person transmission. However, transmission of *Brucellae* species between individuals is not believed to occur, and no specific isolation precautions are needed in patients suspected of having brucellosis. The possibility of contracting brucellosis by inhalation of particles in culture among laboratory workers is significant, and negative-pressure isolation measures and Biosafety Level 3 procedures should be used within laboratories. Healthcare providers should practice universal precautions.

Since a true mass casualty scenario after a *Brucella* attack is unlikely, physicians and other healthcare providers must remain vigilant in identifying trends that may correspond with an outbreak of brucellosis. These trends may only be noted over days to weeks with an increasing volume of otherwise healthy patients with fever and multiple systemic complaints that came on insidiously and have persisted for prolonged time periods.

 ## POSTINCIDENT ACTIONS

Clinicians with a high level of suspicion of a possible *Brucella* attack or confirmatory data of a case of brucellosis should notify the appropriate local, state, and federal public health and law enforcement authorities. Materials and surfaces possibly contaminated by brucellosis patients should be disinfected with 0.5% hypochlorite solution.[1]

 ## MEDICAL TREATMENT OF CASUALTIES

Antibiotic treatment for brucellosis requires multiple agents. Prolonged antibiotic therapy is required to prevent relapse of disease. Most cases can be successfully treated with doxycycline 100 mg twice daily plus rifampin 600 to 900 mg daily for 6 weeks. In more severe cases, streptomycin 1 g intramuscularly daily should be substituted for rifampin during the first 3 weeks.[10] In children, substituting doxycycline with trimethoprim-sulfamethoxazole has been used; however, relapse rates are high when compared with the doxycycline/rifampin regimen.[11]

Although no formal recommendations exist for postexposure prophylaxis, high-risk patients after a *Brucella* attack may be considered to receive a 3-week course of doxycycline and rifampin. Currently, no vaccine is available for brucellosis.

 ## UNIQUE CONSIDERATIONS

Brucellae species are small, gram-negative bacteria that cause a wide spectrum of clinical symptoms and signs in infected humans. Even though they are considered to be a possible bioweapon due to their high virulence when inhaled, *Brucellae* species have a disadvantage when compared with other inhaled bacteria due to their low mortality and prolonged incubation period. This makes the identification of a possible *Brucella* attack extremely difficult. In the event of a *Brucella* attack, the only clue may be the presentation of a large number of healthy individuals over days to weeks with prolonged fevers and a myriad of multisystem complaints. Additionally, providers should be aware that treatment for brucellosis requires multiple antibiotic agents and a prolonged treatment regimen to prevent relapse.

 ## PITFALLS

- Failure to prepare adequate systems to respond to possible terrorist attacks before the attacks occur
- Failure to consider brucellosis as the etiologic factor for persistent fever in patients
- Failure to consider a *Brucella* attack in the setting of a large number of otherwise healthy people who present over days to weeks with a wide range of vague complaints
- Failure to treat cases of brucellosis with multiple agents over a prolonged time period to prevent relapse
- Failure to notify appropriate public health and law enforcement agencies when an outbreak of brucellosis is suspected or confirmed among persons with no exposure to domesticated animals

 ### CASE PRESENTATION

During the past few weeks, both your own emergency department and other departments throughout the city have seen a 20% increase in patient volume. A large number of otherwise healthy individuals are presenting with a wide variety of complaints, most notably fevers and malaise that last for weeks. Public health officials are puzzled and have reluctantly announced that a "viral syndrome" is sweeping the city. On a busy Wednesday morning, you see a 30-year-old graduate student with no medical history who is complaining of fever, fatigue, vomiting, difficulty concentrating, and low back pain. He is unable to tolerate oral fluids, and as a result, he is admitted for dehydration. Persistent low back pain as an inpatient prompts his healthcare providers to perform a bone scan, which reveals evidence of osteomyelitis. Bone cultures taken during debridement have not shown any microorganism growth after 72 hours. Meanwhile, hospitals citywide are getting busier and busier with case of "viral syndromes."

REFERENCES

1. Greenfield RA, Drevets DA, Machado LJ, et al. Bacterial pathogens as biological weapons and agents of bioterrorism. *Am J Med Sci.* 2002;232:299-315.

2. Khan AS, Sage MJ. Biological and chemical terrorism: strategic planning, preparedness, and response. *Morb Mortal Wkly Rep.* 2000;49:1-14.

3. Bellamy RJ, Freedman AR. Bioterrorism. *QJM.* 2001;94:227-34.

4. Franz DR, Jahrling PB, Friedlander AM, et al. Clinical recognition and management of patients exposed to biological warfare agents. *JAMA.* 1997;278: 399-411.

5. Chin J, Asner MS, eds. Control of Communicable Disease Manual. 17th ed. Washington, DC: American Public Health Association; 2000.

6. Young EJ. An overview of human brucellosis. *Clin Infect Dis.* 1995; 21:283-90.

7. Young EJ. Brucella species. In: Mandell GL, Bennett JE, Dolin R, eds. Principles and Practice of Infectious Disease. 5th ed. Vol 2. Philadelphia: Churchill Livingstone; 2000:2386-93.

8. Khan MS, Humayoon MS, Al Manee MS. Epididymo-orchitis and brucellosis. *Br J Urol.* 1989;63:87-9.

9. Al-Harthi SS. The morbidity and morality pattern of brucella endocarditis. *Int J Cardiol.* 1989;25:321-4.

10. Ariza J, Gudiol F, Pallares R, et al. Treatment of human brucellosis with doxycycline plus rifampin or doxycycline plus streptomycin. *Ann Intern Med.* 1992;117:25-30.

11. Lubani MM, Dudin KI, Sharda DC, et al. A Multicenter therapeutic study of 1100 children with brucellosis. *Pediatr Infect Dis J.* 1989;8:75-8.

chapter 106

Coxiella burnetii (Q Fever) Attack

Teriggi J. Ciccone

DESCRIPTION OF EVENT

Q fever is a febrile illness caused by a gram-negative, intracellular rickettsia *Coxiella burnetii*. The name Q fever derives from "Query fever," the original name given to the syndrome first noted among abattoir workers in Australia in the 1930s.[1] *C. burnetii* is maintained in a large natural reservoir within mammals, birds, and arthropods. Natural human infection occurs primarily in persons exposed to livestock including sheep, goats, and cattle. The organism is shed in urine, feces, milk, and birth products from infected livestock, after which aerosolized particles inhaled by the victim result in infection. Placental tissues contain especially high amounts of infectious particles, and persons exposed to parturient livestock are at particularly high risk. Infection can also occur via ingestion of unpasteurized milk from infected animals. Far less commonly, infection can occur through an arthropod vector, particularly ticks. Natural infections occur worldwide, with reports from all continents with the exception of Antarctica. Rarely, infection has occurred with blood transfusions, sexual contact, and transplacental transmission to newborns. Person-to-person transmission has been reported, but is believed to be extremely rare.

C. burnetii is classified as a category B agent by the Centers for Disease Control and Prevention.[2] Although its use in warfare has never been described, military personnel have become infected with *C. burnetii* in endemic areas.[3] The U.S. military stockpiled *C. burnetii* in its biologic arsenal until 1971, when these agents were destroyed.[3,4]

Multiple factors contribute to *C. burnetii's* use as a biologic weapon. This agent is highly virulent, with inhalation of a single particle sufficient to cause disease in some patients.[3,4] Additionally, the spore-like form of *C. burnetii* can survive for weeks to months in the natural environment, resistant to both heat and desiccation, and can spread over large distances while airborne.[3-7] The release of infectious particles within or over a major population center would result in tens of thousands of infections.[7] However, *C. burnetii* infection carries a relatively low fatality rate. In a large case series, Raoult and colleagues reported 13 deaths among 1383 cases of Q fever over 14 years, most frequently from myocarditis,[8] somewhat limit-ing *C. burnetii's* ability to cause a mass-fatality disaster scenario. A biologic attack with *C. burnetii* would more likely cause a "temporarily incapacitating illness."[4]

Infection with *C. burnetii* results in a wide spectrum of human disease. Identification of a biologic attack using aerosolized *C. burnetii* would be difficult for healthcare, public health, and law enforcement officials due to lack of a specific clinical syndrome and a variable incubation period. The most likely scenario for a *C. burnetii* outbreak would involve a cluster of previously healthy persons presenting with a nonspecific febrile illness over days to weeks. Once the diagnosis of *C. burnetii* infection was confirmed in patients without significant risk factors (e.g., exposure to livestock), the possibility of a biologic weapon attack must be considered.

Acute symptomatic infection occurs in 50% to 77% of victims, with asymptomatic seroconversion occurring in nearly all other victims.[8,9] Disease severity is inversely proportional to the amount of inoculum to which the victim is exposed.[3,4] Presumably, a biologic attack with aerosolized *C. burnetii* would expose victims to a relatively high level of inoculum, and thus a greater number of patients with acute disease. A nonspecific febrile illness with fever, chills, malaise, fatigue, anorexia, and headache occurs after an incubation period of 10 to 40 days.[3,4,8] Patients frequently recover from this syndrome without treatment.

Q fever pneumonia occurs in 17% to 50% of cases.[4,8] Patients may complain of cough and pleuritic chest pain. Chest radiographs are most often consistent with an atypical pneumonia, although consolidation and pleural effusion may be found.[10] Frequently, patients will have positive chest radiographic findings without pulmonary symptoms.[11]

Thirty to forty percent of victims will develop hepatitis[4,8] with abdominal pain and tenderness, hepatomegaly, and elevated serum transaminases. Sonographic liver imaging or liver biopsy may reveal a granulomatous hepatitis. Jaundice is a rare finding.[12]

Rarely, endocarditis, myocarditis, meningoencephalitis, and osteomyelitis have been reported, each accounting for about 1% of acute cases of Q fever in a large series of patients.[8] Fatalities from acute Q fever are most often the result of myocarditis. Infection in pregnant women is associated with spontaneous abortion.[8,13]

Chronic Q fever affects up to 23% of patients with *C. burnetii* infection.[8] The most prominent clinical manifestation is endocarditis, affecting 60% to 73% of patients with chronic infection.[8,12] Patients with pre-existing valvular disease and prosthetic valves are at the highest risk.[11] Other chronic syndromes include arterial aneurysms, osteomyelitis, chronic hepatitis, and chronic fatigue syndrome.

Laboratory data are often nonspecific in acute Q fever. Total serum white blood cell count is usually normal. Thrombocytopenia is a common finding. Increased serum transaminase levels are found in a majority of patients. Elevations in erythrocyte sedimentation rate, smooth muscle antibodies, and antiphospholipase antibodies may be found.[12] In chronic Q fever, increases in serum transaminases, creatinine, and rheumatoid factor have been reported.[12]

Diagnosis of *C. burnetii* infection is confirmed by serologic testing. Laboratory methods include complement fixation, indirect fluorescent antibody assays, enzyme-linked immunosorbent assays (ELISA) and macroagglutination and microagglutination. ELISA is regarded as the most sensitive serologic test, with sensitivities greater than 90%.[12] Culture of *C. burnetii*, technically difficult and potentially hazardous to laboratory personnel, is rarely performed.

 PREINCIDENT ACTIONS

General preparation for a possible biologic attack requires that hospitals, emergency departments, public health authorities, and law enforcement officials have disaster plans in place before any attack occurs. A clear chain of command should be established in the event of a disaster that coordinates the actions of these various groups. The volume of patients presenting after such an attack may overwhelm the standard resources of emergency medical services and healthcare facilities, and disaster-based methods of triage should be instituted. Isolation and decontamination procedures should be in place to prevent person-to-person transmission of hazardous substances. Local and regional supplies of critical antidotes and antibiotics should be maintained. Mass-casualty drills should be performed to test the multisystem response to potential biologic attacks and determine where improvements need to be made.

Because person-to-person transmission of *C. burnetii* is thought to be extremely rare, no specific isolation precautions are required. Healthcare workers should practice universal precautions at all times. Laboratory workers handling biologic samples possibly contaminated with *C. burnetii* should work under Biosafety Level 2 precautions, including limited lab access to trained personnel, working in safety hoods with potentially aerosolized materials, and strict protocols for disposal of sharps and autoclaving potentially hazardous materials.

 POSTINCIDENT ACTIONS

Confirmation or suspicion of *C. burnetii* infection in an individual or group without significant exposure to domesticated animals should alert the clinician to the possibility of a biologic attack. Hospital infection control personnel should be consulted. Local, regional, and federal public health and law enforcement officials should be notified. Material and surfaces contaminated with *C. burnetii* should be disinfected with a 0.05% hypochlorite solution.[14]

 MEDICAL TREATMENT OF CASUALTIES

Although most cases of Q fever resolve spontaneously without treatment, antibiotic treatment should be started in confirmed or suspected cases to shorten the course of illness and to reduce the number of complications. Tetracyclines are considered the drug of choice for acute Q fever.[3,4] A standard regimen with 100 mg of doxycycline given twice daily for 14 to 21 days provides adequate coverage for most adults.[12,15] Macrolide and quinolone antibiotics have also been shown to have effect against *C. burnetii*.[3,6] Patients with preexisting valvular heart disease or prosthetic heart valves require a prolonged course of treatment to prevent endocarditis. A combination of doxycycline and hydroxychloroquine (600 mg/d) should be given for 1 year.[14] Treatment of known Q fever endocarditis requires 1 to 3 years of treatment with doxycycline and hydroxychloroquine.[16] In pregnant women with Q fever, treatment with co-trimoxazole during the first two trimesters has

 CASE PRESENTATION

For the past 3 days, emergency departments and emergency medical services throughout the city have been overloaded. A large number of otherwise healthy persons are presenting with complaints of fever, chills, and headache. Many patients have been diagnosed with viral syndromes and atypical pneumonias, then discharged home.

You are treating a young man with similar symptoms who had been seen 3 days before in another emergency department, where he was diagnosed with "viral pneumonia." He now complains of persistent fever, chills, cough, nausea, and mild abdominal pain. His liver is palpable 3 cm below the costal margin, and he has mild right upper quadrant pain. A chest radiograph demonstrates bilateral interstitial infiltrates. Routine blood testing reveals thrombocytopenia and elevated serum transaminases. He is admitted, and on hospital day 2 he begins complaining of mild chest pain. An electrocardiogram reveals nonspecific ST-segment and T-wave changes. Viral myocarditis is suspected. On hospital day 4, an astute infectious disease consultant recommends serologic testing for *C. burnetii* despite the fact that the patient has had no known high-risk exposures. ELISA test results are positive for antibodies to *C. burnetii*. Public health and law enforcement officials are notified, and testing on other patients reveals a large number of Q fever cases, prompting an investigation into a possible biologic attack.

been shown to reduce the incidence of spontaneous abortion,[16] and treatment with macrolides in the third trimester would be appropriate to avoid kernicterus. In children, co-trimoxazole administered at a dosage of 4 mg/kg every 12 hours is a possible treatment regimen. Alternative regimens include doxycycline at 2.2 mg/kg every 12 hours, chloramphenicol 25 mg/kg/day divided every 6 hours, or erythromycin 50 mg/kg/day divided every 6 hours.

A formalin-killed vaccine to *C. burnetii* is available for high-risk personnel such as abattoir workers, veterinarians, and laboratory workers.[3,4] A single vaccination is 95% effective against aerosolized *C. burnetii* and offers protection for up to 5 years.[4]

 ## UNIQUE CONSIDERATIONS

Acute infection with *C. burnetii* causes a nonspecific febrile illness. The time of onset after exposure and the severity of disease are proportional to the amount of inoculum. The ability of *C. burnetii* to cause infection with as few as one infective particle, in addition to the spore-like form's ability to be spread as an aerosol over large distances, make this agent a possible biologic weapon. Release of *C. burnetii* particles over a large population center would result in a high number of casualties over days to weeks. As the clinical syndrome caused by *C. burnetii* infection is relatively nonspecific, healthcare, public health, and law enforcement officials should maintain a high index of suspicion for Q fever when a large number of previously healthy persons without exposure to livestock or other domesticated animals become ill with a febrile illness over a brief time period. The combination of pneumonia with hepatitis should alert the physician to the possibility of Q fever. Once cases of Q fever are confirmed in otherwise low-risk persons, the possibility of biologic attack should be highly considered.

 ## PITFALLS

Several potential pitfalls in response to an attack exist. These include the following:

- Failure to establish disaster plans for a possible biologic attack. Healthcare, public health, and law enforcement systems should have a coordinated plan in place with a clear chain of command before any attack occurs.

- Failure to consider Q fever when a large number of persons present over a brief period of time with non-specific febrile illnesses.
- Failure to consider Q fever in patients with fever, pneumonia, and hepatitis.
- Failure to begin appropriate antibiotic treatment in cases of acute Q fever to prevent more severe chronic forms of disease such as endocarditis.
- Failure to notify appropriate infection control, public health, and law enforcement officials when cases of Q fever are diagnosed or suspected.

REFERENCES

1. Derrick EH. "Q" fever, new fever entity: clinical features, diagnosis, and laboratory investigation. *Med J Aust.* 1937;2:281-99.
2. Khan AS, Sage MJ, Groseclose SL, et al. Biological and chemical terrorism: strategic plan for preparedness and response. *MMWR* 2000;49(RR04):1-14.
3. Byrne WR. Q fever. In: Zajtchuk GR, Bellamy RF, eds. *Textbook of Military Medicine: Part I, Warfare, Weaponry, and the Casualty.* Washington, DC: The Borden Institute; 1997:523-37.
4. Q fever. In: Kortepeter M, Christopher G, Cieslak T, et al, eds. *USAMRIID's Medical Management of Biological Casualties Handbook.* 4th ed. Fort Detrick, Md: U.S. Army Medical Research Institute of Infectious Disease; 2001:33-6.
5. Bartlett JG. Questions about Q fever. *Medicine* 2000;79(5):124-5.
6. Franz DR, Jahrling PB, Friedlander AM, et al. Clinical recognition and management of patients exposed to biological warfare agents. *JAMA* 1997;278(5):399-411.
7. World Health Organization. *Health Aspects of Chemical and Biological Weapons: Report of a WHO Group of Consultants.* Geneva: WHO; 1970.
8. Raoult D, Tissot-Dupont H, Foucault C, et al. Q fever 1985-1998: clinical and epidemiologic features of 1383 infections. *Medicine* 2000;79(2):109-23.
9. Dupuis G, Petite J, Peter O, et al. An important outbreak of human Q fever in a Swiss alpine valley. *Int J Epidemiol.* 1987;16:282.
10. Franz DR, Jahrling PB, Friedlander AM, et al. Clinical recognition and management of patients exposed to biological warfare agents. *JAMA* 1997;278(5):399-411.
11. Marrie TJ. *Coxiella burnetii* (Q fever). In: Mandel GL, Bennett JE, Dolin R, eds. *Principles and Practice of Infectious Diseases.* 5th ed. Philadelphia: Churchill Livingstone; 2000:2043-50.
12. Raoult D, Marrie T. Q fever. *Clin Infect Dis.* 1995;20:489-95.
13. Raoult D, Stein A. Q fever during pregnancy, a risk to women, fetuses, and obstetricians. *N Engl J Med.* 1994;330:371.
14. Greenfield RA, Drevets DA, Machado LJ, et al. Bacterial pathogens as biological weapons and agents of bioterrorism. *Am J Med Sci.* 2002;232:299-315.
15. Centers for Disease Control and Prevention. Q fever—California, Georgia, Pennsylvania, and Tennessee, 2000-2001. *MMWR* 2002;51:924-7.
16. Raoult D, Fenollar F, Stein A. Q fever during pregnancy: diagnosis, treatment, and follow-up. *Arch Intern Med.* 2002;162:701-4.

chapter 107

Rickettsia prowazekii Attack (Typhus Fever)

Vittorio J. Raho And Jonathan A. Edlow

 DESCRIPTION OF EVENT

Historically, the most devastating disease caused by *Rickettsia* bacteria with respect to sheer numbers of human casualties and associated morbidity is epidemic (or louse-borne) typhus (ET). Often rampant during times of war and poverty, plaguing survivors of natural disasters, erupting among prison populations, and even described to be present aboard pirate ships of the eighteenth century, ET has played a significant role throughout recent history.[1,2] Caused by the bacteria *Rickettsia prowazekii* and spread among humans by the body louse, it has been described as an illness that has determined the outcome of major wars. The primary vector of transmission—the body louse—lives in clothes and is supported by conditions of poor hygiene and crowding. As the louse takes a human blood meal, it defecates; as a consequence, it passes bacterial organisms onto the skin of the victim.[3] The local irritation and pruritus stimulates scratching, causing minor trauma and allowing autoinoculation of the microbes. The disease is then spread rapidly from person to person via the infected lice. The illness has also been reported to spread in the form of dried louse feces in an aerosolized route by passing through mucous membranes of the eyes and oropharynx.[3] Other than humans, the only known reservoir for *R. prowazekii* are flying squirrels of the eastern United States, with multiple documented human cases confirmed by the CDC, although the exact mechanism of transmission remains unclear.[4]

Clinical manifestations of ET occur after a 1- to 2-week incubation period and begin with the abrupt onset of extreme exhaustion, severe headache, and high fever. Approximately 5 days after the onset of fever, a maculopapular rash erupts, often beginning on the axillae and upper trunk and spreading to involve the entire body excluding the palms, soles, and face.[5] The rash may evolve over time from macular to papular, and eventually petechial to frank purpura as the course of illness progresses. Also described are photophobia; neurologic manifestations including confusion, delirium, and coma; injected conjunctivae; "dry-brown tongue" changes; and extremity manifestations including gangrenous digits.[3] If untreated, the illness can become severe with vascular collapse, hypotension, renal failure, disseminated intravascular coagulation, pneumonia, and encephalitis, with reported mortality approaching 15% to 40%.[1,6,7]

Early laboratory data are nonspecific and may include marked thrombocytopenia, elevated liver function test results, and normal or decreased white blood cell count.

 PREINCIDENT ACTIONS

Currently, there is no established system for ET surveillance in the United States. Cases are so infrequent that commercial testing is generally unavailable. *R. prowazekii* infection can be confirmed through the use of polymerase chain reaction, serologic testing for immunoglobulin G and M titers, and culture.[8] The most efficient means to identify collected specimens is usually through state public health laboratories for specific CDC molecular testing.

 POSTINCIDENT ACTIONS

If a large-scale attack or outbreak of ET is suspected, several immediate actions may help prevent its spread and decrease mortality. First, proper communication channels must be established; hospitals and emergency departments must set up the proper triage system and isolation rooms necessary to deal with a transmissible infectious illness. Healthcare workers and first responders should take proper body substance isolation precautions. Cleansing of known exposed areas with cyfluthrine has been successfully used in prison outbreaks.[9] Exposed persons who may contain infected lice or dried louse feces should be treated as potential sources of infection and should be decontaminated, isolated, and cleansed. Dusting of exposed persons with permethrin 0.5% powder, and more important, removal and incineration of all clothing and linen articles is required.[9]

 MEDICAL TREATMENT OF CASUALTIES

In all *Rickettsial* infections, antibiotic choice is crucial because the organisms are naturally resistant to all

627

beta-lactams.[10] According to practice guidelines, the current recommended treatment for suspected ET is a single oral 200-mg dose of doxycycline, although most clinicians extend this treatment until patients are afebrile for 72 hours.[11,12] Some authorities recommend 100 mg of doxycycline twice a day for the same duration.[13] Pregnant women and those unable to take tetracycline antibiotics may be treated with 500 mg of chloramphenicol four times a day for the same duration. The remainder of treatment consists of supportive medical care and management of the numerous possible complications of the illness. Postexposure prophylaxis has been successfully used among prison populations,[9] but the decision to treat large numbers of low-risk persons should be made at a public health level. Vaccines have been used successfully by the U.S. military.[14]

 ## UNIQUE CONSIDERATIONS

Most *Rickettsia* bacteria have life cycles that require a strict intracellular existence. They are therefore unable to survive the extracellular environment long enough to be freely transmissible and usually require some means of inoculation through the skin via an arthropod vector. *R. prowazekii*, however, has been reported to spread by the aerosol route and thus has the potential to be manufactured into a bioweapon.

CASE PRESENTATION

On a Thursday afternoon, two men in their 30s who are otherwise healthy and have no chronic medical conditions present from their office downtown to the emergency department after experiencing the rapid onset of high fevers to 104°F, severe exhaustion and weakness, severe headache, myalgias, and nausea and vomiting. The results of their initial workup are nonspecific and include a negative chest radiograph and a negative lumbar puncture, and only thrombocytopenia was noted on the CBC. They are started on empiric antibiotics and admitted to the hospital, as are numerous other people from the same building for similar presentations at other hospitals. The symptoms now include confusion and delirium, and rashes were described beginning on the chest and spreading with purpuric features.

Epidemiologic data months after the outbreak demonstrate a crude mortality rate around 12%, with a total of 196 patients ill—all from the same building complex. When their empiric antibiotic regimens are compared, a strong predictor of mortality appears to be the absence of tetracycline-class antibiotics. It is suspected that a ventilation system attack using an aerosol form of ET was carried out.

 ## PITFALLS

Several potential pitfalls in response to an outbreak of ET exist. These include the following:

- Failure to consider ET as a potential cause of acute, febrile illness during such an outbreak
- Failure to ensure proper decontamination and isolation of suspected exposed persons
- Failure to initiate early empiric therapy when the disease is highly suspected
- Waiting for confirmatory blood test or biopsy results or the presence of a rash before beginning treatment in a suspected case
- Failure to report suspected cases to the state department of public health or affiliated authority for appropriate CDC notification and proper serologic testing
- Failure to alert local and state agencies to a suspected biologic attack when presented with a cluster of unusual and uncommon illnesses
- Failure to use doxycycline in adults and children unless absolutely contraindicated

REFERENCES

1. Centers for Disease Control and Prevention. Viral and Rickettsial Zoonoses Branch Web site. Available at: http://www.cdc.gov/ncidod/dvrd/branch/vrzb.htm.
2. Zinsser H. *Rats, Lice and History*. Boston: Little, Brown;1934.
3. Fauci AS, Braunwald E, Isselbacher KJ, et al. *Harrison's Principles of Internal Medicine*. 14th ed. McGraw-Hill; 1998:1045-7.
4. Reynolds MG, Krebs JW, Comer JA, et al. Flying squirrel-associated typhus, United States. *Emerg Infect Dis*. [serial online] 2003 Oct. Available at: http://www.cdc.gov/ncidod/EID/vol9no10/03-0278. htm.
5. Raoult D, Roux V, Ndihokubwayo JB, et al. Jail fever (epidemic typhus) outbreak in Burundi. *Emerg Infect Dis*. 1997;3:357-60.
6. Watanabe M. An outbreak of epidemic louse-borne typhus in Tokyo 1914: a study on the prevention of epidemics [Japanese]. *Nippon Ishigaku Zasshi*. 2002;48:597-616.
7. Raoult D, Ndihokubwayo JB, Tissot-Dupont H, et al. Outbreak of epidemic typhus associated with trench fever in Burundi. *Lancet* 1998;352:353-8.
8. La Scola B, Raoult D. Laboratory diagnosis of rickettsioses: current approaches to diagnosis of old and new rickettsial diseases. *J Clin Microbiol*. 1997;35:2715-27.
9. Bise G, Coninx R. Epidemic typhus in a prison in Burundi. *Trans R Soc Trop Med Hyg*. 1997;91:133-4.
10. Raoult D, Roux V. Rickettsioses as paradigms of new or emerging infectious diseases. *Clin Microbiol Rev*. 1997;10:694-719.
11. Perine PL, Krause DW, Awoke S, et al. Single-dose doxycycline treatment of louse-borne relapsing fever and epidemic typhus. *Lancet* 1974;2:742-4.
12. Huys J, Kayhigi J, Freyens P, et al. Single-dose treatment of epidemic typhus with doxycycline. *Chemotherapy* 1973;18:314-7.
13. Gilbert DN, Moellering RC, Sande MA. *Sanford Guide to Antimicrobial Therapy*. Hyde Park, Vt: Antimicrobial Therapy; 2004.
14. Woodward TE. Rickettsial vaccines with emphasis on epidemic typhus: initial report of an old vaccine trial. *S Afr Med J*. 1986;Suppl:73-6.

chapter 108

Orientia tsutsugamushi (Scrub Typhus) Attack

Peter B. Smulowitz and Jonathan A. Edlow

DESCRIPTION OF EVENT

Scrub typhus is a febrile illness caused by *Orientia tsutsugamushi*, previously known as *Rickettsia tsutsugamushi*. This bacterial pathogen is a gram-negative coccobacillus, and like other rickettsiae, it is an obligate intracellular bacterium. This tiny parasite is transmitted via the bite of larval stage mites (also known as *chiggers*) of the genus *Leptotrombidium*.

Clinical cases of scrub typhus are exceedingly rare in the United States, limited to travelers returning from endemic areas in eastern and southeastern Asia, India, Pakistan, and northern Australia and its adjacent islands. Focal pockets of infection are created in endemic areas secondary to the chiggers' general ability to feed only once[1] and the mites' preference for certain habitats (e.g., scrub vegetation, forest clearings, riverbanks, grassy regions).[2] Although rodents are the main host for the mites, humans who enter these "mite islands" are at high risk of disease transmission. There may be no risk to humans in nearby areas because chiggers typically stay within several meters of where they hatch.[1]

According to the Centers for Disease Control and Prevention (CDC), travelers and healthcare providers are generally not at risk of becoming infected via exposure to an ill person. Rickettsial species in general are usually not transmissible directly from person to person, although transmission has been documented to occur via blood transfusion.[3] Rickettsial organisms have caused infection via inhalation of laboratory-derived aerosols, suggesting the potential threat of the organisms as an aerosolized bioweapon.[4] The USSR successfully developed *Rickettsia prowazekii* as a biologic weapon during the 1930s and investigated a naturally occurring dormant, stable form that is infectious for long periods of time. During the 1930s and 1940s, the Japanese experimented with both *R. prowazekii* and typhus.[4,5] To date, *O. tsutsugamushi* is not known to have been developed as a biologic weapon. Theoretically, the organism could be spread by aerosol if it were manipulated to enhance its ability to survive in the environment. It may also be spread via the rodent host or the chigger vector. Despite the propensity of the chigger to feed only once, dissemi-nation into a crowded population could result in numerous infections.

Affected persons typically develop clinical symptoms between 6 and 18 days after inoculation by an infected chigger. Before the development of systemic symptoms, patients may develop a red papule at the site of the bite, which later forms a vesicle or ulcerates and forms a black eschar. The incidence of the eschar has been reported to occur in 36% to 88% of cases.[2] The lesion may be associated with regional lymphadenopathy at this time and generalized lymphadenopathy in the next 4 to 5 days. The finding of an eschar in a traveler should raise the possibility of scrub typhus. However, finding this lesion in a domestic patient should raise the possibility of cutaneous anthrax.

The onset of systemic symptoms in scrub typhus is usually sudden, with the most common findings being fever, myalgias, severe headache, and rash. Fever, in early stages up to 104°F to 105°F, is the most common symptom. The rash typically occurs after about 5 days of illness. A macular and papular or occasionally vesicular rash begins on the trunk and spreads to the extremities. Other symptoms occasionally encountered include nausea, vomiting, diarrhea, tremors, delirium, nervousness, slurred speech, deafness, and nuchal rigidity.[1] The disease has even been reported to present as an acute abdominal process.[6]

Serious complications occurring with untreated scrub typhus are predominantly pulmonary. Interstitial pneumonia and pulmonary edema may occur. Up to 22% of patients developed serious pneumonitis.[7] Cardiac involvement is less common, but patients may develop myocarditis or congestive heart failure. Other serious complications include meningitis, encephalitis, disseminated intravascular coagulation (DIC), shock, acute respiratory distress syndrome, and acute renal failure.

No laboratory test is diagnostic in scrub typhus. Most patients have a normal white blood cell count, although both leukopenia and leukocytosis may occur. Patients with severe disease often develop thrombocytopenia. In one series of 47 patients from Taiwan, 77% of patients demonstrated abnormalities of hepatic enzymes, with 6 patients presenting with a picture similar to acute viral hepatitis.[8] Lumbar puncture is also nondiagnostic, usually revealing a lymphocytic pleocytosis; in one series of

27 patients, the white blood cell count ranged from 0 to 110/mm³, with about half lymphocytes.[1]

Diagnosis of scrub typhus is made via serologic studies. The indirect fluorescent antibody test, which detects antibodies to specific antigens of the bacteria, is used most often due to its simplicity, rapidity, and a specificity approaching 99%.[9] The Weil-Felix test, based on cross reactivity between antirickettsial antibodies and *Proteus* antigens, lacks sensitivity and specificity and is not recommended. An enzyme-linked immunosorbent assay, passive hemagglutination assay, dot blot immunoassay dipstick, and polymerase chain reaction have been developed for the diagnosis of scrub typhus. Polymerase chain reaction shows promise in definitively establishing the diagnosis early in the course of infection, when serologic test results may still be negative. It is a relatively rapid test, yielding results in between 6 and 48 hours,[10] but is currently only available in a few specialized centers.

PREINCIDENT ACTIONS

The magnitude of a bioattack using *O. tsutsugamushi* depends on the mode of dissemination: aerosol versus the chigger vector. Populations of patients may present with the eschar or systemic symptoms described. At the phase of illness at which an eschar is present, cutaneous anthrax must be considered. Isolation may be initially required for patients with other symptoms of scrub typhus, which may be similar to the symptoms of bacterial meningitis. Other differential diagnoses to consider include malaria, dengue, leptospirosis, other rickettsial diseases, typhoid fever, endocarditis, tularemia, hemorrhagic fevers, meningococcemia, measles, secondary syphilis, infectious mononucleosis, and rubella.

Transmission of *O. tsutsugamushi* between persons is not believed to occur and poses little risk to healthcare workers.

POSTINCIDENT ACTIONS

Clinicians with a high level of suspicion for a possible scrub typhus attack or confirmatory data of a case of scrub typhus should notify the appropriate local, state, and federal public health and law enforcement authorities. Control of the disease depends on control of the trombiculid mites. Focal areas can be treated with chlorinated hydrocarbons such as lindane, dieldrin, or chlordane, although these may cause secondary environmental problems. Insect repellants and miticides such as *N,N*-diethyl-m-toluamide (DEET) are effective when applied to both clothing and skin, whereas permethrin and benzyl benzoate are effective when applied to clothing and bedding.[11]

MEDICAL TREATMENT OF CASUALTIES

Doxycycline, tetracycline, and chloramphenicol have all been used clinically in treating patients with scrub typhus. Ciprofloxacin and azithromycin have been used successfully with in vitro models, and ciprofloxacin (a rickettsicidal antibiotic with good intracellular penetration), 500 mg given twice a day, was successful in one case study.[12-14] Azithromycin has been suggested as an alternative therapy in pregnant women and children. Doxycycline is the most commonly used treatment for scrub typhus. The regimen consists of 100 mg given orally or IV for 5 to 7 days. Some studies have advocated short-course therapy, consisting of anywhere from 1 to 3 days of treatment, although the 5- to 7-day course is still recommended to prevent relapse of the disease. Relapse may still occur despite proper antibiotic therapy. The two most likely reasons for relapse include treatment during the first 5 days of the disease and the emergence of doxycycline-resistant strains of *O. tsutsugamushi*. In resistant strains, a collection of limited data has demonstrated the utility of adding rifampin to doxycycline.[15,16]

Due to the serotypic heterogeneity of *O. tsutsugamushi*, no effective vaccine has been developed. If an attack with the organism is highly suspected, chemoprophylaxis against potentially exposed persons might be successful with doxycycline 200 mg taken by mouth weekly.[1]

CASE PRESENTATION

A 45-year-old male traveler from Africa presents with his 16-year-old son. Both patients report temperature as high as 103°F, headache, and myalgias. They had recently gone scuba diving in the Torres Straight Islands, off the coast of Northern Australia, and are now visiting the United States. The symptoms have been getting worse since they started about 3 days ago, and the father is worried that both he and his son might have meningitis.

As you are entertaining the possibility of malaria and other tropical diseases, you turn your attention to the son. You immediately notice his toxic appearance. On examination he has conjunctival injection, and his right upper quadrant is mildly tender to palpation. You also notice some tender right inguinal lymphadenopathy, and as you are palpating the lymph nodes you see a black lesion on the right thigh that appears to be an eschar. Wondering whether mosquito bites ever produce an eschar, or whether the father and son might have somehow been exposed to anthrax, you decide to review the possibilities by consulting the CDC.[17]

UNIQUE CONSIDERATIONS

Mass bioattack with the bacteria causing scrub typhus is difficult since the bacteria require the mite vector for dissemination. The larval mites rarely travel far from the place where they hatch, and they usually bite only once. However, focal islands of infection may be created in areas suitable to the mites, and cases have been reported in urban areas of Asia. Scrub typhus should be considered in patients presenting with an eschar or with fever and a rash because early treatment can prevent many of the serious complications of the disease.

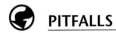 **PITFALLS**

Several potential pitfalls in response to an outbreak of scrub typhus exist. These include the following:

- Failure to consider scrub typhus in a patient with a cutaneous eschar
- Failure to realize that relapse of the disease can occur if treated early in the course or if doxycycline fails (or is not used) to treat resistant strains
- Failure to consider scrub typhus in the setting of high fever and a rash developing in patients within a focal geographic location
- Failure to avoid serious complications of the disease by delaying necessary antibiotic therapy
- Failure to report suspected cases of scrub typhus to the appropriate health and law enforcement agencies

REFERENCES

1. Saah AJ. *Orientia tsutsugamushi* (scrub typhus). In: Mandell GL, Bennett JE, Dolin R, eds. *Principles and Practice of Infectious Diseases.* 5th ed. Philadelphia: Churchill Livingstone; 2000:2056-8.
2. Sexton DJ. Scrub typhus: clinical features and diagnosis. UpToDate online, 2003. Available at: http://www.uptodateonline.com/application/topic.asp?file=tickflea/6173&type=A&selectedTitle=1~7.
3. Centers for Disease Control and Prevention. Travelers' Health Information on Rickettsial Infections. Available at: http://www2.ncid.cdc.gov/travel/yb/utils/ybGet.asp?section=dis&obj=rickettsial.htm&cssNav=browseoyb.
4. Walker DH. Principles of the malicious use of infectious agents to create terror: reasons for concern for organisms of the genus *Rickettsia. Ann NY Acad Sci.* 2003;990:739-42.
5. Azad AF, Radulovic S. Pathogenic Rickettsiae as bioterrorism agents. *Ann NY Acad Sci.* 2003;990:734-8.
6. Yang CH, Young TG, Peng MY, et al. Unusual presentation of acute abdomen in scrub typhus: a report of two cases. *Zhonghua Yi Xue Za Zhi (Taipei).* 1995;55:401-4.
7. Watt G, Parola P. Scrub typhus and tropical rickettsioses. *Curr Opin Infect Dis.* 2003;16:429-36.
8. Yang CH, Hsu GJ, Peng MY, et al. Hepatic dysfunction in scrub typhus. *J Formos Med Assoc.* 1995;94:101.
9. Weddle JR, Chan TC, Thompson K, et al. Effectiveness of a dot-blot immunoassay of anti-Rickettsia tsutsugamushi antibodies for serologic analysis or scrub typhus. *Am J Trop Med Hyg.* 1995;53:43-6.
10. Sugita Y, Yamaka Y, Takahashi K, et al. A polymerase chain reaction system for rapid diagnosis of scrub typhus within six hours. *Am J Trop Med Hyg.* 1993;49:636-40.
11. Sexton DJ. Scrub typhus: treatment and prevention. UpToDate online, 2003. Available at: http://www.uptodateonline.com/application/topic.asp?file=tickflea/6591&type=A&selectedTitle=2~7.
12. Strickman D, Sheer T, Salata K, et al. In vitro effectiveness of azithromycin against doxycycline-resistant and susceptible strains of Rickettsia tsutsugamushi, etiologic agent of scrub typhus. *Antimicrob Agents Chemother.* 1995;39:2406-10.
13. McClain JB, Joshi B, Rice R. Chloramphenicol, gentamicin, and ciprofloxacin against murine scrub typhus. *Antimicrob Agents Chemother.* 1988;32:285-6.
14. Scrub Typhus. Micromedex (diseasedex emergency medicine clinical reviews). Available at: http://10.25.77.24/mdxcgi/display.exe?CTL=C:\www\mdx\mdxcgi\MEGAT.SYS&SET=1C5B94E14BF970B0&SYS=5&T=300&D=328.
15. Panpanich R. Antibiotics for treating scrub typhus. *Cochrane Database Systemic Rev.* 2002;3:CD002150.
16. Watt G, Kantipong P, Jongsakul K, et al. Doxycycline and rifampicin for mild scrub-typhus infections in northern Thailand: a randomized trial. *Lancet* 2000;356:1057-61.
17. Faa AG, McBride WJ, Garstone G, et al. Scrub typhus in the Torres Straight Islands of North Queensland, Australia. *Emerg Infect Dis.* 2003;9:480-2.

chapter 109

Rickettsia rickettsii (Rocky Mountain Spotted Fever) Attack

Vittorio J. Raho and Jonathan A. Edlow

 ## DESCRIPTION OF EVENT

Rocky Mountain spotted fever (RMSF), once known as "black measles" and "black fever" for its associated hemorrhagic rash, has been recognized as the most lethal tick-borne illness in the United States since 1896 when some of the earliest documented outbreaks in Idaho claimed numerous lives.[1,2] Belonging to the group of bacteria called rickettsiae, the etiologic infectious agent of RMSF is *Rickettsia rickettsii*. It is an obligate intracellular bacterium that appears as a gram-negative coccobacillus under proper staining. RMSF is the most recognized and clinically significant rickettsiosis in the United States, with a range of several hundred to over a thousand cases reported annually to the Centers for Disease Control and Prevention (CDC).[3,4] The rickettsiae have a wide distribution and exist naturally in a complex life cycle involving certain hard tick species and their warm-blooded hosts. RMSF-identical illnesses have been reported throughout North, Central, and South America, having local names such as Columbian and Tobia fever.[5] Ticks act as both hosts and vectors by passing the organisms to their progeny transovarially. Wild mammals may become transiently infected when bitten, thus representing another host reservoir for the bacteria.[5] Humans appear to be accidental hosts when bitten by infected ticks and the vast majority of human cases occur in spring and summer months, which represent the peak activity for the tick's reproduction cycle.

The clinical syndrome known as RMSF is a well-described, acute, febrile illness with a reported mortality of up to 30% in the preantibiotic age. Even now, with specific antibiotics and improved supportive care, RMSF still carries a 5% mortality when properly treated. Mortality rises if proper antibiotics are started late in the patient's course, and also in patients who present "out of tick season" or without a rash.[6,7] After inoculation through the skin, the organisms enter the bloodstream via the lymphatics, infecting the vascular endothelium. This infectious vasculitis causes extravasation of plasma, edema, hypovolemia, and ischemia, with secondary thrombosis and platelet consumption. In this manner, multiple organ systems may be affected, and the clinical appearance is either nonspecific or can appear to be focal, depending on what organ system is primarily involved. The classic triad of headache, fever, and rash after tick exposure should raise suspicion of the illness but is only found in, at most, 60% of cases. Severe myalgias are prominent. Gastrointestinal symptoms—nausea, vomiting, abdominal pain, diarrhea, and anorexia—may also predominate. The characteristic rash, which is absent in up to 15% of cases, appears by the third to sixth febrile day as pink macules on the wrists and ankles, progressing to papules and eventually petechiae that characteristically involve the palms and soles.[8] Cardiac dysrhythmias suggesting myocarditis and pulmonary involvement with pneumonitis are a hallmark of higher morbidity.[8] Renal insufficiency is thought to be mostly of prerenal origin caused by the hypovolemic state, although fulminant renal failure requiring hemodialysis is reported. Neurologic sequelae are protean, ranging from focal deficits to florid encephalitis and coma. Headache of varying severity remains by far the most common neurologic manifestation.[9] Each of these various presentations may lead the clinician away from the diagnosis, especially when there is no history of tick bite, which occurs in one third of cases.

Laboratory and radiologic data are relatively unhelpful in aiding the diagnosis. Thrombocytopenia and anemia have been consistently reported in about one third to one half of all cases. Hyponatremia may be noted occasionally, and cerebrospinal fluid evaluation often shows elevated protein and mild pleocytosis. The current preferred method of diagnosing RMSF is through indirect immunofluorescence assay; however, this can only be used later in the course of the illness. The Weil-Felix test has fallen out of favor due to its lack of acceptable sensitivity and specificity compared with more modern testing. Ultimately, physicians must treat patients who may have RMSF based on clinical suspicion and epidemiologic context. Waiting for laboratory confirmation will lead to an increased mortality.

 ## PREINCIDENT ACTIONS

A similar situation exists for all local and state agencies and disaster-management task forces when planning the response to a potential biologic weapons attack. The state's department of public health or a similar organization should ensure the adequate supply of approved equipment for decontamination and isolation procedures. It should provide access to stockpiles of antidotes and antimicrobial agents as needed. Hospital emergency departments in conjunction with local fire and police departments should be conducting random citywide drills to provide feedback and test the integrity of the implemented system.

It is unknown whether RMSF has ever been used as a bioweapon. Considering the natural history of the disease and the relative frailty of the causative organism outside its normal host environment, it seems a daunting task to achieve. Therefore, a biologic attack using *R. rickettsii* is highly unlikely. If it were to occur, clinicians may notice an unusual seasonal or geographic pattern where the diagnosis of RMSF is made. Exposure to infected ticks is the only known risk factor for *R. rickettsii* among humans, and the strong seasonal occurrence is significant. Deviation from the normal pattern of illness may alert the astute clinician to the possibility of an unnatural cluster of cases during an unusual time of year. In this situation, the possibility of bioterrorism should be considered. It should be noted that several epidemiologic studies have shown that approximately 90% of U.S. RMSF cases have occurred between April 1 and September 30, and around 60% of patients had a history of tick exposure.[4]

 ## POSTINCIDENT ACTIONS

Initial response to a bioterrorism event will be local. The success of the response will depend greatly on the efforts of preincident planning. After the event occurs, a number of successive reactions should occur: communication channels must be established, resources need to be activated, teams and leadership structure need to be assembled, and hospitals and emergency departments must initiate and construct proper triage and decontamination sites.

Fortunately, RMSF is not known to be contagious. In addition, there is an inexpensive and effective treatment available for both active disease and for chemoprophylaxis of patients who may have been exposed to a *R. rickettsii* biologic weapon. The difficulty arises in confirmatory diagnostic testing, which is unavailable during the acute phases of the illness. The exception to this is cutaneous tissue biopsy, which is at best about 70% sensitive and only useful in patients presenting with the characteristic rash.[8] The diagnosis remains clinical, and treatment should be instituted early based on the clinician's index of suspicion. Such action might reduce overall mortality as a bioterrorism event unfolds.

In the event of a mass exposure to weaponized *R. rickettsii*, empiric treatment of actual cases with doxycycline should be implemented immediately. Chloramphenicol may be used as an alternative drug but should be used with caution since it may cause aplastic anemia. Prophylactic use of antibiotics should be considered in exposed but asymptomatic patients, although no controlled human studies show whether this is beneficial. From a public health perspective, however, watchful waiting for symptoms would also be a reasonable alternative.

 ## MEDICAL TREATMENT OF CASUALTIES

The current specific recommended treatment for suspected RMSF is 100 mg of doxycycline twice daily for 7 to 10 days or until the patient is afebrile for 48 hours. Although young children (younger than 9 years old) may be susceptible to the adverse bone and tooth-staining effects of the tetracyclines, the known morbidity and mortality of the illness mandates the use of doxycycline in all children unless absolutely contraindicated by allergy or similar reasons.[10-12] Pregnant women and those unable to take tetracycline antibiotics may be treated with chloramphenicol given 50 to 75 mg/kg/day in four divided doses for the same duration.[13] Chloramphenicol carries its own uncommon risks of idiosyncratic aplastic anemia, and blood monitoring should be undertaken accordingly. The remainder of treatment consists of supportive medical care and management of the numerous possible complications of the illness. There are no formal postexposure prophylaxis recommendations, and the decision to treat high-risk persons should be made at a public health level. There is no current vaccine available for RMSF.

CASE PRESENTATION

It is the beginning of March and no influenza cases have been reported in more than 6 weeks. However, your hospital has reported a possible cluster of four young, healthy patients presenting to the emergency department with acute, febrile illness of uncertain etiology. The patients reported fever, headache, and myalgias very similar to influenza but lacking cough or sore throat symptoms. One case fatality from sepsis and apparent encephalitis has occurred among the cluster, and several other patients remain in the intensive care unit. Three of the patients demonstrated diffuse, maculopapular rashes involving the palms and soles that eventually progressed to purpuric lesions.

On further review, the patients had no history of tick exposure or camping trips, no recent travel, and no intravenous drug use. Laboratory cerebrospinal fluid and blood test results have been negative for meningococcemia, HIV, streptococcus species, or other known pathogens to this date. It was determined during the inpatient course that cephalosporins, penicillins, aminoglycosides, and vancomycin were not improving the patients' clinical status. Eventual biopsy of an early skin lesion on the wrist of one of the patients demonstrates intracellular coccobacillary forms within vascular endothelial cells, and an anti-rickettsial antibody titer is 1:128.

UNIQUE CONSIDERATIONS

Rickettsiae, while virulent, are highly adapted to their intracellular environment and exist in a very delicate balance in nature. Their life cycle begins and ends almost entirely within other living organisms. Due to this delicate existence and the apparent need for parenteral inoculation for infection, they are far from the ideal candidate for any bioterrorist attack. A mass exposure would be very difficult to deploy and an unlikely choice for terrorists when other airborne and nonfastidious agents such as anthrax, tularemia, or Q fever exist. If *R. rickettsii* organisms could survive in an aerosolized form in the absence of a tick vector, it is not known whether RMSF could be transferred to exposed victims through inhalation.

 ## PITFALLS

Several potential pitfalls in response to an attack exist. These include the following:

- Failure to consider RMSF as a potential cause of acute, febrile illness, regardless of whether a rash is present
- Failure to initiate early empiric therapy when the disease is highly suspected
- Waiting for confirmatory blood test or biopsy results or the presence of a rash before beginning treatment in a suspected case
- Removing RMSF from the differential diagnosis if a rash is absent
- Failure to report suspected cases to the state department of public health or affiliated authority for appropriate CDC notification
- Failure to alert local and state agencies to a suspected biologic attack when presented with a cluster of unusual and uncommon illnesses such as RMSF

- Using geographic or seasonal exclusion criteria for the diagnosis[2]
- Failure to use doxycycline in adults and children unless absolutely contraindicated

REFERENCES

1. CDC Viral and Rickettsial Zoonoses Branch Web site. Available at: http://www.cdc.gov/ncidod/dvrd/rmsf.
2. Masters EJ, Olson GS, Weiner SJ, et al. Rocky Mountain spotted fever: a clinician's dilemma. *Arch Intern Med*. 2003;163:769-74.
3. Paddock CD, Holman RC, Krebs JW, et al. Assessing the magnitude of fatal Rocky Mountain spotted fever in the United States: comparison of two national data sources. *Am J Trop Med Hyg*. 2002;67:349-54.
4. Dalton MJ, Clarke MJ, Holman RC, et al. National surveillance for Rocky Mountain spotted fever, 1981-1992: epidemiologic summary and evaluation of risk factors for fatal outcome. *Am J Trop Med Hyg*. 1995;52:405-13.
5. Schaechter M, Eisenstein BI, Engleberg NC. *Mechanisms of Microbial Disease*. 2nd ed. Baltimore: Williams and Wilkins, 1993:358-67.
6. Kirkland KB, Wilkinson WE, Sexton DJ. Therapeutic delay and mortality in cases of Rocky Mountain spotted fever. *Clin Infect Dis*. 1995;20:1118-21.
7. Holman RC, Paddock CD, Curns AT, et al. Analysis of risk factors for fatal Rocky Mountain Spotted Fever: evidence for superiority of tetracyclines for therapy. *J Infect Dis*. 2001;184:1437-44.
8. Fauci AS, Braunwald E, Isselbacher KJ, et al. *Harrison's Principles of Internal Medicine*. 14th ed. New York: McGraw-Hill, 1998:1045-7.
9. Helmick CG, Bernard KW, D'Angelo LJ. Rocky Mountain spotted fever: clinical, laboratory, and epidemiological features of 262 cases. *J Infect Dis*. 1984;150:480.
10. Cale DF, McCarthy MW. Treatment of Rocky Mountain spotted fever in children. *Ann Pharmacother*. 1997;31:492-4.
11. O'Reilly M, Paddock C, Elchos B, et al. Physician knowledge of the diagnosis and management of Rocky Mountain spotted fever: Mississippi, 2002. *Ann N Y Acad Sci*. 2003;990:295-301.
12. Donovan BJ, Weber DJ, Rublein JC, et al. Treatment of tick-borne diseases. *Ann Pharmacother*. 2002;36:1590-7.
13. Stallings SP. Rocky Mountain spotted fever and pregnancy: a case report and review of the literature. *Obstet Gynecol Surv*. 2001;56:37-42.

chapter 110

Vibrio cholerae (Cholera) Attack

Milana Boukhman

DESCRIPTION OF EVENT

Cholera is the name given to the severe diarrheal illness caused by the bacterium *Vibrio cholerae*. For purposes of this chapter, the term *cholera* will be used when referring to the symptomatic illness, whereas *Vibrio cholerae* will be used when referring to the organism.

V. cholerae, a Centers for Disease Control and Prevention (CDC) category B bioterrorism agent, is a motile, curved, gram-negative rod that exists in nature independent of a mammalian host and is a normal inhabitant of surface water. Over 99.9% of naturally occurring, waterborne *V. cholerae* organisms are associated with copepods (a zooplankton), a fact that has led to the effective filtering of water through low-tech filters (e.g., eight layers of "sari" cloth in Bangladesh). Although cholera is virtually nonexistent in North America (zero to five cases per year), it is endemic in agrarian areas with poor sanitation such as Asia and Africa. At least 5.5 million cases of cholera occur worldwide each year, with more than 100,000 deaths.

Transmission occurs via the fecal/oral route but also by ingestion of the normal environmental reservoir of *V. cholerae*. Undercooked food, especially shellfish in which the bacteria occur naturally, and "burial ceremonies requiring the handling of intestinal contents" have also been implicated in transmission.[1] Cholera can survive for 24 hours in sewage, about 6 weeks in water containing organic matter, and 16 days in soil. It can withstand freezing for 3 to 4 days but is readily killed by dry heat at 242.6°F (117°C) or boiling.[2] Of the 18 cholera investigations undertaken by the CDC between 1988 and 1998, 4 were in the United States and involved various factors including nursing home patients, imported food, raw fish, or contaminated food on an international flight. In addition to sporadic cases, epidemics sometimes occur, including several during the 1990s in South and Central America.[4]

Only two serotypes of *V. cholerae* cause epidemic disease: the O1 serotype (divided into two groups, El Tor and "classical") and the O139 serotype. Other serotypes cause sporadic cases of gastroenteritis. Recently, the O139 serotype has spread from India and Asia to the Middle East.[5] At this time, there is no known weaponized form of cholera. An attack would most likely occur among persons via a contaminated water or food source.

Infection can occur after the ingestion of as few as 1000 organisms. Infection is more likely in patients who are receiving acid suppression therapy since gastric acid at a pH of less than 2.5 will effectively kill *V. cholerae* organisms. After ingestion, the incubation period is 4 hours to 5 days, with most patients presenting within 2 to 3 days.[2,6,7] Most *V. cholerae* infections are asymptomatic or present with only mild disease. Depending on the serotype, up to 75% of infected persons will remain asymptomatic. Of the other 25%, the majority have a mild diarrheal illness not requiring medical attention, 5% require hospitalization, and 2% develop classic cholera (also known as *cholera gravis*) with voluminous "rice water" stools. The symptoms of cholera gravis include gradual to sudden onset of vomiting, malaise, headache, and intestinal cramping with little or no fever, followed by painless and voluminous diarrhea of rice-water appearance; fluid losses may exceed 5 to 10 liters/day and up to 1 liter/hour of diarrhea is not uncommon. Patients with blood type O are more likely to develop severe disease. The mortality rate in the 2% with cholera gravis is 50% to 75%, giving an overall mortality in infected persons of 1% to 1.5%. Patients can die within 2 to 3 hours of the first signs of illness, although death in untreated patients usually occurs after several days.[8] The mortality risk is increased in children (10 times greater than in adults), the elderly, and pregnant women. There is also an increased risk of fetal death.[9]

Definitive testing for *V. cholerae* is performed relatively easily in the laboratory. Stool cultures should be sent and plated on thiosulfate-citrate-bile salts-sucrose (TCBS) agar or tellurite, taurocholate, and gelatin agar (TTGA). Gram stains of stool may show sheets of curved gram-negative rods. Other rapid diagnostic methods primarily used in epidemiologic studies include the detection of *V. cholera* organisms in stool specimens by polymerase chain reaction and monoclonal antibody-based stool tests.[10]

The most likely scenario for an outbreak would involve a large number of otherwise healthy persons presenting over several days with severe diarrhea/gastroenteritis symptoms and dehydration. Once a few cases of cholera are confirmed, the possibility of biologic terrorism should be considered.

Cholera should be included in the differential diagnosis of all cases of severe watery diarrhea and vomiting, especially those producing severe and rapid dehydration. The possibility of one or more cholera epidemics is a powerful stimulus to the development of needed infrastructure for sanitation and for public health in general, including improvements in sanitation, safer water handling, and public health capacity for surveillance and response to epidemics.

 ## PREINCIDENT ACTIONS

Transmission of cholera-causing species between persons is rare, and no additional precautions beyond universal precautions are needed in patients suspected of having cholera. The possibility of contracting cholera by inhalation is extremely unlikely, and personal protective equipment is not needed.

 ## POSTINCIDENT ACTIONS

If cholera is diagnosed either clinically or by laboratory testing, notify the appropriate local, state, and federal public health and law enforcement authorities. Steps should be taken to identify the source of the contamination and to prevent further spread of infection.

Simple soap-and-water bathing/skin-washing will remove nearly all *V. cholerae* from the skin surface; washing should be performed immediately and often. Chlorine and other antibacterial solutions would provide adequate decontamination of the surfaces of potentially contaminated objects.

Cholera is almost unknown where water supplies are properly disinfected (~100 ppm of chlorine). However, it is tolerant to residual (<2 ppm) chlorine. Water should be boiled if an event warrants necessity of this precaution (e.g., in the event of a water purification infrastructure failure), and all food should be well cooked. Reverse osmosis of water, iodine, chlorine (e.g., chlorine bleach added to drinking water: 2 drops household bleach [5.25%] per liter) or micropore filters can also be used. It is not likely that simple filtering procedures (e.g., sari cloth) would be effective in the event of an epidemic because organisms in purposefully contaminated water would not be associated copepods.

 ## MEDICAL TREATMENT OF CASUALTIES

The course of treatment is decided by the degree of dehydration. Oral rehydration solutions have reduced the mortality rate associated with cholera from over 50% to less than 1%.[5] These solutions take advantage of the fact that sodium and water absorption in the small intestine is facilitated by glucose and occurs even in the presence of cholera toxin. World Health Organization (WHO) recommends a solution containing, per liter of water,[11] 3.5 g of sodium chloride, 2.9 g of trisodium citrate or 2.5 g of sodium bicarbonate, 1.5 g of potassium chloride, and 20 g of glucose or 40 g of sucrose. A number of studies have investigated alternatives to WHO-Oral Rehydration Solution (ORS). ORSs containing rice or cereal as the carbohydrate source may be even more effective than glucose-based solutions in shortening the duration of diarrhea and reducing stool volume.[8,11]

Patients who have lost more than 10% of their body weight from dehydration or who are unable to drink because of vomiting or mental status changes should be started on intravenous rehydration. The ideal solution is lactated Ringer's solution. Normal saline can be used with the realization that bicarbonate and potassium losses are not being replaced. Five percent dextrose in water does not replace sodium, bicarbonate, or potassium losses.

Antimicrobial therapy can also be used in the treatment of cholera but should be viewed as an adjunct to appropriate hydration. Antibiotics reduce the volume of diarrhea by 50% and the duration of *V. cholera* excretion by about 1 day. Thus, antibiotics are cost-effective and generally recommended for severely ill patients (i.e., those with cholera gravis). Antibiotics are given orally when vomiting stops and when initial rehydration is accomplished. Antibiotic susceptibility patterns should guide treatment. Tetracycline and doxycycline are the most commonly prescribed antibiotics. Ciprofloxacin has also been used with equal or greater effectiveness than doxycycline. Risks and benefits need to be weighed when determining treatment in pregnant women and children. Options in children and pregnant women include erythromycin or azithromycin. It is of note that many strains are tetracycline resistant. It is also likely that any organism used as a weapon would be multidrug resistant.

A parenteral killed whole-cell vaccine is available in the United States but provides less than 50% protection for only 3 to 6 months and is not effective for all types of cholera (such as O139).[12] A number of new vaccines are under investigation. In 1999, the WHO recommended that the oral whole-cell/recombinant B subunit (WC/rBS) oral cholera vaccine should be considered for use in preventing cholera in populations at risk of an epidemic within 6 months and not experiencing a current epidemic.[13] Vaccine use during an epidemic is not recommended. Another intuitive option is antibiotic prophylaxis for entire populations. However, this has been shown to be ineffective and should not be used. Since person-to-person transmission does not occur, treating family members is unnecessary. However, if the family is using the same contaminated water source (e.g., in third-world countries or with a breakdown of water treatment in the United States), consider prophylactic use of antibiotics if more than one person in a family becomes infected.

 ## UNIQUE CONSIDERATIONS

The main considerations/problems in the treatment of cholera are (1) ensuring an adequate supply of intravenous fluids if a large population of persons becomes symptomatic and (2) adequately measuring stool output in order to calculate replacement. The first problem can be addressed by using oral rehydration solution in the least sick patients and in all patients who can keep up with fluid output orally. The second problem has been solved in third-world countries using "cholera beds." Cholera beds are stretchers with a hole in them through which the patient stools. The stool is collected in a bucket so that fluid loss can be measured. Cholera beds can be improvised by cutting holes in simple canvas or nylon stretchers or military cots without too much difficulty. Repulsive as it may seem, this setup is very practical and reduces staff time substantially (e.g., time spent getting patients to the commode). Clearly, these would only be used during an epidemic when hospital resources are stretched thin.

 ## PITFALLS

Several potential pitfalls in response to a cholera epidemic exist. These include the following:

- Failure to prepare adequate systems (e.g., hospital beds, personnel, local, state, and federal resources) to respond to possible terrorism attacks before the attacks occur
- Failure to have adequate supplies of the oral and intravenous rehydration solutions and supplies
- Failure to adequately rehydrate patients, instead relying on antibiotic treatment
- Failure to notify appropriate public health and law enforcement agencies when an outbreak of cholera is suspected or confirmed
- Failure to treat patients with oral rehydration solution instead of intravenous hydration, when possible. (An excessive amount of intravenously treated patients will unnecessarily tie up resources needed by sicker patients in the event of a mass-casualty event related to cholera attack.)

REFERENCES

1. Butterton JR. Pathogenesis of *Vibrio cholerae*. In: Rose BD, ed. *UpToDate*. Wellesley, Mass: 2004. Available at: http://www.uptodate.com/index.asp.
2. First reference: *Medical Management of Biological Casualties Handbook USAMIIRD, Feb 2001*. Available at: http://www.nbc-med.org/SiteContent/HomePage/WhatsNew/MedManual/Feb01/TheBlueBook.doc; Medical Issues Information Paper No. IP 3-1-017, March 1998; AFMAN 32-4017, *Civil Engineer Readiness Technician's Manual for Nuclear, Biological, and Chemical Defense*. Available at: http://www.nbc-med.org or http://www.e-publishing.af.mil/pubfiles/af/32/afman32-4017/afman32-4017.pdf or https://ccc.apgea.army.mil/air_force/references.htm or http://www.tpub.com/content/USMC/mcwp3375_web/css/mcwp3375_web_193.htm.
3. David A, Ashford DA, Kaiser RM, et al. *Planning Against Biological Terrorism: Lessons from Outbreak Investigations*. Atlanta, Ga: Centers for Disease Control and Prevention.
4. Tauxe RV, Blake PA. Epidemic cholera in Latin America. *JAMA* 1992;267:1388.
5. World Health Organization. *Cholera: WHO Report on Global Surveillance of Epidemic-Prone Infectious Diseases*. Report No.: WHO/CDS/CSR/ISR/200.1. Geneva: 2000.
6. Goma Epidemiology Group. Public Health Impact of the Rwandan refugee crisis: what happened in Goma, Zaire, in July 1994? *Lancet* 1995;345:359.
7. Lindenbaum J, Greenough WB III, Islam MR. Antibiotic therapy of cholera. *Bull World Health Org.* 1967;36:871.
8. Molla AM, Ahmed SM, Greenough WBI. Rice-based oral rehydration solution decreases the stool volume in acute diarrhea. *Bull World Health Org.* 1985;63:751.
9. Hirschhorn N, Chaudhury AKMA, Lendenbaum J. Cholera in pregnant women. *Lancet* 1969;1:1230.
10. Albert MJ, Islam D, Nahar S, et al. Rapid detection of Vibrio cholerae O139 Bengal from stool specimens by PCR. *J Clin Microbiol.* 1997;35:1633.
11. Ramakrishna BS, Venkataraman S, Srinivasan P, et al. Amylase-resistant starch plus oral rehydration solution for cholera. *N Engl J Med.* 2000;342:308.
12. Centers for Disease Control and Prevention. *Health Information for International Travel 1996-97*. Atlanta, Ga: U.S. Department of Health and Human Services; 1997.
13. World Health Organization. *Potential Use of Oral Cholera Vaccines in Emergency Situations: report of a WHO meeting*. Report No. WHO/CDS/CSR/EDC/99.4. Geneva: WHO; May 12-13, 1999.

chapter 111

Shigella dysenteriae (Shigellosis) Attack

Suzanne M. Shepherd, Stephen O. Cunnion, and William H. Shoff

 ## DESCRIPTION OF EVENT

Recognized since ancient times, shigellosis encompasses a broad spectrum of acute bacterial infectious diseases of the intestinal tract, caused by species of the genus *Shigella*. Shigellae are nonmotile, gram-negative, rod-shaped bacteria. Four groups of shigellae are recognized based on serologic and biochemical differentiation: group A (*S. dysenteriae*), group B (*S. flexneri*), group C (*S. boydii*), and group D (*S. sonnei*). Groups A, B, and C possess multiple serotypes and subtypes. *S. dysenteriae*, type 1, also known as Shiga's bacillus, produces Shiga's toxin and causes the most severe clinical illness, including hemolytic uremic syndrome and toxic megacolon; can harbor R-factor plasmids, conferring resistance to multiple antibiotics; and can produce pandemics with severe clinical illness and a high case-fatality rate in all age groups.[1]

Shigellosis is endemic throughout the world and hyperendemic in developing countries. *S. sonnei* is the predominant isolate in industrialized nations, whereas *S. dysenteriae* and *S. flexneri* are most common in developing countries. The annual worldwide incidence of shigellosis is 200 million cases, most commonly in children 2 to 3 years of age, with an approximate mortality of 650,000.[1] Ten thousand cases of shigellosis are reported in the United States yearly, with particularly high rates of disease noted in daycare centers and custodial centers for the mentally ill and physically challenged.[2] Except for captive primates, humans serve as the only natural host and reservoir for shigellae. Disease incidence is seasonal, peaking in summer. Shigellosis is transmitted via the fecal/hand/oral route under conditions of poor sanitation, crowding, and limited personal hygiene. Less frequently, shigellosis is transmitted via contaminated food and water, including swimming pools, and seasonally via some insects such as houseflies.[3] *Shigella* transmission, primarily *S. flexneri*, is increasingly reported via anal/oral contact in men having sex with men.[4,5]

Both its virulence and short incubation period make *Shigella* a good candidate for use as a bioweapon. Foodborne diseases are a major public health problem in the United States, with a yearly incidence of 60 to 80 million and 500 to 9000 deaths.[6-8] Consequently, identifying an outbreak of shigellosis as an incident of bioterrorism

may initially escape local public health and medical community awareness and surveillance modalities due to the following: (1) the large baseline noise produced by the relatively common occurrence of foodborne and waterborne illness; and (2) the large, often multistate nature of current outbreaks of foodborne disease.

Shigellae are also interesting bioweapon candidates due to their relatively low infectious dose; as few as 10 shigellae may cause disease in humans. This finding supports the clinical observations of the ease with which shigellosis can be transmitted among people via the fecal/hand/oral route during epidemics, particularly in the midst of conditions of crowding and poor sanitation and when poor personal hygiene is practiced among infected victims.[9] The low infectious dose coupled with the short incubation period for *Shigella* infection (1 to 4 days; 1 to 8 days for *S. dysenteriae* type 1) sets the stage for a widespread outbreak in a short period of time when conditions are appropriate. Additionally, since many persons are only mildly ill, they remain in contact with others and can further transmit the infection.[10] Shigellae can infect both immunocompetent and immunosuppressed persons. Finally, shigellae are hardy organisms and may survive for weeks or months in untreated water.[11]

Shigellae are more acid resistant than other bacterial enteropathogens and therefore have higher rates of survival during passage through the stomach, which explains in part their relatively low infectious dose. After a 1- to 4-day incubation period, the spectrum of illness includes asymptomatic infection; mild, watery diarrheal illness similar to that caused by many other bacterial, viral, and protozoal organisms; and classic, severe dysentery, with frequent, small, bloody, mucus-containing stools, tenesmus, significant abdominal cramping, vomiting, high fevers, rigors, and toxemia. Typically, illness progresses through several distinct phases. Initial toxemia, malaise and high fever, and less commonly, seizure activity in children are followed by several hours of watery diarrhea and then dysentery. The terminal ileum and colon serve as the most significant sites of pathology, demonstrating shigellae's ability to invade and reproduce within intestinal epithelial cells, ultimately leading to cell death, with resultant ileal, colonic, and rectal edema and ulceration, hemorrhages, microabscess formation, and a significant inflammatory infiltrate in the lamina propria. Bacteremia is not common, except in patients with AIDS and in malnourished children infected with *S. dysenteriae* type 1. Although all serotypes can cause any type of illness, the *S. flexneri* and *S. dysenteriae* serotypes tend to be associated with more severe illness and *S. sonnei* with more mild illness. Shigellosis may be complicated by severe dehydration in young children. Other complications include the hemolytic uremic syndrome; severe hypoproteinemia in young children, producing an acute kwashiorkor syndrome with edematous extremities[12]; leukemoid reactions (polymorphonuclear leukocyte counts may reach more than 100,000/mm[3]); toxic megacolon and rectal prolapse in young children; and rarely, Reiter's syndrome.

No characteristic features suggest shigellosis on clinical examination. Laboratory data are also nonspecific. The white blood cell count is often elevated, with a left shift on the differential. Stool microscopy for fecal leukocytes usually yields positive results. Patients may develop complications to include the hemolytic uremic syndrome with significant proteinuria and Reiter's syndrome. A specific diagnosis can usually be made within 48 hours by culture of two fresh stool samples on selective and differential media. Of note, *S. dysenteriae* type 1 can be very difficult to culture. In an outbreak investigation, serodiagnosis of serum antibodies to O antigen of specific *Shigella* serotypes can be performed by enzyme-linked immunosorbent assay or passive hemagglutination.

 PREINCIDENT ACTIONS

Preincident actions should focus on public health preparedness, healthcare provider education, and medical surveillance. The Centers for Disease Control and Prevention (CDC) maintain passive national laboratory-based surveillance for shigellae and other foodborne and waterborne pathogens. Rapid statistical analysis of this electronically transmitted information can detect unusual disease clusters by geographic area or time. A passive, physician-based reporting system also provides data to monitor trends. These systems are, however, prone to significant underreporting and lack of timeliness.[7] Realizing this, the CDC designed the Foodborne Diseases Active Surveillance Network (FoodNet) to more precisely determine the incidence of foodborne illness in the United States and to provide a network to identify and respond to new and emerging foodborne diseases.[13] Healthcare providers should remain vigilant in identifying case trends suggestive of a *Shigella* outbreak. Ongoing CDC and World Health Organization funding has focused on the development of a vaccine that is well tolerated, has a broad spectrum, and possesses long-lived immunity.[14]

Emergency department, hospital, and outpatient facilities should all have general disaster plans in place that address bioterrorist attacks and major infectious disease outbreaks, and the plans should be regularly tested.

The importance of staff implementing universal precautions and handwashing procedures should be stressed. Measures should be delineated in these plans for changes in triage guidelines to accommodate a rapid increase in patient census, patient isolation, and procedures to obtain increased antibiotic supplies. These plans should be developed in coordination with those of local, state, and federal emergency medical services and public health and governmental agencies, carefully specifying leadership and decision-making roles.[15]

Ongoing measures to reduce the availability of shigellae for malicious purposes are under development. Congress enacted the Public Health Security and Bioterrorism Preparedness and Response Act of 2002, requiring the U.S. Food and Drug Administration to develop regulations regarding food safety and tracking measures.[16] National collections and hospital and research laboratories are increasingly developing guidelines for the control of access to areas storing microbiologic agents. Freezers and incubators are increasingly secured, with access limited to designated personnel and continuous written records/surveillance maintained of persons entering these areas or handling these materials.[17]

 POSTINCIDENT ACTIONS

Healthcare providers with a high level of suspicion that a possible *Shigella* outbreak is the result of a deliberate action should notify their hospital infection control personnel and their local public health officer and law enforcement authorities. Prepositioning of drug and medical equipment stockpiles may prove critical in responding during very large outbreaks. Appropriate infection control procedures should be strictly enforced. Depending on the nature of the purported attack, materials and surfaces possibly contaminated by *Shigella* should be decontaminated with an appropriate disinfectant solution. During naturally occurring outbreaks of shigellosis, mass antibiotic prophylaxis has not been shown to be useful.[12]

 MEDICAL TREATMENT OF CASUALTIES

The treatment of patients with shigellosis should initially focus on the emergency management of life-threatening complications, supportive measures, and provision of specific antimicrobial therapy. Rapid intravenous access and infusion of crystalloid should be instituted in patients exhibiting signs and symptoms of shock and acidosis. In less critically ill persons, oral rehydration with oral glucose-electrolyte solutions is preferred. Seizure activity in children necessitates monitoring for airway compromise, head and neck trauma, and aspiration. Intravenous benzodiazepine administration can be used for initial seizure control. Accompanying fever can be controlled with antipyretics and ice baths, if needed. Agents that suppress intestinal motility should be used only in conjunction with antibiotic therapy.

Appropriate antibiotics significantly decrease the duration of diarrheal illness, fever, and shigellae excretion. Only a few antibiotics have been proved to be clinically useful, and widespread use of these agents has led to the emergence of resistance to the sulfonamides, tetracycline, and ampicillin. Current treatment options include the use of parenteral ceftriaxone in severely ill children and oral quinolones or trimethoprim sulfamethoxazole. Currently no vaccine is available for shigellosis.

 ## CASE PRESENTATION

Over the past week, your emergency department, which is the major medical center near a large state college, has experienced a significant increase in the number of patients presenting with diarrheal illness. You see a 20-year-old biology student without medical or travel history who presents with malaise, fever, and significant watery diarrhea. She states that most of her friends and others in the biology department have experienced diarrheal illness over the last week. She notes that several persons have been quite ill with fever, cramps, and bloody diarrhea, and some of these students were taken home by their parents. She remembers the onset of illness because it occurred at about the same time that the new biology teaching assistant arrived to replace one who had suddenly departed....

 ## UNIQUE CONSIDERATIONS

Shigella species have an advantage over other potential enteropathogenic bioweapons due to their low infective dose, their short incubation period, and their variety of potential disease presentations. Healthcare providers should be aware of shigellae's ability, especially in those organisms producing Shiga's toxin, to develop resistance to commonly used antibiotics. Furthermore, as relatively common causes of intestinal illness worldwide, the only clue to their use as a bioweapon may be the presentation of a large number of persons with an unusual strain, at an unusual time of year, or in an uncommon setting.

 ## PITFALLS

Several potential pitfalls in response to an attack exist. These include the following:

- Failure to develop, implement, and test emergency response plans that include plans to respond to acts of bioterrorism

- Failure to notify appropriate public health agencies when an outbreak of diarrheal illness is suspected
- Failure to consider *Shigella* as a bioweapon
- Failure to consider *Shigella* in the setting of nondysentery illness
- Failure to monitor *Shigella* for antibiotic resistance.
- Failure to adequately instruct patients on appropriate infection control precautions

REFERENCES

1. Institute of Medicine. Prospects for immunizing against *Shigella* spp. In: *New Vaccine Development: Establishing Priorities; Diseases of Importance in Developing Countries*. Vol 2. Washington, DC: National Academic Press; 1986:329-37.
2. Centers for Disease Control and Prevention. Shigella *Surveillance: Annual Tabulation Summary, 1999*. Atlanta, Ga: U.S. Department of Health and Human Services, CDC; 2000.
3. Cohen D, Green M, Block C, et al. Reduction of transmission of shigellosis by control of houseflies (*Musa domestica*). *Lancet* 1991;337:993-7.
4. Bader M, Pederson AHB, Williams R, et al. Venereal transmission of shigellosis in Seattle–King County. *Sex Transm Dis.* 1977;4:89-91.
5. Centers for Disease Control and Prevention. *Shigella sonnei* outbreak among men who have sex with men—San Francisco, California, 2000-2001. *JAMA* 2002;287(1):37-8.
6. Bennett JV, Holmberg SD, Rogers MF, et al. Infectious and parasitic diseases. In: Amler RW, Dull HB, eds. Closing the Gap: the Burden of Unnecessary Illness. New York: Oxford University Press; 1997; 102-14.
7. Swerdlow DL, Altekruse SF. Food-borne diseases in the global village: what's on the plate for the 21st Century. In: Scheld WM, Craig WA, Hughes JM, eds. *Emerging Infections*. 2nd ed. Washington, DC: ASM Press; 1998:273-90.
8. Jones TF, Pavlin BI, LaFleur BJ, et al. Restaurant inspection scores and foodborne disease. *Emerg Infect Dis.* 2004;10(4):688-92.
9. Green MS, Cohen D, Block C, et al. A prospective epidemiologic study of shigellosis: implications for the new *Shigella* vaccines. *Isr J Med Sci.* 1987;23:811-5.
10. Mohle-Boetani JC, Stapleton M, Finger R, et al. Communitywide shigellosis: control of an outbreak and risk factors in child day-care centers. Am Public Health *Assoc.* 1995;85:812-6.
11. Mitscherlich E, Marth EH. Microbial survival in the environment: bacteria and rickettsiae important in human and animal health, 1984. Berlin: Springer-Verlag; 1984:124-30.
12. Levine MM. Shigellosis. In: Strickland GT, ed. *Hunter's Tropical Medicine and Emerging Infectious Diseases*. 8th ed. Philadelphia: WB Saunders; 2000:319-23.
13. Angulo F, Voetsch A, Vugia D, et al. Determining the burden of human illness from foodborne diseases: CDC's Emerging Infections Program Foodborne Diseases Active Surveillance Network (FoodNet). *Vet Clin N Am.* 1998;14:165-72.
14. Cohen D, Ashkenazi S, Green MS, et al. Double-blind vaccine-controlled randomized efficacy trial of an investigational *Shigella sonnei* conjugate vaccine in young adults. Lancet 1997;349:155-9.
15. Inglesby TV, Grossman R, O'Toole T. A plague on your city: observations from TOPOFF. Clin Infect Dis. 2001;32:436-45.
16. Acheson DWK, Fiore AE. Preventing foodborne disease: what clinicians can do. *N Engl J Med.* 2004;350:437-40.
17. Kolavic SA, Kimura A, Simons SL, et al. An outbreak of *Shigella dysenteriae* type 2 among laboratory workers due to intentional food contamination. *JAMA* 1997;278:396-8.

chapter 112

Salmonella Species (Salmonellosis) Attack

Sumeru Mehta and C. Crawford Mechem

 ## DESCRIPTION OF EVENT

Salmonella organisms are non–spore-forming gram-negative rods of the family Enterobacteriaceae. Salmonellae are primarily pathogens of lower animals. The reservoir of infection in animals constitutes the principal source of nontyphoidal *Salmonella* organisms that infect humans, although transmission may occur from person to person. Salmonellae have been isolated from many animal species including poultry, cows, pigs, turtles, dogs, cats, and many birds.[1]

Salmonella species are classified as category B biologic agents according to the Centers for Disease Control and Prevention (CDC). Criteria for this category include moderate ease of dissemination, a lower mortality rate than category A agents such as anthrax, and the requirement for enhancement of the CDC's diagnostic capacity as well as enhanced disease surveillance. Several category B agents pose a threat to the food supply. *Salmonella*'s potential as a bioterrorism weapon is well established. The most prominent example of the use of *Salmonella* as a bioterrorism agent occurred in 1984 in the Dalles, Oregon, when followers of the cult leader Bhagwan Shree Rajneesh attempted to influence a local election by contaminating salad bars in several local restaurants with *Salmonella* cultures. No deaths resulted, but 751 people were sickened.[2]

In the vast majority of cases, humans acquire salmonellae through the ingestion of contaminated food, milk, or water. Infection has also resulted from the ingestion of contaminated medications, through the administration of intravenous platelet transfusions, and via direct transmission through inadequately sterilized fiber-optic instruments that have been used on patients undergoing upper gastrointestinal endoscopy.[1] Direct fecal/oral spread can also occur, particularly in children.

Salmonella infections occur with greatest frequency in the United States from July through November. A seasonal variation is also seen worldwide, with peak incidence corresponding to warm weather. The majority of reported isolations of *Salmonella* from humans come from sporadic cases; however, epidemiologic investigations of these apparently random events often identify unrecognized outbreaks in larger groups. The largest proportion of *Salmonella* outbreaks occur in the home, with institutional outbreaks (e.g., those affecting hospitals) ranking second.

The development of disease after ingestion of *Salmonella* is influenced by the number and virulence of the organisms ingested as well as individual host factors. In most cases, a large number of bacteria, in the range of 1 million to 1 billion, must be ingested to cause symptomatic infection.[3] In the case of unusually virulent strains or in patients with reduced resistance, symptomatic infection may result from smaller inocula. Factors that predispose persons to infection include underlying immunocompromising diseases, inflammatory bowel disease, malignancy, or use of antacids or histamine-2 blockers.[1] After ingestion of a sufficient number of bacteria, one or more of several clinical syndromes may manifest individually or concurrently. These clinical syndromes include enterocolitis (gastroenteritis), enteric (typhoid) fever, bacteremia, extraintestinal infection, and the chronic enteric or urinary carrier state.

Acute enterocolitis is the most common clinical manifestation of *Salmonella* infection. Nausea and vomiting are the earliest symptoms and develop 6 to 48 hours after ingestion of contaminated food, milk, or water. These are followed by diarrhea, which can range in severity from a few loose stools to fulminant, bloody diarrhea. Diarrhea usually persists less than 7 days but rare cases may continue for several weeks. Fever, when present, usually lasts less than 2 days. Prolonged fever combined with diarrhea should suggest a complication or another diagnosis. Electrolyte and water depletion may be severe, leading to hypovolemic shock in some cases.

Enteric fever produced by *Salmonella* serotypes other than *S. typhi* is called paratyphoid fever. The clinical features of paratyphoid fever are essentially the same as typhoid (see Chapter 113) but with milder symptoms. Signs and symptoms of enteric fever develop after an incubation period of 1 to 2 weeks and include fever, bradycardia out of proportion to the fever, myalgias, arthralgias, headache, hepatosplenomegaly, and rose spots, typically on the anterior chest wall. If the patient is not treated, altered mental status may develop.[1]

Salmonella infection can produce an illness characterized by fever and sustained bacteremia without manifestations of enterocolitis or enteric fever. The clinical syndrome of *Salmonella* bacteremia is characterized

641

by a febrile course lasting for days or weeks. In bacteremia, the organism is isolated from blood, but stool cultures often have negative results. Bacteremia has also been shown to occur in 8% to 16% of infants and children younger than 3 years of age who require hospitalization.[4] The median duration of persistence of *Salmonella* in stool is 7 weeks for patients younger than 5 years and 3 to 4 weeks for older children and adults.

Extraintestinal manifestations of *Salmonella* infection include meningitis, pleuropulmonary disease, endocarditis, pericarditis, arteritis, osteomyelitis, arthritis, hepatosplenic abscess, urogenital tract infections, and soft tissue abscesses. Chronic carriers (i.e., persons who continue to excrete the organism for more than a year after infection) are asymptomatic and unusual in nontyphoidal salmonellosis. Chronic enteric carriers tend to be older and have a much higher incidence of biliary tract disease than the general population.

 PREINCIDENT ACTIONS

Foodborne diseases present a major challenge to public health authorities. Surveillance for acts of terrorism involving the intentional contamination of food or water with a biologic agent is dependent on close cooperation between community clinicians, public health officials, and law enforcement agencies. Clinicians must be able to recognize the unusual disease or disease pattern, order the appropriate laboratory tests and cultures, and report their suspicions or positive culture results to public health officials. The public health officials must then perform an appropriate epidemiologic investigation to identify the source. If a bioterrorism incident is suspected or confirmed, the appropriate law enforcement agencies must be notified. Methods to enhance surveillance include promoting awareness of bioterrorism among the medical community and general public, performing appropriate microbiologic testing in suspected cases, developing a clearly defined reporting system that facilitates early recognition of outbreaks, and promoting interagency cooperation and communication on local, regional, and national levels.[5]

 POSTINCIDENT ACTIONS

Bioterrorism will often resemble a point-source outbreak, with all cases clustering around a single time period. An unusually high incidence may suggest deliberate infection, particularly if several point-source outbreaks occur simultaneously. Several features may suggest that a *Salmonella* outbreak is the result of an act of bioterrorism. These include the following: (1) large numbers of patients seeking care for similar signs and symptoms; (2) unusually high morbidity or mortality, or failure of the infection to respond to standard therapy; (3) multiple clusters of cases of salmonellae in areas that are not geographically contiguous; and (4) a tight cluster of cases with a common point source.[6] If an act of bioterrorism is suspected, the proper authorities should be notified immediately. Information on salmonellosis should also be disseminated to the general public to prevent further transmission of disease, to identify and treat those affected, and to initiate a disease prevention program.

 MEDICAL TREATMENT OF CASUALTIES

The type of syndrome produced by *Salmonella* species influences selection and duration of antimicrobial therapy. Antimicrobial therapy is not indicated in transient intestinal carriers nor in the vast majority of patients with enterocolitis. The most important therapeutic consideration in enterocolitis is fluid and electrolyte replacement. Patients with bacteremia or enteric fever should be treated with appropriate antibiotics, which include ampicillin, trimethoprim-sulfamethoxazole, or chloramphenicol. Recently, the selection of antimicrobial agents has been complicated by the emergence of *Salmonella* strains resistant to multiple antimicrobials.[7] Fluoroquinolones and the third-generation cephalosporins are recommended for use in areas where resistance is common. In 1997, the first recognized outbreak of fluoroquinolone-resistant *Salmonella* infection occurred in the United States.[8] The development of widespread fluoroquinolone resistance among serotypes that commonly cause infection would have serious implications for public health and pose a major obstacle in the response to a bioterrorism incident.

 CASE PRESENTATION

As a local emergency medicine physician in a small rural town, you notice that there has been an unusually high incidence of gastroenteritis among the local high school students in the past few days. You even had to admit an otherwise healthy 17-year-old on your last shift for severe dehydration. You were off yesterday, and this is your first shift since you admitted the young student. On follow-up, you note the patient is still requiring intravenous fluids and is receiving broad-spectrum antibiotics for fever and severe gastroenteritis.

When you begin your shift, three of your first five patients are all young students from the same high school. They present with the same symptoms, including diarrhea, nausea, vomiting, and abdominal pain with cramps, as the young man who was admitted. Along with intravenous fluids and select blood tests, you also decide to request stool cultures because you suspect a foodborne outbreak.

While taking a short dinner break, you overhear on the radio that a recently fired high school cafeteria employee was just arrested for assaulting the high school principal who had fired him. Suddenly, the nurse interrupts your meal because the waiting room is filling up with more high school students and family members, all of whom are afflicted with severe gastroenteritis.

A coordinated investigation involving medical, public health, and law enforcement personnel lead to the arrest of this employee for deliberately contaminating cafeteria food with Salmonella.

UNIQUE CONSIDERATIONS

Salmonellosis is in most cases a disease of morbidity, with an overall mortality rate of 0.4%. However, its appeal as a potential bioterrorism weapon derives from its ability to produce a large number of victims whose care could overwhelm local medical resources. In addition, *Salmonella* is a common pathogen that clinicians encounter routinely, with an estimated 1.4 million cases occurring annually in the United States.[1,9] Therefore, an outbreak of salmonellosis would be less likely to raise concern over an act of bioterrorism than would a rare pathogen such as anthrax. As a consequence, recognition of a deliberate release of *Salmonella* organisms would most likely be delayed, increasing the number of victims and decreasing the likelihood that the perpetrators would be apprehended.

PITFALLS

Several potential pitfalls in response to an outbreak exist. These include the following:

- Failure to educate healthcare providers and the general public on the signs and symptoms of salmonellosis
- Failure of healthcare providers to maintain a high index of suspicion for intentional salmonellosis infection
- Failure to order appropriate laboratory tests, delaying diagnosis
- Failure to treat with appropriate antibiotics and follow up on stool cultures to verify antimicrobial sensitivity
- Administration of antibiotics when they are not indicated, a practice that can lead to the development of antibiotic-resistant strains
- Failure to notify the proper authorities when an outbreak of salmonellosis is suspected or confirmed

REFERENCES

1. Hook EW. *Salmonella* species (including typhoid fever). In: Mandell GL, Bennett JE, Dolin R, eds. *Principles and Practice of Infectious Disease*. 5th ed, vol 2. Philadelphia: Churchill Livingstone; 2000:1700-16.
2. Torok TJ, Tauxe RV, Wise RP, et al. A large community outbreak of salmonellosis caused by intentional contamination of restaurant salad bars. *JAMA* 1997;278:389-95.
3. Hook EW. Salmonellosis: certain factors influencing the interaction of *Salmonella* and the human host. *Bull NY Acad Med*. 1961;37:499.
4. Meadow WL, Schneider H, Beem MO. Salmonella enteritidis bacteremia in childhood. *J Infect Dis*. 1985;152:185-9.
5. Hennessy TW, Hedberg CW, Slutsker L, et al. A national outbreak of *Salmonella enteritidis* infections from ice cream. *N Engl J Med*. 1996;334:1281-6.
6. Keene WE. Lessons from investigations of foodborne disease outbreaks. *JAMA* 1999;281:1845-7.
7. Lee LA, Puhr ND, Maloney EK, et al. Increase in antimicrobial-resistant *Salmonella* infections in the United States, 1989-1990. *J Infect Dis*. 1994;170:128-34.
8. Olsen SJ, DeBess EE, McGivern TE, et al. A nosocomial outbreak of fluoroquinolone-resistant salmonella infection. *N Engl J Med*. 2001;344:1572-9.
9. Mead PS, Slutskur L, Dietz V et al. Food-related illnesses and death in the United States. *Emerg Infect Dis*. 1999;5:607-25.

chapter 113

Salmonella typhi (Typhoid Fever) Attack

Lawrence Proano

 DESCRIPTION OF EVENT

Typhoid fever is a clinical syndrome caused by the bacterium *Salmonella typhi*. These anaerobic, gram-negative, flagellated bacilli possess an antigenic structure comprised of a lipopolysaccharide somatic surface antigen (O) and a flagellar antigen (H). *S. typhi* organisms usually possess a polysaccharide surface antigen (Vi) that coats the O antigen, protecting it from antibody attack.

Salmonella are classified as category B agents by the Centers for Disease Control and Prevention (CDC).[1] This category includes viruses, bacteria, fungi, and toxins that are relatively easy to disseminate, cause moderate morbidity and in most cases low mortality, and require specific enhancement of diagnostic and surveillance capacities for the laboratory to effectively respond during an outbreak. However, unlike the CDC category A agents, typhoid fever has a relatively low mortality rate among immunocompetent hosts, with only about a 10% mortality rate if untreated.[1]

The disease is not the most attractive weapon from a bioterrorism standpoint in that it is difficult to spread efficiently on a wide-scale basis compared with some other organisms, which can be transmitted via the aerosol route. Nevertheless, one should not underestimate the ability to intentionally cause a large outbreak of disease by using the foodborne route of infection.

The potential results of such an attack on the food supply can be inferred from some historic examples of unintentional foodborne disease outbreaks. In 1994, an estimated 224,000 people in the United States were infected during an outbreak of *Salmonella enteritidis*, caused by contamination of pasteurized liquid ice cream that was transported nationally in tanker trucks, resulting in one of the largest foodborne disease outbreaks in U.S. history.[2] In 1985, contamination of pasteurized milk from a dairy plant in northern Illinois resulted in over 170,000 people being infected with an outbreak of *Salmonella typhimurium* that was multidrug resistant.[3]

Due to the lower incidence in the United States, medical and public health officials may not recognize a foodborne attack such as typhoid fever for some time. From 1975 to 1984, the average number of cases of typhoid fever reported annually in the United States was 464. In that period, 57% of cases were in patients aged 20 years or older and 67% of cases were acquired while traveling internationally.[4] The most likely foodborne attack scenario would involve a large number of otherwise healthy persons presenting over days to weeks with vague, multisystem complaints, with some of the cases progressing to more toxic syndromes.

The incubation period of typhoid fever varies from several days to longer than 3 weeks, averaging around 14 days. During the first week there are often nonspecific symptoms such as malaise, anorexia, gradually worsening fever, occasional chills, headache, upper respiratory symptoms, cough, and hearing loss. Patients are often constipated during the first week.

In the second week there is a continuation of fever, often accompanied by a relative bradycardia, diarrhea, vomiting, and a more toxic appearance of the patient. Rose spots, 2- to 4-mm pink papules visible on the torso of fair-skinned persons, are seen in about 50% of patients. Abdominal pain and distension with hepatosplenomegaly may be present.

During the third week the patient becomes increasingly toxic with high fever, delirium, or coma; the so-called typhoid state. Diarrhea may have a "pea-soup" appearance. Multiplication of *S. typhi* in Peyer's patches of the small bowel may result in small bowel hemorrhage or perforation and peritonitis. Sepsis, anemia, leukopenia, pneumonia, and myocarditis may also occur. Death may occur in untreated patients in the third week of illness, usually from gastrointestinal perforation, anemia, toxemia, or occasionally, meningitis. If the patient survives through the fourth week of illness and gastrointestinal complications do not occur, fever, toxemia, and abdominal symptoms abate over a few days.

Complications of typhoid fever are numerous and can occur at any time during the illness, even after a seemingly benign course.[1] Complications may be the presenting symptom or sign rather than the picture of typhoid fever. Complications include small bowel perforation, gastrointestinal hemorrhage, hemolytic anemia (common in patients with G6PD deficiency), typhoidal pneumonia, meningitis, glomerulonephritis, acute renal failure, nephrotic syndrome, arthritis, osteomyelitis, orchitis, hepatitis, acute cholecystitis, and parotitis. Abscesses may occur virtually anywhere in the body as a late complication, most commonly in the liver, spleen, brain, breast, and bone. Deep venous thrombosis and Guillain-Barré syndrome have been reported in association with typhoid fever.

 PREINCIDENT ACTIONS

Adequate preparation for and response to bioterrorism events require coordination of local, state, and federal public safety resources in the United States. Several agencies are involved in detection and epidemiologic investigation of foodborne disease outbreaks, whether intentional or unintentional. These include local and state health epidemiology departments, public health laboratories at the local and state levels, the Council of State and Territorial Epidemiologists, the Association of Public Health Laboratories, and the CDC. The U.S. Food and Drug Administration and the U.S. Department of Agriculture have the primary regulatory authority over food safety, in coordination with state departments of agriculture.[5]

A mass-casualty event resulting from an outbreak of typhoid, or most other foodborne illnesses, is less likely to occur compared with what would be expected from the intentional dissemination of a category A bioterrorism agent. However, smaller-scale attacks are well within the realm of possibility. Therefore, physicians, healthcare workers, and health agency personnel must remain vigilant in identifying trends that may correspond with an outbreak of typhoid, or any foodborne or waterborne illness, whether terrorist related or not. With some diseases, including typhoid fever, these trends may take days or even weeks to develop, and they may involve somewhat nonspecific systemic complaints that evolve over time.

Numerous unintentional foodborne outbreaks are reported every year. Epidemiologic clues to a deliberate, covert act of contamination include the following:

1. The presence of a large epidemic with unexplained morbidity and mortality
2. More severe disease than is usually expected for a specific pathogen or failure to respond to specific therapy
3. Multiple simultaneous or serial epidemics
4. A disease that is unusual for a particular age group
5. Unusual strains or variants of organisms or antimicrobial resistance patterns different from those circulating in the population
6. A similar genetic type among agents isolated from distinct sources at different times or locations

Features that would be suggestive of deliberate contamination might also arise in unintentional outbreaks as well. Confusing matters further, these epidemiologic clues might not necessarily be evident in an outbreak due to deliberate contamination.[1]

 POSTINCIDENT ACTIONS

Clinicians suspicious that an outbreak may represent typhoid fever, even before bioterrorism is suspected, should notify the appropriate local, state, and federal public health and law enforcement authorities. This is the proper course of action, even from a public health perspective, because occasional outbreaks of typhoid fever can occur.

Both state and federal regulatory agencies participate in food-specific aspects of outbreak investigation, especially those related to the tracking of suspected foods and their recall. A trace-back investigation locates the origin of the food vehicle to establish the source of contamination, often by review of the records of vendors, shippers, producers, and processors, and by inspection of their facilities.

Integration of data from the epidemiologic and trace-back investigations is crucial to properly identify the contaminated food and the mode of contamination, underscoring the need for the closest collaboration between epidemiologists, microbiologists, and food-safety officials.[5]

 MEDICAL TREATMENT OF CASUALTIES

Successful treatment of typhoid fever requires rapid diagnosis, antibiotic administration, and supportive care. With prompt treatment, mortality rates have been reduced from between 10% and 15% to between 1% and 4%.[1]

Chloramphenicol is the antibiotic most widely used worldwide for treating typhoid fever. Tetracyclines and aminoglycosides are not effective against *S. typhi*, although they may demonstrate in vitro activity. Ampicillin, amoxicillin, and trimethoprim-sulfamethoxazole have been successfully used to treat this entity. However, in the past decade, flouroquinolones and third-generation cephalosporins have been shown to be as effective as choramphenicol, and in the developed world have largely become the antibiotics of choice. Thus, flouroquinolones would be the recommended agent to treat victims diagnosed with typhoid fever.

Aside from antibiotic administration, general supportive care, hydration, and electrolyte management are important in treating this disease. This is especially important because patients with severe typhoid fever have a limited ability to maintain their nutritional and fluid status.

In addition to antibiotic therapy, studies have clearly demonstrated that corticosteroid administration reduces mortality in patients with severe typhoid fever. It does not appear to increase the incidence of complications, relapse rate, or induction of a carrier state among those treated.

 UNIQUE CONSIDERATIONS

The features of typhoid fever tend to be nonspecific, and a number of other causes need to be considered when encountering febrile illnesses including malaria. Malaria would be the most likely consideration in the tropics but would be far less likely in developed countries such

A notice is posted inviting all 50 workers from the hospital laboratory to the break room to enjoy some free muffins, doughnuts, and coffee. Twenty of the workers respond to the invitation and consume the pastries. Over the next week to 10 days, 17 of the 20 workers become ill with what they initially attribute to a viral illness. Their supervisor notes the cluster of illness among the staff and reports it to the hospital's infection control department.

By the end of the first week, six of the staff members who were ill have visited the hospital's emergency department with fevers, constipation, abdominal pain, and lethargy. Four of these patients require admission and are evaluated for a fever of unknown origin. After admission, two of the four rapidly develop profuse "pea-soup" like diarrhea and become toxic. Three of the four are noted to have hepatosplenomegaly. Blood cultures of all four of these persons are positive for *S. typhi*. The remainder of the staff with similar symptoms is called in for evaluation, cultured, and treated empirically for typhoid fever.

Subsequent investigation of the incident leads to the discovery that a coworker had engaged in an act of foodborne terrorism by intentionally contaminating the pastries with stored bacteria from the laboratory. She subsequently pleads guilty to the charge.

This case presentation may sound apocryphal; however, it is based on a real incident of domestic foodborne terrorism that occurred in 1996 in Dallas, Texas.[6] Although the organism in the actual event was *Shigella dysenteriae*, the consequences could have been much more severe if the agent had been *S. typhi*.

as the United States. Tuberculosis and brucellosis can also mimic typhoid fever. Other illnesses to consider in the differential diagnosis of typhoid fever include dengue fever, endocarditis, typhus, and lymphoproliferative disorders. The tests for typhoid fever do not have a high degree of sensitivity or specificity, and because of the relatively low prevalence of this disease in the United States, it would not likely be an early consideration in the minds of most clinicians.

Nonspecific hematologic and biochemical findings can lend support for the diagnosis of typhoid fever. Leukopenia is common. There is often a modest degree of hyponatremia, as well as a mild transaminitis.

PITFALLS

Several potential pitfalls in response to an outbreak of typhoid fever exist. These include the following:

- Failure to prepare adequate state or local systems to respond to possible terrorist attacks before the attacks occur
- Failure to consider typhoid fever as the etiology for patients who present without diarrheal illness. Early typhoid fever often presents initially with constipation, not diarrhea!
- Failure to consider typhoid fever as a bioterrorism attack in the setting of a large number of people who present over days to weeks with symptoms consistent with this or any foodborne illness
- Failure to notify appropriate public health and law enforcement agencies when an outbreak of foodborne illness is suspected or confirmed

REFERENCES

1. Le TP, Hoffman SL. Typhoid fever [Chapter 15]. In: Guerrant R, Walker D, Weller P, eds. *Essentials of Tropical Infectious Diseases*. Philadelphia: Churchill Livingston, 2001.
2. Hennesy TW, Hedberg CW, Slutsker L, et al. A national outbreak of *Salmonella enteritidis* infections from ice cream. *N Engl J Med*. 1996;334:1281-6.
3. Ryan CA, Nickels MK, Hargrett-Bean NT, et al. Massive outbreak of antimicrobial-resistant salmonellosis traced to pasteurized milk. *JAMA* 1987;258:3269-74.
4. Corales R, Schmitt SK. Typhoid fever. August 11, 2004. Available at: http://www.emedicine.com/MED/topic2331.htm.
5. Sobel J, Khan AS, Swerdlow DL. Threat of a biological terrorist attack on the US food supply: the CDC perspective. *Lancet* 2002;359:874-80.
6. Kolavic SA, Kimura A, Simons SL, et al. An outbreak of *Shigella dysenteriae* type 2 among laboratory workers due to intentional food contamination. *JAMA* 1997;278:396-8.

chapter 114

Burkholderia mallei (Glanders) Attack

Mark A. Graber

DESCRIPTION OF EVENT

Burkholderia mallei is a Centers for Disease Control and Prevention category B biologic agent and causes the disease known as glanders. *Burkholderia mallei* was previously called *Pseudomonas mallei*. It is a non-motile, nonsporulating, obligate aerobic, gram-negative bacillus.[1]

In its natural state, glanders is primarily a disease of horses and other equids (e.g., donkeys, mules), with humans becoming secondarily infected. Because of its impact on equids, glanders has had significant historic, economic, and military effects. In modern times, *B. mallei* was used as a biologic warfare agent in World War I (WWI) with particularly devastating effects on troop and artillery movement on the eastern front. During WWII, civilians and prisoners of war in China were purposefully infected with glanders by the Japanese. Finally, *B. mallei* was used by the former Soviet Union on a limited basis in Afghanistan in the 1980s. Glanders has been all but eradicated in the United States and most developed countries but continues to be a problem in countries still dependent on equids, mainly in Africa and Asia. It is thought likely that antibiotic-resistant strains are being developed as a biologic warfare agent.[1]

The transmission of glanders from equids to humans generally occurs by direct contact with broken skin and mucous membranes, although transmission through intact skin has been reported. The effectiveness of percutaneous transmission is not well documented. Historically, 30% of horses in China were infected with *B. mallei* after WWII but few human cases were reported, suggesting poor transmission. However, the low rate of human cases may reflect reporting problems or a less virulent strain of the bacteria and not the low infectivity of the organism. A second mode of transmission is by inhalation of droplets, either directly from infected patients or equids, or by inhalation of aerosolized laboratory samples. Transmission by droplet is quite efficient, with 46% of those exposed to *B. mallei* in laboratory accidents developing the illness.[2] The number of organisms required for an infectious inoculum in humans is not known. However, in hamsters, inhalation of 1 to 10 aerosolized *B. mallei* organisms is fatal. Rats require a larger inhaled inoculum.[1,3,4] It is the inhalation mode, cou-pled with the ability of *B. mallei* organisms to survive up to a couple of months in favorable conditions, that makes *B. mallei* a potential agent for biologic terrorism.[5]

There are no reported cases of naturally occurring human glanders in English literature since 1949. However, several laboratory-related cases have been reported. Sporadic cases have been reported in Asia and Africa, generally among veterinarians, abattoir workers, or those working closely with horses. Equids (and an occasional infected carnivore) are the only natural reservoir of *B. mallei*. There is no natural occurrence in soil or water. This point is demonstrated by the fact that no isolates of *B. mallei* have been found in Great Britain since WWII. For this reason, *any case of glanders should be considered a bioterrorism event until proven otherwise*.

There are four unique presentations of *B. mallei*: an acute form localized to the skin, a chronic form localized to the skin (also known as "farcy"), a pulmonary form, and a rapidly fatal septic form (Table 114-1). Persons with diabetes and immunosuppressed persons are particularly susceptible to systemic spread. The incubation period for glanders is between 1 and 14 days, with 10 to 14 days being the norm. However, cases have been reported up to 10 years after exposure. The hallmark of systemic glanders (pulmonary and acute sepsis syndromes) is widespread erythroderma or widespread skin pustules and abscesses. Because of the predominance of skin findings, glanders may be mistakenly identified as a systemic staphylococcal infection, etc.[6] *The leukocyte count is often normal or only mildly elevated.* Liver enzymes may be elevated, reflecting hepatic abscess formation.[7]

Historically, a mallein-antigen purified protein derivative (PPD) was used to identify early infection in animals. However, given that the mallein PPD must be injected into the infected organism's palpebral fissure, this method of testing is limited to animals. *B. mallei* can be cultured at 37.5 °C using medium containing 1% to 5% glucose, or 5% glycerol, or both. Meat-infusion nutrient media can also be used. Using these ideal media, the organism can generally be recovered in 48 hours. *Automated bacterial identification systems will often misdiagnose B. mallei as a pseudomonal organism (e.g.,* Pseudomonas fluorescens *or* Pseudomonas putida*).* Gene sequencing can reliably identify *B. mallei*.[8] Enzyme-linked immunosorbent assay and polymerase

TABLE 114-1 PRESENTATIONS OF *B. MALLEI* INFECTION

DISEASE	USUAL INCUBATION	PRESENTATION	LABORATORY/X-RAY	SIGNS	MORTALITY
Pulmonary	10-14 days	Cough, fever, sweats, chest pain, photophobia	Miliary granulomas in lung progressing to consolidation and abscesses, liver and spleen abscesses, and granulomas	Photophobia, lacrimation, hepatosplenomegaly, generalized erythroderma or granulomatous/ necrotic lesions of the skin, adenopathy	90% to 95% if untreated, 40% if treated
Fulminant sepsis	Likely 10-14 days	Sudden-onset fever, rigors, sweats, myalgias, pleuritic chest pain, jaundice, diarrhea	Granulomas in liver and spleen, pulmonary consolidation, nodules and abscesses, mild leukocytosis with left shift or leukopenia	As above	>95% if untreated, 50% if treated
Acute cutaneous	1-5 days	Skin ulceration, swollen lymph nodes, mucopurulent drainage if mucous membrane	Possible systemic dissemination in 2-4 weeks after infection of lymph nodes (possibly sooner)	Nodules, abscesses, ulcers of skin and along lymphatic vessels and subcutaneous tissues	After systemic dissemination: 95% if untreated, 50% if treated
Chronic cutaneous (aka farcy)	Variable	Induration, lymphedema of skin, ulcerations, ropey looking lymphatic vessels with lymphadenopathy	As above	As above	May rarely progress to meningitis; 50% eventual mortality despite treatment

chain reaction tests exist to identify *B. mallei*. However, neither test is widely available. Latex agglutination tests are too nonspecific to be of much use. Finally, a complement fixation test for antibody to *B. mallei* is available. It is considered positive at 1:20 or with a fourfold increase in titer. However, a negative test result does not rule out the disease.[9]

There is no vaccine available for glanders and no prophylactic antibiotic regimens are currently recommended, although this might change in the face of an epidemic. Although person-to-person spread is considered unlikely, isolation is the crux of prevention. Isolation rooms are recommended, if available. At the least, patients should be masked to prevent droplet spread. Standard precautions are recommended for persons caring for patients. These include the use of surgical masks, gloves, face shields, and gowns. Level 3 precautions are recommended for those working with *B. mallei* in the laboratory, and hospital laboratory personnel should be made aware that a potentially dangerous organism is being cultured. The organism is susceptible to heat (55°C), drying, and various disinfectants including benzalkonium chloride, 1% sodium hypochlorite, 70% ethanol, and iodine preparations.[9]

 PREINCIDENT ACTIONS

Preparation should be the same as for any possible bioterrorism event. Additionally, equids should be continuously and closely monitored for the development of glanders. Monitoring, and the destruction of any infected equids, is mandated by law. However, surveillance has likely lapsed given the rareness of the illness. The inclusion of veterinarians in preparation for biologic

emergencies can facilitate early identification of possible outbreaks of this and other diseases (e.g., brucellosis and anthrax).

 POSTINCIDENT ACTIONS

The most important point here is to remove the natural reservoir of *B. mallei* from the population. For this reason, any equids in the area should be tested using the mallein PPD, and those animals testing positive, along with any showing symptoms or signs of *B. mallei,* should be euthanized and disposed of properly. As evidenced by the lack of *B. mallei* infection in developed countries, this approach has been shown to be very effective at removing *B. mallei* from the population and saving animals in the long term.[10] Continued monitoring of the human population is also important given the latency period for developing ganders of up to several years that has been seen after *B. mallei* exposure.

 MEDICAL TREATMENT OF CASUALTIES

Presumed cases should be isolated if possible. There are no trials of antibiotics for glanders in humans; these recommendations reflect those of the *European Union Commission on Preparedness and Response to Biological and Chemical Agent Attacks* as well as other sources. *These recommendations may not apply to the drug-resistant glanders that will likely be used in a bioterrorism event.*

First-line therapy for systemic glanders is imipenem, ceftazidime, or meropenem plus either doxycycline or ciprofloxacin in severe cases. Another option is trimethoprim/sulfamethoxazole (TMP/SMX), 5 to 10 mg/kg (given intravenously or orally) based on the trimethoprim component given every 8 hours. In mild cases of glanders, oral therapy can be tried with TMP/SMX, doxycycline, or amoxicillin/clavulanate. The duration of intravenous therapy should be 2 to 3 weeks. B. mallei *can reactivate and requires prolonged treatment.* For this reason, treatment should be continued with an oral agent. Ciprofloxacin, doxycycline, TMP/SMX, or amoxicillin/clavulanate administered for 60 to 150 days are all good choices. Although there is no consensus, most authors suggest treating for about 24 weeks.[11-14]

CASE PRESENTATION

Two likely scenarios are possible:

1. A 45-year-old man presents with tender lymphadenopathy, fever, chills, and a pustule on the left lower extremity. A presumptive diagnosis of staphylococcal infection with secondary lymphadenitis is made, and the patient is administered a first-generation cephalosporin. Initially the patient appears stable, but 2 weeks later he develops diffuse erythroderma with pustules and an enlarged and tender liver and spleen. Computed tomography reveals granulomas in the liver and spleen.

2. You see multiple patients in your emergency department complaining of cough, fever, and chills during the month of November. A diagnosis of influenza is made. Because influenza A is predominant this season, you administer rimantadine to the patients. The patients become progressively ill, and chest radiographs performed on the second visit reveal evidence of a miliary pattern of granulomas in the lungs. A course of doxycycline and imipenem is begun, the patients are hospitalized, and they do well.

UNIQUE CONSIDERATIONS

Special considerations are noted above and include long-term monitoring of the human population for reactivated or initial disease, removal of any reservoir of *B. mallei* (e.g., culling of equids), and long-term treatment (12 to 24 weeks) with an oral agent to prevent relapse in infected persons.

PITFALLS

Several potential pitfalls in response to an outbreak exist. These include the following:

- Failure to recognize the presentation of glanders
- Failure to monitor equids on an ongoing basis to facilitate prevention and early detection
- Failure to treat infected persons in the long term
- Treatment with inappropriate antibiotics; several antibiotics should be administered when treating glanders since it is likely that organisms released in a bioterrorism event will be multi-drug resistant. Sensitivity testing should always be performed
- Use of inappropriate media for growing the organism
- Misidentification of the organism as a pseudomonal species
- Failure to use proper isolation precautions in the laboratory and clinical settings

REFERENCES

1. U.S. Army Medical Research Institute of Infectious Disease. *USAMRIID's Medical Management of Biological Casualties Handbook.* 5th ed. Fort Detrick, Md: August 2004. Available at: http://www.usamriid.army.mil/education/bluebook.htm.
2. Anonymous. Laboratory-acquired human glanders—Maryland, May 2000. *MMWR* 2000;49:532-5.
3. Lever MS, Nelson M, Ireland PI, et al. Experimental aerogenic *Burkholderia mallei* (glanders) infection in the BALB/c mouse. *J Med Microbiol.* 2003;52(Pt 12):1109-15.
4. Woods DE. The use of animal infection models to study the pathogenesis of melioidosis and glanders. *Trends Microbiol.* 2002;10:483-4.
5. Utrup LJ, Frey AH. Fate of bioterrorism-relevant viruses and bacteria, including spores, aerosolized into an indoor air environment. *Exp Biol Med.* 2004;229:345-50.
6. Rega PP, Batts D, Hall AH, et al. Glanders and melioidosis. April 6, 2005. Available at: http://www.emedicine.com/emerg/topic884.htm.
7. Srinivasan A, Kraus CN, DeShazer D, et al. Glanders in a military research microbiologist. *N Engl J Med.* 2001;345:256-8.
8. Gee JE, Sacchi CT, Glass MB, et al. Use of 16S rRNA gene sequencing for rapid identification and differentiation of *Burkholderia pseudomallei* and *B. mallei. J Clin Microbiol.* 2003;41:4647-54.
9. PATHPORT. PathInfo pathogen information. Virginia Bioinformatics Institute. Available at: http://staff.vbi.vt.edu/pathport/pathinfo/.
10. Blancou J. Early methods for the surveillance and control of Glanders in Europe. *Rev Sci Tech.* 1994;13:545-57.
11. The European Agency for the Evaluation of Medicinal Products, *EMEA/CPMP Guidance Document On The Use of Medicinal Products for Treatment and Prophylaxis of Biological Agents that might be used as Weapons of Bioterrorism,* 2002. Available at: http://www.emea.eu.int/pdfs/human/bioterror/404801.pdf.
12. Heine HS, England MJ, Waag DM, et al. In vitro antibiotic susceptibilities of *Burkholderia mallei* (causative agent of glanders) determined by broth microdilution and E-test. *Antimicrob Agents Chemother.* 2001;45:2119-21.
13. Johns Hopkins Division of Infectious Disease. Johns Hopkins' Antibiotic Guide 2004. Available at: http://hopkins-abxguide.org.
14. Russell P, Eley SM, Ellis J, et al. Comparison of efficacy of ciprofloxacin and doxycycline against experimental melioidosis and glanders. *J Antimicrob Chemother.* 2000;45:813-8.

chapter 115

Burkholderia pseudomallei (Melioidosis) Attack

Sean Montgomery

 ## DESCRIPTION OF EVENT

Melioidosis, also known as *Whitmore's disease,* is caused by the bacterium *Burkholderia* (formerly *Pseudomonas*) *pseudomallei,* a motile, aerobic, non–spore-forming, facultative intracellular gram-negative bacillus.[1] People acquire the illness by inhaling dust or droplets contaminated by the bacteria or when contaminated soil or surface waters come in contact with abraded skin. Clinical cases of melioidosis are uncommon in North America because melioidosis is a disease of tropical climates; it is endemic in Southeast Asia and Northern Australia. In addition, it has been found in the South Pacific, Africa, India, and the Middle East. In the United States, cases range from zero to five each year, predominantly occurring among travelers and immigrants. Melioidosis predominantly occurs during the rainy season in endemic areas.[2] Peak incidence of melioidosis occurs in the fourth to fifth decades of life. It primarily affects people who have an underlying chronic disease, such as diabetes mellitus, renal disease, cirrhosis, chronic lung disease, or those who are otherwise immunocompromised.[3]

Illness from melioidosis can lead to a broad range of manifestations, including acute localized infection, pneumonia, bacteremia, and chronic suppurative infection. Asymptomatic infections are also possible. Melioidosis is highly virulent and has up to a 40% mortality rate in Thailand.[3] The incubation period of melioidosis is not clearly defined but may range from 2 days to many years.

Melioidosis is similar to glanders disease (see Chapter 114) in many respects, but the epidemiology and natural reservoirs of melioidosis are distinct from glanders. The bacteria causing melioidosis can be found in contaminated soil and water and are spread through direct contact. Glanders is typically acquired through contact with infected domestic animals. Both melioidosis and glanders disease have been investigated by the United States and other countries as potential biologic weapons and are classified as category B agents by the Centers for Disease Control and Prevention (CDC). The United States studied these agents as possible biologic warfare weapons in 1943-1944 but did not weaponize them. The former Soviet Union is believed to have been interested in glanders as a potential biologic weapon as well. During World War I, glanders was allegedly used to infect horses and mules destined for delivery to France by German agents.[4] The Japanese are believed to have infected civilians, prisoners of war, and horses during World War II.

Several characteristics make *B, pseudomallei* a potential biologic weapon. The organism can be fairly easily recovered from water and wet soil in rice paddy fields in endemic areas. In northeast Thailand, the organism can be cultured from more than 50% of rice paddies.[5] *B. pseudomallei* grows aerobically on most agar media and produces colonies within 24 hours at 37° C. Biosafety level 3 containment practices are required for laboratory staff when working with these organisms. In addition to being somewhat easily obtained and cultured, *B. pseudomallei* organisms are fairly resilient. They can survive in triple-distilled water for years.[6] If aerosolized and distributed into a densely populated area, the consequences could be potentially devastating. The high mortality of *B. pseudomallei* infections is related to a tendency to develop high bacteremias (>50 cfu/mL).[7] In addition, no effective vaccine currently exists, and successful treatment requires broad-spectrum, potent antibiotics.

Because of the variable presentations of melioidosis, the unpredictable incubation period, and the possibility that many carriers will remain asymptomatic, the medical and public health community may not recognize a bioterrorist attack involving *B. pseudomallei* until the organism is cultured from acutely septic persons. The attack would likely involve aerosolization of media containing *B. pseudomallei* and distributing it over a heavily populated, urban area. Over a period of days to weeks, affected persons would visit healthcare facilities with symptoms ranging from fevers, chills, and cough to fulminant multisystem organ failure. The diagnosis of melioidosis in the absence of travel to an endemic area should be presumed to be evidence of bioterrorism until proven otherwise, and appropriate authorities should be notified.

The outcome of infection with *B. pseudomallei* depends on a balance between the virulence of the organism, the size of inoculum, the point of entry, and the underlying immunologic status of the host. During a bioterrorist event, immunologically compromised hosts and those who received the largest inoculum would likely be the first to manifest symptoms and would develop the most severe illness. Long periods of latency (up to 29 years) have been reported before the disease becomes clinically apparent.[8]

Melioidosis septicemia typically presents with high fever and rigors, although some patients will present with a recurrent fever. About half of patients will have a primary focus of infection, typically in the lung or skin. Patients may develop confusion, jaundice, and diarrhea. They often develop diffuse metastatic foci, acidosis, and shock, and many die within 48 hours. Poor prognostic features include absence of fever, leukopenia, azotemia, and abnormal liver function test results.[3] The disease is characterized by abscess formation.[9] The lung is the most commonly affected organ, and lung abscesses may rupture into the pleural space to cause empyema. The liver, spleen, kidney, and prostate are also common sites for abscess formation. In one third of children with melioidosis in Thailand, the infection was found to present with acute suppurative parotitis.[10] Melioidosis presents as brainstem encephalitis or flaccid paraparesis in 4% of cases from Northern Australia.[11]

Laboratory data may reveal anemia, leukocytosis with neutrophilic predominance, evidence of hepatic and renal impairment, and coagulopathy. An abnormal chest x-ray is found in up to 80% of patients, most commonly with widespread, nodular shadowing.[8] *B. pseudomallei* can be readily cultured from infected sites or the blood.[12] Cultures should be grown on routine blood agar and Ashdown's selective medium. The median time taken to obtain a positive blood culture result is 48 hours. Latex agglutination tests based on monoclonal antibodies to lipopolysaccharide can then be undertaken for definitive identification.[13]

 ## PREINCIDENT ACTIONS

Preparation for a mass-casualty event requires coordination of local, state, and federal officials and resources. Cities, hospitals, and emergency departments should have disaster plans developed and tested before the advent of a terrorist attack. The diagnosis of melioidosis in the absence of travel to an endemic area should be presumed to be evidence of bioterrorism until proven otherwise, and appropriate authorities should be notified. In the event of large numbers of people presenting with symptoms suspicious for a bioterrorist attack, symptomatic persons should be isolated pending further investigation, and the CDC must be rapidly notified.

Healthcare workers must remain vigilant in identifying trends that may correspond with an outbreak of melioidosis. These trends may become apparent over weeks to months, initially involving those with underlying, chronic illness and then possibly spreading to involve otherwise healthy persons presenting with skin infections, pneumonia, and multisystem organ failure. Mechanisms to detect progressively increased emergency department volume and symptom trends should continue to be developed and implemented, and further research into the development of a vaccine against melioidosis is warranted.

 ## POSTINCIDENT ACTIONS

Appropriate federal, state, and local healthcare authorities and the CDC must be notified if any clinician has a high level of suspicion of a melioidosis outbreak or if a confirmed case of melioidosis is diagnosed in an individual without a known history of travel to an endemic area. Implementation of disaster plans may be warranted if several cases are simultaneously reported or emergency department volume is noted to be significantly increased. Mobilization of resources including expansion of intensive care units and release of antibiotic stockpiles may be required.

 ## MEDICAL TREATMENT OF CASUALTIES

Patients presenting with melioidosis septicemia require aggressive supportive care, including hemodynamic and respiratory support and correction of volume depletion and shock. Abscesses should be drained whenever possible. The antibiotics of choice are ceftazidime, imipenem-cilastatin, or meropenem with or without trimethoprim-sulfamethoxazole.[14-17] These should be given in full doses (1 g every 8 hours, or a dose appropriately adjusted for renal function or size) for 2 to 4 weeks, according to the clinical response. This should be followed by a 20-week course of doxycycline (100 mg twice a day) and trimethoprim-sulfamethoxazole (160 mg trimethoprim plus 800 mg sulfamethoxazole twice per day), which has been associated with a lower relapse rate than amoxicillin-clavulanic acid (500 mg amoxicillin/125 mg clavulanic acid three times a day). Prolonged oral antibiotics are needed to prevent relapse, which occurs in up to 23% of patients and is more common in patients who have more severe disease.[17] Other agents with activity against *B. pseudomallei* include

CASE PRESENTATION

Over the past week you have noted an increased volume of patients visiting your emergency department. You see a 28-year-old female with fever and cough. Her examination is notable for a temperature of 40°C, heart rate of 140, respiratory rate of 28, blood pressure of 95/60, and oxygen saturation of 88% on room air. She has diffuse bibasilar crackles on her pulmonary examination and a diffuse pustular rash. Her laboratory results reveal a hematocrit of 24, a white blood cell count of 23 with a neutrophilic predominance, a creatinine level of 2.0, a glucose level of 433, and an international normalized ratio of 2.0. Her chest x-ray reveals widespread, nodular shadowing. Blood cultures are sent for evaluation; the patient is treated with oxygen, insulin, intravenous fluids, and antibiotics; and she is admitted to the intensive care unit. Meanwhile, intensive care units throughout the city are becoming overwhelmed.

ceftriaxone, aztreonam, doxycycline, and ticarcillin-sulbactam. The role of granulocyte colony-stimulating factor, which has also been used as adjunctive treatment in Australia, remains to be determined. Currently, no vaccine exists for melioidosis.

 UNIQUE CONSIDERATIONS

During a bioterrorist event, affected persons would present to healthcare facilities over a period of days to weeks with symptoms ranging from fevers, chills, and cough to fulminant multisystem organ failure. Because of the variable presentations of melioidosis, the medical and public health community may not recognize a bioterrorist attack involving *B. pseudomallei* organisms until the organism is successfully cultured. In addition, *B. pseudomallei* pneumonia could be confused with plague given a similar appearance of stained organisms, and the diffuse, pustular eruption could be confused with smallpox or varicella.[18] Healthcare providers need to be aware that melioidosis should be treated with either ceftazidime, imipenem-cilastatin, or meropenem in the acute phase, and a prolonged antibiotic course is also required to prevent relapse.

 PITFALLS

Several potential pitfalls in response to an attack involving melioidosis exist. These include the following:

- Failure to prepare for potential bioterrorist attacks prior to the event
- Failure to consider melioidosis attack in the context of multiple persons presenting to healthcare facilities over a period of days to weeks with symptoms ranging from fevers, chills, and cough to fulminant multisystem organ failure
- Failure to treat melioidosis with ceftazidime, imipenem-cilastatin, or meropenem in the acute phase, and a prolonged antibiotic course to prevent relapse
- Failure to notify appropriate law enforcement and public health officials in the event of a suspected melioidosis attack or outbreak, or in the event of a confirmed case of melioidosis in a person without a known history of travel to an endemic area

REFERENCES

1. White N. Melioidosis. *Lancet* 2003;361:1715-22.
2. Leelarasamee A, Bovornkitti S. Melioidosis: review and update. *Rev Infect Dis.* 1989;11:413-25.
3. Chaowagul W, White N, Dance D, et al. Melioidosis: a major cause of community-acquired septicemia in northeastern Thailand. *J Infect Dis.* 1989;159:890-9.
4. Horn J. Bacterial agents used for bioterrorism. *Surg Infect.* 2003;4:281-7.
5. Wuthiekanun V, Smith M, Dance D, et al. The isolation of *Pseudomonas pseudomallei* from soil in northeastern Thailand. *Trans R Soc Trop Med Hyg.* 1995;89:41-3.
6. Wuthiekanun V, Smith M, White N. Survival of *Burkholderia pseudomallei* in the absence of nutrients. *Trans R Soc Trop Med Hyg.* 1995;89:491.
7. Walsh A, Smith M, Wuthiekanun V, et al. Prognostic significance of quantitative bacteremia in septicemic melioidosis. *Clin Infect Dis.* 1995;21:1498-500.
8. Dance, D. Melioidosis. In: Cohen J, Powderly W, eds. *Infectious Diseases.* 2nd ed. London: Mosby; 2004:1637-9.
9. Vatcharapreechasakul T, Suputtamongkol Y, Dance D, et al. *Pseudomonas pseudomallei* liver abscesses: a clinical, laboratory, and ultrasonographic study. *Clin Infect Dis.* 1992;14:412-7.
10. Dance D, Davis T, Wattanagoon Y, et al. Acute suppurative parotitis caused by *Pseudomonas pseudomallei* in children. *J Infect Dis.* 1989;159:654-60.
11. Currie B, Fisher D, Howard D, et al. Endemic melioidosis in tropical northern Australia: a 10-year prospective study and review of the literature. *Clin Infect Dis.* 2000;31:981-6.
12. Walsh A, Wuthiekanun V. The laboratory diagnosis of melioidosis. *Br J Biomed Sci.* 1996;53:249-53.
13. Steinmetz I, Reganzerowski A, Brenneke B, et al. Rapid identification of *Burkholderia pseudomallei* by latex agglutination based on an exopolysaccharide-specific monoclonal antibody. *J Clin Microbiol.* 1999;37:225-8.
14. White N, Dance D, Chaowagul W, et al. Halving of mortality of severe melioidosis by ceftazidime. *Lancet* 1989;2:697-701.
15. Simpson A, Suputtamongkol Y, Smith M, et al. Comparison of imipenem and ceftazidime as therapy for severe melioidosis. *Clin Infect Dis.* 1999;29:381-7.
16. Cheng AC, Fisher DA, Anstey NM, et al. Outcomes of patients with melioidosis treated with meropenem. *Antimicrob Agents Chemother.* 2004;48:1763-5.
17. Chaowagul W. Recent advances in the treatment of severe melioidosis. *Acta Trop.* 2000;74:133-7.
18. McGovern T, Christopher G, Eitzen E. Cutaneous manifestations of biological warfare and related threat agents. *Arch Dermatol.* 1999;135:311-22.

chapter 116

Chlamydia psittaci (Psittacosis) Attack

Hans R. House

 DESCRIPTION OF EVENT

Psittacosis, also known as parrot fever, is caused by *Chlamydia psittaci*, an obligate intracellular bacterium. Clinical cases of psittacosis are sporadic and have a worldwide distribution. Approximately 100 to 200 cases are reported annually in the United States.[1] The true incidence, however, is likely higher. Since psittacosis carries a nonspecific presentation and is difficult to culture, many cases go unnoticed or are simply attributed to "atypical pneumonia."

The association of bird ownership or bird exposure with psittacosis is well known. Parrots, parakeets, cockatiels, and canaries are the species most commonly associated with *C. psittaci* infection. More than 130 avian species have been documented as hosts of *C. psittaci*, including pigeons, sparrows, ducks, egrets, chickens, and turkeys.[2] Not all cases of human psittacosis derive from avians; case reports describe transmission from infected sheep, cattle, cats, and dogs.[3,4] Human-to-human transmission has been described, but it is rare.[5]

C. psittaci is categorized as a Centers for Disease Control and Prevention (CDC) class B biologic warfare agent for its potential to spread via aerosol and infect victims with a relatively low mortality rate.[6] The United States, the former Soviet Union, and Egypt have all conducted research into its use as a weapon, but none is known to have deployed it. To date, no known incidents of intentional infection by *C. psittaci* have occurred.[7]

The few incidents of large-scale outbreaks of psittacosis involved the distribution or industrial processing of birds. The largest outbreak, from 1929-1930, involved 750 to 800 cases and was linked to the importation of exotic birds from Argentina to Europe and the United States. Epidemiologic data from the 1970s and 1980s in the United Kingdom, the United States, and Sweden show a direct relationship between increased importation of exotic birds and rising numbers of cases of psittacosis.[8,9] More recent outbreaks occurred in workers at a duck farm and at turkey processing facilities.[10-12]

C. psittaci is usually acquired by inhalation or direct contact with the infectious discharges from infected animals. Infected birds may transmit the disease while asymptomatic, but the greatest number of organisms is expressed during periods of obvious illness (shivering, emaciation, anorexia,

dyspnea, and diarrhea). Since the discharge from the beaks and eyes, feces, and urine are all infectious, feathers and dust in and around the birds' cages become infectious.[13] Aerosolization of infectious material, such as bird excreta, is one possible route of infection that might be attempted in a biologic attack. However, a weaponized agent could also be used. According to Bill Patrick, who headed a component of the U.S. biologic weapons program at Fort Detrick, Md., in the 1950s and 1960s, *C. psittaci* was high on the list to be produced and stockpiled as a biologic weapon just before President Richard Nixon terminated the program in 1969 (Bill Patrick, personal communication, July 30, 2004). The organism, measuring 300 nm in its infectious form (or elementary body), is resistant to drying and may be viable for up to 1 week at room temperature.[14]

After inhalation of *C. psittaci* and establishment of an infection in the epithelial cells of the lower respiratory tract, psittacosis may follow one of two routes of pathogenesis. Direct local invasion of the pulmonary parenchyma results in a disease with a relatively short incubation period (1 to 3 days). More commonly, a primary bacteremia leads to infection of the reticuloendothelial cells of the liver and spleen. This results in an incubation period of 1 week to 15 days.

Based on this bimodal pathogenesis, it can be presumed that a biologic attack on a large population would lead to an epidemic with two spikes in cases. The first, smaller peak would occur only days after the attack, and a second, larger peak may be seen 1 to 2 weeks after the release of the agent.

Cases would probably go unnoticed initially. Although there may be clues on history and physical examination, psittacosis does not have a distinctive presentation; it usually presents as an atypical pneumonia with varying degrees of severity—from an unapparent mild disease to a severe, life-threatening systemic illness and respiratory failure. Untreated, up to 20% of cases may be fatal. With proper treatment, however, the mortality rate is around 1%.

The most common symptoms of psittacosis are cough, fever, headache, and vomiting. Most patients (about two thirds) describe a dry cough with scant sputum. Malaise, anorexia, and diarrhea are also common symptoms. Many other symptoms have been associated with cases of *C. psittaci* infection, including photophobia, tinnitus, ataxia, deafness, sore throat, hemoptysis, epistaxis, and rash.

Typical findings on physical examination include fever, rales, consolidation, and tachypnea.[15,16] Two unusual findings that may alert the examiner to the possibility of psittacosis are splenomegaly and relative bradycardia (a normal heart rate in the presence of a high fever). Many other signs have also been described in reviews of psittacosis cases. These include somnolence, confusion, pleural rub, adenopathy, palatal petechiae, herpes labialis, and Horder's spots. Horder's spots are pink, blanching maculopapular eruptions similar to the rose spots seen in typhoid fever. As the disease progresses, multiple systemic complications may develop (see Postincident Actions).

The most important laboratory finding involves the chest x-ray, which usually demonstrates a variable degree of consolidation. Most often, this consolidation exceeds the clinical severity of the patient. The white blood cell count is usually normal, but often demonstrates a left shift. More than one-half of patients have moderately elevated transaminases levels, and many demonstrate mild hyponatremia.

Although isolation of the organism from the blood in cell culture is possible, it can be difficult and is dangerous for laboratory personnel. The preferred method of diagnosis is by serology; antibodies are measured by complement-fixation (CF) or microimmunofluorescence (MIF) during the acute illness and after recovery. A single convalescent titer of 1:32 in a patient with a compatible clinical picture is considered by the CDC to be a presumptive case. A four-fold rise in titer between acute and convalescent specimens in a consistent clinical setting is defined as a confirmed case. The presence of IgM antibody to *C. psittaci* in either specimen is also considered to be a confirmed case.[17]

 PREINCIDENT ACTIONS

A biologic attack with psittacosis does not necessarily call for unique preparations. As with any potential incident, the emergency department, hospital, and local emergency services should have an integrated disaster response plan. This plan should provide for security and isolation of the treating facility; the triage of potential patients; a mechanism for liberating hospital beds and other treatment space; and the rapid recruitment of local police, fire, and healthcare personnel. Above all, the plan should provide for redundancy in communication methods—the element most commonly deficient in disaster scenarios. This plan should be reviewed and practiced annually.

Person-to-person transmission of psittacosis has been documented, but no specific isolation beyond universal precautions is indicated. The treating hospital should have a sufficient supply of antibiotics (tetracycline or doxycycline [see Medical Treatment of Casualties]) available to initiate therapy in suspected cases. The disaster plan should then include a mechanism for recruiting more doses from local and state suppliers within 1 day. After 48 to 72 hours, the federal stockpiles should be mobilized to the affected area.

The most significant challenge in addressing a *C. psittaci* attack is recognizing the event at all. A large

number of patients presenting with a nonspecific, febrile, respiratory illness would present over 1 to 2 weeks. Such a scenario would probably be interpreted as an influenza outbreak. Establishing a local or statewide syndromic surveillance system might assist in identifying psittacosis and other subtle biologic attacks using nonspecific diseases. A syndromic surveillance system that depends on observed rates of certain symptoms, such as cough, fever, or shortness of breath, would more rapidly detect a psittacosis attack than the conventional public health reporting system. A surveillance system that monitors pharmaceutical sales (such as the National Retail Data Monitor) may also be helpful. It may detect a spike in sales of antipyretics/analgesics or antitussives.

The hospital laboratory should not be expected to culture *C. psittaci*. The CF or MIF test for *C. psittaci* should be readily available. If the local facility cannot provide these tests, it must provide for rapid referral of specimens to the next level in the Laboratory Response Network (LRN). The LRN laboratories are a defined hierarchy of increasingly specialized and sophisticated testing institutions available for the confirmation of suspicious agents.[18] The earlier the outbreak is identified, the sooner specific treatment can be initiated. Early therapy of psittacosis is important to minimize mortality, prevent secondary and recurrent cases, and reduce the rates of systemic complications.

 POSTINCIDENT ACTIONS

If a case of psittacosis has been confirmed, the appropriate local public health authority should be notified (psittacosis is considered a reportable disease). In the event that multiple cases from different households are diagnosed, the possibility of a biologic attack must be considered. Alerting the disaster chain of command up to the federal level would be indicated.

Isolation of patients is not necessary, but decontamination of the affected area may help prevent additional cases. Patients' clothing should be discarded in a safe manner. Any surface possibly contaminated by infectious particles should be disinfected with 70% isopropyl alcohol or a 1:100 dilution of household bleach. Note that *C. psittaci* is susceptible to heat and most detergents, but it is resistant to acid and alkali. Avoid using a vacuum cleaner because it can aerosolize particles; sweep or wet mop the floor after spraying it with a disinfectant. The use of a N95 respirator and disposable protective clothing (gown, gloves, and mask) is advisable for those cleaning infectious dust.

If the outbreak is associated with a known bird population, isolate or cull the birds. Infected avians can be successfully treated with medicated water or feed or can be administered antibiotics. Wash and disinfect all cages or other containment areas.

After the initial acute cases have presented, the affected population can expect sporadic complications of systemic *C. psittaci* infection. In addition to the expected respiratory illness, psittacosis has been known to cause pericarditis, myocarditis, and "culture-negative" endocarditis. Unless the diagnosis is specifically sought, a patient with *C. psittaci* endocarditis might be subjected to repeatedly negative evaluations, delaying definitive therapy and risking valve destruction.

Psittacosis has also been associated with hepatitis and jaundice, glomerulonephritis, hemolytic anemia, pancytopenia, and disseminated intravascular coagulation. A reactive, polyarticular arthritis is seen 1 to 4 weeks after the initial illness. Neurologic complications are common and diverse. Cranial nerve palsies, cerebellar dysfunction, transverse myelitis, confusion, meningitis, encephalitis, and seizures have all been described. The lumbar puncture is usually normal, but the protein level may be greatly elevated.

 ## MEDICAL TREATMENT OF CASUALTIES

Tetracyclines are the treatment of choice for psittacosis. Satisfactory response is seen with oral therapy and doxycycline 100 mg twice per day or tetracycline 500 mg four times per day. Intravenous treatment can be initiated in the severely ill with doxycycline 2.2 mg/kg (up to 100 mg) twice per day. Defervescence is expected after 24 to 48 hours of therapy. Treatment should continue for 10 to 14 days after the fever resolves. Relapses can occur, so adequate duration of therapy is essential. Although in vivo data are lacking, erythromycin is presumed to be the best alternative agent for patients with a contraindication to tetracyclines, such as children and pregnant women. Antibiotic prophylaxis is not specifically addressed by psittacosis infection control guidelines, but preventative therapy for exposed persons (doxycycline 100 mg by mouth once per day) was demonstrated to be effective in at least one outbreak.[19] There is no vaccine for psittacosis in either humans or animals.

 ## UNIQUE CONSIDERATIONS

Psittacosis is an unusual disease that is rarely seen. Every medical student recognizes it as the "pneumonia caused by living with a parrot." But would this disease be considered in a large number of patients who lack a history of exposure to birds? Very little has been written about the use of *C. psittaci* as a biologic weapon, so most would probably consider other agents before testing for psittacosis. Clinical clues to the possibility of psittacosis include a respiratory illness with unusual systemic symptoms and signs. Severe headache, neurologic abnormalities or complications, splenomegaly, or elevated transaminases levels in a patient with x-ray findings consistent with atypical pneumonia should suggest psittacosis as a possible diagnosis.

 ## PITFALLS

- Failure to identify that a biologic attack has occurred; dismissing a spike in respiratory illnesses as a routine influenza outbreak

- Failure to consider psittacosis as a possible diagnosis in a patient who does not have contact with birds
- Failure to directly test for *C. psittaci* by serology in a patient with a history of bird contact or in a group of patients with similar, unexplained cases of "atypical pneumonia"
- Failure to design, practice, and implement a disaster plan to cope with the increase in patient load seen during a biologic attack
- Failure to stock adequate supplies of antibiotics or to request early mobilization of state and federal stockpiles
- Failure to treat infected patients with a sufficient duration of therapy to prevent relapses

CASE PRESENTATION

"Another Z PAK (azithromycin)?" you think, as you write yet another prescription for yet another case of atypical pneumonia. That makes three today alone. Add that to the four from the previous shift and the 12 cases last week, and this is starting to be the worst winter flu season in years. The only problem is that the calendar still reads September. The latest case is a 24-year-old female student complaining of a severe headache, fever, dry cough, sweats, and nausea for 5 days. On physical examination, you find bilateral crackles, splenomegaly, and photophobia, but no meningismus. Her chest x-ray reveals the same bilateral interstitial infiltrates that were seen in the other patients, and her laboratory results include moderately elevated transaminases levels. This prompts you to ask for further history; she denies smoking and alcohol or drug use. She also denies any recent travel, except to the state capital last week for a rock concert. By a strange coincidence, the last patient with pneumonia you treated also mentioned he had been at that particular concert.

REFERENCES

1. Gregory DW, Schaffner W. Psittacosis. *Semin Respir Infect.* 1997;12:7-11.
2. Macfarlane JT, Macrae AD. Psittacosis. *Br Med Bull.* 1983;39:163-87.
3. Schlossberg D. Chlamydia psittaci (psittacosis). In: Mandell GL, Bennet JE, Dolin R, eds. Principles and Practice of Infectious Diseases. 4th ed. New York: Churchill Livingstone; 1995:1693-96.
4. Gresham AC, Dixon CE, Bevan BJ. Domiciliary outbreak of psittacosis in dogs; potential for zoonotic infection. *Vet Rec.* 1996;138:622-3.
5. Ito I, Ishida T, Mishima M, et al. Familial cases of psittacosis: possible person-to-person transmission. *Intern Med.* 2002;41:580-3.
6. U.S. Centers for Disease Control and Prevention. Emergency Preparedness & Response. Available at: http://www.bt.cdc.gov.
7. Davis JA. The looming biological warfare storm. *Air Space Power J.* 2003;17:57-68.
8. Wreghitt TG, Taylor CED. Incidence of respiratory tract chlamydial infections and importation of psittacine birds. *Lancet.* 1988; 8585:582.
9. Reeve RVA, Carter LA, Taylor N. Respiratory tract infections and importation of exotic birds. *Lancet.* 1988;8589:829-30.
10. Hinton DG, Shipley A, Galcin JW, et al. Chlamydiosis in workers at a duck farm and processing plant. *Aust Vet J.* 1993;70:174-6.
11. Hedberg K, White KE, Forfang JC, et al. An outbreak of psittacosis in Minnesota turkey industry workers: implications for modes of transmission and control. *Am J Epidemiol.* 1989;130:569-77.

12. U.S. Centers for Disease Control and Prevention. Psittacosis at a turkey processing plant—North Carolina, 1989. *Morb Mortal Wkly Rep*. 1990;39:460-1.

13. Grimes JE. Zoonoses acquired from pet birds. *Vet Clin*. 1987;17:209-18.

14. U.S. Centers for Disease Control and Prevention. Psittacosis Surveillance, 1975-1984. Atlanta: Centers for Disease Control and Prevention, June 1987.

15. Yung AP, Grayson ML. Psittacosis—a review of 135 cases. *Med J Aust*. 1988;148:228-33.

16. Crosse BA. Psittacosis: a clinical review. *J Infect*. 1990;21:251-9.

17. U.S. Centers for Disease Control and Prevention. Compendium of measures to control Chlamydia psittaci infection among humans (psittacosis) and pet birds (avian chlamydiosis), 2000. *Morb Mortal Wkly Rep Recomm Rep*. 2000;49:RR-8,1-18.

18. Pavlin JA, Gilchrist MJR, Osweiler GD, Woollen NE. Diagnostic analyses of biological agent-caused syndromes: laboratory and technical assistance. *Emerg Med Clin North Am*. 2002;20:331-50.

19. Broholm KA, Bottiger M, Jernelius H, et al. Ornithosis as a nosocomial infection. *Scand J Infect Dis*. 1977;9:263-7.

chapter 117

Escherichia coli O157:H7 (Hemorrhagic *E. Coli*) Attack

Roy Karl Werner

 ## DESCRIPTION OF EVENT

Escherichia coli is a ubiquitous, gram-negative, rod-shaped bacterium that can be located throughout the environment, including water and soil. It is most commonly found as normal flora of the intestinal tract of most mammals, including humans, where it lives to suppress growth of more harmful bacteria. In addition to the enterohemorrhagic *E. coli*, which is of concern as potential biologic weapons, there are four other types of *E. coli* that cause gastrointestinal disease.[1] A detailed discussion of these is beyond the scope of this chapter. However, their characteristics are summarized in Table 117-1.

E. coli O157:H7, an enterohemorrhagic strain, is considered a category B threat by the Centers for Disease Control and Prevention (CDC)[2] since it is easily spread via the fecal-oral route[3] and has moderate morbidity but low mortality. The O157:H7 serotype produces a Shiga-like toxin that can cause a significant inflammatory response within the intestines without direct invasion of cells. The toxin is encoded on a plasmid and can be readily passed from one bacterium to another.[1] This bacterium is quite facile in its ability to obtain new genetic information and incorporate it into its arsenal for defense and infectivity in its hosts. *E. coli* O157:H7 can persist for significant lengths of time in hostile environments and may even require a slightly acidic environment to grow.[4-6] Most *E. coli* O157:H7 outbreaks are linked to fecal-oral transmission due to poor handwashing techniques and unhygienic food handling. Sources of human infection have included, among others, poorly cooked meat (especially hamburger), apple juice, water (including water parks), vegetables and fruit from salad bars, and milk products such as yogurt and unpasteurized milk.[7-11] There are reported cases of aerosolized spread of *E. coli*, usually in sewage, but only under very specific circumstances and conditions.

E. coli O157:H7 can infect anyone, but more severe symptoms are found among patients at the extremes of age or in immunocompromised individuals.[12] The endotheliocidal properties of *E. coli* O157:H7 affect the intestinal endothelium as well as the renal and vascular endothelium, leading to the development of hemolytic uremic syndrome (HUS) and thrombotic thrombocytopenic purpura (TTP).[1,2,7,12-14] *It is noteworthy that other enterohemorrhagic* E. coli *exist with different serotypes. Thus, a bioterrorism attack need not be of the O157:H7 serotype.* For purposes of this chapter, the term *E. coli* O157:H7 will be used since it is the most common serotype, but the reader should understand that the clinical syndrome could be caused by other enterohemorrhagic serotypes as well.

Symptomatic *E. coli* O157:H7 infection affects approximately 75,000 individuals in the United States yearly and was first identified as a human pathogen in 1982 when it was isolated in the stool of individuals who had eaten raw or undercooked meat. In 1993 there was an outbreak from hamburgers served at a regional fast food chain, causing HUS and several deaths.[8,15,16]

The incubation period of *E. coli* O157:H7 is between 3 and 9 days.[6,14] Patients initially complain of symptoms similar to viral gastroenteritis: abdominal cramping with significant abdominal pain and tenderness; flatulence; elevated temperatures; and voluminous, watery diarrhea. The diarrhea eventually becomes bloody; 91% of patients report bloody stools at some time during the course of the disease. This likely overestimates the prevalence of bloody diarrhea since patients with less severe disease likely don't present to physicians. Approximately 30% of symptomatic patients require hospitalization, and the mortality rate is approximately 1%. *Shigella, Vibrio parahaemolyticus, Campylobacter,* and *Salmonella* species; cancerous lesions; ulcerative colitis; incomplete obstruction; gastrointestinal bleeding; and recent antibiotic usage (e.g., for *Clostridium difficile*)[13] should all be included in the differential diagnosis of hemorrhagic diarrhea.

Treatment for *E. coli* O157:H7 infection is limited to supportive measures to prevent dehydration and other complications. The use of antibiotics is contraindicated and has been associated with increased incidence of hemolytic complications.[2,7,13,14,17,18] Antimotility medications are appropriate in afebrile patients *without* bloody diarrhea. Early re-feeding of patients with a lactose-free diet can reduce the duration of diarrhea. The disease is generally self-limited and resolves approximately 1 week after the onset of symptoms.

TABLE 117-1 *E. COLI* CAUSING GASTROINTESTINAL SYMPTOMS

TYPE OF GI DISORDER	SOURCE / GEOGRAPHY	TOXIN	INVASIVENESS	CLINICAL	DIARRHEA
Enterotoxigenic					
Traveler's diarrhea (children and travelers)	Water sources	Cytotoxic heat stable and/or heat labile	None; no cellular changes or bacteremia	No fever, mild dehydration, self-limited illness	Watery, voluminous; originates in proximal small bowel
Enteroinvasive					
Dysentery syndrome (children and adults)	Asia	Shigella-like	Epithelial cells of intestine	Fever, tenesmus, dehydration, abdominal cramps	Blood-tinged with many polymorpho-nuclear lymphocytes
Enteroaggregative					
Children	Less developed countries	Some have a heat stabile	Aggregative adherence	No fever, mild dehydration, self-limited illness	Watery, nonbloody, and persistent
Enteropathogenic					
Children and newborns	Nurseries	None	Adherence, causing effacement	No fever, acute-onset diarrhea in neonates, dehydration	Nonbloody
Enterohemorrhagic					
Children and adults	Foods, raw beef	Shiga-like	Effacement of intestinal mucosa	Vomiting, no fever, nausea, chills, HUS, TTP	First nonbloody, then grossly bloody

HUS, Hemolytic uremic syndrome; *TTP,* thrombotic thrombocytopenic purpura

The most feared sequela of enterohemorrhagic *E. coli* is HUS, a triad of acute renal failure, thrombocytopenia, and microangiopathic hemolytic anemia. This is especially common in infants and children. Patients with the additional findings of fluctuating neurologic symptoms and fever are classified as having TTP. This may be more common in geriatric or infirm populations.[19] Blood urea nitrogen (BUN) should be monitored because an increase may signal extraintestinal endothelial involvement and potential progression to TTP or HUS. Urine should also be monitored for hematuria and/or proteinuria, again suggesting progression to TTP or HUS. Discussion of the treatment of TTP and HUS is beyond the scope of this chapter.

All *E. coli* is easily cultured on sorbitol-MacConkey agar. Laboratory analysis will seldom identify the causative organism unless *E. coli* O157:H7 is specifically sought. *However, the CDC recommends that all stools from patients with bloody diarrhea be screened for the O157:H7 serotype.* Antisera to the O157:H7 antigen can be used to screen isolates. Any isolates that screen positive should be sent to a reference laboratory for further characterization. Isolation of the bacteria is most likely during the first 6 days of diarrhea. Many times the O157:H7 serotype cannot be isolated from even bloody diarrheal stools that commonly have high concentrations of this pathogen.[20,21] Obtaining stool samples from multiple patients will increase isolation yield and assist with characterization of *E. coli* O157:H7 when present. Stool studies should include a search for other etiologic factors of the diarrheal disease, including those previously noted. Multiplex PCR (polymerase chain reaction using multiple primers) studies, fingerprinting, and rapid identification[22,23] studies should be used to assist in determining the specific cause. If *E. coli* O157:H7 is identified, it is mandatory that it be reported to the CDC; this allows centralized monitoring of outbreaks.

 PREINCIDENT ACTIONS

The greatest potential for limiting the impact of a terrorist attack involving the dissemination of *E. coli* O157:H7 is the readiness of the "front-line fighters" of the healthcare system—emergency medical personnel, outpatient clinics, and emergency departments. The presentation of an escalating number of patients with severe diarrheal disease along with similarities in medical, travel, or exposure history should alert medical and public health personnel to the possibility of a nonaccidental exposure.[24]

Continuous water and food production monitoring by the appropriate local, state, and federal agencies as well as routine testing and retesting of in-place barriers to terrorism by Homeland Security task forces[25,26] will also contribute to the safety of citizens.

Computer-aided programs, passive surveillance of foodstuffs, random testing of food processing areas, irradiation and filtration of airborne particles, and tighter control of treatment areas for national food and water supplies are all methods currently in place to decrease the impact of bioterrorism.[24,26] Handwashing and glove use at patient points of contact or before handling foodstuffs are ways spread can be minimized.

 POSTINCIDENT ACTIONS

When an outbreak of *E. coli* O157:H7 infection is suspected, hospital laboratories should be alerted, and

agent-specific cultures of stool samples should be obtained. Stool samples can also be tested for fecal leukocytes,[13,28] although results are not particularly sensitive or specific. Fecal lactoferrin assays have the potential to be beneficial but their utility is also debated; fecal lactoferrin is considered more specific for bacterial causes of diarrhea[29] but cannot help with determining the specific etiologic factor. If the source of the outbreak can be readily identified, it should be contained and eliminated immediately. Foodstuffs in the area should be incinerated to decrease perpetuation of the infection.[30,31] Surface areas can be decontaminated with a 5% to 10% bleach solution.

MEDICAL TREATMENT OF CASUALTIES

Oral rehydration solutions are helpful in patients with *E. coli* O157:H7 infection since most patients have minimal vomiting. The World Health Organization recommends solutions containing: 2.6 g sodium chloride, 2.9 g trisodium citrate dihydrate, 1.5 g potassium chloride, and 13.5 g anhydrous glucose, all dissolved in 1 L of clean water for a total osmolarity of 245 mOsm/L solution.[13,28,32-34] Appropriate infection control practices should be instituted for *E. coli* and include body substance isolation and handwashing. Masks are optional for *E. coli* because airborne spread is inconsequential (unless contaminated feces are aerosolized). Rehydration should include intravenous solutions if oral intake is poorly tolerated or if the patient fails to improve.

UNIQUE CONSIDERATIONS

The relatively benign symptoms of fevers, abdominal cramping, and diarrhea are commonly minimized; therefore, *E. coli* O157:H7 infection is not suspected and thus fecal-oral spread continues before hemorrhagic diarrhea commences or *E. coli* O157:H7 infection is considered. Identification of *E. coli* O157:H7 requires specialized testing that may not be readily available at the local laboratory. Harbingers of a possible bioterrorism event with *E. coli* O157:H7 include a clustering of infectious diarrhea in a previously healthy population, all of whom have similar exposures (e.g., water, food). Travel to an area with a known outbreak of disease should also raise the clinician's level of suspicion.[24,35]

CASE PRESENTATION

A carnival is in town for a July 4th celebration being held at an old farm that was recently converted into a recreational area. There are rides for all ages, games of skill, a large variety foods and fresh vegetables, and tents containing many attractions. Many of the town's people attend the festivities, including significant numbers of the hospital staff. The carnival ends without incident. One week later a number of children seek care at their doctors' offices with complaints of diarrhea and abdominal cramping. Most are sent home with antimotility drugs and prescribed a "BRAT" (bananas, rice, applesauce, toast) diet, and some are given oral antibiotics. There is also an increase in the number of geriatric visits for similar complaints. Three days later, these same people begin presenting to the emergency department due to bloody diarrhea and lethargy. Laboratory analysis is unremarkable, other than for mild leukocytosis and borderline electrolyte abnormalities. Some patients have elevated levels of protein and casts present on urinalysis. Many patients presenting to the emergency department with children or elderly family members are complaining of similar symptoms and easy bruisability. Laboratory studies on these otherwise healthy young adults show renal insufficiency and mild hemolytic anemia. Patients presenting with confusion or weakness are sent for computed tomography of the brain. An emergency medical technician in a town the carnival visited died approximately 2 weeks after the carnival left. She died from complications from treatment of severe dehydration and cerebral vascular accident. A husband and wife, both emergency medical technicians, who worked at a previous site the carnival visited also died after an infant son of theirs died. They all had a similar disease course as described above and had no predisposing factors.

Individuals of a terrorist group obtained part-time employment with the carnival company cleaning animals or common areas. These areas all contained a pressurized watering system used to clean these sections. These areas were theorized to have enormous concentrations of the aerosolized (36) *Escherichia coli* O157:H7 for periods of time throughout the day, usually at times of patron egress through causeways of the carnival. Small Petri dishes were found at the encampment containing genetically identical *E. coli* O157:H7 by multiplex PCR evaluation. After a thorough investigation, the CDC strongly suspects that the carnival was the site of a bioterrorism attack where the perpetrators disseminated *E. coli* O157:H7 via food and water contamination.

REFERENCES

1. Eisenstein BI, Zaleznik DF. Enterobacteriaceae. In: Mandell GL, Bennett JE, Dolin R, eds. Principals and Practice of Infectious Diseases. 5th ed, vol 2. Philadelphia: Churchill Livingstone; 2000:2294-2310.
2. U.S. Centers for Disease Control and Prevention. General and Technical Information. Available at: http://www.cdc.gov/ncidod/dbmd/diseaseinfo/escherichiacoli_g.htm.
3. Todar K. Todar's Online Textbook of Bacteriology. Available at: http://www.textbookofbacteriology.net.
4. Rhee MS, Lee SY, Dougherty RH, et al. Antimicrobial effects of mustard flour and acetic acid against Escherichia coli O157:H7, Listeria monocytogenes, and Salmonella enterica serovar Typhimurium. *Appl Environ Microbiol.* 2003;69:2959-63.
5. Reinders RD, Biesterveld S, Bijker PGH. Survival of Escherichia coli O157:H7 ATCC 43895 in a model apple juice medium with different concentrations of proline and caffeic acid. *Appl Environ Microbiol.* 2001;67:2863-6.
6. Cody SH, Glynn MK, Farrar JA, et al. An outbreak of Escherichia coli O157:H7 infection from unpasteurized commercial apple juice. *Ann Intern Med.* 1999;130: 202-9.
7. U.S. Food and Drug Administration, Center for Food Safety & Applied Nutrition. Foodborne Pathogenic Microorganisms and Natural Toxins Handbook. The Bad Bug Book. Available at: http://www.cfsan.fda.gov/~mow/intro.html.

8. Feng P. Escherichia coli serotype O157:H7: novel vehicles of infection and emergence of phenotypic variants. *Emerg Infect Dis*. 1995;1(2):47-52.

9. U.S. Centers for Disease Control and Prevention. Lake-associated outbreak of Escherichia coli O157:H7—Illinois, 1995. *Morb Mortal Wkly Rep*. 1996;45(21):437-9.

10. U.S. Centers for Disease Control and Prevention. Outbreaks of Escherichia coli O157:H7 infection and cryptosporidiosis associated with drinking unpasteurized apple cider—Connecticut and New York, October 1996. *Morb Mortal Wkly Rep*. 1997;45(21):4-8.

11. U.S. Centers for Disease Control and Prevention. Outbreak of Escherichia coli O157:H7 infections associated with drinking unpasteurized commercial apple juice—British Columbia, California, Colorado, and Washington, October 1996. *Morb Mortal Wkly Rep*. 1996;45(44):975.

12. Guerrant RL, Steiner TS. Principles and syndromes of enteric infections. In: Mandell GL, Bennett JE, Dolin R, eds. Principals and Practice of Infectious Diseases. 5th ed. Vol 1. Philadelphia: Churchill Livingstone; 2000:1080-5.

13. Hamer DH, and Gorbach SL. Infectious diarrhea and bacterial food poisoning. In: Feldman M, Scharschmidt BF, and Sleisenger MH. Editors. Gastrointestinal and Liver Disease. 6th ed. Vol 2. Philadelphia: WB Saunders; 1998:1594-1632.

14. Tauxe RV, Swerdlow DL, Hughes JM. Foodborne disease. In: Mandell GL, Bennett JE, Dolin R, eds. Principals and Practice of Infectious Diseases, 5th ed. Vol 1. Philadelphia: Churchill Livingstone; 2000:1150-65.

15. U.S. Centers for Disease Control and Prevention. Preliminary report: foodborne outbreak of Escherichia coli O157:H7 infections from hamburgers—Western United States, 1993. *Morb Mortal Wkly Rep*. 1993;42(4):85-6.

16. U.S. Centers for Disease Control and Prevention. Update: multi-state outbreak of Escherichia coli O157:H7 infections from hamburgers—Western United States, 1992-1993. *Morb Mortal Wkly Rep*. 1993;42(14):258-63.

17. Weinstein RS, and Alibek K. Shigellosis. In: Biological and Chemical Terrorism—A Guide for Healthcare Providers and the First Responders. New York: Thieme Medical Publishers; 2003:96-7.

18. Weinstein RS, and Alibek K. Biological weapon syndromic cross-references. In: Biological and Chemical Terrorism—A Guide for Healthcare Providers and the First Responders. New York: Thieme Medical Publishers; 2003:13.

19. Richards A, Goodship JA, Goodship TH. The genetics and pathogenesis of haemolytic uraemic syndrome and thrombotic thrombocytopenic purpura. *Curr Opin Nephrol Hypertens*. 2002;11(4):431-5.

20. Osterholm MT, Hedberg CW, Moore KA. Epidemiologic principles. In: Mandell GL, Bennett JE, Dolin R, eds. Principals and Practice of Infectious Diseases. 5th ed. Vol 1. Philadelphia: Churchill Livingstone; 2000:157-9.

21. Gill VJ, Fedorko DP, Witebsky FG. The clinician and the microbiology lab. In: Mandell GL, Bennett JE, Dolin R, eds. Principals and Practice of Infectious Diseases. 5th ed. Vol 1. Philadelphia: Churchill Livingstone; 2000:191-2.

22. Vidal R, Vidal M, Lagos R, et al. Multiplex PCR for diagnosis of enteric infections associated with diarrheagenic Escherichia coli. *J Clin Microbiol*. 2004;42(4):1787-9.

23. Fratamico PM, Bagi LK, Pepe T. A multiplex polymerase chain reaction assay for rapid detection and identification of Escherichia coli O157:H7 in foods and bovine feces. *J Food Prot*. 2000;63(8):1032-7.

24. Burkle FM. Mass casualty management of a large-scale bioterrorist event: an epidemiological approach that shapes triage decisions. *Emerg Med Clin North Am*. 2002;20(2):409-36.

25. Kahn AS, Swerdlow DL, Juranek DD. Precautions against biological and chemical terrorism directed at food and water supplies. *Public Health Rep*. 2001;116(1):3-14.

26. Filoromo C, Macrina D, Pryor E, et al. An innovative approach to training hospital-based clinicians for bioterrorist attacks. *Am J Infect Control*. 2003;31(8):511-14.

27. Brickner PW, Vincent RL, First M, et al. The application of ultraviolet germicidal irradiation to control transmission of airborne disease: bioterrorism countermeasure (practice articles). *Public Health Rep*. 2003;118(2):99-114.

28. Lung E. Acute diarrheal diseases. In: Friedman SL, McQuaid KR, Grendell JH, eds. Current Diagnosis and Treatment in Gastroenterology. 2nd ed. New York: Lange Medical Books/McGraw-Hill; 2003:131-50.

29. Huicho L, Campos M, Rivera J, Guerrant RL. Fecal screening tests in the approach to acute infectious diarrhea: a scientific overview. *Pediatr Infect Dis J*. 1996;15(6):486-94.

30. Bosilevac JM, Arthur TM, Wheeler TL, et al. Prevalence of Escherichia coli O157 and levels of aerobic bacteria and Enterobacteriaceae are reduced when hides are washed and treated with cetylpyridinium chloride at a commercial beef processing plant. *J Food Prot*. 2004;67(4):646-50.

31. Oldfield EC 3rd. Emerging foodborne pathogens: keeping your patients and your families safe. *Rev Gastroenterol Disord*. 2001;1(4):177-86.

32. World Health Organization. 13th Expert Committee on the Selection and Use of Essential Medicines, 31 March to 3 April 2003. Available at: http://whqlibdoc.who.int/trs/WHO_TRS_920.pdf.

33. World Health Organization. WHO Essential Medicines Library. Oral rehydration salts (for glucose-electrolyte solution). Available at: http://mednet3.who.int/EMLib/DiseaseTreatments/MedicineDetails.aspx?MedIDName=235@oral%20rehydration%20salts%20(for%20glucose-electrolyte%20solution).

34. World Health Organization. Oral Rehydration Salts (ORS): A New Reduced Osmolarity Formulation. Available at: http://www.who.int/child-adolescent-health/New_Publications/NEWS/Statement.htm.

35. Weinstein RS, and Alibek K. Basic bioterrorism. In: Biological and Chemical Terrorism—A Guide for Healthcare Providers and the First Responders. New York: Thieme Medical Publishers; 2003:2-12.

36. Teltsch B, Shuval HI, Tadmor J. Die-away kinetics of aerosolized bacteria from sprinkler application of wastewater. *Appl Environ Microbiol*. 1980;39(6):1191-7.

chapter 118

Viral Encephalitides (Alphaviruses) Attack

Matthew Berkman and Kelly J. Corrigan

 ## DESCRIPTION OF EVENT

The Alphaviruses are one of the three families of the arthropod-borne viruses (arboviruses) that can cause encephalitis. Three Alphaviruses currently cause human disease in the United States: the Eastern equine encephalitis (EEE), Western equine encephalitis (WEE), and Venezuelan equine encephalitis (VEE) viruses. All three are transmitted through mosquitoes and can initially present as a flulike illness. The EEE virus is maintained through a bird-mosquito-bird lifecycle. The most important vector is the mosquito *Culiseta melanura*.[1] These mosquitoes are often found in coastal areas and near freshwater swamps. Hence, most U.S. cases have been reported in Florida, Georgia, Massachusetts, and New Jersey. EEE has a high case fatality rate—35% reported by the Centers for Disease Control and Prevention (CDC). Of those who survive, an estimated 35% will have permanent mild to severe neurologic deficits. There have been approximately 200 human cases in the United States since 1964, with two fatalities in August 2004 in Massachusetts.[2]

The closely related WEE has a reported 10% case fatality rate. Like EEE, it is a summertime disease but is found in states west of the Mississippi River and in some western Canadian provinces. It is also maintained by a bird-mosquito-bird lifecycle, with its primary vector the mosquito *Culex tarsalis*. The worst outbreak recorded was 3336 human cases in 1941. Since 1955, a varied range of 0 to 200 cases per year have been reported, with no human cases reported since 1994.[1,2]

VEE is found in South and Central America. It is maintained by a rodent-mosquito lifecycle and claims at least 10 mosquito species as its vector. The fatality rates have been approximately 0.6% in reported outbreaks. Past epidemics include 32,000 human cases in Venezuela from 1962-64, and in 1971, more than 10,000 horses died from a VEE epidemic. Human cases have been sporadic since then.[1,2]

All three of these Alphaviruses can present clinically with nonspecific flulike symptoms, but many may include high fever, headache, photophobia, stiff neck, nausea, and vomiting. In cases of encephalitic invasion, symptoms can progress to confusion, obtundation, seizures, and focal neurologic deficits.

 ## PREINCIDENT ACTIONS

Humans who live in high-risk areas or work or play outside frequently in these areas should be sure to wear mosquito repellant that contains DEET and wear long-sleeved shirts and pants. During outbreaks, outdoor activity should be limited. Widely available vaccines are being developed and are undergoing validity testing.

In preparation for potential biologic terrorist attacks, the Institute of Medicine Committee on Research and Development to Improve Civilian Medical Response recommends that major hospitals conduct mass casualty planning and training and that they have isolation rooms available for infectious diseases; have decontamination capacity; and be fully supplied with drugs, ventilators, and personal protective equipment. The committee also encourages the CDC to keep medical care providers up-to-date on current dangerous biologic materials.[3]

 ## POSTINCIDENT ACTIONS

All cases are to be reported to the CDC. Public health warnings are then issued, and prevention measures are initiated. Eradicating potential arthropod vectors and vaccinating equine reservoirs may help to prevent the spread of encephalitis in the event of a biologic attack.[4]

Since no person-to-person spread is know to be possible, only universal precautions must be maintained in patients infected with one of the arboviruses.[4,5]

 ## MEDICAL TREATMENT OF CASUALTIES

As in the case of most viral illnesses, treatment of the Alphavirus encephalitides consists primarily of supportive care.[2,6-9] Patients suspected of having viral encephalitis should undergo a workup for concomitant meningitis with computed tomography of the head and lumbar puncture and be admitted to the hospital for further serologic testing. The airway should be protected; nutrition, fluids, and electrolytes should be optimized; pyrexia should be aggressively treated; and vigilance in preventing secondary infections should be maintained.[7,9] In the setting of increased intracranial pressure, patients should be managed in the intensive care setting with hyperventilation, head elevation, diuresis, and possibly steroids or intravenous immunoglobulin.[9] Prevention of seizures is important, and consideration for administering temporary anticonvulsant therapy should be given.[2]

Consultation with a neurologist and infections disease specialist is recommended. Neurosurgical consultation may be necessary if a brain biopsy is considered.[8] Although there is no specific medical treatment available for the arboviruses, the use of ribavirin and recombinant interferon alpha is being assessed.[2,8]

Prognosis depends not only on the particular type of arbovirus responsible for the encephalitis, but also on the age and prior health of the individual infected. Children 1 year old or younger and adults 55 years old or older are at increased risk of life-threatening complications.

 UNIQUE CONSIDERATIONS

Although the effects of Alphavirus encephalitis can be devastating with persistent neurologic sequela or death, the vast majority of patients exposed to these viruses will be asymptomatic or present with nonspecific flulike symptoms.[4] An early Alphaviral attack will be difficult to identify and distinguish from routine "viral syndrome" due to the similarity of illness presentation and lack of routine laboratory testing for the viruses.

The viral encephalitides are CDC category B biologic agents, which are moderately easy to disseminate and have low mortality rates. In their natural state, these viruses require arthropod vectors for transmission and have a variable seasonality dependent on the geography, local climate, and virus-specific lifecycle. These qualities make the use of the Alphaviruses as a terrorist agent more difficult to control and disseminate to the general public. That being said, aerosol transmission of a weaponized (manufactured) form of the virus has been demonstrated and would represent the most likely route of mass infection if terrorists were able to produce large amounts of aerosolized virus.[4,9] Other characteristics of the Alphaviruses that lend themselves to weaponization include the ability to inexpensively produce large amounts of stable virus and the potential for genetic manipulation of native viruses.[7]

One possible clue to an Alphavirus attack is a large number of sick or dying equine animals in the vicinity,[9] thus arthropod vector control and vaccinating equine reservoirs may help to prevent the spread of encephalitis during an outbreak.[4]

 PITFALLS

- Failure to notify appropriate public health officials of a diagnosis of viral encephalitis
- Failure to prepare local emergency departments and clinics to respond appropriately in case of an outbreak

- Failure to disseminate medical instructions and training for local communities, as appropriate
- Failure to recognize that reports of sick or dying equine animals in the area may be related to a vector-borne disease

 CASE PRESENTATION

The last few weeks have been hot and rainy, and there has been a moderate increase in the number of otherwise healthy individuals presenting to emergency departments with vague "viral syndrome" complaints. There are also news reports of a large number of equine illnesses in nearby communities. Many patients who were originally sent home with supportive care have returned with worsening mental status, lethargy, and seizures. An elderly patient, who has had a seizure, presents to the emergency department. He was reportedly seen at another hospital 3 days ago for nausea, vomiting, fatigue, low-grade fever, confusion, and headache. Since then his symptoms have become worse, with an inability to tolerate fluids by mouth and increasing agitation and confusion. He has a fever of 101°F, with mild tachycardia and a stable blood pressure.

REFERENCES

1. Markhoff L. Alphaviruses. In: Mandell GL, Bennett JE, Dolin R, eds. Principles and Practice of Infectious Diseases. 5th ed. Philadelphia: Churchill Livingstone; 2000.
2. US Centers for Disease Control and Prevention, Division of Vector-Borne Infectious Diseases. Arboviral Encephalitides. Available at: http://www.cdc.gov/ncidod/dvbid/arbor/index.htm.
3. Katona P. Bioterrorism preparedness: a generic blueprint for health departments, hospitals, and physicians. *Infect Dis Clin Pract.* 2002;11(3):115-22.
4. Rajagopalan S. Deadly viruses. *Top Emerg Med.* 2002;24(3):44-55.
5. Cherry CL, Kainer MA, Ruff TA. Biological weapons preparedness: the role of physicians. *Intern Med J.* 2003;33:242-53.
6. Harwood-Nuss A. The Clinical Practice of Emergency Medicine. 3rd ed. Philadelphia: Lippincott Williams & Wilkins; 2001.
7. Franz DR, Jarhling PB, Friedlander AM, et al. Clinical recognition and management of patients exposed to biological warfare agents. *JAMA.* 1997;278:399-411.
8. de Assis Aquino Gondim F, Oliveira G, Thomas FP. Viral Encephalitis. eMedicine. Available at: http://www.emedicine.com/.
9. Sardesai AM, Brown NM, Menon DK. Deliberate release of biological agents. *Anaesthesia.* 2002;57(11):1067-82.

chapter 119

Tick-Borne Encephalitis Virus Attack

Vittorio J. Raho

 ## DESCRIPTION OF EVENT

Tick-borne encephalitis (TBE) is classically caused by infection with one of two flaviviruses: Russian spring-summer encephalitis virus (RSSEV) or Central European encephalitis virus (CEEV).[1] However, the TBE virus-complex is sometimes extended to include other entities such as Omsk hemorrhagic fever and Kyasanur Forest disease, which are closely related viruses with associated tick vectors.[2] The geographic distribution of TBE includes the former Soviet Union, Central and Eastern Europe, and Asia. TBE viruses are associated with hard-bodied Ixodid ticks, such as *Ixodes persulcatus*, which act as reservoirs for the virus as well as vectors when they infect their hosts, usually small woodland mammals. Humans are accidental hosts and do not participate in the virus's normal reproductive cycle.

In Russia, 5000 to 10,000 cases of TBE are reported annually, with fatalities in the low hundreds.[3] When comparing the two closest subtypes of TBE viruses, RSSEV has a much more virulent clinical course, with reported mortality rates between 20% to 30%.[4,5] RSSEV is sometimes referred to as Far Eastern encephalitis. A recent report of a severe hemorrhagic syndrome not previously described has now been associated with TBE infections in Russia, suggesting that more virulent strains may yet be discovered.[3] Natural outbreaks of TBE coincide with the well-defined periods of tick activity, usually from April to October. Cases have also been documented from human ingestion of raw milk from infected goats.[2,5]

TBE infection manifests clinically across a spectrum of severity, from mild aseptic meningitis to florid meningoencephalitis. After a 1- to 2-week incubation period, patients may experience a biphasic illness with initial symptoms of fever, malaise, myalgia, headaches, nausea, and vomiting that last around 2 to 4 days. After a brief remission of symptoms, between one fourth and one third of patients will develop the manifestations of severe meningoencephalitis, with symptoms of central nervous system dysfunction, including severe headache and meningismus, confusion, lethargy, delirium, convulsions, paralysis, coma, and death.[6] Survivors have a significant rate of neurologic sequelae, including limb paralysis and cognitive deficits.[7] A more rapid and severe course of illness is associated with RSSEV.

Nonspecific laboratory data include leukopenia, thrombocytopenia, and elevated liver function tests and sedimentation rate. During the meningoencephalitis phase, cerebrospinal fluid studies will show lymphocytosis and an elevated protein level.[8] Magnetic resonance imaging has been shown to be superior to computed tomography in identifying tissue inflammation in other forms of viral encephalitis.[9]

 ## PREINCIDENT ACTIONS

Surveillance systems, which acquire data from government sources, hospital emergency room discharge summaries, and state public health networks, can effectively identify unusual clusters of viral syndromes in certain geographic distributions. Epidemiologic analysis may be the only way to detect such an attack, especially since symptoms are so nonspecific and may resemble a myriad of other domestic illnesses.

 ## POSTINCIDENT ACTIONS

Laboratory diagnosis of TBE is usually made using serologic testing, such as IgM enzyme-linked immunosorbent assay or reverse transcriptase PCR (polymerase chain reaction), for detection of viral ribonucleic acid. Laboratory workers should take biosafety precautions to prevent exposure to infectious aerosols.[10] Fortunately, no person-to-person transmission of TBE has been reported. If the attack is via the natural tick-borne route, vector control using repellents such as permethrin may be the most efficient way to thwart an attack once it has been identified. Reports indicate that the TBE virus is neutralized by common disinfectants such as 1% sodium hypochlorite and formaldehyde.[7]

 ## MEDICAL TREATMENT OF CASUALTIES

No specific medical treatment is available for any of these viruses. The management of such patients is dictated by their neurologic and cardiovascular sequelae and may include respiratory support including mechanical ventilation, hemodynamic monitoring, treatment of secondary bacterial infections such as pneumonia, or possible steroid administration to suppress cerebral or spinal edema.

A formalin-inactivated vaccine was introduced in Austria in the late 1970s that confers some degree of immunity to TBE viruses, although it is not currently licensed in the United States.[11] However, researchers have shown promise with naked-DNA (deoxyribonucleic acid) vaccine trials in mice that confer immunity to both the CEEV and RSSEV strains.[12] Postexposure prophylaxis should be considered in high-risk groups.

 UNIQUE CONSIDERATIONS

Flaviviruses are a large group of heterogeneous viruses known for their ability to infect humans through various arthropod vectors. Yellow fever, Japanese encephalitis, and dengue hemorrhagic fever, among others, are well known to the international medical community. TBE has become a significant public health problem in many parts of Europe, as civilization encroaches on wilderness and people engage in more recreational activity in rural areas. TBE may not be as internationally recognized as other flaviviruses and therefore not screened for as often, making it more desirable as a bioweapon. The ability of TBE to infect humans through ingestion is also of concern.

 PITFALLS

- Failure to consider viral encephalitis as a potential cause of acute, febrile illness during such an outbreak
- Failure to properly isolate and inspect patients who may have infected ticks on their body
- Failure to collect blood, cerebrospinal fluid, or tick specimens and send appropriate samples to state public health laboratories
- Failure to take proper respiratory precautions when handling body fluid samples from suspected cases
- Failure to report suspected cases to the state department of public health or affiliated authority for appropriate Centers for Disease Control and Prevention notification and proper serologic testing
- Failure to alert local and state agencies to a suspected biologic attack when presented with a cluster of unusual and uncommon illnesses

REFERENCES

1. Gresikova M, Sekeyova M. Antigenic variation of the viruses belonging to the tick-borne encephalitis complex as revealed by human convalescent serum and monoclonal antibodies. *Acta Virol*. 1987;31:152-7.
2. US Centers for Disease Control and Prevention. Tick-borne Encephalitis. Available at: http://www.cdc.gov/ncidod/dvrd/spb/mnpages/dispages/TBE.htm.
3. Ternovoi VA, Kurzhukov GP, Sokolov YV, et al. Tick-borne encephalitis with hemorrhagic syndrome, Novosibirsk Region, Russia, 1999. *Emerg Infect Dis*. 2003;9(6):743-6.
4. Dumpis U, Crook D, Oksi J. Tick-borne encephalitis. *Clin Infect Dis*. 1999;28(4):882-90 (review).
5. Fauci AS, Braunwald E, Isselbacher KJ, et al. Harrison's Principles of Internal Medicine. 14th ed. New York: McGraw-Hill; 1998:1136-9.
6. Monath TP, Heinz FX. Flaviviruses. In: Fields BN, et al. Fields Virology. 3rd ed. Philadelphia: Lippincott-Raven; 1996:961-1034.
7. World Health Organization. Technical Report Series 889, WHO Expert Committee on Biological Standardization, 48th Report. Geneva: World Health Organization; 1999.
8. Kaiser R, Holzmann H. Laboratory findings in tick-borne encephalitis. Correlation with clinical outcome. *Infection*. 2000;28:78-84.
9. Sampathkumar P. West Nile virus: epidemiology, clinical presentation, diagnosis, and prevention. *Mayo Clinic Proc*. 2003;78:1137-43.
10. US Centers for Disease Control, Office of Biosafety. Classification of Etiologic Agents on the Basis of Hazard. 4th ed. Atlanta: US Department of Health, Education and Welfare, Public Health Service, US Centers for Disease Control, Office of Biosafety; 1974.
11. Kunz C, Heinz FX, Hoffmann H. Immunogenicity and reactogenicity of a highly purified vaccine against tick-borne encephalitis. *J Med Virol*. 1980;6:103-9.
12. Schmaljohn C, Vanderzanden L, Bray M, et al. Naked DNA vaccines expressing the prM and E genes of Russian spring summer encephalitis virus and Central European encephalitis virus protect mice from homologous and heterologous challenge. *J Virol*. 1997;71:9563-9.

CASE PRESENTATION

A 46-year-old man with no significant past medical history and up-to-date vaccinations presents to the emergency department with fevers, chills, myalgia, nausea, and vomiting of 3 days duration. He has had no recent exposures to sick persons, no insect bites, no recent travel, and owns no pets. Other than a fever of 101°F, his vital signs are within normal limits. His physical examination is unremarkable, including a supple neck, clear lungs, and a normal neurologic examination. He is treated with acetaminophen and ibuprofen, tolerates oral fluids, and is sent home with a presumptive viral syndrome. After remaining afebrile and feeling better for several days, his fever recurs to 104°F, and he develops a severe headache, neck stiffness, confusion, and vertigo. He is brought back to the emergency department by ambulance and is noted to be severely lethargic and confused, and he experiences a generalized tonic-clonic seizure. He is given antibiotics for presumed meningitis, and cerebrospinal fluid studies show a lymphocytic pleocytosis and a negative Gram stain. Herpesvirus tests, meningococcus serologies, and blood smears for malaria are negative, and computed tomography of the brain shows no bleeding or abscess. The patient remains unresponsive and intubated in the intensive care unit several days later. Records indicate that in the last month, 142 cases of severe acute viral syndromes of unclear etiology have been reported, with an associated mortality approaching 10%.

chapter 120

Viral Hemorrhagic Fever Virus Attack—Arenaviruses

Sandra S. Yoon

 ## DESCRIPTION OF EVENT

The arenaviruses that cause viral hemorrhagic fevers (VHFs) include the Lassa, Junin, Machupo, Guanarito, and Sabia viruses. The latter four are also known as the New World arenaviruses. They are enveloped, single-stranded ribonucleic acid (RNA) viruses, whose natural host reservoir is the rodent. The rodent species has been identified for each virus except for the Sabia virus. Although its reservoir is unknown, it has caused several natural and laboratory infections. Because these viruses are highly species specific, they determine their endemic geographic distribution—West Africa, Argentina, Bolivia, Venezuela, and Brazil, respectively. Naturally occurring cases are transmitted by infected rodent blood, urine, or feces via aerosol, direct contact, or food contamination. Person-to-person transmission then may occur by direct contact with infected bodily fluids.

The arenaviruses have been classified as category A biologic agents by the Centers for Disease Control and Prevention (CDC).[1] A mortality rate as high as 30%, the relative ease of obtaining and propagating the viruses in cell culture, potential for transmission via the respiratory system, demonstrated person-to-person transmission, and the potential for inducing widespread panic in an affected population all contribute to this classification. Furthermore, these viruses have been produced in large quantities by other countries in the past. Even though person-to-person transmission via the aerosol route has not been proven, it has been suspected in several cases of nosocomial outbreaks involving the Lassa and Machupo viruses.[2]

After initial exposure, the incubation period is typically 3 to 19 days, but it may be as short as 2 to 6 days after parenteral exposure. There have not been any reports of disease transmission during the incubation period. The clinical syndrome of arenavirus hemorrhagic fevers may be difficult, if not impossible, to distinguish from other hemorrhagic fevers or even viral syndromes. The severity of the disease and prognosis are related to the degree of viremia. The virus, in addition to infecting endothelial cells, is thought to induce the release of inflammatory mediators from macrophages, contributing to capillary leak, the hallmark of the disease. Typically, fever, headache, malaise, and myalgia are not sudden in onset as they are for other VHFs. Relative bradycardia and hyperesthesia of the skin may be clues to the diagnosis.

Lassa fever is characterized by the gradual onset of fever, nausea, abdominal pain, severe sore throat, cough, conjunctivitis, ulcerations of buccal mucosa, exudative pharyngitis, and cervical lymphadenopathy, followed by severe swelling of the head and neck, pleural and pericardial effusions, hypotension, and shock. Additional symptoms include retrosternal chest pain, back pain, vomiting, diarrhea, and proteinuria. Deafness may occur, usually in the second to third week of illness.[2-4] The New World hemorrhagic fevers are characterized by gradual onset of fever, myalgia, nausea, abdominal pain, conjunctivitis, flushing of the face and trunk, generalized lymphadenopathy, hypotension, and shock. Epigastric pain, retro-orbital pain, dizziness, photophobia, constipation, and proteinuria may also be present. Hemorrhagic manifestations, such as petechiae, especially in the axilla, and mucous membrane hemorrhages, as well as central nervous system manifestations, such as dysarthria, hyporeflexia, tremors, myoclonic movements, and seizures, are more common than in Lassa fever.[2,3,5,6] Severe manifestations of the disease usually occur during the second week of illness.

Routine laboratory analysis is typically unhelpful in making the diagnosis of VHFs. Laboratory studies may reveal leukopenia, thrombocytopenia, and hemoconcentration. Renal function is generally preserved until late in the course, although proteinuria is commonly present. Liver enzymes may be elevated, and in Lassa fever, aspartate transaminase levels greater than 150 IU/L are associated with higher mortality.[3] Definitive diagnosis requires specialized laboratory studies available at the CDC or the U.S. Army Medical Research Institute of Infectious Diseases (USAMRIID) and include antigen detection by reverse transcriptase polymerase chain reaction (PCR) or enzyme-linked immunosorbent assays (ELISA), IgM and IgG antibody detection by ELISA, and viral isolation. Viral isolation requires a Biosafety Level 4 laboratory and may take several days.[7] The presence of IgM antibody or a four-fold rise in IgG antibody titers is diagnostic;

however, antibodies may not be present until the second week of illness.

 PREINCIDENT ACTIONS

Hospitals should have disaster plans in place and should exercise them frequently. The plans should include methods for coordinating with local, state, and federal authorities and emergency medical services and a method to protect the hospital environment from contamination. Given the constellation of vague symptoms and the challenge of making a diagnosis of VHF, healthcare workers must maintain a high index of suspicion and consider this diagnosis in appropriate patients. Particular attention should be given to patients who have traveled to an endemic region, who have had direct contact with blood or other bodily fluids of a known infected person, or who work in a laboratory that handles the specific viruses.[7] In the event of a bioterrorism attack, these risk factors would be absent. However, one would expect multiple victims with similar symptoms presenting within days of each other.

 POSTINCIDENT ACTIONS

As with any suspected biologic attack, the appropriate local and state public health authorities should be notified.[8] The state authorities are then required to notify the Federal Bureau of Investigation, local law enforcement authorities, and the CDC. Decontamination of patients may be necessary, although this is unlikely in the case of VHFs because symptom presentation lags days to weeks after exposure. Person-to-person transmission via infected bodily fluids is a common and known method of transmission; therefore, specific barrier precautions should be instituted immediately. These include handwashing; double gloving; and the use of gowns, face shields, eye protection, and leg and shoe coverings. Although person-to-person airborne transmission is rare, given the difficulty of differentiating the VHFs, the high mortality, the unknown consequences of massive inoculation that may occur during a bioterrorism attack, and the potential for possible high viral loads, airborne precautions should be instituted as well.[5,7] These include the use of negative air pressure rooms and either an N95 mask or a powered air-purifying respirator.

The hospital's clinical laboratory should be notified as a precaution before sending a potentially infectious specimen. These viruses must be handled in a Biosafety Level 3 laboratory with viral isolations attempts occurring only in Biosafety Level 4 laboratories.[2] Specimens should be hand delivered, not placed in pneumatic tubes. Surfaces or objects contaminated with blood or other bodily fluids, including laboratory equipment, should be disinfected with either 1:100 dilution of household bleach or a U.S. Environmental Protection Agency–registered hospital disinfectant. Bulk bodily fluids can also be treated with bleach before disposal; however, this may damage septic tanks, and the virus is unlikely to survive standard sewage treatment. Linens should be autoclaved, inciner-

ated, or may be washed in hot water with bleach. Laboratory samples of patients with known VHF virus should be pretreated with polyethylene glycol p-tert-octylphenyl ether (Triton X-100) for 5 minutes to reduce the titers of hemorrhagic fever viruses in serum.[6]

 MEDICAL TREATMENT OF CASUALTIES

Medical management of VHF patients consists primarily of supportive care. The antiviral drug ribavirin and, in some cases, convalescent plasma, may be available as a treatment option via an investigational new drug (IND) protocol. Patients should have their fluid balance and electrolytes monitored and corrected, receive adequate analgesia, and have secondary infections aggressively treated. Indwelling lines should be kept to a minimum to prevent damage to already fragile vessels. Aspirin, nonsteroidal antiinflammatory, and other anticoagulant medications, as well as intramuscular injections, should be avoided.

If a VHF is suspected, ribavirin should be given while waiting for diagnostic tests. The dose is 30 mg/kg intravenously once (maximum of 2 g) followed by 16 mg/kg intravenously (maximum 1 g per dose) every 6 hours for 4 days, then 8 mg/kg intravenously (maximum 500 mg per dose) every 8 hours for 6 days. In the event of mass casualties, oral ribavirin may be given at the dose of 2000 mg loading; this is followed for the next 10 days by 600 mg twice a day if the patient weighs more than 75 kg, or 400 mg in the morning and 600 mg in the evening if the patient weighs less than 75 kg. Follow the same dosing guidelines for children, with the exception that for mass casualty settings, oral ribavirin is given at 30 mg/kg loading, followed by 15mg/kg/day divided into twice-daily dosing for 10 days.[2] Ribavirin may be effective in the treatment of Lassa, Junin, and Machupo infections, especially if given within 7 days of disease onset, and it has been suggested for Guanarito and Sabia viruses. The main toxicity of ribavirin therapy is dose-related anemia.[9] Passive immunity using convalescent plasma has been used in the treatment of Junin and Machupo infections, and is suggested in Guanarito infection; however, there have been mixed clinical results.[6]

An effective live attenuated vaccine exists for the Junin virus and has been used in endemic regions of Argentina. Laboratory data suggest that this vaccine may also be effective for the Machupo virus.[3] Postexposure prophylaxis with ribavirin has not been studied in humans. The current recommendations consist of medical surveillance, twice-daily temperature monitoring, and reporting of temperatures greater than 101°F or any symptoms. This should continue for 21 days past the potential exposure.[2]

 UNIQUE CONSIDERATIONS

The arenavirus hemorrhagic fevers are difficult to diagnose. The diagnosis should be considered in patients with temperatures greater than 101°F for less than 3 weeks, who present with severe illness, and who have experienced at least two hemorrhagic manifestations without a known predisposition. If there is any suspicion, ribavirin therapy should be considered and the CDC should be consulted for IND protocol approval. The effect of massive exposure to aerosolized virus has not been studied. In the event of a mass casualty incident, airborne and universal precautions should be followed. Higher levels of viremia are likely to result in greater person-to-person transmission rates. Multiple patients presenting with possible VHF should be clustered in the same part of the hospital.

 PITFALLS

- Failure to have appropriate disaster plans in place
- Failure to consider VHF in the differential of an acutely ill patient with vague complaints

 CASE PRESENTATION

A previously healthy 30-year-old man presents to an emergency department with a 6-day history of fever, headache, myalgia, epistaxis, and diarrhea. His examination is significant for a temperature of 102°F, heart rate of 70, blood pressure of 110/80 mm Hg, dehydration, hyperemic conjunctivae, and an exudative pharyngitis. Laboratory results are significant only for leukopenia (white blood cell count of 4.0), thrombocytopenia (platelet count of 74), and 2+ proteinuria. On further questioning, the patient stated that he recently returned from Venezuela, where he remembered hearing that there was a problem with the growing rodent population.

- Failure to consider ribavirin therapy in a timely manner
- Failure to notify the appropriate authorities and the laboratory
- Failure to practice strict barrier and airborne precautions

REFERENCES

1. US Centers for Disease Control and Prevention. Bioterrorism Agents/Diseases. Available at: http://www.bt.cdc.gov/Agent/Agentlist.asp.
2. Borio L, Inglesby T, Peters CJ, et al. Hemorrhagic fever viruses as biological weapons: medical and public health management. *JAMA*. 2002;287(18):2391-2405.
3. Peters CJ. Arenaviridae. In: Mandell GL, Bennett JE, Dolin R, eds. Principles and Practice of Infectious Disease. 5th ed. Vol 2. Philadelphia: Churchill Livingstone; 2000:1855-62.
4. Isaacson M. Viral hemorrhagic fever hazards for travelers in Africa. *Clin Infect Dis*. 2001;33:1707-12.
5. Charrel RN, Lamballerie X. Arenaviruses other than Lassa virus. *Antiviral Res*. 2003;57:89-100.
6. Harrison LH, Halsey NA, McKee KT, et al. Clinical case definitions for Argentine hemorrhagic fever. *Clin Infect Dis*. 1999;28:1091-4.
7. US Centers for Disease Control and Prevention. Update: management of patients with suspected viral hemorrhagic fever—United States. *Morb Mortal Wkly Rep*. 1995;44(25):475-9.
8. Steinhauer R. Bioterrorism. *RN*. 2002;65(3):48-55.
9. Huggins JW. Prospects for treatment of viral hemorrhagic fevers with ribavirin, a broad-spectrum antiviral drug. *Rev Infect Dis*. 1989;11(Suppl 4):S750-61.

chapter 121

Viral Hemorrhagic Fever Attack—Bunya Virus

Sean Michael Siler

 DESCRIPTION OF EVENT

In general, the hemorrhagic fever viruses, which consist of four families—Filoviridae, Arenaviridae, Bunyaviridae, and Flaviviridae—are seen as emerging pathogens because of the continued intrusion of man into areas where these viruses have developed an ecologic niche. With the increase in international travel, outbreaks caused by these viruses are more widely spread, and it would not be unexpected to see infections in cities with international travelers.

Only the Arenaviridae, which include the etiologic agents of the Argentine, Bolivian, and Venezuelan hemorrhagic fevers and Lassa fever, and the Filoviridae, which consist of the Ebola and Marburg viruses, are classified as Centers for Disease Control and Prevention (CDC) category A biologic agents.[1] Crimean-Congo hemorrhagic fever (CCHF) and Rift Valley fever (RVF) are a subset of the Bunyaviridae viruses that cause hemorrhagic fevers, and although not technically classified as category A agents, they do have the potential to be weaponized and delivered as fine-particle biologic aerosols. Both are a single-stranded ribonucleic acid (RNA) virus, spherical in shape, range from 70 to 120 nm in diameter, and possess a lipid envelope. Bunyaviridae are distributed endemically throughout the world, including Crimea, much of Africa, Iraq, Pakistan, Egypt, Korea, Eastern Europe, Russia, and Scandinavia.[2] CCHF virus is spread by the species of Ixodid ticks, primarily the tick *Hyalomma marginatum*, and occurs widely across Africa, southeastern Europe, the Middle East, and Asia. CCHF also represents a growing threat as bioterrorists seek to weaponize natural pathogens for delivery in populated areas outside the pathogens' endemic regions. The CCHF virus possesses some characteristics that a bioterrorist might find desirable, including the potential for aerosolization and human-to-human transmission; however, it has proven difficult to weaponize.[2] In aerosol form, CCHF is highly contagious, and as technology improves, this agent may become a greater threat. Mortality for Korean and Seoul subspecies is around 15%, and mortality from the Crimean-Congo subspecies ranges from 13% to 50%. Both the young and the old are at increased risk, as are those who have increased opportunity for exposure in the workplace, such as workers in healthcare and agriculture.[2,3]

RVF virus is mosquito-borne illness that causes an acute-onset illness in livestock and wild animals as well as in humans, with an incubation period of 2 to 6 days.[3] Despite high levels of viremia, there have been no reported person-to-person transmissions of RVF. Humans are infected by the bite of an infected mosquito or by direct specimen exposure. Livestock are readily infected and produce high viral titers, which provides a reservoir for mosquitoes to infect humans.[3] RVF has the potential to be used as a bioweapon; it was studied by the U.S. Army in the 1960s but was never weaponized.[3] Mortality is 1%, and there is no sex predilection. High-risk patients include the young and old, farm workers, travelers to endemic areas, and exposure to sick animals or people in the last 21 days. Healthcare workers who treat infected patients are at risk from bodily fluid exposure. Infections from percutaneous exposures have the shortest incubation times and the greatest mortality.[3]

In general, Bunya viruses damage the vascular beds throughout the body, causing increased permeability. CCHF is an influenza-like virus that has a 2- to 12-day incubation period. Initial symptoms include an abrupt onset of fever and chills, headache, myalgia, abdominal pain, nausea, and vomiting. Facial flushing and conjunctival injection are also prominent. A petechial rash starting on the back may extend over the trunk and then to the rest of the body. A hemorrhagic exanthem may begin on the soft palate and uvula. As many as 75% of patients will have hemorrhagic symptoms that begin between days 3 and 7 and include ecchymosis, bleeding from the gums, nose, mouth, uterus, gastrointestinal tract, pulmonary tract, and venipuncture sites. One-half of patients will have hepatomegaly and central nervous system involvement, such as agitation, depression, nuchal rigidity, or coma; central nervous system involvement is associated with a poor prognosis. Multiple organ system failure, severe hemorrhage, and shock can develop, and secondary infections often lead to concomitant sepsis. Death usually occurs between days 5 and 14.[1-6]

RVF leads to the destruction of the infected cell, and patients will have varying degrees of vasculitis and hepatic necrosis. Reduced levels of anticoagulation factors are seen also secondary to disseminated intravascular coagulation (DIC) and hepatic dysfunction. Symptoms include fever, headache, jaundice, retro-orbital pain, and photophobia. RVF may cause retinitis in as many as 10% of individuals, with a rate of blindness of approximately 1%. Fewer than 1% of patients will develop hemorrhagic fever or encephalitis, but the mortality rate is as high as 50% in patients who do.[3,7]

Patients will often have leukopenia and thrombocytopenia, which result in focal inflammatory reactions that produce thrombocytosis. Partial thromboplastin times may be prolonged, but prothrombin times are relatively unaffected. A common pathway for the systemic effects of CCHF is DIC.[8] Transaminase levels are elevated, and hepatic damage is common. Aspartate aminotransferase (AST) is usually raised, and virtually all VHFs distinguish themselves from viral hepatitis because the AST is disproportionately high compared with alanine aminotransferase (ALT). Ratios of AST to ALT may be as high as 11 to 1; the higher the ratio of AST/ALT, the poorer the prognosis. Patients are rarely jaundiced (except in yellow fever), and the bilirubin level is usually normal.[5]

An enzyme-linked immunosorbent assay is available to identify IgM, IgG, or viral antigens in the serum of acutely ill patients. Immunofluorescence assay, complement fixation, and neutralization assays may also be used. These tests are not widely available and often require sending samples to reference laboratory facilities. Isolation and identification often require 3 to 10 days. Electron microscopy of infected tissue also may be helpful in identification. Specimens should be transported only after consultation with the CDC or U.S. Army Medical Research Institute of Infectious Diseases and under very specific biosafety precautions.[6]

 ## PREINCIDENT ACTIONS

Hospitals should have disaster plans in place and run routine drills. The plans should include coordination of local and state authorities and emergency medical services and a method to protect the hospital environment from contamination and exposure to others.

 ## POSTINCIDENT ACTIONS

Report all suspected or confirmed cases to your hospital infection control personnel; laboratory personnel; your public health agency; and, if appropriate, law enforcement personnel. Patients may present as an isolated case or in clusters to one or more hospitals. The clinical situation will dictate when to initiate decontamination procedures. Persons with known or suspected exposures to CCHF or RVF should take a soap-and-water shower and irrigate any potentially exposed mucous membranes.

Extreme heat, detergents, chlorine, formalin, or ultraviolet radiation, including prolonged sunlight, can inactivate viruses. Equipment may be decontaminated with an Environmental Protection Agency–registered hospital disinfectant, or a dilution of household bleach. Care should be taken to ensure solutions are freshly made and correctly applied to allow the disinfectant to completely sterilize the area.[5] Potentially exposed persons should be instructed to check themselves for fever twice daily and to report any temperature of 101°F (38.3°C) or greater or any new symptoms to their physician or public health authority. Surveillance should continue for 21 days, and ribavirin therapy should be considered if either a fever of more than 101°F (38.3°C) or appropriate symptoms are noted. Consultation with the CDC is required since ribavirin would have to be administered under an investigational new drug (IND) protocol.

 ## MEDICAL TREATMENT OF CASUALTIES

Treatment of most viral hemorrhagic fevers is supportive. Patients should be admitted or transferred to facilities capable of providing intensive care for patients in isolation. The early use of vasopressors is often necessary with the goal of minimizing end-organ dysfunction. The most commonly affected areas include the hematologic, pulmonary, and neurologic systems. Extreme care should be used when replacing fluids because the increased vascular permeability often leads to third spacing of fluids.[3] Pulmonary edema is common after aggressive fluid replacement, and patients may require mechanical ventilation. Massive electrolyte shifts are common with aggressive fluid replacement and will need to be closely monitored. Blood component transfusions may be required. Pain and anxiety are also common and should be aggressively managed. Intramuscular injections, venipuncture, and central line placement should be minimized; they carry the same risks as when used with a massively anticoagulated patient. Secondary infections are common, and aggressive antibiotic therapy is often required. Antibiotic selection and dosing should be directed toward the source of the infection, with special consideration being given to any end-organ dysfunction.[3]

Ribavirin is an inhibitor of viral RNA and deoxyribonucleic acid synthesis, and it has been shown to benefit CCHF infections in vitro, in animal studies, and in human case reports.[9,10] The Food and Drug Administration, however, has not officially approved the use of ribavirin for use in viral hemorrhagic fevers, and any use should be administered under an IND protocol. The CDC has recommended the use of ribavirin in suspected or confirmed cases of arenavirus or bunyavirus infection. The initial loading dose is 30 mg/kg (maximum 2 g) IV, followed by 16 mg/kg (maximum 1 g/dose) IV every 6 hours for 4 days, followed by 8 mg/kg intravenously (maximum 500 mg/dose) every 8 hours for 6 days. In a mass casualty setting the CDC recommends a loading dose of 2000 mg orally. This is followed by a 10-day treatment with 600 mg orally twice a day for patients with a body weight greater than 75 kg, or 400 mg every morning and 600 mg every evening for patients with a body weight less than 75 kg. Ribavirin is a category X drug for pregnant women, but the treatment benefit for the mother may outweigh any risk to the fetus.[3] Dosing in pregnancy is the same as for adults. For mass casualty settings, the pediatric dosing recommendations are a loading dose of 30 mg/kg orally, followed by 15 mg/kg per day in two divided doses for 10 days. A pediatric syrup is available for use under an IND application from the manufacturer, Schering-Plough Corp.[3] Steroids have not been shown to improve outcomes.[11] Both live and attenuated vaccines for RFV are under investigation, but none has been approved.[7]

Interferon-alpha given before or just after exposure to RVF has been shown to protect monkeys from viremia and hepatocellular damage, but no human trials have been published to date.[3] After aggressive and early supportive care, most patients will do well and recover, although convalescence may be prolonged.

 ## UNIQUE CONSIDERATIONS

Diagnosis of RVF and CCHF may be quite challenging. The differential diagnosis is quite broad and may include malaria, typhoid fever, leptospirosis, rickettsial infections, relapsing fever, fulminant hepatitis, shigellosis, and meningococcemia. Other noninfectious conditions include acute leukemia, lupus erythematosus, idiopathic or thrombotic thrombocytopenic purpura, hemolytic uremic syndrome, and the multiple causes of DIC. Treatment of RVF and CCHF is largely supportive, but if either is strongly suspected, ribavirin therapy should be considered.

 ## PITFALLS

- Failure to prevent nosocomial spread of infectious material due to a lack of adequate safety precautions or procedures
- Failure to recognize a patient with symptoms consistent with CCHF or RVF with known travel to an endemic area or exposure to persons who have recently traveled to such an area
- Failure to consider the use of a VHF agent in an attack when multiple patients present with symptoms of VHF
- Failure to aggressively treat hypotension with vasopressors
- Failure to use caution with fluid replacement, resulting in third spacing of fluids

- Failure to notify public health and law enforcement officials of suspected or confirmed cases of CCHF or VHF

 ## CASE PRESENTATION

A 39-year-old man presents to an emergency department with 2 days of malaise, nausea, and vomiting and an abrupt onset of fever and chills the previous day. This morning he had two episodes of epistaxis that resolved with direct pressure. The patient also noticed a petechial rash that started this morning. He has a frontal headache and photophobia. He denies any recent illnesses or travel, but notes that several animals in the neighborhood have fallen ill over the past week. On admission and further evaluation, the patient is noted to be in massive hepatic failure. Meanwhile, local surveillance in the emergency department throughout the day notes an increased incidence of patients presenting with "viral syndrome," with several others also commenting that pets and livestock were "not acting right."

REFERENCES

1. Darling R, Catlett C, Huebner K, et al. Threats in bioterrorism I: CDC category A agents. *Emerg Med Clin North Am.* 2002;20(2):273-309.
2. Alai N, Saemi A, Saemi A. Viral Hemorrhagic Fevers. Available at: http://www.emedicine.com/derm/topic880.htm.
3. Borio L, Inglesby T, Peters CJ, et al. Hemorrhagic fever viruses as biological weapons: medical and public health management. JAMA. 2002;287(18):2391-2405.
4. Mayers D. Exotic virus infections of military significance: hemorrhagic fever viruses and pox virus infections. *Dermatol Clin.* 1999;17(1):29-41.
5. McCormick J. Viral hemorrhagic fevers. In: Cohen J, Powderly WG, eds. Infectious Diseases. 2nd ed. St. Louis: Mosby; 2004:1675-8.
6. Artenstein A. Bioterrorism and biodefense. *Infect Dis Clin North Am.* 2001;15(4):99-106.
7. Tsai T, Khan A, McJunkin J: Rift Valley fever. In: Long SS, ed. Principles and Practice of Pediatric Infectious Diseases. 2nd ed. Philadelphia: Churchill Livingstone; 2003:1115.
8. Swanepoel R, Gill DE, Shepherd AJ, et al. The clinical pathology of Crimean-Congo hemorrhagic fever. *J Infect Dis.* 1989;11(Suppl 4):S794-800.
9. Tignor GH, Hanham CA. Ribavirin efficacy in an in vivo model of Crimean-Congo hemorrhagic fever virus (CCHF) infection. *Antiviral Res.* 1993;22(4):309-25.
10. Watts DM, Ussery MA, Nash D, et al. Inhibition of Crimean-Congo hemorrhagic fever viral infectivity yields in vitro by ribavirin. *Am J Trop Med Hyg.* 1989;41(5):581-5.
11. Jahrling P: Viral hemorrhagic fevers. Textbook of Military Medicine. Vol 1. Falls Church, Va: Office of the Surgeon General; 1989.

chapter 122

Viral Hemorrhagic Fever Attack—Filo Viruses

William Porcaro

 ## DESCRIPTION OF EVENT

The Ebola and Marburg viruses are members of the Filoviridae family of viral hemorrhagic fevers, which have the ability to produce a high degree of morbidity and mortality, making them enticing candidates to be used as biologic weapons. The Centers for Disease Control and Prevention (CDC) has classified filoviruses as category A biologic agents because of their high degree of virulence, demonstrated aerosol infectivity, and ability to instill fear and anxiety in the population.[1] Concern exists about terrorist groups obtaining samples of filoviruses from existing laboratory stocks, rogue government agents, or from natural outbreaks. Some researchers have suggested that the Japanese cult group Aum Shinri Kyo, which was responsible for the Sarin subway attack in Tokyo in 1995, sent members to Zaire in the 1990s to obtain samples of the Ebola virus.[2] Viral hemorrhagic fevers are clinical syndromes characterized by acute onset of fevers and generalized symptoms such as malaise, headache, myalgia, and diarrhea. In the majority of victims the syndrome progresses to a bleeding diathesis, septic shock, and multiple organ failure. Russia and the former Soviet Union have produced and stockpiled large quantities of weaponized Marburg and possibly Ebola as recently as the 1990s.[3]

Marburg virus was first discovered in 1967 in Germany and Yugoslavia. African green monkeys, originating from Uganda, were determined to be the source animals that infected laboratory workers. Thirty-two cases were reported, with a 23% mortality rate. The Ebola virus, whose genome is remarkably homologous with the Marburg virus, was first identified in 1976 in Zaire and Sudan when simultaneous outbreaks occurred. In part, because of poor infection control practices, the human impact was devastating, with rapid spread to patients, family members, and healthcare workers. The Ebola-Zaire outbreak involved 318 patients with an 88% mortality rate, and the Ebola-Sudan outbreak affected 284 people with a 53% mortality rate.[4] During the past quarter of a century, there have been numerous outbreaks of Ebola. Different strains of the virus have been identified, and several have been named according to the location of the outbreak.

The filoviruses are enveloped, negative-sense ribonucleic acid (RNA) viruses. They are generally grouped into "Marburg-like" or "Ebola-like" families. Several strains have been characterized in the Ebola family, including Ebola-Zaire, Ebola-Sudan, Ebola-Reston, and Ebola-Cote d'Ivoire. Microscopically, these viruses appear as thread-like filaments that have linear, circular, and U-shaped forms. Each of the viral genomes encodes nine protein products. Some demonstrate immunomodulatory properties, and others cause vascular cell toxicity.[5] To date, the natural reservoirs for the filoviruses have not been discovered.

Both Ebola and Marburg viruses produce similar clinical syndromes. Current epidemiologic evidence suggests that these viruses are spread through direct contact with blood, secretions, or infected tissues. The viruses may also be transmitted via mucosal contact; thus, there is risk of human finger-to-mouth or conjunctiva spread. Although there is no conclusive documented evidence, several human and animal cases have raised some concern for airborne spread of the virus via droplet nuclei.[3,6] Of note, Ebola and Marburg are relatively stable and may retain infectivity for some time at room temperature when exposed to the environment. Previous biologic weapons programs have also succeeded in aerosolizing these viruses and proving aerosol transmission in animal models.[4] The incubation periods are 2 to 21 days for Ebola and 3 to 10 days for Marburg. Because of the possibly prolonged asymptomatic incubation period, the danger of delayed recognition and possible continued dissemination of disease exists. Initial clinical symptoms may include myalgia and arthralgia, fever, nausea and vomiting, abdominal pain, and a rash (petechiae, purpura, and ecchymosis) spreading from the trunk distally. As the hemorrhagic fever progresses, oliguria, hematemesis, melena, pericarditis, encephalitis, acute renal failure, and shock may occur. In severe cases the victim succumbs to disseminated intravascular coagulation.[3,4,7] The classic dermatologic manifestations are quite common since patients generally exhibit a maculopapular rash within 5 days of illness. Although petechiae may be initially apparent, larger patchy lesions generally form and progress to confluent regions. Desquamation may occur and may be the first skin lesion noted in non-Caucasian individuals. Victims may also complain of burning and paresthesias over areas of their skin. The other classic manifestation of viral hemorrhagic fever is bleeding. More than 70% of infected, symptomatic patients suffer from bleeding diatheses. Bleeding may be pronounced and present as melena, epistaxis, hematemesis, hemoptysis, bleeding gums, or puncture sites. The rate of bleeding complication does not appear to differ between survivors and nonsurvivors.[4] Individuals who survive acute viral hemorrhagic fever may be left with long-term sequelae, including arthralgia, uveitis, orchitis, and hearing loss. The virus has been isolated from the urine and seminal fluid of patients who were recovering from the disease up to 3 months after the onset of acute disease.[8]

Specific polymerase chain reaction (PCR) or antibody studies are required to identify infection. These tests are generally only available at specialized laboratories. Reverse transcription-PCR (RT-PCR) has been demonstrated to be effective in the rapid diagnosis of the Ebola virus. Studies have also shown a correlation between disease severity and higher RNA copy levels.[9] The PCR technique has also been used with success in field settings using TaqMan-RT-PCR on a portable SmartCycler during African Ebola outbreaks.[10] The techniques of viral growth in tissue culture followed by electron microscopy and enzyme-linked immunosorbent assay (ELISA) testing have also been used to identify filovirus infection.[11] Immunohistochemical staining of skin biopsies may also prove to be an effective method for identifying infection.[12]

 ## PREINCIDENT ACTIONS

As with any disaster or possible bioterrorism attack, hospitals and emergency departments should have preexisting disaster plans in place that are rehearsed before an event. In suspected cases of filovirus infection/terrorist attack, coordination of local, state, and federal agencies would be required to diagnose and manage the incident. Notably, state departments of public health, the CDC, and the U.S. Army Medical Research Institute of Infectious Diseases (USAMRIID) would need to be involved early in the process of identification and treatment. As always, universal precautions must be practiced. A high level of vigilance must be maintained by healthcare workers when patients present in clusters with febrile illnesses. This vigilance must be even greater if the patient reports recent travel to an area endemic with viral hemorrhagic fever or if there is a report of a recent outbreak. In the event of suspected cases of filovirus infection, facilities must be prepared for proper isolation of the patient, bodily fluids, and specimens. Protective gowns, gloves, high efficiency particulate air (HEPA) face masks, and eye protection should be used by clinical and laboratory personnel because of the theoretical risk of aerosol transmission.

 ## POSTINCIDENT ACTIONS

Level of suspicion for filovirus infection should be high when patients present with the aforementioned signs and symptoms, particularly once there are reports of recent cases or a terrorist attack with viral agents. When there is a high level of suspicion of a filovirus terrorist attack, as previously mentioned, state and federal authorities must be rapidly notified. If there are a limited number of patients, consideration should be given to transferring patients to dedicated Biosafety Level 4 facilities, namely the CDC in Atlanta or the USAMRIID in Fort Detrick, Md. In cases of suspected Ebola or Marburg infection, blood and bodily fluid samples must be handled with extreme caution. No material should be forwarded to the CDC or USAMRIID without prior consultation and arrangement. If a filovirus aerosol attack occurred, victims would begin presenting with illness about 1 week later; at this point, virtually no infectious virus should remain viable in the environment. Patients or staff contaminated with liquids or materials possibly containing a filovirus should be decontaminated via a vigorous hot shower with soap and water. Surfaces or items that may be contaminated should be sterilized with a dilute bleach solution or standard hospital quaternary ammonium or phenol disinfectants. Steam serialization, where applicable, is the most effective method for inactivating filoviruses.[11]

 ## MEDICAL TREATMENT OF CASUALTIES

Unfortunately, treatment for victims of filovirus hemorrhagic fever is largely supportive. As victims progress to disseminated intravascular coagulation and septic shock, usual treatment with blood, clotting products, and vasopressor medications should be instituted. Conventional antiviral agents such as ribavirin have not been shown to have any significant clinical benefit in either in vitro or in vivo studies. Interferon-alpha (INF-a) has shown some success in suppressing filovirus replication in cell culture and some promise in protecting Ebola-infected mice from the illness.[11] Attempts have been made to treat patients by passive immunization through the use of the convalescent blood and serum from recovered filovirus patients. After the transfer of IgG Ebola antibodies to infected patients, a lower mortality rate was observed. However, there were a small number of patients in these studies and questions have arisen about other confounders in their care.[13] Purified IgG from horses hyperimmunized with Ebola-Zaire was shown to protect baboons and guinea pigs from disease when given to them shortly after virus challenge.[14]

A concerted effort to develop an Ebola vaccine is under way. Ebola-related deoxyribonucleic acid, liposome-encapsulated irradiated Ebola virus, and Ebola protein segments are all being studied for possible use as vaccines. Ebola virus-like particles, when injected into mice, allowed the animals to develop Ebola-specific antibodies and conferred protection from the lethal virus.[15]

 ## UNIQUE CONSIDERATIONS

The filoviruses have the potential to be used as devastating biologic weapons. Their high level of virulence and equally impressive mortality rate make them a tempting target for any terrorist organization wishing to obtain a weapon of mass destruction. Initial identification of a viral hemorrhagic fever attack will be difficult given the week-long incubation period and nonspecific signs and symptoms in the initial phase of disease. The high risk of transmission to healthcare providers is another factor that makes this threat even more ominous.

 PITFALLS

- Failure of healthcare personnel to recognize the non-specific signs and symptoms of viral hemorrhagic fever and delayed institution of containment procedures
- Delayed reporting of possible cases of viral hemorrhagic fever to state and federal officials, leading to delay in appropriate diagnostic procedures and isolation of materials and patients
- Failure to practice simple universal precautions, leading to uncontrolled spread of the viral agent
- General public fear and reaction over release of information regarding possible cases of viral hemorrhagic fever

 CASE PRESENTATION

A 25-year-old man presents to a suburban emergency department because he "does not look well." He is febrile, tachycardic, hypotensive, and minimally responsive. Small amounts of blood are noted in his nares and on his gums, and he is still bleeding from several venipuncture sites. His fiancée states that he has been generally unwell for the past few days with low-grade fevers, body aches, and diarrhea. On further questioning, she reports that he returned from a trip to Europe 10 days ago. Given the patient's history, examination findings, and symptoms, the health department is contacted because of the concern for viral hemorrhagic fever. You learn from the health officials that several similar cases have also just been reported in the region.

REFERENCES

1. Rotz LD, Khan AS, Lillibridge SR, et al. Public health assessment of potential biological terrorism agents. *Emerg Infect Dis.* 2002;8:(2):225-30.
2. Kaplan D. Aum Shinrikyo. In: Tucker J, ed. Toxic Terror: Assessing Terrorist Use of Chemical and Biological Weapons. Cambridge, MA: MIT Press 2000; 207-26.
3. Borio L, Inglesby T, Peters CJ, et al. Hemorrhagic fever viruses as biological weapons: medical and public health management. *JAMA.* 2002;287(18):2391-2405.
4. Salvaggio MR, Baddley JW. Other viral bioweapons: Ebola and Marburg hemorrhagic fever. *Dermatol Clin.* 2004;22(3):291-302, vi (review).
5. Takada A, Kawaoka Y. The pathogenesis of Ebola hemorrhagic fever. *Trends Microbiol.* 2001;9(10):506-11.
6. Francesconi P, Yoti Z, Declich S, et al. Ebola hemorrhagic fever transmission and risk factors of contacts, Uganda. *Emerg Infect Dis.* 2003;9(11):1430-7.
7. Easter A. Ebola. *Am J Nurs.* 2002;102(12):49-52.
8. Rowe AK, Bertolli J, Khan AS, et al. Clinical, virologic, and immunologic follow-up of convalescent Ebola hemorrhagic fever patients and their household contacts, Kikwit, Democratic Republic of Congo. *J Infect Dis.* 1999;179(Suppl 1):S28-35.
9. Towner JS, Rollin PE, Bausch DG, et al. Rapid diagnosis of Ebola hemorrhagic fever by reverse transcription-PCR in an outbreak setting and assessment of patient viral load as a predictor of outcome. *J Virol.* 2004;78(8):4330-41.
10. Weidmann M, Muhlberger E, Hufert FT. Rapid detection protocol for filoviruses. *J Clin Virol.* 2004;30:94-9.
11. Bray M. Defense against filoviruses used as biological weapons. *Antiviral Res.* 2003;57(1-2):53-60 (review).
12. Zaki SR, Shieh WJ, Greer PW, et al. A novel immunohistochemical assay for the detection of Ebola virus in skin: implications for diagnosis, spread, and surveillance of Ebola hemorrhagic fever. *J Infect Dis.* 1999;179(Suppl 1):S36-47.
13. Mupapa K, Massamba M, Kibadi K, et al. Treatment of Ebola hemorrhagic fever with blood transfusions from convalescent patients. *J Infect Dis.* 1999;179(Suppl 1):S18-23.
14. Jahrling PB, Geisbert J, Swearengen JR, et al. Passive immunization of Ebola virus-infected cynomolgus monkeys with immunoglobulin from hyperimmune horses. *Arch Virol Suppl.* 1996;11:135-40.
15. Warfield KL, Bosio CM, Welcher BC, et al. Ebola virus-like particles protect from lethal Ebola virus infection. *Proc Natl Acad Sci USA.* 2003;100(26):15889-94.

chapter 123

Viral Hemorrhagic Fever Attack—Flaviviruses

John D. Cahill and James McKinnel

 ## DESCRIPTION OF EVENT

Flaviviruses belong to the family of arboviruses. More than 60 of these viruses are known to exist throughout the world. These viruses share some common features. Most are 40 to 50 nm in diameter and are enveloped, positive-sense, single-stranded ribonucleic acid (RNA) viruses that are transmitted from arthropods, particularly mosquitoes and ticks.[1] Clinically these viruses can cause hemorrhagic fevers and encephalitis. This chapter focuses on those causing hemorrhagic fever: yellow fever, Kyasanur Forest disease, Omsk hemorrhagic fever, and dengue fever. There is at least the potential for these viruses to be manufactured into biologic weapons.

It should be appreciated that in the natural setting, these infections have a wide spectrum of presentation: from mild to severe. From a clinical standpoint, these viruses can present in a similar fashion with findings that may include fever, often biphasic; relative bradycardia; hypotension; bleeding diathesis; petechiae; epistaxis; hemoptysis; hematemesis; melena; hematochezia; and hematuria. Laboratory findings may include leukopenia, thrombocytopenia, hemoconcentration, elevated liver function tests, and prolonged bleeding or prothrombin or activated partial thromboplastin times. Death in infected patients is often secondary to bleeding, shock, and organ failure. The differential diagnosis of these infections is broad and includes influenza, viral hepatitis, gram-negative sepsis, meningococcemia, toxic shock syndrome, rickettsial infections, leptospirosis, typhoid fever, Q fever, malaria, other viral hemorrhagic fevers, collagen vascular diseases, acute leukemia, and platelet disorders.

Yellow fever, Omsk hemorrhagic fever, and Kyasanur Forest disease have been considered by the Working Group on Civilian Biodefense as having some key features that characterize biologic agents that pose particularly serious risks if used as biologic weapons against civilian populations: (1) high morbidity and mortality; (2) potential for person-to-person transmission; (3) low infective dose and highly infectious by aerosol dissemination, with a commensurate ability to cause large outbreaks; (4) effective vaccine unavailable or available only in limited supply; (5) potential to cause panic in the affected population; (6) availability of pathogen or toxin; (7) feasibility of large-scale production; (8) environmental stability; and (9) prior research and development as a biologic weapon.[2] Dengue fever is not considered in this group since initial infection rarely causes hemorrhagic fever and it is not transmissible by small-particle aerosol.[3] Yellow fever was weaponized by the United States offensive biologic weapons program until its cessation in 1969, but it may have been weaponized by North Korea.[3]

The incubation period of *yellow fever* is usually 3 to 6 days, then symptoms of fever, malaise, headache, photophobia, nausea, vomiting, and irritability may occur. Physical examination at symptom onset reveals a patient who is febrile; toxic in appearance; and who has hyperemic skin, injected conjunctiva, coated tongue, and epigastric or hepatic tenderness. Faget's sign, a relative bradycardia with a fever, may be present. After 3 to 5 days, either the patient recovers or enters the next stage of fulminate disease, in which there is extensive hepatic injury with jaundice (hence the name "yellow fever"). Renal failure is not uncommon. A hemorrhagic diathesis may occur, causing epistaxis, oozing at the gums, petechiae, ecchymosis, hematemesis often described as "black vomit," melena, hematuria, thrombocytopenia, and disseminated intravascular coagulation. Myocarditis, encephalopathy, and shock may also ensue. The case fatality rate is 20% to 50%. If one survives, a full recovery can be expected.

The diagnosis of yellow fever may be very difficult in isolated cases; when epidemics occur, physicians are vigilant and the diagnosis is more obvious. In the tropics, the diagnosis is often clinical. A liver biopsy may be performed in an effort to identify the characteristic pathologic changes, such as Councilman bodies and midzonal necrosis. However, the biopsy findings are not absolute and do not exclude the possible diagnosis. Moreover, liver biopsies in yellow fever can be associated with massive hemorrhage. Developed nations have specialized laboratories that can assist in the diagnosis. In such facilities the diagnosis can be made by viral cultures, polymerase chain reaction (PCR), or preferably from enzyme-linked immunosorbent assay (ELISA) tests looking for the IgM rise during acute infection, or IgG later on.[4]

In patients with *Kyasanur Forest disease*, after an incubation period of 3 to 12 days, a severe febrile illness may ensue that may be biphasic in nature. The patient may complain of the acute onset of headache, photophobia, myalgia, upper respiratory symptoms, vomiting, and diarrhea. Physical examination may reveal a febrile patient with a relative bradycardia; hypotension; facial erythema; conjunctivitis; palatal vesicles; lymphadenopathy; hepatosplenomegaly; and manifestations of a bleeding diathesis, including petechiae, epistaxis, hematemesis, hemoptysis, melena, and hematochezia. Patients may develop hemorrhagic pulmonary edema, which is the most common cause of death. The mortality rate may approach 8%.[5] Renal or hepatic organ failure may occur. Between 20% and 50% of individuals will progress to the second stage of the illness after several days of apparent improvement. During this stage, symptoms of encephalitis may appear.[6]

The complete blood count may show leukopenia, hemoconcentration, and thrombocytopenia. Elevation of liver and renal function tests may also be seen. The virus can be directly isolated from blood during the first 12 days of illness. Appropriate laboratory precautions should be taken when handling these samples. Serologic studies are available for IgM and IgG.

In the natural setting, *Omsk hemorrhagic fever* is, fortunately, a self-limited acute infection with only a small minority of patients developing hemorrhagic complications. The mortality rate is 0.5% to 3%. Clinically there is an incubation period of 3 to 7 days and the patient has a presentation similar to that seen in patients with Kyasanur Forest disease; however, there is generally no central nervous system involvement. Diagnosis is made by detecting viral RNA by PCR or by serodiagnosis using ELISA IgM and IgG.

Dengue fever has a global distribution throughout the tropics. The frequency of dengue viral infections has been on the rise since the mid-1950s. Historically, dengue viruses caused sporadic and infrequent epidemics. However, during the last half century, dengue infections have grown to pandemic proportions and patients appear to be presenting with more severe clinical disease. By 1998, 1.5 million cases of dengue fever and dengue hemorrhagic fever from 56 countries marked the first worldwide pandemic. The pandemic in 1998 was followed 3 years later by another worldwide outbreak in 2001. During a span of 50 years, the incidence of dengue viral infection increased approximately 30-fold, affecting approximately 51 million people worldwide per year. In Puerto Rico alone more than $250 million has been spent during the last 10 years in an attempt to deal with the consequences of this disease.[7] The dramatic change in disease epidemiology has been attributed to the population shift from rural to urban centers and the rise in international travel and commerce that characterized the 20th century.

There are four serotypes of dengue virus: DEN-1, DEN-2, DEN-3, and DEN-4. All cause clinical dengue fever. Dengue can be separated from other tropical infectious diseases in that the immunologic response to viral infection is relatively unique. Resolution of the primary infection is thought to produce lifelong immunity to the infecting serotype but only brief protection from the other serotypes. After the transient period of relative immunity, exposed patients become susceptible to secondary infections with other DEN serotypes. It is principally secondary infections, particularly with DEN-2, that are more likely to result in severe disease and dengue hemorrhagic fever.[8] It has been convincingly argued that an antibody-dependent enhancement of secondary infections is responsible for increased viremia and the development of dengue hemorrhagic fever.

Patients with initial infections often present with dengue fever symptoms, whereas those with secondary infections with a different serotype may present with dengue hemorrhagic fever. The incubation period of dengue fever is 2 to 15 days. The classic presentation of dengue fever, or "break bone fever," is a syndrome associated with fever, frontal headache, retro-orbital pain, severe myalgia, and severe arthralgia. Conjunctival injection, pharyngeal irritation, nausea, vomiting, and a fine maculopapular rash that spreads centrifugally may accompany the syndrome. Initially, the fever rises rapidly for 2 to 7 days and may then drop, only to reoccur 24 hours later (hence the name "saddleback fever"). Hepatic transaminase level elevations have been reported in more than 80% of cases, with some reports of fulminant hepatic failure. Transcytopenia can be seen 4 to 5 days into infection, although this is not a universal finding. Although dengue fever is usually a self-limited infection, it can be accompanied by bleeding complications. Severe bleeding, particularly gastrointestinal losses, can be a fatal complication of dengue fever.[9-11]

Dengue hemorrhagic fever is differentiated from dengue fever on the basis of increased capillary leakage of plasma with associated hemoconcentration (hematocrit increase greater than 20%) and thrombocytopenia. Pleural effusions and ascites are possible complications of the microvascular leakage. Sudden extravasation of plasma, typically concomitant with defervescence, is responsible for the circulatory compromise associated with the dengue shock syndrome. The exact pathologic cascade behind microvascular leakage in dengue hemorrhagic fever is unclear but appears to be related to high viral titers causing complement activation and cytokine release, which in turn cause endothelial dysfunction and resulting plasma leakage.[12] Mortality rates may be as high as 50%. Diagnosis is made serologically. The tourniquet test can be used, but it is not disease specific.

 PREINCIDENT ACTIONS

Healthcare providers must maintain a high index of suspicion for these diseases since they are sometimes difficult to diagnosis and since some of these agents may be used as biologic weapons. A clinician's level of suspicion should be increased particularly if a large number of individuals present with a "viral syndrome" or coagulation and bleeding problems. Providers should be familiar with the clinical presentation of these illnesses and the resources available to diagnose and manage infected patients. It should be anticipated that blood products will be in great demand if a large number of patients become infected with these viruses and present for care.

From a public health standpoint, rapid diagnosis would be of utmost importance, since an outbreak of Ebola would be handled very differently from a yellow fever outbreak. Institutions and public health officials should also be prepared to handle mass panic and a large number of psychologic casualties that overwhelm the health-care system. The availability of yellow fever vaccine and a plan for mass vaccination should be anticipated.

 POSTINCIDENT ACTIONS

Since there is no publicly known experience of these viruses being used as biologic weapons, it is not completely clear how infected individuals would present. Standard isolation precautions should be taken by health-care personnel. Potentially exposed contacts should be placed under medical surveillance for several weeks, looking for evidence of fever and signs of viral hemorrhagic fever. Fortunately, in the natural setting, human-to-human transmission has not been reported. If the virus identified is vaccine-preventable, mass vaccination should begin as soon as possible. If viral hemorrhagic fever is suspected, local health officials must be notified to facilitate identification of the agent as well as access to vaccines, in coordination with state and federal health officials.

 MEDICAL TREATMENT OF CASUALTIES

Treatment of all viral hemorrhagic fevers due to flavivirus infection is largely supportive and may include intravenous fluids, vasopressor support, blood products, vitamin K, avoiding nonsteroidal antiinflammatory medications and anticoagulants, and correcting electrolyte imbalances. Although the data are limited, ribavirin has not been shown to be effective in the treatment of flavivirus infection.

Beyond the provision of supportive care to infected patients, management of a yellow fever epidemic involves the institution of preventive measures, including vector control, surveillance, and immunization. A yellow fever vaccination is available. It is a live, attenuated vaccine and has several contraindications, including children younger than 9 months old, pregnancy, and immunosuppression. The vaccine can only be administered at a designated yellow fever center. The vaccination dose is 0.5 mL given subcutaneously in the upper arm. Immunity appears to last at least 10 years after a single dose.

Treatment for Kyasanur Forest disease and Omsk hemorrhagic fever is supportive. In endemic areas, patients should avoid ticks. A formalin inactivated vaccine is available in endemic regions for Kyasanur Forest disease.[13] No vaccine is available for Omsk hemorrhagic fever; however, the tick-borne encephalitis vaccine may offer some cross-protection.[14]

Treatment is of dengue hemorrhagic fever is also supportive. Preventive measures include eradication of mosquito breeding sites and personal protective measures. No vaccine is available; however, several vaccine trials are currently under way.

 UNIQUE CONSIDERATIONS

To date, there is no specific treatment for flaviviral hemorrhagic fevers. Treatment is supportive, although with development of antiviral medications, there may be a role for their use in the future. Several of these diseases are vaccine-preventable, and vaccine trials are under way for dengue fever. Fortunately, unlike some of the other hemorrhagic fevers, the flaviviruses are not known to spread person to person.

 PITFALLS

- Failure to obtain a detailed clinical history, which could result in these illnesses being mistaken for a "flu" or simple viral syndrome
- Failure to obtain careful travel history, including geographic locations, length of trip, activities undertaken, and exposure to mosquitoes or ticks
- Failure to determine the time of onset of symptoms and time of return from travel, since many of these illnesses have a specific incubation period
- Failure to obtain a past medical history that includes previous vaccines
- Failure to maintain clinical suspicion for these viruses when multiple individuals present with similar symptoms outlined in this chapter
- Failure to report suspected hemorrhagic fever cases to the public health officer or department of health

CASE PRESENTATION

The staff physicians at an urban hospital have been overwhelmed by an unusually early onset of the flu this season. The strain seems especially virulent, since several patients have died and the census in the emergency department has increased by 25%. As the week progresses, many of the patients admitted with the "flu" develop gastrointestinal bleeding, necessitating blood transfusions and intensive care unit support. Presenting symptoms of one such 30-year-old male patient include a fever to 101°F, a heart rate of 80, and a blood pressure of 90/50 mm Hg. He has petechiae, is complaining of intermittent epistaxis, and has bloody stools. Laboratory findings include low white blood cell and platelet counts, an elevated hematocrit level, and elevated liver function tests. His bleeding time is prolonged as well.

REFERENCES

1. International Committee on Taxonomy of Viruses. Seventh Report of the International Committee on Taxonomy of Viruses. San Diego, Calif: Academic Press; 2000.
2. Borio L, Inglesby T, Peters CJ, et al. Hemorrhagic fever viruses as biological weapons: medical and public health management. JAMA. 2002;287(18):2391-2405.

3. Peters CJ, Jahrling PB, Khan AS. Patients infected with high-hazard viruses. *Arch Virol Suppl*. 1996;11:141-68.

4. Monath TP. Yellow fever. In: Guerrant RL, Walker DH, Weller PF, eds. Tropical Infectious Diseases. Philadelphia: Churchill Livingstone; 1999:1262.

5. Monath TP. Kyasanur Forest disease. In: Monath TP, ed. The Arboviruses: Epidemiology and Ecology. Vol 3. Boca Raton, Fla: CRC Press; 1998.

6. Pavri K. Clinical, clinicopathological and hematological features of Kyasanur Forest disease. *Rev Infect Dis*. 1989;11(Suppl 4):S854-9.

7. Clark G, et al. Dengue fever. In: CDC Yellow Book. Atlanta: Centers for Disease Control and Prevention; 2003.

8. Vaughn DW, et al. Dengue viremia titer, antibody response pattern, and virus serotype correlate with disease severity. *J Infect Dis*. 2000;181:2-9.

9. Kautner I, et al. Dengue virus infection: epidemiology, pathogenesis, clinical presentation, diagnosis, and prevention. *J Pediatr*. 1997;131:516-24.

10. Hayes EB, et al. Dengue and dengue hemorrhagic fever. *Pediatr Infect Dis J*. 1992;11:311-17.

11. Kalayanarooj S, et al. Early clinical and laboratory indicators of acute dengue illness. *J Infect Dis*. 1997;176:313-21.

12. Lei HY, et al. Immunopathogenesis of dengue virus infection. *J Biomed Sci*. 2001;8:377-88.

13. Broom AK, et al. Kyasanur Forest disease. In: Cook GC, Zumla A, eds. Manson's Tropical Diseases. 21st ed. Philadelphia: Saunders; 2003:748-9.

14. Broom AK, et al. Omsk hemorrhagic fever. In Cook GC, Zumla A, eds. Manson's Tropical Diseases. 21st ed. Philadelphia: Saunders; 2003:751.

chapter 124

Chikungunya Virus Attack

Heather Long

 DESCRIPTION OF EVENT

The chikungunya virus (CHIK) is an alphavirus borne by *Aedes* mosquitoes. The virus is endemic to many tropical and subtropical regions throughout the world, including sub-Saharan Africa, southeast Asia, India, and the western Pacific. The CHIK virus was first isolated from human serum and *Aedes aegypti* mosquitoes in 1953 after an epidemic in Tanzania.[1]

Even though the most common route of transmission is human-mosquito-human, the CHIK virus may also be aerosolized.[2] It is highly infectious, and many laboratory workers have been infected while working with the virus.[3-5] As an agent of biologic terrorism, it would most likely be dispersed as an aerosol or by release of infected mosquitoes.[6] No person-to-person transmission has been documented. To date, there have been no confirmed reports of terrorist acquisition or planned use of this agent. In the event of a CHIK virus attack, a large percentage of the exposed population would be expected to become ill after an incubation period of 2 to 10 days.[2] Illness associated with the CHIK virus is generally self-limited and short-lived; however, it may be temporarily debilitating, and a large number of affected patients would be expected to seek care for fever and severe joint pain. Hospitals with few isolation areas appropriate for screening patients with these presenting complaints may be overwhelmed.

Infection with the CHIK virus is characterized by the triad of fever, maculopapular rash, and arthralgia.[7] Nausea, headache, vomiting, and myalgia are also common. Sudden onset of fever is characteristically the first symptom to appear after an incubation period of 2 to 10 days.[2] Arthralgia is the most prominent symptom, and the word *chikungunya,* translated from Swahili as "that which bends up," refers to this joint pain.[8] Severity ranges from mild weakness and stiffness to excruciating pain. The pain is typically symmetric and involves multiple joints. Previously injured joints and the fingers, wrists, elbows, toes, ankles, and knees are most commonly affected.[6] Joints appear swollen and are tender to palpation. Frequency and severity of symptoms are generally less in children. Complete resolution of all symptoms occurs in most patients after 2 to 5 days; however, about 12% of patients will have a persistent arthropathy

that may last months to years.[5] Persistent arthropathy is associated with high titers of CHIK virus antibodies.[5]

Although not classified as a hemorrhagic virus, hemorrhagic forms of the disease that mimic dengue fever and yellow fever have been reported.[9,10] In some outbreaks of CHIK virus infection, up to 10% of patients were noted to have mild hemorrhage, including petechia, epistaxis, and bleeding gums. Cases of myocarditis and cardiomyopathy after CHIK virus infection have been reported.[11,12] Rare deaths among the elderly and children have been associated with CHIK outbreaks, and the CHIK virus was isolated from one Sri Lankan child who died.[13,14]

Diagnosis of CHIK virus infection in a patient without history of either travel to an endemic area or laboratory exposure to the virus would require a high degree of clinical suspicion. Results from routine laboratory tests are nonspecific. Laboratory confirmation via polymerase chain reaction (PCR) or enzyme-linked immunoabsorbent assay (ELISA) requires submission of serum to either the Centers for Disease Control and Prevention (CDC) or the U.S. Army Medical Research Institute of Infectious Disease (USAMRIID), and results take 2 to 5 days.[6]

 PREINCIDENT ACTIONS

Prehospital services, hospitals, and local and state health departments should have implemented preparedness programs for bioterrorism and mass casualty events. Recognition of a CHIK virus event would require familiarity with the agent as well as a high degree of clinical suspicion. Maintaining a high level of alertness to abnormal patterns is critical to the recognition of any covert bioterrorist attack.

 POSTINCIDENT ACTIONS

All suspected cases of CHIK virus infection should be reported to local and state health departments, who would then notify the CDC. Infection control professionals and laboratory personnel should be notified immediately. Biosafety Level 3 practices should be maintained in handling specimens. If CHIK virus infection is suspected, 10 to 12 mL of serum from the affected patient(s) should be shipped cold or on dry ice in a plastic tube. Public health authorities, in conjunction with the CDC, should aid clinicians in preparing specimens for transport to a reference laboratory. (See "Packaging Protocols for Biological Agents/Diseases" at http://www.bt.cdc.gov/Agent/VHF/VHF.asp.) Laboratory personnel must be alerted to the possibility of small-particle aerosol generation to minimize their risk of infection. With prior notice, the CDC can offer a preliminary laboratory diagnosis after approximately 1 working day.[15]

In its natural state, the CHIK virus is not environmentally stable for long periods. Environmental Protection Agency–registered hospital disinfectants, moist heat, and drying all kill the virus. However, decisions regarding the need for decontamination after an attack should be made after expert analysis of the contaminated environment, the agent used, and the means of distribution. Similarly, contact and respiratory isolation of exposed and infected patients is not believed to be necessary, but specific recommendations should be made after expert analysis. Given that laboratory confirmation may take several days, stricter infection control practices may be warranted until an agent with person-to-person transmission is ruled out. Universal precautions should be taken with all patients.

 ## MEDICAL TREATMENT OF CASUALTIES

The mainstay of treatment of CHIK virus infection is supportive care. Fluid and electrolyte balance should be closely monitored. Nonsteroidal antiinflammatory agents are the first-line therapy for fever and pain. Antiemetics may be required in cases of persistent nausea and vomiting. Antiviral agents, including ribavirin, 6-azauridine, interferon-alpha2b, and glycyrrhizin, alone and in combination, have demonstrated in vitro anti-CHIK activity.[16] Whether any of these agents would be effective in postexposure prophylaxis or treatment remains unstudied. There is currently no U.S. Food and Drug Administration indication for the use of ribavirin after CHIK virus infection. Given the low morbidity and exceedingly rare mortality associated with CHIK virus infection in its natural state, ribavirin should be administered only after expert analysis under an investigational new drug application.[15] There is presently no vaccine for the CHIK virus, but development is on-going; results of a phase II safety and immunogenicity study of a live CHIK virus vaccine were published in 2000.[17]

 ## UNIQUE CONSIDERATIONS

The CHIK virus is highly infectious; a large percentage of people exposed to the agent would be expected to become ill. Illness with the CHIK virus is short-lived but temporarily debilitating and not considered lethal. Because there is no animal reservoir for the virus in Western countries and no person-to-person transmission, it is seen as a "clean" biologic weapon that may be a desirable agent for use against a civilian site.[6]

 ## PITFALLS

- Failure to consider a CHIK virus infection or attack in patients presenting with the nonspecific symptoms of fever, rash, and arthralgia
- Failure to alert laboratory personnel to the possibility of small-particle aerosolization in suspected cases
- Failure to notify local and/or state health departments of suspected cases

 ## CASE PRESENTATION

A 22-year-old woman with no significant past medical history complains of severe bilateral wrist, elbow, and knee pain since waking this morning. The patient had been in her usual state of health until 1 day before presentation when she had a sudden onset of fever and shaking chills while at work. The patient has no rhinorrhea, cough, or sore throat; she complains of headache and nausea but no vomiting or diarrhea. She has no chest or abdominal pain. She denies any sick contacts, trauma or falls, or recent travel. The only medication she takes is oral contraceptives.

Vital signs are as follows: temperature is 39.5°C, heart rate is 120, blood pressure is 118/74 mm Hg, and respiratory rate is 16. The patient appears flushed and in obvious physical discomfort but in no respiratory distress. Her physical examination is remarkable for slight swelling of the knees bilaterally; pain is elicited with active and passive range of motion of the knees, wrists, and elbows bilaterally. There is no warmth or erythema of the joints. Routine laboratory results including white cell count with differential are normal. The erythrocyte sedimentation rate is 40. Aspiration of the left knee joint reveals clear fluid negative for crystals with a white cell count of 200 cells/high-powered field.

REFERENCES

1. Ross RW. The Newala epidemic. III. The virus: isolation, pathogenic properties and relationship to the epidemic. *J Hyg (Lond)*. 1956;54:177-91.
2. Tesh RB. Arthritides caused by mosquito-borne viruses. *Ann Rev Med*. 1982;33:31-40.
3. Shah KV, Baron S. Laboratory infection with chikungunya virus: a case report. *Indian J Med Res*. 1965;53:610-13.
4. Banerjee K, Gupta NP, Goverdhan MK. Viral infections in laboratory personnel. *Indian J Med Res*. 1979;69:363-73.
5. Ramachandra RJ, Singh KRP, Pavri KM. Laboratory transmission of an Indian strain of chikungunya virus. *Current Sci*. 1964;33:235-6.
6. CBWInfo. Factsheets on chemical and biological warfare. Chikungunya fever: essential data. Available at: http://www.cbwinfo.com/Biological/Pathogens/CHIK.html.
7. Brighton SW, Prozesky OW, de la Harpe AL. Chikungunya virus infection. A retrospective study of 107 cases. *S Afr Med J*. 1983;63:313-15.
8. Pfeffer M, Linssen B, Parker MD, et al. Specific detection of chikungunya virus using a RT-PCR/nested PCR combination. *J Vet Med*. 2002;49:49-54.
9. Hammon WM, Rudnick A, Sather GE. Viruses associated with epidemic hemorrhagic fevers of the Philippines and Thailand. *Science*. 1960;131:1102-3.

10. Sarkar JK, Chatterjee SN, Chakravarti SK, et al. Chikungunya virus infection with haemorrhagic manifestations. *Indian J Med Res.* 1965;53:921-5.

11. Maiti CR, Mukherjee AK, Bose B, et al. Myopericarditis following chikungunya virus infection. *J Indian Med Assoc.* 1978;70:256-8.

12. Obeyesekere I, Hermon Y. Myocarditis and cardiomyopathy after arbovirus infections (dengue and chikungunya fever.) *Br Heart J.* 1972;34:821-7.

13. Rao AR. An epidemic of fever in Madras—1964: a clinical study of 4,223 cases at the Infectious Diseases Hospital. *Indian J Med Res.* 1965;53:745-53.

14. Hermon YE. Virological investigations of arbovirus infections in Ceylon, with special reference to the recent chikungunya fever epidemic. *Ceylon Med J.* 1967;12:81-92.

15. Borio L, Inglesby T, Peters CJ, et al. Hemorrhagic fever viruses as biological weapons: medical and public health management. *JAMA.* 2002;287:2391-2405.

16. Briolant S, Garin D, Scaramozzino N, et al. In vitro inhibition of Chikungunya and Semliki Forest viruses replication by antiviral compounds: synergistic effect of interferon-alpha and ribavirin combination. *Antiviral Res.* 2004;61:111-7.

17. Edelman R, Tacket CO, Wasserman SS, et al. Phase II safety and immunogenicity study of live chikungunya virus vaccine TSI-GSD-218. *Am J Trop Med Hyg.* 2000;62:681-5.

chapter 125

Variola Major Virus (Smallpox) Attack

Robert G. Darling

 DESCRIPTION OF EVENT

Smallpox may be responsible for more human deaths throughout history than any other known disease, with estimates that it has killed more than 100 million people since the beginning of recorded history.[1] Smallpox was declared eradicated in 1980 by the World Health Organization, and there have been no cases of smallpox anywhere in the world since 1978. By treaty there are only two official repositories of smallpox in the world today: one repository is at the Russian State Research Center of Virology and Biotechnology in Novosibirsk, Russia, and the other is at the Centers for Disease Control and Prevention (CDC) in Atlanta, Ga. A single case of smallpox should be presumed to be intentional unless it can be shown to be the result of a laboratory accident.

Terrorist use of variola as a biologic weapon could occur under one of several different scenarios. The simplest method might involve obtaining an illicit sample of the virus from a clandestine stock and then exposing a number of unsuspecting victims. These unfortunate individuals would then go about their daily business and serve as vectors for further spread of the disease once they become contagious. This might not be the most efficient manner to spread the infection since most victims become quite ill as symptoms develop and are unlikely to remain ambulatory. The most efficient manner to infect a large number of people would involve the deliberate spread of a weaponized aerosol of the virus.

The incubation period of smallpox averages 12 days, with a range of 7 to 17 days after exposure. Clinical manifestations begin acutely with malaise, fever, rigors, vomiting, headache, and backache; 15% of patients develop delirium. Approximately 10% of light-skinned patients exhibit an erythematous rash during this phase. Two to three days later, an enanthem appears concomitantly with a discrete rash about the face, hands, and forearms.

After eruptions on the lower extremities, the rash spreads centrally to the trunk over the next week. Lesions quickly progress from macules to papules and eventually to pustular vesicles. Lesions are more abundant on the extremities and face, and this centrifugal distribution is an important diagnostic feature. In distinct contrast to varicella, lesions on various segments of the body remain generally synchronous in their stages of development. From 8 to 14 days after onset,

the pustules form scabs that leave depressed depigmented scars upon healing. Although variola concentrations in the throat, conjunctiva, and urine diminish with time, the virus can be readily recovered from scabs throughout convalescence. Therefore, patients should be isolated and considered infectious until all scabs separate.

For the past century, two distinct types of smallpox were recognized. *Variola minor* was distinguished by milder systemic toxicity and more diminutive pox lesions; it caused 1% mortality in unvaccinated victims. However, the prototypical disease, *variola major*, caused mortality of 3% and 30% in the vaccinated and unvaccinated, respectively.[2]

Smallpox must be distinguished from other vesicular exanthems, such as chickenpox, erythema multiforme with bullae, or allergic contact dermatitis. Particularly problematic to infection control measures would be the failure to recognize relatively mild cases of smallpox in persons with partial immunity. An additional threat to effective quarantine is the fact that exposed persons may shed virus from the oropharynx without ever manifesting disease. Therefore, quarantine and initiation of medical countermeasures should be promptly followed by an accurate diagnosis to avert panic.

The usual method of diagnosis is demonstration of characteristic virions on electron microscopy of vesicular scrapings. Under light microscopy, aggregations of variola virus particles, called *Guarnieri bodies,* are found. Another rapid but relatively insensitive test for Guarnieri bodies in vesicular scrapings is Gispen's modified silver stain, in which cytoplasmic inclusions appear black.

None of the aforementioned laboratory tests is capable of discriminating variola from vaccinia, Monkeypox, or cowpox. This differentiation has classically required isolation of the virus and characterization of its growth on chorioallantoic membrane. The development of polymerase chain reaction diagnostic techniques promises a more accurate and less cumbersome method of discriminating between variola and other orthopoxviruses.[3]

 PREINCIDENT ACTIONS

Pre-event preparations should focus on first responder, medical, and public health personnel education. This is particularly important for healthcare providers since an astute clinician will be far more likely to diagnose a first case of smallpox before any surveillance system would lead public health authorities to suspect there is an epidemic in the community. Rapid identification and vaccination of contacts will be the keys to controlling an outbreak of smallpox.

Ideally, all first responders and medical and public health personnel will be vaccinated against smallpox before an outbreak and will have extensively drilled their local smallpox response plans. However, efforts by the CDC in 2003 to vaccinate up to 500,000 volunteers were unsuccessful, largely due to concerns about side effects of the vaccine and a general belief among the public that the threat of terrorist use of smallpox was low. To date the U.S. military has vaccinated more than 600,000 of its personnel with a relatively low rate of complications.[4]

A well-developed, integrated "all-hazards" hospital disaster response plan should be in place and tested regularly. It should include provisions to care for a rapid influx of large numbers of contagious patients. The local plan should be linked to other regional, state, and federal disaster plans.

 ## POSTINCIDENT ACTIONS

A single case of smallpox should be treated as an international public health emergency. Hospital infection control and laboratory personnel; law enforcement authorities, including the Federal Bureau of Investigation; and local, state, and federal public health authorities, including the CDC, must be notified immediately. An epidemiologic investigation to identify all of those potentially exposed must be initiated so that a postexposure vaccination effort can commence. With a mortality rate of 30% and high morbidity, the vaccination risk-benefit ratio shifts markedly in favor of vaccination, even for patients with contraindications to receiving the vaccine. Patients who have been exposed to a smallpox patient should be vaccinated as soon as possible, even up to 5 to 7 days after exposure since the disease may either be prevented or ameliorated.[5]

The smallpox vaccine, using vaccinia virus, is most often administered by intradermal inoculation with a bifurcated needle. The current smallpox vaccine is the Wyeth DryVax, which is a licensed product derived from calf lymph. Future smallpox vaccines will be grown on human cell cultures.[6] Primary vaccinees receive three punctures with the needle; repeat vaccinees receive 15. A vesicle typically appears at the vaccination site 5 to 7 days after inoculation, with associated erythema and induration. The lesion forms a scab and gradually heals over the next 1 to 2 weeks; the evolution of the lesion may be more rapid, with less severe symptoms in those with previous immunity.

Side effects include a low-grade fever and axillary lymphadenopathy. The attendant erythema and induration of the vaccination vesicle is commonly misdiagnosed as bacterial superinfection. More severe vaccine reactions include inadvertent inoculation of the face, eyelid, or other parts of the body; generalized vaccinia; and transient, acute

myopericarditis. Rare, but often fatal, adverse reactions include eczema vaccinatum (generalized cutaneous spread of vaccinia in patients with eczema), progressive vaccinia (systemic spread of vaccinia in immunocompromised individuals), and postvaccinia encephalitis.[7]

Vaccination is contraindicated in the following conditions: immunosuppression; HIV infection; history or evidence of eczema; other active severe skin disorders; during pregnancy; or current household, sexual, or other close physical contact with individuals possessing one of these conditions. In addition, vaccination should not be performed in breast-feeding mothers, in individuals with serious cardiovascular disease or with three risk factors for cardiovascular disease, or individuals who are using topical steroid eye medications or who have had recent eye surgery. Despite these caveats, most authorities state that, with the exception of significant impairment of systemic immunity, there are no absolute contraindications to postexposure vaccination of a person with a confirmed exposure to variola. However, concomitant vaccine immune globulin (VIG) administration is recommended for pregnant and eczematous persons in such circumstances.[8]

VIG is indicated for treating some complications of the smallpox vaccine, including generalized vaccinia with systemic illness, ocular vaccinia without keratitis, eczema vaccinatum, and progressive vaccinia, and should be available when administering vaccine. The dose for prophylaxis or treatment is 100 mg/kg for the intravenous formulation (first line), or 0.6 mL/kg for the intramuscular preparation (second line). Due to the large volume of the intramuscular formulation (42 mL in a 70-kg person), the dose would be given in multiple sites over 24 to 36 hours.

If VIG is not available, cidofovir may be of use for treating vaccinia adverse events. Limited data suggest that VIG may also be of value in postexposure prophylaxis of smallpox when given within the first week after exposure, and concurrently with vaccination. Vaccination alone is recommended for those without contraindications to the vaccine. If more than 1 week has elapsed after exposure, administration of both products, if available, is reasonable.[9]

In the event of a large-scale smallpox outbreak, the controversial issue of quarantine must be considered. Historically, imposition of quarantine was a key element in the eventual control of a smallpox outbreak, but it has been more than 50 years since any such measure has been taken in the United States.

 ## MEDICAL TREATMENT OF CASUALTIES

People who have been exposed to known cases of smallpox should be monitored for a minimum of 17 days from exposure, regardless of their vaccination status; such individuals should be immediately isolated using droplet and airborne precautions at the onset of fever. Strict quarantine of asymptomatic contacts may prove to be impractical and impossible to enforce. A reasonable alternative would be to require contacts to remain at home and to check their temperatures daily.[10] Any fever greater than 38°C (101°F) during the 17 days after exposure to a confirmed case would suggest the development of smallpox. The contact should then be isolated immediately, preferably at home, until smallpox is either confirmed or ruled out and remain in isolation until all scabs separate. Immediate vaccination or revaccination should also be undertaken for all personnel exposed to a clinical case of smallpox. Caregivers should be vaccinated and continue to wear appropriate personal protective equipment regardless of vaccination status. Vaccination with a verified clinical "take," defined as vesicle with scar formation, within the past 3 years is considered to render a person immune to smallpox.

Antivirals for use against smallpox are under investigation. Cidofovir has had significant in vitro and in vivo activity in animal studies.[11] Whether it would offer benefit superior to immediate postexposure vaccination in humans has not been determined. Even though cidofovir is a licensed drug, its use for treating smallpox is "off-label," and thus it should be administered as an investigational new drug. Topical antivirals such as trifluridine or idoxuridine may be useful for treating smallpox ocular disease.

Supportive care is imperative for successful management of smallpox victims; measures include maintenance of hydration and nutrition, pain control, and management of secondary infections.

 UNIQUE CONSIDERATIONS

Smallpox (variola major) is categorized as a category A critical biologic agent by the CDC because of its transmissibility, high morbidity and mortality, ability to cause panic in afflicted populations, and the extraordinary public health measures that would be required to contain an epidemic.[12] Of particular concern with smallpox is evidence that it can be transmitted person-to-person via airborne droplet nuclei. This has been seen among some smallpox patients who have prominent respiratory symptoms.[13]

Significant progress has been made in acquiring enough licensed smallpox vaccine for every American, and work continues on the development of a safer smallpox vaccine with fewer side effects.[6] Recently, Australian researchers have demonstrated an interleukin-2 modified poxvirus that was able to defeat the current smallpox vaccine in an animal model.[14] Research likewise continues on antiviral drugs that could be used to treat smallpox patients, and the drug cidofovir offers some promise.

 PITFALLS

- Failure to recognize a case of smallpox on clinical grounds
- Failure to immediately institute airborne and droplet precautions among patients and hospital staff
- Failure to notify hospital laboratory personnel that clinical specimens may be from a smallpox patient

- Failure to immediately notify law enforcement and public health authorities of a suspected case of smallpox

 CASE PRESENTATION

An 18-year-old male presents with a fever of 104°F, severe cough, a sore throat, a severe backache, and an erythematous maculopapular rash. He has a pulse of 120 that is regular, a respiratory rate of 18, and a blood pressure of 126/88 mm Hg. He appears quite ill. The cutaneous lesions appear all over the patient's body but may be slightly more prominent on the face and arms than on the trunk or lower extremities. The lesions on the face consist mostly of red papules; on the arms they are mostly reddish macules. The lesions all appear about the same stage of development.

REFERENCES

1. Fenner F, Henderson DA, Arita I, Jezek Z, Ladnyi ID. Smallpox and its eradication. Geneva: World Health Organization; 1988.
2. Dumbell DR, Huq F. The virology of variola minor: correlation of laboratory tests with the geographic distribution and human virulence of variola isolates. *Am J Epidemiol.* 1986;123:403-15.
3. Ibrahim M, Lofts R, Jahrling P, et al. Real-time microchip PCR for detecting single-base differences in viral and human DNA. *Anal Chem.* 1998;70:2013-17.
4. Grabenstein J, Winkenwerder W. US military smallpox vaccination program experience. *JAMA.* 2003;289:3278-82.
5. Wharton M, Strikas R, Harpaz R, et al. Recommendations for using smallpox vaccine in a pre-event vaccination program. Supplemental recommendations of the Advisory Committee on Immunization Practices (ACIP) and the Healthcare Infection Control Practices Advisory Committee (HICPAC). *MMWR Recomm Rep.* 2003;52:1-16.
6. Bicknell W, James K. The new cell culture smallpox vaccine should be offered to the general population. *Rev Med Virol.* 2003;13:5-15.
7. Frey S, Couch R, Tacket C, et al. Clinical responses to undiluted and diluted smallpox vaccine. *New Engl J Med.* 2002;346:1265-74.
8. Suarez V, Hankins G. Smallpox and pregnancy: from eradicated disease to bioterrorist threat. *Obstet Gynecol.* 2002;100:87-93.
9. Jahrling PB, Zaucha GM, Huggins JW. Countermeasures to the reemergence of smallpox virus as an agent of bioterrorism. In: Scheld WM, Craig WA, Hughes JM, eds. Emerging Infections 4. Washington, DC: ASM Press; 2000.
10. Henderson D, Inglesby T, Bartlett J, et al. Smallpox as a biological weapon: medical and public health management. Working Group on Civilian Biodefense. *JAMA.* 1999;281:2127-37.
11. De Clercq E. Cidofovir in the therapy and short-term prophylaxis of poxvirus infections. *Trends Pharmacol Sci.* 2002;23:456.
12. US Centers for Disease Control and Prevention. Bioterrorism Agents/Diseases. Available at: http://www.bt.cdc.gov/agent/agentlist.asp.
13. Wehrle PF, Posch J, Richter KH, Henderson DA. An airborne outbreak of smallpox in a German hospital and its significance with respect to other recent outbreaks in Europe. *Bull World Health Organ.* 1970;43:669-79.
14. Jackson R, Ramsay A, Christensen C, et al. Expression of mouse interleukin-4 by a recombinant ectromelia virus suppresses cytolytic lymphocyte responses and overcomes genetic resistance to mousepox. *J Virol.* 2001;75:1205-10.

chapter 126

Influenza Virus Attack

Anna I. Cheh

DESCRIPTION OF EVENT

Influenza is an acute respiratory illness of viral etiology. The influenza virus is a member of the Orthomyxoviridae family. The genome of this enveloped virus contains eight segmented, single-stranded, negative sense RNA. There are three immunologic types: A, B, and C. Type A is the primary pathogen for human disease. Its two surface glycoproteins, hemagglutinin (H) and neuraminidase (N), determine host immunity and subtype designation. Unlike types B and C that reside only in humans, type A also infects birds, pigs, horses, and sea mammals. The gene's segmented nature facilitates genetic reassortment during infection within this broad reservoir. Such genetic shifts (major) or drifts (minor) lead to the genetic diversity of type A.[1] Major antigenic variations underlie the deadly worldwide pandemics, such as that of 1918 and 1957. New concerns regarding disease epidemiology surfaced in 1997 as direct disease transmission from animals to humans caused fatalities in Hong Kong.

Influenza is not classified as a bioterrorism agent by the Centers for Disease Control and Prevention.[2] Among immunocompetent individuals, influenza infection is largely self-limited with low mortality rates. However, several factors support the possible role of influenza in an urban attack. Influenza is highly contagious. Transmission can be via respiratory droplets or fomites.[3] Aerosol transmission of influenza, the method likely used in an attack, takes 27,000 times fewer virion than that required in direct respiratory contact to induce equivalent disease.[4] The incubation period is short, ranging from 18 to 72 hours. A person is contagious within a day after infection and can remain so for a week after becoming symptomatic. Also, the influenza virus is readily available, unlike many other agents that are more difficult to obtain. More worrisome are recent advances that allow infectious agents to be directly produced in the lab without a natural template.[5]

The classic presentation of influenza is the abrupt onset of fever, headache, myalgia, and extreme malaise. The virus targets and reproduces within the ciliated columnar epithelial cells of the respiratory tract.[1] Therefore, signs of both upper and lower respiratory involvement can also be present. Constitutional symptoms are more pronounced during the acute phase encompassing the first 3 to 5 days. The subsequent convalescence phase can last for weeks with lingering respiratory symptoms and malaise, often termed *post-influenza asthenia*.[6]

Complicated influenza has a predilection for individuals with chronic underlying illnesses. High-risk groups include those with cardiovascular or pulmonary disease, diabetes mellitus, renal disease, or immunosuppression. Pneumonia is the complication most responsible for the excess fatalities associated with influenza outbreaks. Other less-common complications include myositis, myocarditis, rhabdomyolysis, and Reye's syndrome. Central nervous system involvement such as encephalitis and aseptic meningitis has also been documented, although a direct relationship has been never clearly established. Viremia is rare.

Diagnosis is often based on clinical presentation. This is especially appropriate within an epidemic. However, during a possible terrorist attack, distinguishing between different viral pathogens will be imperative. Tissue cultures can be obtained within 48 to 72 hours of inoculation.[7] Increasingly, rapid viral diagnostic tests such as enzyme immunoassays (EIA) and PCR are also available for diagnosis. These newer methods, however, cannot be used to identify the responsible subtype strain.

Although common, influenza can still be a formidable foe. Attack rates are between 10% and 20% in the general population but can exceed 50% during pandemics. Institutionalized and close-quartered populations are especially at increased risk. During non-pandemic years, approximately 20,000 annual deaths are attributed to influenza in the United States.[8]

PRE-INCIDENT ACTIONS

Influenza is possibly the most tracked virus in the world. The CDC and the World Health Organization (WHO) Global Influenza Network has in place an extensive worldwide surveillance system (WHO Flunet) to monitor disease activity and identify viral isolates for the development of the annual vaccine. Influenza has the distinct advantage of having this developed immunization infrastructure. Two types of vaccine are currently approved for use in the United States. The trivalent inactivated vaccine contains a killed virus and is safe to use during pregnancy and breastfeeding. The newer trivalent live-attenuated cold-adapted vaccine (LAIV) is administered intranasally.

Effective surveillance and early detection of outbreaks is pivotal for agents such as influenza for which effective prophylaxis and immunization exist.[8] Establishing population immunity to influenza will also aid in distinguishing it from the more deadly biological agents that have a similar initial prodrome.[9] Therefore, increasing immunization rates should be part of a broader strategy against bioterrorism.

POST-INCIDENT ACTIONS

Recognition of an emerging pandemic is aided by influenza's classic presentation and clustering epidemiology. Initiation of a coordinated effort to expedite vaccine development and dissemination will be pivotal. During the initial period following a bioterrorist attack, antiviral agents are another key mechanism of containing morbidity and protecting exposed individuals.[10] Public awareness campaigns regarding measures to reduce transmission and seeking early medical intervention should be quickly instituted to blunt the mortality of an outbreak.[8,11]

MEDICAL TREATMENT OF CASUALTIES

Treatment of influenza is largely supportive. Specific antiviral agents such as amantadine and rimantadine are approved for both the treatment and prophylaxis for influenza A. Newer agents such as oseltamivir and zanamivir are effective for both types A and B. Although not proven to be any more efficacious, these agents are associated with fewer central side effects. Optimal efficacy of all drugs depends on starting the regimen within 48 hours after symptom onset. During possible acute outbreaks, these agents can provide effective chemophylaxis until vaccine-induced immunity can be established in target populations.[10] Constraints on existing medical systems could reach critical levels, pending the extent of the attack.

UNIQUE CONSIDERATIONS

The potential advantage of influenza as a bioterrorism agent is its genetic variation. A variant strain from which wide human immunity does not exist could hold devastating potency.[12] Some experts estimate that a virus of comparable virulence to the 1918 strain could result in 100 million deaths today.[13] Although the self-limiting course of influenza would fail to produce the dramatic and immediate effects that are the aim of terrorist acts, the real impact of an influenza outbreak will be its indirect costs. Modern influenza pandemics have evolved into economic disasters even as medical advances help to avert direct fatalities.[14] For example, 3 million chick-

ens were slaughtered to prevent further transmission of the Hong Kong avian influenza virus in 1997.

Influenza is a virus that impacts certain segments of the population disproportionately. As the population ages and a greater segment live with higher risk morbidities, the impact of a pandemic will also escalate.

 ## PITFALLS

- Failure to consider terrorism during the early phase of a pandemic because of influenza's natural existence.
- Failure to diagnose accurately. The broad spectrum of influenza symptoms often overlaps with many other possible bioterrorism agents. Clinicians should be educated for greater utilization of confirmatory tests and reporting positive cases to a central tracking database.
- Failure to institute mechanisms to ensure adequate supply of antiviral medications, currently unlikely to be able to meet prolonged demand.
- Failure of existing vaccine infrastructure to respond quickly to a novel virulent strain. Currently, a vaccine is almost a year out of date by time of administration.
- Failure to update immunization strategy to better address the unique threats of terrorism.
- Failure to anticipate the social and economic impact of a pandemic outbreak.

 CASE PRESENTATION

In a large metropolitan city, public health officials are baffled by a surge of influenza cases earlier in the winter season than expected. CDC and WHO work overtime to identify the responsible strain, ultimately found to be a novel subtype different than any previously recorded. Nursing homes are virtually emptying out as residents are admitted to hospitals for pneumonia. Even the local colleges are feeling the effects as the school clinics are inundated with students complaining of debilitating myalgia and malaise. Parents pull children from school to avoid exposure. Doctors are flooded by calls from patients frustrated with being unable to fill their amantadine prescription at their local pharmacies. Antiviral medications are being depleted as people wait for the new vaccine to arrive, which is announced to be available in 8 months.

Public health officials predict one of the worst influenza seasons ever in economic costs as more people are calling in sick, productivity is lost, tourism shuts down, and hospital resources are stretched to the breaking point.

REFERENCES

1. Schoch-Spana M. Implications of pandemic influenza for bioterrorism response. *Clin Infect Dis.* 2000;31: 1409-13.
2. Centers for Disease Control and Prevention. Bioterrorism Agents/Diseases. Available at: http://www.bt.cdc.gov/agent/agentlist-category.asp.
3. Rao BL. Epidemiology and control of influenza. *Nat Med J India.* 2003;16:143-8.

4. Madjid M, Lillibridge S, Mirhaji P, et al. Influenza as a bioweapon. *J R Soc Med*. 2003;96:345-6.

5. Cello J, Paul AV, Wimmer E. Chemical synthesis of poliovirus cDNA: generation of infectious virus in the absence of natural template. *Science*. 2002;297:1016-8.

6. Harrison's Internal Medicine On-Line (Chap 190). Available at: www.accessmedicine.com.

7. Covalciuc KA, Webb KH, Carlson CA. Comparison of four clinical specimen types for detection of influenza A and B viruses by optical immunoassay (FLU OIA Test) and cell culture methods. *J Clin Microbiol*. 1999;37:3971.

8. Lutz BD, Bronze MS, Greenfield RA. Influenza virus: natural disease and bioterrorism threat. *J Okla State Med Assoc*. 2003;96:27-8.

9. Irvin CB, Nouhan PP, Rice K. Syndromic analysis of computerized emergency department patients' chief complaints: an opportunity for bioterrorism and influenza surveillance. *Ann Emerg Med*. 2003;41:447-52.

10. Simberkoff MS. Vaccines for adults in an age of terrorism. *J Assoc Acad Min Phys*. 2002;13:19-20.

11. Krug RM. The potential use of influenza virus as an agent for bioterrorism. *Antiviral Res*. 2003;57:147-50.

12. Owens SR. Being prepared: preparations for a pandemic of influenza. *EMBO Reports*. 2001;21:1061-3.

13. Webster RG, Shortridge KF, Kawaoka Y. Influenza: interspecies transmission and emergence of new pandemics. *FEMS Immun Med Microbiol*. 1997;18:275-9.

14. Longini IM, Halloran ME, Nizam A, et al. Containing pandemic influenza with antiviral agents. *Am J Epidemiol*. 2002;159:623-3.

15. Ferguson NM, Fraser C, Donnelly CA, et al. Public health risk from the Avial H5N1 influenza epidemic. *Science*. 2004;304:968-9.

16. O'Brien KK, Higdon ML, Halverson JJ. Recognition and management of bioterrorism infections. *Am Fam Phys*. 2003;67:1927-34.

chapter 127

Monkeypox

John D. Malone

DESCRIPTION OF EVENT

Monkeypox is an orthopox virus, recognized in 1958 in laboratory monkeys. The natural host may be an African squirrel, but the virus can also infect rodents and rabbits. Monkeypox is in the same genus as smallpox *(Variola major and minor)*, *Molluscum contagiosum,* cowpox, and the vaccinia virus. Other non–human associated animal orthopox infections include volepox, skunkpox, raccoonpox, camelpox, and buffalopox. Monkeypox has been endemic in Ghana and Zaire and is associated with the hunting and consumption of infected monkeys and rodents.[1]

In April 2003, six infected African rodents, Gambian giant rats, were imported into the United States. They transferred the monkeypox virus to prairie dog rodents housed in adjacent cages. Within 2 months, human cases were reported in individuals who had been bitten or scratched by the infected prairie dogs.[2] In the outbreak, there were 71 suspected cases and 37 confirmed cases.[3] There was no laboratory-confirmed human-to-human transmission.

The patients presented with fever greater than 38° C and skin lesions. Skin manifestations ranged from nodular swellings in the wound margins to satellite and disseminated lesions. Papules progressed to vesicles and pustules. Significant symptoms include severe chills and sore throat. Lymphadenopathy and tonsillar hypertrophy were present. Along with an intimate rodent animal exposure history, adenopathy is a helpful sign for emergency physicians to differentiate monkeypox from a "flu syndrome" in those with minimal or subtle skin lesions and similar headache, fever, sweats, chills, and cough. Four of the initial eleven cases were hospitalized. The clinical course was self-limited with some central scarring of larger lesions.

With close cooperation of the Centers for Disease Control and Prevention (CDC) and multiple Midwestern state health authorities, the outbreak was controlled through an emergency embargo and quarantine orders against the "importation, sale, distribution, or display of prairie dogs or any mammals that had been in contact with prairie dogs after April 1, 2003."[4] Appropriate and aggressive animal control measures prevented the establishment of monkeypox in the North American rodent population; a vast improvement compared with the his-

tory of the plague bacillus, *Yersinia pestis,* that entered the Southwestern U.S. desert rodent population after a 1900 epidemic in San Francisco.[5]

The skin lesions for monkeypox are identical to those for smallpox: morbilliform, hard and pea sized on an erythematous base, and classically described as dew drops on a rose petal. The rash begins as maculopapular lesions 2 to 5 mm in diameter, progressing through papular, vesicular, pustular, and crust phases over a 14-day period.[6] The lesions are initially located on cooler body parts, particularly the extremities including the palms and soles, and the face. Over the initial days, the lesions spread to the trunk. The initial papules become umbilicated vesicles, with all of the lesions in the same stage at the same time. The skin vesicles are a product of bloodborne viral seeding of the terminal capillaries in the initial viremia. The initial viremia is manifested by the sudden onset of fever, malaise, headache, and severe back pain, and manifested less often with abdominal pain and vomiting.[7]

As for the differential diagnosis of monkeypox, herpes viruses are much more likely to be an etiology of similar skin lesions. The Varicella Zoster Virus (VZV) produces varicella "chickenpox" vesicles that begin centrally on the trunk. The multiple lesions exist in different stages of maturation. VZV may also cause disseminated herpes zoster in an immunocompromised host. A varicella virus direct fluorescent antibody (DFA) test should be available in major emergency departments and initially performed to diagnose this infection. Coxsackievirus commonly occurs in children under 10 years of age in the autumn season. Secondary syphilis (syphilis serology should be positive), erythema multiforme, and drug eruptions can produce less typical vesicular rashes on the palm and soles. Rocky Mountain Spotted Fever, a rickettsial illness, is associated with a spring/summer tick exposure in the Southeastern United States. Meningococcal infection is characterized by rapid progression to shock. Molluscum infection occurs in healthy children and HIV-infected adults; the painless lesions do not cause fever.

Definitive laboratory diagnosis of monkeypox infection is required to ensure that smallpox is not present and for an appropriate public health response. Electron microscopy of vesicular scrapings will identify orthopox viruses by the appearance of an exceedingly large box with rounded corners. Polymerase chain reactions definitively identify the specific species. Tissue from lymph nodes and blood specimens can also be evaluated. Specimen collection instructions are detailed by the CDC.[8]

It is not known whether the monkeypox virus was ever weaponized. However, the process would probably be similar to the method used to weaponize the smallpox virus. Scientists from the former Soviet Union accomplished this. Like smallpox, monkeypox is contagious but less so. If a stable, infectious monkeypox biological aerosol was produced and delivered as a fine particle aerosol under ideal atmospheric conditions over a targeted population, one would expect to see large numbers of casualties presenting at about the same time to local hospitals and doctor's offices with signs and symptoms as described here. The ensuing epidemic and secondary cases would probably not be as severe as one would expect to see if a smallpox weapon was used, since the monkeypox virus is not nearly as contagious as the smallpox virus. Of course, with the genetic engineering techniques that are available today, novel characteristics could be created and infectivity of the virus could be enhanced. There is no evidence to date that this has been attempted.

 PRE-INCIDENT ACTIONS

Emergency departments should have well-rehearsed standard operating procedures to evaluate potentially contagious infectious disease patients using airborne transmission precautions (protective gowns, gloves, HEPA face masks). A small cadre of smallpox-vaccinated healthcare workers should be available to initially evaluate and care for patients with suspected orthopox infection. Along with concerns for patient transmissible bioterrorism agents, such as smallpox, pneumonic plague, and viral hemorrhagic fevers, clinical suspicion is necessary for the more common agents of SARS and rubeola virus in our highly mobile global society.

 POST-INCIDENT ACTIONS

When presented with an initial case of monkeypox, great concerns about the possibility of smallpox are appropriate in this age of ongoing terrorist threats. In contrast to smallpox, monkeypox would be a poor agent for bioterrorism because of a very low mortality rate and respiratory transmission by large droplets that requires direct and prolonged face-to-face contact. Monkeypox is highly unlikely to be able to sustain itself in human communities. However, if suspected, appropriate local and state health authorities must be notified early to assist with agent identification.

 MEDICAL TREATMENT OF CASUALTIES

Supportive therapy with antipyretics and fluids are indicated. Monkeypox has a low lethality (1.5% in a 1996 Democratic Republic of the Congo outbreak) and requires close family contact for transmission. Accumulating expe-

rience in the United States suggests a relatively low risk of person-to-person transmission. According to the CDC, all healthcare settings such as hospitals, emergency departments, and physician offices should have the capacity to care for monkeypox-infected patients and protect health care workers and other patients from exposure.[9] A combination of standard, contact, and droplet precautions, which include gowns, gloves, eye shields, and surgical masks, should be applied in all healthcare settings when concerns for monkeypox exist. Because of a theoretical risk of airborne infection, airborne precautions using N95-rated respirator masks are recommended when possible. A negative pressure room should be used if available. Viremic individuals spread the disease through large respiratory droplets, most likely with the symptoms of cough, pharyngitis, and fever.

Unique Considerations

Smallpox vaccination with the vaccinia virus (Dryvax) is protective against monkeypox infection. The vaccinia virus likely evolved through a reassortment of the cowpox virus and the smallpox virus. During the 2003 monkeypox outbreak, CDC guidelines for vaccination included public health and animal control investigators, healthcare workers caring for monkeypox patients or those who may be asked to care for infected patients, or family members with close contact with someone who was symptomatic with monkeypox. Also included were veterinarians and their technicians who had direct physical exposure to an infected animal. Vaccination up to 14 days after exposure will attenuate or prevent monkeypox illness.

Extensive data from the Department of Defense exist over the safety and efficacy of the "Dryvax" smallpox vaccination.[10] As of July 2005, more than 830,000 individuals have been vaccinated. A causal relationship to one death from a lupus-like illness after both anthrax and smallpox vaccinations has resulted along with 99 cases of myopericarditis with documented complete recovery in 64 cases. Among 27,700 smallpox vaccinated healthcare workers, there were no cases of transmission of vaccinia to a patient. Other investigators have also shown the risk of inadvertent vaccinia transmission from vaccination sites covered by occlusive dressings to be quite low.[11]

Fear and panic are major issues for monkeypox viral infection. Commonality in name with smallpox raises anxieties and misperceptions in the public, patients, and healthcare providers. Significant psychological and economic impacts result. Preliminary knowledge of monkeypox, personal protective equipment, and effective leadership of the healthcare team will ensure appropriate patient care and avoid crisis and closure of emergency departments.

 PITFALLS

- The skin lesions of monkeypox and smallpox are identical.
- Lymphadenopathy, tonsillar hypertrophy, and intimate rodent exposure will assist in differentiating monkeypox from a "flu syndrome."

- Monkeypox has relatively low risk of person-to-person transmission; however, airborne precautions (N95 mask) are recommended.
- A high clinical suspicion and well-rehearsed standard operating procedures are needed to safely evaluate potentially contagious patients.
- Emergency departments should have a cadre of smallpox-vaccinated healthcare workers.

 CASE PRESENTATION

The right index finger of a child has a lesion with a raised border and necrotic center 14 days after a prairie dog bite and 11 days after a febrile illness.[12] Secondary lesions also present on the dorsum of the left hand. The pustules are raised, firm, several millimeters in diameter, and with erythematous flares. One day previously, her mother developed fever, sweats, malaise, and sore throat. The mother has smaller disseminated umbilicated vesicles. The family has multiple animals, including cats, dogs, horses, goats, and donkeys.

REFERENCES

1. Huntin YJF, Williams RJ, Malfait P, et al. Outbreak of human monkeypox, Democratic Republic of Congo, 1996 to 1997. *Emerg Infect Dis*. 2001;7:434-8.
2. Reed KD, Melski JW, Graham MB, et al. The detection of monkeypox in humans in the western hemisphere. *N Engl J Med*. 2004;350:342-50.
3. Cunha BE. Monkeypox in the United States: an occupational health look at the first cases. *AAOHN J*. 2004;52:164-8.
4. CDC. Multistate Outbreak of Monkeypox–Illinois, Indiana, Wisconsin, 2003. *MMWR Morb Mortal Wkly Rep*. 2003;52:537-40.
5. Smith G. *Plague on Us*. New York: The Common Wealth Fund; 1941.
6. DiGiulo DB, Eckburg PB. Human monkeypox: an emerging zoonosis. *Lancet Infect Dis*. 2004;4:15-25. (Review article)
7. Jezek Z, Szczeniowski M, Paluku KM, et al. Human monkeypox: clinical features of 282 patients. *J Infect Dis*. 1987;156:293-8.
8. Centers for Disease Control and Prevention. Interim guidance for collection of diagnostic specimens from persons with suspected monkeypox, June 23, 2003. Available at http://www.cdc.gov/ncidod/monkeypox/diagspecimens.htm.
9. Centers for Disease Control and Prevention. Updated interim infection control and exposure and exposure management guidance in the health care and community setting for patients with possible monkeypox virus infection. Available at: http://www.cdc.gov/ncidod/monkeypox/infectioncontrol.htm.
10. Department of Defense. Smallpox vaccination program (updated September 20, 2005). Available at http://www. smallpox.mil
11. Talbot TR, Ziel E, Doersam JK, et al. Risk of vaccinia transfer to hands of vaccinated persons after smallpox immunization. *Clin Infect Dis*. 2004;38:536-41.
12. Reed KD, Melski J, Stratman E. Index case and family infection of monkey pox from prairie dogs diagnosed in Marshfield, WI, Marshfield Clinic May-June 2003. Available at: http://www.research.marshfieldclinic.org/crc/monkeypox.asp.

chapter 128

Hantavirus Pulmonary Syndrome

Bonnie H. Hartstein and Curtis J. Hunter

 ## DESCRIPTION OF EVENT

Hantavirus pulmonary syndrome (HPS) is characterized by rapidly developing non-cardiogenic pulmonary edema, which develops after infection with rodent-borne *Hantavirus*. Early recognition of HPS is essential as the initial flu-like symptoms of malaise, fever, and muscle aches can progress to shock and complete respiratory failure within a few days.[1] Although hantavirus has not been weaponized or used for bioterrorism to date, it is recognized by the Centers for Disease Control and Prevention (CDC) as a category C agent, an emerging pathogen that could be engineered for mass exposure in the future because of its presumed ease of production and dissemination, and potential for high morbidity and mortality.[2] A genus of the family Bunyaviridae, *Hantavirus* was first isolated in Korea in 1978 as the culpable agent in the Old World disease known as hemorrhagic fever with renal syndrome (HFRS), an acute prostrating febrile illness with renal failure and shock.[3,4] In 1993 a mysterious clinical entity causing fever, rapid respiratory failure, and cardiopulmonary dysfunction killed 29 people in the southwestern United States.[5] Linked by genetic sequencing to a previously unknown *Hantavirus* species but lacking the renal and hemorrhagic manifestations, the disease was named hantavirus pulmonary syndrome and changed the recognized spectrum of hantavirus disease.

Over 20 different sero/genotypes of *Hantavirus* have been identified, each maintained in nature by a single unique rodent species. Human infection occurs through inhalation of aerosolized virus shed in rodent saliva, urine, and feces, or by direct inoculation via rodent bites.[4] The primary causative agent of the largest outbreak in the United States, the Sin Nombre virus, is carried by the deer mouse, Peromyscus maniculatas. Other hantaviruses know to cause HPS in the United States include the New York, Black Canal, and Bayou viruses hosted by the white-footed mouse (Peromyscus leucopus), the cotton rat (Sigmodon hipidus), and the rice rat (Oryzomys palustris). The rodent reservoir of the Seoul virus, Rattus norvegicus, thought to have been brought by cargo ship to the Western Hemisphere from Europe, has caused the only cases of HFRS documented in the United States.[6] Nearly all of the United States falls within range of one or more hantavirus-carrying rodent species, all of which cause HPS.

The incubation period for human hantavirus infections is documented from 4 to 42 days, with an average range of 12 to 16 days.[7] HPS progresses through four clinical phases: prodrome, pulmonary edema and shock, diuresis, and convalescence.[8] The initial prodrome lasts for 3 to 6 days and is characterized by malaise, myalgia, fever, tachypnea, and gastrointestinal symptoms such as nausea, vomiting, diarrhea, or abdominal pain. In 10% of cases the abdominal pain is reported to be severe enough as to mimic appendicitis.[1] Presenting symptoms may overlap with more common viral infections, challenging early recognition by healthcare workers. One study attempting to quantify a clinically distinct constellation of symptoms suggests excluding patients with rapid Influenza A proven infection from consideration and that the presence of sore throat or nasal symptoms and the finding of an injected pharynx are less likely to be associated with HPS.[9]

The subsequent cardiopulmonary phase is heralded by the acute onset of non-cardiogenic pulmonary edema.[10] Clinically, patients have progressive cough and shortness of breath. On the cellular level, significant capillary leak in pulmonary endothelial cells occurs.[7,10] The time interval from the development of dyspnea to the need for ventilator support is reported to be within 1 to 6 hours, underscoring the extremely rapid progression of respiratory collapse.[1,8] Other signs include hypoxia and copious amber-colored non-purulent secretions with secretion protein/serum protein ratio greater than 80%.[5,11]

Specific laboratory and radiographic findings that are suggestive of HPS assist in diagnosis and should raise clinical suspicion. A peripheral blood smear triad of thrombocytopenia, leukocytosis with left shift, and circulating immunoblasts are unique to HPS in North America.[11] Elevated lactate levels, and hemoconcentration up to 77% that corrects to anemic levels after fluid resuscitation, are observed.[12] Radiographically HPS is distinguished by the central location of infiltrates rather than the peripheral pattern typically seen in ARDS and the lack of focal consolidation common in most pneumonias.[9]

The sepsis syndrome observed in HPS features a diminished cardiac index and normal or elevated systemic vascular resistance, which is the opposite of that typically seen in sepsis.[13] Hypotension, which may be seen initially, is a result of low cardiac stroke volume resulting from inadequate left ventricular preload exacerbated by myocardial depression and is usually marked by hemoconcentration.

Death rates range between 50% and 70% with cardiogenic shock and pulseless electrical activity as the proximate cause.[5] Survivors of the cardiopulmonary phase recover quickly with a spontaneous diuresis occurring 2 to 5 days after the onset of pulmonary edema, usually facilitating extubation within 1 week of initiating ventilator support. Convalescence ensues with minor residual respiratory impairment.[8]

Identification of the virus is achieved through serologic testing in the acutely ill for IgG and IgM antibodies to viral nucleocapsid proteins.[1] ELISA assays are available at most state public health laboratories or by state health department referral at CDC.[6] Because of the time delay before results are obtained, a recombinant immunoblot assay in the form of a test strip is being evaluated.[1]

 ## PRE-INCIDENT ACTIONS

Exposure of individuals or groups to hantavirus might occur naturally as a result of increased exposure caused by an environmental change such as increased rodent food production or decreased rodent predator population, or because of a planned bioterrorist attack. Similar to the epidemic that heralded the discovery of HPS in the southwestern United States in 1993, individuals or groups of people can be exposed through contact with contaminated material. Increased rodent population or high-risk activities such as cleaning enclosed rodent-infested areas can lead to infection.

Disaster scenarios, either naturally occurring or as a result of terrorism, that displace populations, disrupt the sanitation infrastructure, or create living conditions where people are forced to reside in makeshift structures or sleep on the ground significantly increase the risk of hantavirus exposure. Risk reduction suggestions published by the CDC serve as a useful guide to mitigate risks. Actions to reduce exposure to rodents involve securing food and trash in rodent-proof containers; keeping items that attract rodents such as garbage cans, woodpiles, and bird feeders far from human dwellings; and using raised cement foundations in new construction of outbuildings or shelters.[14]

Hantavirus is recognized as an emerging pathogen for bioterrorism because of its relative ease of transmission and high mortality. Dissemination would most likely occur via aerosolization of infectious particles released over populated areas. Bioterrorists might use low-flying aircraft, munitions, or indoor contamination through air ducts to initiate exposure.

 ## POST-INCIDENT ACTIONS

Suspicious patterns of disease presentation would be the first clue that an HPS outbreak had occurred at the hands of bioterrorists. An understanding of the demographic distribution of naturally occurring hantavirus infection allows the healthcare professional to recognize unusual variations and to suspect bioterrorist activity. Infection caused by hantavirus and rodent hosts not recognized in the United States, an infectious disease consistent with HFRS in the New World, and disease in nonendemic areas or in patients with no travel history should all raise suspicion of an unnatural or deliberate infection. Virus isolation, genotyping, and comparison to known national and world prevalence data could unveil irregular geographic incidence patterns.

Cases of natural hantavirus have generally occurred in young adults and previously healthy persons because exposure occurred during activities like farming, cleaning, or camping.[5] An attack generated by terrorism with infectious particles in high concentration on the ground or in soil in densely populated areas might affect children, who are smaller and shorter, in greater proportion than observed naturally. Also, an increase in disease incidence without a rise in the endemic rodent population or in persons not exposed to rodents should raise suspicion.

Universal precautions and respiratory isolation of affected individuals is recommended. Although person-to-person transmission is generally not recognized, during one hantavirus outbreak in Argentina, five health care workers involved in treating HPS patients may have contracted disease without known exposure to rodents.[3]

 ## MEDICAL TREATMENT OF CASUALTIES

Supportive care is the mainstay of treatment for HPS. Volume replacement must be cautious and conservative because of the potential for significant pulmonary capillary leak. Pulmonary artery occlusive pressures higher than 10-12 mmHg are associated with significant pulmonary edema. Classic to HPS is a shock state characterized by decreased cardiac output and increased systemic vascular resistance, although frank hypotension is also observed. Use of inotropic agents such as dobutamine should usually be accompanied by judicious volume resuscitation. Despite the presence of severe pulmonary edema, adequate oxygenation can usually be maintained with mechanical ventilation and high levels of positive end-expiratory pressure.[1]

Further studies on the treatment of HPS are needed to assess the role of immunologic therapy and inflammatory mediators on vascular function, as well as the use of antiviral agents such as ribavirin, which has been shown to reduce mortality in HFRS.[6] It is also conceivable that some added benefit could be achieved by applying the principles of early goal-directed therapy, which is showing some promise among patients with sepsis.

 ## UNIQUE CONSIDERATIONS

The importance of rapid recognition of HPS and the need for widespread dissemination of information between other health care institutions and health departments is the key to effective management. Since nearly all infected patients become ventilator dependent, the prospect of a mass casualty situation caused by HPS could prove catastrophic unless adequate intensive care unit capabilities were mobilized and appropriately staffed to augment local healthcare facilities.

 PITFALLS

- Failure to rapidly recognize the symptoms of HPS and to disseminate information to other health care institutions and health departments

 CASE PRESENTATION

A 24-year-old male presents to the emergency department of a small community hospital with a chief complaint of flu-like symptoms and cough. He states that 3 days ago he awoke with a headache, general malaise, vomiting, diarrhea, and crampy abdominal pain, which he initially attributed to a hangover and food poisoning. Over the following days the symptoms persisted and worsened. Most concerning to him is a dry cough with amber-colored sputum that started last night, kept him from sleep, and prevented him from his normal routine of running in the morning. He states he just returned from a trip to White Sands Proving Ground, Arizona where he participated in a commemorative marathon honoring military troops killed in combat. He states that two of his close friends who also participated in the event are developing the same symptoms. His vital signs are pulse 86, respiratory rate 22, blood pressure 112/78, temperature 101.4°F, and pulse oximetry 99% on room air. A chest radiograph reveals early interstitial edema with Kerley B lines and peribronchial cuffing. The patient begins to complain of dyspnea and the pulse oximetry continues to decline despite switching to a non-rebreather mask with high flow oxygen. A portable chest radiograph reveals significantly worsening pulmonary edema and the patient is electively sedated and intubated for respiratory failure.

- Failure to recognize respiratory failure and initiate appropriate ventilatory support
- Failure to prepare for significant numbers of patients requiring ventilator support
- Failure to judiciously manage fluid balance and cardiovascular status

REFERENCES

1. Simpson SQ. Hantavirus pulmonary syndrome. *Heart Lung.* 1998;27:51-7.
2. Moran GJ. Threats in bioterrorism II: CDC category B and C agents. *Emerg Med Clin North Am.* 2002;20:311-30.
3. McCaughey C, Hart CA. Hantaviruses. *J Med Microbiol.* 2000; 49:587-99.
4. Chapman LE, Khabbaz RF. Etiology and epidemiology of the Four Corners hantavirus outbreak. *Infect Agents Dis.* 1994;3:234-44.
5. Levy H, Simpson SQ. Hantavirus pulmonary syndrome. *Am J Respir Crit Care Med.* 1994;149:1710-3.
6. Doyle TJ, Bryan RT, Peters CJ. Viral hemorrhagic fevers and hantavirus infections in the Americas. *Infect Dis Clin North Am.* 1998;12:95-110.
7. Butler JC, Peters CJ. Hantaviruses and hantavirus pulmonary syndrome. *Clin Infect Dis.* 1994;19:387-95.
8. Jenison S, Koster F. Hantavirus pulmonary syndrome: clinical, diagnostic, and virologic aspects. *Semin Respir Infect.* 1995; 10:259-69.
9. Moolenaar RL, Dalton C, Lipman HB, et al. Clinical features that differentiate hantavirus pulmonary syndrome from three other respiratory illnesses. *Clin Infect Dis.* 1995;21:643-9.
10. Graziano KL. Hantavirus pulmonary syndrome: a zebra worth knowing. *Am Fam Physician.* 2002;66:6.
11. Duchin JS, Koster FT, Peters CJ, et al. Hantavirus pulmonary syndrome: a clinical description of 17 patients with a newly recognized disease. *N Engl J Med.* 1994;330:949-55.
12. Zakik SR, Greer PW, Coffield LM, et al. Hantavirus pulmonary syndrome, pathogenesis of an emerging infectious disease. *Am J Pathol.* 1995;146:552-79.
13. Hallin GW, Simpson SQ, Crowell RE, et al. Cardiopulmonary manifestations of hantavirus pulmonary syndrome. *Crit Care Med.* 1996;24:252-8.
14. Mills JN, Corneli A, Young JC, et al. Hantavirus pulmonary syndrome—United States: updated recommendations for risk reduction. *MMWR* 2002;51:RR-9.

chapter 129

Hendra and Nipah Virus Attack (Hendra Virus Disease and Nipah Virus Encephalitis)

Kelly J. Corrigan

 ## DESCRIPTION OF EVENT

Both the Hendra virus and the Nipah virus belong to the same subfamily, *Paramyxoviridae*. They have both been identified in various zoonotic disease outbreaks in Southeast Asia and Australia within the past 10 years. Formerly known as the equine Morbillivirus, Hendra virus was the first to be identified and has been implicated in three separate disease outbreaks in Queensland, Australia between 1994 and 1999. It was first isolated in 1994 following an outbreak of severe respiratory disease in both horses and humans in Brisbane, Queensland, Australia.[1-3] Out of 21 horses infected in the first outbreak, 14 died. Three human infections resulting in two deaths have been reported as a result of the Hendra virus. These individuals reportedly had severe flu-like symptoms and others have presented with severe, often fatal, pneumonia. Encephalitis-like clinical signs have also been reported. The primary source of the Hendra virus appears to be the black fruit bat, with birds having been implicated as carriers of the deadly virus as well.[4,5]

The Nipah virus is genotypically similar to the Hendra virus, and they both belong to a new genus within the family *Paramyxoviridae*.[6] Nipah has been implicated in outbreaks of encephalitis in Malaysia in 1998 and 1999. Investigations of these outbreaks concluded that the pigs and humans were likely infected with Nipah via the respiratory route. In April 1999, 100 fatal encephalitis cases were reported in Malaysia.[7] Nipah was identified as the cause, and pigs were the primary source. However, Nipah does not appear to be transmitted from person to person.

Nipah-infected patients present with fever, headache, dizziness, vomiting, and altered mental status.[8] Autonomic instability is also a common sequelae of infection that suggests brain stem involvement. Some patients who have undergone magnetic resonance imaging demonstrate widespread microinfarctions of the CNS, which are presumably the result of small vessel disease.[8] This is supported by direct evidence from human autopsies that have revealed systemic CNS thrombotic occlusions and microinfarctions in victims of Nipah virus infection.[9] The Centers for Disease Control and Prevention (CDC) has conclusively identified both of these viruses and has developed serologic tests to detect both IgG and IgM antibodies to Hendra and Nipah.[6] Both IgG and IgM antibodies can be detected in blood and cerebrospinal fluids.[10]

 ## PRE-INCIDENT ACTIONS

In preparation for potential chemical and biological terrorist attacks, the Committee on Research and Development to Improve Civilian Medical Response recommends that major hospitals conduct mass-casualty planning and training; designate isolation rooms available for infectious diseases, create decontamination capacity, and be fully supplied with drugs, ventilators, and personal protective equipment.[11] The committee also encourages the CDC to keep medical care providers up to date on current dangerous biologic materials and promotes advance notice from law enforcement agencies regarding potential terrorist incidents. The CDC must maintain a containment level 4 laboratory in order to run the appropriate tests that identify Nipah and Hendra, without risking further human infection.

 ## POST-INCIDENT ACTIONS

Suspicion of an outbreak of Hendra or Nipah virus infection should be reported to the proper authorities (local public health and CDC) immediately so that appropriate diagnostic and response measures can be taken. Isolation of the viruses, as previously mentioned, should only be done in a biosafety level 4 containment laboratory located at either The United States Army Medical Research Institute for Infectious Diseases (USAMRIID) or the CDC.[6] Human-to-human transmission is not known. Infected patients should be treated by following standard precautions.

Infected animals apparently excrete the Hendra virus through their urine, therefore, in order to prevent further transmission of Hendra virus, it is recommended that horse stables follow strict hygiene guidelines.[4] Nipah outbreak control has been accomplished in Malaysia through the mass culling of hundreds of thousands of potentially infected pigs and by banning the importation of pigs into the country. Other efforts include educational programs directed at farmers and a national surveillance program to monitor for outbreaks of disease.[1]

 ## MEDICAL TREATMENT OF CASUALTIES

Supportive therapy should be initiated as appropriate, including airway management and ventilatory support. Previous work has demonstrated the drug ribavirin to be effective against both Hendra and Nipah viruses in vitro.[2] A trial of ribavirin in 140 patients infected with Nipah virus, with 54 of these patients serving as the control, showed 32% mortality in the ribavirin group compared with 54% mortality in the control group.[12] Given the low side effect profile of ribavirin in the acute treatment setting, ribavirin should be seriously considered in Nipah virus victims as well as Hendra virus infections, since they are similar sub-types.

The dosing of ribavirin is 30 mg/kg IV once (maximum of 2 g) followed by 16 mg/kg IV (maximum 1 g/dose) every 6 hours for 4 days, then 8 mg/kg IV (maximum 500 mg/dose) every 8 hours for 6 days. In the event of mass casualties, oral ribavirin may be given at the dose of 2000 mg loading, followed by 600 mg twice a day if greater than 75 kg, and 400 mg in AM, 600 mg in PM if less than 75 kg for 10 days. Children follow the same dosing guidelines, with the exception that oral ribavirin is given at 30 mg/kg loading, followed by 15 mg/kg/day divided into twice-daily dosing for 10 days.[6]

Research continues on the development of vaccine against Nipah virus infection.[3]

 ## UNIQUE CONSIDERATIONS

Since Hendra virus infection may resemble severe influenza and since Nipah-infected patients present with symptoms similar to meningitis and encephalitis, suspicion for infection with these organisms will largely be based on an appropriate history. Hendra virus has been diagnosed only in humans who were exposed to secretions and bodily fluids of infected horses. Human Nipah infections were identified mostly in humans exposed to infected pigs; however, the World Health Organization has received recent reports of infections among children in Bangladesh who had no known exposure to swine.[5] The fruit bat is suspected as the primary source in these cases, but the specific mode of transmission remains to be identified. No human-to-human transmission has been reported. Both Hendra and Nipah virus have short incubation periods and high mortality.

 ## PITFALLS

- Failure to suspect Hendra or Nipah when the history suggests these as a possible etiology.

- Failure to immediately report suspicious cases to the CDC for definitive diagnostic studies in a level 4 biocontainment laboratory.
- Failure to consider treatment with ribavirin in the acute setting.

 ## CASE PRESENTATION

A 41-year-old male presents to the emergency department with a 5-day history of flu-like symptoms, fever, cough, and now shortness of breath. He denies headache, rash, nausea, vomiting, diarrhea, or abdominal pain. He has no known medical problems and no HIV risk factors. He cleans horse stables for a living and a new shipment of horses came in 2 weeks ago from Australia. A co-worker has been complaining of some of the same symptoms since yesterday. His vital signs are: temperature 102.1 °F, heart rate 110, blood pressure 123/79, respiratory rate 24, and room air oxygen saturation of 93%. His chest radiograph shows a small right lower lobe infiltrate.

REFERENCES

1. CDC: Morbidity and Mortality Weekly Report. Update: Outbreak of Nipah Virus: Malaysia and Singapore, 1999. April 30, 1999.
2. CDC: Hendra virus disease and Nipah virus encephalitis. November 26, 2003.
3. Guillaume V, Contamin H. Loth P, et al. Nipah virus: vaccination and passive protection studies in a hamster model. *J Virol.* 2004;78(2):834-40.
4. Chong HT, Kunjapan SR. Nipah encephalitis outbreak in Malaysia, clinical features in patients from Seremban. *Can J Neurol Sci.* 2002;29(1):83-7.
5. Das P. Infectious disease surveillance update. *Lancet Infect Dis.* 2004;4(4):657.
6. Brown D, Lloyd G. Zoonotic viruses. In: Cohen and Powderly: Infectious Diseases. Philadelphia: Elsevier; 2004, pp 2095-109.
7. Moran GJ. Threats in bioterrorism II: CDC category B and C agents. *Emerg Clin North Am.* 2002;20(2):311-30.
8. Nipah Virus. In: Gershon. Krugman's Infectious Diseases of Children, ed 11. St Louis: Mosby; 2004.
9. Wong KT. A golden hamster model for human acute Nipah virus infection. *Am J Pathol.* 2003;163(5):2127-37.
10. Hendra and Hendra-Like (Nipah) Viruses. In: Mandell. Principles and Practice of Infectious Diseases, ed 5. London: Churchill Livingstone; 2000.
11. Institute of Medicine, Committee on Research and Development Needs for Improving Civilian Medical Response to Chemical and Biological Terrorism Incidents. Pre-Incident Communication and Intelligence and Medical Communities. In: Chemical and Biological Terrorism. National Academy Press, 1999, pp 29-34.
12. Chong HT, Kamarulzaman A, Tan CT, et al. Treatment of acute Nipah encephalitis with ribavirin. *Ann Neurol.* 2001;49(6):810-3.

chapter 130

SARS-CoV Attack (Severe Acute Respiratory Syndrome)

Suzanne M. Shepherd, Stephen O. Cunnion, and William H. Shoff

 DESCRIPTION OF EVENT

The events unfolding between November 2002 and June 2003, which heralded the advent of severe acute respiratory syndrome (SARS), effectively demonstrated one significant downside of globalization and air travel: the ability to rapidly disseminate lethal respiratory infections worldwide. Although SARS was a natural biologic pandemic, it tested the global medical community's ability to recognize and rapidly respond to a potential covert biologic weapon attack. Dispersion of a previously unknown biologic agent produced illness after a relatively short incubation period, when victims had already dispersed to five continents. Effective medical response depended upon the ability of astute clinicians, not sophisticated electronic surveillance, to identify the case cluster announcing the presence of a new illness.

Although many details regarding SARS-CoV, its origin, spreading mechanisms, full extent of illness, and effective management remain to be elucidated, much has already been determined. SARS-CoV, a novel *Coronavirus* species, produces a rapidly progressive atypical pneumonia. Coronaviruses are a family of enveloped, single-stranded RNA viruses that produce disease in several animal species, including humans. Seroepidemiologic data suggest that SARS-CoV originated as an animal virus, with live game animal markets hypothesized to be the potential site of recent interspecies transmission.[1-3] Isolation of SARS-CoV from several species, including the palm civet (*Paguma larvata*), suggests a wide range of host hiding places for SARS between human epidemics. SARS-CoV is the cause of SARS, as it satisfied all four of Koch's postulates. Reverse transcriptase polymerase chain reaction (RT-PCR) and virus isolation demonstrated virus from lung biopsy specimens, feces, urine, and respiratory secretions in SARS patients, but not controls. Seroconversion to SARS-CoV was shown in ill patients. Experimental cynomolgus macaque infection with SARS-CoV produced pneumonia pathologically similar to SARS in humans.[4-9] No vector has been identified.

Several SARS-CoV characteristics make it an interesting bioweapon candidate. Its unique RNA-dependent RNA polymerase allows for ready mutation and potential adaptation. It shows moderate transmission, with two to four secondary cases, and *occasional "super-spreader" events, involving transmission to multiple individuals.* Within months, more than 8000 individuals were infected and 774 individuals died in 26 countries on five continents. SARS-CoV has an incubation period of 2 to 10 days (median 4-7 days; range 2-14 days). Although mild and asymptomatic cases have been documented, they are uncommon and do not appear to contribute to infection spread. SARS-CoV is stable, surviving for many days in feces and for 1 or more days on hard surfaces.

The primary mode of transmission is via direct or indirect mucous membrane contact with infectious respiratory droplets or fomites.[10] Fecal-oral transmission may be an important secondary means, as virus is found in large quantities in stool and profuse, watery diarrhea is not uncommon.[5,11,12] Transmission is not described before clinical illness onset, which corresponds with peak viral load at day 12 to 14 of symptoms. As such, early patient isolation may facilitate transmission prevention.[11] Transmission occurs with close patient contact, with passage to casual contacts being unusual. Transmission is facilitated by aerosol-generating procedures in medical settings. Seasonality is suspected but remains to be elucidated.

SARS affects individuals of all age groups and immune status, although children appeared less severely affected in the 2003 epidemic. Infected individuals initially experience fever, myalgias, and chills. Cough is common early, but tachypnea and shortness of breath are more prominent later in the illness. The elderly may not present with fever but may manifest decreased appetite and malaise.[13] Upper respiratory symptoms are uncommon, perhaps serving as one clinical clue differentiating a cluster of epidemiologically linked SARS patients from those with other atypical pneumonias. Pulmonary findings, such as rales, occurred in less than one third of SARS cases, and often did not correlate clinically with chest radiography (CXR) findings.[7,14] Twenty percent of patients had prominent gastrointestinal symptoms, including watery diarrhea. CXR findings appear to correlate with the rapidity at which patients require hospitalization. The most common initial findings on CXR are ground-glass opacifications or focal consolidations of the peripheral, subpleural lower lung fields. In 67% of patients with an initially normal CXR, findings appear on subsequent high-resolution chest tomography (HRCT). Pleural effusions, mediastinal lymphadenopathy, and cavitation are rare.[16] One third of SARs patients showed improvement, with defervescence and radiographic resolution over several weeks. In the remainder, fever persisted and progressive shortness of breath, hypoxia, tachypnea, increasing auscultative findings, and often diarrhea were noted. Serial radiography, or HDCT, revealed progression to multifocal unilateral or bilateral air-space consolidation, and often non-iatrogenic pneumomediastinum. Approximately 20% to 30% of patients require intensive care. Death is usually due to respiratory failure and/or multiple organ failure, sepsis, or accompanying cardiac decompensation. Later lung findings include diffuse alveolar damage, edema, hyaline membrane formation, pneumocyte desquamation, giant cells, a high viral load, and an inflammatory infiltrate.[6,14,17] Mortality risk factors, determined by multivariate regression analysis, include advanced age, co-morbid cardiovascular disease and diabetes, and high neutrophil and lactate dehydrogenase levels on presentation.[17,18] Between 6% and 20% of recovered patients have some residual respiratory impairment.[3]

Clinical manifestations are nonspecific. In one study, the WHO case definition was shown to be 96% specific but only 26% sensitive.[3] Laboratory data are nondiagnostic; however, lymphocytopenia is common and thrombocytopenia may be noted. Alanine aminotransferase, lactate dehydrogenase, and creatine kinase levels may be elevated. Although RT-PCR has been shown to be diagnostic in respiratory and fecal specimens, and viral RNA is detectable in serum and urine, the CDC and WHO do not deem RT-PCR currently reliable to rule out SARS infection.[19] Lower respiratory tract specimens are the most useful but place healthcare providers at the most risk of transmission via aerosol generation.[20] Seroconversion 21 to 28 days after symptom onset (whole-virus immunoassay via IFA or ELISA) remains the gold standard to confirm SARS infection.[21]

 ## PRE-INCIDENT ACTIONS

Pre-incident actions focus on preparedness, healthcare provider education, and surveillance. Active syndromic surveillance for fever and respiratory symptom clusters should occur. Research focuses on improving testing sensitivity earlier in illness and on finding effective antiviral and immunomodulating agents.[21]

Emergency department, hospital, and outpatient facilities should have disaster plans in place that address bioterrorist attack/major infectious disease outbreaks, and they should regularly conduct mock attacks. The importance of incorporating travel, immigration, and contacts into routine history-taking must be reinforced. Facilities should upgrade isolation and ventilation systems, using increased air flow in clustered negative pressure rooms. Strict staff universal precautions, frequent

and thorough hand-washing, and the use of properly fitting N95 respiratory masks must be stressed.[22] Measures should be delineated for changing triage guidelines to accommodate rapid increases in patient census; isolating patients; and safely holding large numbers of ill and infectious patients in the likely advent of hospital overloading. These plans, developed in coordination with those of local, state, and federal EMS, public health and government agencies should specify leadership and decision-making roles.[23] Policies regarding restricted public gatherings, contact quarantine, and prepared quarantine facilities, if individuals will not maintain home quarantine, should be in place.[24,25] The possibility of contracting SARS-CoV by particle inhalation from laboratory culture is significant, and negative pressure measures and BSL-3 procedures within laboratories should be used.[26]

 ## POST-INCIDENT ACTIONS

Healthcare providers entertaining a high level of suspicion for a possible SARS-CoV attack should notify hospital infection control, the administrator on duty, and the local public health officer. Appropriate local, state, and federal public health and law enforcement authorities should be involved. In the healthcare area, provision of adequate supplies and reinforcement of patient isolation, mask placement, and thorough hand-washing precautions should be enforced immediately and strictly. Healthcare provider use of N-95 mask, eye protection, gown, shoe covers, and gloves must be enforced; adequate equipment ensured; and clearly marked biohazardous waste receptacles placed to facilitate use and disposal. Rooms, materials, and surfaces possibly contaminated by SARS-CoV patients should be disinfected appropriately with hypochlorite solution. Aerosol-generating procedures, such as intubation and bronchoscopy, if necessary, should be performed by highly experienced staff under the most strict infection control precautions. Exclusion from duty should be considered for exposed unprotected healthcare workers, with temperature and symptom monitoring. Visitors should be excluded from contact with suspected SARS-CoV patients and their close contacts.[25]

 ## MEDICAL TREATMENT OF CASUALTIES

Treatment of SARS-CoV patients focuses on emergency management of life-threatening complications and ventilatory support. Interventions to manage profound hypoxemia should be instituted, including intubation, sedation, paralysis, lung recruitment maneuvers, and high-frequency, low–tidal volume and inflation pressure ventilator management.[28] To date, no efficacious antiviral or antiinflammatory drugs are identified.[3,27] Current research focuses on candidate antiviral agents and vaccine development. If patients are not sick enough to warrant admission, they should be sent home, with strict guidelines regarding activity restriction and hospital return if symptoms worsen.[12,25]

UNIQUE CONSIDERATIONS

SARS-CoV has several potential advantages over other respiratory biologic weapons because of its clinical similarity to other common atypical pneumonias, its relative stability, and its spread potential by large droplets, stool, and on fomites. Its unique RNA-dependent RNA polymerase allows for mutation and adaptation to adverse conditions. SARS-CoV release into a community could produce a large number of casualties in a relatively short period and allow widespread dispersion of infected individuals before symptoms manifest. Potential disadvantages of SARS-CoV use include the lack of transmission before clinical illness onset, suggesting that early patient isolation may facilitate transmission prevention and its apparent uncommon transmission to casual contacts. An aerosolized SARS-CoV attack would most likely occur in a large urban setting transportation hub, allowing significant spread over large population areas globally. Identification of SARS-CoV as the cause, without the obvious epidemiologic clue of an outbreak in another country, would be delayed because of its clinical similarity to other atypical pneumonias during respiratory virus season.

 PITFALLS

- Failure to prepare, and frequently test, a system's ability to respond to potential terrorist attacks in advance
- Failure to notify appropriate public health agencies when an outbreak of atypical lower respiratory illness is suspected
- Failure to ask an appropriate travel, immigration, and exposure history
- Failure to adequately isolate patients suspected of having SARS
- Failure of medical staff to use appropriate respiratory and contact precautions

 CASE PRESENTATION

A 25-year-old student presents with fever and malaise for 2 days and increasing cough today and has right-sided rales on pulmonary examination. The patient is requesting a chest radiograph and a prescription for azithromycin, which has "worked in the past." A travel history discovers that she just returned 8 days ago from visiting her cousin in Singapore. She states that her cousin is proud of his job, testing antiviral agents against SARS-CoV, and she toured the facility and was introduced to his co-workers.

REFERENCES

1. Enserlink M. Clues to the animal origins of SARS. *Science* 2003;300:1351-5.
2. Wenzel RP, Edmond MB. Listening to SARS: Lessons for infection control. *Ann Int Med.* 2003;139(7):592-3.
3. Peiris JSM, Yuen KY, Osterhaus ADME, et al. Current concepts: The severe acute respiratory syndrome. *N Engl J Med.* 2003; 349(25):2431-41.
4. Peiris JS, Lai ST, Poon LL, et al. Coronavirus as a possible cause of severe acute respiratory syndrome. *Lancet* 2003;361:1319-25.
5. Drosten C, Gunther S, Preiser W, et al. Identification of a novel coronavirus in patients with severe acute respiratory syndrome. *N Engl J Med.* 2003;348:1967-76.
6. Ksiazek TG, Erdman D, Goldsmith CS, et al. A novel coronavirus associated with severe acute respiratory syndrome. *N Engl J Med.* 2003;348:1953-66.
7. Poutanen SM, Low DE, Henry B, et al. Identification of severe acute respiratory syndrome in Canada. *N Engl J Med.* 2003;348:1995-2005.
8. Rota PA, Oberste MS, Monroe SS, et al. Characterization of a novel coronavirus associated with severe acute respiratory syndrome. *Science* 2003;300:1394-7.
9. Marra AM, Jones SJ, Astell CR, et al. The genome sequence of the SARS-associated coronavirus. Available at: http://www.cdc.gov/ncidod/sars/factsheetcc.htm.
10. Peiris JSM, Chu CM, Cheng VCC, et al. Clinical progression and viral load in a community outbreak of coronavirus-associated SARS pneumonia: a prospective study. *Lancet* 2003;361:1767-72.
11. Cheng PKC, Wong DA, Tong LKL, et al. Viral shedding patterns of coronavirus in patients with probable severe acute respiratory syndrome. *Lancet* 2004;363:1699-700.
12. Masur H, Emmanuel E, Lane HC, Severe acute respiratory syndrome: providing care in the face of uncertainty. *JAMA* 2003;289(21):2861-3.
13. Li G, Zhao Z, Chen L, et al. Mild severe acute respiratory syndrome. *EID* 2003;9(9):360-4.
14. Lee N, Hui D, Wu A, et al. A major outbreak of severe acute respiratory syndrome in Hong Kong. *N Engl J Med.* 2003;348:1986-94.
15. Hsueh PR, Cheng HH, Shiou Hwei Y, et al. Microbiologic characteristics, serologic responses, and clinical manifestations in severe acute respiratory syndrome, Taiwan. *EID* 2003;9(9):367-70.
16. Nicolaou S, Al Nakshabandi NA, Muller NL. Radiologic manifestations of severe acute respiratory syndrome. *N Engl J Med.* 2003; 348:2000-1.
17. Lew TWK, Kwek T-K, Tai D, et al. Acute respiratory distress syndrome in critically ill patients with severe acute respiratory syndrome. *JAMA* 2003;290:374-80.
18. Chan JW, Ng CK, Chan YH, et al. Short term outcome and risk factors for adverse clinical outcomes in adults with severe acute respiratory syndrome (SARS). *Thorax* 2003;58:686-9.
19. Centers for Disease Control and Prevention. Severe acute respiratory syndrome and coronavirus testing-United States, 2003. Available at: http://www.cdc.gov/mmwr/preview/mmwrhtml/mm5214a1.htm.
20. Cheng P, Tsang OT, Chau NT, et al. Coronavirus-positive nasopharyngeal aspirates as predictor for severe acute respiratory syndrome. *EID* 2003;9:1381-7.
21. Hui DSC, Sung JJY. Severe acute respiratory syndrome. *Chest* 2003;124(1):12-5.
22. Seto WH, Tsang D, Yung RW, et al. Effectiveness of precautions against droplets and contact in prevention of nosocomial transmission of severe acute respiratory syndrome (SARS). *Lancet* 2003;361:1519-20.
23. Inglesby TV, Grossman R, and O'Toole T. A plague on your city: observations from TOPOFF. *Clin Infect Dis.* 2001;32:436-45.
24. Mitka M. SARS thrusts quarantine into the limelight. *JAMA* 2003;290:1696-8.
25. Centers for Disease Control and Prevention. Interim guidance on infection control procedures for patients with suspected severe acute respiratory syndrome (SARS) and close contacts in households. Available at: http://www.cdc.gov/ncidod/sars/factsheetcc.htm.
26. Heymann DL, Aylward RB, Wolff C. Dangerous pathogens from the laboratory: From smallpox to today's SARS setbacks and tomorrows polio free world. *Lancet* 2004;363:1566-7.
27. Rubenfeld GD. Is SARS just ARDS. *JAMA* 2003;290(3):397-9.
28. Mazulli T, Farcas GA, Poutanen SM, et al. Severe acute respiratory syndrome-associated coronavirus in lung tissue. *EID* 2004;10:20-30.

chapter 131

Staphylococcal Enterotoxin B Attack

Robert G. Darling

 DESCRIPTION OF EVENT

Staphylococcus aureus produces a number of exotoxins including staphylococcal enterotoxin B (SEB). Such toxins are referred to as *exotoxins* because they are excreted from the organism that synthesizes them. Because they normally exert their pathologic effects on the gastrointestinal tract, they are also called *enterotoxins*. SEB causes a markedly different clinical syndrome when inhaled than it characteristically produces when ingested. Significant morbidity is produced in persons who are exposed to this toxin by either portal of entry to the body.

SEB is one of the most common causes of food poisoning. It is a pyrogenic toxin that commonly causes food poisoning in humans when improperly handled foodstuffs are contaminated with *S. aureus*, which in turn produces and releases SEB into the food that is subsequently ingested, causing illness. Often these outbreaks occur in a setting such as a picnic or other community event due to common source exposure in which contaminated food is consumed. Although an aerosolized SEB toxin weapon would not likely produce significant mortality, it could render a significant percentage of an exposed population clinically ill for 1 to 2 weeks.[1] The demand on the medical and logistical systems could be overwhelming. For these reasons, SEB was one of several biologic agents stockpiled by the United States during its biologic weapons program, which was terminated in 1969.[2]

Staphylococcal enterotoxins are proteins produced by coagulase-positive staphylococci. Up to 50% of clinical isolates of *S. aureus* produce exotoxins. They are produced in culture media and also in foods when there is overgrowth of the organism. SEB is one of at least seven antigenically distinct, moderately stable enterotoxins that have been identified. SEB causes symptoms in humans when inhaled at doses at least 100 times less than the lethal dose that would be sufficient to incapacitate 50% of those exposed.[1] This toxin could also be used to sabotage food or small-volume water supplies.

Staphylococcal enterotoxins belong to a class of potent immune stimulants known as bacterial superantigens.[3] Superantigens bind to monocytes at major histocompatibility complex type II receptors rather than the usual antigen-binding receptors. This leads to the direct stimulation of large populations of T-helper lymphocytes while bypassing the usual antigen processing and presentation pathway. This induces a brisk cascade of proinflammatory cytokines (such as tumor necrosis factor, interferon, interleukin-1, and interleukin-2), with recruitment of other immune effector cells and relatively deficient activation of counter-regulatory immune inhibitory mechanisms. This results in an intense inflammatory response that injures host tissues. Released cytokines are thought to mediate many of the toxic effects of SEB.[4]

Symptoms of SEB intoxication begin after a latent period of 3 to 12 hours after inhalation, or 4 to 10 hours after ingestion. Symptoms include nonspecific flu-like symptoms (e.g., fever, chills, headache, myalgias) and specific clinical features dependent on the route of exposure. Oral exposure results in predominantly gastrointestinal symptoms: nausea, vomiting, and diarrhea. Inhalation exposures produce predominantly respiratory symptoms: nonproductive cough, retrosternal chest pain, and dyspnea. Gastrointestinal symptoms may accompany respiratory exposure due to inadvertent swallowing of the toxin after normal mucociliary clearance of toxin-containing secretions from the respiratory tract.

Respiratory pathology is due to the activation of proinflammatory cytokine cascades in the lungs, leading to pulmonary capillary leak and pulmonary edema. Severe cases may result in acute pulmonary edema and respiratory failure.[5] Fever may last up to 5 days and range from 103° to 106°F, with variable degrees of chills and prostration. The cough may persist up to 4 weeks, and patients may not fully recover for 2 weeks.

Physical examination in patients with SEB intoxication is often unremarkable. Conjunctival injection may be present, and postural hypotension may develop due to fluid losses. Chest examination yields unremarkable results except in the unusual case in which pulmonary edema develops, when rales may be heard on auscultation. The chest x-ray also generally has normal results, but in severe cases increased interstitial markings, atelectasis, and possibly overt pulmonary edema or adult respiratory distress syndrome may occur.

 PREINCIDENT ACTIONS

It is essential that hospitals have a well-developed emergency response plan that is regularly exercised by hospital staff and is well integrated into community, state, and federal emergency response plans. There should be robust plans in place to expand patient care facilities to accommodate large numbers of sick patients who self-refer or who arrive by ambulance. At the present time, there is no vaccine available for human use to protect against aerosol exposure to SEB; however, studies in animals are promising, and human trials may begin soon.[6]

 ## POSTINCIDENT ACTIONS

Identifying aerosolized SEB as the cause of a mass-casualty event will be difficult unless the healthcare provider considers exposure to this toxin early in the course of the event. One must maintain a high index of suspicion. The differential diagnosis for patients presenting with a febrile respiratory illness is quite large and involves most respiratory pathogens including many bacteria and viruses. Diagnosis of SEB intoxication is based on clinical and epidemiologic features. The symptoms of SEB intoxication may be similar to several respiratory pathogens such as influenza, adenovirus, and mycoplasma. Persons experiencing any of these symptoms might present with fever, nonproductive cough, myalgias, and headache. The epidemiologic pattern of the illness outbreak is an important clue for determining the causative agent of, as well as the circumstances leading to, the epidemic (i.e., a naturally occurring or biologic attack). SEB attack would cause cases to present in large numbers over a very short period of time, probably within a single 24-hour period. Naturally occurring pneumonias or influenza would involve patients presenting over a more prolonged interval of time. Persons with naturally occurring staphylococcal food-poisoning would not exhibit pulmonary symptoms. Because it is not an infection, SEB intoxication tends to plateau rapidly to a fairly stable clinical state, whereas inhalational anthrax, tularemia pneumonia, or pneumonic plague would all continue to progress if left untreated. Tularemia and plague, as well as Q fever, would be associated with infiltrates on chest radiographs. Other diseases, including hantavirus pulmonary syndrome, *Chlamydia pneumonia* infection, and chemical warfare agent inhalation (e.g., mustard and phosgene) should also be considered.

Laboratory confirmation of SEB intoxication includes antigen detection enzyme-linked immunosorbent assay) and electrochemiluminescence on environmental and clinical samples and gene amplification techniques (polymerase chain reaction to detect staphylococcal genes) on environmental samples.[7] SEB may not be detectable in the serum by the time symptoms occur; regardless, a serum specimen should be drawn as early as possible after exposure. SEB accumulates in the urine and can be detected for several hours after exposure. Therefore, urine samples should also be obtained and tested for SEB. Respiratory secretions and nasal swabs may demonstrate the toxin early (within 24 hours of exposure). Because most patients will develop a significant antibody response to the toxin, acute and convales-

cent sera should be drawn for retrospective diagnosis. Nonspecific findings include a neutrophilic leukocytosis, an elevated erythrocyte sedimentation rate, and chest x-ray abnormalities consistent with pulmonary edema.

Once a mass-casualty situation is recognized as a possible bioterrorism event, the hospital's emergency plan should be activated. Simultaneously, public health and law enforcement officials should be notified. An epidemiologic investigation should begin immediately.

Standard precautions are sufficient because SEB intoxication is not contagious and secondary aerosol production is unlikely. Decontamination with soap and water is sufficient.

 ## MEDICAL TREATMENT OF CASUALTIES

Supportive care is the current mainstay of treatment. Attention to oxygenation and hydration is essential. Most patients' conditions will quickly stabilize after the acute phase of the illness; rarely, some patients may develop acute pulmonary edema requiring intubation and mechanical ventilation.

 ### CASE PRESENTATION

Thirteen patients suddenly present to your emergency department after attending a major football bowl game earlier in the day. There was national interest in the game, and the press covered the event heavily on both radio and television. The national terrorism threat level had not changed from "elevated" prior to the game, and there was no unusual terrorist "chatter" being reported by the Department of Homeland Security.

Most of the patients presenting for care are young college students. All attended the bowl game that afternoon. Several are in acute respiratory distress. All have fever and cough. You immediately suspect some sort of toxic exposure. As you begin administration of supplemental oxygen and monitoring of several of the sicker patients, you begin to consider the differential diagnosis. You attempt to gather additional history and learn that nothing out of the ordinary occurred during the game. One of the students tells you there was an "awesome" halftime show involving a flight demonstration by a number of small airplanes that flew over the stadium performing aerobatics. One plane appeared to be producing more smoke than the others, and for a moment some thought the plane might be experiencing an engine malfunction, but when it continued to fly normally, this idea was dismissed.

Suddenly the phone rings. You are told by your local emergency medical systems director that hundreds of patients are requesting ambulance transport to your facility.

 ## UNIQUE CONSIDERATIONS

SEB toxin is one of the most ubiquitous toxins in nature and, in its natural state, is one of the most common causes of food poisoning. However, respiratory disease caused by exposure to an SEB aerosol is never a natural event and will almost certainly be due to either a laboratory accident or bioterrorism.

The U.S. government weaponized SEB in the 1960s and investigated its use on the battlefield as an incapacitating agent.[2] The toxin was especially attractive because of the extremely small doses required to cause incapacitating illness in soldiers. The incapacitating dose, or effective dose to produce 50% casualties (ED_{50}), was found to be 0.0004 µg/kg; the lethal dose (LD_{50}) was estimated to be 0.02 µg/kg. Both measurements were taken in terms of the inhalational route.[2]

Ingestion of SEB toxin causes classic food poisoning: nausea, vomiting, and diarrhea without fever. Aerosol exposure produces a far different clinical picture consisting of fever, headache, severe respiratory distress, and sometimes nausea, vomiting, and diarrhea. The gastrointestinal symptoms seen after aerosol exposure are most likely due to the swallowing of toxin from respiratory tract secretions and are not likely to be as severe as those seen in primary gastrointestinal SEB exposure.

Prophylactic administration of an investigational vaccine protects laboratory animals against aerosol exposure and is nearing transition for study in humans.[6] However, it is not currently available for clinical use.

 PITFALLS

Several potential pitfalls in response to an SEB attack exist. These include the following:

- Failure to consider aerosolized SEB as the potential cause for large numbers of patients presenting with an acute febrile respiratory illness

- Failure to notify laboratory personnel of a suspected case of SEB intoxication and failure to collect appropriate clinical specimens to aid in the diagnosis, including nasal swabs and urine
- Failure to notify appropriate law enforcement and public health authorities in the event of a suspected biologic attack

REFERENCES

1. Hursh S, McNally R, Fanzone J Jr, Meshon M. *Staphylococcal Enterotoxin B Battlefield Challenge Modeling with Medical and Non-Medical Countermeasures*. Technical Report MBDRP-95-2. Joppa, Md: Science Applications International Corp; 1995.
2. Textbook of Military Medicine. Part I: Medical Aspects of Chemical and Biological Warfare. Available at: http://www.nbc-med.org/SiteContent/HomePage/WhatsNew/MedAspects/Ch-31electrv699.pdf.
3. Ulrich RG, Bavari S, Olson M. Bacterial superantigens in human diseases: structure, function and diversity. *Trends Microbiol.* 1995; 3:463-8.
4. Stiles BG, Bavari S, Krakauer T, et al. Toxicity of staphylococcal enterotoxins potentiated by lipopolysaccharide: major histocompatibility complex class II molecule dependency and cytokine release. *Infect Immun.* 1993;61:5333-8.
5. Mattix ME, Hunt RE, Wilhelmsen CL, et al. Aerosolized staphylococcal enterotoxin B–induced pulmonary lesions in rhesus monkeys (*Macaca mulatta*). *Toxicol Pathol.* 1995;23:262-8.
6. Coffman JD, Zhu J, Roach JM, et al. Production and purification of a recombinant staphylococcal enterotoxin B vaccine candidate expressed in *Escherichia coli. Protein Expr Purif.* 2002;24:302-12.
7. USAMRIID's *Medical Management of Biological Casualties Handbook*. 5th ed. August 2004. Fort Detrick, Md. Available at: http://www.usamriid.army.mil/education/bluebook.htm.

chapter 132

Clostridium botulinum Toxin (Botulism) Attack

Gary M. Vilke

 ## DESCRIPTION OF EVENT

Botulinum toxin has been used by terrorists as a bioweapon, although unsuccessfully, on several occasions. *Clostridium botulinum* was obtained from soil and cultivated, and the toxin was then collected. The attacks likely failed due to faulty microbiologic techniques, deficient aerosol-generating equipment, or internal sabotage.[1] As with many biologic agents, it is not likely that a terrorist attack using botulinum toxin will be reported or even noticed at the time it occurs.

There is a variable delay before the effects of botulinum toxin poisoning become clinically apparent, depending on the route of exposure, with as little as 2 hours before onset of symptoms and up to a week or more after ingestion. Patients will initially present with prominent bulbar palsies including blurred vision, mydriasis, diplopia, ptosis, and photophobia. Dysarthria, dysphonia, and dysphagia also tend to present early in the clinical course. Patients will be afebrile with a clear sensorium and, as symptoms progress, will develop progressive, symmetrical, descending skeletal muscle paralysis to the point of respiratory failure when muscles of respiration become involved.

 ## PREINCIDENT ACTIONS

Background knowledge of *C. botulinum*, the bacterium that produces botulinum toxin, is critical if diagnosis and treatment are to be rendered in a timely manner to prevent significant casualties from an exposure, either accidental or intentional. Botulinum toxins compose a family of neurotoxic proteins produced and secreted by the anaerobic bacteria *C. botulinum*. There are seven serotypes, A through G, that are produced by different strains of the bacteria, all acting by similar mechanisms and with slight variations in their effects. Although technical factors would make such dissemination difficult, a single gram of crystalline toxin effectively weaponized and aerosolized would kill more than 1 million people.[1] These toxins are the most poisonous substances known

with an oral dose lethal to 50% of an exposed population (LD_{50}) estimated to be 1 ng/kg.[2] This lethality is consistent in laboratory animals whether the toxin is given by the subcutaneous, intravenous, or intraperitoneal route. The inhalational route appears to have less toxicity, with the human LD_{50} for inhalation estimated at 3 ng/kg.[3]

Botulinum toxin's site of action is within the presynaptic nerve terminal of the neuromuscular junction and cholinergic autonomic synapses. Botulinum toxin is a simple dichain polypeptide that consists of a 100-kd "heavy" chain joined by a single disulfide bond to a 50-kd "light" chain. The toxin's light chain is a Zn^{++}-containing endopeptidase that cleaves one or more fusion proteins, which blocks acetylcholine-containing vesicles from fusing with the terminal membrane of motor neurons, thereby preventing the presynaptic release of acetylcholine.[4] This disrupts cholinergic neurotransmission, generating the clinical findings of bulbar palsies, skeletal muscle weakness, and paralysis. Inhibition of acetylcholine release also causes dry mucous membranes, as is seen in anticholinergic poisoning. Although nerve agent poisoning also causes muscular paralysis, the cholinergic finding of copious secretions typically differentiates it from botulism.

If an intentional exposure threat is identified by intelligence, botulinum toxin vaccines can be considered for use. The vaccine is developed by treating the toxin with formalin, destroying its toxicity, but maintaining its antigenic properties. The toxoid protects against serotypes A through E and is administered at 0, 2, and 12 weeks, followed by annual booster doses. Eighty percent of patients receiving the vaccine will develop protective titers at 14 weeks, but almost all will not have any measurable titer just before receiving the first booster dose.[5] The 1-year booster dose will result in a robust response in almost all patients. Clinical experience with the vaccine in many persons, mostly military personnel, reflects that it is safe and effective. A recombinant vaccine is also in developmental stages.[6]

It is also important to identify the local source of any botulinum antitoxin that can be required so that it can be located quickly if it is needed.

POSTINCIDENT ACTIONS

Postincident actions include early diagnosis and initiation of treatment. With the presentation of a single patient, the diagnosis can be challenging. The classic presentation is an acute, symmetric, descending flaccid paralysis with bulbar musculature involvement in an afebrile patient. Multiple cranial nerve palsies are always associated with symptomatic botulism exposures. However, the clinical presentation is often confused early with other neuromuscular disorders, such as myasthenia gravis, Guillain-Barré syndrome, or tick paralysis.[7] In the evaluation of such a patient, the edrophonium (Tensilon) test for myasthenia gravis may have transiently positive results for botulism. Electromyelography testing characteristically shows normal nerve conduction velocity and sensory nerve function, small amplitude motor potentials, and an incremental response (facilitation) to repetitive stimulation. The cerebral spinal fluid analysis in patients with botulism is normal. Laboratory testing is of little utility in the clinical diagnosis of botulism.

Diagnosis is confirmed with a mouse bioassay neutralization test, which demonstrates botulinum toxin in bodily fluids or blood. This test is available at the Centers for Disease Control and Prevention (CDC) and a number of state and municipal public health laboratories. Samples used for this assay can include serum, stool, gastric aspirate, vomitus, and suspected contaminated foods. Serotyping of the botulinum toxin is by neutralization of the bioassay with the appropriate botulinum antisera (serotypes A through G). Because a terrorist attack is a criminal event, it is important to treat all laboratory samples collected as evidence, maintaining an appropriate chain of custody between collection and delivery to the testing agency. Serum samples must be obtained before therapy with antitoxin because it nullifies the diagnostic mouse bioassay. The mouse bioassay can detect as little as 0.03 ng of botulinum toxin and usually yields results in 1 to 2 days.[8] Fecal and gastric specimens can also be anaerobically cultured, with results typically available in 7 to 10 days. Toxin production by culture isolates is then confirmed by the mouse bioassay.

If a respiratory route of exposure is suspected, then persons in the area where the patient was exposed should wear full-face respirators to protect themselves from residual aerosolized toxin. Environmental persistence of botulinum toxin is difficult to determine after an initial release. Conditions such as weaponization techniques, humidity, temperature, wind, and size of aerosol particles will determine the rate of atmospheric dissipation. The toxin does not penetrate intact skin, so special protective clothing is not necessary for caregivers. Botulism is not contagious and is not transmitted person to person.

Local and state health authorities must be notified quickly for several reasons. They assist in obtaining botulinum antitoxin to treat current patients and to arrange for assay tests to confirm the toxin. Additionally, health authorities assess the route of exposure and initiate tracking of other potential victims who may benefit from early intervention. If a terrorist attack is suspected, local, state, and federal law enforcement and emergency management agencies must be notified as early as possible. This will facilitate criminal investigations and initiate activation of federal response assets, such as the Strategic National Stockpile, if needed.

The toxin is heat sensitive; therefore decontamination of equipment can be accomplished by heating to 85°C for 10 minutes or using a 0.1% hypochlorite bleach solution.

 ## MEDICAL TREATMENT OF CASUALTIES

The two main treatment modalities available for managing botulism patients are supportive therapy and antitoxin treatments. Treatment of botulism is largely supportive, including ventilatory support if respiratory failure develops. Some patients may be mildly affected, whereas others may become completely paralyzed, appear comatose, and require months of ventilatory support. The rapidity of onset and the severity of paralysis depend on the amount of toxin absorbed into the circulation. Symptoms of foodborne botulism may begin as early as 2 hours or as long as 8 days after ingestion of toxin.[8] The time to onset of inhalational botulism in humans was approximately 72 hours after exposure in the three known cases reported of inhalational botulism from small amounts of reaerosolized toxin.[9]

Supportive therapy involves mechanical ventilation when appropriate, and often long-term enteral feeding is necessary. In patients who do not require mechanical ventilation but have some degree of respiratory insufficiency, reverse Trendelenburg's position of 20 to 25 degrees with cervical stabilization on a rigid mattress is reported to potentially improve ventilation and respiratory excursion by reducing entry of oral secretions into the airway and by suspending more of the weight of the abdominal viscera from the diaphragm.[1] Up to 20% of patients involved in foodborne outbreaks require mechanical ventilation, and more than 60% of children suffering infant botulism require ventilation.[10,11] Repeated bedside spirometry is used to assess diaphragmatic function. Indication for intubation is a vital capacity less than 12 to 15 mL/kg.

Antibiotics have no role in most cases of acute botulism; however, it is often recommended that patients suffering from wound botulism be treated with penicillin to eliminate the source of the toxin.[12] Patients with botulism are prone to secondary infections, particularly pneumonia. If antibiotics are required for secondary infections, aminoglycosides and clindamycin are contraindicated because they can exacerbate neuromuscular blockade.[13,14] Activated charcoal has no reported effect in foodborne botulism.

Unlike nerve agent exposures that involve excess acetylcholine at the neuromuscular junction due to inhibition of acetylcholinesterase, botulism is caused by a lack of acetylcholine in the synapse. Therefore, pharmacologic treatments such as atropine are relatively contraindicated and could worsen the symptoms.

Beyond supportive therapy, the mainstay of treatment rests with the early use of botulinum antitoxin. Early administration of passive neutralizing antibody is critical,

702 TOXINS

so that the agent might bind with circulating toxin before it becomes tissue bound. Antitoxin will minimize subsequent nerve damage and severity of disease but will not reverse existent paralysis.[15] Antitoxin should be administered to patients with neurologic signs of botulism as soon as possible and must not be delayed for laboratory confirmatory testing. In the United States, botulinum antitoxin is available from the CDC via state and local health departments. There are three forms of the vaccine available. The licensed trivalent equine antitoxin contains neutralizing antibodies against botulinum toxin types A, B, and E, which are the most common causes of naturally occurring human botulism. It is provided in a single 10-mL vial that provides 5500 to 8500 IU of each type of specific antitoxin, is diluted at a ratio of 1:10 in normal saline, and is given as a slow intravenous infusion. This product has all of the side effects of any equine serum product, including anaphylaxis and serum sickness. An investigational heptavalent (ABCDEFG) antitoxin held by the U.S. Army could be used to cover for additional serotypes.[16] Although it is said to be despeciated by cleaving the Fc fragments from the horse immunoglobulin G molecules, approximately 4% of equine antigens still remain. A monovalent human type A antitoxin is available for infant botulism from the State of California Department of Health Services.

Use of the equine antitoxin requires skin testing for horse serum sensitivity prior to use. This is performed by injecting 0.1 mL of a 1:10 sterile dilution of antitoxin intradermally and observing for 20 minutes. The skin test result is considered positive if there is any of the following: fever or chills; hypotension with a drop of 20 mm Hg in the systolic and diastolic blood pressures; hyperemic skin induration > 0.5 cm; nausea and vomiting; shortness of breath or wheezing; or skin rash or generalized itching. If any of these reactions occur, desensitization should be performed and allergy specialist consultation is advised. Even if the skin test result is negative, anaphylaxis may still occur unpredictably. If no allergic reactions occur, then the dose of 10 mL of antitoxin is given as a single intravenous dose in saline over 20 to 30 minutes. Pretreatment with intravenous diphenhydramine 50 mg and possibly an H2 blocker is recommended as well as having epinephrine immediately available in case an anaphylactic reaction does occur.

Recovery results from new motor axon twigs that sprout to reinnervate paralyzed muscle fibers—a process that, in adults, may take weeks or months to complete.[17]

 UNIQUE CONSIDERATIONS

Four routes of exposure to botulism exist. Intestinal and wound botulism result from the production of botulinum toxin in devitalized tissue in a wound or the intestine. Neither is usually considered to be from an act of bioterrorism. However, foodborne botulism can be either natural or intentional, and the aerosolized route is highly likely to be intentional. No cases of waterborne botulism have ever been reported.[18]

The rapidity with which patients present largely depends on the route of exposure and the dose absorbed. Symptoms may not appear for several days if the toxin is inhaled at lower concentrations, but they may appear earlier if inhaled at higher concentrations or if absorbed by ingestion. With ingestion, the course from onset of symptoms to respiratory failure has progressed in less than 24 hours.

There is no indication that treatment of children, pregnant women, and immunocompromised persons with botulism should differ from standard therapy.[1] Children and pregnant women have received equine antitoxin without apparent short-term adverse effects; however, the risks to fetuses of exposure to equine antitoxin are unknown.[19-22] A human-derived neutralizing antibody, Botulism Immune Globulin, decreases the risk of allergic reactions that are associated with equine botulinum antitoxin, but use of this investigational product is limited to suspected cases of infant botulism.[23]

 PITFALLS

Several potential pitfalls in response to a botulism attack exist. These include the following:

- Failure to consider the diagnosis of botulism in a patient presenting with descending paralysis
- Failure to notify local and state health authorities as soon as possible to access botulism antitoxin in an expedited fashion
- Failure to make the clinical diagnosis of botulism if multiple patients present with bulbar and cranial nerve palsies and a descending paralysis
- Exacerbation and prolongation of neuromuscular blockade with use of aminoglycosides and clindamycin in patients with botulism

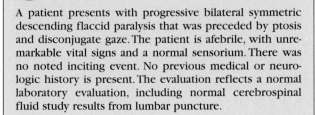

CASE PRESENTATION

A patient presents with progressive bilateral symmetric descending flaccid paralysis that was preceded by ptosis and disconjugate gaze. The patient is afebrile, with unremarkable vital signs and a normal sensorium. There was no noted inciting event. No previous medical or neurologic history is present. The evaluation reflects a normal laboratory evaluation, including normal cerebrospinal fluid study results from lumbar puncture.

REFERENCES

1. Arnon SS, Schechter R, Inglesby TV, et al. Working Group on Civilian Biodefense. Botulinum toxin as a biological weapon: medical and public health management. *JAMA* 2001;285:1059-70.
2. Gill DM. Bacterial toxins: a table of lethal amounts. *Microbiol Rev.* 1985;21:654-5.
3. McNally RE, Morrison MB, Berndt JE, et al. *Effectiveness of medical defense interventions against predicted battlefield levels of botulinum toxin A.* Vol 1. Joppa, Md: Science Applications International Corporation; 1994:3.
4. Montecucco C, ed. Clostridial neurotoxins: the molecular pathogenesis of tetanus and botulism. *Curr Top Microbiol Immunol.* 1995;195:1-278.

5. Middlebrook JL. Contributions of the U.S. Army to botulinum toxin research. In: Das Grupa B, ed. *Botulinum and Tetanus Neurotoxins and Biomedical Aspects.* New York: Plenum Press; 1993:515-9.

6. Byrne MP, Smith LA. Development of vaccines for prevention of botulism. *Biochimie* 2000;82:955-66.

7. Schantz EJ, Johnson EA. Properties and use of botulinum toxin and other microbial neurotoxins in medicine. *Microbiol Rev.* 1992;56:80-99.

8. Terranova W, Breman JG, Locey RP, et al. Botulism type B: epidemiological aspects of an extensive outbreak. *Am J Epidemiol.* 1978;108:150-6.

9. Holzer VE. Botulism from inhalation. *Med Klinik.* 1962;57:1735-8.

10. St Louis ME, Peck SH, Bowering D, et al. Botulism from chopped garlic: delayed recognition of a major outbreak. *Ann Intern Med.* 1988;108:363-8.

11. Schreiner MS, Field E, Ruddy R. Infant botulism: a review of 12 years' experience at the Children's Hospital of Philadelphia. *Pediatrics.* 1991;87:159-65.

12. Bleck TP. *Clostridium botulinum* (botulism). In: Mandell GL, Bennett JE, Dolin R, eds. *Mandell, Douglas and Bennett's Principles and Practice of Infectious Diseases.* 6th ed. Philadelphia: Churchill Livingstone; 2005:2822-8.

13. Santos JI, Swensen P, Glasgow LA. Potentiation of *Clostridium botulinum* toxin by aminoglycoside antibiotics: clinical and laboratory observations. *Pediatrics* 1981;68:50-4.

14. Schulze J, Toepfer M, Schroff KC, et al. Clindamycin and nicotinic neuromuscular transmission. *Lancet* 1999;354:1792-3.

15. Tacket CO, Shandera WX, Mann JM, et al. Equine antitoxin use and other factors that predict outcome in type A foodborne botulism. *Am J Med.* 1984;76:794-8.

16. Hibbs RG, Weber JT, Corwin A, et al. Experience with the use of an investigational F(ab')$_2$ heptavalent botulism immune globulin of equine origin during an outbreak of type E botulism in Egypt. *Clin Infect Dis.* 1996;23:337-40.

17. Duchen LW. Motor nerve growth induced by botulinum toxin as a regenerative phenomenon. *Proc R Soc Med.* 1972;65:196-7.

18. Centers for Disease Control and Prevention. *Botulism in the United States 1899-1996: Handbook for Epidemiologists, Clinicians, and Laboratory Workers.* Atlanta, Ga: Centers for Disease Control and Prevention; 1998.

19. Weber JT, Goodpasture HC, Alexander H, et al. Wound botulism in a patient with a tooth abscess: case report and literature review. *Clin Infect Dis.* 1993;16:635-9.

20. Keller MA, Miller VH, Berkowitz CD, et al. Wound botulism in pediatrics. *Am J Dis Child.* 1982;136:320-2.

21. Robin L, Herman D, Redett R. Botulism in a pregnant woman. *N Engl J Med.* 1996;335:823-4.

22. St Clair EH, DiLiberti JH, O'Brien ML. Observations of an infant born to a mother with botulism. *J Pediatr.* 1975;87:658.

23. Krishna S, Puri V. Infant botulism: case reports and review. *J Ky Med Assoc.* 2001;99:143-6.

chapter 133

Clostridium perfringens Toxin (Epsilon Toxin) Attack

Lynne Barkley Burnett

DESCRIPTION OF EVENT

Because of their relative ease of manufacture, capability to be deployed without a sophisticated delivery system, and capacity to kill or injure significant numbers of people, biologic weapons have been termed the "poor man's nuclear bomb."[1] As the former head of a secret bioweapons research program said, "A small container of pathogens could kill a million people. It's hard enough to secure fissile materials, which are large and easy to detect. How do you begin to control a substance that looks like nothing more than sugar?"[2]

Bioterrorists may use microorganisms that produce one or more toxins, biologically active proteins that are antigenic but do not grow or reproduce. In the case of a toxin bioweapon, it is the poison produced, rather than the microorganism that produced it, that is weaponized and is harmful.[3]

Epsilon toxin is one of numerous toxins produced by bacteria of the genus Clostridium that cause pathologic medical conditions including botulism, tetanus,[4] "gas gangrene," and food poisoning.[5,6] Clostridia are gram-positive, nonencapsulated, spore-forming, fermentative, catalase-negative bacilli.[7] Of approximately 90 species, fewer than 20 are known to be associated with clinical illness in humans.[6]

Clostridium perfringens, which may well be the most common bacterial pathogen,[6] has five strains designated types A through E,[5] elaborating more than 20 toxins.[8] In humans, type A is notorious for producing alpha-toxin and causing clostridial myositis and myonecrosis, also known as gas gangrene. During World War II, at the infamous Unit 731, the Japanese tested the intentional contamination of shrapnel or fléchettes with C. perfringens to increase the likelihood of wound infection[9]—something modern-day terrorists might find attractive if explosive devices were used.

Epsilon toxin, the most potent clostridial toxin after botulinum and tetanus neurotoxins,[4] is a permease enzyme made by C. perfringens types B and D.[5] These are commensal organisms whose primary host is sheep, although they are occasionally isolated from other herbivores such as goats and cattle[10] and, rarely, humans.[11] In a natural infection in herbivores, a large dose of epsilon toxin results in increased intestinal permeability, facilitating entry of C. perfringens from the gut into the blood with hematogenous spread to all organs.[12] As a biologic weapon, epsilon toxin could be manufactured via fermentation of C. perfringens or genetically combined with a producer microorganism that could express the cloned gene for the toxin.[13-15] Indeed, the gene producing epsilon toxin has been cloned[16] and genetically combined with Escherichia coli.[2] After freeze-drying, it was placed into a sealed glass cylinder, inserted into a toothpaste tube along with a few grams of cooling gel to ensure a stable temperature, and transported into the United States. This was done to provide proof to government officials of a top secret project carried out by South Africa to develop bioweapons, such as anthrax, plague, salmonella, botulinum, and epsilon toxin, that have been genetically altered to make them harder to detect and to treat.

The literature is bereft of reports of human illness caused by this toxin,[10] but a brief examination of its natural history readily demonstrates why epsilon toxin is designated a category B biologic agent by the U.S. Centers for Disease Control and Prevention (CDC).[17] Epsilon toxin is not taken up into cells and does not appear to have any intracellular activity.[12] Its putative mechanism of action is cell membrane pore formation, producing wide, nonselective diffusion channels permeable to hydrophilic solutes, including potassium, sodium, and other ions.[10,12] This disrupts the vascular endothelium, causing widespread osmotic alterations with extravasation of serum proteins and red blood cells and massive edema[18] involving the brain,[19] kidneys, lungs,[18] and liver.[20] Subserous and subendocardial hemorrhages are also often seen.[21] At a cellular level, formation of membrane pore complexes[22] causes ion loss from cells, with a rapid decrease in intracellular potassium, a rapid increase in intracellular chloride and sodium, and a slower increase in intracellular calcium.[12] The efflux of intracellular potassium causes plasma membrane blebbing, cell swelling, lysis,[10] and cell death.[12]

In animal studies, epsilon toxin administered intravenously accumulates preferentially in the brain, where pathologic changes are characterized by focal-to-diffuse[4] liquefactive necrosis and, secondary to damage of vascular endothelial intercellular junctions,[7] perivascular proteinaceous edema in the internal capsule, thalamus, cerebellar white matter[19] and meninges.[7] It appears likely that, at high doses, the neurotoxicity of epsilon toxin is due to stimulation of neurotransmitter release from glutamatergic and dopaminergic neurons.[4] It is thought that the toxin binds to presynaptic glutamatergic nerve fibers, inducing excessive release of glutamate, resulting in postsynaptic dendritic damage and pyramidal cell death. Epsilon toxin also accumulates in the kidney,[18] where necrosis of the renal cortex ("pulpy kidney disease") may occur.[7,21]

These pathologic effects in animals manifest clinically as cerebral edema,[19] pulmonary edema,[5] pericardial fluid collections,[10] and diarrhea, with severe abdominal cramping and abdominal distention.[13] Onset of neurologic signs[19]—including ataxia, trembling,[20] nervousness, opisthotonos, seizures, agonal struggling,[10] and hyperesthesia—may be observed within 2 to 60 minutes after intravenous injection in calves.[19] Surviving animals can have residual neurologic deficits resulting from focal symmetric encephalomalacia.[20] Epsilon-toxin toxicity results in hyperglycemia and glycosuria[21] due to altered hepatic metabolism of glycogen[20] and a stress response caused by cerebral edema that initiates catecholamine release and activation of adenylate cyclase.[21]

The anticipated primary routes for mass dissemination of epsilon toxin would be as an aerosol[10] or in foodstuffs or water. Epsilon toxin is taken up from the gut in naturally occurring disease in animals; thus, food contamination might be the most natural avenue for a terrorist attempt to cause human disease. In an aerosol toxin attack, the presumption is that the agent cloud retains its harmful potential for 8 hours.[3] To use epsilon toxin as an effective aerosolized biologic weapon, terrorists would need to manufacture a respirable aerosol of the purified toxin,[23] with particles ranging from 0.5 to 5 microns—the "ideal" droplet size for absorption into the circulatory system via the inhalational route. Particles within this size range remain airborne for a prolonged period of time and are optimal for being carried to the distal airways, where retention and absorption of a toxin biologic weapon is maximized. Similarly, aerosolized *infectious* biologic agents (e.g., anthrax spores) achieve their highest rates of infection in the distal airways.[3] However, unlike the spores of *Bacillus anthracis*, there is no evidence that spores of clostridia can be aerosolized to produce disease. Studies in sheep, goats, and mice[5] suggest the most likely effects on humans following inhalation could be damage to pulmonary vascular endothelial cells, resulting in high-permeability pulmonary edema, with hematogenous spread and damage to the kidneys, heart, and central nervous system.[10] Although such spread results in pulmonary edema, renal failure, shock, and multisystem organ failure,[5] the central nervous system is the primary target of epsilon toxin.[4]

Further speculation on the clinical presentation in humans might include central nervous system manifestations such as weakness, dizziness, ataxia, and neurologic dysfunction.[24] Pulmonary manifestations include respiratory irritation, cough, bronchospasm, dyspnea,[19] adult respiratory distress syndrome, and respiratory failure.[24] Cardiovascular abnormalities include tachycardia, hypotension, or hypertension.[11] Gastrointestinal distress including nausea, vomiting, and diarrhea may also be seen.[24]

Pancytopenia is a late complication resulting in bleeding, increased susceptibility to bruises, and immunosuppression. Initial laboratory studies might reveal anemia caused by intravascular hemolysis, thrombocytopenia, elevation of serum aminotransferase levels, and hypoxia.[25]

The estimated lethal dose via inhalation is 1 µg/kg.[10] Onset of illness is anticipated to be within 1 to 12 hours of exposure.[13,24] Death can occur within 30 to 60 minutes of symptom onset in affected animals[20]; thus, the abrupt onset of clinical illness could eventuate rapidly in death.[10]

Clinical acumen, tempered by an appreciation of the context of the presentation, facilitates appropriate reporting, definitive diagnosis, and response to a biologic weapon attack using epsilon toxin.[26] Diagnosis of an epsilon-toxin attack would have to be based on clinical and epidemiologic grounds, possible confirmation by growth of *C. perfringens* in culture (only true if the actual organism [*C. perfringens*] were used in the attack; if the attacker used epsilon toxin, there is nothing to culture because it is a poison, not a live infectious organism), or identification of toxin via polymerase chain reaction genotyping[5] or immunoassay.[23] Swabs of the nasal mucosa,[23] acute serum, and possibly tissue samples should be collected as soon as possible[27] in cooperation with the local or state health department or the CDC and sent to an appropriate reference facility[25,27] via the laboratory response network. They must be properly packaged to preserve their biologic structure and/or activity. Because these samples are also evidence of a crime, they must be transported in a manner that maintains an appropriate chain of custody.

 PREINCIDENT ACTIONS

Terrorist attacks are unpredictable, may vary in size, occur in multiple sites simultaneously or be conducted sequentially, and will likely overtax resources at every level of response: local, state, and national.[1] Thus, while there are no preincident steps to be taken insofar as epsilon toxin is specifically concerned, it is essential that emergency medical response (EMS) agencies, hospitals, and healthcare professionals proactively plan, organize, train, and obtain the supplies necessary for responding to terrorist incidents involving biologic agents.

 POSTINCIDENT ACTIONS

It may be unclear whether the initial cases of an infectious disease outbreak are the result of a natural occurrence or an act of hostility. Thus, all apparent infectious disease outbreaks should be approached as possible bioterrorist attacks until proven otherwise. Implications of such a posture for clinical practitioners include the immediate reporting of suspicious or clustered syndromes to local, state, or federal public health officials for investigation; immediate implementation of respiratory protection and/or body fluid precautions for all responders; and recognition that biologic samples and other materials (e.g., clothing), as well as laboratory results, have potential forensic, as well as clinical, relevance. Therefore, appropriate steps must be taken to preserve their evidentiary value.[26]

Toxins are easier to remove by decontamination than are live organisms.[3] Use of soap and water is the recommended approach.[13,23] There is no known *person-to-person* spread of epsilon toxin by air.[5] Direct contamination of consumables, such as water, food,[19,24] or medications,[3] is a possible route of dissemination and would be difficult to detect prior to the onset of illness because it is unlikely that appearance, taste, or smell would be significantly affected. Epsilon toxin is dermonecrotic[8] and can be transmitted via contaminated wound discharge[24]; thus, body fluid precautions should be observed.

 ## MEDICAL TREATMENT OF CASUALTIES

The biggest challenge faced by EMS, emergency department, and community medical practitioners after a terrorist attack may well be the psychological trauma that may affect most of the population.[1] Insofar as epsilon toxin is concerned, there are no vaccines, antitoxins,[5] antidotes,[24] or specific treatment[25] for humans, although *C. perfringens* epsilon toxoid has been prepared for use in animals.[28,29] Supportive medical care, including airway management[24] and fluid replacement, with particular attention paid to electrolyte status because of potassium loss, would be the mainstay of therapy.[13] Critical care in an intensive care unit setting, including mechanical ventilation and vasopressors, may be needed for the treatment of multisystem organ failure and shock.[5]

If weaponized and aerosolized *C. perfringens* were the biologic agent disseminated (as opposed to weaponized purified epsilon toxin), high-dose penicillin might be indicated, although a primary role for antibiotic therapy has not been established.[5] A study of guinea pigs with gas gangrene (caused by clostridial alpha toxin) showed that protein synthesis inhibitors were more effective inhibitors of cell wall–active toxins than were antimicrobial agents with a different mechanism of action,[6] with penicillin plus clindamycin considerably more efficacious than penicillin alone. There are also reports that rifampin stopped the lethal intoxication of the toxin microcystin in animal models when administered within 15 to 30 minutes of exposure to the agent.[14]

Adjunctive hyperbaric oxygen therapy for gas gangrene is based on blocking production of alpha toxin at a partial pressure of oxygen level of more than 250 mm Hg.[29] However, use of hyperbaric oxygen and its effect on the production of epsilon toxin have not been reported.

 ## UNIQUE CONSIDERATIONS

Children who have been infected with epsilon toxin are more likely to decompensate if not monitored carefully and treated appropriately and are at greater risk from many bioterrorism agents. For example, aerosolized agents create special risks for pediatric patients. Compared with adults, their larger minute ventilation volume may result in the inhalation of a larger relative dose of an aerosolized agent and a more rapid onset of illness. Furthermore, children may absorb more of a given substance before its clearance from the respiratory tract. In addition, the breathing zone of children is closer to the ground, where many heavier-than-air aerosols may settle. Children are also at greater risk from agents that cause vomiting and diarrhea because they dehydrate easily and possess less physiologic reserve than adults. Thus, agents that cause minor symptoms in adults may precipitate hypovolemic shock in an infant.[1]

 ## PITFALLS

Several potential pitfalls in response to an epsilon toxin attack exist. These include the following:

- Absence of familiarity with weapons of mass destruction on the part of medical personnel, public health officials, and disaster planners is a pitfall.[1] All healthcare providers are essential to community preparedness for a terrorist incident.[26]
- Failure to recognize a bioterror incident early in its presentation may compromise the removal or decontamination of the agent, the appropriate medical care of casualties, and the criminal investigation to apprehend those responsible.[26]
- Failure to consider *C. perfringens* epsilon toxin in the differential diagnosis of an outbreak of a gastrointestinal or neurologic syndrome can also lead to a less-than-optimal response.

REFERENCES

1. Redlener I, Markenson D. Disaster and terrorism preparedness: what pediatricians need to know. *Disease-A-Month*. 2004;50:6-40.
2. Warrick J, Mintz J. Lethal legacy: bioweapons for sale. *Washington Post*. April 20, 2003:A01. Available at: http://www.washingtonpost.com.
3. Biological Weapons. Chapter 4 in: *The Medical NBC Battlebook*. The U.S. Army Center for Health Promotion and Preventive Medicine. USACHPPM Tech Guide 244; 2000:4-1-40.
4. Miyamoto O, Minami J, Toyoshima T, et al. Neurotoxicity of *Clostridium perfringens* epsilon-toxin for the rat hippocampus via the glutamatergic system. *Infect Immunol*. 1998;66:2501-8.
5. Lucey DR. A guide to the diagnosis and management of 17 CDC category B bioterrorism agents ("Beware of Germs"). Washington Hospital Center. April 10, 2003. Available at: http://bepast.org/docs/posters/BEWARE%20OF%20GERMS%20Category%20B%20page%201%2023-04-03.pdf.
6. Lorber B. Gas gangrene and other *Clostridium*-associated diseases. In: Mandell GL, Bennett JE, Dolin R, eds. *Principles and Practice of Infectious Disease*. 5th ed. London: Churchill Livingstone, Inc.; 2000:2549-61.
7. Anaerobic infections. Veterinary Pathobiology 331 Lectures. College of Veterinary Medicine, University of Illinois at Urbana-

The speed of the patient's decompensation had impressed everyone. A 28-year-old man, whose personal papers identified him as a foreign national, had been found alone, having apparently collapsed on his kitchen floor. His landlady had called 9-1-1 when she heard a loud sound, as if something heavy hit the floor, and there was no answer to her ringing of his doorbell or her telephone calls.

Police arrived on the scene at approximately 7:31 AM. The landlady reported the patient and his roommate had been making noise all night, something unusual for them. Initially, she said, her impression was that they were "making something...or cleaning," given the repeated sounds of objects being moved, water running, etc. Then, as the sounds of movement subsided, she noticed a lot of coughing—she wasn't sure whether it was one or both of them—with the coughing increasing in frequency and intensity as daylight approached.

She further informed the police that the patient shares the apartment with a male roommate of approximately the same age. Both are from the same country, and both work at the convention center, a venue that will be packed with 50,000 people for tonight's collegiate basketball championship.

On entering the apartment the police officer found, in addition to the patient, several empty boxes and multiple plastic containers—some empty, some partially filled. The officer assessed the patient, found him to be alive, and summoned paramedics, who arrived at 7:38 AM. Because of fluid on the floor, possibly used in an attempt to clean up some kind of spill, emergency personnel had to be careful they didn't slip as they worked in the kitchen. A fan was blowing, and the mist created by the fan was making them wet. Although it was cool in the apartment, they opted to keep the fan on because it helped dissipate the odors of vomitus, urine, and feces emanating from the patient.

Examination revealed a male with snoring respirations, mild bilateral wheezing, and rales on auscultation of the lungs; sinus tachycardia at a rate of 126 per electrocardiogram; blood pressure 144/82; Glasgow Coma Scale score of 6 (E1V1M4); pupils that were equal and reactive bilaterally at 4 mm; and pale, cool, wet skin. Paramedics intubated the patient, confirmed correct tube position, and ventilated him with 100% oxygen. They also inserted a large-bore intravenous tube and administered glucose and naloxone, without effect. His wet, soiled clothes were removed and he was covered with a blanket before being taken to the ambulance.

The patient arrived at the emergency department at 8:05 AM, his clinical condition having markedly deteriorated since first assessed by paramedics 27 minutes earlier. The patient was in clinically obvious pulmonary edema, and he was hypotensive with muffled heart sounds. The patient was placed on a ventilator and a second intravenous tube was inserted. A bedside ultrasound revealed pericardial fluid.

While preparations were being made to perform a pericardiocentesis, the patient's cardiac rhythm changed to pulseless electrical activity. Resuscitation efforts lasting approximately 30 minutes, including pericardial decompression, were unsuccessful and the patient died. Lines and tubes were left in situ, the patient's body was moved to a holding room, and a call was placed to the medical examiner's office. Because of the patient's atypical presentation and rapid death, you agreed with the emergency department nurse who suggested that local public health officials be notified as well.

The medicolegal death investigator is the first to respond 3 hours after the patient's death. He indicates that he needs to interview you and also asks that you have the paramedics and police return to the hospital, so that all the interviews can take place in one location. You respond that you will have a nurse call the paramedics' dispatch center, as well as the police. However, at that very moment, you happen to see both paramedics walking through the emergency department doors. The difference in their appearance from that observed earlier, when bringing the patient to the emergency department, is striking. Both paramedics appear ill, have obvious wet coughs, and one paramedic seems to have an unsteady gate you had not previously noticed. On seeing you, the other paramedic says, "Doc, something's got to be going on here!"

Champaign. Available at: http://www.cvm.uiuc.edu/courses/vp331/AnaerobesandAnaerobiosis/.

8. Songer G. Clostridia causing enteric disease. Lecture notes: Pathogenic bacteriology. Veterinary Science and Microbiology, The University of Arizona. Available at: http://microvet.arizona.edu:16080/courses/mic420/classnotes.html.

9. Mangold T, Goldberg J. *Plague Wars: The Terrifying Reality of Biological Warfare.* New York: St. Martin's Griffin; 1999:14-28.

10. Greenfield RA, Brown BR, Hutchins JB, et al. Microbiological, biological, and chemical weapons of warfare and terrorism. *Am J Med Sci.* 2002;323:326-40.

11. Structural studies on epsilon toxin from *Clostridium perfringens.* Research in the School of Crystallography. Birkbeck College, The University of London. Available at: http://people.cryst.bbk.ac.uk/~bcole04/epsilontoxin.html.

12. Petit L, Maier E, Gibert M, et al. *Clostridium perfringens* epsilon toxin induces a rapid change of cell membrane permeability to ions and forms channels in artificial lipid bilayers. *J Biol Chem.* 2001;276:15736-40.

13. *Clostridium perfringens* epsilon toxins: essential data. CBWInfo.com. Available at: http://www.cbwinfo.com/Biological/Toxins/Cper.html.

14. Franz DR. Defense against toxin weapons. In Sidell FR, Takafuji ET, Franz DR, eds. *Medical Aspects of Chemical and Biological Warfare.* Washington, DC: Office of the Surgeon General at TMM Publications, Department of the Army, United States of America; 1997:608, 616.

15. Takafuji ET, Johnson-Winegar A, Zajtchuk R. Medical challenges in chemical and biological defense for the 21st century. In Sidell FR, Takafuji ET, Franz DR, eds. *Medical Aspects of Chemical and Biological Warfare.* Washington, DC: Office of the Surgeon General at TMM Publications, Department of the Army, United States of America; 1997:682.

16. Minami J, Katayama S, Matsushita C, et al. Lambda-toxin of *Clostridium perfringens* activates the precursor of epsilon-toxin by releasing its N- and C-terminal peptides. *Microbiol Immunol.* 1997;41:527-35.

17. Agrawal AM, O'Grady NP. Biological agents and syndromes. In: Farmer JC, Jiminez EJ, Talmor DS, et al, eds. *Fundamentals of Disaster Management.* Des Plaines, Ill: Society of Critical Care Medicine; 2003:72.

18. Structural studies on the epsilon toxin from *Clostridium perfringens.* Birkbeck College, The University of London. Available at: http://people.cryst.bbk.ac.uk/~toxin/cproj/eps.html.

19. Epsilon toxin of *Clostridium perfringens*. Ames, Ia: Center for Food Security and Public Health, Iowa State University College of Veterinary Medicine; 2003. Available at: http://www.scav.org/Epsilon-toxin%20Fact%20Sheet.htm.

20. Williamson L. *Clostridium perfringens* type D: young ruminant diarrhea. LAMS 5350 Large animal digestive system. Available at: http://goatconnection.com/articles/publish/article_38.shtml.

21. Kit for the detection of *Clostridium perfringens* epsilon toxin in biological fluids or culture supernatants. Available at: http://64.233.161.104/search?q=cache:6Nd61xZ_t4MJ:www.biox.com/Epsilon.htm+kit+for+the+detection+of+clostridium+perfringens+epsilon+toxin+in+biological+fluids+or+culture+supernatants&hl=en.

22. The channel-forming ε-toxin family. Transport Classification Database. University of California San Diego. Available at: http://tcdb.ucsd.edu/tcdb/tcfamilybrowse.php?tcname=1.C.5.

23. Franz DR. *Defense Against Toxin Weapons*. Fort Detrick, Md: US Army Medical Research Institute of Infectious Diseases; 1997.

24. *Clostridium perfringens* toxins. Bioterrorism Treatment Guidelines. Illinois Department of Public Health. Available at: http://www.idph.state.il.us/Bioterrorism/pdf/bioterrorismcards.pdf.

25. *Clostridium perfringens* toxins. *NATO Handbook on the Medical Aspects of NBC Defense*. Virtual Naval Hospital: FM8-9. Available at: http://www.vnh.org/MedAspNBCDef/2appb.htm.

26. Bogucki S, Weir S. Pulmonary manifestations of intentionally released chemical and biological agents. *Clin Chest Med*. 2002;23:777-94.

27. *Clostridium perfringens*. USAF pamphlet on the medical defense against biological weapons. Available at: http://www.gulflink.osd.mil/declassdocs/af/19970211/970207_aadcn_015.html.

28. Titball R, Mainil J, Duchesnes C, et al, eds. Protein toxins of the genus *Clostridium* and vaccination. In: Genus *Clostridium*. Concerted Action QLK2-CT2001-01267. Liege, Belgium: Presse de las faculte de Medecine Veterinaire de l'Universite de Liege; 2003. Available at: http://www.genusclostridium.net/scbooklet2.pdf.

29. Van Unnik AJM. Inhibition of toxin production in *Clostridium perfringens* in vitro by hyperbaric oxygen. *Antonie Leeuwenhoek Microbiol*. 1965;31:18;181-6.

chapter 134

Marine Toxin Attack

Wende R. Reenstra

 DESCRIPTION OF EVENT

Marine toxins are poisons of biologic origin that may be used as chemical weapons. These toxins are produced by a variety of organisms ranging from small microbes to fish and snails. These toxins are not infectious. Exposure to the toxins either by invenomation, ingestion, or inhalation may lead to a death through paralysis of cardiac or respiratory muscles.

Several marine toxins discussed here are further classified as neurotoxins. These toxins can interfere with the transmission of the nerve impulse by blocking specific ion channels. The neurotoxins vary in mechanism of action. The concentration of the exposure to the toxin is not indicative of its effects. Several toxins can cause seizures or paralysis in nanomolar concentrations, others may cause gastrointestinal upset or blindness in much larger concentrations.

Three of the marine toxins classified as neurotoxins are saxitoxin, conotoxin, and tetrodotoxin. The fourth toxin—palytoxin—exerts its effects on all cell membranes and is not classified as a neurotoxin.

 PREINCIDENT ACTIONS

As in other toxin attacks a robust public healthcare system is of most benefit in the preincident phase. Hospitals should have disaster plans that would be adaptable to a toxin attack and the subsequent surge of patients demonstrating the characteristic symptoms of the marine toxins. Adequate resuscitation equipment, including mechanical ventilators, should be part of the preparation of such an attack.

 POSTINCIDENT ACTIONS

Emergency medical providers should recognize a rise in the number of patients exhibiting the characteristic parasthesias and progressive paralysis seen in marine toxin exposure. Once a trend is recognized, notification should be made to local and regional public health departments and adequate supplies to handle large numbers of symptomatic patients should be gathered. Rising numbers of symptomatic patients should be an indicator of a potential terrorist attack using a marine toxin agent, especially in areas where such toxins are not commonly seen (e.g., inland regions). Once an attack is suspected, notification of law enforcement on the local and federal level should follow.

 MEDICAL TREATMENTS OF CASUALTIES

Saxitoxin

Saxitoxin is one of the family of neurotoxins that cause paralytic shell fish poisoning (PSP). This toxin is soluble in water and stabile at high temperatures.[1] The toxin is made by small organisms called dinoflagellates, which contaminate shellfish (clams, scallops, oysters). The toxin is also produced by blue green algae. The algae may grow rapidly, producing blooms called "red tides." Human ingestion of filter-feeding crabs and lobsters or shellfish results in an intoxication.[1-4]

Saxitoxin binds to voltage-gated sodium channels on nerve fibers and muscle cells. The binding of the toxin blocks conduction of the nerve impulse. General symptoms of saxitoxin poisoning are neurologic and respiratory paralysis.[1-3]

Clinical Features

General: There is an initial latent period varying from 30 minutes to several hours following ingestion, before the onset of neurological symptoms.

Cardiovascular: There are no specific cardiovascular effects although in laboratory animals, saxitoxin caused hypotension and conduction defects.

Respiratory: Respiratory distress from muscular paralysis may occur up to 12 hours after intoxication. The respiratory paralysis may lead to death.[1,5]

Gastrointestinal: Gastrointestinal symptoms may appear hours to days after ingestion. These symptoms may include nausea, vomiting, abdominal pain, and diarrhea.[1,5]

Other: A tingling and burning sensation, initially occurring around the mouth and lips, is usually the first symptom. The numbness may be on the hands and spread over the chest and abdomen.[1,5] These symptoms may progress, with difficulty walking and arm and leg weakness.[1,5] Involuntary movements and tremors may occur.[1]

There are no specific antidotes for saxitoxin poisoning.[1] Treatment is symptomatic. If oral ingestion is suspected, emptying the stomach via emetic or gastric lavage is recommended. Intubation and mechanical ventilation with monitoring to support respiration may be necessary.[1] Routine laboratory studies are not helpful. Diagnosis is confirmed by detection of the toxin in food, water, or environmental samples.[5,6]

Saxitoxin is water soluble and therefore can be easily aerosolized. It is toxic by both inhalation and ingestion.[1]

Conotoxin

The venom of the cone snail is composed of small substances termed conotoxins. There are more than 2000 peptides identified[7] that lead to a complex set of symptoms. The toxins are heat stable but are inactivated by the disinfectants glutaraldehyde and formaldehyde.[7]

The conotoxins mechanism of action can be divided into pre- and post-synaptic pathways. The presynaptic conotoxin blocks the release of acetylcholine.[5,8] The postsynaptic conotoxin inhibits sodium, potassium, and calcium channels and blocks muscular contraction.[5] The toxicity of the venom is thought to result from the additive effects and not the concentration of the toxin.

Clinical Features

General: The onset of symptoms is almost immediate upon injection. Common symptoms include localized pain, swelling, numbness, and ischemia at the injection site.[5,7] The numbness, swelling, and tingling may spread rapidly from the injection site to involve the entire body.[5,7]

Cardiovascular: No specific cardiac effects are seen.

Respiratory: Progressive weakness, droopy eyelids, headache, abdominal pain, and difficulty breathing, may occur. Death results from respiratory paralysis.[5,7]

Gastrointestinal: Stomach cramps and nausea are common effects.

Other: The clinical course is characterized by rapid onset and deterioration for the first 6 to 8 hours.[7] This is followed by improvement, and complete recovery may take 4-6 weeks.[5,7]

Diagnosis is by clinical signs and symptoms, and there are no laboratory tests available. Treatment is to immobilize the limb or site of envenomation. Pressure dressings should be applied and pain medication and tetanus prevention provided.[7] Intubation and mechanical ventilation may be necessary to support breathing.[5,7]

Conotoxins are very small, stable toxins that theoretically may be weaponized and disseminated as aerosols. A search of the open scientific literature regarding their inhalation toxicity found no publications.[7] They are poisonous by injection.

Tetrodotoxin

Tetrodotoxin is one of the best characterized marine toxins because of its involvement in fatal food poisoning.

The toxin is named from the pufferfish family (Tetraodontidae), where it has been found to be concentrated in the liver and other organs.[9,10] The toxin can also be found in the Blue Ringed Octopus, Parrot fish, crabs, newts, and algae.[2,5,9-11]

The toxin is made by a bacterium that forms a symbiotic relationship with the animals.[5,12] Tetrodotoxin is a neurotoxin that interferes with transmission of the nerve impulse at the nerve-muscle junction.[5,12] The toxin is heat stable and can be soluablized in acetic solutions.[5,12] This toxin specifically blocks sodium channels on the nerve cell and inhibits transmission of the impulse.[2,5,12] The target molecular channels are thought to be very similar to saxitoxin.[9]

Clinical Features

General: The first symptom is increasing numbness and tingling in the face and around the mouth.[12] These may extend to the extremities or become generalized.[5,12]

Cardiovascular: Hypotension and cardiac arrhythmias may occur.[5,12]

Respiratory: There is increasing respiratory distress. The victim usually exhibits difficulty breathing and cyanosis. Paralysis increases and convulsions, mental impairment, and cardiac arrhythmia may occur.[5,12]

Gastrointestinal: Autonomic effects such as headache, diaphoresis, and chest pain may occur and gastrointestinal symptoms such as nausea, diarrhea, and/or vomiting may develop.[5,12]

Other: A coagulation disturbance, which is an occasional complication, may lead to bleeding into the skin and mucosa, formation of blood blisters, and peeling of the skin. The neurologic involvement may start as muscular twitching and proceed to complete skeletal muscle paralysis, interfering with speech and swallow.[10,12] The pupils, after initially constricting, may become fixed and dilated.[12] The victim may be completely paralyzed but conscious. Untreated, the death rate is 50-60% in some studies.[5,12] Death usually occurs within 4 to 6 hours, with a known range of about 20 minutes to 8 hours.[10,12] Management is supportive and standard management of poison ingestion should be employed if intoxication is by the oral route. These include gastric lavage or emetics, particularly after control of the airway has been obtained. Intubation and mechanical ventilation may be required in severe intoxication.[5,12]

After weakness has become apparent, the treatment is symptomatic (e.g., maintenance of respirations, monitoring of vital signs and electrolytes).[5,10,12] Because of the likelihood of consciousness being maintained with complete paralysis, periodic administration of a tranquillizer is recommended along with continuous reassurance.[10,12]

Relatively little is known about TTX as a possible toxin weapon. A company in Japan is known to produce the toxin.[12] It is not known to be made in large quantities that could be used in weapons, and little or nothing has been published about its inhalational toxicity.[12]

Palytoxin

Palytoxin is one of most potent marine toxins known. It was isolated first from corals located in the South

Pacific.[13,14] Originally it was thought that the toxin was made by the corals; now, however, it is known that the toxin is made by a dinoflagellate (a small single-celled organism) and the corals concentrate the toxin.[2,8,13] It is estimated that the lethal dose for a human is less than 5 μg.[3,10,13,14] Palytoxins are stable in seawater and alcohols.

Extensive pharmacological research has determined that palytoxin is not a neurotoxin.[13,15] It instead acts at the cellular membranes to make them porous to charged molecules such as sodium, potassium, and calcium.[13,15] Without the gradients of these ions, the cells are unable to function or maintain the cell shape.[14,15]

Clinical Features

General: Symptoms are rapid, with death occurring within minutes.[13]

Cardiovascular: Initial symptom may be chest pain from constriction of the cardiac blood vessels. This may lead to cardiac ischemia and death of cardiac tissue. This may be seen on the EKG as peaked T waves or ST segment elevation.[13] The next symptom may be the loss of consciousness as unstable blood pressure, particularly episodes of low blood pressure, reduce blood flow to the brain.[13]

Respiratory: There may be difficulty breathing, with symptoms of wheezing. This again may be due in part to constriction of blood vessels in the lungs.

Gastrointestinal: There are no specific gastrointestinal effects.

Other: Hemolysis (breakdown of blood cells) may occur as the cell membranes become permeable to various ions, the red blood cells swell and the membranes rupture. This results in decreased oxygen carrying capacity. Death is thought to result from decreased oxygenation.[13]

There are no known therapeutics for Palytoxin poisoning. Relatively is little is known about Palytoxin as a possible toxin weapon. It is not known to be made in large quantities that could be used in weapons and little or nothing has been published about its inhalational toxicity.[13]

In summary these toxins act on a variety of sites. Table 134-1 summarizes their specific effects.

TABLE 134-1   SPECIFIC EFFECTS OF MARINE TOXINS

TOXIN	ORIGIN	EFFECT
Conotoxin	Marine snail	Blocks voltage-sensitive calcium channels; blocks voltage-sensitive sodium channels; blocks ACh receptors
Palytoxin	Soft coral	Activates sodium channels, ATPase
Saxitoxin	Dinoflagellate	Blocks voltage-sensitive sodium channels
Tetrodotoxin	Puffer fish	Blocks sodium channels

ACh, acetylcholine; *ATPase,* adenosine triphosphatase.

 UNIQUE CONSIDERATION

Marine toxins should be considered when a number of patients present with the characteristic parasthesias and paralysis. It is highly unusual to have large numbers of such patients, particularly in non-coastal regions, and therefore a terrorist attack should be suspected when this is seen. Early intervention with supportive care, including mechanical ventilation if needed, can be lifesaving.

 PITFALLS

Several potential pitfalls in response to a marine toxin attack exist. These include the following:

- Failure to prepare adequate systems to respond to possible terrorist attacks before an attack occurs
- Failure to consider marine toxins as the cause for paralysis in patients
- Failure to consider a marine toxin attack in the setting of a large number of otherwise healthy people presenting over several hours with acute paralysis
- Failure to rapidly support the respiratory system with urgent intubation and mechanical ventilation
- Failure to notify appropriate public health and law enforcement agencies when marine toxin exposure is suspected or confirmed among persons with no aquatic environment exposure or seafood ingestion

 CASE PRESENTATION

As an emergency physician in a small hospital outside of Chicago, you begin to see several patients during the first hours of your shift complaining of numbness and tingling in their face and mouth. During the next 3 hours you have four more patients present with the same symptoms while your original patients begin showing signs of respiratory distress. After intubating the patients in respiratory distress, you begin to suspect there may be more than just a coincidence occurring. You pick up the phone to make a call to your local Department of Public Health, only to find out a hospital 20 miles away is also seeing a surge in patients with similar symptoms.

REFERENCES

1. Saxitoxin: essential date. Available at: http://www.cbwinfo.com/Biological/Toxins/Saxitoxin.html.
2. Yasumoto T, Murata M. Marine toxins. *Chem Rev.* 1993;93:1897-909.
3. Tu A, ed. *Handbook of Natural Toxins: Marine Toxins and Venoms.* Marcel Dekker, 1988.
4. Mines DM, Stahmer S, Shepherd S. Poisonings: Food, Fish, Shellfish. *Emerg Med Clin North Am* 1997;15:157-77.
5. Edmonds C. In: *Dangerous Marine Creatures: a Field Guide for Medical Treatment.* Best Publishing; 1995.
6. Edmonds C, Lowry C, Pennefather J, eds. Diving and Subaquatic Medicine, ed 3. Butterworth-Heinemann; 1997.

7. Conotoxins: essential data. Available at: http://www.cbwinfo. com/Biological/Toxins/Conotox.html.
8. Halstead BW. In: Poisonous and Venomous Marine Animals of the World, rev ed 2. Darwin Publications; 1988.
9. Kao C, Levinson SR, eds. *Tetrodotoxin, Saxitoxin and the Molecular Biology of the Sodium Channel.* New York: The New York Academy of Sciences; 1986.
10. Hall S, Strichartz G, eds. *Marine Toxins, ACS Symposium series.* Washington DC: American Chemical Society; 1990.
11. Underman AE, Leedom JM. Fish and shellfish poisoning. *Curr Clin Top Inf Dis.* 1993;13:203-25.
12. Tetrodoxin: essential data. Available at: http://www.cbwinfo.com/ Biological/Toxins/TTX.html.
13. Palytoxin: essential data. Available at: http://www.cbwinfo.com/ Biological/Toxins/Palytoxin.html.
14. Moore RE, Scheuer PJ. Palytoxin: a new marine toxin from a coelenterate. *Science* 1971;172(982):495.
15. Haberman E. Palytoxin acts through Na+,K+-ATPase. *Toxicon* 1989;27:1171-87.

FURTHER RECOMMENDED READING

1. Velez P, Sierralta J, Alcagaga C, et al. A functional assay for paralytic shellfish toxins that uses recombinant sodium channels. *Toxicon* 2001;39:929-35.
2. Benton BJ, Rivera VR, Hewetson JF, Chang FC. Reversal of saxitoxin-induced cardiorespiratory failure by a burro-raised alpha-STX antibody and oxygen therapy. *Toxicol Appl Pharmacol.* 1994; 124:39-51.
3. Bove A, ed. *Bove and Davis' Diving Medicine.* WB Saunders; 2004.

chapter 135

T-2 Toxin (Trichothecene Mycotoxins) Attack

Frederick Fung

 ## DESCRIPTION OF EVENT

The 1972 Biological and Toxin Weapons Convention is a major international treaty to control biologic and chemical warfare that prohibits state parties from developing, producing, and testing biologic and toxic weapons.[1,2] However, with the expansion of terrorism, the possibility of using mycotoxins as a chemical weapon exists. In reality, there are three likely attack scenarios using T-2 mycotoxin as an agent of terrorism:

1. Product tampering: substantial human and economic damages caused by product tampering, such as the cyanide contamination of Tylenol in 1984, could happen. Use of T-2 mycotoxin to contaminate premade consumer products may be the most plausible attack scenario.
2. A second scenario is the use of T-2 mycotoxin as part of state-sponsored bioterrorism against a discrete population, group, or region.
3. The third scenario is related to food industry contamination: food, especially in the dairy industry (e.g., milk transported by tanker truck) is vulnerable to biologic and chemical attack. An attack on the food industry could cause local outbreaks of disease within hours or days, as well as enormous economic damage.

Trichothecenes (Fig. 135-1) are a large group of sesquiterpenoid chemicals characterized by a tetracyclic 12,13-epoxy ring commonly known as the 12,13-epoxytrichothecene and are classified into four groups. Group A includes T-2 toxin and diacetoxyscirpenol. Group B includes 4-deoxynivalenol and nivalenol. Many *Fusarium* species produce group A and B trichothecenes. *Baccharis megapotamica* produces the group C trichothecene baccharin. Group D mycotoxins include roridins produced by *Myrothecium roridum*, verrucarin produced by *Myrothecium verrucaria,* and satratoxins produced by *Stachybotrys atra*.[3]

It is important to point out that the more common and potent trichothecenes are produced by *Fusarium* species. There are nearly 150 toxins produced by fusaria and related fungi. They infect wheat and other grains that are important as sources of human food.

They are highly resistant to heat. T-2 toxin has been the most extensively studied. All trichothecenes are mycotoxins, whereas some mycotoxins belong to other chemical groups and are not trichothecenes.

T-2 is rapidly absorbed from the gastrointestinal (GI) tract. Although there are no human data on absorption through inhalational or dermal exposure, in vitro and animal studies have shown that trichothecenes are poorly absorbed through intact skin.[4] Trichothecenes undergo deepoxidation and glucuronidation, resulting in less toxic metabolites. The elimination half-life is estimated at 1.6 ± 0.5 hours after intravenous injection of the toxin in a canine model.[5] Another model using swine and cattle showed a half-life of 13 and 17 minutes, respectively.[6] T-2 does not require metabolic activation to exert its toxicity. The presence of the reactive electrophilic 12,13-epoxide moiety accounts for a rapid onset of its toxicity. The mechanism of toxicity involves inhibition of protein and DNA synthesis.[7] They also produce general cytotoxicity by inhibiting the mitochondrial electron transport system.[8] The 12,13-epoxide of the trichothecenes is essential for the toxicologic activity. The deepoxidation of T-2 in mammalian systems results in loss of toxicity.[9]

The dose of trichothecene needed to cause symptoms in humans is unknown. There is great variability in the toxicity of these compounds in animal studies. The dose of trichothecenes that will be fatal to 50% of an exposed population ranges from 0.5 to 300 mg/kg, depending on the route of administration and animal model used.[10]

T-2 is a potent blistering agent. Purified trichothecenes have been investigated because of their potential use in chemical warfare. T-2 toxin was implicated in the "yellow rain" attacks in Southeast Asia. However, further investigations have been inconclusive.[11]

Acute pulmonary hemorrhage in infants was purportedly associated with residential exposure to *Stachybotrys chartarum* and other toxigenic fungi. A detailed analysis of this report was conducted by the Centers for Disease Control and Prevention, which found methodologic shortcomings and concluded that the association was not confirmed.[12]

FIGURE 135–1. Structure of T-2 and HT-2. Trichothecenes: T-2 (R1 = OAc) and its metabolite HT-2 (R1 = OH).

An early report indicates that direct contact with trichothecenes produced irritant contact dermatitis after skin exposure.[13] Mild to moderate abdominal pain has been reported to develop within 15 minutes to 1 hour after ingestion of foods contaminated with significant levels of trichothecenes. Throat irritation and diarrhea have also been frequently described after ingestion. GI tract symptoms usually resolve within 12 hours.[14,15]

After a presumed T-2 attack, four clinical stages have been suggested.[16] The first stage includes irritation and inflammation of the GI mucosa, leading to abdominal pain, vomiting, and diarrhea, which may last 3 to 9 days. The second stage occurs on days 10 to 14 after exposure and is a latent period; symptoms are not prominent, but progressive anemia, thrombocytopenia, and leukopenia with relative lymphocytosis develop. The third stage occurs over the ensuing 3 to 4 weeks. Clinically, patients may show petechial hemorrhages on their skin and mucous membranes, and a hemorrhagic diathesis from mucous surfaces occurs. Varying degrees of necrotic lesions may develop in the GI tract or larynx, and generalized lymphadenopathy may appear. Blood abnormalities become more severe, and the erythrocyte sedimentation rate is elevated. Infections and sepsis during this stage are usually fatal. The fourth is the convalescence stage, when there is a rebound in the white blood count, the necrotic lesions of the mucous membranes resolve, and the patient recovers completely. The current weight of scientific evidence does not support a causal relationship between purported inhalation exposure to fungi capable of producing trichothecenes in the indoor environment and specific health effects.[17]

High-performance liquid chromatography, gas chromatography, and liquid chromatography mass spectrometry[18,19] have been used for trichothecene analysis in human blood and urine. However, these methods have not been validated by or used in sound epidemiologic studies. Serologic testing for antibodies specific to toxigenic fungi does not provide accurate information on exposure to trichothecenes or mycotoxins because the immunoglobulin is directed toward fungal antigens, not mycotoxins. Concerns on cross-reactivity in laboratory assays exist between *S. chartarum* antigens and fungi that are commonly found in outdoor environments.[20] Abnormalities in lymphocyte subset analysis have been reported in some studies, but consistent and specific findings have not been identified. The most appropriate diagnostic test to evaluate hematologic and immune status associated with trichothecene exposure is a complete blood count (CBC) with white blood cell differential.

PREINCIDENT ACTIONS

Hospital, emergency department, and ambulatory care facilities should have general disaster plans in place in the event of mycotoxin attack. The plan should be well thought out, should include an "all-hazards" approach, should be robust enough to respond to large numbers of victims, and should be tested by periodic and realistic exercises involving all essential personnel. The early detection of illness outbreaks requires surveillance systems that are capable of finding and validating the diagnosis and providing a means of communication between clinicians and health departments.[21] This would require coordination of local, state, and federal public health and safety resources. In the event of a large number of patients seeking medical care in a short timeframe, emergency medical services, hospital, and ambulatory care facilities need to be mobilized in a coordinated and expeditious fashion. Isolation and decontamination procedures should be in place and triage and decontamination personnel trained well before an attack occurs. Since most physicians and healthcare providers, as well as first responders, may not be familiar with mycotoxin attack, close contact with local poison control center or local health department may be important to identify and treat the initial cases.

POSTINCIDENT ACTIONS

Medical providers should maintain a high level of suspicion for possible mycotoxin attack should there be a sudden increase in the number of patients with similar symptoms and histories. Appropriate local, state, and federal public health and law enforcement authorities will need to be notified. Materials (e.g., clothing), bodily fluids, and surfaces possibly contaminated by mycotoxins should be decontaminated with 10% bleach (sodium hypochlorite) solution. Proper environmental sampling may be necessary for mycotoxin identification and documentation. Further epidemiologic investigations in collaboration with state or local health authorities may be necessary. CBC and liver function tests are recommended. Analysis of blood or urine samples may provide information concerning the metabolites of the mycotoxin. All samples should be stored and shipped using strict chain of custody procedures to preserve their evidentiary value.

MEDICAL TREATMENT OF CASUALTIES

There are no specific antidotes for trichothecene or T-2 poisoning. Standard supportive care is indicated for symptomatic cases after removal from the exposure and decontamination. These measures should include management of the airways, breathing, and circulation.

Supplemental oxygen can be given, if indicated. Contaminated clothing should be removed before skin decontamination occurs. The skin can be effectively decontaminated within minutes after T-2 exposure through washing with an aqueous soap solution. Polyethylene glycol 300 (PEG 300) is also effective at removing large doses of T-2 toxin from the skin.[22] An animal model has shown dexamethasone may improve survival after low- and high-dose exposure to T-2 toxin.[23] T-2 toxin is tightly adsorbed onto activated charcoal and has been associated with improved survival when administered with oral or parenteral doses of T-2 toxin in a mouse model.[24] These findings suggest that activated charcoal may decrease toxin absorption from the GI tract and may possibly enhance elimination of toxin via enterohepatic circulation. Although human data are lacking, a single dose of activated charcoal is probably warranted after acute trichothecene ingestion.

Laboratory testing should include serial CBC and differential evaluations for thrombocytopenia, anemia, and effects on the various white blood cell lines. The development of significant immune suppression, including pancytopenia, warrants neutropenic precautions and antibiotic coverage for fevers. After ingestion, careful examination of the oral mucous membranes and GI tract is warranted to evaluate for the presence of petechial, necrotic, or ulcerative lesions. In cases of airway compromise due to blistering effects of inhaled T-2 mycotoxin, patients should be monitored in a critical care setting with aggressive airway management readily available.

 CASE PRESENTATION

A previously healthy man comes to the emergency department complaining of blisters on his hands and the exposed skin of his neck and face that began to appear after he went jogging through a park a day prior. He also complains of nausea, vomiting, diarrhea, and abdominal pain but denies fever or chills. He also reports weakness, severe dizziness, and shortness of breath. Blood tests reveal that his white blood cell count is normal, but his lymphocyte count appears to be on the low side. On examination, there is evidence of extreme redness to his eyes, nose, and throat. There are a few hemorrhagic petechia noted on his trunk, arms, face, and oral mucosa. A general blood chemistry panel shows normal liver and kidney function. Due to his severe vomiting and diarrhea, he is hospitalized and treated with intravenous fluids. The next day, the local news media reports that an additional 50 people had been hospitalized or treated in local emergency departments for similar symptoms.

 UNIQUE CONSIDERATIONS

Although skin blistering may be produced by dermal exposure to T-2, T-2 is most toxic when ingested. An attack using an aerosolized T-2 weapon is unlikely to produce sufficient inhalational dosages to cause significant morbidity or mortality.[25] The most probable sign that a T-2 toxin or related mycotoxins attack has occurred may be the presentation of a large number of previously healthy persons over a course of hours to days with non-specific and systemic symptoms.

 PITFALLS

Several potential pitfalls in response to a mycotoxin attack exist. These include the following:

- Failure to prepare adequate plans, to perform realistic training exercises, and to develop emergency response systems to respond to a possible terrorist attack before the incident occurs
- Failure to consider mycotoxin as the cause for non-specific, as well as systemic, symptoms in previously healthy patients
- Failure to consider mycotoxin attack in the setting of a large number of otherwise healthy people presenting over hours to days with a similar range of general as well as specific complaints
- Failure to notify appropriate public health, safety, and law enforcement authorities when a possible biochemical agent attack is suspected, especially when animals are affected along with people
- Failure to provide basic supportive medical care when a patient is suspected to have undergone exposure to a biochemical warfare agent

REFERENCES

1. Zilinskas RA. Verifying compliance to the biological and toxin weapons convention. *Crit Rev Microbiol.* 1998;24:195-218.
2. Zilinskas RA. Terrorism and biological weapons: inevitable alliance? *Perspect Biol Med.* 1990;34:44-72.
3. Fung F, Clark RF. Health effects of mycotoxins: a toxicological overview. *J Tox Clin Tox.* 2004;42:1-18.
4. Kemppainen BW, Riley RT. Penetration of [H]T-2 toxin through excised human and guinea pig skin during exposure to [H]T-2 toxin adsorbed to corn dust. *Food Chem Toxicol.* 1984;22:893-6.
5. Barel S, Yagen B, Bialer M. Pharmacokinetics of the trichothecenes mycotoxin verrucarol in dogs. *J Pharm Sci.* 1990;79:548-51.
6. Beasley VR, Swanson SP, Corley RA, et al. Pharmacokinetics of the trichothecene mycotoxin, T-2 toxin, in swine and cattle. *Toxicon* 1986;24:13-23.
7. Ueno Y. Mode of action of trichothecenes. *Ann Nutr Aliment.* 1977;31(4-6):885-900.
8. Khachatourians GG. Metabolic effects of trichothecene T2 toxin. *Can J Physiol Pharmacol.* 1989;68:1004-8.
9. Yoshizawa T, Sakamoto T, Kuwamura K. Structure of deepoxytrichothecene metabolites from 3-hydroxy HT-1 toxin and T-2 tetraol in rats. *Appl Environ Microbiol* 1985;50:67-9.
10. World Health Organization. *WHO Environmental Health Criteria 105. Selected Mycotoxins: Ochratoxins, Trichothecenes, Ergot.* Geneva: World Health Organization; 1990.
11. Marshall E. Yellow rain: filling in the gaps. *Science* 1982;217:31-4.
12. Update: Pulmonary hemorrhage/hemosiderosis among infants—Cleveland, Ohio, 1993-1996. *Morb Mort Wkly Rep.* 2000;49:180-4.
13. Drobotko VG. Stachybotryotoxicosis: a new disease of horses and humans. *Am Rev Soviet Med.* 1945;2:238-42.
14. Wang ZG, Feng JN, Tong Z. Human toxicosis caused by moldy rice contaminated with Fusarium and T-2 toxin. *Biomed Environ Sci.* 1993;6:65-70.
15. Bhat RV, Beedu SR, Ramakrishna Y, et al. Outbreak of trichothecene mycotoxicosis associated with consumption of mould-damaged

wheat production in Kashmir Valley, India. *Lancet* 1989; 1(8628):35-7.

16. Stahl CJ, Green CC, Farnum JB. The incident at Tuol Chrey: pathologic and toxicologic examinations of a casualty after chemical attack. *J Forensic Sci.* 1985;30:317-37.

17. Hardin BD, Kelman BJ, Saxon A. Adverse human health effects associated with molds in the indoor environment. ACOEM evidence-based statement. *J Occup Environ Med.* 2003;45:470-8.

18. Gilbert J. Recent advances in analytical methods for mycotoxins. *Food Additive Contam.* 1993;10(1):37-48.

19. Yagen B, Sintov A. New sensitive thin-layer chromatographic-high-performance liquid chromatographic method for detection of trichothecene mycotoxins. *J Chromatogr.* 1986;356:195-201.

20. Halsey J. Performance of a Stachybotrys chartarum serology panel. Abstract of presentation at the Western Society of Allergy, Asthma and Immunology Annual Meeting. *Allerg Asthma Proc.* 2000;21:174-5.

21. Buehler JW, Hopkins RS, Overhage JM, et al. Framework for evaluating public health surveillance systems for early detection of outbreaks. *MMWR* 2004;53(RR05):1-11.

22. Fairhurst S, Maxwell SA, Scawin JW, et al. Skin effects of trichothecenes and their amelioration by decontamination. *Toxicology.* 1987;46:307-19.

23. Fricke RF, Jorge J. Beneficial effect of dexamethasone in decreasing the lethality of acute T-2 toxicosis. *Gen Pharmacol.* 1991; 22:1087-91.

24. Fricke RF, Jorge J. Assessment of efficacy of activated charcoal for treatment of acute T-2 toxin poisoning. *J Toxicol Clin Toxicol.* 1990;28:421-31.

25. Ciegler A. *Mycotoxins: A New Class of Chemical Weapons.* Department of Defense, Washington DC: NBC Defense and Technology International; 1986:52-7.

chapter 136

Ricin Toxin from *Ricinus communis* (Castor Beans) Attack

Angela C. Anderson

 ## DESCRIPTION OF EVENT

Ricin is a potent biologic toxin derived from the castor bean plant *Ricinus communis*. After pressing for castor bean oil, 1% to 5% of the bean's dry weight is comprised of ricin.[1,2] It is three to five times more toxic than the nerve agent VX. Although ricin is thought to be 1000-fold less toxic than botulinum toxin, it remains an important consideration as a potential terrorist weapon because it is stable in ambient conditions, readily available, and easily produced in mass quantities.[2] Ricin is technically difficult to disseminate in concentrations high enough to be an effective weapon of mass destruction. However, its potential use in smaller-scale terrorist attacks cannot be ignored. Ricin is classified by the Centers for Disease Control and Prevention (CDC) as a category B agent (i.e., an agent that is moderately easy to disseminate and causes moderate morbidity and low mortality).

R. communis is indigenous to Africa but can be found worldwide and can be purchased via the Internet. It grows wild in the southwestern United States and other parts of the world. The plant is cultivated commercially for the production of castor oil, which is used as an industrial lubricant, as a medical purgative and laxative, and as an additive in paints, shampoos, and cosmetics. Major producers include India, China, and Brazil. Castor oil contains no ricin because of the extraction process.

Extraction of ricin toxin from the oil is a relatively simple procedure that involves using hexane or carbon tetrachloride and the process of chromatography. During the extraction, the ricin-rich *resin* portion of the plant is separated from the non–ricin-containing *oil* portion. Any ricin remaining in commercially produced oil is heat inactivated. The ricin-rich resin that remains is known as castor meal or "waste mash" and contains 5% to 10% (dry weight) ricin. The maximum amount of ricin that can be extracted from a single bean is approximately 10 mg.[3] Active ricin toxin can be produced in the form of a liquid, a crystal, or a dry powder.

Ricin exerts its effects by inhibiting protein synthesis. It belongs to a group of poisons known as A-B toxins. These toxins have a moiety (the B chain) that binds to cell surfaces and another moiety (the A chain) that enters the cell and promotes catalytic activities that result in cell death. Bacterial toxins in this group include Shiga's toxin, diphtheria toxin, pseudomonas exotoxin A, and cholera toxin. Similar plant toxins are abrin, modeccin, and viscumin (from mistletoe).[4,5] The ricin B chain binds to cell-surface glycoproteins and glycolipids that have a terminal galactose residue.[4,6] Reticuloendothelial cells are particularly susceptible because they bear surface receptors to which ricin can bind. Once bound, ricin uses the cell's intracellular transport pathways to travel to ribosomes in the cytosol.[4,7] The ricin A chain then removes a specific adenine residue from ribosomal ribonucleic acid (rRNA): the 28s rRNA subunit.[6,8] Inactivation of the 28s ribosomal subunit blocks protein synthesis, which leads to cell death. Damage to endothelial cells results in extravascular fluid and protein leakage and tissue edema, which is known as *vascular leak syndrome*.

Clinical ricin poisoning requires ingestion, inhalation, or injection of a sufficient amount of the toxin. A summary of human clinical presentations is listed in Table 136-1. Contamination of food or water supplies or commercial products would be likely methods by which *oral* ricin poisoning would occur. Ingestion is the least toxic route because gastrointestinal absorption of ricin is poor and it is partially deactivated by passage through the stomach. Ricin toxin is complexed within the matrix of the castor bean, and intact beans pass through the gastrointestinal tract with little or no toxic effect. To cause significant toxicity by the oral route, the beans must be chewed or crushed to facilitate ricin release.

Lethal oral doses vary greatly between animal species. The dose of ricin that will be fatal to 50% of an exposed population (LD_{50}) in laboratory mice is 20 mg/kg with a time to death of 85 hours after intragastric administration.[2] The National Institute for Occupational Safety and Health Registry of Toxic Effects of Chemical Substances lists 2 mg/kg as the lowest published oral lethal dose in humans.[9]

Symptoms of mild ricin poisoning by ingestion include nausea, vomiting, abdominal pain/cramping, and diarrhea (often bloody), typically within 10 hours of ingestion. Moderate to severe toxicity causes significant fluid loss due to vomiting, diarrhea, hemorrhage, and third spacing of fluids into the tissues of the gastrointestinal tract with

TABLE 136-1 SUMMARY OF HUMAN CLINICAL PRESENTATIONS

EXPOSURE ROUTE	SYMPTOMS
Mild ingestions	Nausea, vomiting, abdominal pain and cramping
Moderate to severe ingestions	Extravascular fluid extravasation with resultant tachycardia, hypotension and mental status change, renal and hepatic failure
Inhalational exposure	Allergic symptoms including conjunctival irritation, rhinitis and bronchospasm. Cough dyspnea, chest tightness, and arthralgias
Intravenous exposure	Flu-like symptoms and extravascular fluid extravasation leading to pulmonary edema, hypotension, and renal insufficiency
Intramuscular/Subcutaneous injections	Local necrosis, weakness, myalgias, nausea, hepatorenal failure, cardiorespiratory failure

resultant tachycardia, hypotension, oliguria, and possibly mental status change. Renal failure and hepatic failure have also been reported.

Fatality rates from ricin ingestion are low, ranging from 2% to 6%. Ingestion of fatal doses of ricin results in rapid onset of symptoms (less than a few hours). In these cases, death usually occurs within 36 to 72 hours of exposure. Autopsy findings include multifocal mucosal ulcerations and hemorrhages of the stomach and small intestine, mesenteric lymph node necrosis, hepatic necrosis, splenic inflammation, and nephritis.[10]

The ability to deliver ricin via the *inhalational* route is limited by two variables: (1) the estimated amount of ricin required to kill 50% of the people in a 100 km^2 area is significant: 8 metric tons[11]; and (2) to cause significant ricin inhalation, one must succeed at the technically difficult task of aerosolizing the toxin into particles less than 5 μm.[10] With these facts in mind, the toxic dose of ricin by inhalation is significantly less than that required for ingestion: 3 mcg/kg (in mice).[2]

The only human data regarding ricin inhalation come from reports of workers occupationally exposed to castor bean *dust*, which can be a potent allergen. Susceptible patients present with conjunctival irritation, rhinitis, urticaria, and possible bronchospasm.[3]

Human studies regarding inhalation of *aerosolized* ricin are sparse. In the 1940s, unintentional sublethal exposures led to fever, chest tightness, cough, dyspnea, diaphoresis, and arthralgias.[10] Symptoms appeared within 4 to 8 hours of exposure and did not progress to severe illness or death. Mice exposed to the aerosol LD$_{50}$ of ricin (14 mcg/kg) developed an alveolar influx of inflammatory cells (predominantly neutrophils), pulmonary edema, type 2 pneumocyte hyperplasia, and peribronchovascular fibroplasias.[12] Bronchoalveolar lavage (BAL) revealed pulmonary inflammation with an increase in BAL protein.[12] Rats exposed to lethal ricin concentrations developed necrotizing interstitial and alveolar inflammation and edema, as well as fibropurulent pneumonia.[2,13] These changes were delayed 8 or more hours after exposure.[2,12] Immunohistochemical evaluation revealed that ricin binds to bronchiolar cilia, alveolar macrophages, and alveolar lining cells.[2,12] Death occurred 36 to 48 hours after exposure. It is likely that dose, duration of exposure, and particle size will affect clinical presentation and symptom progression.

Much of the information regarding *intravenous* ricin exposures is derived from persons with cancer who are treated with ricin as a means of targeting and killing tumor cells. Research evaluating the use of ricin as a chemotherapeutic agent evolved from the concept of replacing the binding moiety of ricin (the B chain) with a moiety that could recognize and bind cancer cell surface proteins (such as an antibody directed against cancer antigens). Administration of intravenous ricin immunotoxin in cancer patients at low doses (18 to 20 mcg/kg) has caused a flu-like illness (i.e., nausea, vomiting, fatigue, and muscular pain).[14] Intravenous ricin immunotoxin at a dose of 30 mg/kg/day for 7 days caused fatal vascular leak syndrome.[14,15] In fact, the dose-limiting adverse effect in ricin antitumor immunotherapy appears to be the development of the vascular leak syndrome.[16,17] This syndrome is characterized by hypoalbuminemia, pulmonary edema, renal insufficiency, cardiac failure, and hypotension.[17]

Intramuscular and *subcutaneous* injections of ricin can cause local necrosis, weakness, myalgias, nausea, dizziness, hepatorenal failure, cardiorespiratory failure, and death. The lowest published lethal dose from subcutaneous injection in a human is 43 mcg/kg.[9]

Dermal ricin exposures are unlikely to cause significant toxicity if the skin is intact. It is unknown whether the addition of a solvent will increase dermal absorption. *Ocular* exposure of ricin in rabbits has caused severe inflammation and pseudomembranous conjunctivitis.[18]

 PREINCIDENT ACTIONS

Currently there is no approved immunization or prophylactic agent against ricin. Most studies involve mice exposed to aerosolized ricin after immunization by various routes. Poli and colleagues[19] found that treating mice with *aerosolized* specific anti-ricin immunoglobulin (Ig) G 1 hour prior to aerosolized ricin exposure improved survival and greatly reduced the lung pathology. Yan and others[20] demonstrated that *intranasally* administered microsphere-encapsulated ricin toxoid protected mice against lethal doses of aerosolized ricin. *Oral* administration of microencapsulated ricin toxoid induced IgG and IgA antibodies within 7 weeks and provided complete protection against death from aerosolized ricin exposure.[21] Smallshaw and colleagues[22] experimented with a recombinant *intramuscular* vaccine; they induced a single mutation of the ricin A chain at the site thought to cause vascular leak syndrome. These vaccines protected mice against 10 times the LD$_{50}$ of ricin without the toxicity associated with the vascular leak syndrome. *Parenteral* administration of ricin toxoid improves survival but is only partially protective against lung damage caused by aerosolized ricin.[19]

The U.S. Department of Defense has submitted an investigational new drug application to the Food and Drug Administration (FDA) for the purpose of conducting ricin vaccine trials in humans. The administration of vaccine may prove to be protective; however, with the exception of the aerosolized vaccine by Poli and colleagues,[19] most animal studies thus far have found that vaccination must take place weeks before ricin exposure to be effective.

 POSTINCIDENT ACTIONS

The regional poison control center (1-888-222-1222), local health and law enforcement agencies, and federal authorities should be notified if ricin use is suspected. Ambulances, environmental surfaces, and equipment should be cleaned with 0.1% sodium hypochlorite solution (i.e., household bleach) or soap and water. Contaminated articles should be disposed of in a sealed plastic bag placed inside another sealed plastic bag.

 MEDICAL TREATMENT OF CASUALTIES

Currently, there is no antidote for ricin poisoning. Additionally, there are few evidence-based data to direct the management of ricin-exposed casualties. Mouse studies evaluating the use of a monoclonal antibody to neutralize ricin toxicity are promising but have yet to obtain FDA approval.[23] Consequently, management options must be extrapolated from animal studies and previous experience with similar toxins.

The course of medical management is partially determined by the route of ricin exposure. All healthcare providers, regardless of the exposure route encountered by the patient, should use standard universal precautions including a disposable gown, disposable nitrile gloves, and respiratory and eye protection.

Ricin Ingestion

Gastric decontamination will likely be unsuccessful and unnecessary if intact, unchewed beans have been ingested. A single dose (adults, 50 g; children, 1 g/kg) of activated charcoal should be administered if the airway is protected. Fluid losses and cardiovascular instability should be treated with fluid resuscitation and vasopressors. Electrolytes, liver and renal function, hematocrit count, and white blood cell count should be monitored. Gastrointestinal blood losses should be treated with follow-up stool guaiacs, hemoglobin and hematocrit measurements, and blood transfusions as necessary. Ricin is a large (66-kDa) globular protein that is not dialyzable, therefore there is no role for hemodialysis in ricin poisoning except in the setting of renal failure.

Exposure to Aerosolized Ricin

Contaminated clothing and jewelry should be removed; this can potentially reduce additional patient contamination by as much as 90%[10] and may prevent contamination of the emergency department, its staff, and other patients. Pulmonary effects, such as airway edema and necrosis and noncardiogenic pulmonary edema, should be treated supportively and aggressively. Continuous positive airway pressure or endotracheal intubation and ventilation may be necessary to manage pulmonary edema. Fluid and electrolyte abnormalities should be treated with intravenous fluid resuscitation and repletion of electrolytes. Allergic reactions should be treated with beta-2 adrenergic agonists, steroids, and antihistamines.

Parenteral Exposure

Routine burn and wound care can be used to treat local necrosis. Analgesia should be provided as necessary, as should replacement of fluids and electrolytes. Healthcare providers should watch for signs of systemic toxicity such as hepatic and renal failure. Cardiopulmonary collapse can be treated with vasopressors and ventilatory support.

Dermal/Ocular Exposure

If ricin has been dispersed in a powder form, skin decontamination at the scene is preferable. Contaminated clothing and jewelry should be removed, and skin should be washed with soap and water. It is unlikely that ricin will be absorbed to any significant extent through *intact* skin; however, it is prudent to decontaminate patients to prevent secondary contamination of healthcare providers and equipment. The eyes of patients with ocular exposures should be irrigated with tepid water for at least 15 minutes.

 CASE PRESENTATION

Over the course of a few days, 10 patients present to local emergency departments complaining of nausea, vomiting, and bloody diarrhea. Within hours of presentation, patients experience severe fluid losses with associated tachycardia and hypotension requiring significant fluid resuscitation. Two days after presentation, many patients develop evidence of hepatic and renal failure. Routine stool and blood cultures all have negative results. All but two patients recover completely with supportive therapy. Further investigation revealed that all 10 patients had been at a small company picnic where they had ingested the same beverage. The beverage was sent to a laboratory response network, which found evidence of the ricin by fluorescence immunoassay. The presence of ricin was confirmed by the CDC. The amount of ricin ingested by each person, based on personal accounts of the patients before death, was approximately 2 mg/kg or greater.

UNIQUE CONSIDERATIONS

Ricin is stable at ambient temperatures. It can be detoxified by exposing it to temperatures of 176°F (80°C) for 10 minutes or 122°F (50°C) for 1 hour.[24]

In 1999, the CDC established the Laboratory Response Network (LRN) to test for substances that could potentially be used in a terrorist event. Each of the 50 states has a state department of health laboratory called the *public health laboratory*. There are also other national, military, hospital-based, and state-based laboratories within this network. Suspicious samples of potentially toxic agents should be sent to an LRN reference laboratory. These laboratories currently can test for ricin by either of two methods: (1) time-resolved fluorescence immunoassay in which antibodies that bind to ricin are used; and (2) polymerase chain reaction, which searches for DNA of the gene that produces ricin protein. If a sample is found to contain ricin by a LRN reference laboratory, the sample is then sent to the CDC for additional testing, archiving, or storage. (Information on shipping procedures can be found at http://www.bt. cdc.gov/labissues/index.asp.) At present, testing can only document or confirm exposure. Testing results are not immediately available; therefore, its use as a diagnostic tool to aid in clinical decision-making is limited.

Ricinine is an alkaloid derived from the leaves and seeds of the castor bean plant. Recently, Darby and colleagues[25] developed a method using matrix-assisted laser desorption/ionization time-of-flight mass spectrometry and electrospray liquid chromatography/mass spectrometry to screen for and identify ricinine in samples. Thus far, tests for ricinine are not available for clinical use.

Ricin is very immunogenic. Circulating antibodies develop 2 weeks after exposure. Therefore, patients surviving at least 2 weeks after exposure can be tested for a humoral immune response.

Further information can be obtained from the following sources: the CDC Public Response hotline (1-888-246-2675); and the CDC Emergency Preparedness and Response Web site (http://www.bt.cdc.gov); the Agency for Toxic Substances and Disease Registry (1-888-422-8738); and the CDC's "Chemical Agents: Facts About Personal Cleaning and Disposal of Contaminated Clothing" (http://www.bt.cdc.gov/planning/personalcleaning facts.asp).

 PITFALLS

Several potential pitfalls in response to a ricin attack exist. These include the following:

- Exposure may mimic gastroenteritis or the flu.
- Ingestion can cause symptoms easily confused with iron, arsenic, or colchicine poisoning.
- Clinical presentation can mimic ingestion of bacterial pathogens such as salmonella and shigella.

- Inhalational ricin exposure may mimic infectious agents including community-acquired pneumonia, influenza, anthrax, Q fever, and pneumonic plague.
- Ricin inhalation may mimic inhalation of other toxins such as products of combustion from burning Teflon and Kevlar, nitrogen oxides, and phosgene.
- Patients may be exposed to more than one toxin, making the constellation of clinical symptoms confusing.

REFERENCES

1. Savino D. *CDI Factsheet: Ricin*. Washington DC: Center for Defense Information; 2003.
2. Franz D, Jaax N. Ricin toxin. In Zajtchuk R. ed. *Medical Aspects of Chemical and Biological Warfare*. Falls Church, Va: Office of the Surgeon General, Department of the Army; 1997:631-42. Available at: http://www.bordeninstitute.army.mil/cwbw/default_index.htm.
3. Bradberry S, Dickers KJ, Rice P, et al. Ricin poisoning. *Toxicol Rev*. 2003;22:65-70.
4. Sandvig K, Grimmer S, Lauvrak SU, et al. Pathways followed by ricin and Shiga toxin into cells. *Histochem Cell Biol*. 2002;117:131-41.
5. Doan L. Ricin: mechanism of toxicity, clinical manifestations, and vaccine development. A review. *J Toxicol Clin Toxicol*. 2004;42:201-8.
6. Olsnes S, Kozlov J. Ricin. *Toxicon* 2001;39:1723-8.
7. Poli MA, Rivera VA, et al. Aerosolized specific antibody protects mice from lung injury associated with aerosolized ricin exposure. *Toxicon* 1996 Sep;34(9):1037-44.
8. Kende M, Yan C, et al. Oral immunization of mice with ricin toxoid vaccine encapsulated in polymeric microspheres against aerosol challenge. *Vaccine* 2002 Feb 22;20(11-12):1681-91.
9. *Ricin TRECS#:VJ2625000*. Washington DC: National Institute for Occupational Safety and Health: Registry of Toxic Effects of Chemical Substances; 2002.
10. Daniels K, Schier J. Recognition, management and surveillance of ricin-associated illnesses. Public Health Practice Program Office, Webcast WC 0-0-4-8. Atlanta, Ga: Centers for Disease Control and Prevention; December 30, 2003. Available at: http://www.phppo.cdc.gov/phtn/webcast/ricin/RicinScript.rev.07-14-04.htm.
11. Shea D, Gottron F. *Ricin: Technical Background and Potential Role in Terrorism*. Washington DC: Congressional Research Service. Library of Congress; 2004.
12. DaSilva L, Cote D, Roy C, et al. Pulmonary gene expression profiling inhaled ricin. *Toxicon* 2003;41:813-22.
13. Darby SM, Miller ML, et al. Forensic determination of ricin and the alkaloid matter is ricinine from castor bean extracts. *J Forensic Sci*. 2001 Sep;46(5):1033-42.
14. Fodstad O, Kvalheim G, Godal A, et al. Phase I study of the plant protein ricin. *Cancer Res*. 1984;44:862-5.
15. Fidias P, Grossbard M, Lynch TJ Jr. A phase II study of the immunotoxin N901-blocked ricin in small-cell lung cancer. *Clin Lung Cancer*. 2002;3:219-22.
16. Baluna R, Coleman E, Jones C, et al. The effect of a monoclonal antibody coupled to ricin A chain-derived peptides on endothelial cells in vitro: insights into toxin-mediated vascular damage. *Exp Cell Res*. 2000;258:417-24.
17. Baluna R, Sausville EA, Stone MJ, et al. Decreases in levels of serum fibronectin predict the severity of vascular leak syndrome in patients treated with ricin A chain-containing immunotoxins. *Clin Cancer Res*. 1996;2:1705-11.
18. Grant E, ed. *Toxicology of the Eye*. 3rd ed. Springfield, Ill: Charles C. Thomas; 1986.

chapter 137

Aflatoxin Attack (*Aspergillus* Species)

Frederick Fung

 ## DESCRIPTION OF EVENT

Aflatoxins are metabolites produced by certain strains of the fungi *Aspergillus flavus* and *Aspergillus parasiticus*. They were discovered during a disease epidemic in Great Britain that wiped out more than 100,000 turkeys in 1960. The source of the illness was traced to aflatoxin-contaminated turkey feed made of moldy Brazilian peanuts. Eventually it was discovered that all crops and foodstuffs, including corn, rice, wheat, barley, and nuts, can contain naturally occurring mycotoxins.[1]

There are several aflatoxins and their metabolites (such as AFB_1, AFG_1, AFM_1) that are capable of producing human disease.[2] Aflatoxins are named by their fluorescence under ultraviolet light as blue (AFB) or green (AFG) as well as other analytic characteristics. Aflatoxins M (AFM), where M denotes milk or mammalian metabolites, are secreted in the milk of animals exposed to aflatoxins. There are two broad categories of aflatoxins according to their structures: aflatoxins B_1 and M_1 are within the difurocoumarocyclopentenone series (Fig. 137-1), and aflatoxin G_1 is of the difurocoumarolactone series (Fig. 137-2).

Exposure to aflatoxins is typically via ingestion of contaminated foodstuff. Dermal exposure results in slow and insignificant absorption.[3] Inhalational exposure in humans has not been studied. In vitro metabolism studies have shown the following metabolic reactions for AFB_1: reduction produces aflatoxicol (AFL); hydroxylation produces AFM_1; hydration produces AFB_{2a}; and epoxidation produces AFB_1-2,3-epoxide. The epoxide is the most reactive metabolite and is thought to be responsible for both the acute and chronic toxicity of AFB.[4] In an Indian report, ingestion of an estimated 2 to 6 mg/kg/day of aflatoxin over 1 month produced hepatitis, with some fatalities.[5] However, a suicide attempt by acute ingestion of 1.5 mg/kg of pure aflatoxin resulted only in nausea, headache, and rash.[6]

The liver is the primary target of toxicity and may lead to hepatic failure. Early symptoms of hepatic injury from acute poisoning include abdominal pain, anorexia, malaise, and low-grade fever.[7] Icterus and jaundice develop within several days, followed by abdominal distention, vomiting, ascites, and edema.[8] Mortality rates from acute aflatoxicosis range from 10% to 76%.[7] The chronic effects of aflatoxins are primarily carcinogenesis resulting in hepatocellular carcinoma. Laboratory tests of liver function confirm the extent of hepatic injury in acute aflatoxicosis. Elevated aspartate and alanine aminotransferase levels frequently exceed 5000 IU/liter. Bilirubin levels are also increased. Acute jaundice and death have been recently reported in an outbreak of aflatoxin poisoning in Kenya.[9] In cases of liver failure, elevation of the prothrombin time, metabolic acidosis, and hypoglycemia are the characteristic signs.[10] Pathologically, there is extensive centrilobular necrosis in the perivenular zone (zone 3) extending to periportal zones (zone 1) with giant cell infiltration and cholestasis.[11]

The 1972 Biological and Toxin Weapons Convention is a major international treaty seeking to control biologic warfare. It prohibits state parties from developing, producing, stockpiling, and testing biologic and toxic weapons.[12,13] However, with the expansion of terrorism, the use of mycotoxins as weapons is a real threat. Possible attack scenarios include the following:

1. Product tampering: Substantial human and economic damage could result from consumer product tampering such as the cyanide poisoning of Tylenol in 1984.[13] Tampering by spiking premade consumer products with mycotoxins may be the most plausible attack scenario.
2. Chemical weaponry: A second scenario is large-scale terrorism using aflatoxins as chemical weapons against a population group or region, such as the Anfal Operations against the Kurds of Northern Iraq.
3. Food tampering: Another scenario is an attack on food industries. The dairy industry is especially vulnerable to biochemical agents, probably because of the nature of manufacturing process and the reliance of animal feeds that could be contaminated with biochemical (mycotoxins) agents.[13] Such an attack would cause local outbreaks of disease within hours or days. In September 2004, the Hungarian government pulled paprika off the market due to excessive levels of aflatoxin detected in much of their product.[14]

 ## PREINCIDENT ACTIONS

Hospitals, emergency departments, and ambulatory care facilities should have general disaster plans in place to

FIGURE 137–1. Structures of AFB$_1$ and AFM$_1$ (see text).

AF	R
AFB$_1$	H
AFM$_1$	OH

FIGURE 137–2. Structure of AFG$_1$.

respond to a biochemical (mycotoxin) attack. Early detection of a biologic or chemical weapon attack requires a surveillance system that is capable of finding and confirming the diagnosis and serving as a means of communicating this information between clinicians and health departments in a timely fashion.[15] Current syndromic surveillance appears to be directed more toward respiratory and flu-like illness, although several monitor gastrointestinal illness.[16] Efforts should be made to include hepatitis syndromes in such monitoring efforts. This would require coordination of local, state, and federal public health and safety resources. In the event of an attack, emergency medical services, hospitals, and ambulatory care facilities need to be mobilized to care for potentially large numbers of patients seeking medical care in a short timeframe. Decontamination and triage procedures should be in place, and personnel properly trained, before an attack occurs. Since most physicians, healthcare providers, and first responders are not likely to be familiar with the characteristics of an aflatoxin terrorist attack, close contact with the local poison control center or local health department may be important in identifying the initial cases.

 POSTINCIDENT ACTIONS

Medical providers should include aflatoxin toxicity in the differential of acute hepatitis. Appropriate local, state, and federal public health agencies and law enforcement authorities need to be notified. Aflatoxin-contaminated materials, body fluids, and surfaces should be decontaminated with a 10% bleach (sodium hypochlorite) solution. Bleach should not be used to decontaminate patients. Proper sampling by a qualified industrial hygiene profes-

sional may be necessary for aflatoxin identification and evidence documentation. Further epidemiologic investigations in collaboration with state or local health services may be necessary. Complete blood count and liver function tests are recommended. Analysis of blood or urine samples may provide information concerning the metabolites of the mycotoxin.

 MEDICAL TREATMENT OF CASUALTIES

Treatment of acute aflatoxin exposure requires identification of and removal from the source of exposure. Activated charcoal is recommended in cases of recent ingestion. Aggressive supportive management, especially for acute liver failure, is indicated in all suspected cases. Hemodialysis and hemoperfusion are not expected to enhance elimination. Although there is no known antidote, N-acetylcysteine (NAC) may have a protective effect against aflatoxin carcinogenesis by increasing intracellular glutathione levels.[17] An animal model[18] found reduced hepatic injury when NAC was coadministered with high daily doses of AFB$_1$; however, efficacy in humans has not been demonstrated.

 CASE PRESENTATION

There are several reports from Asia and Africa that suggest acute poisonings secondary to aflatoxins resulting from ingestion of a large amount of toxin over a short period of time. A typical presentation is as follows:

Two young children are taken to the local hospital emergency department from the neighborhood village. Patient's family members inform the emergency department physician that they have all consumed corn from a local farmers market. Over the last 5 days, the children developed swelling of their lower extremities, abdominal pain, vomiting, and diarrhea, but no fever. Further history reveals that the adults experienced similar but milder symptoms. On examination, the patients are lethargic. Also present is slight jaundice with an enlarged liver that is tender to palpation. The next day, it is reported in the news media that an additional 30 children have been admitted to surrounding hospitals and more than 100 adults and children have been seen in local ambulatory care clinics for similar but milder symptoms. They all report eating corn and fruits purchased from a local farmers' market. Laboratory testing of the initial two young children reveals elevated liver aminotransferase levels, low blood glucose, and elevated blood ammonia levels. These two patients fully recover after 1 week of supportive care and intravenous fluids.

 UNIQUE CONSIDERATIONS

Diseases caused by mycotoxins such as aflatoxins are most effective when they are ingested. Aflatoxin attack using an aerosolized mechanism is unlikely to produce sufficient levels to cause significant morbidity or mortality.[19]

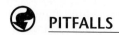

Several potential pitfalls in response to an aflatoxin attack exist. These include the following:

- Failure to prepare adequate systems to respond to possible terrorist attacks before an incident occurs
- Failure to consider aflatoxin as the cause for nonspecific as well as systemic symptoms of acute hepatitis
- Failure to consider aflatoxin attack in the setting of a large number of otherwise healthy people presenting over hours and days with a wide range of general and specific complaints
- Failure to notify appropriate public health, safety, and law enforcement authorities when a biochemical agent attack is suspected, especially when animals fall sick along with people
- Failure to collect specimens for identification of aflatoxins
- Failure to provide basic supportive care when a patient is suspected to have been exposed to a biochemical warfare agent

REFERENCES

1. Pitt JI, Basilico JC, Abarca ML, et al. Mycotoxins and toxigenic fungi. *Med Mycol.* 2000;38(suppl 1):41-6.
2. Fung F, Clark RF. Health effects of mycotoxins: a toxicological overview. *J Tox Clin Tox.* 2004;42:1-18.
3. Riley RT, Kemppainen BW, Norred WP. Penetration of aflatoxins through isolated epidermis. *J Toxicol Environ Health.* 1985;15:769-77.
4. Hsieh DPH, Wong JJ. Metabolism and toxicity of aflatoxins. *Adv Exp Med Biol.* 1982;126(B):847-63.
5. Patten RC. Aflatoxins and disease. *Am J Trop Med Hyg.* 1981;30:422-5.
6. Willis RM, Mulvihill JJ, Hoofnagle JH. Attempted suicide with purified aflatoxin. *Lancet* 1980;1(8179):1198-9.
7. Ngindu A, Johnson BK, Kenya PR, et al. Outbreak of acute hepatitis caused by aflatoxin poisoning in Kenya. *Lancet* 1982;1:1346-8.
8. Krishnamachari KA, Bhat RV, Nagarajan V, et al. Hepatitis due to aflatoxicosis: an outbreak in Western India. *Lancet* 1975;1:1061-3.
9. Nyikal J, Misore A, Nzioka C, et al. Outbreak of aflatoxin poisoning: Eastern and central provinces, Kenya, January–July, 2004. *MMWR* 2004;53(34):790-3.
10. Olson LC, Bourgeois CH Jr, Cotton RB, et al. Encephalopathy and fatty degeneration of the viscera in northeastern Thailand: clinical syndrome and epidemiology. *Pediatrics* 1971;47:707-16.
11. Chao TC, Maxwell SM, Wong SY. An outbreak of aflatoxicosis and boric acid poisoning in Malaysia: a clinicopathological study. *J Pathol.* 1991;164:225-33.
12. Zilinskas RA. Verifying compliance to the biological and toxin weapons convention. *Crit Rev Microbiol.* 1998;24(3):195-218.
13. Zilinskas RA. Terrorism and biological weapons: inevitable alliance? *Perspect Biol Med.* 1990;34:44-72.
14. Greenberg G. Hungarian government temporarily prohibits sale of paprika. November 3, 2004. Available at: http://list.mc.duke.edu/cgi-bin/wa?A2=ind0411&L=occ-env-med-l&F=&S=&P=2429.
15. Buehler JW, Hopkins RS, Overhage JM, et al. Framework for evaluating public health surveillance systems for early detection of outbreaks. *MMWR* 2004;53(RR05):1-11.
16. Bravata DM, McDonald KM, Smith WM, et al. Systemic review: surveillance systems for early detection of bioterrorism-related diseases. *Ann Intern Med.* 2004;140:910-22.
17. De Flora S, Bennicelli C, Camoirano A, et al. In vivo effects of *N*-acetylcysteine on glutathione metabolism and on the biotransformation of carcinogenic and/or mutagenic compounds. *Carcinogenesis* 1985;6:1735-45.
18. Valdivia AG, Martinez A, Damian FJ, et al. Efficacy of N-acetylcysteine to reduce the effects of aflatoxin B1 intoxication in broiler chickens. *Poult Sci.* 2001;80:727-34.
19. Ciegler A. *Mycotoxins: A New Class of Chemical Weapons.* 1986 NBC Defense and Technology International, Department of Defense, Washington DC: April 1986:52-7.

chapter 138

Coccidioides immitis Attack (Coccidioidomycosis)

James F. Martin and Jill A. Grant

 ## DESCRIPTION OF EVENT

Coccidioidomycosis is a specific disease, caused by the fungus *Coccidioides immitis*. It was first defined as a syndrome in 1892 and shown to be a fungal infection in 1900. This disease is known as San Joaquin Valley fever, or valley fever, due to its native location in the San Joaquin Valley of California, Arizona, New Mexico, Texas, and Utah, as well as in Mexico and portions of Central and South America. There are approximately 25,000 clinically significant cases defined per year in the United States, with 75 deaths per year attributed to the illness.[1-3] In 2001, the Arizona Department of Health reported 43 cases per 100,000 population, representing an increase of 186% since 1995.[3] Although there are endemic areas, with the majority of long-term residents demonstrating evidence of prior *C. immitis* infection, those areas often experience intermittent sharp seasonal increases in the number of cases, demonstrating the infectivity of the disease as well as its capability for mutation.

C. immitis exists as both a saprophyte and a parasite at different times during its life cycle. It is in the saprophytic stage in which it grows in soil as a mold with septate hyphae. It is initially spread by airborne spores, with epidemics often occurring after large-scale soil disturbances such as earthquakes, excavations, or storms. Once disturbed, these hyphae are broken off, forming arthroconidia, which in turn become airborne. The parasitic phase occurs if an animal or human inhales the arthroconidia, which become lodged in the pulmonary alveoli. It is here that they grow into multinucleate spherules, producing thousands of uninucleate endospores, each of which can give rise to a new spherule. The endospores have been shown to spread in a suitable host within the lung or through the bloodstream. Dissemination through the bloodstream has been shown to lead to deposition in perihilar, peritracheal, and cervical lymph nodes. Multisystem involvement can include skin and soft tissue infection, joint and bone infection, and meningitis.

The majority of symptoms are pulmonary. In the 40% of acutely exposed persons displaying symptoms, the most common are cough, shortness of breath, chest pain, and sputum production, along with systemic symptoms of fever, sweating, anorexia, weakness, and arthalgias.[1] These symptoms may last for several weeks, with spontaneous resolution. The average otherwise healthy person infected with *C. immitis* misses an average of 1 month of school or work.[1] If the disease becomes disseminated, multiple sites can be affected.[4] The most common extrapulmonary site is the skin, with superficial maculopapules, keratotic nodules, verrucous ulcers, and subcutaneous fluctuant abscesses being found.[2] The pus may be described as "gel-like." These lesions have a predilection for the nasolabial fold. Erythema multiforme and erythema nodosum may occur, more commonly in female patients. Erythema nodosum may be the initial presentation and reflects a heightened immune response. These patients rarely go on to disseminate.[2] The triad of fever, erythema nodosum, and arthralgias is called *desert rheumatism*.[2] Bone and joint infections may occur, in the company of dramatic effusions and synovial involvement, with dissemination. Joint lesions are unifocal in 90% of cases. The knee is the most commonly affected joint, followed by the ankle.[1,2] Coccidioidal meningitis is the most life-threatening of manifestations, with mortality approaching 90% at 12 months if untreated.[1,2] Usually the basilar meninges are involved, and presenting symptoms include fever, headache, vomiting, and altered mental status. Complications include hydrocephalus, cerebral vasculitis, and focal intracerebral coccidioidal abscesses.[2] Neurosurgical consultation may be urgent, for shunting or incision and drainage.

Diagnosis of coccidioidomycosis may be difficult and challenging, primarily due to a failure to consider the disease outside its endemic areas.[5] A specific travel history is usually necessary in nonendemic areas to prompt suspicion of the diagnosis.[6] Skin testing results become positive after the initial onset of symptoms in most patients with primary infections; anergy, however, is common in progressive disease.[1] Routine laboratory tests are not specific, although the erythrocyte sedimentation rate is usually elevated and the eosinophil counts are often increased.[7]

Culture and serologic testing are the most commonly available tests, although direct microscopic examination of tissue samples is deemed safest. The mycelial form of the fungus has minimal growth requirements, growing after 3 to 7 days on most mycologic or bacteriologic media under aerobic conditions and at most temperatures.[1,2] Mature colonies can have a myriad of appearances and are very highly infectious to laboratory workers.[1] In histopathology specimens, a mature spherule with endospores is pathognomonic of infection and is easily recognizable on wet mounts using potassium hydroxide or Calcofluor white.[8] Spherules also can be easily seen with multiple staining techniques,[1] particularly with periodic acid-Schiff. The organism can often be seen in, or grown from, pus, sputum, and body fluid aspirates.[1] Serologic testing is almost entirely based on immunoglobulin (Ig) M and IgG antibodies. False-positive test results are rare.[1] IgM is detected transiently in 75% of acutely infected persons 1 to 3 weeks after onset of symptoms due to primary infection and may last 3 to 4 months. Complement-fixing IgG appears later after the acute infection and disappears in 6 to 9 months if symptoms resolve.[8] Persistently elevated IgG antibody is observed in disseminated disease.

In the case of *C. immitis* meningitis, cerebrospinal fluid (CSF) cultures are usually negative in 85% of early cases.[1] The CSF will show an elevated pressure, a marked mononuclear pleocytosis, low glucose level, and high protein level.[1] A positive result of an IgG test of the CSF confirms the diagnosis.[2] Imaging studies are nonspecific but can aid in the diagnosis. Chest radiology may delineate cavities and granulomas. Magnetic resonance imaging may be useful to examine the brain for signs of meningitis or abscesses.[2] Radionuclide bone scanning may delineate bone lesions.

Coccidioidomycosis would appear to make a poor biologic weapon. Most immunocompetent patients are asymptomatic, with only 40% of infected persons displaying any type of symptom. Among those who are symptomatic, the most common form is an upper or lower respiratory tract infection, which usually resolves without specific therapy and can last up to 3 or 4 weeks and still go undiagnosed. Extrapulmonary manifestations have much higher morbidity and mortality but occur in only 0.5% of cases, may take up to a year to develop, and occur in subpopulations of immunocompromised persons with defects in delayed hypersensitivity, pregnant women in their third trimester, infants, or patients of Filipino, African American, or Mexican descent who are genetically predisposed to disseminate the disease. The organism is almost entirely contained in the "Western Hemisphere," with an estimated majority of those Americans who are living in the endemic areas already showing signs of prior exposure or infection. Thus, if the fungus were used as a weapon of mass destruction, a minority of the population would be symptomatic, with most symptoms resolving in a few weeks. In those few persons who do have life-threatening infections, it will usually occur in minority populations and could take up to a year to develop.

There are, however, some facts that demonstrate the potential lethality of coccidioidomycosis if used as a biologic weapon. First, each year, 25,000 new cases are diagnosed, and 75 deaths occur annually. These deaths almost always occur in those persons suffering from disseminated disease. The most common dissemination is to the skin, closely followed by the meninges. If meningitis occurs, the 12-month mortality is 90% if not treated. Even with appropriate treatment, mortality rates from fulminant infections remain high. It is estimated that, even with our most advanced treatment, neurologic involvement by coccidioidomycosis has a 70% to 80% death rate. Hence, there is a significant mortality of the disseminated disease.

Second, the fungus has a very high virulence, with only a single *C. immitis* arthroconidium required to produce pulmonary infection.[2] However, devastating outbreaks have been demonstrated when coccidioidomycosis has been specifically grown in the laboratory setting, such as in the case of hospital laboratory personnel attempting to diagnose a patient. This occurrence demonstrates the increased virulence of the spore form of the organism when being grown in the laboratory. Add to this fact the apparent capability to mutate, and a potentially devastating biologic weapon could be developed.

Third, healthcare workers may not initially recognize a coccidioidomycosis attack. With the majority of patients asymptomatic, and those who are symptomatic displaying a nonspecific upper respiratory infection, initial cases may be ignored or diagnosed with a self-limited viral disease. Three to 4 weeks is the incubation period for the pulmonary manifestations, so a delay from the initial exposure may be present. For the sickest patients, an even longer incubation period of up to 1 year may be evident, further complicating the diagnosis and increasing the morbidity in the specific population of infected persons with the highest mortality. Although there has been no documented incidence of person-to-person spread through air droplets, the infectivity of these long-incubation patients is unknown. Use of *C. immitis* as a weapon could therefore cause a subtle increase in the workload of the healthcare system over time.

The most likely scenario of a *C. immitis* attack would consist of a large urban population with a large number of persons presenting over a few weeks with a nonspecific upper respiratory infection. Minority populations; pregnant women; infants; and immunocompromised patients, such as those with HIV, those having received organ transplant; and patients taking steroids would be the worst affected. An effective attack would require a large target population localized in a specific area that could be inoculated with airborne particles. Although evidence of prior infection may already be present in much of the population, a dramatic increase in clinical cases should alert healthcare workers, and once positive diagnoses are made, a biologic attack should be considered. The population should be followed up for as long as 1 year after the incident for evidence of chronic severe infection; this requirement in itself will increase the load on the healthcare system and could increase public fear, as those exposed would constantly worry that they might develop delayed and serious illness.

 ## PREINCIDENT ACTIONS

In endemic areas, coccidioidomycosis can only be prevented by occupationally preventing susceptible persons from working in high-risk situations; therefore, in these specific areas, focused educational programs for construction and agricultural workers should be in place, as well as for students, military personnel, and healthcare workers. Documented cases of mass infection with *C. immitis* show occurrence in one of three ways: (1) recent visit to an endemic area; (2) reactivation of a prior infection; or (3) exposure to spores brought out of an endemic area.

Hospitals, emergency departments, and outpatient facilities should each have a disaster response plan in place. Coordination of local, state, and national public health and public safety resources are required in the event of a mass-casualty situation such as biologic warfare. Both emergency medical services and hospital triage systems may need to be altered to account for the influx of patients with specific treatment requirements—in this case, respiratory ailments. Universal precautions should be in place, even though person-to-person transmission of coccidioidomycosis has never been documented.[9] Diagnosis of the index case may be difficult, again, mainly due to a lack of suspicion for the agent in nonendemic areas. Special and specific care needs to be taken with the culturing of *C. immitis*: namely, specialized training for laboratory technicians, universal precautions, Biosafety Level 3 procedures, and negative pressure rooms. Cultures should be planted on slants rather than on culture slides. Physicians should be trained to highlight their suspicions for coccidioidomycosis when submitting culture specimens from suspect patients.

A real coccidioidomycosis attack or a major natural outbreak is unlikely; however, healthcare providers need to be aware of the disease and keep it on the differential diagnosis list. The possibly long incubation period, nonspecific complaints, and multiple organ involvement may make initial diagnosis extremely difficult. Universal precautions need to be in place, as well as a surveillance system that can recognize a trend in patient syndromes. With documentation of trends over time, a specific index incident may be able to be identified.

 POSTINCIDENT ACTIONS

Healthcare providers with suspicion of, or a clear demonstrated case of, coccidioidomycosis need to contact specific public health officials because coccidioidomycosis became a nationally reportable disease in 1995.[3] Also, any medical providers or disaster response teams that may come into contact with an infected party or a putative exposure location should be notified and screened. Such responders may include any hospital or clinic worker or physician who treated patients from a specific location, as well as emergency medical services, police, or fire personnel; clean-up crews; those working for the Red Cross and other relief organizations; and the military.

Disinfection of surfaces possibly contaminated with arthroconidia should be carried out with standard disinfectants or antiseptic agents.

 MEDICAL TREATMENT OF CASUALTIES

Of the endemic fungal infections, coccidioidomycosis is the most resistant to therapy.[10] The treatment and care of the primary respiratory infection is controversial, primarily due to the lack of controlled clinical trials.[1,2] For the majority of patients, care should include symptomatic treatment and careful reexamination to ensure the resolution of symptoms. Follow-up radiology to monitor the resolution of pulmonary findings is also recommended. The goal of this approach is to monitor resolution in the event of not using antifungal therapy. Historically, initial pulmonary manifestations have a 95% spontaneous resolution rate. However, some authorities propose rapid and high-dose antifungal medications at the time of diagnosis for unusually severe infections or with comorbid conditions such as organ transplantation, HIV infection, diabetes, or steroid use. The severity of the disease should be estimated, with the following characteristics kept in mind: symptoms that persist longer than 2 months; weight loss greater than 10%; greater than 3 weeks of night sweats; infiltrates involving greater than 1 lung; development of anergy to skin tests; prominent or persistent hilar adenopathy; Filipino, African American, or Mexican ethnic background; pregnant female patients in their third trimester; or an antibody test result demonstrating antibody to *C. immitis* in a titer greater than 1:16.[2]

For persons with severe infections, the two treatment options consist of surgical debridement or chemotherapy. Surgery should be determined on a case-by-case basis and is an option in the case of extensive bone or skin involvement. The theory behind the use of debridement is that the spherule wall (1) is a strong stimulus for inflammation, (2) cannot be degraded by the body, and (3) cannot be cleared by macrophages.[2] Thus, continued tissue damage can occur until the spherule is physically removed. Also, pulmonary cavities have been shown to react poorly to chemotherapy.[1,2]

In cases of disseminated disease, chemotherapy should always be initiated.[1] Chemotherapy is achieved with either amphotericin B or antifungal azoles (ketoconazole, fluconazole, itraconazole).[1,2,10,11] Although known for potent side effects, amphotericin B is preferred due to the more rapid onset when compared with the azoles. Also, whereas the azoles as a group are categorized as pregnancy class C, amphotericin B is a class B agent. Standard precautions and monitoring with the medications should be performed. Amphotericin B is administered for a total of 2 months, or until the disease becomes inactive. Although the azoles are taken orally, and thus better tolerated, they are currently not approved for this use by the U.S. Food and Drug Administration. Efficacy seems to be similar between the two classes of drugs, but frequent relapses have shown that therapy with the azoles needs to be continued for 6 months.[1,2,10] Future treatment may involve novel azole agents (e.g., posaconazole, voriconazole), caspofungin (an echinocandin that inhibits glucan synthetase), or sordarin derivatives (drugs that specifically inhibit fungal protein synthesis).[10]

CASE PRESENTATION

You have a follow-up visit with a patient who was initially seen 1 week ago in the emergency department by one of your peers. He is an elderly diabetic man, and his initial complaints were fever, night sweats, and vague upper respiratory complaints of a productive cough, sputum production, and shortness of breath. He states he was in his usual state of health until this past week, with his only unusual activity being 4 weeks ago when he was a guest at an archaeologic dig in New Mexico. When an initial workup yielded negative results, he was treated for a viral respiratory infection and discharged home.

The patient returns today with the continuation of his initial complaints, but now he complains of a rash over his entire body, pain and swelling in his right knee, difficulty concentrating, and a persistent irritating headache. While reviewing the charts of the emergency department, you notice that there have been at least 10 other patients with similar symptoms in the past week, with seemingly the worst affected being a pregnant woman and a renal transplant patient.

UNIQUE CONSIDERATIONS

Coccidioidomycosis is a fungal infection that usually causes self-limited upper respiratory or febrile illnesses, but which, when disseminated, can cause life-threatening extrapulmonary disease. Its manifestations are similar to many common nonspecific illnesses and thus may elude diagnosis when the diagnosis is not sought. Although it is considered a possible biologic weapon due to the high virulence of the arthroconidia and severe mortality of the disseminated disease, *C. immitis* would likely make a poor bioweapon due to the fact that it is not a virulent infection in normal hosts. Terrorists would need to either find a way to cause immune suppression in a normal population in advance of seeding the infection or target a compromised host population. More important are its very long incubation period, that 60% of infected persons are asymptomatic, and that the majority of patients spontaneously recover. The use of coccidioidomycosis as a biologic weapon would be ineffective, and the identification of infected persons would be extremely difficult; a natural outbreak is far more likely but poses similar diagnostic pitfalls. The main points to remember are to keep this organism in the differential diagnosis and remember that appropriate therapy requires a multidisciplinary approach, using symptomatic therapy, antifungal chemotherapy, and surgery to produce the best outcome.

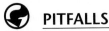

PITFALLS

Several potential pitfalls in response to an attack exist. These include the following:

- Failure to have a disaster response plan
- Failure to consider coccidioidomycosis as a possible cause in patients with mild symptoms
- Failure to adequately diagnose persons suspected of having the disease process
- Failure to adequately treat patients with both surgical options as well as antifungal agents
- Failure to have adequately prepared and trained laboratory capabilities
- Failure to notify laboratory workers of a high suspicion for coccidioidomycosis in submitted specimens, so that they may take appropriate precautions to limit their own exposure
- Failure to notify and screen possibly infected persons who were involved with the index incident
- Failure to notify local, state, and federal agencies in the instance of a suspected case

REFERENCES

1. Stevens D. Current concepts: coccidioidomycosis [review article]. *N Engl J Med.* 1995;332:1077-82.
2. Riauba L. Coccidioidomycosis. Emedicine Web site. July 15, 2002. Available at: http://www.emedicine.com/derm/topic742.htm.
3. Centers for Disease Control and Prevention. Leads from the *Morbidity and Mortality Weekly Report*, Atlanta, Ga: Increase in Coccidioidomycosis:Arizona, 1998-2001. *JAMA* 2003;289:1500-2.
4. Galgiani J. Coccidioidomycosis: a regional disease of national importance. Rethinking approaches for control. *Ann Intern Med.* 1999;130:293-300.
5. Arsura E, Kilgore W. Miliary coccidioidomycosis in the immunocompetent [case series]. *Chest* 2000;117:404-9.
6. Standaert SM, Schaffner W, Galgiania JN, et al. Coccidioidomycosis among visitors to a *Coccidioidomycosis immitis*–endemic area: an outbreak in a military reserve unit. *J Infect Dis.* 1995;171:1672-5.
7. Galgiani JN. Coccidioidomycosis. In: Remington JS, Swartz MN, eds. *Current Clinical Topics in Infectious Diseases*. Vol. 17. Malden, Mass: Blackwell Sciences; 1997:188-204.
8. Walsh TJ, Chanock SJ. Diagnosis of invasive fungal infections: advances in non-cultural systems. In: Remington JS, Swartz MN, eds. *Current Clinical Topics in Infectious Diseases*. Vol. 18. Malden, Mass: Blackwell Sciences; 1998:127-8.
9. Centers for Disease Control and Prevention. Leads from the *Morbidity and Mortality Weekly Report*, Atlanta, Ga: Coccidioidomycosis – United States, 1991-1992. *JAMA* 1993;269:1098-9.
10. Deresinki S. Coccidioidomycosis: efficacy of new agents and future prospects [review article]. *Curr Opin Infect Dis.* 2001;14:693-6.
11. Galgiani JN, Catanzaro A, Cloud GA, et al. Comparison of oral fluconazole and itraconazole for progressive, non-meningeal coccidioidomycosis: a randomized, double-blind trial. *Ann Intern Med.* 2000;133:676-86.

chapter 139

Histoplasma capsulatum Attack (Histoplasmosis)

Carol L. Venable and Elizabeth L. Mitchell

 ## DESCRIPTION OF EVENT

Histoplasma capsulatum, the organism responsible for histoplasmosis, is a dimorphic fungus that is endemic to many parts of the world, most notably the United States and Latin America. *H. capsulatum* spores are present in soil, especially soil that has been contaminated by bird or bat excrement.[1] In the Americas, histoplasmosis is found primarily in the regions of the Ohio, St. Lawrence, Mississippi, and Rio Grande river systems.[2] Humans come into contact with aerosolized spores of *H. capsulatum* when they engage in occupational or recreational activities in endemic areas. Construction or demolition work, bridge cleaning or repairs, farming, gardening, and exploring caves are all high-risk activities for infection.[2] In the endemic region, skin testing demonstrates that a majority of the population has had prior infection with *H. capsulatum*, and up to 25% of patients with acquired immunodeficiency syndrome (AIDS) in these areas will have active disease.[3]

Histoplasmosis has numerous clinical manifestations. The majority of infected persons are asymptomatic, which complicates the identification of outbreaks of this disease. When present, symptoms usually begin within 1 or 2 weeks of exposure.[2] The most common clinical form of disease from *H. capsulatum* is acute pulmonary histoplasmosis, which typically presents with fever, fatigue, dry cough, and headaches.[1] Acute pulmonary histoplasmosis tends to be self-limited and often resolves on its own over the course of 2 to 3 weeks.[4] The disease may be so mild that affected patients may not seek medical attention. More severe or prolonged cases may prompt patients to visit clinics or emergency departments. Less commonly, patients will present with severe respiratory failure and, in these cases, acute pulmonary histoplasmosis can be fatal if not rapidly diagnosed and treated.[5] Other, more chronic forms of histoplasmosis exist, such as chronic lung disease from *H. capsulatum* in patients with preexisting emphysema, but these disease manifestations do not have relevance to acute outbreaks or attacks.

In patients with AIDS, hematologic malignancies, transplants, or some other source of immunocompromise,

there is a much greater risk of developing disseminated histoplasmosis, the manifestation of *H. capsulatum* that affects almost every organ system and is also potentially fatal.[5] Infants and elderly persons may manifest this form as well, even in the setting of an apparently healthy immune system.[1] Disseminated disease may progress rapidly and may present as dysfunction of the reticuloendothelial system, shock, and multiorgan system failure.[5] In immunocompetent patients who are not at the extremes of age, disseminated histoplasmosis is less common and more indolent. It may present as a fever of unknown origin without many other associated symptoms.[5]

Despite having some virulent disease manifestations, there is no evidence that *H. capsulatum* has ever been weaponized. Although its spore form might lead one to believe that it could be easily manipulated, in fact, there are several features of the organism that make it difficult to use as an intentional biologic weapon. First, in areas where *H. capsulatum* is endemic, a significant percentage of the population has at least partial immunity to histoplasmosis, having been previously exposed at some level.[2] This lowers the likelihood that a biologic attack would cause widespread, severe disease in these areas. Second, the toxic exposure limits for *H. capsulatum* are not known, making it difficult for an aggressor to know what level of concentration to produce for use as a weapon.[2] Finally, histoplasmosis causes a broad spectrum of disease, the majority of which is nonfatal, self-limited, and treatable. Even in AIDS patients with disseminated disease, antifungal therapy has reduced the mortality to less than 25%.[4]

One can hypothesize, however, a variation on an intentional disaster scenario in which *H. capsulatum* would inadvertently become a biologic weapon. If an explosive device detonated in an area with soil containing *H. capsulatum*, there is a high likelihood that histoplasmosis could be a secondary cause of morbidity and mortality in victims or rescue workers who inhale the spores. Again, the prior consideration of partial immunity would hold for people living in the endemic area. However, if the soil contained a high enough spore concentration and was dispersed widely enough by the explosion, large numbers of people might still be at risk for significant infections.

729

A far more likely disaster scenario would be a completely unintentional exposure. In the past, unintentional exposures and the subsequent outbreaks they have caused have originated from a number of different sources. In Acapulco, Mexico, in the spring of 2001, the source of *H. capsulatum* that infected hundreds of American travelers is thought to have been the soil in the utility shaft adjacent to a central stairway in a major tourist hotel.[6] In Nicaragua in October 2003, several tourists were infected during a visit to a bat-infested cave.[7] Outbreaks have been reported in Tennessee, Kentucky, Indiana, Michigan, and several other states in which people cleaned, constructed, or demolished bridges or buildings that were surrounded with soil contaminated by bat or bird excrement.[3,8-10] Many of these outbreaks theoretically could have been predicted, and prevented, if the workers or their employers had considered the risks of manipulating potentially contaminated soil and either decontaminated the area first or used protective gear.

Diagnosis of histoplasmosis requires having a high clinical suspicion and obtaining a thorough travel and occupational history. The differential diagnosis is extensive and includes atypical pneumonia, influenza, tuberculosis, sarcoidosis, and other fungal diseases. Physical examination may be unrevealing, although in disseminated disease, patients may have hepatosplenomegaly or lymphadenopathy. Routine laboratory test results are likely to be normal in cases of acute pulmonary histoplasmosis. Disseminated disease may be associated with pancytopenia, as well as elevated liver function test results. Chest radiographs in cases of acute pulmonary histoplasmosis may be normal or may show reticulonodular infiltrates, often with hilar or mediastinal lymphadenopathy. The majority of cases of disseminated disease yield abnormal chest radiographs, also with interstitial or reticulonodular infiltrates.[5]

Cultures, fungal stains, serologies, and antigen detection permit the laboratory diagnosis of *H. capsulatum*. Cultures can detect between 80% and 90% of cases of disseminated disease but have a much lower sensitivity for acute pulmonary histoplasmosis.[11] In addition, they may take several weeks of growth before they turn positive.[5] This makes culture suboptimal in an outbreak setting. Serologic tests can be performed either by immunodiffusion or complement fixation technology, of which the complement fixation is the more sensitive although less specific test.[2] The serologic tests have a sensitivity of greater than 90% for acute pulmonary histoplasmosis, although their sensitivity for disseminated disease is lower.[12] The difficulty with these tests is that up to 6 weeks may be required before the serology yields positive results. In addition, positive serologic test results may be due to prior infections or infections caused by other fungi.[5] Despite these limitations, complement fixation is a viable option for detecting acute pulmonary histoplasmosis in outbreaks, especially in patients with severe disease, because the test has a much better sensitivity in highly symptomatic patients.[12]

Urine antigen testing is the test of choice in the majority of patients during an outbreak. It has a turnaround time of 1 to 2 days and has a sensitivity of approximately 90% in patients with disseminated disease and approximately 75% in patients with acute pulmonary histoplasmosis.[12] Serum antigen testing can also be performed but is less sensitive than urine antigen testing. Like the serologic tests, antigen testing has the potential drawback of cross-reaction with other fungal agents.[11] The only other test as rapid as antigen testing is tissue fungal stain, which can be used if tissue is obtained from a patient—for example, from a transbronchial or bone marrow biopsy. The accuracy of fungal stain results is dependent, however, on a given laboratory's skills in distinguishing among different types of fungal organisms.[5]

 PREINCIDENT ACTIONS

Histoplasmosis has a wide range of disease severity. Patients are likely to present to clinics, urgent care centers, and emergency departments with this disease. Rapid identification of an outbreak, therefore, requires a preexisting system of coordination among ambulatory care centers, emergency departments, and state or national public health authorities. Healthcare providers, especially those in endemic areas, need education about possible presentations of outbreaks and specific instructions as to the best way of reporting any suspected cases.

If there were any threat of an explosion of a building in an area endemic for histoplasmosis, steps could be taken to eradicate *H. capsulatum* as a secondary threat. For example, obvious targets such as skyscrapers, bridges, and major government buildings could have soil testing performed in the area surrounding them. Any soil with significant concentrations of *H. capsulatum* could then be treated with a 3% solution of formalin, which inactivates the spores.[13,14] This would eliminate at least the threat of an inadvertent biologic disaster in the unfortunate case of an explosion. A similar approach is recommended, and has been used in the past, in the setting of building construction, demolition, and cleaning.[2]

 POSTINCIDENT ACTIONS

Histoplasmosis is not transmitted from one human to another.[2] Therefore, isolation of potentially infected patients is not necessary. The two critical postincident actions that need to be taken are as follows: (1) rapid identification of *H. capsulatum* as the cause of the outbreak and (2) decontamination of any remaining *H. capsulatum* spores. Diagnosis can be performed by any of the methods listed above, but, in general, serologic and urine antigen testing will be the most useful modalities in an outbreak.

Soil testing around the presumed site of an outbreak, along with subsequent formaldehyde decontamination of any *H. capsulatum*–containing soil, is critical for preventing continued exposures and infections. Investigators involved in outbreaks need to wear appropriate protective gear when evaluating possible sites of exposure. In particular, powered, air-purifying respirators with full face piece are optimal. These should be used along with disposable clothes and shoe coverings.[2]

MEDICAL TREATMENT OF CASUALTIES

Not all cases of histoplasmosis require treatment, and in a disaster setting, antifungal agents must be restricted to those patients most in need. In the setting of acute pulmonary histoplasmosis without acute respiratory failure, treatment should only be given to patients who fail to improve after experiencing symptoms for 1 month. Oral itraconazole at a dosage of 200 mg daily for 6 to 12 weeks can be used in this group. For immunocompetent patients with severe manifestations of acute pulmonary histoplasmosis (e.g., requiring a ventilator), the treatment of choice becomes amphotericin B administered at a dosage of 0.7 mg/kg/day. Prednisone (60 mg) taken daily for 2 weeks may be used in conjunction with amphotericin B in immunocompetent patients, although the data studying this are limited. After discharge from the hospital, the patient's treatment can be maintained on itraconazole (200 mg) taken once or twice daily to complete a 12-week antifungal course.[4]

Patients with disseminated histoplasmosis are subdivided for treatment purposes into persons with AIDS and those without AIDS. Patients with AIDS undergo a total of 12 weeks of therapy with amphotericin B (0.7 mg/kg/day) followed by itraconazole (200 mg twice daily) on discharge home. Patients who never require hospitalization can be treated with itraconazole (200 mg) three times daily for 3 days followed by twice daily for a total of 12 weeks. After the initial 12 weeks, a life-long maintenance regimen of itraconazole (200 mg) once or twice daily is recommended.[4]

Patients with disseminated histoplasmosis who do not have AIDS are treated with amphotericin B (0.7 to 1.0 mg/kg/day) if they require hospitalization. The amphotericin B can be switched to oral itraconazole once the patient defervesces. Itraconazole (200 mg) once or twice daily can be continued for 6 to 18 months for completion of therapy. Duration of treatment can be determined by serial measurement of *H. capsulatum* antigen concentrations.[4]

UNIQUE CONSIDERATIONS

Low mortality and a vast range of disease manifestations make outbreaks of *H. capsulatum* difficult to detect. In addition, histoplasmosis resembles many other pulmonary and infectious diseases. Patients may not be identified as part of an outbreak unless a careful occupational, recreational, and travel history is obtained. A history of close contacts, especially those who went on the same trip or participated in the same job, may also be extremely helpful in diagnosis.

PITFALLS

Several potential pitfalls in response to a histoplasmosis attack exist. These include the following:

- Failure to consider histoplasmosis as a possible cause of secondary morbidity and mortality in natural disasters or explosions in areas in which *H. capsulatum* is endemic
- Failure to obtain a complete occupational and travel history in patients presenting with nonspecific pulmonary complaints
- Failure to consider histoplasmosis as a possible diagnosis during influenza season or during known outbreaks of other pulmonary illnesses
- Failure to consider decontamination or protective gear for *H. capsulatum* as a protective option when attempting to evaluate the site of a possible outbreak
- Failure to consider in advance the importance of decontamination of soil containing *H. capsulatum* surrounding buildings, bridges, and other structures that could be threatened by explosions or that are scheduled for cleaning, construction, or demolition

CASE PRESENTATION

A 30-year-old male construction worker in Tennessee presents to his primary care physician (PCP) in December with the chief complaint of having had a dry cough for the past 2 weeks. He is an otherwise healthy man with no history of any lung disease. During a review of systems, he notes that he has had some headaches, mild fatigue, and low-grade, subjective fevers. He denies any exposure to tuberculosis or any risk factors for human immunodeficiency virus. He states that none of his family is sick but that several of his coworkers have had "the flu." He says that a couple of them are actually in the hospital, but he does not have any further details. The results of his lung examination are unremarkable, but because of the duration of the cough, the PCP obtains a chest radiograph, which is notable for diffuse reticulonodular infiltrates bilaterally.

On reinterviewing the patient and focusing on occupational history, the PCP learns that he and his coworkers have been tearing down an old building previously infested with bats. They started the demolition process about 3 or 4 weeks prior. There are approximately 100 workers at the site. The PCP then contacts the state health department with her concerns about a possible outbreak of histoplasmosis. The health department instructs her to obtain serologic and urine antigen testing for *H. capsulatum* at that visit. She instructs the patient to return for antifungal therapy if he has worsening symptoms at any point or still has his current symptoms in 2 more weeks.

REFERENCES

1. Cano MVC, Hajjeh RA. The epidemiology of histoplasmosis: a review. *Semin Respir Infect*. 2001;16:109-18.
2. Centers for Disease Control and Prevention. Histoplasmosis: protecting workers at risk, revised guidelines for preventing histoplasmosis. National Institute for Occupational Safety and Health; 1997;97-146. Available at: http://www.cdc.gov/niosh/97-146.html.
3. Wheat LJ. Histoplasmosis in Indianapolis. *Clin Infect Dis*. 1992;14(suppl 1):S91-9.
4. Wheat J, Sarosi G, McKinsey D, et al. Practice guidelines for the management of patients with histoplasmosis. *Clin Infect Dis*. 2000;30:688-95.

5. Wheat LJ, Kauffman CA. Histoplasmosis. *Infect Dis Clin North Am.* 2003;17:1-19.

6. Morgan J, Cano MV, Feikin DR, et al. A large outbreak of histoplasmosis among American travelers associated with a hotel in Acapulco, Mexico, Spring 2001. *Am J Trop Med Hyg.* 2003;69:663-9.

7. Weinberg M, Weeks J, Lance-Parker S, et al. Severe histoplasmosis in travelers to Nicaragua. *Emerg Infect Dis.* 2003;9:1322-5.

8. Jones TF, Swinger GL, Craig AS, et al. Acute pulmonary histoplasmosis in bridge workers: a persistent problem. *Am J Med.* 1999;106:480-2.

9. Centers for Disease Control and Prevention. Histoplasmosis—Kentucky, 1995. *MMWR* 1995;44:701-3.

10. Stobierski MG, Hospedales CJ, Hall WN, et al. Outbreak of histoplasmosis among employees in a paper factory: Michigan, 1993. *J Clin Microbiol.* 1996;34:1220-3.

11. Williams B, Fojtasek M, Connolly-Stringfield P, et al. Diagnosis of histoplasmosis by antigen detection during an outbreak in Indianapolis, Ind. *Arch Pathol Lab Med.* 1994;118:1205-8.

12. Wheat LJ. Laboratory diagnosis of histoplasmosis: update 2000. *Semin Respir Infect.* 2001;16:131-40.

13. Tosh FE, Weeks RJ, Pfeiffer FR, et al. The use of formalin to kill Histoplasma capsulatum at an epidemic site. *Am J Epidemiol.* 1967;85:259-65.

14. Bartlett PC, Weeks RJ, Ajello L. Decontamination of a *Histoplasma capsulatum*-infested bird roost in Illinois. *Arch Environ Health.* 1982;37:221-3.

chapter 140

Cryptosporidium parvum Attack (Cryptosporidiosis)

Miriam John and Carol Sulis

 ## DESCRIPTION OF EVENT

Human cryptosporidiosis is a disease caused by the protozoan cryptosporidium, an obligate intracellular parasite. *Cryptosporidium parvum* is the most common species in humans, but other species have been identified in immunocompromised hosts. The human pathogen *C. parvum* (genotype 1) and the bovine pathogen *C. parvum* (genotype 2) are the most important agents in human disease.[1] Reservoirs for *C. parvum* include humans; domesticated animals such as cows, goats, and sheep; and wild animals, such as deer and elk. Tyzzer and Clarke discovered cryptosporidia in the stomach of a mouse in 1907. The first human case was reported in 1976 in a child with diarrhea. Since 1982, and the beginning of the AIDS epidemic, cryptosporidia have been increasingly recognized as a cause of diarrheal illness in both immunocompromised and immunocompetent human hosts. Cryptosporidiosis is the leading cause of diarrhea due to protozoal infections worldwide.[2]

C. parvum is classified by the Centers for Disease Control and Prevention (CDC) as a category B bioterrorism threat agent and, more specifically, as a water safety threat. Cryptosporidia are highly infectious enteric pathogens that are resistant to chlorine, are small and difficult to filter, and are ubiquitous in many animals, making them a persistent threat to the U.S. water supply.[3] *C. parvum* is also a hardy organism that can survive for 18 months at 4°C in surface water and for 2 to 6 months in groundwater.[4] Oocysts have been found in 87% of untreated water samples tested in the United States and Canada.[5] Cryptosporidia are resistant to common water disinfection techniques such as chlorination, treatment with sodium hypochlorite, and filtration (if the filter pore size is greater than 1 micron).[1] A recent study of 66 water treatment plants in 14 states and one Canadian province showed that 27% of filtered water samples contained *Cryptosporidium* oocysts.[4]

Cryptosporidium infection occurs after ingestion of fecally contaminated food or water. Transmission can also occur directly from animal to person or person to person. The infectious form of *C. parvum* is the thick-walled 4- to 6-micron oocyst.[1] The dose at which 50% of those

exposed become infected ranges from 10 to 300 oocysts.[5] Ingested oocysts undergo excystation in the upper small intestine after being exposed to reducing conditions, proteolytic enzymes, and bile salts. Sporozoites invade the intestinal brush border epithelial cells and mature into merozoites, leading to inflammation, villous blunting, malabsorption, and diarrhea. Merozoites undergo sexual reproduction to produce thin-walled oocysts, which continue autoinfection in the host, or thick-walled oocysts, which are excreted and can then infect other hosts.[3,5] *Cryptosporidium* infection can be found at rates of 2.2% to 6.1% in immunocompetent persons with diarrhea in industrialized and developing countries, respectively. HIV-positive persons with diarrhea showed *Cryptosporidium* infection in 14% to 24% of cases in industrialized and developing areas, respectively.[3,6]

There have been numerous well-documented outbreaks of cryptosporidiosis in the United States. Most are waterborne outbreaks due to contamination of drinking water or recreational water, such as swimming pools or wading pools. There were approximately one dozen documented outbreaks of cryptosporidiosis in the United States between 1993 and 1998. The largest waterborne outbreak in U.S. history occurred in March and April 1993 in Milwaukee, Wisc., and affected an estimated 403,000 persons. This constituted a 52% cryptosporidiosis attack rate among those served by the South Milwaukee water works plant. Person-to-person spread has also been documented in institutions such as daycare centers and hospitals and may be especially difficult to control because infectious oocysts may be excreted for up to 5 weeks after diarrheal illness ends.[3,6]

The clinical manifestations of *C. parvum* infection are largely host dependent. In an immunocompetent host, cryptosporidiosis is primarily an intestinal disorder with a 1- to 2-week incubation period followed by symptoms of watery diarrhea, abdominal cramps, anorexia, nausea, vomiting, and possibly a low-grade fever. The disease is self-limited, with an average duration of 9 to 12 days. The main risk is dehydration. In the immunocompromised host, cryptosporidiosis can be an acute dehydrating diarrheal syndrome or a chronic diarrheal and wasting syndrome. Patients with CD4 counts greater than 180 cells/mm³ tend to have the self-limited syndrome. *Cryptosporidium* infection of biliary and pancreatic ducts leading to cholangitis or acalculous cholecystitis has been documented in patients with CD4 counts less than 50 cells/mm³.[1,5] There are also infrequent reports of pulmonary and tracheal cryptosporidiosis in immunocompromised hosts, which manifests as cough with low-grade fever, usually accompanying severe intestinal illness.[2]

Diagnosis of *C. parvum* is made using modified acid-fast staining on unconcentrated fecal smears. However, cryptosporidiosis is likely underdiagnosed in industrialized countries because relatively few laboratories routinely process stool ova and parasite specimens for cryptosporidium or other acid-fast enteric pathogens. Direct fluorescence antibody (DFA), enzyme-linked immunosorbent assay, and polymerase chain reaction testing are more sensitive and less user dependent than routine acid-fast testing, but these are newer and less commonly available.[1,5]

 ## PREINCIDENT ACTIONS

Since cryptosporidia are ubiquitous and persistent in the environment and highly transmissible, these organisms are well suited to be used in a covert biologic attack. Mortality in a bioattack would be low, except among immunocompromised patients, but morbidity could be extremely high, especially since there can be person-to-person transmission of cryptosporidiosis. Physicians, particularly those working in emergency departments, must remain vigilant to distinguish cryptosporidiosis from routine viral gastroenteritis. Large numbers of persons can be affected in an outbreak and may seek medical attention because of the frequency of stools (average of 12 to 15 per day), prolonged course of diarrheal illness (average of 9 to 12 days), or severity of illness if the person is immunocompromised.[5] Patients with suspected cryptosporidiosis should undergo laboratory analysis of stool samples including modified acid-fast staining or DFA to confirm the diagnosis. Examples of pre-event public health surveillance might include monitoring the volume of antidiarrheal medication sold, monitoring HMO and hospital logs of patient chief complaints, or monitoring the incidence of diarrhea in nursing homes or daycare centers.[7]

To protect against widespread outbreaks, the public water supply should be monitored closely. Water filtration and flocculation techniques that can eradicate oocysts are not routinely performed at many plants. Waterborne outbreaks have occurred even when the water supply met required turbidity levels. Methods such as reverse osmosis, membrane filtration, ozone treatment, or irradiation can eradicate infectious oocysts from the water supply but are not cost-effective. Ozone treatment is likely the most effective chemical means of inactivating *Cryptosporidium* oocysts.[3]

 ## POSTINCIDENT ACTIONS

Public health authorities should be notified when cryptosporidia are confirmed by laboratory analysis of a stool sample. If an outbreak is suspected, an epidemiologic investigation involving appropriate public health authorities should be initiated promptly to identify the source of the outbreak and to rapidly institute corrective measures. In addition to standard precautions in hospitals, contact precautions should be instituted for diapered children and incontinent adults. Rigorous handwashing by hospital staff is necessary to prevent nosocomial spread. Public health authorities would likely issue a boil-water advisory if the public water supply were contaminated. Information and education about *Cryptosporidium* species should be provided to the general public and should include instructions specific to immunocompromised groups. Boiling water is the most certain method of eradicating *Cryptosporidium* oocysts. Use of microstraining water filters capable of removing particles less than or equal to 1 micron, or using sterile water, can also reduce the risk of cryptosporidiosis.[7-9]

 ## MEDICAL TREATMENT OF CASUALTIES

There is no definitive therapeutic agent that eradicates cryptosporidiosis. The disease is self-limited in immunocompetent hosts requiring only supportive care and monitoring hydration and volume status. The disease is often sufficiently severe in immunocompromised hosts to warrant specific therapy, even though currently available therapeutic options have limited efficacy. The most commonly used medications are paromomycin and azithromycin. Paromomycin, a poorly absorbed aminogly-

CASE PRESENTATION

In late July, an urban emergency department in a major metropolitan city begins to see a large number of otherwise healthy small children with prolonged courses of diarrhea, abdominal cramps, and vomiting. An astute physician notes that all the children she has treated belong to the same daycare center. She notifies local public health authorities about these cases. Their investigation yields similar findings in numerous emergency departments in the city. The investigation also shows that numerous immunocompetent and immunocompromised adults are also experiencing this illness. Public health authorities request that stool samples be analyzed for cryptosporidia, in addition to routine ova and parasites. This testing yields many stool samples with a positive modified acid-fast stain for cryptosporidia.

The CDC and Environmental Protection Agency also become involved in the epidemiologic investigation. Water sample analysis from water treatment plants yields a heavy *Cryptosporidium* oocyst concentration at a municipal water plant that serves the daycare center and many other regions of the city. As control measures to quell the cryptosporidiosis outbreak, public health authorities change residents in the affected area to an alternative water supply, issue a boil-water advisory, and continue water sample analysis. The hunt for the source of the water contamination continues.

coside, has been shown to decrease stool frequency and oocyst excretion at doses of 2 g/day. It is approved in liquid formulation for pediatric use. Nitazoxanide, a nitrothiazole benzamide compound, has been shown to reduce both diarrhea and oocyst shedding in controlled trials conducted in Mexico; however, it is not currently approved by the Food and Drug Administration for use in the United States. Immune reconstitution in HIV disease, using highly active antiretroviral therapy (HAART), results in decreased stool frequency, weight gain, and fecal oocyst clearance. However, there is rapid relapse after discontinuation of HAART, suggesting that cryptosporidial infection had been suppressed rather than cured.[1]

 ## UNIQUE CONSIDERATIONS

C. parvum is a small, highly infectious and transmissible protozoan. These features make it a possible bioweapon and water safety threat. Although there is low mortality, there is substantial morbidity associated with cryptosporidiosis. A *Cryptosporidium* attack will be extremely difficult to identify and distinguish from routine viral gastroenteritis due to the similarity of illness presentation and lack of routine laboratory stool testing for *C. parvum*. Therefore, healthcare providers must be vigilant while treating diarrheal illness, especially in immunocompromised patients. Without appropriate supportive care and institution of paromomycin treatment, cryptosporidiosis can lead to high mortality levels in immunocompromised populations.

 ## PITFALLS

Several potential pitfalls in response to a cryptosporidiosis attack exist. These include the following:

• Failure to consider cryptosporidiosis as the cause of diarrheal illness

• Failure to request specific laboratory analysis of stool samples for *C. parvum*
• Failure to aggressively treat immunocompromised patients with diarrheal illness
• Failure to notify public health authorities about suspected or confirmed cases of cryptosporidiosis
• Failure to notify public health authorities about a suspected or confirmed cluster of patients with diarrheal illness

REFERENCES

1. Kosek M, Alcantara C, Lima A, et al. Cryptosporidiosis: an update. *Lancet Infect Dis.* 2001;1:262-9.
2. Butt A, Aldridge K, Sanders C. Infections related to the ingestion of seafood. Part II: parasitic infections and food safety. *Lancet Infect Dis.* 2004;4:294-300.
3. Guerrant RL. Cryptosporidiosis: an emerging, highly infectious threat. *Emerg Infect Dis.* 1997; 3:51-7.
4. Balbus J, Lang M. Is the water safe for my baby? *Pediatr Clin North Am.* 2001;48:1129-52.
5. Katz D, Taylor D. Parasitic infections of the gastrointestinal tract. *Gastroenterol Clin North Am.* 2001;30:797-815.
6. Chen X, Keithly JS, Paya CV, et al. Cryptosporidiosis. *N Engl J Med.* 2002;346:1723-31.
7. Addiss D, Arrowood M, Bartlett M, et al. Assessing the public health threat associated with waterborne cryptosporidiosis: report of a workshop. *MMWR* 1995;44:1-19.
8. Bongard J, Savage R, Dern R, et al. Cryptosporidium infections associated with swimming pools—Dane County, Wisconsin. *MMWR* 1994;43:561-3.
9. Weber DJ, Rutala WA. Cryptosporidiosis. *N Engl J Med.* 2002; 347:1287.

chapter 141

Introduction of Explosions and Blasts

Michael I. Greenberg and Dziwe W. Ntaba

 DESCRIPTION OF EVENT

Physics of Blast Injury

Although the exact physical parameters of bomb explosions are typically not known at the time of a given event, a basic understanding of the effects of blast wave physics can allow an estimation of the respective spectrum of blasts.[1]

An explosive blast is essentially an intense exothermic reaction generated by triggering a rapid chemical conversion of a solid or a liquid into a gas.[1-3] The resulting compressed energy release leads to detonation and a massive increase in local pressure.[4] Conventional explosive devices are typically categorized into two broad categories: "ordinary explosives" and "high explosives." *Ordinary explosives* include materials such as propellants (e.g., gunpowder) and are designed to release energy relatively slowly.[2] *High explosives* (e.g., trinitrotoluene [TNT]) are designed to detonate very rapidly, typically within only a few microseconds.[5]

As a consequence of the phase transformation mentioned above, a "pressure pulse" rapidly expands into the surrounding medium at speeds exceeding the speed of sound.[6] This expanding pressure pulse moves, as a blast wave, in all directions. The leading edge of this blast wave is known as the "blast front."[1,5] As the blast front spreads, it slows down and loses strength.[7]

The potential for a given explosive to cause injury is related to the concept of *overpressure*. Blast overpressure represents the increased pressure, in excess of atmospheric pressure, associated with a blast. It is a dynamic phenomenon wherein a highly pressurized cascade superheats air molecules with which it interacts, propelling the blast wave at supersonic speeds.[6] When the blast front encounters an object, it causes a virtually instantaneous rise in the atmospheric pressure from an ambient static pressure to a peak overpressure.[1,4,7] The duration of overpressure is typically less that 100 milliseconds (ms) for conventional explosive devices, but may exceed 100 ms for other events such as nuclear detonations.[1] With continued expansion of gases from their point of origin, the ambient pressure at a fixed point subsequently and exponentially drops below predetonation levels, temporarily creating a relative vacuum known as *underpressure*. Eventually, the blast wave deteriorates and forms acoustic waves.[6]

Substantial overpressure may impart a force of impact known as a "shock wave," which possesses a characteristic termed *brisance*, or shattering effect.[1,5] The magnitude of the shock wave at the blast front, known as *positive phase impulse*, is an important factor determining the severity of blast-related injury.[5,7] Other factors include the duration of overpressure and the medium in which it is propagated.[1] Underpressure associated with a particular explosion generates a "blast wind," which may attain speeds in excess of 800 miles/hour.[4,5] Whereas overpressure is the major force generating primary blast injury (PBI), underpressure forces are the principle mechanisms involved in producing secondary and tertiary blast injury.

Specific characteristics of the environment in which an explosion occurs are important modulators of blast effect.[1,6] Explosions occurring in an open space are associated with peak pressures and overpressure durations related to both the size and nature of the explosive charge, as well as to the distance from detonation.[1,7] Explosions in confined spaces involve reflecting surfaces that cause an extended duration of overpressure and lead to very complex wave patterns.[1] If a pressure wave is reflected from a solid object, the pressures generated from the reflecting surfaces may be more than 20 times that of the incident wave.[5,7] Consequently, a blast wave capable of causing only minor blast injury in an open space may be lethal for victims in closed spaces.[1,7] This explains the popularity of the terrorist use of explosive devices inside confined spaces such as buses. Water, due to its incompressible properties, generates a greater speed of wave propagation, and the incident wave in underwater explosions conserves energy over distance and time. The lethal radius around an explosion in water is approximately three times what it would be in air.[5,7]

Physiology of Blast Injury

The clinical spectrum of blast injury is usually described as involving primary, secondary, tertiary, and quaternary or miscellaneous blast injury. Combinations of these may also occur.

PBI is a direct result of blast overpressure forces.[1,5,6,8] Overpressure forces tend to damage air-containing organs or those made up of tissues with internal varying densities such as the ear, lungs, intestine, and brain.[6] Experimental studies conducted in the early 1940s showed that PBI of internal organs involves direct conduction of forces derived from a blast wave coming in contact with external bodily surfaces.[5]

The mechanism of blast injury, or *blast load*, can be further subdivided to include concepts of irreversible work, inertial effects, spalling, and implosion.[2,4,5] *Irreversible work* results when blast loading results in extreme pressure differentials. The resultant external force creates two forms of stress on the body known as a *stress wave* and a *shear wave*, both of which are propagated into underlying tissues.[3-6,9] The potential for injury induced by the stress wave is directly related to the peak amplitude. Damage caused by the shear wave is related to velocity.[10] *Inertial effects* may occur when two adjacent objects of different densities are acted on by the same force.[7] The lighter object accelerates faster than the denser object, creating a shearing stress at the boundary between the two.[4,5,11]

Spalling is the tendency of a boundary between two media of different densities to disrupt when a compression wave in the denser medium is reflected at the interface.[7,11] When the components of a blast wave interact with a fluid-filled organ, the velocity and potential for injury are intensified.[4,5] *Implosion* is defined as the forceful compression of a gas bubble by a shock wave in a liquid medium resulting in the pressure within the bubble rising higher than the initial compressive pressure.[7] This leads to a disruptive reexpansion of tissue.[4,5,11]

The cumulative damage of blast overpressure forces can be illustrated by examining pulmonary PBI. Blast waves tend to strike the torso in a manner similar to any form of blunt trauma.[1] Inward displacement of the chest wall causes compression of air within the lung parenchyma at a rate that is slower than the compression of the hollow respiratory tracts (inertial effects).[3,4] This leads to a contained system within the air sacs that can generate internal pressures that match or exceed the initial blast overpressures.[5] Compression and reexpansion (implosion) of the alveoli causes a form of lung injury similar to adult respiratory distress syndrome (ARDS), which is then complicated by disruption of the alveolar-capillary membrane (spalling) and potential introduction of air emboli into the vascular space.[3,4,12]

Secondary blast injury results from so-called missile effects generated by an explosion and has the broadest potential range of injury with regard to distance from the detonation site. Objects accelerated by the energy of an explosion may cause blunt and/or penetrating injuries.[5] Blast-related debris may include fragments originating from the casing of the charge (shrapnel) or secondary fragments such as pieces of glass, wood, stones, and other materials.[1] Skin and clothing may offer protection from debris at long ranges. Tiny particles of dust may be embedded in the skin, producing a discoloration known as "dust-tattooing."[1]

Tertiary blast injury results from deceleration forces after a victim's body has been set in motion by the pressure and high winds of an explosion.[1] Once a victim's body is in motion, it is at risk of injuries sustained from striking and/or being impaled with stationary objects.[5] The following survivor's recollection of an explosion in Northern Ireland presents a sobering account of body displacement:

"... as I started to pull the door open, there was a terrific noise. It was a tremendous whoosh. It was a similar noise made by a pool of petrol being ignited, only much magnified. Accompanied by this, I was aware of a great deal of debris and glass flying about. I was thrown up sideways towards the southern wall of the bar. This was as if by a terrific amount of pressure, not unlike the forces rendered by a very large sea wave. I was thrown sideways for a distance of about 6 feet..."[1]

Quaternary, or miscellaneous, blast injury is a broad category of injury including thermal and chemical burns, inhalational exposure, and crush-related trauma. Flash burns may result from heat generated by the initial explosion.[4] Conventional thermal burn injury may result from the release of hot gases, secondary fires in the surrounding environment, and contact with hot dust-laden air.[1] Chemical exposures result from the release of chemicals in the surrounding environment along with the inhalation of dust, chemically complex smokes, and carbon monoxide.[1,13] Crush injury may result in the event of structural collapse of a building after an explosion.

HISTORICAL CONTEXT

Increasing Prevalence and Lethality of Explosive Devices

An accident in the early twentieth century demonstrated to the world the potential for death and destruction from an explosive blast. In 1917 two ships, the *Imo* and the *Mont Blanc*, collided in Halifax Harbor, Nova Scotia. Their cumulative cargoes included 35 tons of benzene, 2300 tons of picric acid, 10 tons of gun cotton, 200 tons of TNT, and 300 rounds of ammunition.[14] The collision resulted in the largest manmade, non-nuclear explosion in history. Casualties reportedly included over 2000 deaths and 9000 injuries. One of the ships was reportedly blown a mile into the air. Approximately 2.5 km of the city was leveled, and the blast shattered windows 100 km away.[14]

Current events suggest that we are in the midst of a growing epidemic of terrorist bombings worldwide. The first documented terrorist bombing was probably in 1587, in Antwerp, Belgium, where 7 tons of gunpowder was used to destroy a bridge on the River Schelt.[14] There was a 10-fold increase in terrorist bombings around the world between 1968 and 1980, with 5075 events documented between 1973 and 1983.[14] From 1980 to 1990, 12,216 bombings and suspicious explosions occurred in the United States alone.[14]

Prognostic Factors and Critical Mortality Rates

An instructive terrorist explosive attack occurred in 1983 in Beirut, Lebanon, where the U.S. Marine Corps barracks was bombed using an ammonium nitrate–based explosive device with an equivalent of roughly 6 tons of

TNT. The blast resulted in the near complete collapse of a four-story building with 234 immediate deaths (68% of all victims).[14] Several first responders were killed by sniper fire from waiting terrorists carrying out a "second hit" tactic. Most of the survivors had noncritical injuries; however, 19 survivors (17%) did suffer critical injuries, and seven of these initial survivors ultimately died. Six of the seven late deaths were among victims who were rescued and treated more than 6 hours after the blast.[14] Conversely, among all initial survivors rescued within 4 hours (n = 65), only one died. The reported causes of mortality in this event included the following: (1) head trauma as the cause of immediate death (71%) and late death (57%); (2) chest trauma as the cause of overall death (29%) (rare among survivors); and (3) burns as the cause of overall death (29%).[14]

Analysis of this event provides important lessons regarding the medical response to explosive device detonation. Most striking is the effect of early and aggressive resuscitation as a key prognostic factor for long-term survival. However, expeditious evacuation and treatment must be balanced with the danger to personnel when terrorists make use of secondary devices meant to kill responder personnel.[14] Other lessons include the clear impact of both explosive magnitude and building collapse on survival and the importance of anatomic site and nature of injury as prognostic factors. In an excellent review discussing the medical response to terrorist bombings, Frykberg[14] proposed the use of a "critical mortality rate" (the death rate only among those critically injured) as an appropriate measure when calculating vital statistics for a terrorist event. Since overall mortality rates may be falsely diluted by the number of noncritical survivors, the critical mortality rate more accurately describes those victims actually at risk for death.

Triage Efficacy

A major terrorist event in Buenos Aires, Argentina, occurred when the Argentine Israeli Mutual Association (AMIA) was bombed in 1994. This explosion involved the detonation of ammonium-nitrate material (430 lb TNT-equivalent), leading to the complete collapse of a seven-story building. There were 286 casualties reported, with 82 (29%) immediate deaths.[14,15] In the immediate aftermath of the explosion, the closest hospital emergency department (ED) faced rapid overcrowding by ambulatory survivors and medical personnel offering to help. Of the 204 survivors, 40 were eventually hospitalized, 7% (n = 14) in critical condition, among whom 4 later died. These figures represent a 3.4% overall mortality rate and a 29% critical mortality rate.[15]

Among survivors, 58% (n = 50) of those who visited the ED suffered minor injuries, 12 of whom were admitted. Moderate injuries were reported among 19% (n = 16) of survivors presenting to the ED, with 13 ultimately admitted. Major injuries were reported among 21% (n = 18) of presenting patients, 12 of whom were sent directly to the operating room or intensive care unit; seven later died.[15] A total of five survivors were extricated from rubble, two of whom later died. Only five patients underwent laparotomy, and hepatic lacera-

tions were found in two of these. Three patients were found to have pneumothorax, and two others showed bilateral infiltrates consistent with PBI of lung.[15]

The AMIA bombing demonstrated that hospitals in close proximity to a major explosion suffer rapid and early overcrowding of their EDs with patients who have sustained minor and moderate injuries. This illustrates the need for disaster management plans that emphasize appropriate and effective triage to be carried out both in the field and at the ED entrance.

A retrospective analysis of triage efficiency in the AMIA bombing showed only one case of "under-triage" and four cases of "over-triage."[15] Frykberg[14] has demonstrated a linear correlation between critical mortality and the rate of over-triage in a series of terrorist bombings. He concluded, "[I]n mass casualty settings, over-triage can be as deadly as under-triage." Kluger[10] has suggested that a designated triage physician "guide medical teams as to the appropriate evaluation algorithms, considering the type of explosion (closed space vs. open space), explosive, and [presence of] metal projectiles... [and] on the proper use of auxiliary diagnostic modalities and the proper sequence of transferring patients to the operating rooms."

Building Collapse

Another example of a terrorist explosion resulting in a building collapse was the bombing of the Alfred P. Murrah Federal Building in Oklahoma City, Oklahoma, in 1995. In this incident, an ammonium nitrate–based bomb exploded with the equivalent of two tons of TNT, causing 759 total casualties with a 21% immediate mortality rate (n = 162).[16] Fourteen percent of survivors (n = 83) were hospitalized, of which 52 were critically injured. Five of these later died (representing a 9.6% critical mortality rate).[16] As with the AMIA bombing, the highest mortality and most severe morbidity in Oklahoma City occurred among victims who were located in collapsed portions of buildings at the time of blast.[16]

There were 506 survivors of the Oklahoma City bombing. The injury pattern among survivors included 85% who suffered soft tissue injuries, including lacerations, abrasions, contusions, and puncture wounds.[16] Among survivors, 210 (35%) were reported to have musculoskeletal injury, with 60 patients suffering from fractures and/or dislocations and the remainder suffering from various sprains and/or strains. Smaller numbers of patients had severe soft tissue or musculoskeletal injuries.[16]

Head injuries were reported in 80 survivors, with 44% of these hospitalized (n = 35).[16] Severe head injury was reported in eight patients, with four open skull fractures, two subdural hemorrhages, and two depressed skull fractures. Of 59 reported ocular injuries, there were nine ruptured globes, four of which were accompanied by detached retina.[16] Internal organ injuries included four patients with intra-abdominal injury (lacerated spleen, kidney, liver, and partial bowel transection), four patients with ARDS, six patients with pneumothorax (four closed, one open, one hemopneumothorax), and three patients with pulmonary contusions.[16]

Severe burns (up to 70% body surface area) were reported in nine survivors, seven of whom were hospitalized. Four of these patients were near the point of detonation at the time of the blast.[16] Auditory damage was found in 35% of survivors by self-report (n = 210), but only 78 of these patients had a documented medical diagnosis of auditory damage. Tympanic membrane perforation (unilateral or bilateral) was reported in 22 patients. Tinnitus, vestibular injury, or otalgia was reported in 12 patients.[16]

The majority of survivors of the Oklahoma City bombing incurred injuries caused by flying glass, other debris, and collapsed ceilings. A review of this event by Mallonee and colleagues[16] suggests that the role of building collapse and flying glass should be a consideration in future building designs and in retrofitting of existing buildings. In addition, the National Research Council has published recommendations on blast hardening technologies.[17]

Open Air versus Confined Space

Another important variable affecting the pattern of injury involves the occurrence of blast within a confined space. Leibovici and colleagues[18] compared open air (OA) versus confined space (CS) terrorist bombings in Israel. This was a review of 297 victims from four separate events—two OA bombings and two bus bombings. The explosive devices used and victim density in proximity to each bomb were similar in all four incidents. The authors compared PBI, significant penetrating trauma, and injury severity score between the OA group and the CS group. A higher incidence of mortality and a greater severity of morbidity was reported from CS explosions, compared with a higher total volume of injuries in the OA settings.[18] In addition, a higher incidence of PBI was seen in the CS group. These findings may be due to unique blast wave behavior within the relatively small confined spaces of buses.[18]

The two OA explosions in this review occurred at a bus station and a marketplace. Of the 15 fatalities in the OA group, only one died after admission to hospital. The two CS explosions reviewed both happened on buses, and there were fewer total casualties but a significantly higher mortality rate (Table 141-1). Of the 46 fatalities in the CS group, five died after admission to the hospital, all from injuries that were secondary to pulmonary PBI.[18]

There was a similar incidence of mild injury in both the OA and CS groups, with an injury pattern that included psychological stress, auditory damage with intact tympanic membrane (TM), and minor penetrating/musculoskeletal trauma. However, among the severely injured patients in both groups, the OA population had a lower overall injury severity and more favorable initial clinical presentation than those in the CS comparison group.[18]

Published reports of predominantly outdoor bombings tend to show consistent patterns of mostly noncritical injuries with relatively low immediate and late death rates. A review by Adler and others[2] discussed terrorist bombings occurring between 1975 and 1979, in Jerusalem, Israel. Various locales included 19 OA (e.g., seashore, street, marketplace) and five CS settings (bus, other public transport). Of the total 511 casualties, 340 were evacuated to an ED with 272 hospital admissions, three of which later died of their injuries. Injury severity was recorded using an Abbreviated Injury Scale (AIS), with results showing 87% "light," 3% "medium," and 10% "severe" injuries at presentation in the ED.[2]

These reviews clearly describe an increased mortality for victims of CS bombings. Survivors of CS bombings suffer from more severe injuries, as well as burns with a larger surface area compared with survivors from OA bombings. CS victims have a higher incidence of PBI than OA victims, particularly pulmonary PBI. Leibovici and colleagues[18] postulated that the mechanism of increased mortality and severity of injury among CS explosions was linked due to the relatively sustained and markedly increased amplitude of overpressure (generated by comparatively similar explosive charges) as a result of reflective phenomenon within the confined spaces. The more extensive and severe burns in the CS group were thought to be due to containment of an initial fireball generated on detonation within the closed space. Conversely, the OA group showed a larger number of total casualties because these explosions were not contained within a closed space, therefore bomb fragments and other shrapnel were ejected to a considerable distance, with a capacity to injure more people.[18] Other important lessons included the observation that the AIS score established in the ED was a valid prognostic factor when used to triage patients. Specifically, ED use of AIS scores correlated very well with subsequent and more detailed injury severity score on follow-up.[2]

MEDICAL TREATMENT OF CASUALTIES

The most common injury patterns seen among explosion survivors are due to secondary and tertiary blast injury.[19] The incidence of PBI varies according to explosive charge, proximity of the victim to the blast, and the

---

TABLE 141-1 CHARACTERISTICS OF OPEN AIR (OA) VERSUS CONFINED SPACE (CS) BOMBINGS

SETTING	MORTALITY RATE	PULMONARY PBI	AUDITORY PBI	GI PBI	VICTIMS ADMITTED TO HOSPITAL	BURNS: BSA AFFECTED
OA (n = 209)	7.8%	6.8%	12.1%	0%	13.1%	18.3%
CS (n = 93)	49.5%	57.6%	40.4%	3.8%	59.6%	31.4%

PBI, primary blast injury; GI, gastrointestinal; BSA, body surface area.

environment in which it occurs.[3,13] However, given the general lack of familiarity with the assessment and management of PBI among U.S. civilian medical personnel, the following discussion will emphasize PBI at the expense of the more commonly encountered mixture of secondary and tertiary blast injury.

Anatomically, the structures at greatest risk for PBI are the auditory system, thorax, and abdomen.[11,13,19,20] The greatest potential for avoiding preventable deaths due to PBI lies in the appropriate treatment of thoracic PBI. Although injuries to the central nervous system (CNS) and extremities may involve some contribution from PBI, most of the injury burden to these areas results from the secondary and tertiary forms of blast injury. Survivors of explosions that occur in confined spaces or underwater may manifest a higher incidence of PBI.[3,18] Most severely injured survivors of blasts have multiple injuries.[10]

Primary Stabilization

As with any trauma patient, initial management begins with conventional priorities outlined in the advanced trauma life support protocols, which have been well described elsewhere. There are, however, several important caveats unique to the stabilization of a patient with suspected PBI. These include the potentially harmful consequences of prehospital intubation and the need for cautious fluid resuscitation. The potential for prehospital pain relief to mask latent abdominal PBI may be a valid concern.[21] Wherever possible, blast victims should be kept at rest because some reports describe an increase in mortality in victims undergoing strenuous activity after an explosion.[7,13]

Auditory Injury

The ear is the organ most frequently injured by an explosion.[9] However, auditory PBI is frequently overlooked in the context of more serious co-existing injuries during mass-casualty scenarios.[6] The auditory system is uniquely predisposed to PBI because the TM acts as an efficient means for transmitting pressure waves to the middle and inner ear.[3,7] Auditory PBI rarely requires emergent intervention, and the important considerations involve recognition and appropriate referral to reduce long-term morbidity.[9] All survivors of blast should have an otologic assessment and audiometry at some time in their aftercare.[3,6]

Symptoms of auditory PBI include tinnitus, otalgia, and a feeling of aural fullness.[9] Perforation of the TM is a hallmark of auditory PBI and is typically seen as multiple "punched out" lesions or radial lacerations.[6] The pars tensa is usually involved.[3,5,7] Other signs include hearing loss, blood and/or debris in the ear canal, and disruption of the ossicles.[13] The presence of tinnitus and hearing loss may be initially profound; however, these findings are usually self-limited and both improve quickly.[3] Prolonged duration of these symptoms may be seen in survivors of blast occurring in confined spaces.[9]

Vertigo is uncommonly due to auditory PBI, and its presence should prompt evaluation for neurologic injury.[6,13] The complication of perilymph fistula should be considered in a patient with vertigo and sensorineural hearing loss, particularly if these findings are fluctuating. This is the only component of auditory PBI requiring prompt surgical treatment (i.e., emergent tympanotomy and fistula repair).[3] Cholesteatoma may be a late complication (12 to 48 months) of TM perforation.[3,6,22]

Eighty percent of TM perforations heal spontaneously, and nonoperative management is appropriate for most cases.[3,6,9,13] Large perforations may warrant surgical repair, but elective tympanoplasty can safely be delayed for up to 12 months with good outcomes.[3] Antibiotics are not indicated unless underlying infection is suspected.[6]

It is important to note that TM perforation correlates poorly with PBI involving other organ systems and should not be used as a marker of latent PBI elsewhere in the body.[3] In a study of 647 survivors of explosion, 9.3% had blast lung in the absence of TM rupture.[8] Furthermore, of those survivors with *isolated* TM rupture at initial presentation, none went on to develop PBI of the lungs or intestine.[8] Current evidence suggests that patients presenting with TM perforations in the absence of clinical features of other blast injuries, and with a chest radiograph having a normal appearance, may be safely discharged after 6 hours of observation.[8]

Thoracic Injury

PBI has been shown to be a major cause of death in patients who survive initial resuscitation from blast injury.[4,12] PBI involving the respiratory system can lead to a constellation of findings known as "blast lung."[1,7,13] Blast lung injury (BLI) involves pulmonary hemorrhage, edema, and associated disruption of alveolar architecture leading to air embolism.[3,11,12] Gross lesions can range from scattered or multifocal petechiae to large confluent hemorrhages involving an entire lung.[3,6] Certain regions of the lung tend to be more severely affected, including lung parenchyma proximal to the mediastinum and in the costophrenic angles.[4] Bruising of the intercostal spaces has also been observed and paradoxically called *rib markings*.[3,6] Pleural and subpleural hemorrhages tend to be bilateral but are usually more extensive on the side facing the source of blast.[5,6] Recent studies show that the prognosis from BLI is significantly improved with aggressive treatment.[12,23] Victims of explosions within confined spaces are at considerably greater risk of BLI.[12]

The etiology of BLI may be associated with disruption of alveolar membranes and interalveolar septa via implosion and spalling caused by the blast wave leading to shearing of the lung parenchyma from vascular structures with subsequent hemorrhage into the distal branches of the respiratory tree.[1,3-6,12,13] These changes cause a ventilation-perfusion mismatch and reduced compliance resulting in hypoxia and increased work of breathing.[3,5,13]

Traumatic alveolar-capillary fistulae may form, and air may be introduced into blood vessels leading to air embolism.[3,12] Carotid artery doppler ultrasound studies have demonstrated showers of intravascular bubbles in blast-injured animals for up to 30 minutes after exposure, suggesting that PBI can affect the CNS.[7,20] Ultrastructural damage of type II epithelial cells may disrupt surfactant production and further exacerbate pulmonary injury.[3,6]

Progressive pulmonary insufficiency has been described in many patients with BLI and is thought to be due to the cumulative effect of several mechanisms including blast effects, inhalation injury, hypovolemic shock, sepsis, aspiration and/or aggressive fluid resuscitation.[6] Clinically, the pulmonary function of patients with BLI resembles pulmonary contusion and ARDS with symptoms including dyspnea, difficulty completing sentences in one breath, cough, hemoptysis, and chest pain.[3,5,7] Clinical findings associated with BLI include tachypnea with rapid, shallow breathing; poor chest wall movement (due to decreased compliance); dullness to percussion; decreased air movement; hemopneumothorax; subcutaneous emphysema; and retinal artery emboli.[3,5,6,11,24] The diagnosis is suspected on clinical grounds and is subsequently confirmed with radiographs. Signs and symptoms usually develop within hours after an explosion but may be delayed as long as 24 to 48 hours.[3,12]

Chest radiography is required for all patients exposed to blast forces to gauge the initial severity of injury and to monitor progression. Diffuse pulmonary opacities may develop within a few hours and will become maximal within 24 to 48 hours. They typically occur in a "butterfly distribution" of bilateral patchy infiltrates.[25] Any changes that develop after 48 hours will most likely be due to complications such as ARDS or pneumonia.[13] Other radiologic findings may include hemopneumothorax, pneumomediastinum, subdiaphragmatic free air, subcutaneous emphysema, and foreign body impaction.[13,25] Computed tomography (CT) of the chest is not currently part of the routine evaluation, but some authors suggest a role for it in select patients because CT has shown a higher sensitivity than x-ray in the detection of early parenchymal lesions in patients with non–blast-related pulmonary contusion. CT may be useful in predicting which patients will require mechanical ventilation.[3]

Although the general management of BLI is similar to that of pulmonary contusion and ARDS, the relatively higher risk of significant barotrauma (i.e., alveolar rupture, systemic air emboli, and pneumothorax) in patients incurring BLI is a critically important feature.[3,12,23] Persistent observations show that the use of positive pressure ventilation, especially high levels of positive end-expiratory pressure, increases the risk of and/or the exacerbation of pulmonary barotrauma and should therefore be avoided whenever possible.[6,13,23,26] Furthermore, patients with BLI may be at increased risk of pulmonary complication related to overly aggressive fluid resuscitation.[3,6,26]

Various strategies aimed at ameliorating these risks have shown some success, including (1) permissive hypercapnia with a reduction of tidal volume and peak inspiratory pressure, (2) use of intermittent mechanical ventilation and continuous positive airway pressure to facilitate reversion to spontaneous breathing as soon as possible, and (3) prophylactic insertion of chest tubes.[3,6,12,13,18,23,26] Patients with unknown neurologic status pose a particular challenge for the use of permissive hypercapnia because of concerns regarding increased intracranial pressure. Some authors recommend bilateral tube thoracostomy for pulmonary PBI patients requiring aeromedical evacuation.[3,6] The use of dual-lumen endotracheal tubes (i.e., independent lung ventilation) or high-frequency jet ventilation is recommended for patients with bronchopleural fistulae.[5,12]

Case reports have shown that high-frequency jet ventilation provides adequate oxygenation, whereas superimposed low-frequency positive pressure ventilation can improve ventilation with the lowest possible airway pressures.[12] Expeditious use of hyperbaric oxygen therapy has been shown to reduce mortality in animal models and has been recommended in humans with BLI, although convincing evidence supporting this practice in humans is lacking.[6,13,26] Extracorporeal membrane oxygenation has been used, but this modality is controversial.[3,18,23,26]

A retrospective study of patients sustaining BLI from explosions on civilian buses in Israel established that the first 24 hours after injury constitute a critical period for effective management.[12] These authors proposed that a BLI severity score (BLISS) may be useful in the initial stabilization phase to direct treatment and predict outcome. The BLISS is derived from objective signs of hypoxemia, chest radiograph findings, and the presence of bronchopleural fistula.[12] Based on the initial BLISS, none of the patients in this study who were classified as mildly injured went on to develop any form of lung injury. Of those classified as moderately injured, 33% went on to develop ARDS. All those classified as severely injured either developed ARDS or later died.[12]

Most importantly, this study showed that aggressive and complex interventions, guided by stratification of BLI severity, can lead to dramatic improvements in outcome. A follow-up study showed that most patients who survive BLI will regain good lung function within 1 year, although most of the patients involved were relatively young and healthy.[27]

Cardiovascular Injury

In addition to conventional causes of hemodynamic instability seen in trauma patients, there are special factors particular to the management of victims with suspected blast injury. Although there are numerous reports of changes in heart rate and blood pressure that are thought to be due to effects of PBI, much of what is known about the PBI of the cardiovascular system has been gleaned from experimental studies in animal models.[5] Beginning in World War I, it was observed that "men subjected to the concussion of large shells often developed a condition of shock that was unrelated to obvious trauma since no external wounds were visible."[6]

A World War II study of 200 casualties assessed *immediately* after blast exposure showed that more than 25% of them had heart rates of less than 60 bpm and that over 90% had heart rates of less than 80 bpm. This review also found that hypotension was nearly universal, with blood pressures of 80 to 90 mm Hg (systolic) and 40 to 50 mm Hg (diastolic) being common.[28] The bradycardia observed after blast exposure has been consistently reproduced in animal studies and may be a vagal effect as experiments have shown the bradycardia can be prevented with bilateral vagotomy.[28,29]

Irwin and colleagues[29] proposed that vagally mediated cardiovascular changes in humans are initiated by the so-called pulmonary defensive reflex. This reflex acts when acute pulmonary congestion and edema lead to fluid shifts in the lung, stimulating pulmonary C-fibers and triggering increased cholinergic activity with consequent systemic effects. This mechanism is supported by the clinical observation of brief periods of apnea after blast exposure, followed by rapid shallow respirations.[3,24] This phenomenon has been observed in experimental blast injury models using artificial stimulation of pulmonary C-fibers.[29]

The hypotension observed in the World War II study has also been reproduced in animal simulations. Several studies have reported a greater than 50% decrease in mean arterial pressure in animals immediately after blast exposure, with spontaneous resolution over time.[6,11,30]

Clinically, the contribution of these various mechanisms for cardiovascular PBI may be complicated by co-existing factors such as hemorrhage. Given the importance of judicious fluid administration (including blood products) for appropriate cardiorespiratory resuscitation, in the context of potentially exacerbating soft tissue injury with suboptimal fluid resuscitation, invasive monitoring to guide therapy is often necessary.[2,3,13,26] Colloid solutions are generally the resuscitation fluid of choice.

Various electrocardiographic changes have been observed immediately after blast and are also thought to be due to blunt thoracic trauma and/or coronary air emboli.[6,29] These may include atrioventricular and bundle branch blocks, nonspecific ventricular ectopy, low-voltage QRS complexes, and T-wave and ST-segment abnormalities. Blast-induced electrocardiographic changes typically revert to normal sinus rhythm within a few minutes but may deteriorate into sustained dysrhythmias, including lethal ventricular arrhythmias. Ischemic changes may also occur due to complications of air emboli.[6,29]

Abdominal Injury

Nonlethal abdominal PBI is almost exclusively found in gas-containing organs and is likely caused by forces including shearing, spalling, and implosion. Solid organ damage may present as subcapsular hematomas or lacerations of the liver, spleen, and kidney.[3,6,7] These injuries are thought to be due to acceleration-deceleration caused by either the initial effects of the blast wave and/or from secondary and tertiary mechanisms of injury.[5,13] The incidence of intestinal PBI may be higher in victims of underwater or CS explosions.

The classic lesions of intestinal PBI involve small, multifocal intramural hematomas. These are morphologically similar to those caused by blunt abdominal trauma.[31] Initial bleeding in submucosal regions may range from scattered petechiae or large confluent hematomas.[3,6] Partial- or full-thickness lacerations may occur and may lead to immediate or delayed perforation of the bowel.[5] Since the ileocecal region and colon are the most likely areas to contain gas, these areas are the most prone to perforation during blast exposure.[2,6,7]

Since it is relatively uncommon, intestinal PBI presents a particular diagnostic challenge. Signs and symptoms of intestinal PBI include abdominal or testicular pain, nausea, vomiting, tenderness, absence of bowel sounds, and other peritoneal signs. Initial evaluation may be complicated by the overall acuity of a multiply injured patient or prior administration of pain-control medication.

Gastrointestinal injury may be delayed as long as 48 hours after initial blast exposure.[6] However, this may be more often due to latent injury with delayed perforation as opposed to delayed diagnosis.[21] No reliable clinical predictors exist to help clinicians determine which patients may progress to delayed perforation.[6]

Abdominal CT, ultrasound, and diagnostic peritoneal lavage have been shown to be useful modalities for the evaluation of intestinal PBI.[5,12] Kluger[10] reported that diagnostic peritoneal lavage is particularly useful when treating blast injuries involving abdominal wall penetration by multiple metal projectiles. Colonoscopy has been suggested for the surveillance of large bowel contusions. But given the potential for iatrogenic perforation, colonoscopy may be ill advised in the post-blast period.[3] Indications for urgent laparotomy are similar to those established for blunt abdominal trauma.[3]

Musculoskeletal/Extremity Injury

Most blast injuries involving the musculoskeletal system are due to secondary and tertiary blast injury. There are numerous reports of traumatic amputation in blast victims that are thought to be due to PBI, but these injuries are rare among survivors.[3] Blast-related amputations often traverse the proximal third of the tibia but rarely traverse joints such as the ankle and knee. This anatomic distribution may reflect an initial disruption of soft tissue and bone by the incident shock wave, followed by completion of the amputation by other components of overpressure forces.[32]

In an extensive review, Covey[33] discussed important considerations in the physical examination of blast injuries of the musculoskeletal system. He highlighted the following: "(1) fragments do not always travel in straight lines, (2) small tissue wounds may be associated with extensive internal injury, (3) entry wounds in the buttocks, thighs, or peritoneum can be associated with intra-abdominal injury, (4) a high degree of suspicion for compartment syndrome should be maintained, and (5) an entry wound in the groin, or hematoma elsewhere may mean major vascular injury."

The conventional military approach to small fragment wounds has involved treating penetrating wounds in an aggressive fashion with early exploration, debridement, and delayed primary closure.[33,34] However, recent evidence suggests that a more conservative approach may be appropriate provided that bacterial colonization is prevented with appropriate antibiotic coverage.[34] Bowyer[34] reported success with a conservative approach when the following criteria were met: (1) involvement of soft tissue only with no breach of pleura or peritoneum and no major vascular involvement and (2) an entry or exit wound of less than 2 cm in maximum dimension that was (3) not frankly infected and (4) not caused by a mine blast.

Although successful in wartime, nonoperative treatment of fragment wounds remains controversial. Microbial threats to fragment wounds include *Clostridium* species and *Pseudomonas* species for severely contaminated and high-grade open fractures.[33] Appropriate antimicrobial coverage should be administered and tetanus immunization addressed. Primary closure of blast wounds greatly increases the risk of infection; therefore delayed primary closure is performed once the wound is clean and granulation tissue has appeared.[33]

CNS Injury

CNS injury from explosions is an important entity because secondary and tertiary injuries to the head are common and are leading causes of immediate (71%) and delayed mortality (52%).[3,14] Arterial air emboli may cause secondary damage to the CNS and are important causes of immediate death among blast victims.[6,13] Although PBI of the CNS is poorly understood, there is increasing evidence that this mechanism may be a factor. Anxiety and adjustment reactions are nearly universal among survivors of explosions. Posttraumatic stress disorder (PTSD) is to be expected in victims and their families as well as in the responders and medical providers who care for them.

Signs and symptoms of CNS PBI include headache, vertigo, ataxia, seizures, altered mental status, retinal artery emboli, tongue blanching, and anterograde or retrograde amnesia.[2] If any of these findings are present, immediate administration of adequate oxygen therapy is appropriate. Expeditious administration of hyperbaric oxygen may be helpful for suspected CNS PBI. Previous recommendations of placing the patient in Trendelenburg's position to avoid complications of arterial air emboli should be abandoned; the left lateral decubitus position with the head down is instead recommended.[13] There have been several reports of transient motor paralysis with sensory preservation that may be due to blast effects on peripheral nerves.[20,29]

PTSD may also have an organic basis linked to CNS PBI. Cernak and others[35] have speculated that behavioral alterations observed in the posttraumatic period, in the absence of structural changes, may be due to a variety of chemical alterations in the CNS after blast exposure. They report a substantially increased incidence of PTSD in patients after blast exposure. Mental health referral for blast victims is indicated for general counseling and surveillance of serious postincident morbidity. Critical incident stress debriefing sessions for providers are recommended.

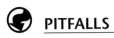 **PITFALLS**

A variety of pitfalls may be encountered when evaluating and managing survivors of blast injury incidents.

Perhaps the most critical issue in mass-casualty scenarios involves meeting the requirement for precise and effective triage. Several scoring systems with proven effectiveness have been developed or adapted for use in evaluating blast injury patients (e.g., AIS and BLI scores).[2,12]

Physicians and emergency medical systems that traditionally err on the side of over-triage in everyday operations must understand the direct relationship between over-triage and increased mortality observed in terrorist events.[14] Understanding the epidemiology of past explosion scenarios will help providers allocate resources appropriately. For example, survivors of CS explosions will present with a much higher incidence of PBI than survivors of OA explosions, who tend to have predominantly fragmentation injuries.[3,12]

Experience shows that auditory injuries are commonly underestimated or overlooked during initial evaluation. The possibility of missing latent gastrointestinal injuries with the potential for delayed perforation must be kept in mind. Patients who are exposed to a significant blast with subsequent depressed mental status or after taking narcotic analgesics are at increased risk of missed diagnoses. Some authors recommend that such patients be observed for at least 48 hours and undergo serial abdominal examinations.[7,21]

Providers should anticipate a high incidence of psychological stress after an explosion and should make appropriate management referrals to minimize long-term morbidity and loss of productivity among survivors.

Overly aggressive fluid resuscitation, which may be complicated by failure to recognize transient PBI-induced cardiovascular changes (e.g., hypotension, bradycardia), is an important pitfall. However, concomitant soft tissue injuries and burns requiring intensive fluid resuscitation are common. Therefore, meticulous attention to fluid balance and judicious use of fluid infusions are of paramount importance. Invasive monitoring is considered the standard of care in patients with suspected pulmonary PBI who require fluid management.

The use of positive pressure ventilation in suspected pulmonary PBI is a well-established hazard due to the risk of progressive respiratory failure and air embolism. Patients who have incurred BLI reportedly do not tolerate anesthesia well, so regional or spinal anesthesia should be considered whenever possible.[7,13,26] Although oxygen administration is indicated in all patients with signs of respiratory distress or air embolism, oxygen toxicity may result. Dilation of the pulmonary vasculature in response to supplemental oxygen may exacerbate pulmonary hemorrhage.[6]

REFERENCES

1. Cooper G, Maynard R, Cross N, et al. Casualties from terrorist bombings. *J Trauma.* 1983;23:955-67.
2. Adler J, Golan E, Golan J, et al. Terrorist bombing experience during 1975-79: casualties admitted to the Sharre Zedek Medical Center. *Israel J Med Sci.* 1983;19:189-93.
3. Horrocks C. Blast injuries: biophysics, pathophysiology, and management principles. *J R Army Med Corps.* 2001;147:28-40.

4. Mellor S. The relationship between blast loading to death and injury from explosion. *World J Surg.* 1992;16:893-98.

5. Wightman J, Gladish S. Explosions and blast injuries. *Ann Emerg Med.* 2001;37:664-78.

6. Guy R, Glover M, Cripps N. The pathophysiology of primary blast injury and it's implications for treatment. Part I: the thorax. *J R Nav Med Serv.* 1998;84:79-86.

7. Philips Y. Primary blast injuries. *Ann Emerg Med.* 1986; 15:12;1446-50.

8. Leibovici D, Gofrit O, Shapira S. Eardrum perforation in explosion survivors: is it a marker pf pulmonary blast injury? *Ann Emerg Med.* 1999;34:168-72.

9. Cohen J, Ziv G, Bloom J, et al. Blast injury of the ear in confined space explosion: auditory and vestibular evaluation. *Israel Med Assoc J.* 2002;4:559-62.

10. Kluger Y. Bomb explosions in acts of terrorism: detonation, wound ballistics, triage and medical concerns. *Israel Med Assoc J.* 2003;5:235-40.

11. Irwin R, Lerner M, Bealer J, et al. Cardiopulmonary physiology of primary blast injury. *J Trauma.* 1997;43:650-55.

12. Pizov R, Oppenheim-Eden A, Matot I, et al. Blast injuries from an explosion on a civilian bus. *Chest* 1999;115:165-72.

13. Argyros GJ. Management of primary blast injury. *Toxicology.* 1997;121:105-15.

14. Frykberg ER. Medical management of disasters and mass casualties from terrorist bombings: how can we cope? *J Trauma.* 2002;53:201-12.

15. Biancolini C. Argentine Jewish community institution bomb explosion. *J Trauma.* 1999;47:728-32.

16. Mallonee S, Shariat S, Stennies G, et al. Physical injuries and fatalities resulting from the Oklahoma City bombing. *JAMA* 1996; 276:382-7.

17. National Research Council. *Protecting Buildings from Bomb Damage: Transfer of Blast Effects Mitigation Technologies from Military to Civilian Applications.* Washington, DC: National Academy Press; 1995.

18. Leibovici D, Gofrit O, Stein M, et al. Blast injuries: bus versus open-air bombings—a cooperative study of injuries in survivors of open-air versus confined-space explosions. *J Trauma.* 1996; 41:1030-35.

19. Hadden W, Rutherford W, Merrit J, et al. The injuries of terrorist bombing: a study of 1532 consecutive patients. *Br J Surg.* 1978;65:525-31.

20. Guy R, Glover M, Cripps N. The pathophysiology of primary blast injury and it's implications for treatment. Part III: injury to the central nervous system and the limbs. *J Roy Nav Med Serv.* 2000;86:27-31.

21. Paran H, Neufeld D, Shwartz I, et al. Perforation of the terminal Ileum induced by blast injury: delayed diagnosis or delayed perforation? *J Trauma.* 1996;30:472-75.

22. Kronenberg J, Ben-Shoshan J, Wolf M. Perforated tympanic membrane after blast injury. *Am J Otolaryngol.* 1993;14:92-4.

23. Sorkine P, Szold O, Kluger Y, et al. Permissive hypercapnia ventilation in patients with severe pulmonary blast injury. *J Trauma.* 1998;45:35-8.

24. Cernak I, Savic J, Dragan I, et al. Blast injury from explosive munitions. *J Trauma.* 1999;47:96-103.

25. Shaham D, Sella T, Makori A, et al. The role of radiology in terror injuries. *Isr Med Assoc J.* 2002;4:564-7.

26. Weiler-Ravell D, Adatto R, Borman J, et al. Blast injury of the chest. *Israel J Med Sci.* 1975;11:268-74.

27. Hirshberg B, Oppenheimer-Eden A, Pizov R, et al. Recovery from blast lung injury: one year follow up. *Chest* 1999;116:1683-8.

28. Barrow DW, Rhoads HY. Blast concussion injury. *JAMA* 1944;125:900-2.

29. Irwin R, Lerner M, Bealer J, et al. Shock after blast wave injury is caused by vagally mediated reflex. *J Trauma.* 1999;47:105-10.

30. Guy R, Kirkman E, Watkins P, et al. Physiologic response to primary blast. *J Trauma.* 1998;45:983-87.

31. Cripps N, Glover M, Guy R. The pathophysiology of primary blast injury and it's implications for treatment. Part II: the auditory structures and then abdomen. *J Roy Nav Med Serv.* 1999;85: 13-24.

32. Hull J. Traumatic amputation by explosive blast: pattern of injury in survivors. *Br J Surg.* 1992;79:1389-92.

33. Covey DC. Blast and fragment injuries of the musculoskeletal system. *J Bone Joint Surg Am.* 2002;84:1221-34.

34. Bowyer GW. Management of small fragment wounds: experience from the Afghan border. *J Trauma.* 1996;40(suppl 3):S170-2.

35. Cernak I, Savic J, Zunic G, et al. Involvement of the central nervous system in the general response to pulmonary blast injury. *J Trauma.* 1996;40:S100-4.

chapter 142

Explosions: Conventional

Robert Partridge

 ## DESCRIPTION OF EVENT

Explosions occur when solid or liquid material is rapidly transformed into a gas with sudden energy release. High explosives, such as trinitrotoluene (TNT) or other nitrate compounds, detonate very rapidly and release large amounts of energy capable of causing blast injuries as well as severe structural damage. Conventional explosions and blasts occur as a result of unintentional civilian incidents (e.g., explosive detonation during ship or truck transport), intentional and unintentional detonation of military ordinance, and terrorist attacks. Powerful explosions have the potential to inflict many different types of traumatic injuries on humans, but such injuries can vary depending on the type and amount of explosive agent, the location of the victims (inside or outside), and whether the blast occurs on air or water.

Conventional explosions cause physical trauma by three mechanisms. *Primary* blast injury (PBI) results from the damage to human tissue from the sudden change in atmospheric pressure that propagates from the explosion (i.e., blast wave). *Secondary* blast injury occurs as debris accelerated by the blast strikes the victim, causing blunt or penetrating trauma. *Tertiary* blast injury occurs as the body of the victim is thrown onto the ground or into fixed objects as a result of the blast. In addition, *quaternary* injury can occur from inhalation of smoke or hot gases, carbon monoxide poisoning, fire, or structural collapse.

The damage caused by PBI is a type of barotrauma that primarily affects gas-containing organs—the lungs, ears, and gastrointestinal tract. The degree of tissue injury is directly related to the magnitude and duration of the maximum overpressure of the blast wave. Most victims of primary blast lung injury are killed immediately, often as a result of massive coronary or cerebral air embolism. Other immediate deaths are attributed to severe multisystem injury due to secondary and tertiary blast injury. The majority of survivors will experience trauma caused by secondary, tertiary, or quaternary blast injury.

PBI must be considered in all victims exposed to an explosion, even if there are no external signs of injury. Severe pulmonary manifestations include hemorrhage, barotrauma, and arterial air embolism, and gastrointestinal manifestations would include hemorrhage and hollow viscous perforation. Of the small number of survivors with lung PBI, deaths may occur by progressive pulmonary insufficiency. These lesions appear similar to pulmonary contusion, both radiographically and pathologically.[1,2]

Indoor detonations or explosions within a vehicle appear to cause more severe PBIs than open-air bombings because the blast wave is magnified rather than dissipated as it is reflected off the floor, walls, and ceiling.[3,4] The type of explosion and victim location at the time of the blast must be considered when managing blast injury.

 ## PREINCIDENT ACTIONS

Conventional explosions can occur anywhere, at any time, with variable numbers of casualties. For these reasons, there is little a person can do to prepare for a conventional explosion. However, communities can be prepared for such an event. Other than safety and law enforcement measures designed to prevent an explosion, the most effective preincident actions involve establishing an effective security, rescue, and medical infrastructure.

One of the major determinants of mortality from conventional bombings is the availability of medical resources at the disaster scene. Explosions occurring in or near major cities with established prehospital systems, emergency departments, and advanced trauma care would be expected to have lower mortality rates than remote areas or areas with less advanced medical systems and longer rescue and transport times. Medical management of blast victims is also enhanced if help is available beyond the community affected and if there is an ability to transfer victims to other medical facilities. In addition, the panic, chaos, and emotional trauma of large conventional explosions can worsen morbidity and mortality. A plan for prompt leadership; coordination of security, rescue, and medical agencies involved in the disaster; and a preexisting plan for rapid rescue, disposition, and treatment of casualties can reduce this risk.[3,5-8]

 ## POSTINCIDENT ACTIONS

Previous disasters involving conventional explosions have demonstrated that safety and protection of first responders and medical personnel is the most important

745

initial action. In both terrorist bombings and other non-military explosions, scene safety is the first priority for all responders, because of the risk of being struck by falling or unstable debris or becoming victims of a secondary explosion.[7] Keeping medical personnel away from the scene of an explosion reduces their risk of injury from such events. Because first responders are trained to rescue and help victims, any secondary explosion and incapacitation of these persons would greatly impair subsequent rescue efforts.[9]

Immediately after a blast, rescue, police, and emergency medical services (EMS) personnel will be the first to care for casualties. Responders should not enter the blast scene until the incident commander has declared the area safe. Most victims will have traumatic injuries resulting from secondary and tertiary blast injury. EMS personnel should observe standard trauma protocols for management of these injuries.

EMS personnel should assess casualties for PBI. A careful assessment of the scene can give clues to the potential for PBI. The presence of a crater or a building collapse are indicators of high blast strength. An assessment of crater size and structural damage and the location and time of the explosion may be useful in estimating the number of casualties and the likelihood of PBI. Blast peak overpressures in unobstructed open-air explosions are directly related to the explosive force of the blast and inversely proportional to the distance from the explosion.[10] The further away a person is from a blast, the less likely he or she is develop severe PBI. The location and position that victims were in at the time of the blast should be noted. Reflected blast waves are even more likely to cause PBI. Solid surfaces that can reflect blast waves create a zone of very highly pressurized air as the blast wave is reflected back on itself.[11,12] Rigid shields between a person and an explosion may reduce the risk of secondary blast injury but may not prevent significant PBI.[13,14] Victims in close proximity to an explosion may have PBI only, and may initially appear uninjured. Because physical activity after PBI can result in a poorer outcome, EMS personnel must ensure that these persons are not physically active until evaluation and observation for PBI is complete.

Injuries sustained from underwater PBI are different than those in open-air blasts. Because blast waves are reflected back underwater from the water-air surface boundary and interact with direct blast waves, greater blast loads are transmitted to the more deeply submerged parts of the victim. If a victim is submerged in a vertical position, particular concern should be raised for the possibility of PBI in the lower segments of the lungs or gastrointestinal tract. PBI to the bowel, including acute or delayed presentations of bowel perforation in addition to lower gastrointestinal bleeding, may occur in partially submerged victims of underwater blasts.[2,15]

MEDICAL TREATMENT OF CASUALTIES

Management of casualties after a blast event initially involves gathering as much information as possible to assess the potential for PBI, including the force of the blast, victim location inside or outside, whether the blast took place in air or submerged underwater, and whether there was any postevent strenuous activity. A thorough trauma evaluation is mandatory for all victims of explosive blasts. Standard trauma management for secondary and tertiary injury will be familiar to prehospital personnel, emergency physicians, and traumatologists, so this section will focus on management of PBI and other injuries commonly occurring in blast victims.

The most critically injured patients after an exposure to a conventional blast succumb to their injuries at the scene. For those patients killed immediately after an explosion, death results from head injuries, PBI of the lung, abdominal injuries, or chest injuries.[16,17] Among survivors, non–life-threatening injuries including fractures, soft tissue injuries, and blast injuries to ears and eyes are common.[1,5,7,16,18] Of those who survive a conventional explosion, only very few will have severe chest and abdominal injuries, including blast lung. These injuries should be recognized as prognostic markers of severity, and it is important to identify and treat them early because surviving patients with such injuries have a significantly increased mortality rate.

Evaluation of prior blast injuries indicates certain patterns of morbidity and mortality from which conclusions about future events may be drawn. Immediate deaths appear to be related to the strength of the explosion, an associated building collapse, or a blast location that is indoors. The Beirut bombing in 1983 illustrates some important principles of medical management of casualties after an explosion. Most survivors had noncritical injuries, and for those critically injured, death occurred days to weeks later. Most of these deaths (86%) occurred in victims who were rescued and treated more than 6 hours after the blast event. A short interval between blast event and treatment and early aggressive resuscitation are good prognostic factors for survival.[16,19]

Pulmonary PBI may have an acute or delayed presentation. Patients with acute pulmonary PBI will present with chest pain, dyspnea, and tachypnea with rapid and shallow respirations, dry cough, wheezing, and hemoptysis. Breath sounds will be diminished on the affected side, making the diagnosis of PBI difficult unless pneumothorax, hemothorax, and pulmonary contusion have been excluded. Inspiratory rales, dullness to percussion, and poor chest wall expansion may also be present.[1] A chest radiograph is mandatory for all patients with respiratory difficulty or suspected PBI or chest trauma. Computed tomography (CT) scans of the chest may be useful to detect small pneumothoraces or pulmonary contusions, both of which may not be well visualized on a plain radiograph of the chest.

Massive hemoptysis resulting from PBI can be managed by preferentially intubating the unaffected lung with a cuffed endotracheal tube, thus protecting the function of that side. Patients with PBI of the lung may have concurrent pneumothorax, tension pneumothorax, or hemothorax. Emergent decompression with a tube or needle thoracostomy is indicated.[20] Patients with pulmonary PBI who are not having ventilatory problems are at risk for hypoxemia and should be managed with high-flow oxygen through a non-rebreather mask or continuous positive airway pressure. Patients able to ventilate spontaneously reduce their risk for arterial gas embolism. It has been suggested that patients requiring mechanical ventilation should be managed with low ventilatory pressures and permissive hypercapnia to reduce the risk of air embolism.[21,22]

Air embolism resulting from PBI may cause coronary vessel occlusion with subsequent myocardial infarction or cerebral infarction with altered mental status or stroke symptoms. Other organ systems may also be affected. Coronary artery air embolism after PBI can be difficult to diagnose but should be suspected in any blast victim who has electrocardiographic evidence of a myocardial infarction or is in shock with all other likely reasons for shock excluded. A head CT scan is mandatory in any patient with altered mental status, seizures, or focal neurologic deficits. Air embolism should be managed with hyperbaric oxygen therapy. Transferring patients to hyperbaric chambers may be problematic, given the risks of worsening the condition during aeromedical transportation and patient deterioration due to worsening pulmonary PBI.

The abdominal evaluation for PBI should focus on the search for perforation and the signs of lower gastrointestinal hemorrhage and shock. The presentation and diagnosis of these conditions as well as diagnosis may be delayed. Diagnostic peritoneal lavage (DPL) is indicated in hemodynamically unstable patients with abdominal findings. Ultrasonography of the abdomen may be considered in patients with suspected intra-abdominal trauma or hypotension and may be especially valuable in managing mass-casualty incidents. Abdominal CT scanning in stable patients to detect abdominal injury due to PBI may be useful in detecting small gastrointestinal perforations or hemorrhage. An abdominal CT scan performed after a DPL may have false-positive results because air and fluid will have been introduced into the peritoneum during the DPL procedure.[1]

Tympanic membrane (TM) rupture is a relatively common injury as a result of blast waves. Patients with TM rupture may have acute pulmonary PBI but are unlikely to have delayed-onset pulmonary PBI. The absence of TM rupture is important because such patients are unlikely to develop pulmonary PBI.[23]

Patients who appear stable but may be at risk for delayed PBI—including those in close proximity to the blast, knocked unconscious, or who felt the blast wave hit them—should be admitted for observation. Patients who have abdominal pain or tenderness, even if initial studies have normal results, may develop life-threatening bowel complications and should also be admitted.[20]

Patients can be discharged home if they have no chest complaints, normal chest radiographs, and no evidence of hypoxia, provided they have been observed at least 6 hours. The risk of pulmonary PBI is low in these patients, and onset of any PBI-related complications in such patients should present slowly. These patients can safely return to the hospital for a secondary evaluation. Additionally, patients with TM rupture

only may also be discharged home because they do not appear to be at risk of delayed-onset pulmonary PBI.[24] These patients should be given standard instructions on care of ear perforations and provided with otolaryngologic follow-up.

CASE PRESENTATION

There are numerous historical examples of conventional explosions. There were over 12,000 explosive or bombing incidents in the United States between 1980 and 1990.[25,26]

You are working in the emergency department of a medium-sized port city. A fire aboard a cargo ship on a weekday afternoon results in a massive response by city and regional fire departments. A large crowd of curious onlookers forms, and a major police and security effort is made to cordon off the area. Suddenly, the ship's load of ammonium nitrate fertilizer explodes, destroying the ship, collapsing two nearby buildings, igniting fires, and hurling debris for more than a mile. There are hundreds dead at the scene, including rescue and security personnel, and there are over 1000 survivors.

As the rescue effort begins and victims begin to flood local and regional healthcare centers, the challenge for healthcare providers is to identify and manage those with PBI while also evaluating and managing a larger number with varying degrees of trauma resulting from secondary, tertiary, and quaternary blast injury.

UNIQUE CONSIDERATIONS

Conventional blasts are unique because blast waves can cause PBI in persons physically separated from the epicenter of the explosion. Blast waves travel around walls and can be magnified traveling down corridors. Persons in enclosed spaces frequently have the highest incidence of PBI regardless of whether the explosion occurred within that space or outside it.[14,21,27] The risk of PBI also increases as the volume of the enclosed space decreases. Persons located next to walls or in corners at the moment of the blast are also more likely to sustain PBI.[12] Persons wearing body protection, such as Kevlar, at the time of the blast, may be protected against secondary blast injury from flying objects but are still at risk for PBI. These garments transmit and may even amplify blast waves, so it should not be assumed that a blast victim wearing body protection has no PBI even if he or she has no secondary blast injury.[28]

Persons protected from secondary blast injury, either by a physical structure, body armor, or water may have sustained PBI. Because their injuries are not as immediately apparent as those with external injuries from secondary blast injury, they may still be active and helping with the relief effort in the aftermath of the blast. Strenuous activity after PBI may result in poorer outcome. EMS and other medical personnel on the scene must ensure that apparently uninjured persons in close proximity to an explosion do not engage in physical activity.

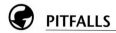

The most significant pitfall in the evaluation of blast victims is failing to consider PBI in a person exposed to an explosion, whether near or far from the blast, indoors or outdoors, or in air or water.

REFERENCES

1. Argyros GJ. Management of primary blast injury. *Toxicology* 1997;121:105-15.
2. Huller J, Bazini Y. Blast injuries of the chest and abdomen. *Arch Surg*. 1970;100:24-30.
3. Cooper GJ, Maynard RL, Cross NL, et al. Casualties from terrorist bombings. *J Trauma*. 1983;23:955-67.
4. Leibovici D, Gofrit ON, Stein M, et al. Blast injuries: bus vs. open-air-bombings—a comparative study of injuries in survivors of open-air versus confined space explosions. *J Trauma*. 1996;41:1030-5.
5. Brismar B, Bergenwald L. The terrorist bomb explosion in Bologna, Italy, 1980: an analysis of the effects an injuries sustained. *J Trauma*. 1982;22:216-20.
6. Rignault DP, Deligny MC. The 1986 terrorist bombing experience in Paris. *Ann Surg*. 1989;209:368-73.
7. Mallonee S, Shariat S, Stennies G, et al. Physical injuries and fatalities resulting from the Oklahoma City bombing. *JAMA* 1996;276:382-387.
8. Ammons MA, Moore EE, Pons PT, et al. The role of a regional trauma system in the management of a mass disaster: an analysis of the Keystone Colorado chairlift accident. *J Trauma*. 1988;28:1468-71.
9. Stein M, Hirshberg A. Medical consequences of terrorism: the conventional weapon threat. *Surg Clin North Am*. 1999;79:1537-52.
10. Stuhmiller JH, Phillips YY, Richmond DR. The physics and mechanisms of primary blast injury. In: Bellamy RF, Zajtchuk R, eds. *Conventional Warfare: Ballistic, Blast and Burn Injuries*. Washington, DC: Office of the Surgeon General of the US Army; 1991:241-70.
11. Iremonger MJ. Physics of detonations and blast-waves. In: Cooper GJ, Dudley HAF, Gann DS, et al, eds. *Scientific Foundations of Trauma*. Oxford, UK: Butterworth-Heinemann; 1997:189-99.
12. Yelverton JT. Blast biology. In: Cooper GJ, Dudley HAF, Gann DS, et al, eds. *Scientific Foundations of Trauma*. Oxford, UK: Butterworth-Heinemann; 1997:200-13.
13. Wiener SL, Barrett J. Explosions and explosive device-related injuries. In: Wiener SL, Barrett J, eds. *Trauma Management for Civilian and Military Physicians*. Philadelphia: Saunders; 1986:13-26.
14. Mellor SG. The pathogenesis of blast injury and its management. *Br J Hosp Med*. 1988;39:536-9.
15. Paran H, Neufeld D, Shwartz I, et al. Perforation of the terminal ileum induced by blast injury: delayed diagnosis or delayed perforation? *J Trauma*. 1996;40:472-5.
16. Frykberg ER, Teppas JJ, Alexander RH. The 1983 Beirut Airport terrorist bombing: injury patterns and implications for disaster management. *Am Surg*. 1989;55:134-41.
17. Pyper PC, Graham WJH. Analysis of terrorist injuries treated at Craigavon Area Hospital, Northern Ireland, 1972-1980. *Injury*. 1982;14:332-8.
18. Frykberg ER, Tepas JJ. Terrorist bombings: lessons learned from Belfast to Beirut. *Ann Surg*. 1988;208:569-76.
19. Rignault DP. Recent progress in surgery for the victims of disaster, terrorism and war. *World J Surg*. 1992;16:885-7.
20. Wightman JM, Gladish SL. Explosions and blast injuries. *Ann Emerg Med*. 2001;37:664-78.
21. Pizov R, Oppenheim-Eden A, Matot I, et al. Blast lung injury from an explosion on a civilian bus. *Chest*. 1999;115:165-72.
22. Sorkine P, Szold O, Kluger Y, et al. Permissive hypercapnia ventilation in patients with severe pulmonary blast injury. *J Trauma*. 1988;45:35-8.
23. Mellor SG. The relationship of blast loading to death and injury from explosion. *World J Surg*. 1992;16:893-8.
24. Leibovici D, Gofrit ON, Shapira SC. Eardrum perforation in explosion survivors: is it a marker of pulmonary blast injury? *Ann Emerg Med*. 1999;34:168-72.
25. Slater MS, Trunkey DD. Terrorism in America: an evolving threat. *Arch Surg*. 1997;132:1059-66.
26. Karmy-Jones R, Kissinger D, Golocovsky M, et al. Bomb-related injuries. *Mil Med*. 1994;159:536-9.
27. Katz E, Ofek B, Adler J, et al. Primary blast injury after a bomb explosion on a civilian bus. *Ann Surg*. 1989;209:484-8.
28. Cooper GJ, Townend DJ, Cater SR, et al. The role of stress waves in thoracic visceral injury from blast loading: modification of stress transmission by foams and high density materials. *J Biomech*. 1991;24:273-85.

chapter 143

Explosions: Fireworks

Craig Sisson

 ## DESCRIPTION OF EVENT

This chapter will address the preparation for and response to an explosion involving fireworks. Most formal fireworks displays follow strict safety guidelines meant to predict and prevent major complications. According to the American Pyrotechnics Association, only 3% of all fireworks injuries are related to public fireworks displays. In contrast, it is hard to predict and control the behavior of persons associated with the production and distribution of fireworks. There are multiple reports of large-scale explosions in fireworks factories around the world. This scenario is the focus of the chapter.

Carelessness around fireworks can lead to an explosive event. In Lima, Peru, on Dec. 29, 2001, more than 1100 tons of fireworks were concentrated in the Mesa Redonda shopping area. A fire then developed, resulting in close to 300 deaths and 357 injuries.[1] Chen and colleagues[2,3] analyzed retrospective data from 339 patients involved in fireworks factory explosions from January 1987 to December 1999. They report a 13% mortality rate among victims, a significant percentage when compared with other causes of burns during the same period.

Black powder, the basic component of fireworks, has not changed much since its invention by the Chinese approximately 1000 years ago. Historically, it is composed of saltpeter, charcoal, sulfur, and small amounts of water.[4] Black powder is considered a "low explosive" and burns by a process known as deflagration.[5] Compared with high explosives (e.g., TNT), the chemical reaction is relatively slow and releases energy over a longer period of time. However, if the reaction is enclosed within a contained space, pressure can build rapidly, leading to an explosion. This property makes black powder very useful as a propellant, eventually giving it the nickname *gunpowder*. The current classification system for explosive materials was developed by the U.S. Department of Transportation. Fireworks are included in this classification system under divisions 1.3 and 1.4, which include large display fireworks and "common" publicly available fireworks, respectively.

 ## PREINCIDENT ACTIONS

Perry and Lindell[6] describe four key steps that a community must take to prepare for a disaster involving a large-scale fireworks explosion: vulnerability analysis, capability assessment, plan development, and coordinated training exercises. The most vulnerable population in a fireworks disaster are those persons working inside the factory or storage facility and those found in close proximity to it. How easily can rescue teams access the site? How much and what kind of material is stored at the site? Where are the nearest first responders located? How far is it to the closest medical facility? Where is the nearest burn center? Are the surrounding buildings residential, commercial, or industrial? Do the citizens, first responders, and medical community know about this facility? How advanced are the safety systems found at the facility? Are the materials being stored properly? Is a protocol in place so that any change at the site is adequately communicated to those who would respond to an event? All of these factors will affect *vulnerability*.

The *capabilities* of the responding parties must be analyzed to determine whether the community is prepared to respond to an event. A hospital may be located close to the potential disaster site but lack personnel and equipment to deal with a large volume of burn victims. Airway control is very important, and responders experienced in recognition of airway compromise and definitive airway management should have priority on the scene and in patient transport.

The *planning* stage requires the collaborative effort of the local government, fire department, police, emergency medical systems, medical community, citizens, and site owners. A *network of communication* must be built so that all parties will be informed of changes in both vulnerability and capability. Finally, organized exercises must be performed to maintain the proper level of preparedness.

 ## POSTINCIDENT ACTIONS

In the immediate aftermath of a fireworks incident, the appropriate medical facilities and response personnel should be dispatched through predetermined communication pathways. This ensures that information and resources are distributed in the most organized and effective way. Medical facilities must be made aware of potential trauma and burn victims so that space may be allocated and appropriate equipment and personnel made available. In the Mesa Redonda fireworks disaster, the local hospitals lacked adequately experienced personnel and were quickly depleted of intravenous fluids, antibiotics, and analgesics.[1] In 1999, the Jahn Foundry in Springfield, Mass, exploded and within 5 minutes the first victims arrived at Baystate Medical Center. The Baystate emergency department was full at the time, necessitating reorganization.[7]

The initial responders to a fireworks storage facility explosion should be cautious. One should assess the scene immediately for any potential further danger to the victims and rescuers.[8] The American Pyrotechnics Association instructs that emergency responders should never attempt to fight a fire that involves a building used in the manufacture of fireworks.[9] The main goal should be removal and treatment of victims and prevention of secondary fires away from the initial site. The surrounding community should be evacuated immediately and triage and treatment areas set up at a safe distance from the disaster site. All nonambulatory patients should be transported to triage areas for evaluation.

MEDICAL TREATMENT OF CASUALTIES

The majority of reports in the medical literature on fireworks injuries involve individual use of class 1.4 fireworks. Reports of large-scale fireworks disasters and the wounds they cause are very rare. The mortality rate associated with fireworks factory explosions is variable and depends on many factors. A study by Navarro-Monzonis and others[10] reports a mortality of 47% in casualties of industrial gunpowder explosions. A 13-year retrospective study by Chen and colleagues[2,3] demonstrates a 13% overall mortality rate with greater than 50% mortality in those with inhalation injury. The injuries seen in the survivors were a combination of burns, blast injuries, trauma, and inhalation injury.[3] In comparison with other blast injury disasters, fireworks disasters have a higher incidence of thermal injury. The burns characteristically involve a large total body surface area, and the majority of the burns are deep dermal or full thickness.[1-3,10] Wounds found in casualties close to the blast may be severely contaminated with gunpowder residue.[3] The primary explosion of gunpowder in combination with smoke generated by secondary fires makes inhalation injury a common finding.[1-3]

For the initial treatment of burn victims, remove all of the patients' clothing to prevent further thermal or chemical injury. Jewelry and watches should also be removed to prevent a tourniquet effect from tissue swelling. First responders must evaluate the ABCs (i.e., airway, breathing, circulation) of each victim, taking time only to perform interventions that are immediately required on salvageable patients.[11,12] Airway is a very important aspect of

management given the high incidence of inhalation injury and risk of blast lung injury. Indications for immediate definitive airway management include voice hoarseness, brassy cough, and stridor.[13] If a patient was in an enclosed space or has facial burns or carbonaceous sputum, early definitive airway management should be considered. Early tracheostomy is the preferred option for long-term management of ventilated patients.[2]

Intravenous access and aggressive intravenous hydration with normal saline or lactated Ringer's solution should be a priority. These patients will require extensive fluid resuscitation given the frequency of deep dermal and full-thickness burns, large burn surface area, inhalation injury, and potential delays in treatment.[13-17] The Parkland formula may underestimate the fluid requirement and should only be used as a starting point for resuscitation. A urine output of 0.5–1.0 mL/kg/hour, a heart rate of less than 120 and a clear sensorium can be used as end points for resuscitation in adults.[14] For children, a goal urine output of 1.0 mL/kg/hour and age-appropriate heart rate should be maintained.[13]

To decrease the temperature of the burned skin, cool tap water or a water-soaked towel should be used.[12] Ice should be avoided because it can cause decreased circulation to already damaged tissue. Nguyen and colleagues[18,19] report that cooling the burn wounds helps prevent progression to deep partial-thickness or full-thickness burns and reduces future complications. Medical providers must use sterile dressings to cover the wounds and wrap blankets around the patient to keep them warm. The principle is to keep the wounds cool and the patient warm.

Primary, secondary, and tertiary blast injuries can be found in fireworks disaster patients.[3,10] However, there are limited data available on blast injury resulting from large-scale explosion of stored gunpowder. Therefore, many of the treatments recommended in this text will be inferred from similar large-scale events. Primary blast injury is more severe when the victim is exposed to the blast wave overpressurization while inside an enclosed space.[20-24] Leibovici and others[23] make a specific comparison between open-air and enclosed-space explosions, showing an increased incidence of primary blast injury, more severe injuries, and higher mortality rate in enclosed-space explosions. Intuitively, victims who are located in the collapsed portions of buildings are far more likely to die.[25,26] Most fireworks today are still made by hand inside enclosed buildings. One can expect a high incidence of immediate death of victims in close proximity to the initial blast.[23,24]

A rapid and complete secondary survey of all patients will prevent missed associated injuries. Chen and colleagues[2] report 10% of burn victims to have an associated injury. The most common in decreasing frequency were limb fracture, blast lung injury, fractured rib with hemopneumothorax, and tympanic membrane rupture. The incidence of associated injuries among those who survived versus those who died was 5% and 48%, respectively. Leibovici and colleagues[23] report psychological stress, tinnitus, mild hearing loss, minor penetrating trauma, and simple fractures as associated injuries for patients not requiring hospital admission in open-air bombings.

Patients should be provided with adequate analgesia after initial stabilization, either in the prehospital setting or in the emergency department. Once a patient has reached the hospital, aggressive early debridement of devitalized tissue and topical antimicrobial treatment should begin as soon as possible.[14,15] Foreign bodies, such as paper fireworks covers and shrapnel from the blast, can increase the risk of infection and should be removed.[10] Chen and others show that 68% of victims required surgery with an average of 2.7 surgeries per patient.[3] There is a high risk of barotrauma in blast lung injury patients requiring mechanical ventilation.[22,24] They also show decreased mortality in patients undergoing early tracheostomy and subsequent mechanical ventilation.[2] Sepsis, multiple organ failure, hypovolemic shock from inadequate resuscitation, and pulmonary infection were common causes of death in hospitalized patients.[2] Long-term management of these patients requires an experienced intensive care specialist, preferably within a burn unit setting.

UNIQUE CONSIDERATIONS

Fireworks contain various chemical compounds and elements for the purpose of producing colored spectacles. One of these chemicals is elemental phosphorus. Elemental phosphorus is used in the military in various weapons due to its unique chemical properties. There are three allotropic forms of phosphorus: white, red, and black.[27] White phosphorus is sometimes included in the manufacture of fireworks. It burns spontaneously at 34°C, producing a bright greenish light, copious amounts of white fumes, and a garliclike odor. A wound that is smoking white and exuding a garliclike odor is characteristic of this substance. When placed in contact with oxygen, white phosphorus is oxidized to phosphorus pentoxide, which then combines with water to form phosphoric acid. This chemical sequence releases heat into the environment, causing burns. The phosphoric acid formed lowers the pH of tissues, causing chemical burns.[28] This chemical reaction sequence will continue until all of the phosphorus has reacted or until the phosphorus is deprived of its oxygen fuel.

When an explosion occurs with a device containing white phosphorus, immediate steps must be taken to stop the chemical reaction. Treatment should focus on wound irrigation, phosphorus neutralization, and wound debridement.[29] The victim's clothing should be removed immediately to prevent any retained phosphorus particles from burning through to the skin or igniting the clothing. Once the clothing has been removed, the wounds should be washed with large amounts of water. This will cut off the oxygen supply and cool the wound to below the ignition temperature, effectively stopping the reaction.[27,29-31] Before transport, the wounds should be covered with saline–soaked gauze to prevent them from drying and spontaneously igniting again. Oily dressings should not be used because white phosphorus is lipid–soluble and may penetrate into tissues.[28,29]

Once at the hospital, prompt debridement of all wounds is necessary to remove retained phosphorus particles. A Wood's lamp causes retained phosphorus to fluoresce, aiding in removal.[31] A second option is to wash the wound with a 1% copper sulfate solution, which reacts with elemental phosphorus and covers the particles with dark-colored copper phosphate. This easily

CASE PRESENTATION

On December 29, 2001, more than 1100 tons of fireworks were being stored in the Mesa Redonda market in Lima, Peru. The market was stocked for a busy sales season during the Christmas and New Year's fireworks celebrations. The streets were coated with a film of gunpowder left from careless transport of packaged fireworks. At 6:30 PM, a vendor ignited a firework for demonstration that in turn ignited nearby displays, leading to a chain of explosions lasting 2 hours.[1] Within minutes, five city blocks were consumed in flame and smoke; nearly 300 people were killed and over 300 more wounded.

The majority of fireworks injuries involve young males. In Mesa Redonda, 70% of the victims were women and children. Many of the bodies were found in groups of 15 to 30, presumably clustering in areas thought to be safe. Gulati and colleagues[1] described the collapse of a high-voltage electrical transformer that crushed 40 people and electrocuted 27 others. Local hospitals treated 357 patients, 263 were treated for burns with 143 admissions for thermal injury.[1] Seventy percent of admitted burn patients had involvement of greater than 20% of their total body surface area. The majority of the burns were second and third degree, and stores of fluids, antibiotics, and analgesics were quickly depleted.[1] Inadequate fluid resuscitation due to fluid shortages led to acute renal failure in a number of patients. The majority of victims suffered some degree of smoke inhalation, and 16% of admitted burn patients had inhalation injury requiring ventilation.

It took 8 hours for firefighters and police officers to bring the blaze and surrounding chaos under control. The stores and houses were built close together and constructed of a highly flammable mix of straw and mud. Combined with the wind and the large amount of gunpowder present, the fire and smoke spread with devastating speed. The streets were very narrow, and many of the buildings lacked windows and emergency exits. The streets were packed with vendors and shoppers at the time of the disaster. Electrical wires were not protected and dangled over the streets, posing another threat to victims and rescue workers. The fire departments were poorly funded, and much of their equipment was old and in need of replacement. There were not enough ambulances available in the area and access to victims was difficult. Most local hospitals were at or near capacity when the disaster occurred. Additionally, patients began arriving at hospitals around 8:00 PM, during staff shift changes, which added to the confusion.

The production, importation, and sale of fireworks was banned by the president of Peru after this disaster.[1]

identifies sites that need further debridement and theoretically may slow the oxidation process. One concern is that copper itself is toxic and has never been shown to improve wound healing over normal saline washes alone.[28-30] As a result of phosphorus absorption, rapid changes in serum calcium and phosphorus levels can occur. Animal models have linked this to cardiac electrical abnormalities with increased risk of sudden death.[32] Therefore, continuous telemetry should be initiated for the patient, and his or her serum calcium and phosphorus levels should be monitored. Phosphorus absorption may also damage the kidneys and liver and cause other systemic effects.[27,33]

Magnesium and aluminum powders and pellets are also used in the production of fireworks. The chemical reactions are similar, producing a brilliant white light, intense heat, and loud noise effects if ignited in the presence of oxygen. Magnesium has an ignition temperature of 623°C and burns at roughly 3600°C. Once the oxygen source is removed, the reaction will stop.[34] Magnesium can react with oxygen, nitrogen, carbon dioxide, and water. The reaction with carbon dioxide produces magnesium oxide and carbon, and the reaction with water produces magnesium oxide and hydrogen gas. These reactions are important information for first responders. Applying water to a fire containing magnesium will increase the severity of the fire.[35] Hydrogen gas will be liberated and ignite, with the potential for a secondary explosion. Metal-extinguishing powders, such as graphite powder, powdered talc, and powdered sodium chloride present in class D fire extinguishers must be used to fight these fires.

All explosions can spread flaming debris, but fireworks are unique. Many class 1.4 fireworks are designed as self-propelled projectiles. Class 1.4 fireworks, although not at risk of initiating an explosive event, can spread fire throughout the storage facility and surrounding environment. They can also cause a projectile injury during the initial stages of a fire similar to secondary blast injuries but preceding an explosion. This may inhibit a person's ability to evacuate the site and put that person at risk for more severe injury.

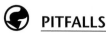 PITFALLS

Several potential pitfalls in response to a fireworks disaster exist. These include the following:

- Failure to stop the burning process
- Not performing ABCs with early definitive airway management
- Failure to complete secondary survey; other types of trauma can kill faster than burns
- Failure to remember: fluids, fluids, fluids
- Attempting to extinguish fire in a fireworks warehouse; instead, all persons should be evacuated
- Inadequate pain management
- Failure to establish triage areas a safe distance from primary event site

REFERENCES

1. Gulati S, Cruz R, Milner S. The fireworks tragedy of Peru. *J Burns Surg Wound Care*. December 11, 2003. Available at: http//www.journalofburnsandwounds.Com/volume02/volume02_article 22.pdf.
2. Chen X, Wang Y, Wang C, et al. Gunpowder explosion burns in fireworks factory: causes of death and management. *Burns* 2002; 28:655-8.
3. Chen X, Wang Y, Wang C, et al. Burns due to gunpowder explosions in fireworks factory: a 13-year retrospective study. *Burns* 2002; 28:245-9.
4. Russell M. *The Chemistry of Fireworks*. Cambridge, UK: Royal Society of Chemistry; 2000.
5. Bailey A, Murray SC. The explosion process: detonation shock effects. In: *Explosives, Propellants, and Pyrotechnics*. London: Brassey; 1989:21-47.
6. Perry R, Lindell M. Preparedness for emergency response: guidelines for the emergency planning process. *Disasters*. 2003; 27: 336-50.
7. Leslie CL, Cushman M, McDonald GS, et al. Management of multiple burn casualties in a high volume ED without a verified burn unit. *Am J Emerg Med*. 2001;19:469-73.
8. Delaney J, Drummond R. Mass casualties and triage at a sporting event. *Br J Sports Med*. 2002;36:85-8.
9. National Council on Fireworks Safety. Available at: http//www.fireworksafety.com/home.htm.
10. Navarro-Monzonis A, Benito-Ruiz J, Baena-Montilla P, et al. Gunpowder-related burns. *Burns* 1992;18:159-61.
11. Bar-Joseph G, Michaelson M, Halberthal M. Managing mass casualties. *Curr Opin Anaesthesiol*. 2003;16:193-9.
12. Allison K, Porter K. Consensus on the prehospital approach to burns patient management. *Emerg Med*. 2004;21:112-4.
13. Monafo W. Initial management of burns. *N Engl J Med*. 1996; 335:1581-6.
14. Tang H, Xia Z, Lui S, et al. The experience in the treatment of patients with extensive full-thickness burns. *Burns* 1999; 25:757-9.
15. Rose J, Herndon D. Advances in the treatment of burn patients. *Burns* 1997;23:S19-26.
16. Navar P, Saffle J, Warden G. Effect of inhalation injury on fluid resuscitation requirements after thermal injury. *Am J Surg*. 1985;150:716-20.
17. Cancio L, Chavez S, Alvarado-Ortega M, et al. Predicting increased fluid requirements during the resuscitation of thermally injured patients. *J Trauma*. 2004;56:404-14.
18. Nguyen N, Gun R, Sparnon A, et al. The importance of immediate cooling—a case series of childhood burns in Vietnam. *Burns* 2002;28:173-6.
19. Nguyen N, Gun R, Sparnon A, et al. The importance of initial management: a case series of childhood burns in Vietnam. *Burns* 2002;28:167-72.
20. Wrightman J, Gladish S. Explosions and blast injuries. *Ann Emerg Med*. 2001;37:664-78.
21. Frykberg E. Medical management of disasters and mass casualties from terrorist bombings: how can we cope? *J Trauma*. 2002; 53:201-12.
22. Gans L, Kennedy T. Management of unique clinical entities in disaster medicine. *Disaster Med*. 1996;14:301-26.
23. Leibovici D, Gofrit O, Stein M, et al. Blast injuries: bus versus open-air bombings—a comparative study of injuries in survivors of open-air versus confined-space explosions. *J Trauma*. 1996; 41:1130-5.
24. Pizov R, Oppenheim-Eden A, Matot I, et al. Blast lung injury from an explosion on a civilian bus. *Chest* 1999;115:165-72.
25. Mallonee S, Shariat S, Stennies G, et al. Physical injuries and fatalities resulting from the Oklahoma City bombing. *JAMA* 1996; 276:382-7.
26. Biancolini C, Del Bosco C, Jorge M. Argentine Jewish community institution bomb explosion. *J Trauma*. 1999;47:728.
27. Chau T, Lee T, Chen S, et al. The management of white phosphorous burns. *Burns* 2001;27:492-7.
28. Summerlin W, Walder A, Moncrief J. White phosphorous burns and massive hemolysis. *J Trauma*. 1967;7:476-84.

29. Konjoyan T. White phosphorus burns: case report and literature review. *Mil Med*. 1983;148:881-4.
30. Eldad A, Simon G. The phosphorous burn: a preliminary comparative experimental study of various forms of treatment. *Burns* 1991;17:198-200.
31. Davis K. Acute management of white phosphorous burn. *Mil Med*. 2002;167:83-4.
32. Bowen T, Whelan T, Nelson T. Sudden death after phosphorus burns: experimental observations of hypocalcemia, hyperphosphatemia and electrocardiographic abnormalities following production of a standard white phosphorus burn. *Ann Surg*. 1971;174:779-84.
33. Ben-Hur N, Giladi A, Neuman Z, et al. Phosphorus burns: a pathophysiological study. *Br J Plast Surg*. 1972;25:238-44.
34. Mendelson J. Some principles of protection against burns from flame and incendiary munitions. *J Trauma*. 1971;11:286-94.
35. Madrzykowski D, Stroup W. *Magnesium Chip Fire Tests Utilizing Biodegradable, Environmentally Safe, Nontoxic, Liquid Fire Suppression Agents*. Gaithersburg, Md: Underwriters Laboratories Inc; 1995.

chapter 144

Suicide Bomber

Jeffry L. Kashuk and Shamai A. Grossman

 DESCRIPTION OF EVENT

An unprecedented wave of terror has captivated world attention for several years, increasing in magnitude with daily warnings.[1,2] Not unlike other disease outbreaks in world history, this terror epidemic knows no borders and strikes innocent civilians during their most productive years of life. The objective of terrorists is to kill and maim as many citizens as possible; hence, dense population centers and locations where the public congregate are emphasized targets.

Differences have been noted between bombs prepared by terrorists and those of traditional warfare. Operating on more limited budgets, terrorists have discovered methods of packing bombs with nails, metal bolts, and similar objects so as to inflict maximum injury. These bombs are created so as to be easily transportable, usually hidden on the body of the terrorist who carries out the suicide mission. Other bombs are prepared in small, contained, transportable packages or in automobiles.

Blast injury patterns have classically been described based on wartime injuries, with limited survivors requiring medical care.[1-4] In contrast, civilian urban bomb explosions result in many patients simultaneously arriving at the hospital alive despite the devastating nature of their injuries. These patients may present with an extraordinarily varied constellation of clinical patterns.

Virtually all patients exposed to the blast front will incur primary blast injury. The immediate blast front is dissipated from the explosion center based on forces of spalling, acceleration, and implosion mechanisms. Primary blast injuries classically result in injuries to air-containing structures.[4] More than 50% of patients exposed to a blast of greater than 50 psi will suffer tympanic membrane perforation. This injury can be used as sign of blast exposure and may be a harbinger of coincident injuries. Primary blast lung injury may not be readily apparent and should be carefully considered in such a scenario. Delayed infiltrates in blast injury are common in primary blast lung injury and may be difficult to differentiate from lacerated lung resulting from secondary blast mechanisms. Primary blast head injury appears to have a higher mortality than other conventional head injuries, most probably due to the tremendous force of the exposure and associated injuries.

Blast lung versus lacerated lung represents another clinical challenge. Whereas lacerated lung may result from secondary blast injury due to penetrating sheer forces, blast lung injury serves as the classic injury pattern of bomb explosions. Although both mechanisms may commonly manifest as pneumothorax, hemothorax is less common in classic blast lung injury. Both may develop significant respiratory difficulties, with persistent air leaks requiring creative ventilator techniques. However, in the early phase of injury, fluid management may be quite different; blast lung injury requires restrictive management whereas lacerated lung injury requires resuscitative therapy. Repair of a lacerated lung may occasionally require operative therapy—most commonly, tractotomy or oversew for hemorrhage control. In contrast, blast lung injury treatment is physically non-operative.

The secondary blast effect results from flying shards of glass, metal, and other explosive objects that inflict injury are similar to classic penetrating patterns. Benign-appearing skin wounds may signal underlying severe injury due to the penetration of metal bolts, pellets, and nails.

Terrorists know that maximum death and injury can be accomplished by bringing the explosive content to closed spaces. There is a direct correlation between the location of a blast and survivability. Open, closed, and sealed spaces result in differential injury patterns based on the standard categories of blast injury.[5] Mortality appears to be highest in super-closed spaces such as buses. Explosions on buses result most commonly in the highly lethal tertiary blast front (i.e., Mach stem effect), where the human body may be propelled via a supercharged blast front against stationary objects, resulting in immediate amputation or death. Such patients typically arrive at the hospital with agonal breathing and extensively burned, mangled extremities. Survival for these persons is rare.

Quaternary blast injuries are burn injuries perpetrated by the highly flammable surrounding area of the explosions. These burn patterns may include all types of classical burn injuries, including inhalation, chemical, and contact burns.

PREINCIDENT ACTIONS

The multidimensional injury pattern, a complex of injuries that occur simultaneously in the same patient, seems unique to bomb explosions.[5-7] Patients now arrive at the hospital alive who, in previous war settings, would have died of their extensive blast injuries. Although well-established trauma protocols such as advanced trauma life support remain the gold standard against which one should gauge treatment plans, this injury pattern has resulted in new dilemmas that demand a reassessment of established techniques to improve preparedness, treatment, and survival.

The management of mass-casualty events demands strict adherence to established protocols and superb coordination of available manpower and medical resources, which are commonly stressed to the maximum.[5,6,8,9] Given recent world events, many protocols are in evolution with plans for a high level of preparedness. Despite this, the sheer volume of injured patients encountered in such events may challenge even the most experienced institution. In addition, refinements in protocols and improvements in techniques are always in evolution as greater experience is gained.[8-10]

Triage protocols for mass-casualty events are different from other trauma situations. Virtually all local and regional hospital facilities are recruited to handle the sheer volume of injured patients.

 ## POSTINCIDENT ACTIONS

Care for the sickest patients should begin immediately. The initial clinical issue in these events is the lack of diagnostic capabilities. Patients who are triaged to smaller facilities for stabilization may require transfer to a trauma center for more definitive care.

 ## MEDICAL TREATMENT OF CASUALTIES

As with all critically ill patients, emergency care of casualties of a suicide bombing begins with evaluation of the ABCs: airway, breathing, and circulation. Once an airway has been secured and breathing and circulation established, the primary and secondary physical examination should proceed.

In evaluating the multidimensional injury pattern with associated abdominal visceral injury, certain patterns have been noted. There appear to be more diffuse and associated injuries necessitating meticulous abdominal exploration. This may be particularly difficult in the midst of a multicasualty event involving other injured patients who are waiting to enter the operating room.[8,10,11] An intensive and persistent search for injury must be undertaken, with the underlying mechanisms of both blunt and penetrating injuries being kept in mind.

Diagnostic peritoneal lavage (DPL), first described almost 40 years ago, has returned as the most important diagnostic tool in mass-casualty events.[5,7] It can be rapidly performed at the bedside and provides immediate diagnostic information to accompany triage decisions in mass-casualty events. In the absence of other diagnostic maneuvers or bedside ultrasound, this minimally invasive technique is valuable in the acute evaluation of the injured, as well as for follow-up evaluation after the tertiary survey. In patients presenting with delayed injuries, DPL has sometimes been the only test to have positive results. In some cases, these injuries appeared after a computed tomography (CT) scan with initial negative results. A high index of suspicion must be maintained when multiple shrapnel pieces are identified on radiograph or fluoroscopy. Visceral blast injuries may occur from multiple wounding mechanisms. Primary or tertiary blast injury may cause slow dissection along tissue planes, resulting in delayed peritonitis. In contrast, missile trajectory of secondary blast injury may parallel classic penetrating injury that is described in stab or gunshot wounds.[6] Due to the potential for multiple mechanisms of action, a minimum of 5000 red blood cells/ml as a lower-level threshold for DPL in blast visceral injury has been suggested.[5]

Prioritization of CT scan and ultrasound must be established because these tests must be reserved for immediate, life-threatening, decision-making protocols. Usually, CT scan is available for only the most severe head injuries to support immediate interventional decisions.

Total body fluoroscopy should be used liberally to identify all potential projectiles. Routine mapping of such findings is mandatory for documentation and future reference. Bedside ultrasound is of limited use. An obviously positive examination result may expedite diagnosis of hemothorax or hemoperitoneum; however, in many situations ultrasound may not be available due to the volume of injured patients competing for limited resources. Expert clinical judgment is demanded in such scenarios.

Because of delayed injury presentation, previous negative examination results require careful reevaluation. Blast injuries may develop exponentially over time, resulting in injuries that are missed initially. For this reason, the tertiary survey has assumed a renewed level of importance in these events. If this examination suggests potential missed injury, further tests such as ultrasound or CT may be available and appropriate as soon as the majority of casualties have been admitted and routed through triage.

 ## UNIQUE CONSIDERATIONS

When a complex of injury patterns occur simultaneously in the same patient, as described, this has been termed the *multidimensional injury pattern*.[5-7] This subgroup of patients is not predicted adequately by the classic injury severity score system. Parameters such as length of hospital stay, length of stay in the intensive care unit, and mortality appear significantly different than other groups of patients, emphasizing the unique nature of this subgroup.

The management of multidimensional injury can be contrasted with that of other, conventional traumatic injury. Due to the multiple wounding mechanisms, the

A 45-year-old man was a bystander in a bus explosion. The patient was triaged to the closest facility along with 45 other multiple-injured patients. The initial emergency department evaluation noted a Glasgow Coma Scale score of 3 with bilateral hemopneumothoraxes. The patient was promptly endotracheally intubated with concomitant placement of bilateral chest tubes and moderate blood return.

An examination of the patient then revealed a perforation of the right eye, a periorbital laceration, peppering of the facial region and scalp, and an extensive laceration of the scalp. The initial abdominal examination revealed a soft and scaphoid abdomen. On closer inspection, a small round wound was noted in the left lower quadrant. A skeletal survey disclosed that the left arm had a comminuted humoral fracture with active bleeding; this was controlled with a pressure dressing. In addition, a 30% body surface area burn encompassing the chest, abdominal wall, and lower extremities was noted, as were multiple lacerations to both legs.

Due to lack of neurosurgical coverage, the patient was prepared for transfer to a level I trauma center (to occur in approximately 40 minutes). Before the transfer, bedside abdominal ultrasound was normal. In addition, CT scan of the head, chest, and abdomen revealed moderate cerebral swelling and multiple shrapnel injuries with metallic spheric balls throughout the body but no penetration of the chest or abdominal cavity.

The patient arrived in the trauma center with stable vital signs. A small spherical ball was noted in the right lower chest area. There was concern that this ball could have traversed the abdominal cavity from the left lower quadrant abdominal wound previously noted. Despite the otherwise normal abdominal examination results, the Focused Assessment with Sonography for Trauma (FAST) examination was repeated. Although this ultrasound had negative results, a DPL was then found to have a positive result of 5000 red blood cells/ml. Further evaluation noted the absence of a pulse in the right hand distal to the injury.

Multiple surgical teams were mobilized. Personnel from the plastic surgery and ophthalmology departments worked on the facial region. The right eye required enucleation. Vascular surgery and orthopedics personnel treated the extremity injuries. A transection of the left brachial artery with comminuted humorous fracture was treated with a temporary arterial shunt. External fixation was placed over the fracture. Abdominal exploration (via the burned abdominal wall) disclosed lacerations of the sigmoid colon, small bowel (mid jejunum), a tear of the right diaphragm, and grade 2 injury of the right lobe of the liver.

An ulnar nerve injury required reconstruction. One week of mechanical ventilation was required for blast lung injuries, and early tracheostomy was performed. Neurosurgical follow-up confirmed resolution of the brain swelling, and the patient regained full neurologic function with rehabilitation.

sional injury will often require the careful coordination of multiple surgical teams. This translates into the need for a large operating space to accommodate the teams who may need to be working simultaneously.

PITFALLS

Several potential pitfalls in response to a suicide bomber attack exist. These include the following:

- Coordination of manpower and medical resources by protocol are the most important requirements for bombing events.
- The combined clinical scenario of head injury, burns, blast lung, and intra-abdominal or thoracic injury may create extreme difficulties in decision-making for surgery as well as critical care management.
- Due to the vast number of victims, CT scanning equipment may be available only for the most obviously severe injuries.
- Constant clinical vigilance is required to time interventional modalities in the case of combined head and other injuries.
- Healthcare providers must be wary of profound acidosis and hypothermia. Aggressive warming mechanisms must be used, and the potential for developing coagulopathy must be recognized.[11]

REFERENCES

1. Frykberg ER. Medical management of disasters and mass causalities from terrorist bombings: how can we cope? *J Trauma.* 2002;53:201-12.
2. Fryberg ER. Principles of mass casualty managed following terrorist disasters. *Ann Surg.* 2004;239:319-21.
3. Mellor SG, Cooper GJ. Analysis of 828 serviceman killed or injured by explosion in Northern Ireland 1970-84. The Hostile Action Casualty System. *Br J Surg.* 1989;76:1006.
4. Katz JE, Ofek B, Adler J, et al. Primary blast injury after a bomb explosion in a civilian bus. *Ann Surg.* 1989;209:484-8.
5. Kluger Y, Kashuk J, Mayo A. Terror bombings: mechanisms, consequences, and implications. *Scand J Surg.* 2004;93:11-4.
6. Kluger Y. Bomb explosions in acts of terrorism: detonation, wound ballistics, triage, and medical concerns. *Isr Med Assoc J.* 2003;5:235-40.
7. Kluger Y, Sofer D, Mayo A, et al. Bomb explosions in acts of terrorism—from explosion to medical concerns. Presented at the American Association for the Surgery of Trauma, Annual Meeting. Minneapolis, Minn: September 11, 2003.
8. Almogy G, Belzsberg H, Mintz Y, et al. Suicide bombing attacks: update and modification to the protocol. *Ann Surg.* 2004;239:319-21.
9. Einav S, Fridenberg Z, Weissman L, et al. Evacuation priorities in mass casualty terrorism related events: implications for contingency planning. *Ann Surg.* 2004;239:304-10.
10. Peleg K. Patterns of injury in hospitalized terrorist victims. *Am J Emerg Med.* 2003;21:258-62.
11. Pelez K, Aharouson, Daniel L, et al. Gunshot and explosion injuries: characteristics, outcomes, and implications for care of terror—related injuries in Israel. *Ann Surg.* 2004;239: 311-8.

likelihood that these patients will require some type of surgical intervention is high. Such multiple injuries result in difficult challenges in diagnosis, decision-making, and treatment. Providing care to a patient with multidimen-

chapter 145

Vehicle-Borne Improvised Explosive Devices

Michael I. Greenberg, Michael Horowitz, and Rachel Haroz

 ## DESCRIPTION OF EVENT

Vehicle-borne improvised explosive devices (VBIEDs) may be used in two general logistical scenarios. They can be used as assassination devices targeting an individual or group of persons or as a weapon intended to damage or destroy a specific target. VBIEDs have been used to attack "high-profile" targets such as specific buildings or targets with symbolic and/or logistical importance. "Soft" targets, or those having inadequate security protection, may also be targeted with the aim of causing substantial casualties in an area where many people are gathered.[1] As an assassination device, VBIEDs may be predeployed with the goal of destroying the occupants of the vehicle in which the device has been installed. As an explosive delivery device, the entire vehicle becomes a bomb that can be used against groups of people, buildings, or other targets. In most instances, a VBIED attack involves a single, high-profile event that cannot be readily predicted. However, detailed preplanning for such an eventuality is essential to maximize the effectiveness of a coordinated medical response. VBIEDs are associated with widely varying casualty and mortality rates. The 1993 World Trade Center bombing resulted in approximately 1000 persons injured, whereas the 1998 bombing of the U.S. Embassy in Nairobi, Kenya, injured more than 4000 persons.[2,3]

VBIEDs provide a readily available delivery system: the vehicle itself. The explosive devices contained therein may be assembled in a safe and remote location prior to delivery to the intended target. Defense against the deployment of a VBIED is exceedingly difficult because the explosive device is easily concealed and precise target prediction is difficult. Trucks used as VBIEDs may have a dual purpose of being able to carry a very large load of explosive material coupled with the potential mechanical ability and power to penetrate and breach protective barriers. In some cases, separate assault vehicles may be used to break through protective barriers, thus allowing unencumbered access to the vehicle containing the VBEID. VBIEDs may combine a variety of combustible chemicals and explosives as well as radiologic materials and devices.

No specific vehicle type has been associated with VBIEDs; however, terrorists usually choose vehicles that are common to and widely available in a given geographic region as well as vehicles possessing routine access to the intended target. Vehicles of virtually any size can be used as VBIEDs. However, the size of the vehicle used may depend on the nature and size of the explosive device being used. In the 1993 World Trade Center attack, approximately 1200 lb of improvised explosives were positioned in a rental van reported stolen by one of the perpetrators. Various large vehicles including limousines, sports utility vehicles, small trucks, delivery vehicles, ambulances, and minivans may have special attraction to be used as VBIEDs, based on their relatively large storage capacity. An example of selective vehicle use for specific access to a target is the use of limousines, which may convey the appearance of authority, thus facilitating access to specific locations within buildings or to facilities generally denied to the public.

 ## PREINCIDENT ACTIONS

Although intelligence reports may help to protect against VBIED use in many cases, those who wish to use VBIEDs may often evade preemptive detection. Law enforcement techniques for detection and preemption against VBIEDs are beyond the scope of this discussion. However, response preplanning is a key preincident action and must include coordination between police, firefighters, emergency medical services (EMS) personnel, public works officials, structural engineers, local elected officials, and others. Relationships must be preestablished and roles precoordinated, including who will have overall authority on the scene and who will be the medical authority.

Immediately after a VBIED incident, many competing priorities may emerge. These include rescuing the casualties, securing the area and controlling access, searching for a secondary explosive device, determining whether there is a need for evacuation of the surrounding area, preserving the crime scene, directing traffic to allow easy access/egress to emergency vehicles, and preventing further injury. Something as simple as a passing train could shake already damaged buildings, causing further collapse or fall of debris.[4,5] Careful preplanning may allow the adverse effects of such factors to be quickly addressed and corrected.

Communication is a key element that requires careful preplanning. The medical authority at the scene must be able to communicate with the scene commander, EMS on-scene (including the EMS dispatcher at the staging area), and local hospitals. The medical commander will need information from all of these sources to properly allocate resources. Information from hospitals regarding patient load and remaining available resources will be vital, allowing the medical commander to direct patients appropriately. Information from the scene commander allows for casualty estimates that will influence the amount and type of personnel that need to be called to the scene. The medical commander must also be provided with constant updates from the triage area at the scene to be aware of needs for resupply. In short, the medical commander will require overall situational awareness to effectively direct medical resources both at the scene and at local hospitals.[1,6-9]

It is important to remember that, in the event that the major trauma center for an area is a target or is quickly overrun by casualties, a large number of patients may flood some of the smaller surrounding hospitals.[6,10]

Few factors correlate with patient survival that can be influenced in the case of a car or truck bomb. Factors influencing survival that are not in the medical planner's control include the size of the explosion, the patterns of injury, the number of casualties, and the time of the day of the attack. Some factors important to survival over which a medical planner may have influence include having a well-rehearsed plan, being educated so as to improve triage efficiency, striving to have a minimum interval from injury to treatment, and ensuring that there is a sufficient number of competent medical staff that can be made available if an event occurs.[11,12] As every car bomb incident will be unique, it is vital that the medical plan allows for contingencies. After the Oklahoma City truck bombing, the medical triage/treatment area needed to be moved three times after it was initially established because of threats of another bombing.[9]

 POSTINCIDENT ACTIONS

The overall emergency response will, in most locales, be initiated by police officers, who are usually first on the scene. Firefighters, EMS personnel, and other public safety responders will be expected to follow local response protocols. It is of critical importance that the initial responders survey the overall situation before becoming actively involved in the rescue because the danger of unstable buildings and the potential for the detonation of secondary devices will be high. In addition, the area should be surveyed for the presence of radiation by first responders because the use of radiologic dispersion devices must be considered.[13] Those on the higher echelons of medical control will need to be made aware of the nature of the event and should receive an initial estimate of the number of casualties. EMS supervisors should alert area hospitals and begin to determine what resources will need to be deployed to the scene of the incident.

Police and/or military bomb units or hazardous materials teams will need to survey the scene to assess the risk for secondary devices while EMS responders initiate rescue efforts and treat casualties. This may engender a variable degree of risk for first responders, as it is likely that the scene will not be completely secured prior to the start of the rescue operation.

Triage and treatment operations should follow local preestablished protocols. A covered and protected area, out of view of the survivors, should be designated as a morgue. Also, a possible air evacuation site can be determined, although there may be substantial amounts of loose debris that could become dangerous during helicopter operations.[1,4,8]

The flow of casualties from the scene should be as regulated as possible by one medical commander who has a good overall situational awareness both at the scene and at the area hospitals. The goal will be to send less-injured patients to hospitals that are farther from the scene to conserve resources at the closer hospitals for the more seriously injured patients. Real world incidents have demonstrated that the majority of patients bring themselves to the closest hospital by car, by foot, or via public transit.[1,7,9]

Area hospitals will need to activate individual mass-casualty plans. These plans should include the ability to triage patients away from the emergency unit. It is vital that the typical earlier arrival of less-injured patients not interfere with the later treatment of more critically ill patients. Over-triage (i.e., referring patients for potentially serious injuries when only relatively minor injuries exist) at the scene may also result in a hospital being overwhelmed with less-injured patients.

 MEDICAL TREATMENT OF CASUALTIES

The epidemiology of VBIED incidents may be useful in predicting the patterns and numbers of injuries expected in future events. The literature regarding VBIED attacks reveals predictable patterns, including the fact that many injuries in survivors are relatively minor.[13,14] For example, after the Oklahoma City bombing there were 759 casualties; of these, 167 died, 83 were hospitalized, and 509 were treated and released.[15] The greatest risk for death after the detonation of a VBIED is building collapse. It is estimated that 95% of the deaths associated with the Oklahoma City bombing were secondary to blunt trauma consequent to the collapse of the building.[9]

Other factors influencing the mortality rate include an open versus closed blast environment.[16-18] A closed environment leads to greater overall mortality, increased risk of blast injury, more severe injuries among survivors, and a higher risk of significant burns.[19] Most studies of VBIEDs do not report large numbers of survivors with blast-related injuries. This is likely due to the fact that those close enough to the blast to experience these injuries do not survive the initial explosion. Most survivors therefore sustain injuries from secondary blast effects, including injuries from loose material or fragments propelled by the blast.[16] This epidemiology may be helpful not only during medical preplanning, but also in providing the receiving facility with important predictors of what to expect in the immediate aftermath of an event involving VBIEDs.

The literature is also helpful in planning what supplies are critical in the initial treatment of casualties. The most heavily used supplies in past events were reported to include antibiotics, narcotics, bandages, and tetanus toxoid.[7,20] The most common injuries observed after a VBIED detonation are soft tissue injuries as well as hearing loss, fractures, and musculoskeletal injuries. The most profound challenge to medical resources of the hospital involves the emergency department, where adequate staffing is essential to ensure a proper flow of casualties.[7,20] In addition, an increased demand on the radiology services may occur. Thus, in the early hours after an event, the indications for radiology studies may need to be limited to the most critical injuries.[21]

In some cases, the mode of arrival may give a clue as to injury severity, and it is important to remember that the initial group of presenting patients will generally have only minor injuries. This phenomenon was evident after the World Trade Center bombing in 1993, the Oklahoma City bombing, and the Nairobi Embassy bombing. After the 1993 World Trade Center bombing, just 450 of 1040 patients were transported by EMS, and after the Oklahoma City bombing EMS transported only 33% of patients seen in area hospitals.[1,7] Those patients transported by EMS were much more likely to require hospital admission.[7]

Studies of VBIED events have highlighted the importance of triage both at the scene and at receiving hospitals. It is critical for those performing triage to quickly identify critically injured yet salvageable patients and to initiate treatment. Over-triage is common after VBIED incidents. Even physicians with extensive experience in trauma triage may find it difficult to identify patients with certain blast injuries on initial triage assessment.[21] Specific clinical findings may be helpful. Tympanic membrane rupture may be a subtle sign of blast injury in some cases. However, the presence of an intact tympanic membrane does not ensure that a patient has not sustained a significant blast injury.[16] Although over-triage places an increased strain on hospital resources, an over-triage rate of 50% is necessary to avoid the less desirable scenario of under-triage (i.e., categorizing a critically injured patient into a delayed treatment category). Frykberg and Tepas[14] evaluated 14 terrorist bombing incidents and found an average over-triage rate of 59%. In general, accurate and efficient triage is an important factor in patient survival.

 UNIQUE CONSIDERATIONS

VBIED explosions stand apart from other explosions because they are, unfortunately, relatively common, unpredictable, and frequently perpetrated by terrorist groups. As numerous domestic and international VBIED incidents have demonstrated, morbidity and mortality are

 CASE PRESENTATION

At 10:30 AM, a truck carrying approximately 2 tons of explosives detonates in the center of a city's financial district. The explosion results in the collapse of a portion of a 12-story office building and damages buildings in a 24-block radius. Within minutes several EMS units arrive at the scene, and over the next 30 minutes coordination begins between police, fire, and EMS personnel at the scene. Incident command is established per preplanned protocols, and specific areas are designated as casualty treatment and triage sites. The incident area is cordoned off, and rescue efforts begin. Large numbers of people are exiting buildings and police are directing them to safe locations. Hospitals in the immediate vicinity activate their individual disaster plans, and all local emergency departments are quickly inundated with patients. Most victims arrive at area emergency departments on foot or via private vehicle.

Communications from the scene of the explosion to the local hospitals offer limited details of initial casualty estimates. During the course of the day, nearly 700 patients are evaluated at area hospitals as a result of the explosion; of these, 580 patients are treated and released, 12 patients die en route to the hospital or within the first 24 hours, and 115 are admitted to the hospital for further care and/or observation.

high. Another risk to consider with VBIEDs is the potential to use these devices as a dispersal mechanism for various hazardous materials. For example, the bombing of the World Trade Center in 1993 may have involved a cyanide compound, which the perpetrators hoped would be dispersed into the building ventilation system after the explosion. It is not clear whether cyanide was used during this attack; however, it is clear that the terrorists involved possessed cyanide and had plans to use chemicals in conjunction with future explosive devices.[22]

 PITFALLS

One potential pitfall in responding to a VBIED attack is the failure to consider the risk of a secondary explosion after the initial explosion. Secondary explosive devices may be designed to kill and injure emergency responders both at the scene as well as at the hospital. It is important to note that secondary devices may be located near the epicenter of the original blast as well as at other locations. An example of the use of a secondary device deployed at a location remote from the original blast was the Thiepval barracks bombing incident.[12] In this incident, a second car bomb was deployed and timed to target the local medical treatment facility at a time when arriving patients and medical personnel would be present. Medical treatment facilities must be mindful of this tactic and should have protocols in place to protect against such an eventuality.

A second potential pitfall in responding to such an attack is the failure to consider that a VBIED explosion may be used to disperse hazardous materials.

REFERENCES

1. Maniscalco PM. Terrorism hits home. *Emerg Med Serv.* 1993; 22:31-2, 34-7, 40-1.
2. Hollander D. Mairobi bomb blast-trauma and recovery. *Trop Doct.* 2000;30:47-8.
3. U.K. Security Service (MI5). Vehicle Bombs. Available at: http://www.mi5.gov.uk/print/Page42.html.
4. Cabinet Office Civil Contingencies Secretariat. *Dealing with Disaster.* Revised 3rd ed. June 2003. Available at: http://www.ukresilience. info/contingencies/dwd/index.htm.
5. Hillier T. Bomb attacks in city centers. September 1994. Available at: http://www.emergency.com/carbomb.htm.
6. Doyle C. Mass casualty incident integration with pre-hospital care. *Emerg Med Clin North Am.* 1990;8:163-75.
7. Hogan DE, Waeckerle JF, Dire DJ, et al. Emergency department impact of the Oklahoma City terrorist bombing. *Ann Emerg Med.* 1999;34:160-7.
8. Jacobs Jr LM. An emergency medical system approach to disaster planning. *J Trauma.* 1979;19:157-62.
9. Maningas PA, Robison M, Mallonee S. The EMS response to the Oklahoma City bombing. *Prehospital Disaster Med.* 1997;12:80-5.
10. Frykberg ER. Principles of mass casualty management following terrorist disasters. *Ann Surg.* 2004;239:319-21.
11. Hodgetts TJ. Lessons from the Musgrave Park hospital bombing. *Injury* 1993;24:219-21.
12. Vassallo DJ, Taylor JC, Aldington DJ, et al. Shattered illusions: the Thiepval Barracks bombing, 7 October 1996. *J R Army Med Corps.* 1997;143:5-11.
13. Frykberg ER, Tepas III JJ, Alexander RH. The 1983 Beirut airport terrorist bombing injury patterns and implications for disaster management. *Am Surgeon.* 1989;55:134-41.
14. Frykberg ER, Tepas III JJ. Terrorist bombings lessons learned from a Belfast to Beirut. *Ann Surg.* 1988;208:569-76.
15. Greenberg M. Routine screening for environmental radiation by first responders at explosions and fires. *Ann Emerg Med.* 2003; 41:421.
16. Mellor SG, Cooper GJ. Analysis of 828 servicemen killed or injured by explosion in Northern Ireland 1970-84: the hostile action casualty system. *Br J Surg.* 1989;76:1006-10.
17. Mallonee S, Shariat S, Stennies G, et al. Physical injuries and fatalities resulting from the Oklahoma City bombing. *JAMA* 1996; 276:382-7.
18. Arnold JL, Halpern P, Tsai MC, et al. Mass casualty terrorist bombings: a comparison of outcomes by bombing type. *Ann Emerg Med.* 2004;43:263-73.
19. Cooper GJ, Maynard RL, Cross NL, et al. Casualties from terrorist bombings *J Trauma.* 1983;23:955-67.
20. Adler J, Golan E, Golan J, et al. Terrorist bombing experience during 1975-9 casualties admitted to the Shaare Zedek medical center. *Isr J Med Sci.* 1983;19:189-93.
21. Hirshberg A, Stein M, Walden R. Surgical resource utilization in urban terrorist bombing: a computer simulation *J Trauma.* 1999; 47:545-50.
22. Parachini JV. The world trade center bombers, 1993. In: Tucker JB, ed. *Toxic Terror: Assessing Terrorist Use of Chemical and Biological Weapons.* Cambridge, Mass: MIT Press; 2000:185-206.

chapter 146

Rocket-Propelled Grenade Attack[*]

Marshall Eidenberg

INTRODUCTION

Rocket-propelled grenades (RPGs) have been used in combat since World War II, with the American bazooka and German Panzerfaust. All RPGs share one common element: a shaped charge in the warhead designed to penetrate armor.[1] In one attack in Vietnam, RPGs caused 12% of casualties.[2] More recently, in Operation Iraqi Freedom, RPGs caused 14.5% of battlefield injuries.[3] RPGs have been used to bring down helicopters and have been mass fired, reminiscent of American Civil War battles, to attack armored vehicles. Current examples are the American light antitank weapon (LAW) rocket and AT4 and the Russian-made RPG-7. The RPG-7 has a maximum range of 920 meters, at which time it self-explodes (4.5 seconds from firing). As a result, this weapon is sometimes used as a form of anti-aircraft artillery against slow, low-flying, or hovering helicopters.

There is a second class of weapons that physically resembles RPGs, called enhanced blast weapons (EBWs). They also made their debut in World War II. The Soviet-made Katyusha and German Nebelwerfer were the first. EBWs rely primarily on blast overpressure and secondarily on heat for their effects. Confined spaces intensify the blast effect by reflection of the pressure waves from interior surfaces. Current examples are the Russian TBG-7V (which is fired from the RPG-7 launcher) and the Chinese RPO-A.[4,5]

 ## DESCRIPTION OF EVENTS

Shaped-charge warheads cause a mix of wound patterns including thermal, blast, and ballistic trauma. The shaped charge forces a jet of super hot material through armor. These wounds have been described as similar to those caused by a blowtorch. The explosion will cause blast injury, discussed in greater detail below, and fragments of the RPG and spall (i.e., fragments of the vehicle or building hit by the RPG) from the target can cause ballistic damage with perforations and lacerations.[6]

The EBWs cause injuries from the compressive effects of the shock waves transmitted to the victim (i.e., primary blast injury). The lungs and all air-filled organs are most vulnerable to blast overpressure, and injury to these organs increases the risk of mortality. Internal organs such as the intestines, heart, liver, and kidneys are also susceptible to damage from primary blast injury. The most likely result will be the crushing or rupture of the organ, which can lead to rapid loss of blood, accumulation of body fluids, or eventual peritonitis. Air embolism can also occur in coronary and cerebral vasculature. Pneumothoraces may also result from primary blast injury.

Secondary blast injuries result from limited fragmentation of the warhead as well as the debris displaced by the blast. In open areas this is limited. In enclosed areas like buildings, debris is usually present, which increases the likelihood of these injuries. Typical secondary blast injuries are perforations of the body, fractures, injuries to the eyes (from dirt or dust), and lacerations. Unless a vital organ is damaged, rapid blood loss is the primary danger from this type of injury.

Tertiary blast injury results from the blast throwing the casualty. Typical injuries are blunt trauma, fractures, and amputated limbs. Again, rapid blood loss is the major danger.

 ## PREINCIDENT ACTIONS

Aside from having a well-developed and rehearsed disaster response plan, there are no specific preplanning actions to be taken. Body armor helps cut down on secondary injuries from fragmentation but may enhance primary blast injuries in enclosed spaces.[4,5]

 ## POSTINCIDENT ACTIONS

Prehospital trauma life support becomes the primary care at the point of wounding. Simple life-saving skills are necessary to treat airway, breathing, and circulatory problems of persons with these types of wounds. Prehospital personnel should document injuries that occurred within an enclosed space to highlight the possibility of blast overpressure injuries when the casualty

---

[*]Disclaimer: The opinions or assertions contained herein are solely those of the author and do not represent the views of the Army Medical Department or the Department of Defense.

reaches the emergency department. Postincident actions include notification of the trauma team and activation of the hospital's mass-casualty plan. Plans should be in place for casualties who may have unexploded ordinance embedded in their bodies, are still alive, and require care. These weapons can be handled relatively safely during removal from patients, but they will need ultimate disposal by the "bomb squad." Police bomb disposal personnel should be involved if there are any unexploded RPGs or EBWs retained in the patient's body. Other considerations consist of mobilization of type O-positive and O-negative blood. The police department and hospital security personnel should be used for crowd control and media control.

 ## MEDICAL TREATMENT OF CASUALTIES

Treatment for both RPGs and EBWs are essentially the same as that of any other injury. The primary survey, airway, breathing, and circulation issues must be addressed first. Traumatic injuries are treated in the same way as any other casualty. Frequently, these patients have a multiple modality injury—burn, blast, and fragmentation (foreign body). Recent information from Operation Iraqi Freedom indicates that RPGs are the leading cause of multiple site injury.[3]

Blast injuries are relatively difficult to diagnose in the prehospital setting and can take time to reveal themselves, especially in the case of chest and abdominal blast injuries. Injuries to the torso and abdomen may have no external symptoms and may initially be indistinguishable from benign causes of respiratory distress, such as hyperventilation, breathlessness, and agitation due to stress reaction. More subtle signs of primary blast injury include deafness, bleeding from the ears, chest or abdominal pain, confusion, and difficulty breathing. Suspected blast casualties should be transported by stretcher because exercise has been shown to worsen pulmonary problems.[7]

Inappropriate use of intravenous fluids in patients with primary blast injury can cause rapid development of pulmonary problems due to pulmonary contusion (i.e., blast lung). Fluids should not be withheld for

resuscitation but should be used based on clinical parameters such as level of consciousness, urine output, and peripheral pulses. This is slightly different than the current advanced trauma life support guidelines, which recommend the rapid infusion of 2 liters of isotonic crystalloid.[8]

 ## UNIQUE CONSIDERATIONS

Remember that these patients who have been caught in an RPG attack have incurred multiple mechanisms of injury. In addition, these are high–kinetic-energy military weapons, especially compared with civilian modes of wounding, and the amount of energy transfer and tissue damage is likely to be greater.

The RPO-A EBW uses isopropyl nitrate as an energetic material in the warhead. Isopropyl nitrate can be absorbed into the skin, ultimately causing formation of methemoglobin.[9] Isopropyl nitrate is also a carcinogen. Ordinarily, isopropyl nitrate is a clear fluid, but it may have been dyed pink for ease of identification during maintenance. If a pink fluid is present when the RPO-A malfunctions, avoid contact with this fluid.

 ## PITFALLS

Several potential pitfalls in response to an RPG attack exist. These include the following:

- As with every trauma patient, finding the first injury necessitates the search for the second, third, etc. Responder should not stop looking until the patient has had the tincture of time to unmask the more subtle injuries.
- The anxious patient with no apparent injuries may still have sustained injuries to his or her lungs or abdomen. Rule out the medical causes (e.g., primary blast injury) for this anxiety before obtaining a psychiatry referral.
- Large-volume intravenous fluid resuscitation should be avoided. Healthcare providers should treat for shock, but titrate volumes based on mental status, urine output, and peripheral pulses.

REFERENCES

1. Bellamy RF, Zajtchuk R. The weapons of conventional land warfare and Assessing the effectiveness of conventional weapons. In: Bellamy RK, Zajtchuk R, eds. *Textbook of Military Medicine: part I*. Volume 5, Conventional Warfare: Ballistic, Blast and Burn Injuries. Washington DC: U.S. Office of the Surgeon General, Department of the Army; 1991:27, 66, 68.
2. Wound Data and Munitions Effectiveness Team. Evaluation of wound data and munitions effectiveness in Vietnam. Alexandria, Va: U.S. Defense Documentation Center of the Defense Logistics Agency; 1970:Vol. 3, Table 4, p. C-7, Table D. 10-3, p. D-19.
3. Dunemn KN, Oakley CJ, Gamboa SR, et al. *Profile of Casualties Treated in US Army Medical Treatment Facilities During Operation Iraqi Freedom: 10 March-30 November 2003*. Washington DC: Center for AMEDD Strategic Studies; 2004:1-98.
4. Grau LW, Smith T. A 'crushing' victory: fuel-air explosives and grozny 2000. *The Marine Corps Gazette*. Aug 2000;84(8):30.

5. The threat from blast weapons. *The Bulletin, for Soldiers by Soldiers, The Canadian Army Lessons Learned Centre.* 2001; 7-3:1-10.

6. Dougherty PJ. Armored vehicle crew casualties. *Mil Med.* 1990;155:417-20.

7. Hamit HF, Bulluck MH, Frumson G, Moncrief JA. Air blast injuries: report of a case. *J Trauma.* 1965; 5:117-24.

8. Bellamy RF. The nature of combat injuries and the role of ATLS in their management. In: Zatjuk R, ed. *Combat Casualty Care Guidelines.* Washington DC: U.S. Office of the Surgeon General, Department of the Army; 1991:9-19.

9. Safety (MSDS) data for isopropyl nitrate. October 27, 2003. Available at: http://ptcl.chem.ox.ac.uk/MSDS/IS/isopropyl_nitrate.html.

chapter 147

Conventional Explosions at a Mass Gathering

Franklin D. Friedman

 DESCRIPTION OF THE EVENT

The magnitude and severity of primary injuries from a blast explosion are determined by proximity, the quantity and type of explosive, and whether the explosion occurs in an open or enclosed space.[1,2] Naturally, when an explosion occurs in the midst of a large gathering of people, other factors that strongly affect overall morbidity and mortality include access of rescuers to the injured and the personnel and resources available to care for an overwhelming number of victims in the immediate aftermath.

The increasing prevalence of terrorism and insurgency over the last three decades has increased our understanding of the types of injuries caused by blast in the civilian environment—injuries once seen only on the battlefield—as well as the predictors of survival and management techniques for such incidents.[3-5] By the time victims of these injuries reach the hospital, primary blast injuries are uncommon because, so often, they result in immediate death.[6] Because they are so rare, and because a bombing often results in so many casualties converging on a single institution, many physicians and other healthcare workers with no prior expertise in trauma or disaster management may be pressed into service to care for trauma patients.[7]

Although many articles in the medical literature describe the effects of blast injuries,[8-11] and others describe medical planning and care for mass gatherings[12-15] (i.e., mass "gatherings of potential patients"[16]), few combine both topics.[17-20] As late as 2002, a 25-year review of the literature pertaining to mass gatherings did not reference a single article describing a terrorist incident at a mass gathering, or even discuss the topic.[11] Most articles concerning healthcare planning for mass gatherings, in fact, ignore the risk of a major traumatic event such as a bombing, instead focusing on environmental or medical emergencies. An incident in which 60,000 spectators are exposed to an exploding bomb demands a different response.

Fortunately, very few incidents of intentional or accidental explosions have occurred, affecting large gatherings such as sporting or entertainment events (e.g., the

Atlanta Olympics in 1996 and Bali in 2002). Many of the terrorist bombings from which we have learned about injury patterns occurred in other settings (e.g., U.S. barracks in Beirut in 1983, the Alfred P. Murrah Federal Building in 1995, the World Trade Center in New York in 1993, the Madrid train in 2004, numerous attacks in Israel). By extrapolating from what is known about the nature of explosion injuries, the outcome of explosions that have affected many victims, and the strategies developed to provide medical care at major events, one can build a workable strategy to care for persons with these injuries.

The *medical usage rate* (generally reported as numbers of patients per 10,000 in attendance) at a mass gathering is rarely greater than 50 at a spectator event, and it is most often related to weather. By stark contrast, one author documents a mortality of 7.8% for open-air and 49% of closed-space bombings, although these do not refer to mass gatherings with several thousand persons in attendance.[2]

 PREINCIDENT ACTIONS

Preparation for conventional explosions at a large gathering is best when it is preventive, rather than reactive. The best preparations depend on making conditions unfavorable for the bomber and designing structures that are fire resistant, are less likely to collapse, and offer easy egress in the event of an explosion. Measures can be taken, as in the London Underground, to remove waste receptacles in which an explosive device may be hidden. Similarly, although inconvenient, inspecting backpacks and the trunks of vehicles for those entering events have become a necessary precaution.

The importance of repeated drilling of all the facets of a hospital and a region's disaster plan must not be underestimated. After the bombing at the 1996 Atlanta Olympics, Atlanta emergency medical services leaders attributed pre-event training and drills practiced during 5 years leading up to the event as the principal reason why their response went well.[19] All 111 injured patients were evacuated to the area hospitals within just 32 minutes of the explosion.[19] To best prepare for a conventional bombing at a mass gathering, perform a drill involving a scenario with a large surge of trauma victims, mixing both critically ill and lightly injured victims.

 POSTINCIDENT ACTIONS

The potential volume of patients with both critical and noncritical injuries is the greatest risk to successful management of an explosion at a mass gathering. Establishing effective triage, both at the scene and again at the receiving hospitals, will prevent overwhelming limited resources and ensure that the most seriously injured patients are identified rapidly and sent to appropriate medical facilities.

Virtually all civilian bombings constitute a criminal act. Therefore, any material from the explosives found on or inside of victims is evidence that may be useful to investigational authorities in solving the crime. Salvaged clothing may contain identifiable explosive residue. Even corpses may yield important clues; consider performing postmortem radiographs to identify shrapnel. Expect to continue to work with law enforcement personnel after an incident, especially in matters such as evidence collection and serving as witnesses as the examining healthcare providers.

After treatment of casualties is completed, how should outcomes be assessed? Data points of interest include injury severity scores, specific injuries, morbidity, mortality, and location of persons with respect to the explosive device. By publishing data such as these, and lessons learned, it may be possible to improve the response to the next bombing incident.

 MEDICAL TREATMENT OF CASUALTIES

When caring for victims of a conventional bombing at a mass gathering, keep in mind the convergence of two types of disaster: injuries unique to conventional explosives and caring for the surge of many simultaneously injured patients. Those close to the actual explosion often will die or suffer serious injuries, but the majority of casualties will receive relatively minor injuries, frequently from flying debris.[21] The other traumatic injuries likely seen will be those related to stampede from those trying to escape or burns from a resulting fire. Despite the variety of serious injuries unique to blast injuries, the most common injuries among blast survivors involve standard penetrating and blunt trauma.[22]

The major medical challenge in caring for the victims of bombs, in addition to the multiple simultaneous casualties, is to identify those who are seriously injured but salvageable and to realize that they will be mixed in with a large number who are lightly injured or psychologically traumatized.[1] Children are particularly at risk for the damages inflicted by bomb explosions, yet the physical clues of injury may be less apparent, particularly to rescuers mainly accustomed to treating adults.[23] Large numbers of children may also be present at certain mass gatherings. Details concerning the nature, type, and care

of injuries common to conventional explosions are described in other chapters in this section.

In addition to the actual explosions, the other two principal injury-causing features of this attack were the collapse of the Sari Club (a largely open-sided building), which trapped patrons, and the ignition of a huge fire that was apparently caused by exploding gas cylinders. Care of the injured was compromised by a limited medical infrastructure in Kuta; although it has one of the best hospitals in Bali, the care offered there is still rudimentary.[27] Many of the foreign nationals were evacuated to Australia and Singapore. Sixty-one patients were transferred to Royal Darwin Hospital in Australia, 28 of whom had major trauma including "severe burns, missile injuries from shrapnel, limb disruption, and pressure-wave injury to ears, lung, and bowel."[28]

In Bali, beyond the limitations of caring for so many burned and otherwise injured patients, untrained volunteers performed much of the initial mortuary care. Tourists took on the daily responsibility of bringing ice to a makeshift morgue. Unfortunately, they also combined victims' remains in single bags, commingling DNA and making some identification impossible. Three unidentified bodies were cremated subsequently.[26]

💡 UNIQUE CONSIDERATIONS

Responding to a conventional explosion at a mass gathering is unlike treating either a small number of victims from an explosion or the typical patients presenting from a large event (usually medical complaints, minor injuries, or environmental-related problems). A carefully placed explosive device at a major indoor event can result in hundreds or potentially thousands of casualties suffering assorted trauma, including burns. Triage, both at the scene and again at the receiving hospitals, is one of the most crucial aspects of the response to prevent overwhelming limited resources. Keep in mind that, unlike a medical emergency, at a sports event, the EMTs prepositioned in the stadium may be among the victims when a bomb explodes.

Delay of care for those truly in need (i.e., those requiring chest decompression, mechanical ventilation, operative exploration) while methodically evaluating and bandaging every patient with an abrasion will mean lives lost. The effective disaster response, as for any surge of trauma patients, will rely on a variety of caregivers pressed into service to treat minor injuries,[7] while senior, experienced emergency providers perform rapid triage, directing casualties to appropriate sites for care.

 ## PITFALLS

Several potential pitfalls in responding to an explosion at a mass gathering exist. These include the following:

- Over-triage could rapidly overwhelm hospitals, resulting in the needless death of casualties who otherwise might have been saved.
- Failure to consider the possibility of additional explosive devices after the initial detonation can needlessly result in additional casualties.
- Failure to rapidly institute an orderly means to perform triage, both in the field and at hospitals, will result in unnecessary chaos. A military processing station model should be the ideal.

REFERENCES

1. Stein M, Hirshberg A. Medical consequences of terrorism. *Surg Clin North Am*. 1999;79: 1537-52.
2. Leibovici D, Gofrit ON, Stein M, et al. Blast injuries: bus versus open-air bombings—a comparative study of injuries in survivors of open-air versus confined-space explosions. *J Trauma*. 1996;41: 1030-5.
3. Frykberg ER, Tepas JJ 3rd. Terrorist bombings, lessons learned from Belfast to Beirut. *Ann Surg*. 1988;208:569-76.
4. Biancolini CA, Del Bosco CG, Jorge MA. Argentine Jewish community institution bomb explosion. *J Trauma*. 1999;47:728-32.
5. Pahor AL. The ENT problems following the Birmingham bombings. *J Laryngol Otol*. 1981;95:399-406.
6. Boffard KD, MacFarlane C. Urban bomb blast injuries: patterns of injury and treatment. *Surg Annu*. 1993;25:29-47.
7. Fisher D, Burrow J. The Bali bombings of 12 October 2002: lessons in disaster management for physicians. *Int Med J*. 2003;33:125-6.
8. Phillips YY. Primary blast injuries. *Ann Emerg Med*. 1986; 15: 105-9.
9. Mallonee S, Shariat S, Stennies G. Physical injuries and fatalities resulting from the Oklahoma City bombings. *J AMA* 1996; 276: 382-7.
10. Wightman JM, Gladish SL. Explosions and blast injuries. *Ann Emerg Med*. 2001;37:664-78.
11. Gibbons AJ, Farrier JN, Key SJ. The pipe bomb: a modern terrorist weapon. *J R Army Med Corps*. 2003;149:23-6.
12. Milsten AM, Maguire BJ, Bissell RA. Mass-gathering medical care: a review of the literature. *Prehospital Disaster Med*. 2002; 17: 151-62.
13. Michael JA, Barbera JA. Mass gathering medical care: a twenty-five year review. *Prehospital Disaster Med*. 1997;12:305-12.
14. Arbon P, Bridgewater FHG, Smith C. Mass gathering medicine: a predictive model for patient presentation and transport rates. *Prehospital Disaster Med*. 2001;16:150-8.
15. Nordberg M. EMS and mass gatherings. *Emerg Med Services*. 1990;19:46-56, 91.
16. Butler II WC, Gesner DE. Crowded venues: avoid an EMS quagmire by preparing for mass gatherings. *J Emerg Med Serv*. 1999; 24:62-5.
17. Severance HW. Mass-casualty victim "surge" management: preparing for bombings and blast-related injuries with possibility of hazardous materials exposure. *N C Med J*. 2002;63:242-6.
18. Frykberg ER. Medical management of disasters and mass casualties from terrorist bombings: how can we cope? *J Trauma*. 2002;53:201-12.
19. Feliciano DV, Anderson GV, Rozycki GS, et al. Management of casualties from the bombing at the Centennial Olympics. *Am J Surg*. 1998;176:538-43.
20. Brismar BO, Bergenwald L. The terrorist bomb explosion in Bologna, Italy, 1980: an analysis of the effects and injuries sustained. *J Trauma*. 1982;22:216-20.
21. Kennedy TL, Johnston GW. Civilian bomb injuries. *BMJ*. 1975;1:382-3.
22. Explosions and blast injuries: a primer for clinicians. *Mass Preparedness and Response*. Available at: http://www.bt.cdc.gov/masstrauma/explosions.asp.
23. Waisman Y, Aharonson-Daniel L, Mor M, et al. The impact of terrorism on children: a two-year experience. *Prehospital Dis Med*. 2004;18:242-8.
24. Bonner R. Bombing at resort in Indonesia kills 150 and hurts scores more. *New York Times on the Web*. October 13, 2002. Available at: http://travel2.nytimes.com/mem/travel/article-page.html?res=9F06E7DA103AF930A25753C1A9649C8B63.
25. Mydans S. Terror in Bali: The aftermath—survivors of Indonesia blast are left stunned and searching. *The New York Times on the Web*. October 14, 2002. Available at: http://travel2.nytimes.com/mem/travel/article-page.html?res= 9C02E4D9113AF937A25753-C1A9649C8B63.
26. 2002 Bali terrorist bombing. *Wikipedia*. Available at: http://en.wikipedia.org/wiki/2002_Bali_terrorist_bombing.
27. Watts J. Bali bombing offers lessons for disaster relief. *Lancet* 2002;360:1401.
28. Palmer DJ, Stephens D, Fisher DA, et al. The Bali bombing: the Royal Darwin Hospital response. *Med J Aust*. 2003;179:353-6.

chapter 148

Conventional Explosion at a Hospital

Donald MacMillan

 DESCRIPTION OF EVENT

Although a highly unlikely event, a hospital explosion and its impact on the infrastructure, patients, staff, and the community must be considered. The hospital setting is rich in flammable and toxic materials, making it a potentially hazardous environment. The ever-increasing use of hazardous materials, nuclear agents, and toxic substances makes most medical centers vulnerable to explosions.[1] Although there is a paucity of reports of hospital explosions in the literature, the increasing frequency of terrorist events makes such an event more likely.[2] The experience gained from damage to healthcare facilities by earthquakes and terrorist incidents provides some insight into how to respond to this type of emergency. This chapter will discuss the types of explosions that may affect a hospital, and the associated injuries will be described. Potential pitfalls and successes from similar events will also be discussed. All will be considered in the context of the Incident Command System (ICS).

Conventional explosions in hospitals are exceedingly rare. When a hazard vulnerability analysis is performed, the probability of such an event would be given a low score; however, the impact of the event on the institution warrants a high score, making the overall score low to intermediate. Explosions can result from either a terrorist event or an internal mishap, such as a ruptured gas line. No matter the source, the result is essentially the same.

A terrorist incident will most likely involve the detonation of an improvised explosive device. These devices come in a variety of shapes and sizes, ranging from small pipe bombs composed of metal pipe and rapidly burning gunpowder to large truck bombs like the one used to destroy the Alfred P. Murrah Federal Building in Oklahoma City in 1995. Secondary devices, which are devices timed to detonate after the primary explosion, must be considered. Although they failed to function as intended, the suspects in the Columbine High School shooting in 1999 had many secondary devices, which were designed to maim and kill emergency responders.[3] Secondary devices were also used in the Centennial Park bombing at the 1996 Atlanta Olympics as well as the Atlanta abortion clinic bombing in 1997. Until the source of the explosion can be identified, the presence

of secondary devices must be considered. Unlike terrorist bombings, explosions caused by flammable gases or liquids may continue to burn, resulting in secondary explosions that can cause further damage to the structure. The storage of compressed gases, including oxygen and air, can be the source of an explosion at a healthcare facility.

No matter what the source of the explosion, damage to the building can include the structural components or infrastructural components (e.g., ventilation, water supply, and sprinkler systems). Fires ignited from the initial explosion can generate injured patients, even among those who avoided injury in the initial event. Damage to anything other than a small confined area requires the consideration of a partial or facility-wide evacuation.

 PREINCIDENT ACTIONS

An ICS is the foundation of the hospital's emergency operations plan. Repeated drills using the ICS are a must. An ICS is an organized system of command and control that allows the user to employ procedures for organizing personnel, facilities, equipment, and communications during an emergency response. A full discussion of the ICS can be found in Chapter 30. Table 148-1 briefly outlines the immediate tasks of the sector chiefs.

 POSTINCIDENT ACTIONS

The Incident Commander will determine when the incident is over or determined to be under control and when to discontinue or contract the ICS. The incident may be turned over to the top-ranking police or fire agency during the investigative phase. The primary function is to restore the hospital to its preincident state. Partial restoration of services may begin as soon as the building is deemed structurally sound and certain patients may be returned to their beds or the hospital can start accepting new patients. The determination of whether severely damaged structures can be repaired or will have to be razed must be addressed. After the 1994 Northridge, Calif, earthquake, four of the eight hospitals that evacuated patients because of that disaster required demolition.[4]

TABLE 148-1 IMMEDIATE TASKS OF SECTOR CHIEFS IN EMERGENCY RESPONSE

TITLE	TASKS TO CONSIDER
Incident Commander	1. Activate Emergency Operations Center. 2. Set agenda for status report by sector chiefs (i.e., operations, logistics, planning and finance). 3. Assign liaisons to coordinate with responding agencies. 4. Assign a public information officer 5. Prepare staff for extended operations. 6. Determine whether patient evacuation will be required.
Logistics Sector Chief	1. Determine the structural integrity of the affected building and advise the Incident Commander. 2. Secure the utilities, including medical gases. 3. Ensure adequate supplies to treatment area. 4. Activate emergency communications plan.
Planning Sector Chief	1. Consider alternative care sites. 2. Secure transportation for patients to alternative care sites. 3. Ensure accurate patient tracking. 4. Develop a plan for convergent volunteerism.
Operations Sector Chief	1. Organize triage and treatment of all casualties. 2. Ensure continued care of all unaffected patients.
Finance Sector Chief	1. Immediately track all costs associated with response, recovery, and mitigation of event.

Immediate real-time cost tracking may become important for reimbursement. The finance officer should work closely with outside agencies, including the institution's insurance carrier, to provide accurate costs. This must include personnel costs as well as replacement costs for material. Determining what types of disaster relief or grant money will be available and how best to access these funds will assist the institution in returning to its preincident condition.

In the event the source of the explosion is unknown and possibly the result of a terrorist attack, the facility also becomes a crime scene. Evidence preservation and limited access to the scene are critical. Jurisdictional issues, particularly with law enforcement agencies, may become complicated. All agencies should understand that safety issues take priority, but responders should try to minimize their impact on the scene. Working with these agencies during drills and appreciating one another's roles and capabilities will greatly enhance the working relationship and allow both missions to be accomplished in overlapping time frames.

Finally, since hospitals have large amounts of hazardous and radioactive material, patient decontamination may be required. Contaminated patients cannot enter the general population without first being decontaminated. Depending on the location of the explosion and the damage sustained, the hospital's own decontamination facility may be unavailable. Even if the facility is undamaged, the personnel who usually provide decontamination may be unavailable. Contamination with radioactive material has some special considerations. Working closely with the hospital physicist or the radiation safety officer will greatly enhance decontamination efforts. In addition, educating staff about radioactive decontamination will reduce the anxiety of treating these patients.

Although explosions at hospitals are rare, they must be considered during the hazard vulnerability analysis. The best way to prepare for these and all types of events is to implement an Incident Command–based hospital emergency management plan. This plan should be exercised frequently and should involve as many community agencies as possible. This experience will be invaluable no matter what type of emergency disrupts the function of a hospital.

Medical Treatment of Casualties

Victims of a conventional explosion at a hospital will have the myriad of injuries seen in blasts and structure collapse. The care of these victims will follow those guidelines described thoroughly in Chapters 141, 142, and 162. In a hospital setting, however, some casualties may have underlying medical conditions for which they are being hospitalized. The management of such patients should also take into account these underlying conditions.

 CASE PRESENTATION

An explosion and fire occurs at 11 PM in the main power plant of a large inner-city hospital, severely damaging that part of the hospital structure. An adjacent building with inpatient wards on seven floors, including the emergency department, operating rooms, and medical and surgical intensive care units, is damaged from the explosion. The backup power supply initiates, then fails after 1 minute and another explosion. Electrical power is lost throughout the hospital. All of the lights as well as some ventilators and monitors turn off, elevators stop, and communications cease. As first responders arrive, one section of the hospital is enveloped in flames, and the remainder of the hospital is in complete darkness. Inside, hospital staff in every unit frantically attempt to locate patients in the dark, rescue patient and staff victims of the explosion and fire, assist those whose ventilators have failed, and begin the evacuation procedure.

UNIQUE CONSIDERATIONS

There are unique considerations with hospital explosions. The first is operating in an oxygen-rich environment. The potential for increase in fire is directly related to the amount of oxygen available from ruptured medical gas lines. It should be an absolute top priority of the operations sector chief to have the oxygen lines shut down as soon as possible. This may mean shutting down the entire facility until the affected area of the building can be isolated.

Whether the explosion is due to a terrorist event or is an accident, there is an increased potential for the dispersal of radioactive material. Contamination will add a level of complexity to the management of the incident because decontamination will have to be executed in consultation with the facility's radiation safety officer. If the explosion is the result of a terrorist event, the involvement of law enforcement personnel adds yet another level of complexity. To ensure that potential radiation contamination is considered, the radiation safety officer should be notified whenever the emergency operations plan is implemented. He or she is a staff officer or liaison to the Incident Commander and needs to be incorporated into the operations plan. The Incident Commander can quickly dismiss him or her if the officer's services are not required, or the officer can be reassigned to the operations sector as needed.

The risk of evacuating patients from a structure that is potentially unstable must be considered. These risks include moving unstable patients through an environment that is immediately dangerous to life and health. If the building is damaged similar to what was seen in Oklahoma City, technical rescue experts will be required and the evacuation will be lengthy. Sheltering in place also has its risks, including turning a potentially stable structure into an unstable one as a result of any secondary explosions. The important point to determine is whether a patient is going to be exposed to greater risk during evacuation than he or she would if sheltered in place.

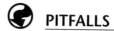 **PITFALLS**

Several potential pitfalls exist in responding to an explosion at a hospital. These include the following:

- Lack of an ICS-based emergency operations plan
- Failure to participate with local agencies that will respond in the event of an explosion
- Operating outside the ICS, allowing "freelancing" to occur
- Not incorporating ICS into all facets of drills, tabletop scenarios, and events
- Not getting to know all of the responders' capabilities and limitations before an event occurs

REFERENCES

1. Aghababian R, Lewis CP, Gans L, et al. Disasters within hospitals. *Ann Emerg Med.* 1994;23:771-7.
2. Hodgetts TJ. Lessons from the Musgrave Park Hospital bombing. *Injury* 1993;24:219-21.
3. Administration UF. *Wanton Violence at Columbine High School.* 1999.
4. Schultz CH, Koenig KL, Lewis RJ. Implications of hospital evacuation after the Northridge, California, earthquake. *N Engl J Med.* 2003;348:1349-55.

Conventional Explosion in a High-Rise Building

Ryan Friedberg

 ## DESCRIPTION OF EVENT

High-rise buildings are architectural wonders that shape the skylines of many cities across the United States. Explosions in high-rise buildings were essentially unheard of until 1993, when these structures became targets of terrorism. Until then, healthcare workers in the United States had no experience with mass casualties from explosions in high-rise buildings.

There have been three large-scale attacks on high-rise buildings in the United States since 1993. The first was the bombing of the World Trade Center in New York in 1993. This event resulted in six deaths and 1042 injuries.[1] The second attack was in Oklahoma City in 1995, when a truck bomb exploded adjacent to the Alfred P. Murrah Federal Building. This attack killed 167 persons and injured more than 750 persons.[2] The most recent attack, and the worst single act of terrorism in the history of the United States, was the attack on the World Trade Center towers in New York on Sept. 11, 2001. The actual death toll from this attack is unknown. There have been 1527 identified bodies, but it is believed that the actual death toll is between 2726 and 2742 persons.[3,4] Thousands of persons suffered injuries from the attack, and 1103 were treated in hospitals for their injuries.[5] The attack has changed the way people in the United States live and created an urgent need not only to attempt to prevent another such attack, but also to prepare for the possibility of future attacks on high-rise buildings.

There are many different types of explosives that terrorists may attempt to detonate in high-rise buildings. High explosives, including trinitrotoluene (TNT), composite C4, and ammonium nitrate are powerful enough to cause building collapse. However, the explosions and resulting fires from massive amounts of less-explosive aviation fuel in the World Trade Center attack resulted in the greatest structural failure in human history. Trauma after an explosion in a building can be categorized into primary, secondary, and tertiary blast injury. Primary blast injuries are due to the direct effect of the pressure wave on the victim.[6] The most sensitive organ affected by the primary blast is the ear.[7] Other systems that are affected include the respiratory, circulatory, and digestive systems, as well as the eye and orbit.

Secondary blast injuries are incurred due to objects propelled by the blast. These projectiles can be very significant in a high-rise building explosion and may extend far beyond the distance of the initial blast effect. These fragments that become projectiles can be both large and small and can cause both penetrating and blunt injuries.

Tertiary blast injuries occur when a person is propelled by the blast against another structure. These are typically blunt injuries including soft tissue injuries, lacerations, head injuries, and fractures. Less commonly seen are flash burns and thermal injuries.

Crush injuries are common if a building explosion results in structural collapse, and these frequently cause immediate death. In the Oklahoma City bombing, 97% of fatalities were immediate, and most were killed in the building collapse.[2] This was also true in the World Trade Center attack.[3] The risk of building collapse and resultant high fatality rates distinguish explosions in high-rise buildings from other types of explosions. Medical personnel are unlikely to care for victims crushed in a high-rise collapse because survival is rare.

 ## PREINCIDENT ACTIONS

Prevention is the most effective method of reducing morbidity and mortality in the aftermath of an explosion in a high-rise building. In addition to the obvious goal of preventing such an explosion in the first place, constructing high-rise buildings that can withstand an explosion without structural failure should significantly reduce mortality. Other safeguards will help to prevent secondary and tertiary injuries.

Currently, significant focus is being placed on design guidance, including site location, layout, building envelope and interior, and on the mechanical and electrical systems used in high-rise construction. When designing a new building, design guidance is provided for limiting or mitigating the effects of terrorist attacks. It is beyond the scope of this chapter to discuss each of these methods. The U.S. Federal Emergency Management Agency's Web site (http://www.fema.gov) extensively describes each of these strategies in their risk management series as of December 2003.

Another critical element to have in place in the aftermath of a building explosion is a disaster plan that involves all medical and rescue personnel of a given area. Any city or large community must have a well-rehearsed disaster plan in place in case of a mass-casualty event.

 POSTINCIDENT ACTIONS

Immediately after a conventional explosion in a high-rise building, there are three phases that need to be addressed. The first is the prehospital management, followed by the emergency department management, and finally, in-patient hospital management of the victims. Each of these will be addressed in this section.

The prehospital management starts with the activation of the mass-casualty alert that makes local, state, and federal agencies as well as all medical personnel aware of a disaster event. The first aspect of the disaster that needs to be addressed is the scene itself. Secondary explosive devices designed to explode on a delay, and directed at the personnel trying to rescue the victims, are unfortunately very common in terrorist attacks.[8] The safety of the remaining structure must also be assessed. Building collapse is always a significant risk during a bombing, and it is never acceptable to lose rescue workers when attempting to save victims. Once the building is as secure as possible, it is of utmost importance to quickly triage the victims according to standard protocols and determine which of them has life-threatening injuries.

Prehospital and emergency department staff must be prepared to triage patients appropriately, as the more severely injured patients are not usually the first wave of patients seen. Scene triage and separate emergency department triage may be necessary to direct patients to the most appropriate venue for care and maximize use of resources.

Prehospital personnel should expect to see familiar injuries including blunt, penetrating, and thermal injuries. After an explosion, all medical personnel need to maintain a high index of suspicion for primary blast injury. It is very important to evaluate the scene while performing rescue operations. Presence of a crater, injuries to closer victims, and building collapse are important observations regarding blast strength. Likewise, assessment of damaged objects near a casualty situation might yield a gross estimate of the pressures that existed in the vicinity. For example, shock waves able to rupture a tympanic membrane are about the same needed to shatter automobile glass.[9]

It is also important to get a quick history. Phillips and Zajtchuk[10] recommend the following questions when evaluating a bombing casualty:

- What type of ordinance was used? How large was the explosion?
- Where was the casualty located with respect to the blast?
- Did the blast occur inside an enclosed space, such as a room or vehicle?

- What was the casualty's activity after exposure?
- Were fires or fumes that might lead to an inhalation injury present?
- What was the orientation of the casualty's head and body in relation to the blast?

Prehospital medical personnel should be ready to perform life-saving interventions, including intubations, resuscitations, field amputations, and chest decompressions, although the most common procedures performed are spinal immobilizations, field dressings, and intravenous fluid administration.[11] Prehospital personnel should also be well equipped for the extrication of victims after complete or partial building collapse. Extricating these victims as quickly as possible greatly improves their chance of survival.

The second phase of treatment occurs in the emergency department. It is very important for medical control to direct the prehospital personnel to the most appropriate emergency department. Designated trauma centers should receive the most severely injured patients, even if they are not the closest hospital. Once the patient reaches the emergency department, the emergency staff needs to be prepared for the many types of injuries occurring in a blast. Emergency staff must be prepared for victims to arrive by all modes of transportation, most of whom will have only minor injuries. In the Oklahoma City bombing, Hogan and colleagues[11] report that 55% of victims came by private vehicle whereas only 33% came by emergency medical services transport; 80% were discharged that day.

As soon as hospitals are made aware of an explosion, emergency staff must mobilize the equipment necessary to treat numerous victims. This includes wound care trays, tetanus immunizations, antibiotics, fracture care, endotracheal tubes, thoracostomy tubes, cricothyroidotomy trays, and medications for conscious sedation, rapid sequence induction, and advanced cardiac life support. It is also the role of the emergency physician to ensure that the hospital disaster plan goes into effect. This includes making sure trauma teams are aware of any incoming patients and that the hospital is ready to accommodate the many injured patients that will need rapid admission to the hospital. This will improve throughput in the emergency department and create space in the emergency department for incoming wounded. Preparing for this type of disaster includes drilling the plan by hospital staff, and the plan should be well known by all staff members. The importance of adequate communication from the scene and prehospital providers to hospitals and emergency departments about the number of victims and types of injuries cannot be overstated.

 MEDICAL TREATMENT OF CASUALTIES

The treatment of casualties after an explosion in a high-rise building can be very challenging due to the different types of injuries seen and the pattern in which injured persons arrive at healthcare facilities. Healthcare professionals should be prepared for all three types of blast injuries as well as flash injuries, thermal burns, and crush injuries.

It is very important to properly triage patients who arrive from a blast event. The most common injuries are superficial, including abrasions and lacerations, and these patients are often the first group to present for care. The emergency physician must always be aware of the potential for primary blast injury and internal injuries that may present with delayed symptoms. When patients are examined, standard trauma protocols should be followed. For those patients with seemingly minor injuries, it is still necessary to do a thorough examination of the entire body. This will decrease the risk of missing an injury or any sign of an internal injury. Blast injuries differ from many other types of injuries because serious injuries may not manifest themselves immediately, particularly with primary blast injury, and careful observation of the patient is often necessary. Primary blast injury may result after any explosion but is amplified when it occurs in a building due to the enclosed surroundings. The management of primary blast injuries is discussed in more depth in earlier chapters in this section.

Secondary blast injuries are caused from projectiles due to the blast. These types of injuries make high-rise building explosions different from other conventional blasts. With many of the high-rise buildings today made with significant amounts of glass and steel, projectiles traveling at a high speed are very dangerous. It is these types of injuries that are most often seen in the emergency department. This is because the shrapnel that comes from a high-rise building can reach victims well outside the reach of the primary blast zone. During the Oklahoma City bombing, glass laceration injuries occurred as far as 10 blocks from the explosion. The most important thing to remember when treating patients with lacerations is to rule out other more serious injuries. Once more serious injuries have been ruled out, lacerations should be treated as time and resources allow. Delayed closure should be used if resources aren't available to treat both the critically ill and those with minor injuries. Injury to the eye often results from secondary blast injuries and should not be overlooked. Of the surviving victims of the Oklahoma City bombing, 8% sustained eye injuries, including lid lacerations, open globe injuries, orbital fractures, corneal abrasions, retinal detachment, and intraocular foreign bodies.[12]

The most worrisome type of secondary blast injury is the penetrating injury. Every part of the building and its contents has the ability to become shrapnel moving at high velocity. Victims with penetrating injuries should be treated promptly and with the involvement of the surgical trauma team. As with all penetrating injuries, the practitioner should be ready to treat hemorrhagic shock. In a stable patient, deep penetrating shrapnel should only be removed in a safe, controlled environment, usually the operating room.

Penetrating injuries are obvious; however, blunt trauma must not be overlooked. Blunt trauma can occur from secondary or tertiary blast injury after a high-rise explosion. Severe entrapment or crush injuries are rare

in survivors but may be seen in the emergency department. Patients with crush injuries are at risk for amputation, compartment syndrome, and rhabdomyolysis. These patients should be treated according to standard trauma protocols. Flash burns and thermal injuries are usually superficial injuries and should be treated with standard burn care.

CASE PRESENTATION

It is 9:30 AM, and you are the only attending physician working at the only level one trauma center in a small rural city. You receive a call from emergency medical services alerting you that there was just a large explosion from the ground floor of a commercial bank building. The building is made mostly of steel and glass. It is 22 stories high, and there are approximately 650 persons in the building. You are providing medical control for the paramedics.

What do you tell them? What do you need to do immediately with regard to your emergency department and hospital staff? Who else should be notified? What type of injuries do you expect to see, and what special equipment will you need to treat these injuries?

 UNIQUE CONSIDERATIONS

Preparing for a conventional bombing in a high-rise building is a difficult task because of the large variety of injuries seen and the great numbers of victims. Unique to these types of attacks is the pattern in which patients arrive. The first wave of patients is usually the furthest from the blast. These are usually secondary blast injuries, most of which are minor. The second wave of patients is usually the most critical. Another consideration in the explosion of a high-rise explosion is the presence of toxic substances, which may necessitate decontamination of victims and rescuers. A final consideration is emergency department patient flow. A triage system needs to be in place that will properly direct the large flow of injured victims.

 PITFALLS

Several potential pitfalls in response to an explosion in a high-rise building exist. These include the following:

- Failure to make sure the building is secure and safe for rescue personnel
- Failure to have a rehearsed disaster plan in place for a mass-casualty incident involving an explosion in a high-rise building
- Underestimation of the severity of injuries sustained by victims as a result of a conventional explosion in a high-rise building

REFERENCES

1. Federal Bureau of Investigation Bomb Data Center. *General Information Bulletin 96-1: 1996 Bombing Incidents*. Washington, DC: US Department of Justice; 1996.
2. Mallonee S, Shariat S, Stennies G, et al. Physical injuries and fatalities resulting from the Oklahoma City bombing. *JAMA* 1996;276:382-7.
3. Schwartz SP, Li W, Berenson L, Williams RD. Deaths in World Trade Centers Terrorist Attacks: September 11th, 2001. *MMWR* 2002;51:16-8.
4. Hirschkorn P. New York reduces 9/11 death toll by 40. October 29, 2003. Available at:. *www.cnn.com/2003/US/ Northeast/ 10/29/wtc.deaths*
5. Centers for Disease Control and Prevention. Rapid assessment of injuries among survivors of the terrorist attack on the World Trade Center—New York City, September 2001. *MMWR* 2002;51:1-5.
6. Phillips YY. Primary blast injuries. *Ann Emerg Med*. 1986;15:1446-50.
7. Adler OB, Rosenberger A. Blast injuries. *Acta Radiol*. 1988;29:1-5.
8. Boffard KD, Macfarlane C. Urban bomb blast injuries: patterns of injury and treatment. *Surg Ann*. 1993;25:29-47.
9. Wightman JM, Gladish SL. Explosions and blast injuries. *Ann Emerg Med*. 2001;37:6.
10. Phillips YY, Zajtchuk JT. The management of primary blast injury. In: Bellamy RF, Zajtchuk R, eds. *Conventional Warfare: Ballistic, Blast, and Burn Injuries*. Washington, DC: Office of the Surgeon General of the US Army; 1991:295-335.
11. Hogan DE, Waeckerle JF, Dire DJ, et al. Emergency department impact of the Oklahoma City terrorist bombing. *Ann Emerg Med*. 1999;34:160-7.
12. Mines M, Thach A, Mallonee S, et al. Ocular injuries sustained by survivors of the Oklahoma City Bombing. *Ophthalmology* 2000;107:837-43.

chapter 150

Conventional Explosion at a Nuclear Power Plant

Michelle McMahon-Downer

 ## DESCRIPTION OF EVENT

Since the attack on the World Trade Center in New York City on Sept. 11, 2001, there has been increased worldwide concern over the safety of nuclear power plants. In the United States, there are over 100 such plants.[1] Security has been heightened around nuclear power plants. Barricades are in place and armed guards are present.[2] All commercial nuclear power plants in the United States house the reactor core in a thick stainless steel vessel within a concrete building.[3] Nonetheless, studies have shown that if a jet aircraft crashed into a nuclear reactor and only 1% of its fuel ignited after impact, the resulting explosion could compromise the integrity of the reactor core containment building. Thus, these reactor core containment buildings, although designed to withstand impacts, are certainly destructible and vulnerable to large-scale explosions. Nuclear power plants harbor additional radioactive materials in the form of spent fuel pools. The spent fuel pools are housed in corrugated steel buildings, which are much more vulnerable to attack than the reactor core containment structure.[4]

An example of a conventional explosion at a nuclear power plant took place at Chernobyl Nuclear Power Plant in 1986. An accidental steam explosion during a safety test destroyed the reactor core. An atmospheric plume of radioactive substances was released into the environment during the explosion and fire.[5] Approximately 600 persons were hospitalized within a week due to injuries and ailments linked to the Chernobyl explosion.[6] Two died the first day as a result of trauma, combined with thermal burns and irradiation.[7] One hundred thirty-four persons were confirmed to have acute radiation sickness. Twenty-eight of those with acute radiation sickness died within the first 3 months, and 14 died in subsequent years.[8] Nineteen of the 28 who died in those first 3 months had severe radiation skin injuries that complicated their course of treatment in the hospital.[7]

At the time of the explosion, approximately 100,000 persons lived within a 30-km radius around Chernobyl Nuclear Power Plant. When the explosion occurred, radioactive substances were released into the atmosphere and continued to do so for 10 days, until the fire was finally contained. Winds and rainfall distributed the radioactive substances throughout the northern hemisphere, with the highest concentration around the power plant in the former U.S.S.R. Contamination of the area around the power plant was patchy in that distribution of the fallout depended largely on where it happened to rain. The volatile radioisotopes of iodine and cesium were the most important in terms of health risk.[6] Radioactive iodine has a half-life of just 8.05 days, but radioactive cesium has a half-life of approximately 30 years.[5,7] A total of 350,400 persons were resettled due to concerns over contamination caused by the Chernobyl explosion.[5]

Long-term effects of exposure to radiation, mainly carcinogenesis, are being seen in the population affected by the Chernobyl explosion. A clear association has been made between exposure to radiation and thyroid cancer, especially in children.[5] An increase in the incidence of leukemia in Russian clean-up workers has been seen, and Ukrainian scientists have indicated that there is an increase in other solid cancers (e.g., breast, lung, urologic) among the inhabitants of contaminated areas and clean-up workers.[8]

 ## PREINCIDENT ACTIONS

Each nuclear power plant is required to have an emergency response plan, as are the local and state government agencies in which the power plant is housed. Some federal agencies have emergency response plans in the event of a power plant explosion.[1] Control and command procedures must be clarified before an incident occurs, as must organizational responsibilities. Assessment of type and quantity of materials and equipment needed, along with decontamination plans and healthcare worker protection, should be addressed. Location of Geiger meters and other radiation survey instruments should be posted along with reference material on what the various readings mean in terms of patient care. An adequate supply of potassium iodide to combat exposure to radioactive iodine should be available for the entire affected population.[3]

Each community surrounding a nuclear power plant should have a designated person who makes decisions about evacuation and other issues concerning the potentially exposed population. Communication during the incident is of vital concern, and emergency communication systems must be tested in advance.[3] There are two emergency planning zones—the first is within a 10-mile radius of the event, where the threat of direct radiation is highest, and the second is within a 50-mile radius, where the radioactive plume is the biggest threat to residents. A warning system, such as sirens or flashing lights, is required to be provided by the nuclear power plant to alert all inhabitants within a 10-mile radius of an event. Each year, the nuclear power plant is required to distribute emergency information materials to all people who live within a 10-mile radius so that, in the event of an explosion, the public in the vicinity of the plant are prepared.[1]

Every hospital, regardless of the proximity to a nuclear power plant, should have a radiation control officer. This officer is responsible for monitoring all patients and medical personnel with radiation counters, supervising clean-up of the potentially radioactive waste, and devising a plan to minimize contamination. Training for physicians to prepare for a disaster involving radiation exposure is offered by the Radiation Emergency Assistance Center/Training Site, which can be contacted by phone at 1-865-576-1005.[3]

The World Health Organization suggests that the general population, particularly those in the vicinity of nuclear power plants, be prepared for a nuclear incident. One recommendation is that they become aware of possible solid shelter areas in the local area. A second is to have disaster supplies on hand; these include food and water for 3 to 5 days, a first-aid kit, respiration protection, flashlights and batteries, a battery-operated radio with extra batteries, and stable iodine.[9]

 POSTINCIDENT ACTIONS

Immediately after a conventional explosion at a nuclear power plant, the local emergency personnel will be activated. The disaster area must be designated as safe for these personnel to enter. Geiger counters and other devices used to detect radiation should be used. If the level is 0.1 Gy/hour or above, emergency personnel should not enter the area and should return to the control point until further notice. Specialized protective equipment is needed to enter the area safely.

As with any mass-casualty event, on-scene triage should be performed. Those with life-threatening injuries are to be taken directly to the hospital.[3] For these patients, emergency personnel are to use gloves and gowns, remove the patients' clothes, cover their hair with surgical caps if available, and wrap the patients in sheets for transport. Simply removing the clothes reduces the patient's contamination by approximately 80%.[10] Those who are uninjured or suffering from minor injuries should be relocated upwind, and decontamination should be performed. Decontamination in these situations consists of removing the victim's clothes and placing them in hazardous material bags and washing

the person's skin and hair with soap and warm water.[11] All those with nausea, vomiting, diarrhea, or rash should be referred to the emergency department for evaluation of possible acute radiation syndrome.[3]

In mass-casualty situations, approximately 80% of victims are decontaminated at hospitals; thus, the hospital facility must be prepared to decontaminate patients both inside and outside the emergency department.[10] For those whose conditions are stable, decontamination should be done immediately, and if possible, it should be done outside of the hospital. Those who must be brought into the emergency department immediately should be treated in an area roped off from the rest of the department. Hospital personnel should wear disposable clothing, gowns, gloves, and shoe covers when treating these patients.[12]

The radiation control officer is responsible for monitoring the exposure of hospital staff. Personnel involved with care of contaminated patients should wear dosimeters to monitor radiation exposure.[10] The dose limit for persons providing emergency services other than lifesaving actions is 5 rem per event, whereas for lifesaving activities the recommended maximum dose is 25 rem per event. In the event of a disaster, the recommended limit increases to 150 rem per event.[3]

The U.S. Federal Bureau of Investigation is the lead federal agency during crisis management, that is, during the period when the focus is on ensuring that there is no further threat and establishing the site of attack as a crime scene. The Federal Emergency Management Agency takes the lead during consequence management, where the focus is on limitation of damage, protection of the public, decontamination, and disposal of the radioactive material. These two agencies will be lead coordinating organizations and should be contacted with questions. Also, the Radiation Emergency Assistance/Training Site should be contacted with any concerns via telephone (1-865-576-1005) or via their interactive Web site (http://www.orau.gov/reacts).[3]

 MEDICAL TREATMENT OF CASUALTIES

A conventional explosion at a nuclear power plant will lead to a variety of injuries. Blast, thermal burns, and smoke inhalation will be responsible for most immediate deaths. Radiation injuries will include whole-body or localized exposure (i.e., irradiation) and internal deposition of radioactive substances (i.e., contamination).[12]

Whole-body irradiation by gamma rays can lead to acute radiation syndrome. The most susceptible cells to radiation damage are rapidly dividing cells such as those in the intestinal mucosa and bone marrow.[3] However, with massive irradiation, even the central nervous system, with its relatively low cellular turnover rate, will show the effects.[12] The degree of whole-body radiation exposure is estimated using clinical signs and symptoms, the minimal lymphocyte count within the first 48 hours, the severity of thrombocytopenia and reticulocytopenia, and cytogenic studies looking for chromosomal abnormalities in bone marrow and red blood cells.[3,12] Lymphocytes are the most radiosensitive cells in the blood, and a substantial dip is apparent within the first 8 to 12 hours.[13]

The faster the fall and the lower the nadir of lymphocytes, the greater the whole-body radiation dose.[3] Furthermore, the sooner the onset of signs and symptoms for each phase of radiation illness, the greater the whole-body irradiation.[1] Nausea, vomiting, diarrhea, and rash are the first presentation after gamma irradiation. Later, the clinical manifestations of acute radiation syndrome are related to the level of leukocytes and platelets (Table 150-1). Fever, infections, and hemorrhaging occur. Also, with sloughing of the intestinal mucosal surface, mucositis and enteritis occur.[3]

In addition to the whole-body, uniform irradiation discussed above, the skin is susceptible to local radiation injury. The distribution tends to be nonuniform, and the skin radiation dosage absorbed is estimated to be 10 to 20 times greater than the bone marrow doses. The signs of a radiation burn are very similar to those of a thermal burn, with the difference being that the signs of radiation burns appear after a period of days in contrast to thermal burns, where the results appear immediately.[3] In the Chernobyl explosion, a period of primary erythema was seen in the first few days, followed by a 3- to 4-day period of latency. In severe cases, secondary erythema and the full extent of the burn manifested as early as 5 to 6 days and as late as 3 weeks in milder cases. The most frequent locations early on were the wrists, face, neck, and feet. As time went on, burns were also seen on the chest and back, and later on the knees, hips, and buttocks.[12] Vascular insufficiency can develop at any time after the radiation exposure, even years later, with necrosis occurring. Treatment includes control of pain, vasodilator therapy, and prophylaxis against infection.[3] Surgery and plastic surgery consultants should be involved because extensive debridement, skin grafting, and amputation are often required.[14] Burns to the eyelids and eyes are often seen, requiring ophthalmology consultation.

Internal contamination occurs through inhalation, ingestion, and absorption through open wounds. Inhalation can lead to radiation pneumonitis. Early bronchopulmonary lavage may be helpful in removing some of the radioactive contaminants. Chronic low-level inhalation of radioactive substances is more common and was seen among those involved in the clean-up efforts from the Chernobyl explosion. Radiation fibrosis was seen, and treatment with interferon was of some benefit.[12]

Ingestion of radioactive substances is either treated with specific antidotes and/or general measures to decrease absorption, both of which should be instituted as soon as possible after exposure. Specific antidotes include blocking agents that saturate a tissue with a nonradioactive element, thus reducing the uptake of the radioisotope, and chelating agents that bind metals into complexes, preventing tissue uptake and allowing urinary excretion.[12] As in all poisonings, the local or regional poison control center should be contacted.[3]

Contaminated wounds should be rinsed with saline until the Geiger meter reads no evidence of radioactive material. If the patient has received a dose of whole-body radiation that leads to decreased lymphocyte count (above 1 to 2 Gy to the bone marrow), the wound should be closed as soon as possible to decrease the chance of the wound serving as a portal of entry for infection.[3] Surgical debridement is necessary for the usual indications of dirt and nonviable tissue as well as for continued high readings of radioactive contamination despite saline rinses.[12]

 CASE PRESENTATION

The result of a conventional explosion at a nuclear power plant is directly related to the strength and location of the explosion. A large bomb released directly on a nuclear power plant will be tantamount to exploding an atomic bomb. Radioactive contamination will last longer because nuclear power plants house more long-life radioactive substances than do atomic bombs. A smaller explosion, or one that does not hit the structure directly but damages the core or coolant systems, will lead to a core meltdown.[2] The amount of radiation released into the environment will depend on the severity of damage to the containment structure from the explosion.

TABLE 150-1 CLINICAL MANIFESTATIONS AND TREATMENT OF GAMMA RADIATION EXPOSURE

DOSE (GY)	SYMPTOMS	LYMPHOCYTE NADIR	TREATMENT
>30	Hypotension, high fever, mental status change, syncope, seizures	<100	Palliative
>10	Immediate nausea, vomiting, diarrhea	<100	Palliative
4-10	Delayed (by hours) nausea, vomiting, diarrhea	100-499	Protective isolation, TPN, gut sterilization, hematopoietic growth factors, antimicrobials
2-4	Delayed (by days) nausea, vomiting, or no symptoms	500-999	Antiemetics, pain control, fluids, close monitoring
<1 Gy	Less than 10% with delayed (by days) nausea and vomiting	>1000	Symptomatic care

TPN, Total parenteral nutrition.

UNIQUE CONSIDERATIONS

A conventional explosion at a nuclear power plant differs from all other explosions because of the risk of radiation exposure, illness, and death to large populations. Decontamination is imperative and must be undertaken on a massive scale. Psychosocial issues are very important after the release of radioactive material occurs. The possibility of exposure elicits fear, with common stress reactions. Symptoms can also mimic those of radiation exposure such as nausea, vomiting, and rash. The psychosocial effects can be quelled by communication with the general public in an honest and open manner about the event and the short-term and long-term health risks.[3]

 PITFALLS

Several potential pitfalls in response to an explosion at a nuclear power plant exist. These include the following:

- Many of the victims most severely affected by radiation exposure are emergency personnel and those who were involved in clean-up activities.
- In the event of a conventional explosion at a nuclear power plant, radiation-safe and contaminated areas must be identified. Those with the proper personal protective equipment would be able to enter the designated contaminated area and bring patients to emergency personnel located in the designated radiation-safe areas. Once the patients are removed from the area of high radiation and are decontaminated, they no longer pose a significant risk to healthcare workers using universal precautions.[3]

REFERENCES

1. *Are You Ready? A Guide to Citizens Preparedness*. Washington, DC: Federal Emergency Management Agency; 2002.
2. Chernobyl: Ten Years After, Causes Consequences, Solutions. Greenpeace International; 1996. Available at: http://archive.green peace.org/comms/nukes/chernob/read24.text.
3. Mettler F, Volez G. Current concepts: major radiation exposure: what to expect and how to respond. *N Engl J Med*. 2002; 346: 1554-61.
4. Helfand I, Forrow L, Tiwari J. Nuclear terrorism. *BMJ* 2002; 324: 356-9.
5. UNDP/UNICEF. *The Human Consequences of the Chernobyl Nuclear Accident: A Strategy for Recovery*. New York: United Nations; 2002.
6. United Nations Scientific Committee on the Effects of Atomic Radiation. *Exposures from the Chernobyl Accident: UNSCEAR Report to the General Assembly, with Specific Annexes*. New York: United Nations; 1988.
7. United Nations Scientific Committee on the Effects of Atomic Radiation. *Acute Radiation Effects in Victims of the Chernobyl Accident: UNSCEAR Report to the General Assembly, with Specific Annexes*. New York: United Nations; 1988.
8. *Fifteen Years After the Chernobyl Accident. Lessons Learned: Executive Summary of an International Conference, Kyiv, April 18-20, 2001*. Minsk, Belarus: Committee on the Problems of the Consequence of the Catastrophe at the Chernobyl Nuclear Power Plant; 2001.
9. *Health Protection Guidance in the Event of a Nuclear Weapons Explosion*. Geneva, Switzerland: World Health Organization; 2003.
10. Blackwell T. Weapons of mass destruction. In: Marx J, Hockberger R, Walls R, eds. *Rosen's Emergency Medicine: Concepts and Clinical Practice*. 5th ed. St Louis, Mo: Mosby, Inc; 2002:2616-49.
11. *What You Should Know if There is an Attack Involving Radioactive Materials*. Fact Sheet no. 16. Washington State Department of Health; 2002.
12. Markovchick V. Radiation injuries. In: Marx J, Hockberger R, Walls R, eds. *Rosen's Emergency Medicine: Concepts and Clinical Practice*. 5th ed. St Louis, Mo: Mosby, Inc; 2002:2056-63.
13. Goans R, Holloway E, Berger M, et al. Early dose assessment in criticality accidents. *Health Phys*. 2001;81:446-9.
14. Aslan G, Terzioglu A, Tuncali D, et al. Consequences of radiation accidents. *Ann Plast Surg*. 2004;52:325-8.

chapter 151

Tunnel Explosion

Patrick Zelley

DESCRIPTION OF EVENT

The importance of tunnels in modern travel cannot be overestimated. Multiple uses including transportation across mountainous terrain, under waterways, and through urban areas make tunnels an invaluable component of modern travel. These same aspects also make tunnel disasters a particularly costly event for many reasons, not the least of which are the challenges inherent to providing medical assistance to victims of a tunnel disaster.

Over the years, there have been many documented incidents of tunnel disasters resulting from numerous causes, which illustrate the devastating consequences. In the year 2000, a deadly tunnel fire resulted in the death of 155 passengers on a shuttle train in Kitzsteinhorn, Austria. Another tragic tunnel disaster occurred in Mont Blanc, France, in 1999 with 39 deaths in a 10-car accident. But although these examples demonstrate terrible outcomes of tunnel tragedies, they do not come close to the scale of disaster associated with a large-scale tunnel explosion.

In the changing world we live in, an obvious source of tunnel explosions is the risk related to international terrorism. Traditionally, explosive weapons used by terrorists have been of limited size, usually a few kilograms, resulting in a low mortality rate of approximately 5%. However, due to advanced technology and more elaborate planning, there is the potential for much greater damage. There are three primary factors that increase the risk of morbidity and mortality: larger explosive devices, confined space, and structural collapse. All three of these are possibilities in a tunnel explosion.[1]

Although terrorist activity is certainly a realistic possibility, there are many other potential causes of tunnel explosions that must be considered. Construction accidents involving tunnels have occurred. For example, in 1995 a gas explosion in an underground railway in Daegu, South Korea, claimed the lives of 101 people and injured another 143. In 1919, a dynamite explosion in the Baltimore Tunnel, a mining tunnel in Wilkes Barre, Pennsylvania, claimed the lives of 92 people. Other possible causes are tanker truck explosions and multicar accidents.

Tunnel explosions represent a significant challenge to emergency personnel due to many unique characteristics. The purpose of this chapter is to understand the broad scope of preparedness that is essential to a successful emergency response.

PREINCIDENT ACTIONS

In addition to normal disaster preparation, there are some key areas that deserve specific attention when preparing for the possibility of tunnel explosion. Due to the huge variety of tunnel locations, it is common for multiple hospitals and rescue teams to serve the area of a tunnel explosion. An integrated response plan that maximizes the effectiveness of triage, treatment, disposition, and evacuation must be prepared as much as possible in advance. This response plan must be constructed with the ability to adjust from the plan based on actual events. In past mass-casualty incidents, including the bombing of Centennial Park at the Atlanta Olympics in 1996 and the bombing of the World Trade Center in 1993, adhering to a coordinated response plan represented a great challenge. With so many hospitals involved in the recovery process, effective coordination and communication was essential before, during, and after the incidents to effectively make use of all available resources.

There are additional communication challenges associated with tunnel explosions due to the complexities of tunnel design. With multiple entry and exit sites, several control points will be required. Walkie-talkies, cell phones, and landlines should all serve a role in establishing effective communication. In addition, site flags should be used to explain the purpose of each organizational area in both English and Spanish. Translators should be available, both on site and by phone correspondence.

Tunnel explosions are associated with an increased risk of smoke and toxin exposure. Tunnel explosions may involve nuclear, biologic, or chemical toxins in transport for peaceful purposes or criminal acts. Equipment readiness should address the extensive need for respiratory equipment, not only to aid victims suffering from inhalation injuries, but also to prevent similar injuries in the response teams. It is also important for assistance teams to wear proper protective equipment to limit additional injuries, including nuclear, biologic, and chemical protective gear. Therapeutic agents, including atropine, pralidoxime chloride, oral prophylactic antibiotics, and potassium iodide should be available to treat victims as well as healthcare providers who may be exposed.

Readiness for a possible tunnel explosion includes preparation of site maps to determine the best locations for command posts and triage sites. As was previously stated, multiple entry and exit points increase the need for multiple control points. As a result, it is vital to have accurate maps available in advance of the incident. Finally, transportation plans must include alternative methods of travel due to the high likelihood that a tunnel explosion will result in delays for land travel.

 ## POSTINCIDENT ACTIONS

The effective use of law enforcement is vital for many reasons. Site security is an essential and often overlooked aspect of disaster response planning. A cordoned area should be established as quickly as possible to keep victims from leaving the disaster scene without assessment and to prevent injuries to outsiders who may enter the disaster area. It is also important to set up a release point for equipment and personnel both into and out of the disaster scene. This will help with control of resources. Quick distribution of information concerning the site layout should occur as rapidly as possible among the response team members to prevent improper use of resources. Security should not only be considered at the site of the explosion but also at the receiving hospitals because they are a prime target for secondary explosions when the initial disasters are intentional.

A major post-event challenge that exists with tunnel explosions is related to the multiple access/egress points that may exist. As a result, multiple primary triage points must be established at different sites to limit the obstacles that may exist between different points. For example, a subway explosion would involve multiple underground-to-surface exit stairways that would allow injured passengers to exit at several locations. If triage personnel are not located at or near each of these sites, there is the potential for significant delays in disposition of victims, as well as the increased likelihood that victims will leave the scene without evaluation. This can result in uneven distribution of injured persons to local hospitals and can also increase the risk of morbidity and mortality in those with delayed symptoms. At each of these triage sites, there should also be treatment stations for immediate administration of medical assistance.

A large percentage of patients treated in hospital facilities will arrive at the emergency department by foot, taxi, or other nonemergency transportation method. This results in further administrative difficulties and an exacerbation of over-triage, reducing the effectiveness of hospital resources. For this reason, establishing an external triage site at the receiving facilities is important as an initial triage area for those who have not been previously assessed, and to facilitate secondary triage of patients who have arrived under their own power. Quickly identifying serious injuries in this group is essential because time is of the essence for those who may suffer from previously unrecognized serious injuries. In addition, these external triage sites should quickly direct victims in need of decontamination to isolated decontamination sites to avoid further exposure to others and contamination of medical facilities.

 ## MEDICAL TREATMENT OF CASUALTIES

Blast injuries are responsible for the majority of the victims after tunnel explosions. The incidence of primary blast injury correlates directly to blast size and proximity to the blast, while correlating indirectly to the amount of open space surrounding the blast.[1] In tunnels, it is important to consider the effects of an explosion in the confined longitudinal space of the tunnel with respect to the frequency and severity of injuries expected. In general, primary blast injuries are most likely to occur with victims located closest to the explosion due to the dissipation of shock waves with progression away from the blast source. However, the confined tunnel space increases reflection of blast forces and, therefore, increases the frequency of primary blast injury. In addition, the reflection of shock waves can increase the destructive potential by 2 to 20 times that of the incident wave, thereby increasing the severity of primary blast injuries.[2]

Secondary injury is the result of hurled objects causing blunt or penetrating trauma. This involves soft tissue, orthopedic, and head injuries, with traumatic head or limb amputations occurring in those closest to the blast source.[3] Tertiary injury is the result of two broad causative factors: the physical displacement of victims (those hurled from the blast source) and the structural collapse of buildings or tunnel walls (crush injuries) as a result of the force of the blast.

Quaternary injury is a collection of other injuries resulting from the blast.[1] This includes thermal injury (hot gases and secondary fires), inhalation injury (dust, smoke, carbon monoxide, and chemicals) and water injury (underwater tunnels).[3] Quaternary injuries are likely to be increased in tunnel explosions because the length of the confined space may make it difficult to escape, prolonging exposure, and persons in the tunnel far from the explosion may still be exposed to smoke and gases that vent from the tunnel.

Primary blast injury to the lung or gastrointestinal (GI) blast injury may occur as a result of a tunnel explosion. GI blast injury is more common when victims are submerged or partially submerged in water. A secondary underwater explosion in an underwater tunnel that flooded from the primary blast raises the possibility of underwater blast waves striking victims while submerged and may result in GI blast injury. Blast injury to the GI system can result in hemorrhage and shock or perforation. Because it is the major site of intestinal gas accumulation, the colon is the most common site of GI blast injury.[3] Physical evidence of GI blast injury includes absent bowel sounds, bright red blood from the rectum, guarding, rebound tenderness, abdominal pain, nausea, vomiting, diarrhea, and tenesmus.[4] This nonspecific presentation makes it necessary to maintain a high index of suspicion for GI blast injury.

The risk of extensive bleeding makes fluid and blood transfusions vital to maintenance of cardiovascular stability before definitive surgical care. Due to the limitations of computed tomography scans in the recognition of hollow viscous injury, judicious use of more invasive diagnostic procedures, including diagnostic peritoneal lavage and laparotomy, should be used to maximize treatment success.[4]

Secondary and tertiary blast injuries include a huge variety of typical and atypical traumatic injuries. Due to the large amount of fragmented materials projected from the blast site in tunnels, a large number of soft tissue injuries, penetrating injuries, head injuries, and traumatic amputations are to be expected. Secondary, tertiary, and quaternary injuries resulting from tunnel explosions should be managed according to standard treatment protocols.

CASE PRESENTATION

It's rush hour in the city of Boston and the Ted Williams Tunnel is bumper to bumper across the entire 1.6-mile span of the underwater passageway. In the middle of the tunnel sits a yellow rental truck that is packed to capacity with high-explosive materials, waiting for ignition at the hands of the driver. As the stop-and-go traffic proceeds, he nears the halfway point that was the planned marker for detonation. He takes his foot off the break and advances 15 feet before the traffic stops him again. The truck comes to a halt, he puts his head down as his last thoughts go through his mind, and then he pushes the button. The contents of his vehicle are blown in all directions, creating a shock wave that passes abruptly through the length of the tunnel to both its front and its rear. The cars surrounding the explosion are launched violently in opposite directions toward the nearest exit point from the tunnel. As if chasing the pressure wave, a rush of flames covers the distance at a slower pace with thick, black smoke furling closely behind it.

As those surviving the initial blast come staggering out of their vehicles, they face the first of their many challenges—smoke is everywhere. It is pitch black, and they struggle to find enough oxygen to breathe. Chaos ensues as people attempt to determine the direction toward help. As the first rescue vehicles converge on the exit points, hundreds of people—some appearing well, others obviously injured—struggle for safety and assistance.

UNIQUE CONSIDERATIONS

Tunnel explosions increase the risk of primary blast injury because the explosion occurs within a confined space, which magnifies the intensity of the blast wave. Tunnel explosions also increase the risk of quaternary injury. Thermal injuries and toxic inhalations are common, with increased incidence in direct proportion to proximity to the blast source. The extent and severity of these injuries

depends greatly on the explosives, chemicals, and materials present at the site of the blast, as well as each victim's proximity to the blast and duration of exposure.[3]

Multiple triage sites must be established because there are often many different ways out of a tunnel, including stairs to the surface, ventilation shafts, connections to separate tunnels for traffic moving in the other direction, and the obvious entrance and exit points.

Body armor increases the severity of primary blast injuries. A high index of suspicion for severe primary blast injury should be maintained when caring for injured tunnel or subway security personnel.[4]

 PITFALLS

Several potential pitfalls in response to a tunnel explosion exist. These include the following:

- As with other explosions, the major pitfall after a tunnel explosion is failure to recognize primary blast injury in victims who are asymptomatic or have only mild symptoms. Victims of primary blast injury who sustain minimal secondary and tertiary injuries may be inappropriately triaged based on initial evaluation.
- Due to the often delayed symptoms of blast injuries, it is important to recognize associated physical examination findings which may signify otherwise occult injury. These findings include tympanic membrane rupture, hypopharyngeal petechiae or ecchymosis, retinal artery air emboli, and subcutaneous emphysema.[4]
- Because the explosion occurs in a confined space, the risk of blast lung is greater in tunnel explosions than in open-air explosions. In addition, the risk of gastrointestinal injury is greater in underwater tunnels due to the risk of secondary explosions occurring after the influx of significant volumes of water.

REFERENCES

1. Horrocks C, Brett S. Blast injury. *Curr Anaesth Crit Care*. 2000; 11:113-9.
2. Frykberg E. Medical management of disasters and mass casualties from terrorist bombings: how can we cope? *J Trauma*. 2002;53:201-12.
3. Wightman J, Gladish S. Explosions and blast injuries. *Ann Emerg Med*. 2001;37:664-78.
4. Argyros G. Management of primary blast injury. *Toxicology* 1997;121:105-15.

chapter 152

Liquefied Natural Gas Explosion

Michael I. Greenberg

 DESCRIPTION OF EVENT

Natural gas is composed primarily of methane, with small quantities of other hydrocarbons, as well as water, carbon dioxide–, nitrogen–, oxygen–, and sulfur-containing compounds.[1-5] If natural gas is cooled to less than −259°F, most impurities present are removed and the natural gas is transformed into a clear liquid. This colorless and odorless material is known as *liquefied natural gas* (LNG). LNG is a cryogenic material. That is to say, it will remain in the liquid state if kept at adequately low temperatures. This liquid form of natural gas, in itself, is a noncorrosive and relatively harmless substance. It is important to note that LNG is lighter than water and thus will float on the surface if spilled in water.

LNG in itself is not an explosive material and when properly stored will not combust spontaneously. However, if converted to a vapor, LNG can become suddenly explosive, especially if it is released into a closed space. However, it is explosive only if it exists within a specific "flammable range" of 5% to 15% of an air mixture.[1-5] Similarly, LNG may be combustible if LNG vapor in the same concentration range (5% to 15%) contacts air that is relatively warm in temperature. If a large volume of LNG is spilled into water at a rapid rate, a so-called rapid phase transition may occur, and heat is rapidly transferred from the water to the much colder LNG. This results in very rapid transformation of LNG from its liquid state to a gaseous state. This transformation may result in the release of a large amount of energy and a substantial risk of explosion may develop. Obviously, if such an explosion were to occur, it could pose a serious hazard to buildings and people in areas near the explosion. If such a scenario took place in a port area in relative proximity to populated areas, a major disaster threatening life and property could result.

Under certain circumstances, LNG is considered to be a potentially hazardous material that embodies a few important safety concerns including cold-related skin injury, the creation of oxygen-poor environments, and explosion/incendiary risks.[1-5] The extremely cold temperatures at which LNG must be stored makes it a direct cryogenic hazard. Although the results of fleeting contact between LNG and human skin may be relatively benign, more extended contact may cause serious local cold injury to the skin. An LNG vapor cloud may facilitate the formation of an oxygen-poor environment with the potential for asphyxia by virtue of its ability to displace oxygen. This is may be a special hazard if LNG is released into a closed or relatively closed space. Finally, LNG vapor clouds may ignite within the portions of the cloud where the flammability characteristics necessary (concentrations of 5% to 15%) are present. However, even under these circumstances, a source of ignition is required for a conflagration to take place.

Of special concern with regard to LNG as a potential hazard is a spill or release of LNG on a large body of water such as a lake or the ocean (as opposed to land). Under these circumstances, effective containment of the spill would be difficult or impossible, and LNG would evaporate rapidly, forming a vapor cloud with the potential for explosion and fire. This situation could result from a terrorist attack against an LNG tanker at or near a port or harbor. If attacked in a manner that resulted in the spill of a large quantity of LNG with a source for ignition (e.g., the detonation of an improvised explosive device, bomb blast, or air attack against a tanker hull), the results could be devastating.

 PREINCIDENT ACTIONS

The most important preincident actions with regard to LNG transport are the protection of LNG tankers and LNG storage facilities from terrorist attack.

LNG is typically transported by double-hulled tanker ships. These vessels are specifically designed to accommodate the very low storage temperatures necessary to maintain LNG in its liquid state. In addition, all LNG transport tankers are required to be compliant with rigorous federal and international regulations promulgated by such agencies as the U.S. Coast Guard, the U.S. Department of Transportation, and the International Maritime Organization.[6-8]

On land, LNG is usually stored at fixed facility receiving terminals. There are currently only four LNG receiving terminals in the continental United States, and only three of these terminals (Boston, Savannah, Ga, and Lake Charles, La) are operational.[5] The U.S. Coast Guard regulations require that a 2-mile "moving safety zone" surround any LNG tanker ship entering Boston Harbor. This regulation mandates that Boston's Logan Airport be shut down whenever an LNG tanker enters or leaves the harbor. Coast Guardsmen board all LNG tankers before their arrival in Boston Harbor and provide continuous monitoring of cargo transfers from these LNG tankers during off-loading operations.[5-9] These are examples of extraordinary measures that have been implemented due to concern for the destructive potential that an explosion and fire involving an LNG tanker would cause.

Although the majority of all LNG transport is done by tanker ships, some lesser amounts of LNG are transported over ground in tanker trucks. LNG is also transported from Canada and within the United States via pipeline. The transport of LNG over land engenders some of the same concerns as those described for waterborne transport of this material.

Catastrophic accidents involving LNG receiving terminals have been modeled.[4] These simulations provided conservative estimates of the projection of downwind effects after the catastrophic loss of a four-tank LNG storage vessel and predicted a downwind spread of intense heat.[4] These models emphasize the potential damage involved in an LNG catastrophe.

First responders working in areas that may store, receive, or transport LNG should be aware of the potential hazards and should train for hazardous materials incidents that may involve LNG.

 ## POSTINCIDENT ACTIONS

Actions following an explosion and conflagration resulting from an accident or terrorist attack depend, in part, on the location of the incident. If an incident involved an LNG tanker on the high seas, damage and loss of life would probably be limited to the ship itself and its crew. However, if an incident occurred in or near a port or at a fixed storage facility, the degree of property destruction, human injury, and death could be considerable. A fire resulting from the explosion and ignition of LNG could be extremely difficult to control, particularly in cases involving the phenomenon known as *burn back*, in which the entire transported load of LNG combusts. In this situation, the resultant fire may burn uncontrolled until the supply of LNG that was fueling the fire was fully consumed by the burning process.[8,10,11]

 ## MEDICAL TREATMENT OF CASUALTIES

As in virtually all hazardous materials incidents, removal of victims or potential victims from the scene is of paramount importance. In the event of skin contact with LNG, treatment requires immediate removal of the material from the skin and the initiation of standard therapies for cold injury, including immediate rewarming of cold-injured skin or digits by immersion in warm water. Persons exposed to oxygen-poor environments induced by the creation of an LNG vapor cloud may require cardiopulmonary resuscitation after removal from the environment. First responders entering such environments must use adequate respiratory protection with external supplied air. Persons who may be injured or burned in an explosion involving LNG should be evaluated and treated using standard trauma and burn protocols.

CASE PRESENTATION

A double-hulled tanker ship transporting LNG collides with a smaller cruise ship carrying 1500 passengers in a fog-laden port just after dusk. For reasons that are unclear, all navigational aids on the tanker failed and the U.S. Coast Guard was not accompanying the vessel as it made its way into port, as regulations require. The collision takes place less than a mile from the harbor of a large east coast city. A large tear in the hull of the tanker develops and LNG leaks out, vaporizing soon after contact with sea water. Reports indicate that people are in the water and the cruise ship is aflame. Shortly after the initial reports of the collision, a large explosion occurs in the harbor, and early reports indicate that a fireball has enveloped both ships. There are buildings ashore that have been destroyed by the blast. Substantial loss of life and property is predicted based on the earliest reports from the scene of the incident.

A large-scale disaster is declared and federal, state, county, and city medical, hazardous material, law enforcement, military, and public service personnel and resources are mobilized. Prearranged protocols are launched in response to the disaster, including the curtailing of all sea and air transport within 500 miles of the incident. The response to this incident lasts 10 days and the multilevel legal, sociologic, and medical ramifications extend for many years.

 ## UNIQUE CONSIDERATIONS

The excellent safety record for LNG is somewhat unique among potentially hazardous materials. International transport of LNG via tanker ship began in 1959, and since that time there have been no reports of serious explosions at sea or in port.[5] However, since 1944 approximately 13 important incidents at onshore LNG terminals have been documented. One accident occurring in Algeria in 1977 and another at Cove Point, Maryland, in 1979 each resulted in at least one fatality.[5] In 2004, a fire at the LNG processing facility in Skikda, Algeria, resulted in the death of approximately 27 workers with injuries sustained by an additional 74 persons.[9] Although these data illustrate an excellent safety record for the LNG industry, they also emphasize that LNG is a potentially hazardous material that can cause a major disaster.

 ## PITFALLS

Confusing LNG with liquefied petroleum gas (LPG) or compressed natural gas (CNG) is a common mistake.[5] LPG is a mixture of propane and butane in a liquid state at room temperatures and moderate pressures. LPG is highly flammable and requires storage away from sources of ignition and in a well-ventilated area, so that any leak may disperse safely away from populated areas. An additive, mercaptan, is usually mixed in to give LPG a distinctive and unpleasant smell, making leaks readily detectable. The concentration of the added mercaptans is such that an LPG leak can be detected when the concentration is below the lower limit of flammability.

LNG also differs from the material known as CNG.[5] CNG is a form of pressurized natural gas and is usually the same composition as pipeline-quality natural gas. CNG is often misrepresented as the only form of natural gas that can be used as vehicle fuel. However, LPG and LNG may also be used as transport fuels.

REFERENCES

1. Fialka J, Gold R. Fears of terrorism crush plans for liquefied gas terminals. *Wall Street J.* May 14, 2004:A1.
2. Fay JA. Model of spills and fires from LNG and oil tankers. *J Haz Mater.* 2003;B96:171-88.
3. Gerasimov VE, Kuz'menko IF, Peredel'skii VA, et al. Introduction of technologies and equipment for production, storage, transportation, and use of LNG. *Chem Petroleum Eng.* 2004;40:31-5.
4. Havens J. *Maintaining Security in an Era of Heightened Awareness.* GTI New Frontiers in LNG Shipping Conference, London, 2002.
5. Institute for Energy, Law & Enterprise. *Introduction to LNG: An Overview on Liquefied Natural Gas, its Properties, the LNG Industry, Safety Considerations.* Houston: University of Houston, 2003.
6. Lehr W, Simecek-Beatty D. Comparison of hypothetical LNG and fuel oil fires on water. *J Haz Mater.* 2004;107:3-9.
7. *Natural Transportation Safety Board Report: Columbia LNG Corporation Explosion and Fire, Cove Point, Md: October 6, 1979.* NTSB-PAR-80-2, April 16, 1980.
8. Parfomak P. *Liquefied Natural Gas (LNG) Import Terminals: Siting, Safety and Regulation. CRS Report for Congress.* January 2004.
9. Kemezis P. Algeria blast has officials rethinking LNG safety. *Engineering News Record.* 2004;252:17.
10. Shook B. *Despite Recent Explosion, BP and Shell Expanding LNG Efforts. Natural Gas Week.* New York: February 13, 2004.
11. U.S. Bureau of Mines. *Report on the Investigation of the Fire at the Liquifaction, Storage, and Regasification Plant of the East Coast Gas Co., Cleveland, Ohio, October 20, 1944.* February 1946.

chapter 153

Liquefied Natural Gas Tanker Truck Explosion

Jonathan M. Rubin

 DESCRIPTION OF EVENT

The explosion of a liquid natural gas tanker is a boiling liquid expanding vapor explosion (BLEVE). A BLEVE occurs when a pressurized liquid evaporates rapidly, leading to explosion of the tank containing the liquid. Either mechanical damage to the tank shell or intense heat from a fire outside the tank causes the liquid to evaporate. In the case of fire, the extreme heat weakens the walls of the tank, the tank is unable to withstand the rising pressure within, and the tank fails.[1] In either case, the resulting explosion leads to a blast wave, fireball, and flying tank fragments. BLEVEs typically occur within 8 to 30 minutes of the start of a fire, with an average of 15 minutes.[2] This time can be significantly shorter inside a tunnel.[3] Damage to the tank (as with impact in a traffic crash) usually results in immediate BLEVE. Relief valves that are located on the top of the tanker truck are designed to vent vapor to reduce pressure in the vapor space of the tank but may not function properly if the tanker is on its side, as in a traffic crash. In this situation, the valves will vent liquefied natural gas (LNG) and will not reduce the pressure inside the tank.

 PREINCIDENT ACTIONS

Safety standards and codes related to LNG and propane have been established by the American National Standards Institute, the National Fire Protection Association (NFPA), and the American Society of Mechanical Engineers. These standards address safety issues related to tank design and manufacturing, relief valves, transportation, and fire and hazardous materials response. In addition, federal agencies such as the U.S. Department of Labor and the U.S. Department of Transportation have established rules and regulations pertaining to the transportation of LNG and other flammable gases. Educational programs sponsored by the National Propane Gas Association and the NFPA have also raised the awareness of emergency responders about appropriate decisions in managing LNG incidents. These efforts are all intended to enhance the safe transport of LNG and to ensure the enaction of the appropriate emergency response to an incident involving an LNG

tanker. In fact, since 1993 only three significant BLEVE incidents have occurred in the United States and Canada[4] (Table 153-1).

At the incident scene, truck placards and color schemes can be used to identify tanker contents. The type of flammable gas as well as the size of the tank are important considerations for the Incident Commander. The size of a BLEVE depends on the weight of the container pieces and how much liquid vaporizes when the container fails.[2] The condition of the tank must also be evaluated; structural damage and the presence of fire are essential considerations. Besides the type of fuel present, an additional consideration during scene assessment is the incident location. A BLEVE inside a tunnel or other closed space results in more devastating effects than one occurring in an open area. If fire is present at the incident scene, the decision to evacuate the scene may be more prudent than committing firefighting personnel to extinguish the fire. This decision must be based on the length of time the fire has been burning and knowledge of the usual time course for BLEVE occurrence. The potential for a BLEVE should be considered any time there is direct flame impingement on an LNG tank, when venting through relief valves is not adequate to relieve the rising pressure.[2]

 POSTINCIDENT ACTIONS

Once a BLEVE occurs, the resulting explosion typically burns up the fuel source, causing a large fireball. At this point the fire usually burns itself out as the fuel source is consumed, but extinguishing the fire may be necessary. The containment and clean-up of leaked, unburned fuel may also be required, although LNG typically evaporates quickly. Casualties with burns and/or explosion injuries will necessitate field triage and treatment as well as transport to the hospital.

 MEDICAL TREATMENT OF CASUALTIES

Injuries occurring in conjunction with a BLEVE fall into two categories: burns and thermal injuries, and trauma

TABLE 153-1   SIGNIFICANT NORTH AMERICAN BLEVE INCIDENTS, 1993–2004

DATE	LOCATION	DESCRIPTION	CASUALTIES
June 27, 1993	Ste. Elizabeth de Warwick Quebec, Canada	1055-gallon propane storage tank	4 fatalities, 7 injured
October 2, 1997	Burnside, Ill	1000-gallon propane storage tank	2 fatalities, 2 injured
April 9, 1998	Albert City, Ia	18,000-gallon propane storage tank	2 fatalities, 7 injured

from fragments thrown from the explosion. Standard medical care for these injuries is appropriate. The potential for exposure to a leaking fuel source before the BLEVE also exists. In this case, patients will require decontamination and evaluation for potential toxic effects.

CASE PRESENTATION

At 5:00 PM, a fully loaded tanker truck carrying LNG jack-knifes on an interstate highway and is struck by two vehicles traveling at a high rate of speed in the adjoining lanes. One of the vehicles crashes into the midsection of the tanker and bursts into flames. The fire subsequently engulfs the tanker and 12 minutes later it explodes, creating a large fireball and sending multiple large fragments up to 200 feet from the crash site. The driver of the tanker truck is able to escape unharmed, but multiple casualties result from the fire and projectiles.

UNIQUE CONSIDERATIONS

Projectiles from a BLEVE are a major hazard. A Queens University study showed that projectiles are dispersed more than 300 feet away from an exploding tank.[2] Failure to take this into consideration can greatly increase the number of casualties and fatalities at the incident scene.

PITFALLS

Past practice was based on the belief that debris fragments only come from the ends of the tank. BLEVE research and experience have shown that this is not accurate: any part of the tank can break and become a projectile. The U.S. Department of Transportation now recommends that emergency responders stay away from tanks engulfed in fire.[5]

REFERENCES

1. Herrig Brothers Propane Tank Explosion. *CSB Investigation Digest*. June 23, 1999. U.S. Chemical Safety and Hazard Investigation Board, Washington, DC.
2. Albert City, Iowa. *NFPA: Alert Bulletin*. 1998;98:1. National Fire Protection Association, Quincy, MA.
3. Ciambelli P. The risk of transportation of dangerous goods: BLEVE in a tunnel. *Ann Burns Fire Disasters*. 1997; 10: 241-47.
4. National Propane Gas Association. Propane emergencies training-program. Available at: http://www.propanesafety.com.
5. U.S. Department of Transportation. *North American Emergency Response Guidebook 2000*. Washington, DC.

chapter 154

Petroleum Distillation/Processing Facility Explosion

David C. Lee and Henry C. Chang

 ## DESCRIPTION OF EVENT

The petroleum industry concentrates on the process of obtaining and refining crude oil into usable compounds (i.e., gasoline or petrol, other fuel oil, plastics, polymers). Crude oil or crude petroleum is a liquid or semisolid mixture of mainly hydrocarbons that often contain sulfur, nitrogen, and oxygen, as well as metals such as iron, vanadium, nickel, and chromium. As crude oil is refined into fuels and gasoline, other useful products that are not fuels can also be manufactured (e.g., lubricants and asphalt for road paving). There are more than 4000 different petrochemical products, but those that are considered as basic products include ethylene, propylene, butadiene, benzene, ammonia, and methanol. The main groups of petrochemical end products are plastics, synthetic fibers, synthetic rubbers, detergents, and chemical fertilizers.

The chemical constitution of crude oil varies widely, and they can also vary in consistency from a light volatile fluid to a semisolid substance. Crude oil can be classified into three broad chemical groups: aliphatic/paraffin compounds with saturated hydrocarbon chemical structures, naphthalene-type compounds with saturated cyclic chemical structure, and aromatic compounds. Crude oil may also be categorized as asphalt base, paraffin base, or mixed base. Crude oil may be a sweet crude or a sour crude. Sweet crude oils have less than 5 ppm of hydrogen sulfide, and sour crude oils have significantly more hydrogen sulfide; drilling site wellhead concentrations of hydrogen sulfide may range from 50,000 to 180,000 ppm.[1,2]

Refining crude oil can be grouped by several stages, each with certain characteristics, and disasters have occurred in all stages:

1. Obtaining and extracting crude oil, often by heavy machinery drilling and pumping, usually in an isolated area.
2. Transporting crude oil, often involving large volumes.
3. Refining, usually requiring heat and multiple other potentially toxic chemicals.
4. Transporting end products of refinement, usually through populated centers.

In the extraction phase, subterranean crude oil must be obtained by means of wells. Typically, an exploratory well, known as the wildcat, is dug. Once oil is located, full-scale drilling commences. Oil drilling is a complex and risky process involving exposure to high temperatures and pressurized systems. Usually, the petroleum from a new well will come to the surface under its own pressure. Later, the crude oil must be pumped out or forced to the surface by injecting water, gas, or air into the deposits. Many of these wells are located in isolated areas of extreme environmental conditions that challenge the most modern transportation systems. Additionally, exposures to toxic gases released from the initial contact with oil field deposits frequently occur.[3,4]

In the second stage of transportation, crude oil must be transported from extraction site to refineries. The main methods of transporting crude oil and natural gas from the oil fields to refineries are usually by ocean tanker or by pipelines.

Thirdly, the processes involved in petroleum refining consist of three basic steps: distillation, conversion, and treatment. Fractional distillation involves using the difference in boiling point to separate the hydrocarbons in crude oil, and the process typically occurs in a vacuum distillation column. A large amount of heat is expended during this stage. As the distillate exits the column, it often requires further processing to make other fractions and to convert crude into basic petrol and other useful chemicals.

Conversion involves three main processes: cracking, unification, and alteration. Cracking is the most widely used conversion method and is the process for breaking down larger molecules into smaller ones. Unification is the process of combining smaller molecules to make larger ones. Finally, alteration is the process of rearranging various molecules to make the desired hydrocarbon product. These processes typically involve the use of significant amounts of heat, as well as additional hydrogen source and a catalytic unit.

Finally, the distillate undergoes finishing treatments to make it into products that meet specific requirements. Such processes can include solvent extraction, dewaxing, and hydrogenation. Distillated and chemically processed fractions are further treated to remove impurities, such as organic compounds containing sulfur, nitrogen, oxygen, water, dissolved metals, and inorganic salts. Treating is usually done by passing the fractions through the following methods:

1. A column of sulfuric acid removes unsaturated hydrocarbons (those with carbon-carbon double bonds), nitrogen compounds, oxygen compounds, and residual solids (e.g., tars, asphalt).
2. An absorption column filled with drying agents removes water.
3. Sulfur treatment and hydrogen-sulfide scrubbers remove sulfur and sulfur compounds.

Finally, the refined products are transported to the consumer. Because of this, many refineries are located near large-population centers. Large customers, like airports, are supplied directly from the refinery by pipelines. A disaster at a refinery may involve a nearby high-volume consumer like a petrochemical plant or a power station. Smaller consumers, like gasoline stations, are supplied by a road tanker originating from terminals, which act as storage depots and distribution centers. The terminals are supplied by rail or pipeline if they are inland or by coastal tanker if they are on the coast or a river estuary.

POTENTIAL HAZARDS

The main process of the petroleum industry is to obtain and convert a relatively flammable product to a highly flammable one. Thus, the majority of deaths reported in the petroleum industry disasters are caused by explosive blast injuries and burns (see Table 154-1 and Chapters 141 and 155).

EXPOSURES

The petroleum industry makes use of various chemicals in the process of refining crude oil. These include chlorine, chromium-containing corrosion inhibitors, and biologic additives. Byproducts of the refining process can also cause significant toxicity. These include carcinogenic polyaromatic hydrocarbons such as benzene. Hydrogen sulfide is another byproduct that can cause significant injury and is produced in the drilling and refining processes. Hydrogen sulfide gas has been reported to be a significant problem of oil fields in Alberta, Canada, due to its high concentration of sulfur.[5]

 ## PREINCIDENT ACTIONS

The first order of action is to confirm the site of the disaster. Although the majority of disasters reported are from explosions and burns, various parts of the petrochemical refining process are susceptible to specific scenarios. Disasters occurring in the process of obtaining crude oil often occur when an oil well ignites. Oil wells are often distant from major population centers. On the other hand, refineries are often close to major population centers. In the former scenario, healthcare workers may have to deal with getting to a remote location such as an offshore oil rig.[4] In the latter situation, healthcare workers must address the demands of the local community.

The materials involved in an explosion must also be identified. Many refineries use and store toxic compounds. Hydrofluoric acid is a compound found ubiquitously in the refining process. It is lethal substance and is toxic on contact to the lungs, skin, and eye. It is often in liquid form but turns into gas quickly. In significant releases of hydrofluoric acid, prehospital care providers will require personal protective devices (see Chapter 36). Treatment of injuries caused by hydrofluoric acid exposure often require unique antidotes, such as calcium-containing dermal, inhalational, and intravenous treatments.[6,7]

Another order of business is to identify blast-resistant portable buildings. These buildings are structures developed to provide temporary safe haven to personnel from the potential hazards associated with the petroleum industry. They are designed to resist the explosive forces that can cause sliding and overturning of buildings during a blast. They are also designed to be easily sealed and airtight to provide a shelter during a toxic gas release. They are often the size and shape of shipping containers and are positioned to be easily accessed by personnel. During disasters, healthcare personnel should identify and seek out these structures to locate potential victims and also to provide shelter if secondary incidents occur.[8]

 ## POSTINCIDENT ACTIONS

After the explosion of a petroleum distillation or processing facility, possible contaminants must be identified. A disaster at an eastern European oil storage depot was reported to cause significant environmental contamination of heavy metals (e.g., lead, arsenic, cadmium, nickel, chromium, and copper), polyaromatic hydrocarbons, and polychlorinated biphenyls.[9-11]

Identify and address psychological issues of victims, healthcare workers, and the community. Many of the reported disasters in the oil industry have involved a significant number of patients with burns, and there are multiple documented reports of significant effects on the mental health of healthcare workers.[7,12-20]

 ## MEDICAL TREATMENT OF CASUALTIES

Disasters at petroleum facilities typically involve exposure to blast injuries and high-temperature burns (see Chapters 141 and 155). Additionally, exposures to toxic chemical fumes via inhalation or dermal contact are also common.

TOXIC CHEMICAL EXPOSURES

Chemical exposures in a petroleum refinery are common. Hydrofluoric acid is a relatively common toxic

TABLE 154-1 MAJOR DISASTERS IN THE PETROLEUM INDUSTRY SINCE 1970 AS REPORTED BY THE UNITED NATIONS ENVIRONMENT PROGRAMME

CAUSE OF ACCIDENT	YEAR	LOCATION	PRODUCTS INVOLVED	NUMBER OF FATALITIES	NUMBER OF INJURED	NUMBER OF EVACUATED
Transport accident	1994	Zurich, Switzerland	Gasoline		7	120
Oil platform eruption	1979	Gulf of Mexico	Crude oil			
Explosion	1979	Phang-Nga, Thailand	Oil	50	15	
Explosion	1988	Monterrey, Mexico	Gasoline	4	15	10,000
Explosion	1983	Dhulwari, India	Gasoline	41	100	
Explosion	1979	Galveston Bay, USA	Crude oil	32		
Explosion	1980	Africa	Crude oil	36		
Explosion	1971	Czechowice, Poland	Oil	33		
Explosion (marine transport)	1979	Bantry Bay, Ireland	Oil, gas	50		
Explosion (marine transport)	1979	Istanbul, Turkey	Crude oil	52	>2	
Explosion (storage)	1988	Chihuahua, Mexico	Oil		7	15,000
Explosion (transport)	1988	Canada, at sea	Gasoline	29		
Explosion and fire	1991	Lake Charles, USA	Petroleum	3	12	
Explosion (refinery)	1991	Sweeny, USA	Petroleum		2	
Explosion (refinery)	1994	Pembroke, UK			26	
Explosion (refinery)	1990	Chalmette, USA	Flammable gas			
Explosion (refinery)	1991	Coatzacoaloas, Mexico	Chlorine	2	122	
Explosion and fire (oil platform)	1988	North Sea, UK	Oil, gas	167		
Fire	1972	Doraville, USA	Gasoline	2	161	
Fire	1990	Chtaura, Lebanon	Fuel oil		45	
Fire	1983	Dhurabari, India	Oil	76	>60	
Fire	1985	Padaval, India	Gasoline	>43	82	
Fire	1979	Caribbean Sea, Tobago	Crude oil	26		
Fire (fuel storage)	1990	Denver, USA	Kerosene			
Fire (road transport)	1994	Onitsha, Nigeria	Fuel oil	60		
Fire (refinery)	1991	Beaumont, USA	Hydrocarbons			
Fire (refinery)	1991	Port Arthur, USA	Petroleum			
Fire (refinery)	1990	Ras Tan, Saudi Arabia	Kerosene, benzene	1	2	
Fire (refinery)	1988	Bombay, India	Oil	35	16	
Explosion and fire	1983	Pojuca, Brazil	Gasoline	42	>100	>1,000
Explosion and fire (refinery)	1995	Cilacap, Indonesia	Gas			
Leak (oil terminal)	1986	Northville, USA	Gasoline			
Leak (pipeline)	1981	San Francisco, USA	Oil, PCBs			30,000
Release	1993	Remeios, Columbia	Crude oil	430		
Release	1994	Houston, USA	Crude oil		<70	12,000
Release (storage)	1988	Floreffe, USA	Diesel oil			
Release	1974	Mizushima, Japan	Oil			
Explosion	1993	Nam Khe, Vietnam	Petrol	47	48	
Transport accident (road)	1997	Stanger, South Africa	Petroleum	34	2	
Transport accident (ship)	1980	Rome, Italy	Oil	25	26	
Release (storage)	1978	Sendai, Japan	Crude oil	21	350	
Explosion (storage)	1982	Tacoa, Venezuela	Fuel oil	>153	500	40,000
Explosion (storage)	1983	Corinto, Nicaragua	Fuel oil		17	25,000
Transport accident (transhipment)	1975	Marcus Hook, USA	Crude oil	26	35	
Transport accident (transhipment)	1985	Algeciras, Spain	Oil	33	37	
Transport accident	1985	Tamil Nadu, India	Gasoline	60		
Transport accident	1998	Yaoundi, Cameroon	Petroleum products	220	130	
Transport accident	1995	Madras, India	Fuel oil	100	23	
Leakage (storage)	1984	Denver, USA				2,500
Explosion (pipeline)	1984	Cubatao, Brazil	Gasoline	89		
Fire (oil platform)	1980	Alaska, USA	Oil	51		

PCBs, polychlorinated biphenyls.
Data from United Nations Environment Programme. Awareness and Preparedness for Emergencies on a Local Level Disasters Database. Available at: *http://www.uneptie. org/pc/apell/disasters/lists/disasterloc.ht* (accessed October 2005).

chemical that requires specific treatments and antidotes. Patients should be immediately removed from the area and be evaluated for signs of respiratory decompensation as a result of pulmonary edema, pneumonitis, pulmonary hemorrhage, or systemic toxicity. Administering 2.5% or 3% calcium gluconate inhalational solution by nebulizer as a therapy has been suggested for respiratory exposures. Treatment of hydrofluoric acid dermal injury consists of immediate irrigation with copious amounts of water for at least 15 to 30 minutes, removal of all blisters because they may harbor fluoride ions, and calcium gluconate (2.5%) gel applied to the debrided skin surface. Systemic toxicity from hydrofluoric acid exposure can cause dysrhythmias and hypocalcemia, thus warranting cardiac and electrolyte monitoring. A 10% calcium gluconate solution should be administered intravenously or intra-arterially in patients exhibiting significant hydrofluoric acid systemic toxicity.

Ammonia is another compound that is found throughout the refining process. Ammonia is widely used as a cleaning agent and as a coolant. The release of ammonia causes injury to the patient in two ways: (1) because of its low freezing point (−33°C), frostbite injury occurs to any skin in direct contact; and (2) ammonia vapors readily dissolve in the moisture of the skin, eyes, and mucosa, causing chemical burns through liquefaction necrosis. Exposures require prompt irrigation of the eyes and skin with water and management of inhalation injury.

 ## CASE PRESENTATION

A mist develops after a pipe rupture at an oil refinery. Multiple workers at the plant begin complaining of cough, sore throat, and difficulty breathing. Disaster plan management is implemented, and emergency medical services are called into action. Plant supervisors notify personnel that the pipe delivers hydrofluoric acid. Prehospital healthcare workers are notified to use personal protective equipment. Patients are treated with nebulized calcium gluconate solutions, and the evacuation of potential personnel and the surrounding community is initiated.

The pipe is later repaired, and the hydrofluoric acid spill is contained and dissipates.

 ## UNIQUE CONSIDERATIONS

A common scenario in a petroleum industry disaster is the explosion of oil and gasoline drums. Bak and colleagues[21] reported a series of incidents where these containers were inappropriately handled. The typical scenario was that in which a worker attempted to divide or cut through a presumably empty 55-gallon drum with a grinder or a blowtorch. These drums often contain residual quantities of flammable material in liquid or vapor form. Once the container is penetrated, the metal drum explodes. Nearby workers suffer from significant trauma from projectiles, the blast force, and burns.

 ## PITFALLS

Many different and potentially toxic chemicals are used throughout a petrochemical refinery. When a refining column is damaged as in an explosion, lighter components are released. These hydrocarbons composed of fewer carbon and hydrogen atoms vaporize, leaving behind a heavier, less volatile fraction. Gasoline contains relatively high proportions of toxic and volatile hydrocarbons, such as benzene (which is known to cause cancer in humans) and hexane (which can affect the nervous system). Gasoline and kerosene releases are exceptionally hazardous due to their high flammability. Crude oils and semirefined products such as diesel and bunkering oils may contain cancer-causing polycyclic aromatic hydrocarbons and other toxic substances. These differing chemicals have various thresholds for combustion, and multiple explosions can occur at differing times. This poses a serious threat to healthcare workers who arrive on the scene after the initial incidents.

REFERENCES

1. Snodgrass WR. Petroleum industry. In: Greenberg MI, Phillips SD, eds. *Occupational, Industrial, and Environmental Toxicology.* 2nd ed. St Louis, Mo: Mosby; 2003.
2. U.S Environmental Protection Agency. Types of petroleum oil. 2004. Available at: http://www.epa.gov/oilspill/oiltypes.htm.
3. Yapa PD, Zheng L, Chen F. A model for deepwater oil/gas blowouts. *Mar Pollut Bull.* 2001;43:234-41.
4. Leese WL. Some medical aspects of North Sea oil industry. *Scott Med J.* 1977;22:258-66.
5. Gabbay DS, De Roos F, Perrone J. Twenty-foot fall averts fatality from massive hydrogen sulfide exposure. *J Emerg Med.* 2001;20:141-4.
6. Trevino MA, Herrmann GH, Sprout WL. Treatment of severe hydrofluoric acid exposures. *J Occup Med.* 1983;25:861-3.
7. Dayal HH, Brodwick M, Morris R, et al. A community-based epidemiologic study of health sequelae of exposure to hydrofluoric acid. *Ann Epidemiol.* 1992;2:213-30.
8. Harrison BF. Blast resistant modular buildings for the petroleum and chemical processing industries. *J Haz Mater.* 2003;104:31-8.
9. Skrbic B, Miljevic N. An evaluation of residues at an oil refinery site following fires. *J Environ Sci Health Part A Tox Hazard Subst Environ Eng.* 2002;37:1029-39.
10. Skrbic B, Novakovic J, Miljevic N. Mobility of heavy metals originating from bombing of industrial sites. *J Environ Sci Health Part A Tox Hazard Subst Environ Eng.* 2002;37:7-16.
11. Attias L, Bucchi AR, Maranghi F, et al. Crude oil spill in sea water: an assessment of the risk for bathers correlated to benzo(a)pyrene exposure. *Cent Eur J Public Health.* 1995;3:142-5.
12. Hull AM, Alexander DA, Klein S. Survivors of the Piper Alpha oil platform disaster: long-term follow-up study. *Br J Psychiatry.* 2002;181:433-8.
13. Alexander DA. Burn victims after a major disaster: reactions of patients and their care-givers. *Burns* 1993;19:105-9.
14. Campbell D, Cox D, Crum J, et al. Initial effects of the grounding of the tanker Braer on health in Shetland. The Shetland Health Study Group. *BMJ.* 1993;307:1251-5.
15. Crum JE. Peak expiratory flow rate in schoolchildren living close to Braer oil spill. *BMJ.* 1993;307:23-4.
16. Dayal HH, Baranowski T, Li YH, et al. Hazardous chemicals: psychological dimensions of the health sequelae of a community exposure in Texas. *J Epidemiol Community Health.* 1994;48:560-8.
17. Palinkas LA, Petterson JS, Russell J, et al. Community patterns of psychiatric disorders after the Exxon Valdez oil spill. *Am J Psychiatry.* 1993;150:1517-23.
18. Qiao B. Oil spill model development and application for emergency response system. *J Environ Sci (China).* 2001;13:252-6.
19. Qiao B, Chu JC, Zhao P, et al. Marine oil spill contingency planning. *J Environ Sci (China).* 2002;14:102-7.
20. Li J. A GIS planning model for urban oil spill management. *Water Sci Technol.* 2001;43:239-44.
21. Bak B, Juhl M, Lauridsen F, et al. Oil and petrol drum explosions: injuries and casualties by exploding oil and petrol drums containing various inflammable liquids. *Injury* 1988;19:8-5.

chapter 155

Introduction to Fires and Burns

Marianne E. Cinat and Victoria M. Vanderkam

Burn injuries are commonly seen in disasters. In addition to being associated with structure fires, they may also occur in conjunction with explosions; wild land fires; plane, train, or automobile crashes; or other serious events. Injuries may be the result of flame, flash, chemicals, or electricity. More recently, there has been increased concern about nuclear, biologic, and chemical warfare disaster management, all of which can result in significant burn injury to a large number of victims. Burn injury can involve only the skin or may have an inhalational component resulting from heat exposure to the face and upper airway or from smoke inhalation causing damage to the distal airways and bronchial tree. Burn injury with inhalation may result in rapid loss of airway and shock. Immediate triage and resuscitation are essential to survival and optimal outcomes. Many authors have described burn injuries associated with major disaster. Recent events and lessons learned will be reviewed.

CURRENT PRACTICE

Preincident Action: Disaster Planning

Firefighters, rescue workers, and emergency medical personnel should have a good working knowledge of the treatment of burns. Disaster preparedness in a specific geographic area should include a plan to triage burn victims to burn centers in the area that are equipped for and experienced in handling critically injured patients. Burn care should be prioritized as a curriculum item for instruction to emergency medical services (EMS) workers including emergency medical technicians, paramedics, and firefighters. All EMS responders should be aware of the nearest burn center as well as nearest receiving centers. Collaboration among burn centers should be proactive. Working relationships among centers with specific plans and transfer agreements will be effective in ensuring the triage and early care of burn victims. Burn centers must be prepared to receive multiple burn patients that may have other associated injuries.

Prehospital Management of the Incident

The American Burn Association (ABA) endorses the Advanced Burn Life Support course curriculum. A section of this course is devoted to the management of multicasualty burn incidents as well as scene safety with fire hazards.[1] Excerpts of this course are provided in Boxes 155-1, 155-2, and 155-3. Organizational components for incident management by all responding units are listed in Box 155-1.

The triage area should have adequate lighting and be located in an area where the triage officer can visualize the entire scene. It should be located away from hazards, at a site between the scene of the incident and transport vehicles. Four treatment categories are recommended and are summarized in Box 155-2.

Stabilization in the field is managed by EMS using protocols and communication with base hospitals. Airway control is the top priority. The airway should be established and maintained with endotracheal intubation based on local protocols. In general, burn patients without other injuries typically do not go into shock within 60 minutes from the time of injury, even if no treatment is provided.[1] Therefore, a burn victim who develops shock soon after an incident should be evaluated immediately for underlying injury, occult hemorrhage, respiratory failure, or other causes of shock (e.g., cardiac, neurologic).

Masellis and others[2] provide guidelines for the general public regarding immediate first aid in the care of burn victims. They are as follows:

1. Maintain self-control—don't panic.
2. Protect yourself.
3. Reduce the activity of the fire.
4. Extract and transfer victims to open air if possible.
5. Extinguish burning clothing.
6. Remove burning clothing.
7. Provide emergency treatment of burns.

   a. Thermal burns: Leave blisters intact. Cool the burn for up to 10 minutes. Avoid hypothermia. Cover body with dry, clean sheet. Avoid ointments or other medications.
   b. Chemical burns: Flush the exposed area with water thoroughly. Collect detailed information about the chemical agent, and be prepared to provide this information to the emergency medical personnel.
   c. Electrical burns: Remove the source of electricity and protect the airway.

BOX 155-1 BURN DISASTER MANAGEMENT

A. The medical command post should:
  1. Be established in a safe area.
  2. Serve as the communication center for dispatch and medical control.
B. Security and hazard control:
  1. Should minimize risks of injury to rescuers and onlookers.
  2. Is coordinated at the medical command post.
  3. Are the responsibility of all members of the rescue team.
  4. Should ensure crowd and hazard control.
C. A communication center at the medical command post should:
  1. Communicate patient information to incident managers, including the number of victims and their condition.
  2. Ensure casualty distribution to appropriate facilities.
  3. Communicate to the receiving facility the number of casualties and treatment provided.

Reproduced from *Advanced Burn Life Support–Pre-Hospital Course Manual.* Chicago: American Burn Association; 2001:19–20, with permission.

BOX 155-2 TRIAGE TREATMENT CATEGORIES

1. Immediate care (red)
   a. Burns >20% TBSA in patients aged 10 to 50 years
   b. Burns >10% TBSA in patients aged <10 or >50 years
   c. Inhalation injury
   d. Chemical injury
   e. Electrical injury
   f. Associated, life-threatening injuries
2. Delayed care (yellow)
   a. Burns <20% TBSA in patients aged 10 to 50 years
   b. Full-thickness burns of <5% TBSA
   c. Sunburn or first-degree burn
3. Minor category (green)
   a. Minor injuries; no emergency care required
4. Deceased (black)
   a. Survival unlikely

Reproduced from *Advanced Burn Life Support–Pre-Hospital Course Manual.* Chicago: American Burn Association; 2001:20–1, with permission.

Masellis and colleagues[2] also recommend guidelines for trained personnel regarding the initial management of burn victims. They are as follows:

1. Immediate triage of seriously ill victims
2. Inspection of the upper airway
3. Qualitative assessment of the burns
4. Quantitative assessment of the burns
5. Intravenous resuscitative therapy
6. Analgesic therapy
7. Hospital transfer

To appropriately triage burn victims in a mass-casualty incident, emergency medical personnel must be able to accurately assess the severity and extent of the burns along with the signs of inhalation injury. Outcomes

BOX 155-3 PRINCIPLES OF SCENE SAFETY WITH FIRE HAZARDS

1. In the presence of a major fire, the emergency vehicles should be located a safe distance from the scene. The safe area may vary depending on the type of incident and scene assessment.
2. Before entering a burning structure, rescue personnel should have proper knowledge of and training in the following:
   a. the utilization of approved protective clothing
   b. the use of self-contained breathing apparatus
3. The rescuer must be knowledgeable and skilled in rescue techniques from a burning structure.

Reproduced from *Advanced Burn Life Support–Pre-Hospital Course Manual.* Chicago: American Burn Association; 2001:17, with permission.

after burn injury are negatively affected when care is delayed. Rapid triage and treatment are essential to survival. Specific parameters that should be measured in the field and reported to the hospital include the following:

- Severity of burns
- Extent of burns (total body surface area [TBSA])
- Status of inhalation injury
- Etiology of injury
- Symptoms of shock

Assessing the Severity of Burns

Burn wounds have classically been described as being first, second, third, or fourth degree. Recently, however, this classification has changed to reflect the anatomic thickness of the skin layer involved. Specifically, wounds are now classified as superficial, partial-thickness, or full-thickness burns.

First-degree burns, or *superficial burns*, involve only the epidermis. They are not included when calculating the TBSA burned for use in fluid resuscitation. This category of burn is usually caused by a brief exposure to heat or ultraviolet radiation from the sun (i.e., sunburn). First-degree burns are painful and appear as reddened skin without blistering.

Second-degree burns, or *partial-thickness burns*, involve the entire epidermis and part of the dermis. Superficial partial-thickness burns appear bright red with blister formation and a moist surface. They are extremely painful to touch, especially once blisters are broken, and they blanch with pressure, demonstrating brisk capillary refill.

Third-degree burns, or *full-thickness burns*, involve all layers of the skin (i.e., epidermis, dermis, and dermal appendages). They may appear charred, mottled, pale, waxy, yellow, brown, or nonblanching red. They are firm, dry, and leathery.

Fourth-degree burns, or *subdermal burns*, extend through the skin into the subcutaneous tissues and may involve underlying, bone, muscle, and associated structures. Tissue appears charred, firm, dry, and leathery; mummification may also be apparent. These wounds are insensate.

Assessing Extent of Burn

The extent of burn wounds is reported as the percentage of TBSA burned. When calculating TBSA burn for fluid resuscitation, only second-, third-, and fourth-degree burns are used in the calculation.

The "rule of nines" is the classic way of calculating the TBSA[3] (Figure 155-1). The body surface is divided into areas that equal 9%. When all the body areas are summed they equal 99%, with the remaining 1% attributed to the genitalia and perineum. This is an efficient method of calculating the extent of a burn, but is less accurate in children under the age of 10 years, especially infants, due to the difference in body proportions.

For small or irregular burns, the TBSA can be calculated by using the patient's palm (including the fingers) to represent approximately 1% of his or her TBSA.[4]

Identifying Inhalation Injury

The likelihood of inhalation injury is increased in patients with facial burns, soot in the oropharynx, or singed nasal hairs. Inhalation injuries can be divided into supraglottic and infraglottic categories. Supraglottic inhalation injury is the most common. It can result from thermal or chemical sources and causes injury to the upper air passages and supraglottic structures. Rapid airway edema and occlusion can occur.[1] Signs and symptoms of supraglottic inhalation injury include hoarseness, a change in phonation, stridor, and difficulty breathing. In unresuscitated patients, supraglottic edema may be delayed until fluid resuscitation is well under way. Because of this risk of delayed airway obstruction, early intubation is recommended to prevent airway occlusion and the need for a surgical airway.

Infraglottic inhalation injury almost always occurs due to chemical injury of the airways and lung parenchyma. Direct damage to the epithelium of the airways occurs because of inhaled noxious chemicals (e.g., aldehydes, sulfur oxides, and phosgenes). The factors that increase the extent of injury are prolonged exposure to such chemical gases (seen in patients found unconscious at the scene) and smaller size of gas particles. These factors cause the smaller airways and terminal bronchi to be affected. This toxin inhalation can lead to respiratory failure with prolonged intubation and ventilatory support. Inhalation injury leading to pulmonary failure should be anticipated in a victim with a history of smoke exposure in an enclosed space and with subsequent loss of consciousness.

Etiology of Injury

Information regarding the cause of the fire and subsequent burn are helpful to the treating physician. Information should be obtained at the scene and then communicated to the receiving hospital personnel. Information that is pertinent to treatment includes whether the incident occurred indoors or outdoors. Indoor incidents are very likely to result in inhalation injury. Treatment of the burn wound may vary depending on the cause or agent involved (e.g., flame, electrical, chemical).

Symptoms of Shock

Decreased level of consciousness, decreased blood pressure, increased heart rate, and decreased peripheral perfusion are all classic indicators of shock. In patient with burns, adequate blood pressure may be maintained for some time due to release of catecholamine after the burn occurs. These substances constrict blood vessel and act to maintain the blood pressure.

Emergency Department Assessment and Treatment

Initial assessment of a burn victim follows the same priorities as for any injured patient. Airway management is the top priority in a major burn with inhalation injury and is the first priority in the emergency department (ED) triage area. Respiratory support and fluid resuscitation must take place concurrently. Although intravenous access through unburned skin is preferred, access through burned skin is acceptable if necessary. Central lines or femoral access may be required. Circulatory compromise must be identified early. Any jewelry or circumferential devices should be immediately removed because profound swelling during burn resuscitation can result in these devices functioning as tourniquets, leading to circulatory compromise. Escharotomies may be required for circumferential full-thickness burns to the chest or extremities but should be performed at a burn center under the supervision of a burn surgeon. Neurologic deficits and mental status should be accu-

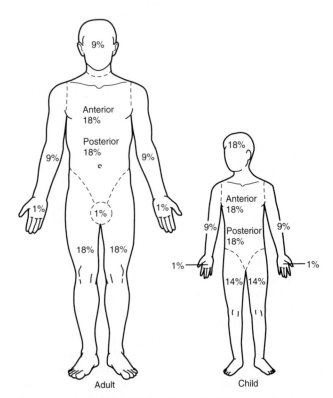

FIGURE 155-1. The rule of nines.

rately assessed and recorded. The patient should be fully exposed to allow appropriate assessment of burn depth and extent. However, the patient should then be immediately covered with a warm dry sheet to prevent hypothermia. During assessment and resuscitation, it is important to avoid hypothermia and maintain the patient's body temperature. This can be accomplished by liberal use of warm blankets, increasing the temperature of the room, warming intravenous fluids, and warming the ventilator circuit for intubated patients.

Fluid resuscitation should be initiated using the burn consensus formula of 2 to 4 cc/kg/%TBSA burned.[1] Once calculated, half of this volume is given in the first 8 hours after the burn injury; the second half is given in the next 16 hours. This formula should only be used as a guide for initial volume resuscitation rates. Rates can be adjusted hourly to maintain a urine output of 0.5 cc/kg/hour in adults and 1.0 cc/kg/hour in children.

Analgesia and sedation are needed, and the patient should be monitored on an ongoing basis. Once the initial priorities are managed and the patient's condition is stabilized, he or she is moved to an intensive care unit for ongoing care.

 ## UNIQUE CONSIDERATIONS

Arturson[5] analyzes a series of 14 fire disasters that occurred between 1973 and 1990. Details of these disasters are summarized in Table 155-1. This study demonstrates that indoor fires result in fewer survivors than outdoor fires, with six times more injuries reported from the latter. In the study, actual hospital admissions were 20 times higher after outdoor incidents. Indoor fires are more likely to result in the rapid death of those who cannot escape, due to hypoxia and inhalation of toxic chemicals. Relatively few admissions were seen

after indoor fire disasters in the Arturson study. Survivors of indoor disasters were typically a result of less severe burns (i.e., <30%) or inhalation injury. Outdoor incidents resulted in larger numbers of hospital admission with more severe injuries. Patients with large TBSA burns (>70%) are more likely to be encountered in outdoor disasters. Triage should involve getting the most severely burned persons to specialized burns beds. Minor burns can be triaged to medical personnel in nonburn facilities if necessary. The outcomes noted in this review are attributed to inhalation of smoke and poisonous compounds.

 ## PITFALLS

Leslie and colleagues[6] provide an informative report of management of a multiburn casualty at an ED in Massachusetts without a burn unit that provided insight into potential problems. In this disaster, 11 burn victims were brought to Baystate Medical Center after a foundry explosion.

Their retrospective review of this event resulted in a number of recommendations for both field triage and for hospitals. In respect to triage, it is recommended that the first ambulance to arrive at the scene become the dedicated triage unit. A method of triage should be preplanned by the EMS and hospital systems in each particular geographic area. A proactive plan maximizes assessment and allows for rapid relay of information to the receiving hospital. This in turn allows hospital personnel to make early decisions regarding staffing and allocation of resources. The importance of providing as much information as possible regarding the causative agents was stressed. In this example, the causative agent was phenolic resin. There was a delayed recognition of the possibility of toxic exposure to the

TABLE 155-1   DESCRIPTION OF 14 DISASTERS CAUSING MASS BURN CASUALTIES, 1973-1990

INCIDENT	DATE	DESCRIPTION
Indoor Disasters		
Summerland, UK	August 2, 1973	Fire in leisure complex
Dublin, Ireland	February 14, 1981	Fire in discotheque
Cardowan, UK	January 27, 1984	Coal mine in explosion
Manchester, UK	August 22, 1985	Fire in aircraft on runway
King's Cross, UK	June 24, 1988	Fire in underground station
Piper Alpha, UK	July 6, 1988	Fire on oil platform
Scandinavian Star (SCA), Skagerak	April 7, 1990	Fire in ferry
Outdoor Disasters		
Nakivubo, Uganda	January 13, 1973	Petrol tanker crash in market place
Los Alfaques, Spain	July 11, 1978	LPG tanker crash at campsite
Bangalore, India	February 7, 1981	Circus fire
San Juanico, Mexico	November 19, 1984	Explosion in LPG plant
Bradford, UK	May 11, 1985	Fire in football stadium
Ramstein, Germany	August 28, 1988	Plane crash at air show
Bashkir, Soviet Union	June 4, 1989	Natural gas explosion causing a train crash

LPG, Liquefied petroleum gas.
Modified from Arturson C: Analysis of severe fire disasters. In: Masellis M, Gunn SWA, eds. *The Management of Mass Burn Casualties and Fire Disaster*. Dordrecht, The Netherlands: Kluwer Academic Pub; 2002:24–33, with permission.

resin. While the possibility was remote, the real potential for contamination of the entire treatment area remained.

Lessons learned in the ED included the need for a clearly demarcated command center with a large whiteboard to be used for patient documentation. Information including patient identification, injuries, and transfer status should be made readily accessible in this format. A team captain who will make all important decisions should be designated. Further, the need for large amounts of warm intravenous fluids, humidified gases for inhalation, warming blankets, and radiant heat sources are absolutely necessary; this was not appreciated early on. Hospital personnel reported difficulty in controlling ambient temperatures in the ED where rooms could not be enclosed, and this made core body temperatures difficult to maintain.

Dunbar[7] reports on the Rhode Island nightclub fire that resulted in 200 injuries and 100 deaths. The author, an emergency room nurse, was present at the receiving ED in a hospital with a burn center. Activation of the Hospital Emergency Incident Command System allowed an orchestrated response that enabled the staff to meet their goals of providing life-sustaining procedures and comfort measures. They received 67 victims, admitted 43 patients, and intubated 22 of them in a matter of hours. Areas they identified for improvement were family support and control of traffic congestion around the ED. They are currently working on a system to better support families during a disaster. Traffic congestion will be minimized in future disasters by implementation of an alternate route for employees returning to the hospital.

Several authors have reviewed the September 11, 2001, World Trade Center disaster in New York City as it pertains to burns and disaster planning.[8-10] These reports cite the importance of having a hospital incident command center and proactive disaster plan in place. Other factors that had a positive impact on outcomes were early mobilization and organization of the workforce and consistent methods of patient care among all practitioners.[9] Several important issues were identified. Medical teams were dispatched to the scene within hours of the attack. This placed these persons at risk for illness and injury. Secondly, the hospital was not equipped to handle nuclear, biologic, or chemical weapon casualties. Finally, many volunteers responded to the hospital to assist, but there was no system in place to verify the credentials of these people. These issues have resulted in the reassessment of disaster planning. It is interesting to note that Kirschenbaum and others[8] found that the mix of injuries corroborated the findings of Arturson described earlier. A large number of victims were seen, but there were a small percentage of victims who had severe injuries.

The increased incidence of large disasters with multiple casualties has initiated the discussion of how best to manage these types of events and the resulting patient populations. Mackie[11] has suggested that medical personnel should not be dispatched to the disaster scene. Doing so puts healthcare workers at risk of personal injury. Similar opinions were documented by reviewers of the 2001 World Trade Center disaster.[8] While this is a debated issue, it seems that there is growing consensus that burn assessment teams should be hospital based versus scene based. He further recommends that national associations should work to develop and refine disaster plans that are appropriate to their regions.

To this end, the ABA has made major strides following the New York City World Trade Center attack in developing a national response to fire/burn disasters. The ABA has identified burn centers and burn beds across the country. Via e-mail, this system can be activated as necessary to respond to major burn disasters. It is estimated that 350 to 500 beds could be filled during a disaster. This system would require judicial movement of patients to verified regional burn centers from the burn center nearest the disaster rather than the movement of trained personnel. Consensus of the ABA board after an evaluation of the Sept. 11, 2001, disaster response is that local burn nursing corps will yield greater efficiency when remaining stationary, rather than transferring personnel to overloaded burn centers.[12]

SUMMARY

In summary, the effective management of a fire disaster involving multiple burn victims requires quick action on the part of the EMS. Expert triage with clear communication to the base is essential to the rapid movement of patients that is so critical to the positive outcome for the burn patient. Hospital EDs that are prepared for disaster with efficient means of communication and prioritization will optimize the outcome of the victims of a multicasualty disaster.

REFERENCES

1. *Advanced Burn Life Support-Pre-Hospital Course Manual.* Chicago: American Burn Association; 2001.
2. Masellis M, Ferrara MM, Gunn SWA. Immediate assistance and first aid on the spot in fire disaster education of the public and self-sufficiency training. In: Masellis M, Gunn SWA, eds. *The Management of Mass Burn Casualties and Fire Disaster.* Dordrecht, The Netherlands: Kluwer Academic Pub; 2002:121-32.
3. Lund CC, Browder NC. The estimation of areas of burns. *Surg Gyn Obstet.* 1944;79:352.
4. Sheridan RL, Petras L, Basha G, et al. Planimetry study of the percent of body surface represented by the hand and palm: sizing irregular burns is more accurately done with the palm. *J Burn Care Rehab.* 1995;16:605-6.
5. Arturson C. Analysis of severe fire disasters. In: Masellis M, Gunn SWA, eds. *The Management of Mass Burn Casualties and Fire Disaster.* Dordrecht, The Netherlands: Kluwer Academic Pub; 2002:24-33.
6. Leslie CL, Cusman M, McDonald GS, et al. Management of multiple burn casualties in a high volume ED without a verified burn center. *Am J Emerg Med.* 2001;19:469-73, 2001.
7. Dunbar JA. The Rhode Island nightclub fire: the story from the perspective of an on-duty ED nurse. *J Emerg Nurs.* 2004;30:464-6.
8. Kirschenbaum L, Keene A, O'Neill P, et al. The experience at St. Vincent's Hospital, Manhattan on September 11, 2001: preparedness, response, and lessons learned. *Crit Care Med.* 2005;33:S48-52.

9. Rolls JA, Bauer G, Bessey PQ, et al. September 11, 2001—a physician's experience [abstract]. *J Burn Care Rehabil.* 2002;23:S107.

10. Yurt RW, Bessey PQ, Bauer G, et al. The World Trade Center disaster: one burn center's experience [abstract]. *J Burn Care Rehabil.* 2002;23:S107.

11. Mackie DP. Mass burn casualties: a rational approach to planning. *Editorial Burns.* 2002;28:403-4.

12. Jordan MH. "9/11 This is Not a Drill!" *J Burn Care Rehabil.* 2004; 25:15-24.

chapter 156

Structure Fire

Deborah Gutman

 ## DESCRIPTION OF EVENT

Each year, 2 million fires are reported to U.S. fire departments. Based on 2000 data from the National Fire Incident Reporting System, fires in structures account for approximately 30% of all fires, but they cause nearly 76% of property loss, approximately 72% of fatalities (3500 annually), and nearly 82% of injuries (19,600 annually) resulting from fires. Structure fires occur in homes, assembly buildings, office buildings, schools, stores, businesses, manufacturing facilities and plants, and many other structures. Almost all *fatal* structure fires occur in residential structures.

In residential structures, kitchens are the most common fire location, with bedrooms being the second. Among nonresidential structures, the majority of fires occur in storage facilities (30.9%), followed by businesses (19.8%), assembly structures (14.1%), and manufacturing (9.9%), with the leading cause being arson.[1] Although there is no seasonal pattern for fires in general, more structure fires take place in the winter, with the lowest percentage taking place in the summer. The highest percentage of structure fires occur between 5:00 and 6:00 PM.

The fire and subsequent collapse of the World Trade Center in New York City on September 11, 2001, has raised consciousness regarding high-rise fires and firefighting tactics. High-rise fires are inherently more difficult for the fire service. By nature of the buildings' height, smoke movement in high-rise structures is very different than those in other structures. Temperature gradients result in varying pressures throughout the structures and allow for uncontrolled movement of smoke and flame (known as the *stack effect*).[2] The air-conditioning and heating vents and other utilities in some high-rise structures service multiple levels and can facilitate the spread of smoke and flame through a building, injuring occupants who are floors away from the fire itself. Elevators stall or shut down (elevators failed at 59 of 179 major high-rise fires), fire radios don't function above certain floors because the structural steel interferes with radio communication, fire ladders are too short, and civilians may jump to their death.[3] In an emergency, the movement of people out of the building is particularly difficult.

A high-rise structure fire is usually defined as a fire in a structure that is five stories or taller, although this defi-

nition may vary by jurisdiction. Unlike the World Trade Center fire, the majority of high-rise fires occur in apartment buildings; 6% occur in hospitals, 4% in hotels, 3% in dormitories, and 3% in offices. Three-quarters of high-rise fires take place in residential structures. However, residential high-rise death rates are half as common as those of residential structures in general. More people are available in a high-rise building than in a single-family home to alert residents of a fire and to assist with an evacuation. Also, most building codes require hardwired smoke alarms in high-rise buildings. A smoke alarm activates in 69% of residential high-rise fires compared with 38% of all residential structure fires. Similar to other residential fires, the leading cause of all high-rise fires is cooking (38%), but cause patterns vary by property type.

 ## PREINCIDENT CONSIDERATION

The United States has made significant progress in reducing the number of fire deaths through the widespread use of smoke detectors, fire sprinkler systems, stricter fire codes, and changes in lifestyle, including decreased smoking.[4] However, three-quarters of fire deaths and nearly 60% of fire injuries occur in structure fires where no alarm is present, or where an alarm was present but failed to operate.[5] Preventive measures are usually lacking in all investigated fires and training of personnel is rare, in particular, with regards to communications. Fire safety plans should be in place and inspections kept up to date. Firefighters must be familiar with the construction of local buildings and have access to the layout of local buildings. People should also learn the emergency evacuation procedures of the office buildings they work in and the stores and businesses they frequent.

Experience with burn disasters has suggested that one of the most important features early in a burn disaster is effective communication between prehospital personnel, local hospitals, and specialized burn centers allowing for expert triage of the severely burned patient. Appropriate patient triage involves both promptness of care as well as level of care and appropriate hospital destination. Triage becomes essential to the use of limited resources such as air evacuation, burn beds, ventilators, and operating rooms. Expert triage may even reduce the need for burn beds. In one review of 14 severe fire disasters, they found that victims from structure fires had less severe burns and more significant risk from inhalation injuries.[6,7]

There is often a very small time window for establishment of effective communication between the scene and all area hospitals to accomplish this triage. In the Coconut Grove fire in Boston in 1942, the first casualties arrived 15 minutes after the fire started. It is estimated that one casualty arrived at Boston City Hospital every 11 seconds for a total of more than 300 patients in 2 hours.[8] The time elapsed between notification and arrival of patients after a burn disaster is brief for most hospitals, and some reviews have suggested that numbers of victims are often underestimated. Many large structural fires or high-rise fires occur in major cities, and there is a major response from city rescue agencies with most victims evacuated from the site within 30 minutes. Apart from ambulances, many patients will be transported by private cars, taxis, and even buses and will simultaneously arrive to the emergency department, overloading its capacity. In fire disasters, the massive arrival of burn patients in a specialized burn unit will quickly paralyze its capacity to accept and care for patients.

A central command center at the site would assist with the assessment of available burn beds and resources (e.g., ventilators) at each of the area hospitals and match the distribution of patient types and severity to each hospital, thereby shifting the major burden for triage away from nearby hospitals. The disaster system needs to establish, in advance, procedures for prioritizing and coordinating both ground and air medical evacuation of patients to specialized burn centers to prevent the need for many interhospital transfers and competition for limited air flight services to burn centers.

This emphasizes the need for the development of improved information systems/networks as part of disaster planning. For example, in New York State after the September 11, 2001, World Trade Center attack, the State Department of Health implemented an enhanced statewide system known as the Hospital Emergency Response Data system that allows hospitals to communicate over a Web-based secure system during a crisis.[9] The U.S. Army has developed an automated e-mail system that queries participating burn centers each morning regarding bed and resource capacity. These types of systems would facilitate appropriate triage and use of specialized burn centers.

 ## POSTINCIDENT CONSIDERATIONS

Fire causes panic in its victims, and their actions then may serve to worsen the damages. Some people trapped in a burning high-rise building who cannot be reached will leap to their deaths. It can be anticipated that persons who are not trapped will try to go to the aid of trapped victims, putting themselves in harm's way. In the 1911 fire at the Triangle Shirtwaist Company in New York, some trapped victims chose to leap to their deaths from windows on the eighth and ninth floors. One hundred forty-six people leapt to their deaths, were burned, or crushed

to death in the panic. The potential for secondary traumatic injuries in survivors who leap to safety or reenter burning buildings should be taken into account.

 ## MEDICAL TREATMENT OF CASUALTIES

The first 72 hours of burn care constitutes the resuscitation phase. The actions composing appropriate medical treatment follow:

1. Remove the victim from the source of the burn, taking care not to become a victim yourself. Rescuers must assess the situation and must be able to protect themselves from flames, fumes, toxic gases, falling masonry, and other hazards to their personal safety. All rescuers at the scene of a fire should use protective clothing and devices. Ventilation and cooling systems must be turned off, and any fixed extinguishing equipment should be turned on. To extinguish a victim's clothing, throw the person to the ground and wrap him or her in a blanket. Cut away belts, sleeves, and tight clothing with care; remove rings, bracelets, and other constricting items. Do not violently tear off clothing that may adhere to burned skin.

2. Check the patient's vital signs, check for other associated trauma, and stop any bleeding.

3. Evaluate the patient's airway. Involvement of the upper airways should be suspected in the presence of face and neck burns. Look for carbonaceous sputum and singed nasal hairs. The more serious the thermal damage, the more rapidly the patient needs airway management. Treat with oxygen and orotracheal intubation as necessary. Have a high suspicion for inhalational injuries. In structure fires, many new synthetic polymers are used for furniture, upholstery, carpets, bedding, and curtains, and these yield combustion products such as carbon monoxide, cyanide, phosgene, hydrogen chloride, and nitrogen oxides. These noxious gases may be additive. Autopsies after the Stardust nightclub fire in Dublin, which killed 48 people, showed that 80% of victims had a carbon monoxide level higher than 50%. In the 1990 Nagasakiya supermarket fire in Osaka, Japan, the dead bodies were covered with soot but not badly burned. Of 14 blood specimens, 8 showed carbon monoxide levels over 50%, and in 10 cases the cyanide level was higher than 3.0 μg/mL, which is believed to be a lethal concentration. Hyperlacticacidemia is an excellent indicator of cyanide intoxication, and an initial plasma lactate greater than 10 mmol/L is a sure indication of toxicity. The use of amyl nitrite pearls in unconscious patients with inhalation injury should be seriously considered in the prehospital setting. In the hospital, serum should be sent for measurement of carbon monoxide, lactate, and cyanide levels.

4. Make a qualitative and quantitative assessment of victim's burns. Use the rule of nines for adults (9% for each upper limb and for the head, 18% for each lower limb and for the front and back of the thorax) or the rule of palms (size of patient's palm is equal to 1% of the body surface area [BSA]). In children, the head is 20% of BSA.

5. Start intravenous resuscitation therapy if the burned surface exceeds 15% to 20% BSA in an adult or 15% in a child. Use physiologic fluids such as normal saline or Ringer's lactate solution. If intravenous therapy is impossible, the victim should sip water containing a little salt. If there are no veins visible, a venous cutdown may be necessary. The fluid requirements for the first 4 hours can be calculated as 0.5 cc/kg for each percent of BSA.

6. Use analgesia therapy liberally. For severe pain, intravenous morphine can be titrated to effect.

7. Perform bladder catheterization to monitor urine output.

8. Institute burn treatment. Cover burned tissue with clean sterilized wet sheets. Cooling reduces burn depth, edema, and pain. If more than 2 hours have elapsed since the accident, it may be necessary to perform emergency escharotomy for deep circumferential burns that involve the neck, thorax, or limbs and hands. Do not burst blisters or remove the epidermis. Do not cool for longer than 20 minutes, and stop if patient begins to shiver. Use care with cooling children and the elderly. Use clean plastic bags to wrap burned hands and feet, and do not apply any constrictive dressings.

9. Reexamine the patient. Detection of additional injuries may have to be delayed until this point.

10. Make decisions regarding hospital transfer. Basic resuscitative measures should be taken before secondary air transport. If smoke inhalation is suspected, a preflight chest radiograph and an arterial blood gas should be done. If a pneumothorax is diagnosed or suspected, a chest tube must be placed prior to flight, nasogastric and urinary catheters must be placed and the balloon filled with fluid, not air. Plastic bottles must be used for fluids and blood, and parenteral infusions must be provided through a large-bore catheter.

 CASE PRESENTATION

It is 2 AM on a winter morning. You are the attending physician on duty in a level I trauma center, and you receive a call from a local EMS personnel notifying you of 100 potential burn victims from an ongoing fire at a local nightclub.

What else do you need to know? What do you do to prepare?

 UNIQUE CONSIDERATIONS

There are certain populations and fire situations that deserve additional discussion. In the case of structure fire fatalities, 25% of deaths occur in persons older than 64 years, and 16% of deaths occur in children under the age of 10 years. Children may not respond appropriately to fire; they may hide or not tell adults about the situation. Even in the presence of working smoke detectors, children may not react properly and usually need adult

rescuers to help them get out of a burning building. From ages 3 to 5 years, children are more likely to play with matches, lighters, or candles and start fires if left unsupervised. Nationally, among children younger than the age of 6 years who die in residential fires, one-third are due to children playing with matches or fire. Efforts to teach match and lighter safety to children and parental education regarding child supervision would be worthwhile in preventing child fire deaths.[10]

Older Americans also represent a high-risk group. Over the age of 65 years, fire death rate exceeds that of the national average.[11] Smoking is the leading cause of fire deaths among older adults, and cooking is the leading cause of injuries. Cooking injuries occur due to accidental igniting of loose-fitting clothes or forgetting to turn off a burner or leaving food on the stove. Disabilities including vision, hearing loss, and impaired mobility impair their ability to escape a fire.

Among all structure fires, nightclub fires in the United States are proportionately few in number (0.3%). However, over-capacity crowds at nightclubs create the potential for high numbers of casualties in the event of a fire; therefore, when these types of fires occur, they attract national media attention. Local jurisdictions that do not routinely inspect nightclubs or do not enforce existing safety regulations, coupled with the exemption of small clubs from installing sprinkler systems, increase the potential for a fatal nightclub fire. Oftentimes, the exits are locked or blocked. The detection of the fire is slowed, and alarms are often delayed. Nightclubs pose a challenge for fire prevention and public safety.

 PITFALLS

Several potential pitfalls in response to a structure fire exist. These include the following:

• Not instituting strict fire prevention codes and inspections and not implementing public safety campaigns can result in unnecessary injury. Fire disasters are preventable and avoidable, and most of them are man-made.

• If no on-scene triage officer is designated, a "scoop and run" practice will put significant burden on receiving hospitals for secondary triage of burn patients to specialized burn units and will create competition for limited aeromedical resources.

• Inadequate advance planning for use of limited resources such as aeromedical transport and specialized burn facilities is another potential pitfall.

• Not suspecting and treating for toxic inhalants and associated trauma in an unconscious fire victim can lead to avoidable exacerbation of injury from fire disaster.

REFERENCES

1. U.S. Fire Administration. Non-Residential Structure Fires in 2000. Topical Fire Research Series, Volume 3. Federal Emergency Management Agency; 2004. Available at: http://www.usfa.fema.gov/inside-usfa/nfdc/pubs/tfrs.shtm.

2. U.S. Fire Administration. High-rise Fires. Topical Fire Research Series, Volume 2. Federal Emergency Management Agency; 2002. Available at: http://www.usfa.fema.gov/inside-usfa/nfdc/pubs/tfrs.shtm.

3. Rayman G. Disaster foreshadowed: deputy warned of high rise fires in 1995 article. October 31, 2001. Available at: http://www.newsday.com.

4. American Academy of Pediatrics. Reducing the number of deaths and injuries from residential fires. *Pediatrics* 2000;105:1355-7.

5. U.S. Fire Administration, National Fire Data Center. All Structure Fires in 2000. Topical Fire Research Series, Volume 3. Federal Emergency Management Agency; 2004. Available at: http://www.usfa.fema.gov/inside-usfa/nfdc/pubs/tfrs.shtm.

6. Arturson C. Analysis of severe fire disasters. In: Masellis M, Gunn SWA, eds. *The Management of Mass Burn Casualties and Fire Disasters*. Boston, Dordrecht, London: Kluwer Academic Publishers; 1992.

7. Mackie DP, Koning HM. Fate of mass burn casualties: implications for disaster planning. *Burns* 1990;16:203-6.

8. Saffle JR. The 1942 fire at Boston's Cocoanut Grove nightclub. *Am J Surg*. 1993;166:581-91.

9. Berman MA, Lazar EJ. Hospital emergency preparedness: lessons learned since Northridge. *N Engl J Med*. 2003;348:1307-8.

10. Shai D, Lupinacci P. Fire fatalities among children: an analysis across Philadelphia's census tracts. *Public Health Reports*. 2003;118:115-26.

11. U.S. Fire Administration. Older Adults in Fire. Topical Fire Research Series, Volume 1. Federal Emergency Management Agency; 2001. Available at: http://www.usfa.fema.gov/inside-usfa/nfdc/pubs/tfrs.shtm.

chapter 157

Wilderness/Forest Fire

John Moloney

DESCRIPTION OF EVENT

Fire is a natural phenomenon that has been a part of our ecosystem for millions of years.[1] Fire in an area not inhabited may have environmental and ecologic consequences, but the fire per se does not have health and medical consequences. These only arise when there is an interaction between the fire and the infrastructure of human civilization.

Prior to the ability of the human race to light fires, most forest fires were due to lightning strikes. Lightning strikes the earth an average of 100 times per second, or over 3 billion times per year.[2] Fires caused by lightning are, on average, less severe than human-caused fires. Lightning tends to strike at the tops or ridges, where there is often higher humidity, lower temperatures, and less fuel.

Naturally occurring fires cannot occur in all environments. Some parts of the globe are too wet or too sparsely vegetated.[4] Due to the importance of fire in agriculture, humans have historically chosen to live in fire-prone areas. Burning kills the local flora and soil microfauna, leaving a cleared space in which to plant crops. Farmers would allow a field to lie fallow for a season, after which they burn it to regenerate the area.[4] A recent study has identified a substance in smoke that stimulates the germination of many plant species.[5]

As greater proportions of the population began to live in towns and cities, fire began to be seen as an enemy. Fire could easily spread from forest to town, and then from house to house. There have been a number of large fires involving the interface between forest and urbanization that have had large costs in terms of lives lost and economic costs. Federal agencies of the U.S. government spent $3 billion suppressing 170,000 fires over the 2-year period from 2002 to 2003.[6]

More and more people are choosing to live in forested areas that are susceptible to fire. The qualities that people value in this environment (e.g., dense forests providing a sense of seclusion and screening from the neighbors) are the same qualities putting them at risk.[7]

Ninety percent of fires in the United States are caused by humans and their activities.[3] Accidental causes include the use of faulty machinery (e.g., chain saws), which release sparks. Other causes include discarded cigarettes, burning of leaves and other garden debris, and children playing with matches. Loss of control of an intentionally lit fire can be another contributor. This may include campfires or fires used for fuel reduction of firebreak formation. A certain percentage of fires are deliberately lit for various reasons. The South Wales Fire and Rescue Service estimated that 98% of the 5239 grass and forest fires it attended in 2001–2002 were deliberately lit.[3] In May 2000, the U.S. Park Service deliberately lit a fire to clear brush at the Bandelier National Monument. After getting out of control, the fire burned for 2 weeks, destroying 200 homes and 47,000 acres of forest.[8]

PREINCIDENT ACTIONS

Management of forest resources can reduce the likelihood and impact of fire. Controlled burning can be used to reduce fuel levels or to create buffer strips or firebreaks. These controlled burns should be carried out in low-hazard periods, such as the cooler months of the year.

Local communities in areas at risk for forest fires need to take preventive action to minimize the risk of fire involving their properties. Long-term issues include setting up firebreaks around housing and other buildings and prohibiting vegetation from growing up to the edge of structures. Potential fuel for fires (e.g., fuel for farm machinery, piles of dry firewood) should not be stored next to housing. Buildings should be kept in a good state of repair, with the guttering clear of leaves and other flammable debris. Local governments can designate areas to be used as fire refuges (e.g., sporting grounds), to which residents can evacuate if needed. In the time prior to the fire season, fuel loads can be assessed and reduced if appropriate.

Visibility on the roads can be impaired by smoke, roads may be blocked by fire or falling trees, and there may be high numbers of emergency vehicles on the road. The lack of effective traffic management during the Berkeley Hills Tunnel Fire in California in 1991 is said to have directly contributed to loss of life.[9] In contrast, 26,000 people were evacuated in 2 hours from the Laguna Beach area in 1993. This evacuation included planning for separate fire service access and civilian egress.

Communities and individuals in areas of high fire risk should develop a personal fire plan. These plans should include a considered opinion about whether, in high-risk conditions, to stay in the area to defend the house or to leave the area early. The decision to evacuate when the fire is very close can be a deadly decision. The plan should include notification of relatives of where you will be and a plan for children and pets. The plan could also include neighbors who, due to age or illness, are less able to care for themselves. At times of high risk, such as hot dry summer days with winds from dangerous areas predicted, fire action plans should be invoked. An example of a fire plan can be accessed at: http://www.cfa. vic.gov.au/residents/living/index.htm.

If fire does invade an area, actions can be taken to further minimize risk to life and property. Appropriate clothing will reduce the risk from radiant heat. As a fire approaches, people should move to the inner parts of the house away from windows and the radiant heat. Garden hoses, which may be used to put out small fires after the main fire front has passed, may be damaged by the main fire front, so these should be protected.

Michael Rhode[9] undertook a review of incident command of fires at the interface between wild land and the urban environment. He noted that command decisions and actions could and should be preplanned, both for firefighter safety and efficiency. He reviewed the response to six fires in California between 1990 and 1996. The initial command post locations were inadequate. Command posts burned in three of the six fires. In all fires, public volunteerism proved unmanageable. Communications centers and fire radio systems were overwhelmed. Before an incident, local emergency managers can develop and communicate strategies and tactics for managing the incident. Planning of evacuation routes and fire refuges should be communicated to the local population as well as emergency managers.

 POSTINCIDENT ACTIONS

In many emergency situations, the postincident actions aim to gain control of the incident, and then to safely and effectively respond to it. With wilderness fires, effective control of the fire may not be possible for days or weeks. During this time, effective and efficient incident management must occur.

As is often seen in emergency situations, maintenance of command can be difficult. This is especially so if the incident is spread geographically and there are impaired communications. In the 1993 fires around Malibu, 20 separate entrapments of firefighters occurred. These resulted from actions independent of command.[9]

Forest fires may cause displacement of people from their homes or even from their areas of residence, often with minimal time to prepare for the evacuation. Other areas may become isolated due to road closures. This may affect the ability to provide routine medical care and pharmaceuticals, regardless of any increase in requirements related to the fire. Local plans should include methods for provision of this routine care to isolated communities or people.

Persons managing healthcare facilities and prehospital medical services may not be able to access extra staff because these staff may either be protecting their homes[10] or unable to safely travel to their place of work. Because most wilderness fires will continue for hours, days, or weeks, provision of adequate staffing levels, with adequate rest breaks, will stretch the personnel resources of many institutions.

Management of the media in the postincident phase is crucial. Media, particularly the radio and television, can provide up-to-date information to communities over a large area. In the case of radio, this can also include members of the community who are not at home, as they are moving, or after they have reached a refuge.

 MEDICAL TREATMENT OF CASUALTIES

Common medical complaints in patients who have been involved in forest fires include smoke inhalation, bronchospasm, heat-related injuries, and burns. After the fires around Canberra, Australia, in 2003, there were 233 presentations to the emergency department of The Canberra Hospital (Table 157-1).

Poor air quality was a major contributing factor for the increase in patients presenting for healthcare after the San Diego fires in 2003.[10]

Important in the initial management of burns is the decision about where patients should be managed. Patients with burns can be managed in an ambulatory setting, a general hospital, or a specialized burns unit. Factors affecting this decision include the size and thickness of the burn, location of burns (e.g., face, perineum), comorbidities, and extremes of age.

TABLE 157-1 PRESENTING COMPLAINTS OF EMERGENCY DEPARTMENT PATIENTS FOLLOWING THE CANBERRA, AUSTRALIA FIRE OF 2003

CONDITION	PRESENTATIONS	ADMISSIONS
Breathing problems/ smoke inhalation	65	10
Eye problems (irritation, ulcer, foreign bodies)	43	0
Trauma (falls and motor vehicle)	45	6
Burns	24	10
Medication issues*	21	0
Accommodation and chronic disease†	5	5
Other	30	5
Total	233	36

Adapted from Richardson DB, Kumar S. Emergency response to the Canberra Bushfires. *Med J Australia*. 2004;181:40-2.
* Supply of usual medications required by people unable to return home. These included insulin, antipsychotics, antihypertensives, and home oxygen.
† Persons with chronic disease requiring emergency accommodation.

It is Christmas Day, 2001, and 5000 firefighters are fighting more than 70 fires in the area around Sydney, Australia. Winds at speeds of 90 kph make control difficult. Major highways are closed, stranding motorists, many of whom are holidaymakers commencing their summer vacation. Three thousand people are evacuated from the Royal National Park. Conditions deteriorate over the next few days, with fierce winds and temperatures of 39°C (102°F).

More than 1.2 million acres of bushland burned over the next week. This is approximately 50% larger than Rhode Island. Half of the fires were suspected to be the result of arson. Many of the arsonists were aged 9 to 16 years.[11,12]

The NSW Health Counter Disaster Unit managed the health response. One thousand five hundred clients were evacuated from 9 aged-care facilities. More than 10,000 persons evacuated from their homes received assistance. Ten disaster medical teams were deployed, and some of these went into communities isolated by road closures. There were two reported deaths.[13]

 ## UNIQUE CONSIDERATIONS

Wilderness fires are unique among disasters. It is possible to predict, in most cases, when the conditions are suitable for a fire to develop. Preventive actions, such as fuel reduction, can reduce the impact of a fire on the population.

Wilderness fires are ongoing events, with the potential to continue to spread to adjacent areas or to commence somewhere else. Most other disasters that cause "trauma," with the exception of war-like activities, have a beginning and an end to "new" injuries. They also have a well-localized geography.

Another unique consideration of wilderness fires is their ability to destroy or threaten healthcare facilities at a time when these facilities are needed to manage casualties.

 ## PITFALLS

Several potential pitfalls in response to a wilderness fire exist. These include the following:

- Failure to prepare adequate systems to respond to large numbers of low-acuity patients (e.g., those with smoke inhalation or ocular foreign bodies)

- Failure to consider unavailability of staff to respond due to personal involvement in an incident or restricted ability to travel
- Failure to prepare adequate systems to deliver commonly used pharmaceuticals to members of the population displaced from their homes or communities
- Failure to consider that health facilities may be directly threatened by the fire or smoke
- Failure to appreciate that wilderness fires are an ongoing incident that may last for days to weeks and that may change rapidly
- Failure to appreciate the extent of a burn injury; this may result in inadequate fluid resuscitation, or triage to an appropriate facility

REFERENCES

1. Wildland Fires: A Historical Perspective. U.S. Fire Administration. Topical Fire Research Series, Volume 1. Issue 3, October 2000. Available at: http://www.usfa.fema.gov/downloads/pdf/tfrs/v1i3-508.pdf
2. Ainsworth J, Doss TA. *Natural History of Fire and Flood Cycles.* Santa Barbara, Calif: University of California; 1955.
3. South Wales Fire Service Available at: http://www.fire-tan.org.uk/Fire_Safety/index.html.
4. Pyne S. The long burn. *Whole Earth Mag.* Winter 1999. Available at http://www.wholeearthmag.com/ArticleBin/292.html.
5. Flematti GR, Ghisalberti EL., Dixon KW, Trengove RD. A compound from smoke that promotes seed germination. *Science* 2004; 305(5686):977.
6. National Interagency Fire Center. Boise, Idaho. Available at http://www.nifc.gov/stats/wildlandfirestats.html.
7. Williams J. Managing fire-dependent ecosystems: we need a public lands policy debate. *Fire Management Today.* 2004;64:6-11.
8. Fairbanks Museum & Planetarium. Available at: http://www.fairbanksmuseum.org/CMS100Sample_CF/uploadedfiles/fire_in_the_forest.pdf.
9. Rhode MS. Fires in the wildland—urban interface: best command practices. *Fire Management Today.* 2004;64:27-31.
10. Hoyt KS, Gerhart AE. The San Diego County wildfires: perspectives of healthcare. *Disaster Management Response.* 2004;2:46-52.
11. Available at: http://www.disasterrelief.org/Disasters/020104 Ausfires4/index.html.
12. Richardson, I. The bushfires around St Albans: the worst bushfires in NSW. Xmas 2001-Jan 2002. Available at: http://www.saintalbans.org.au/xmas_2001_firesummary.html.
13. Cooper D, Flynn M, Hills M, et al. New South Wales bushfires 2001-2002: catastrophe averted [abstract]. Presentation at 13th World Congress for Disaster and Emergency Medicine. *Prehosp Disaster Med.* 2002;17:s29.

chapter 158

Tunnel Fire

Daniel L. Lemkin and Wade Gaasch[*]

 DESCRIPTION OF EVENT

People have been constructing tunnels for thousands of years. Tunnels have been created under rivers, through mountains, and beneath cities. Engineering marvels, they displace huge amounts of earth and still support enormous weight above them.

Society has become dependent on tunnels as a vital component of our transportation system, allowing movement of vehicular traffic, subways, and rail cars. The volume of traffic in major U.S. metropolitan areas is enormous. For example, more than 42 million people traveled through Baltimore's Fort McHenry tunnel in 2003.[1] Subway systems weave a complex network of tunnels beneath most large metropolitan areas. Although less visible to the public, rail systems are still very active and use many tunnels in both urban and rural settings. Freight train tunnels lack hazardous materials restrictions, and in many cases, adequate ventilation or fire-suppression systems.[2] Train fires have much greater destructive potential, which is made worse by absent safety systems.[3] Persistently high levels of traffic combined with flammable and hazardous materials cargo make tunnel fires almost inevitable. The increasing threat of terrorism makes an intentional tunnel fire or explosion even more likely and potentially more disastrous than an accidental event.

One of the greatest challenges in coping with tunnel fires is early recognition that every tunnel's construction and features are substantially different. Technology and materials have changed appreciably over the years, so crews that respond to tunnel emergencies face a wide range of possible scenarios. Most older tunnels were excavated using drills, dynamite, and substantial manual labor. Many were constructed using horseshoe geometry and lined with brick and mortar. Modern tunnels are generally round and lined with steel and concrete. They are carved from the earth using enormous hydraulic tunnel-boring machines, which create clean cylindrical tubes in which reinforced liners have been placed. These variances in construction materials and geometry

call for different types of systems for evacuation, ventilation, and fire suppression.

After ensuring responder safety, the first priority during a tunnel fire is to evacuate all of the people trapped inside. In large roadway tunnels and subway systems, this could mean the evacuation of hundreds or thousands of people.[4] Rail tunnels used for passenger trains may rival or supersede subway passenger levels. If used strictly for freight, trains commonly travel with only a two- or three-person crew. Because construction varies greatly, so do escape routes and protocols.

Many older tunnels consist of single-tube construction, whereas most modern roadway tunnels are built in connected pairs. Lengthy single-tube tunnels constructed for passenger traffic often have escape route stairways that provide access to the surface. Paired tunnels usually contain cross-tunnel adits,[5] that is, air-tight passageways connecting the two tubes. The adits are usually recognized as doorways lining one side of a tunnel spaced at regular intervals. Sometimes labeled, sometimes not, these doorways provide essential refuge to motorists from rapidly expanding smoke and heat. If these doorways are left closed, the paired tunnel serves as a parallel escape route with a separate air supply and shielding from heat. If left open, the adits will permit contamination of the unaffected tunnel.

Subway tunnels may be single or paired and vary with regard to cross-tunnel ventilation. They also contain an additional hazard for escaping passengers—the electrified third rail. These rails generally operate on direct current at around 750 volts. During an emergency, electrified rails should be shut off. There are many separate segments of electrified rail, however, and the possibility of failing to remove power from an occupied portion of track is certainly plausible. This presents a significant danger to both passengers and rescuers. Rescuers should be provided with "hotsticks" (voltage detectors) and trained in their use to ensure track is de-energized before working in close proximity. The track should be rechecked repeatedly and always treated as if energized to minimize the chance of electrocution. If staffing permits, dedicated personnel should be assigned to continuously monitor tracks for electricity. This provides a greater level of safety for crews and evacuating passengers.

*Technical consultants for this chapter were William Shives, Battalion Commander, Baltimore City Fire Department, and Scott C. Gorton, Assistant Director, Field Services, Hazardous Materials Systems, CSX.

803

Once fires ignite, large plumes of smoke and super-heated gas rapidly fill a tunnel's confined spaces.[6] Within minutes, victims could be overcome with smoke at temperatures over 1000°F. To provide a safe environment for escaping motorists and passengers, tunnel engineers have designed and instituted various types of ventilation systems. The most simple is a longitudinal system. Air is injected into a tunnel at one end, where it travels within the same compartment as passenger traffic, exiting the other end. Depending on the system, air flow is driven by supply fans or pulled by exhaust fans. In most systems, a combination of both types operates in a push-pull fashion. When a fire is identified, manual or automated systems activate the fans to direct plumes of smoke and heat away from the majority of people. If these systems can generate adequate air velocities in the tunnel, they provide a temporary safe environment on the supply side of the fire. However, the exhaust side becomes significantly more dangerous because of a "burner effect"[5] generated by winds blowing past fires with superheated exhaust fumes. People trapped on the exhaust side of a fire in a longitudinal ventilated tunnel will succumb rapidly from intense heat and smoke exposure. In systems of this type, the fans can generally be reversed to direct exhaust in either direction.

However, this feature may not be effective. Tunnels have a natural air flow perpetuated by the flow of traffic. As vehicles travel through a tunnel, air is pushed along with them. This creates a "piston-effect" that can take several minutes to diminish, even after traffic stops. Depending on the capacity and location of supply and exhaust fans, the natural air flow may be too strong to overcome. Attempts to do so would result in an increase in turbulent flow within the tunnel and dispersion of superheated gases and smoke. Testing of such systems is imperative to prevent disastrous results during a real fire. Longitudinal ventilation systems are used in many older tunnels, as well as subway, rail, and smaller vehicular tunnels.

Another method, the transverse-ventilation system, is used in many large metropolitan vehicular tunnels. In these systems, the circular tunnel tube is divided into three horizontal sections. The portion used by commuters occupies the center section. Two large semicircular sections remain hidden from sight but serve several important purposes. Contained in these sections are communications antennae, a water-drainage system, and a supply and exhaust ventilation system. Large buildings stationed near both entrances house enormous fans that funnel air through the tunnels via large cement conduits. The Holland tunnel is ventilated with 84 such fans. The Fort McHenry tunnel's 4 tubes are ventilated with 24 much larger fans. The supply of air is generally delivered at curb level through vents placed along either side of the traffic lanes. Exhaust fumes are suctioned through vents in the steel-plate ceiling and blown out of stacks located in the ventilation buildings. These systems generally have much greater air flow capacity and have been shown to function quite effectively in real fire situations. Unlike longitudinal flow systems, transverse-flow ventilation has not been shown to exacerbate fires or create dangerous conditions for escaping motorists. Modern systems are incorporating adjustable dampers that focus exhaust air flow over or surrounding a fire to further speed evacuation of smoke and superheated gases.

Once ventilation is addressed and evacuation is ensured, fire suppression activities take precedence. The decision of whether to enter a tunnel to attack a fire is neither a simple one nor one that should be made hastily. There is no way to know with certainty what hazards exist at the source of a tunnel fire. Hazardous materials restrictions exist for most vehicular tunnels, but the same restrictions do not apply to most rail tunnels. Although laws are in place, it is quite possible that trucks may knowingly or unknowingly transport hazardous materials through restricted tunnels. The threat of terrorism brings with it unpredictability and the potential for intentional secondary explosive devices. While tunnels are designed to withstand fires of great intensity, most are not designed to withstand large explosions. Great care should be exercised when entering a tunnel with the intent of suppression. If available, material safety data sheets carried by all carriers should be inspected. All freight train conductors carry a "consist," which contains a detailed accounting of all rail car locations on the train, their contents, hazard potential, and specific instructions on suppression.

Not all flammable materials respond well to water. Powdered sodium, for example, when exposed to water, will combust spontaneously in a massive exothermic reaction. The rail industry has many hazardous materials specialists on staff. Their expertise and that of local and regional experts should be requested for evaluating hazards before blindly attacking a fire. At a minimum, all responders should have access to and familiarity with the Department of Transportation's *Emergency Response Guidebook,* which lists most industrial hazards, their placard identification numbers, and suppression information.

Although tunnels are confined spaces, they affect a much broader area. As the fire burns, smoke accompanied by possibly toxic gases will be released out of the tunnel ends or ventilation buildings. This should be monitored continuously for possible community hazards. If the potential for toxic releases is recognized, early consideration and planning for resident evacuation should be undertaken. There are many other less emergent but significant consequences of tunnel fires. Closure of major vehicular or subway routes can cause major traffic delays. These delays could be prolonged if significant damage has occurred and requires repair. Prolonged rail disruption could significantly affect a region's industrial and commercial viability. In addition, tunnels are often lined with communications and Internet data cables. Fires often destroy these lines and can cause significant disruption of telecommunications traffic on a regional or national scale.[7]

 ## PREINCIDENT ACTIONS

Prior to an incident, all emergency operations plans should be amended to address specific hazards associated with fires and explosions. They should specifically address evacuation, ventilation, and fire suppression for all tunnels located in a given jurisdiction. Because each tunnel's construction is different, it is imperative that emergency operations personnel become familiar with each tunnel's infrastructure. Site visits and training operations should be coordinated with tunnel officials. These training sessions serve many purposes, including hazard analysis, validating operating procedures, identifying and correcting flaws, testing communications equipment, and improving relationships between agencies. Ventilation systems and water-delivery systems should be tested on a regular basis. Because of the hazardous materials potential, a network of specialists who can respond to any significant event should be formed. Personnel and agencies that should be included are the Department of the Environment, the Environmental Protection Agency, railroads, industrial hygienists, toxicologists, structural tunnel engineers, and the Department of Public Works. This list is not all inclusive and will likely vary by jurisdiction and local risk potential.

 ## POSTINCIDENT ACTIONS

The primary goal after recognition of a tunnel fire is evacuation of trapped passengers or motorists. Rapid coordination with tunnel control center officials can help locate the fire and direct appropriate application of ventilation to provide a safe environment for evacuating people. Rapid identification of possible hazardous materials should be sought before the initiation of conventional fire-suppression activities. Most tunnel fires involve single vehicles and do not represent a significant threat to other motorists or the tunnel; larger trucks and fires involving flammable liquids can present a much greater hazard. A rapid but informed and methodical approach is warranted when dealing with unknown hazards in a confined space such as a tunnel. If the fire represents anything other than a simple event, the prearranged emergency hazardous materials network should be activated and involved in decision-making.

 ## MEDICAL TREATMENT OF CASUALTIES

Most injuries occurring as a result of a tunnel fire will be related to smoke inhalation. If people are able to escape the fire by crossing over to an adjacent tube, they may avoid potentially fatal exposure to smoke and superheated gases. Any people trapped on the exhaust side of a substantial fire once longitudinal ventilation has been initiated will likely not survive. Rescuers should concentrate on rapid evacuation of motorists and passengers to a safe location outside the tunnel. Rescue operations should focus on checking abandoned vehicles and subway cars for people unable to ambulate to safety. Depending on the size of the tunnel and the number of casualties, a mass-casualty incident may be declared. Emergency medical services personnel should follow standard Incident Command System protocols for triage and transportation of the injured. Burn centers and centers with hyperbaric capabilities may be warranted in some circumstances.

 ### CASE PRESENTATION

A call comes over the radio that smoke is coming from the mouth of a local railroad tunnel[8]. On arrival, the firefighters see copious amounts of black smoke rising from the tunnel. They don self-contained breathing apparatus and walk into the tunnel carrying 2 1/2-inch dry lines. The railroad engineer and conductor run up to the fire officer and recommend they not enter until reviewing the consist. Several hazardous rail cars are identified, including sulfuric acid, ethylene oxide, tripropylene, and anhydrous ammonia. All suppression activities are halted and personnel removed from the tunnel. The hazardous materials team is notified and arrives with gas-sampling devices. The railroad dispatches its hazardous material experts, and a team of industrial hygienists, toxicologists, and engineers is consulted.

Smoke is seen emanating from the other end of the tunnel, which is located in a heavily populated area. A major highway bridge is located within 1/8 mile from the tunnel entrance. Rush hour traffic is starting to build. Initial sampling notes no toxic gas release. The mayor shows up and asks, "What is going on?" What are you going to tell him?

UNIQUE CONSIDERATIONS

Tunnel fires present numerous unique challenges that make emergency response dangerous and, at times, frustrating. Access to the fire is often hampered by several factors. Because of the confined space and dense smoke, visibility will likely be nonexistent. Many tunnels are quite long, and depending on the tunnel, a reliable water supply may not be available close to the fire. Once a fire breaks out, people will abandon their vehicles, obstructing the tunnel and making access by any means other than walking impossible. Firefighters will have great distances to cover by foot, reducing their available air from self-contained breathing apparatuses once they reach the fire.

Other conditions make suppression activities very dangerous. The confined space makes rapid evacuation impossible, and usually there are no areas of refuge should the fire flash over or explode. If flammable liquids are extinguished, their vapors remain volatile and could saturate the tunnel, creating a dangerous explosive condition. In Swiss tunnel fire simulations using an abandoned rail tunnel, a gasoline fire spontaneously exploded 19 minutes after it was initially extinguished by sprinklers.[2] Another factor complicating suppression activities is the development of dangerous steam clouds within the tunnel. Without effective means of escape, application of water to intensely burning fires can create a hazard to firefighters and evacuating people far greater than the fire itself.

 ## PITFALLS

Several potential pitfalls in response to a tunnel fire exist. These include the following:

- Failure to familiarize operations personnel with specific tunnel features, systems, and hazards
- Inappropriate application of the ventilation system, which can endanger evacuating people and complicate suppression activities
- Failure to test the capacity of ventilation and standpipe systems prior to a fire
- Failure to coordinate a network of hazardous materials specialists who can respond and aid in hazard analysis, mitigation, and clean-up
- Premature suppression activities before potential hazards are identified
- Delay in the application of appropriate ventilation and fire suppression
- Delay in the recognition of hazardous condition and public notification or evacuation
- Failure to verify that abandoned vehicles are empty and do not contain viable nonambulatory patients.

REFERENCES

1. "The Fort McHenry Tunnel, A Toll Facility of The Maryland Transportation Authority" (*Informational Flyer*) The Maryland Transportation Authority, Office of Media and Customer Relations. Baltimore, Maryland. 2004.

2. Bajwa C. *An Analysis of a Spent Fuel Transportation Cask Under Severe Fire Accident Conditions*. ML022340066. Washington, DC: Spent Fuel Project Office, U.S. Nuclear Regulatory Commission; 2002.
3. Styron HC. *CSX Tunnel Fire, Baltimore, MD*. USFA-TR-140. Technical Report Series, U.S. Fire Administration, Federal Emergency Management Agency. July 2001.
4. Facts at a glance. Chicago: Chicago Transit Authority; 2004. Available at: http://www.transitchicago.com/welcome/overview.html#a.
5. Hay RE. *Prevention and Control of Highway Tunnel Fires*. Publication no. FHWA-RD-83-032 U.S. Department of Transportation, Federal Highway Administration – Office of Bridge Technology. May 2000. National Technical Information Service, Springfield, VA 22161.
6. CFD (Computational Fluid Dynamics) analysis of fire growth and smoke spread in tunnels. ARUP Fire Safety Engineering for Tunnels. Website: http://www.arup.com/fire/skill.cfm?pageid=4383
7. *Media Advisory—Keynote: The Internet Performance Authority*. San Mateo, Calif: Keynote Systems, Inc; 2001.
8. National Transportation Safety Board Advisory. *Investigation into the Derailment of CSX Train L41216 in Howard Street Tunnel, Baltimore, Maryland, August 7, 2001*. Washington, DC. Website: http://www.ntsb.gov/pressrel/2001/010807.htm. Media Contact: Keith Holloway, (202) 314-6100.

chapter 159

Gunshot Attack: Mass Casualties

Leon D. Sanchez and Jason Imperato

 DESCRIPTION OF EVENT

In 2001 there were 20,308 homicides in the United States, 11,348 of which involved firearms.[1] Gunshot injuries include violence-related, accidental, and self-inflicted injuries.[2] The majority of these injuries are caused by handguns. Although most gunshot attacks involve only one victim, there have been several well-publicized cases in which multiple persons were killed and injured in a single event.

Firearms include two basic types: rifled firearms and shotguns. A rifled firearm (i.e., pistol or rifle) has spiral grooves in its barrel. When the cartridge is fired, the burning of the powder generates gas in a contained space, and the pressure generated by the gas propels the bullet forward. The bullet accelerates while inside the barrel, reaches its maximum speed upon exit (muzzle velocity), and heads toward its target. As the bullet enters tissue, it will begin to tumble and deform. Depending on the makeup of the bullet and the properties of the tissue through which it travels, it may expand, fragment, or remain in one piece.[3-6]

Shotguns differ from rifles and pistols in that they have a smooth barrel that discharges hot gases, wad, and either multiple projectiles or a single projectile (rifled slug). Shot charges containing multiple projectiles spread out from the muzzle in a conelike pattern. The distance from the muzzle of the shotgun to the point of impact of the projectiles is a key determinant of the magnitude of injury. At short range (less than 6 m), the shot charge containing multiple projectiles results predominantly in a single-hole wound (diameter of less than or equal to 6 cm) that communicates with a deep underlying wound with massive tissue destruction. At this short range, soft tissue impact deforms the individual pellets, increasing their original cross section with a concomitant increase in tissue crush or hole size. The multiple pellets result in severe disruption between the multiple wound channels. A gradual decrease in the amount of pellet deformation and tissue destruction occurs as the distance of the impact range increases. When the impact range exceeds 7 m, the multiple projectiles result in numerous discrete wounds that are not associated with underlying massive tissue destruction.[3]

Shotguns also can discharge rifled slugs that are designed for killing larger animals. The muzzle velocity of rifled slugs (487 m/sec) is approximately half that of nonexpanding, fully jacketed rifle projectiles. The rifled slug does not hold the point orientation that it has as it is propelled from the muzzle of the gun, but drifts toward a sideways orientation as it moves toward the target. The rifled slugs experience a 25% decrease in velocity as the impact range increases from 5 to 45 m. At short range (less than or equal to 45 m), the slug deforms on striking the tissue, thereby enhancing the size of the permanent and temporary cavities.

 PREINCIDENT ACTIONS

Hospital, emergency department, and outpatient facilities should all have general disaster plans in place in the event of an attack. Mass-casualty events require coordination of local, state, and federal public safety resources. Both emergency medical service (EMS)- and hospital-based triage systems may need to be altered in the event of a large number of patients seeking medical care within a brief period of time. Healthcare providers should practice universal precautions. In the event of multiple casualties, triaging of the victims at the scene and on arrival to the hospital will be necessary. Protocols for the triaging of the victims are part of a properly prepared disaster plan. Disaster plans should be in place and personnel should be familiar with the plans so that when an event does occur, a minimum of confusion will ensue.

 POSTINCIDENT ACTIONS

First responders and EMS personnel should confirm the scene is safe before evaluating casualties at the site of the event. If a large number of casualties are identified and a disaster needs to be declared, the proper channels must be notified and triage protocols instituted. Receiving hospitals should be given as much advance notice as possible to ensure that hospital personnel will be ready to handle the influx of patients. The need for psychological help for victims, bystanders, and personnel responding to the scene should not be forgotten.

CLINICAL PRESENTATION

Tissue is injured by a bullet via two mechanisms: tissue crush and tissue stretch. These two mechanisms correspond to the permanent and temporary cavities created by passage of the projectile.[4,7] As the bullet travels through tissue, it will crush tissue that is directly in its path. This is the primary method of injury from gunshot wounds. The most important determinant of injury is the tissue the bullet crushes. The tissue that is crushed corresponds to the permanent cavity formed by the bullet. Injury created by the temporary cavity becomes more important with higher-energy bullets (see Chapter 160).

 ## MEDICAL TREATMENT OF CASUALTIES

Initial evaluation of persons with gunshot wounds is similar to that of any multiple-trauma victim, with initial evaluation of the ABCs (i.e., airway, breathing, circulation), followed by the secondary survey and ongoing monitoring, including vital signs, electrocardiographic monitoring, and pulse oximetry. The focus of the examination is the detection of penetrating or perforating injuries. A careful examination of the patient including the back, under the hair, the axillae, and the gluteal fold will help identify injuries. Radiographs of the areas the bullet is thought to have traversed are indicated to identify the position of the projectiles. Laboratory studies should be ordered as clinically indicated.

Evaluation, resuscitation, and ongoing management should proceed as for any other multitrauma victim in both the prehospital setting and the emergency department. The management of gunshot wounds is best conducted in consultation with a trauma surgeon. If adequate resources are unavailable, the decision to transfer the patient should be made early in the course of treatment.

Wounds that may have crossed the mediastinum require a thorough evaluation, even in the stable patient. In this setting, injury to the aorta, heart, pericardium, and esophagus must be ruled out. Patients who present with unstable vital signs or become unstable during evaluation should receive bilateral chest tubes. The presence of pericardial tamponade should also be considered; using bedside ultrasound is a fast way to identify cardiac tamponade. Surgical exploration is often indicated in these patients.[5]

Patients with penetrating gunshot wounds to the abdomen require exploratory laparotomy, even in the presence of stable vital signs. Stable patients with back or flank wounds can be evaluated by computed tomography and observation, but these patients may also benefit from surgical exploration. This decision must be made in conjunction with the trauma surgeon.

Injuries to the extremities require evaluation of the distal neurovascular status. A bullet does not need to transect a vessel to cause injury. The development of compartment syndrome resulting from swelling of the injured area should be considered. Angiography is indicated if arterial injury is suspected. Fractures from a gunshot wound should be treated as open fractures with early administration of antibiotics. Debridement of devitalized soft tissue is often necessary.[5]

Penetrating gunshot wounds to the head are often not survivable. For patients with this type of injury who arrive at the hospital alive, consultation with a neurosurgeon is indicated. Injuries to the spine can occur even when the bullet does not actually pass through the vertebral canal. Use of steroids is not indicated for penetrating cord injuries. Additionally, the presence of a central nervous system injury should not delay assessment for the presence of thoracoabdominal injuries that can be rapidly fatal.

CASE PRESENTATION

On a sunny afternoon at 11:10 AM on Tuesday, April 20, 1999, Dylan Klebold and Eric Harris arrived in separate vehicles at Columbine High School in Littleton, Colorado. Although the arrival of these students may not have been unusual, the events that followed would shock the nation.

Around 11:14 AM, the boys carried two 20-lb propane bombs in duffel bags and placed them near tables in the school cafeteria, then returned to their cars. When the bombs failed to ignite, the pair began to prepare for the next stage of their attack.

Klebold, wearing cargo pants and a black T-shirt with the word "wrath" written on the front, was armed with a 9-mm semiautomatic handgun and a 12-gauge double-barrel sawed-off shotgun. Harris, wearing dark pants and a white T-shirt that read "natural selection" was armed with a 9-mm carbine rifle and a 12-gauge pump sawed-off shotgun. Both wore black trench coats to conceal their weapons and their utility belts filled with ammunition. They also carried a backpack and duffle bag full of homemade bombs.

At 11:19 AM, Klebold and Harris entered the school and started firing at students outside the school cafeteria. The students continued to fire at their peers in the cafeteria, the hallways, and later in the school library. Local, state, and federal authorities including police, healthcare workers, and SWAT teams were dispatched to the scene. From 12:02 to 12:05 PM, the two students fired toward the police and paramedics who had arrived at the scene and waited outside the school as students frantically fled the dangers from inside the school. Finally, the Columbine massacre ended at 12:08 PM when Klebold and Harris pointed their guns to their heads and shot themselves.

In the most devastating school shooting in U.S. history, a total of 12 students, 1 teacher, and the 2 killers were dead, and 21 others were injured.

 ## UNIQUE CONSIDERATIONS

Gunshot wounds must be reported to the appropriate authorities. In most cases, shootings become the subject of a criminal investigation by law enforcement authorities. Therefore, the medical record and patient property should be preserved as evidence. If patient clothing is cut, care should be used to avoid cutting through portions a bullet might have gone through. Any material that needs to be saved for law enforcement authorities should be placed in paper bags because plastic bags will trap moisture, and this can degrade evidence. The location of all wounds identified should be recorded in the medical record, including comments on the presence of any powder residue observed surrounding the wound. It is often difficult to differentiate entrance from exit wounds. Although it is often thought that the smaller wound must be the entrance wound, this is not always true. If a bullet is recovered, avoid making any markings on the sides of the bullet because this will interfere with forensic evaluation of rifling patterns.[3] Any marking of recovered bullets that may be necessary for the preservation of chain of custody should be at the nose or base.

 PITFALLS

Several potential pitfalls in response to a gunshot attack exist. These include the following:

- Allowing EMS personnel to enter the scene before it is secured
- Failure to have a disaster plan in place prior to the event
- Failure to involve a trauma surgeon early in the management of the patient
- Failure to consider transfer of the patient to another facility
- Delays in the evaluation of stable patients with thoracoabdominal injuries

REFERENCES

1. National Center for Health Statistics. *Vital Statistics Mortality Data, Underlying Cause of Death Detail, 2001.* U.S. Department of Health and Human Services, Public Health Service, Centers for Disease Control and Prevention; Atlanta; 2001.
2. Weapon Related Injury Surveillance System. *Weapon Related Injury Update Oct 1999.* Massachusetts Department of Public Health, Bureau of Health Statistics, Research and Evaluation; Boston; 1999.
3. Di Maio V. *Gunshot Wounds.* CRC Press LLC; Boca Raton, Fla; 1999.
4. Fackler ML. Ballistic injury. *Ann Emerg Med.* 1986;15:1451-5.
5. Swan KG. Missile injuries: wound ballistics and principles of management. *Milit Med.* 1987;152:29-34.
6. Zajychuck R, ed. *Textbook of Military Medicine.* Part I, Volume 5. Conventional warfare: ballistics, blast and burn injuries. TMM Publications, Washington, D.C.; 1989.
7. Fackler ML. Wound ballistics: a review of common misconceptions. *JAMA* 1980;259:2730.

chapter 160

Sniper Attack

Jennifer E. DeLaPena and Leon D. Sanchez

 ## DESCRIPTION OF EVENT

A sniper is a concealed, usually skilled shooter who fires at exposed persons. These attacks typically occur using powerful high-energy, military-style assault rifles. These rifles have the capability of being fired semiautomatically or automatically. Semiautomatic weapons fire as quickly as one can pull the trigger, whereas automatic weapons continue to fire until the trigger is released. Assault rifles are becoming more available to the public.[1]

Rifles are the most powerful of the three main types of firearms: rifles, shotguns, and handguns.[1] When a cartridge is fired, the burning of the powder generates gas in a contained space, which generates the pressure that propels the bullet forward. The bullet accelerates while inside the barrel and reaches its maximum speed upon exit (known as *muzzle velocity*). Military-style rifles have long barrels and are therefore able to accelerate to higher muzzle velocities.[1-5]

The majority of bullets in use today are at least partially jacketed. The jacket is a layer of harder metal that surrounds what is typically a lead core. This allows bullets to reach greater muzzle velocities; without the jacket the lead bullet would be stripped at higher velocities, quickly fouling up the firearm's barrel.[5] Military-style bullets are fully jacketed, whereas bullets for sale to civilians usually have the lead core exposed at the tip (soft point), which can be modified into different varieties of hollow-point bullets. The exposure of lead at the tip will cause the softer lead to deform much more than a fully jacketed bullet on entry into tissue. Hollow-point bullets are designed so as to expand as they penetrate tissue. The injury patterns of fully jacketed and hollow-point bullets will be different, although the claims that soft or hollow-point bullets cause more tissue destruction are not consistently borne out.

 ## PREINCIDENT ACTIONS

In light of the recent sniper attacks in the Washington, D.C. area, confusion and panic may ensue if a sniper attack were to occur. Emergency departments should have disaster plans and protocols in place to handle such events. Personnel should be familiar with the plans in order to minimize confusion. This may require coordination of local, state, and federal public safety resources.

Healthcare providers should always practice universal precautions. In the event of multiple victims and casualties, protocols for triaging victims must be used. These protocols are an important part of the disaster plan, and hospital personnel should be familiar with them.

 ## POSTINCIDENT ACTIONS

For prehospital personnel and first responders, it is important that the scene be secured and declared safe before the victims are approached and the casualties evaluated. If patients are awake, they should be asked how many shots they heard and any other information they have relating to the event, such as their position and that of the assailant and the weapon or weapons used. Gunshot wounds must be reported to the appropriate authorities.

There should be close communication with emergency medical services personnel and the receiving hospitals to give as much lead time as possible for healthcare facilities to prepare for casualties. It is also important to be prepared to offer psychological help for victims and their families.

CLINICAL PRESENTATION

Injuries from a gunshot are the product of two mechanisms: tissue crush and tissue stretch. As the bullet travels through tissue, it will crush tissue that is directly in its path, and this results in a permanent cavity. This is the primary method of injury from most gunshot wounds. Passage of the projectile at a high rate of speed also displaces tissue surrounding the direct path away from the path of the projectile. As this tissue stretches away from the path, a temporary tissue cavity is formed. This is a more significant mechanism of injury with higher-velocity bullets, such as those encountered in a sniper attack.[3,6]

The degree of tissue stretch and the size of the temporary cavity that is formed vary depending on the elastic properties of the injured tissue. Elastic tissues such as muscle, skin, and lung are good energy absorbers. Their elastic properties allow them to maintain a lot of their structure and function, even after temporary cavitation. Inelastic tissue, including liver, heart, and brain, will be fractured and rendered nonviable to a much greater degree by a temporary cavity.[5]

Since the brain is encased in a solid container (the skull), brain tissue is even more susceptible to injury from temporary cavitation than other inelastic tissue. The solid container prevents tissue displacement during tissue cavitation, resulting in increased pressure inside the skull as a bullet penetrates. This pressure can only be relieved either through the entrance or exit wounds. The brain is also very sensitive to structural disruption. This combination makes high-velocity gunshots to the head very destructive.

 ## MEDICAL TREATMENT OF CASUALTIES

Initial evaluation of persons with gunshot wounds in the prehospital setting and the emergency department is similar to that of any trauma victim. Initial assessment of the ABCs (i.e., airway, breathing, circulation) should be followed by the secondary survey and ongoing monitoring of vital signs. The focus of the examination is the detection of penetrating or perforating injuries. All clothing should be removed, and careful examination for entrance and exit wounds must include the back, under the hair, the axillae, the perineum, and the gluteal fold. Radiographs can be useful to identify the position of bullets. Radiographs and laboratory studies should be ordered when clinically indicated. Evaluation and treatment of gunshot wounds are best conducted in consultation with a trauma surgeon. Patients should be stabilized and transferred as quickly as possible if appropriate resources are unavailable where they are being treated.

Injury to the aorta, heart, pericardium, and esophagus must be suspected when wounds cross the mediastinum. These wounds require a thorough evaluation, even in stable patients. Surgical exploration is often indicated in these patients. Those who present with unstable vital signs or who become unstable during evaluation should receive bilateral chest tubes, and the presence of pericardial tamponade should be considered. Ultrasound is a fast way of identifying cardiac tamponade.[4]

Patients with gunshot wounds to the flank or back can be evaluated by computed tomography and observed if their conditions are stable. The decision to observe a patient must be made in conjunction with a trauma surgeon because these patients may benefit from surgical exploration. Patients with gunshot wounds to the abdomen require exploratory laparotomy.

Gunshot wounds to the extremities may cause neurovascular damage and fractures. Neurovascular function should be assessed carefully. There should be close monitoring for the development of compartment syndrome from swelling of the injured area. Angiography is indicated whenever arterial damage is suspected. High-velocity wounds should be debrided and closed secondarily. Fractures from a gunshot wound are considered open fractures, and early antibiotics should be instituted.[4]

Evaluation of gunshot wounds to the head should be done in consultation with a neurosurgeon. These injuries are often not survivable. Spinal cord injuries can result from direct penetrating injuries, but the spine can be injured by temporary cavitation even in the absence of direct passage of the bullet through the vertebral canal. Steroids are not indicated in direct penetrating injury to the spinal cord. Although injuries to the central nervous system can be distracting to the physician, it is important not to delay the assessment and treatment of thoracoabdominal injuries.

 ## CASE PRESENTATION

The Beltway Sniper attacks took place during 3 weeks of October 2002 in the eastern United States. Ten persons were killed and three others critically injured in and around the Baltimore-Washington, D.C. metropolitan area. The attacks were carried out with a Bushmaster XM-15 semiautomatic .223 caliber rifle, the civilian equivalent of the U.S. military's M-16 assault rifle, at a range of 50 to over 100 yards.

The sniper attacks began October 2, 2002, with a series of five fatal shootings in 15 hours in Montgomery County, Maryland, a suburban county north of Washington. The attacks continued for the next 3 weeks in the Washington, D.C., metropolitan area, filling residents of the region with fear. The shootings occurred at gas stations, supermarkets, restaurants, and schools in a rough circular pattern around Washington. The victims were apparently selected at random, crossing racial, gender, and socioeconomic categories.

During the period of the attacks, the North American media devoted enormous amounts of airtime and newspaper space to news of each new attack. By the middle of October 2002, all-news television networks were providing live, ongoing coverage of each new attack.

On October 24, 2002, John Allen Muhammad and Lee Boyd Malvo were found sleeping in their car, a blue 1990 Chevrolet Caprice, at a Maryland rest stop, and were arrested on federal weapons charges. A 223-caliber weapon and tripod were found in a bag in Mr. Muhammad's car. Ballistics tests later conclusively linked the seized rifle to 11 of the 14 bullets recovered from earlier attacks. In March 2004, Muhammad was sentenced to death and Malvo to life imprisonment for the attacks.

 ## UNIQUE CONSIDERATIONS

Gunshot wounds must be reported to the appropriate authorities. Special care must be taken because the medical record and patient property often become evidence. Paper bags should be used to collect material to be saved for law enforcement because plastic bags can trap moisture, resulting in damage to the evidence. If a bullet is recovered and it must be marked, this should be done at the nose or base rather than the side. Marking the side will interfere with the evaluation of rifling patterns. Care should be taken during clothing removal to avoid cutting through portions of clothing that a bullet might have gone through. The location of all wounds identified should be recorded in the medical record, with comment on the presence of any powder residue observed surrounding the wound. Attempts to differentiate between entrance and exit wounds are often an educated guess. The smaller wound is often thought to be the entrance wound, but this is not always the case.[2]

 PITFALLS

Several potential pitfalls in response to a sniper attack exist. These include the following:

- Failure to ensure that a scene is secure prior to approaching victims
- Failure to fully examine the patient and identify multiple injuries
- Failure to consult a surgeon early in the management of the patient
- Failure to consider transfer to another facility
- Failure to fully evaluate stable patients with thoracoabdominal injuries

REFERENCES

1. Barach E, Tomlanovich M, Nowack R. Ballistics: a pathophysiologic examination of the wounding mechanisms of firearms, Part I. *J Trauma*. 1986;26:225-35; Part II. *J Trauma*. 1986;26:374-83.
2. Di Maio V. *Gunshot Wounds*: Practical Aspects of Firearms, Ballistics, and Forensic Techniques. Boca Raton, Fla: CRC Press LLC; 1999.
3. Fackler ML. Ballistic injury. *Ann Emerg Med*. 1986;15:1451-5.
4. Swan KG. Missile injuries: wound ballistics and principles of management. *Milit Med*. 1987;152:29-34.
5. Zajychuck R, ed. *Textbook of Military Medicine*. Part I, Volume 5. Conventional warfare: ballistics, blast and burn injuries. Falls Church, VA: TMM Publications; 1989.
6. Fackler ML. Wound ballistics: a review of common misconceptions. *JAMA* 1980;259:2730.

chapter 161

Grenade and Pipe Bomb Injuries

Charles Stewart

 ## DESCRIPTION OF EVENT

Recent terrorist events have featured an increasing use of explosives. The weapon of choice of these terrorists is often the grenade, pipe bomb, or explosive-containing vest. Other terrorists will use a rocket-propelled grenade that was originally designed to cheaply defeat armor.

Pipe Bombs

The design of a pipe bomb is quite simple: it consists of a piece of pipe that is filled with explosives. The end caps for the pipe are used to contain the explosives and the force of the explosion. The fragments of the exploding pipe are propelled by the explosion and can cause lethal injury at a considerable distance. Since pipe comes in many sizes and materials, the shape and size of the pipe bomb is quite variable. These devices often either contain scrap metal or may be wrapped in scrap metal to increase the number of fragments and consequent injuries.

Pipe bombs can be carried in a satchel, briefcase, or backpack. The Centennial Park terrorist explosive device activated during the 1996 Olympics in Atlanta was a backpack containing pipe bombs.

Grenades

In World War II, the grenade was a cast-iron segmented oval shape designed to fit the thrower's hand. This is often called the "pineapple" grenade because of its shape. After the Vietnam War, the U.S. army deployed an egg-shaped grenade that was created by wrapping scored steel wire around a high-explosive core. This wire would fragment much more reliably and in smaller pieces than the older cast-iron bodies. This design has been copied and improved and is widely available throughout the world. The U.S. M26 grenade weighs 425 g and has a fuse delay of 5 seconds. The average throwing distance is about 40 m. Its blast radius is 10 m, with a killing distance of 5 m and a wounding distance of up to 25 m. Other countries have developed a cylinder-shaped grenade with attached handle, "the potato masher"

design. These are similar in performance and specifications to the US grenade.

Two special forms of grenade have evolved that are now widely dispersed, and an emergency physician may encounter casualties produced by their effects. These are the rifle grenades designed to project the grenade beyond the soldier's ability to throw and the antitank grenade, which has evolved into the rocket-propelled grenade discussed below.

Other types of grenades are also produced, but most of these have lesser wounding potential. These include concussion grenades (i.e., flash-bang grenades), illuminating grenades, smoke grenades, incendiary grenades, and chemical or gas grenades. These are often cylinder-shaped containers.

Rifle Grenades

The grenade launcher has evolved into a weapon that projects a grenade with good accuracy for about 200 m. First used during the Vietnam War, the M79 grenade launcher resembles a short, fat (40 mm), breech-loading, break-open, single-shot shotgun. The military also designed a grenade launcher that clamps onto the infantryman's M16 rifle that uses exactly the same ammunition as the M79 weapon. Numerous similar designs for these weapons are used by military forces of both North Atlantic Treaty Organisation and former Warsaw Pact nations. Comparable devices are often used by police forces to project riot-control agents, "nonlethal" beanbag rounds, and smoke. Multiple different rounds exist for both military and civilian grenade-launching weapons, and an emergency physician may well encounter patients injured by these devices. The grenade rounds contain about as much explosive and cause as much damage as the more common baseball grenade.

Rocket-Propelled Grenades

The need for an antitank weapon that could reliably penetrate enemy armor has been present since the tank was first used in World War I. One solution to this problem was to upsize the grenade and to mount it atop a rocket, creating the rocket-propelled grenade (RPG). Many countries manufactured these devices by the millions and sold the inexpensive RPG to hundreds of rebel and terrorist groups. The former Soviet RPG launcher is reloadable. The United States distributes a similar light antitank weapon (the M72 LAW or the M136 AT4) that is not reloadable. The RPG is designed to defeat the armor on a tank and carries substantially more explosive material than any other device discussed in this chapter. See Chapter 146 for a more detailed discussion of RPGs.

Clinical Presentation

Trauma caused by explosions traditionally has been divided into the injury caused by the direct effect of the blast wave (primary injuries), the effects caused by other objects that are accelerated by the explosive wave (secondary injuries), the effects caused by movement of the victim (tertiary injuries), and miscellaneous effects caused by the explosion or explosives.

The victims of primary blast injury almost always have other types of injury, such as penetrating wounds from flying debris or blunt trauma from impact on immovable objects.[1] The number of victims of primary blast injury due to a grenade, pipe bomb, or suicide vest will likely not be large since the quantities of explosives contained are small. (A suicide vest is an improvised explosive device to be worn as a vest, a waist belt, or a backpack. Suicide bombs are covered in detail in Chapter 144.) The topic of primary blast injury is covered in Chapters 141 and 142.

With both grenades and pipe bombs, secondary blast injuries are both the most common and the intended injury mechanism. Terrorist devices often have additional objects such as nails, nuts, and bolts added to the explosive mixture to increase the effects of secondary blast injury. Military devices such as grenades are designed in such a way as to increase the number of fragments flung by the explosion. The penetrating injuries occur most often in the exposed areas such as the head, neck, and extremities.

Tertiary blast injuries are caused when the victim's body is propelled into another object by blast winds.[2,3] This is unlikely to occur from the relatively small amounts of explosives found in a grenade. It may be possible to note these effects with the larger amount of explosive in an RPG, pipe bomb, or suicide vest.

 PREINCIDENT ACTIONS

It is difficult, indeed, to plan for the consequences of an explosive device that can be carried in a backpack, briefcase, or even in a pocket. The use of these devices in the United States has not been common, but given the evolving worldwide political climate, such events could occur. Emergency physicians are increasingly likely to see the effects of these devices and must be prepared to treat the victims of these explosive hazards.

 POSTINCIDENT ACTIONS

The predominant injury found after an explosion of a grenade or pipe bomb will be penetrating trauma from fragment wounds. Those who are quite close to the blast may sustain either primary blast injury or traumatic amputations. An explosion that occurs in a confined space (e.g., vehicles, mines, buildings, subways) is associated with greater morbidity and mortality.

Field Medical Care

The following are important points regarding appropriate field medical care of patients sustaining injuries from a grenade or pipe bomb explosion.

- Appropriate initial care is similar to regular trauma care.
- Rapid evacuation increases the chance of survival.
- Do not attempt definitive care in triage.
- Arterial bleeding from traumatic amputations should be controlled with tourniquets until the area is entirely safe and the patient can have definitive care.
- Do not attempt extensive resuscitation in the field.
- Cardiopulmonary resuscitation at the scene of a mass-casualty event is not indicated.

 MEDICAL TREATMENT OF CASUALTIES

Most of the injuries seen after the explosive in a grenade or pipe bomb detonates are blunt, penetrating, and thermal trauma that is well known to prehospital providers, emergency physicians, and trauma surgeons.[4] Much of this trauma involves soft tissue, orthopedic, or head injuries.[5-7] The appropriate approach to the patient with blast-related injury from grenades or pipe bombs is therefore the same as any other trauma victim.

The first and most important step of management is to assess life support needs and ensure that the patient has an adequate airway, appropriate ventilation, and adequate circulation. As noted above, use of tourniquets can buy time to evacuate the victim to a safe area where appropriate care can be rendered.

A thorough physical examination should be then performed. Most of the wounds will have been caused by fragments from the device or metal surrounding the device.

There are few screening studies that are of any benefit in the casualty with primary blast injury. Indeed, for these smaller devices, studies should be directed toward the effects of multiple penetrating fragments. A seemingly small abrasion or wound may mask the entrance wound for a substantial fragment. The physician should also remember that blast fragments may be traveling up to five times as fast as a military bullet.

A chest radiograph should be obtained in all patients who have been near a significant explosion. If the patient is not wearing body armor, presume there are fragments in the chest until a chest radiograph proves to be negative for both pneumothorax and intrathoracic fragments. A chest radiograph may also show fragments or free air under the diaphragm, signifying hollow viscus rupture in the abdomen. Long-bone films are indicated in traumatic amputation or if wounds are found in a patient's extremities.

A computed tomography (CT) scan of the head, chest, or abdomen should be obtained if the history or physical examination suggests pathology in these areas. If the patient is unconscious, these CT studies are not optional. There is about an 80% rate of infection when fragment wounds are sutured. All debris that is flung by the explosion is not radiopaque, and the wise provider should carefully explore injuries and consider CT, ultrasound, or magnetic resonance imaging of wounds to evaluate for radiolucent foreign bodies.

The only laboratory study that is useful is serial hemoglobin determinations. These appear to be of use in evaluating patients who have severe bleeding. The data can be used as a guide for blood transfusion requirements.

Hypotension in blast injury victims can be due to several mechanisms:

- blood loss due to wounds (otherwise not related to the cardiovascular system); this is particularly common with traumatic amputations and the multiple fragments sustained at close range from a modern fragmentation grenade
- blood loss due to gastrointestinal hemorrhage
- blood loss due to intraabdominal solid organ rupture
- hypotension from compression of vessels and heart by pneumothorax
- hypotension due to the cardiovascular effects of an air embolism
- hypotension due to vagal reflexes

The disposition of these patients depends on the injury sustained by each victim. Those who were close to the center of the explosion should be considered for observation for at least 24 hours, even if they have no obvious injuries.

CASE PRESENTATION

You are listening to a professional football game in your emergency department. A newscaster reports a loud explosion at about the 50-yard line. Cameras show an RPG that streaked over them and impacted in the crowd on the other side of the field. You realize, as an employee of the closest hospital to the event, that your facility is going to be receiving substantial casualties in the next few minutes. You activate your disaster plan and prepare for the casualties that you will be getting.

The television shows emergency medical services (EMS) providers moving to the area to provide care to the victims as you make your first phone calls contacting the hospital supervisor and administrator. Horrified, you watch as a hot dog vendor pulls out a second RPG and aims it at the ambulance rally point. The casualties will now include EMS providers.

 UNIQUE CONSIDERATIONS

Expect that the most severely injured patients will arrive after those who are less injured. The less injured often skip emergency medical services and proceed directly to the closest hospitals. For a rough prediction of the "first wave" of casualties, double the first hour's casualty count.

Ensure that physical activity of the victims is minimized after the blast explosion; exertion after the blast explosion can increase the severity of primary blast injury. This was seen in World War II in cases of some blast casualties who appeared well but died after vigorous exercise.[8]

 PITFALLS

Secondary Devices

Remember to check all victims for weapons, booby traps, and explosives. It is quite common for a bomber to become a victim of his own device. It is also common for a secondary device to be concealed under a casualty. Frequently, this secondary device is a grenade with the pin removed, so that disturbing the body will allow the spoon to fly off and the grenade to arm and explode.

Abrupt Decompensation

If a patient with a blast lung injury abruptly decompensates, the clinician should presume that the patient has a tension pneumothorax and treat accordingly. This is particularly true when the patient has thoracic fragment wounds from a grenade or pipe bomb.

Blast Lung

If the clinician does not consider the possibility of primary blast injury, it may further complicate the patient's care. This entity is covered elsewhere in another chapter.

Air Transportation

The potential from pneumothorax that results from grenade or pipe bomb explosion can be exacerbated by evacuation. Regardless of the altitude and distance of the flight, casualties with evidence of pneumothorax must have a chest tube placed. Evacuation aircraft should fly at the lowest possible altitude.

REFERENCES

1. Cernak I, Savic J, Ignjatovic D, et al. Blast injury from explosive munitions. *J Trauma*. 1999;47:96-103.
2. de Candole CA. Blast injury. *Can Med Assoc J*. 1967;96:207-14.
3. Stuhmiller JH, Phillips YY, Richmond DR. The physics and mechanisms of primary blast injury. In: Bellamy RF, Zajtchuk R, eds. *Conventional Warfare: Ballistic, Blast, and Burn Injuries*. Washington, DC: Office of the Surgeon General of the United States Army; 1991:241-70.

4. Weiner SL, Barrett J. Explosions and explosive device-related injuries. In Weiner SL, Barrett J (eds): *Trauma Management for Civilian and Military Physicians*. Philadelphia: Saunders; 1986: 13-26.

5. Hadden WA, Rutherford WH, Merrett JD. The injuries of terrorist bombing: a study of 1532 consecutive patients. *Br J Surg*. 1978; 65:525-31.

6. Mallonee S, Shariat S, Stennes G, et al. Physical injuries and fatalities resulting from the Oklahoma City Bombing. *JAMA* 1996;276:382-7.

7. Frykberg ER, Tepas JJ, Alexander RH. The 1983 Beirut Airport terrorist bombing: injury patterns and implications for disaster management. *Am Surg*. 1989;55:134-41.

8. Hutton JE Jr. Blast lung: history, concepts, and treatment. *Curr Concepts Trauma Care*. 1986;9:8-14.

chapter 162

Introduction to Structural Collapse (Crush Injury and Crush Syndrome)

Pier Luigi Ingrassia, Alessandro Geddo, Francesca Lombardi, and Francesco Della Corte

 ## DESCRIPTION OF EVENT

Crush injuries are commonly seen in disasters and they are often found in victims of collapsed structures, which may result from earthquakes, hurricanes, tornados, bombings, and other large-scale events. Crush syndrome is the systemic manifestation of rhabdomyolysis caused by prolonged continuous pressure on muscular tissue[1,2]; in particular, it is a reperfusion injury as a result of traumatic rhabdomyolysis.

Crush syndrome was first described in the English literature by Bywaters and Beall.[3] They described several patients who were trapped under the rubble of buildings bombed in the United Kingdom and who subsequently died of acute renal failure (ARF). The clinical features typically seen with crush syndrome are predominantly a result of traumatic rhabdomyolysis and subsequent release of muscle cell contents. The mechanism behind crush syndrome is increased permeability of the sarcolemmal membrane resulting from pressure or stretching. As the sarcolemmal membrane is stretched, sodium, calcium, and water leak into the sarcoplasm, trapping extracellular fluid inside the muscle cells. In addition to the influx of these elements, the cell releases potassium and other toxic substances such as myoglobin, phosphate, and urate into the circulation.[4-6] Injury to other cells may release: lactic acid, histamine, leukotrienes, peroxides, free radicals of oxygen, superoxides, lysozymes, and enzymes (such as like creatine phosphokinase).

These events may result in hypovolemic shock, hyperkalemia, metabolic acidosis, compartment syndrome, and ARF. The ARF is caused by a combination of hypovolemia with subsequent renal vasoconstriction, metabolic acidosis, and the insult of nephrotoxic substances such as myoglobin, urate, and phosphate. Compartment syndrome occurs when injured skeletal muscle contained within fascia-bound compartments develops swelling due to increased fluid uptake by injured muscle cells. Once the compartment pressure exceeds capillary perfusion pressure (at about 30 mm Hg), the tissue inside the compartment become ischemic and compartment syndrome develops.

Major earthquakes often result in a substantial number of crush syndrome injuries, the victim of which develop rhabdomyolysis and pigment-induced ARF. The incidence of crush syndrome has been estimated at a minimum of 2% to 5%. Approximately 50% of patients with crush syndrome will develop ARF, and of these, 50% will need dialysis.[5]

 ## PREINCIDENT ACTION

Emergency physicians, general practitioners, surgeons, and pediatricians should be familiar with the diagnosis and management of crush injuries and crush syndrome. As part of disaster preparedness to treat these patients, simple portable medical kits for on-scene treatment of patients with crush injury should be organized. These kits should contain materials and means to treat at least five critically ill patients and also maps and telephone numbers of all medical-aid centers in the region to which patients should be moved as soon as possible, theoretically within the first hour.[7]

The medical-aid centers would be identified at no more than an hour's walk from any location to ensure accessibility even if the road transportation system failed. Sites might include schools, gymnasiums, fire stations, and hospitals and should be located near potential helicopter landing zones for patient evacuation and delivery of supplies and equipment.

Since crush syndrome is a common cause of death in large-scale events, hemodialysis facilities and their capacity should be identified in advance.

After a disaster, challenges in communication should be anticipated. Therefore, one of the first priorities must be to establish an independently powered short-wave communication network. The hospitals, especially emergency departments and intensive care units, must be prepared to receive multiple critically ill patients.

Triage practices are of vital importance during a mass-casualty disaster. The Simple Triage and Rapid Treatment system is internationally suggested to categorize patients according to the severity of their illness and priority to evacuation.[8]

 POSTINCIDENT ACTION

It is critically important that medical and rescue personnel coordinate their efforts in caring for victims of crush injury. Serious morbidity and mortality can occur with delay in treatment of a crush victim. Aggressive medical treatment of patients before and during extrication will help prevent renal and cardiac complications of crush injury.

Since the crush syndrome is the second most important reason for increasing morbidity and mortality, triage guidelines must incorporate this into patient assessments to facilitate the strategic use of hemodialysis resources.

In the field, disaster medical personnel can obtain relevant physiologic parameters from crush victims that do not require any specific devices. An initial field triage model for determining which patients may require early intervention for crush syndrome could consist of the following three factors:

- pulse rate
- delay of response activity (>3 hours)
- macroscopic urine findings

A second triage model, applied in healthcare facilities, could be composed of other parameters, including the following laboratory tests:

- Tachycardia (> 120/minute)
- Macroscopic abnormal urine findings
- White blood cell count
- Hyperkalemia

Hemodialysis machines and filters, together with nephrologists, nurses, and technicians, should arrive within 24 to 36 hours as national and international resources are mobilized. Emergency dialysis units should be set up in easily accessible areas to avoid problems of transportation for those patients who may have other serious injuries requiring major surgery. On-scene doctors treating disaster victims can consult with remote renal experts using telemedicine or Internet linkages for advice on treating particularly complex cases. Decisions about which type of dialysis modalities to use should take into account the hypercatabolic state of the victims, the degree of electrolyte disturbances, the presence of polytrauma and bleeding tendency, as well as specific geographic and local conditions, transport problems, and other logistic difficulties. Conventional hemodialysis allows for efficient solute removal, treatment of multiple patients, and application without anticoagulants.

Peritoneal dialysis is difficult to administer in patients with abdominal trauma and often is inefficient for removal of potassium and other catabolic metabolites. It might offer temporary help, however, especially during disaster scenarios where conventional hemodialysis equipment is not ready available.[9]

 MEDICAL TREATMENT OF CASUALTIES

The treatment of crushed casualties should begin as soon as they are discovered. Attention should be given to the possibility of concomitant injury such as fractures, solid organ damage, or spinal injury. Intravenous access should be obtained with large-bore intravenous catheters, and the patient should receive fluid as soon as possible.[10-12] Multiple intravenous lines are necessary because these patients require large fluid volumes and individual intravenous lines may be dislodged during extrication. Normal saline is an appropriate initial choice for intravenous fluid resuscitation. A saline infusion of 1000 to 1500 mL/hour should be initiated during extrication. When a urine flow has been established, a forced mannitol-alkaline diuresis up to 8 L/day should be maintained (urine pH > 6.5). Once the patient reaches the hospital, 5% dextrose should be alternated with normal saline to reduce the potential sodium load. Since large volume of intravenous fluids may not be available in the first 2 days after a major incident, it is reported that hypertonic saline is also safe and effective in a variety of trauma patients.[13] Placement of a Foley catheter is also recommended to have accurate measurements of urine output.

Alkalinization increases the urine solubility of acid hematin and aids in its excretion. This may protect against renal failure and should be continued until myoglobin is no longer detectable in the urine. In addition to its protective effect as an osmotic diuretic, mannitol also is an effective scavenger of oxygen free radicals and may help reduce the reperfusion-related components of this injury by this mechanism.[4,6]

At hospital admission, electrolytes, arterial blood gases, and muscle enzymes should be measured. Performing a simple dipstick test on the urine for hemopositivity in the mildly injured patients can diagnose subclinical rhabdomyolysis and can be useful in identifying this critical condition. If these patients are discharged because of a limitation of facilities, they should be advised to check the color and the volume of their urine daily and to watch for other symptoms of ARF such as weight gain and edema.[1]

The outcome of the renal victims of catastrophic earthquakes is influenced by the type of trauma, concomitant events, and complications observed during the clinical course as well as epidemiologic features such as age, distance to reference hospitals, and time elapsed between disaster and admission to reference hospitals.[14] The earlier one starts intravenous therapy, the better the chance of preventing ARF. When fluid therapy is delayed for 6 hours after extrication, ARF is almost ensured. If the desired urinary output cannot be achieved, the use of diuretics, preferably furosemide, should be considered. The majority of crush injury victims who do not receive intravenous therapy early enough and who do not respond to forced alkaline diuresis go on to develop renal failure and the requirement for hemodialysis.[15]

There are case reports of hyperbaric oxygen improving the outcome of victims of crush injury.[16,17] The use of this modality is obviously limited in disaster situations because of lack of access to hyperbaric chambers.

CASE PRESENTATION

You are the physician of an emergency medical services ambulance. You are attending a victim of building collapse. You have already assessed the patient's airway, breathing, and circulation, and you are coordinating with rescue personnel. Which is your next priority?

- Notify 9-1-1 dispatch center and obtain directions.
- Consider amputation as soon as possible.
- Use tourniquets as a treatment of wounds.
- Obtain multiple intravenous lines and start fluid infusion.
- Perform field fasciotomy.

Note: To obtain multiple intravenous lines, reduce the possibility of the lack of intravenous access during extrication procedures and allow intravenous effusion of larger amounts of normal saline to prevent ARF and hemodialysis.

 UNIQUE CONSIDERATIONS

There is no doubt that the majority of deaths occur immediately after structural collapse or a catastrophic event, such as an earthquake.[18] And among those still alive, short-term mortality dramatically increases as the time the persons are buried under the rubble lengthens. During the first few hours, a not inconsiderable number are still alive. After 24 hours the survival curve starts to fall more steeply, and after 5 days all those not recovered are dead. Disaster medical plans should comprise a medical care chain in which casualties receive life-supporting measures at the accident scene, with subsequent transport to hospital for more definitive care within a few hours of their rescue. The development of crush syndrome after crush injury is preventable and treatable. Crush injury patients may present with few signs or symptoms; hence, medical personnel must maintain a high index of suspicion in treating crush victims.

 PITFALLS

Several potential pitfalls in response to a structural collapse exist. These include the following:

- Failure to plan evacuation routes prior to an event
- Failure to know who is in command of disaster operations within your local area

- Delayed treatment after the victim extrication
- Delay in starting intravenous fluids
- Low index of suspicion for crush injuries
- Failure to continue the monitoring of patients with a high risk for ARF

REFERENCES

1. Sever MS, Erek E, Vanholder R, et al. Clinical findings in the renal victims of a catastrophic disaster: in the Marmara earthquake. *Nephrol Dial Transplant.* 2002;17:1942-9.
2. Visweswaran P, Guntupalli J. Rhabdomyolysis. *Crit Care Clin.* 1999;15:415-28.
3. Bywaters EGL, Beall D. Crush injuries with impairment of renal function. *BMJ* 1941;1:427-32.
4. Better OS. Rescue and salvage of casualties suffering from the crush syndrome after mass disasters. *Military Med.* 1999; 164:366-9.
5. Erek E, Sever MS, Serdengeçti K, et al. An overview of morbidity and mortality in patients with acute renal failure due to crush syndrome: the Marmara earthquake experience. *Nephrol Dial Transplant.* 2002;17:33-40.
6. Smith J, Greaves I. Crush injury and crush syndrome: a review. *J Trauma.* 2003;54:S226-30.
7. Schulz CH, Di Lorenzo RA, Koenig KL, et al. Disaster medical direction: a medical earthquake response curriculum. *Ann Emerg Med.* 1991;20:470-1.
8. Benson M, Koenig KL, Schultz CH. Disaster triage: START, then SAVE—a new method of dynamic triage for victims of a catastrophic earthquake. *Prehospital Disaster Med.* 1996;11:117-24.
9. Vanholder R, Sever MS, Erek E, et al. Rhabdomyolysis. *J Am Soc Nephrol.* 2000;11:1553-61.
10. Better OS, Stein JH. Early management of shock and prophylaxis of acute renal failure in traumatic rhabdomyolysis. *N Engl J Med.* 1990;322:825-9.
11. Better OS and Rubinstein L. Management of shock and acute renal failure in casualties suffering from crush syndrome. *Ren Fail.* 1997;19:647-53.
12. Noji EK. Prophylaxis of acute renal failure in traumatic rhabdomyolisis. *N Engl J Med.* 1990;323:550-1.
13. Vassar MJ, Fisher RP, O'Brien PE, et al. A multicenter trial for resuscitation of injured patients with 7.5% sodium chloride: the effect of added dextran 70: the Multicenter Group for the Study of Hypertonic Saline in Trauma Patients. *Arch Surg.* 1993; 128:1003-11.
14. Sever MS, Erek E, Vanholder R, et al. Lessons learned from the catastrophic Marmara earthquake: factors influencing the final outcome of renal victims. *Clin Nephrol.* 2004;61:413-21.
15. Castañer Moreno J. Insuficiencia renal aguda postraumática. *Rev Cubana Med Milit.* 1999;28:41-8.
16. Siriwanij T, Vattanagomgs V, Sitprija V. Hyperbaric oxygen therapy in crush injury. *Nephron* 1997;75:484-5.
17. James PB. Hyperbaric oxygen treatment for crush injury. *BMJ* 1994;309:1513.
18. Pointer JE, Michaelis J, Saunders C, et al. The 1989 Loma Prieta earthquake: impact on hospital patient care. *Ann Emerg Med.* 1992;21:1228-33.

chapter 163

Train Derailment

J. Scott Goudie

 DESCRIPTION OF EVENT

Railroads provide a vital means of transportation for both passengers and industrial products. The high-volume and varied nature of cargo carried means that railway disasters are an ever-present risk that make possible a wide variety of situations, as demonstrated by past events:

- a high-speed passenger train derailment in the rural Southwest[1]
- a train derailment and hazardous material spill in rural North Dakota[2]
- a collision of two commuter trains in Chicago[3]
- a freight train derailment with subsequent hazardous material spill and fire in downtown Baltimore[4]

Each situation presents its own unique problems, whether it is a remote accident scene, a high-volume of patients, or a hazardous material spill potentially affecting those on the train, those living nearby, and emergency personnel responding to the scene.

Although most railway disasters are unintentional, arising either from human error or equipment failure, railways remain prominent targets for terrorism, as demonstrated by the Madrid subway bombings in March 2004. The many miles of railroads crossing the United States make it extremely difficult to provide security for every stretch of track, thus providing a potentially soft target for terrorists.

 PREINCIDENT ACTIONS

To respond effectively to a train derailment, hospitals, emergency departments, emergency medical services, and fire departments should all develop disaster response plans for mass-casualty and hazardous material disasters. These plans must also be supported by the proper equipment and training with regular tabletop and live disaster drills. A well-established system of communication and coordination between all local emergency services is vital, as well as maintaining points of contact with regional, state, and federal disaster response agencies.

A hazard assessment should be performed to identify the potential for railway disasters in a community based on the number of railways, the population density adjacent to the rails, the volume of rail traffic, the characteristics of rail services (e.g., subway, high-speed commuter, industrial freight, hazardous waste), and vulnerable facilities adjacent to the railways (e.g., schools, nursing homes, hospitals, apartment complexes, military bases) that may create unique problems for an emergency response.

 POSTINCIDENT ACTIONS

Initial priority should be given to the extraction, triage, transport, and treatment of the victims. Remote railway locations can present difficulties in reaching the scene, necessitating use of aeromedical assets in addition to land-based responders. Once at the scene, it is vital to do the following: (1) perform a rapid assessment to identify any potential hazardous material spills and (2) establish an incident commander and command center in a secure location. If the potential for a hazardous material contamination has not been determined, the information regarding the contents on board the train should be available, along with their material safety data sheets from the managing railroad company.

On-scene triage of victims according to an established system, such as the Simple Triage and Rapid Treatment system, allows for prioritizing medical evacuation of victims back to the medical center according to severity of injury.[5] The transportation of victims may include all traditional assets such as ground ambulances and aeromedical transports, as well as "lifts of opportunity" that may present themselves such as buses, police or fire vehicles, and military transport. Identification and tracking of the victims after their extrication and evacuation is vital and may be accomplished by triage tag number if no further identification is available on the scene. Definitive identification must be pursued at the time of presentation at the medical centers, for both the living and the deceased, to ensure all victims are recovered and accurately identified.

Early contact and coordination with state, regional, and national organizations such as the National Transportation Safety Board and the Federal Emergency Management Agency are essential in providing an appropriate response to a large-scale railway disaster. Local resources can rapidly be exhausted, thus necessitating outside aid such as from a National Guard unit or a disaster medical assistance team.

All railway disasters are potentially crime scenes and must be approached as such throughout the response. Extrication of victims is of paramount importance; however, attention must be paid to not destroy any potential evidence. In the case of a terrorist attack, there is also the potential for secondary devices targeted at the emergency responders.

Coordination of early statements and releases to the press should be handled through a single entity, whether it is the public affairs office of the hospital, the local police or fire department, or an outside agency; for instance, Amtrak manages all public affairs information and press releases for any accidents involving their trains.[1]

 ## MEDICAL TREATMENT OF CASUALTIES

Passengers will present with a broad spectrum of traumatic injuries, ranging from simple lacerations and fractures to severe head injuries and deceleration injuries (e.g., aortic or mesenteric avulsions). Patterns of injury may vary greatly depending on the passenger's location (e.g., seated versus standing, forward- versus rear-facing seats) at the time of the injury:

- Standing patients have a higher incidence of neck and craniofacial injuries.[6]
- Seated patients have a higher incidence of thoracoabdominal injuries, with those in forward-facing seats having a greater potential for facial injuries and deceleration injuries.[7]

In prolonged extrications, victims may also be suffering from crush syndrome and effects from exposure such as hypothermia or hyperthermia. There may also be a substantial number of burn or blast injuries, depending on the presence of combustible materials onboard the train or due to terrorist explosives.

Traumatic injuries to passengers and railway workers will often be the primary medical challenge; however, in cases of hazardous material exposures, the potential for exposure and illness extends to include rescue workers and residents living near the disaster. After trauma, the most frequent injuries sustained by railroad employees are respiratory irritation, nausea, vomiting, and headache—all suggestive of hazardous material exposure.[8] Residents near the derailment and first responders are most likely to present with respiratory, dermatologic, or ophthalmic complaints due to exposure.[4] Proper use of personal protective equipment for rescue workers, decontamination of both victims and rescuers upon leaving the scene, and evacuation of any residents nearby can all minimize the effects of a hazardous material spill.

Be prepared for a significant number of psychological casualties presenting both immediately and delayed.[9] These victims may present with either psychological complaints, somatic symptoms, or both. Posttraumatic stress disorders have been identified in both train passengers as well as nearby residents after a major train derailment.[10] Establishment of a critical incident support center to pro-

vide stress management, chaplain services, and psychological support for victims and families, as well as first responders, is helpful in minimizing the short- and long-term psychological sequelae after a railway disaster.

 ## CASE PRESENTATION

On a weekday afternoon, the call comes into the emergency department of the county's only community hospital that there has been a reported train derailment in a small outlying town approximately 40 miles away. Initial reports state that a freight train with six workers on board has derailed adjacent to an elementary school and that there is a large fire burning on scene. Local fire and emergency medical systems crews are rolling onto the scene and requesting medical direction.

What are your next moves? How would your response be different if it had been a high-speed commuter train with 100 passengers on board?

 ## UNIQUE CONSIDERATIONS

Train derailments are unique in the diversity of potential problems for responders. A derailment may occur in an urban environment with the subsequent risk of injury to the many people living and working nearby, or it can present in an isolated, rural location thus causing delays in response to the accident. The number of casualties can vary from only a handful of railway workers to hundreds of passengers on board a commuter rail. The possibility of hazardous material exposure exists in every train derailment, which may delay extrication of victims as well as present serious problems for rescue workers and those nearby. For a disaster response plan to be effective in the event of a train disaster, it must take into account all of these diverse possibilities.

 ## PITFALLS

Several potential pitfalls in response to a train derailment exist. These include the following:

- Failure to develop and practice a disaster response plan
- Failure to coordinate response with other agencies
- Failure to recognize hazardous material release
- Failure to maintain integrity of a crime scene for investigators
- Failure to address positive identification of both victims and deceased
- Failure to communicate with the public regarding risk and need for evacuation

REFERENCES

1. Jenkins BM. Protecting surface transportation systems and patrons from terrorist activities. *MTI Report*. 1997;97:20–7.

2. National Transportation Safety Board. Railroad Accident Report, NTSB # RAR-04-01. Washington, DC: 2004. Available at: http://www.ntsb.gov/publictn/2004/RAR0401.htm.

3. National Transportation Safety Board. Railroad Accident Brief, NTSB # RAB-04-07. Washington, DC: 2004. Available at: http://www.ntsb.gov/publictn/2004/RAB0407.htm.

4. Hsu EB, Grabowski JG, Chotani RA, et al. Effects on local emergency departments of large-scale urban chemical fire with hazardous materials spill. *Prehospital Disaster Med*. 2002;17:196–201.

5. Super G, Groth S, Hook R. *START: Simple Triage and Rapid Treatment Plan*. Newport, CA: Hoag Memorial Hospital Presbyterian; 1994.

6. Cugnoni HL, Finchman C, Skinner DV. Cannon Street rail disaster: lessons to be learned. *Injury* 1994;25:11–3.

7. Ilkjaer LB, Lind T. Passengers' injuries reflected carriage interior at the railway accident in Mundlestrup, Denmark. *Accid Anal Prev*. 2001;33:285–8.

8. Orr MF, Kaye WE, Zeitz P, et al. Public health risks of railroad hazardous substance emergency events. *J Occup Environ Med*. 2001;43:94–100.

9. Hagstrom R. The acute psychological impact on survivors following a train accident. *J Trauma Stress*. 1995;8:391–402.

10. Chung MC, Easthope Y, Farmer S, et al. Psychological sequelae: posttraumatic stress reactions and personality factors among community residents as secondary victims. *Scand J Caring Sci*. 2003;17:265–70.

chapter 164

Subway Derailment

Jason Dylik and David Marcozzi

 DESCRIPTION OF EVENT

Subways are a common means of mass transit found in many urban settings. Subways are essentially electrified trains that can transport hundreds or even thousands of people per train. Since the subway runs on a track, instead of freely on the road, derailment can present a host of problems, ranging from a thump barely noticed by passengers to catastrophic failure resulting in massive injury and death. One of the worst accidents in subway history occurred in New York City on November 1, 1918, when an inexperienced dispatcher (filling in for striking motormen) entered a tunnel too fast and caused the wooden train to derail. The train struck a wall, killing 97 people and injuring 200. This incident led to the Brooklyn Rapid Transit Company going out of business a month later.[1,2] Subways have become considerably safer in the years that have followed, but accidents including derailments may still occur. Operator error remains the most common cause of derailment.[3] Intentional sabotage of tracks or cars can also lead to derailment. On March 11, 2004, 191 people were killed and more than 2000 injured when 10 bomb explosions occurred simultaneously on 4 commuter trains in Madrid, Spain.[4]

The location of these events can present unique challenges for emergency responders. Subways may travel underground, on elevated platforms, or on bridges over bodies of water, gorges, and ravines. An underground subway derailment necessitates evacuation of the train in a dark tunnel with possibly a long walking distance to access points. During an above-ground derailment, train cars may tip over. Train derailment from an elevated railway may result in the train falling off the bridge entirely. Passengers and emergency responders risk falling off the elevated railway as well. Elevated railways passing over water present the additional hazard of drowning and exposure to cold for victims falling into the water. A common hazard to all electrified train accidents is the ever-present risk of electrocution that can result on contact with the third rail, which runs along the track in many subway systems and conducts several

hundred volts of direct current, providing power to the train. Contact with the third rail can be fatal.

 PREINCIDENT ACTIONS

Hazard vulnerability analysis by hospital disaster planners should include a survey of subway or train stations located in the vicinity of the hospital. Any past rail accidents that have occurred within the hospital catchment area should be carefully reviewed to determine whether there are "danger zones" where future accidents may be more likely to occur. The kinetic energy of a traveling train is proportional to the number of cars (mass) and the velocity. The higher the kinetic energy, the greater the risk of injury to passengers in the event of a derailment event.[5] An estimate of the potential number of injuries that could result from a theoretical rail accident can be made by multiplying the number of cars per train traveling through local stations and rail routes by the passenger capacity of each car. If the potential number of patients that could result from such a rail accident exceeds the capacity of local prehospital and hospital resources, multiagency disaster plans should be developed for this scenario.

 POSTINCIDENT ACTIONS

Because of the variety of potential disaster scenes after a subway accident, the responder must pay particular attention to scene safety issues. Adequate resources should be mobilized to address the specific scenarios faced and preconceived evacuation plans for the victims should be implemented. After victim rescue operations, assessment of the rail bed must be made to determine structural integrity before reestablishment of service along that route. Train cars must likewise be inspected to determine future usability.

Debriefing with emergency responders should be undertaken by senior members of involved agencies and other trained personnel from specialized organizations after any rescue operation to understand any difficulties that may have been encountered during the rescue and recovery operations.

MEDICAL TREATMENT OF CASUALTIES

Multiple types of casualties may be encountered in victims of rail accidents. In low-speed derailments, musculoskeletal injuries such as ankle and wrist injuries, and injuries due to falls are predominantly seen. In high-speed derailments, deceleration forces may be significant, with a resulting spectrum of traumatic injuries similar to that seen in other patients with high-speed blunt trauma. High-speed derailments occurring in tunnels may result in collision with tunnel support posts or stanchions, which may remain intact but cause passenger cars to collapse.[6,7] Fire, with smoke and release of toxic gases, may complicate injuries resulting from blunt trauma.[4]

Rail accident scenes are prone to multiple hazards of which emergency responders must be aware and must take precautions to avoid. Live electrical wires or the train's electrified third rail present the risk of electrocution leading to burns and respiratory and cardiac arrest. Fire in a subway tunnel can result in low oxygen levels and the presence of toxic fumes. If fire is present, effective suppression must take place before rescue attempts can be made. There may be a risk of falling debris or collapse of on-scene structures and train cars, as well as the potential that rescuers and victims could fall from elevated railways.

When scene safety is insured, victims should be evacuated from the accident zone as quickly as possible to minimize further risk from on-scene hazards and to allow for appropriate triage, on-scene treatment, and transportation to hospital. High-angle rope rescue techniques may be needed in some cases of elevated railway accidents. The scenario of needing to apply spinal immobilization and extricate hundreds of patients on long boards presents an enormous technical and logistical challenge to emergency responders. In this scenario, deployment of physicians to the field to evaluate and clinically clear patients without evidence of cervical spine injuries can significantly expedite the safe extrication of patients at risk for cervical spine and other injuries.

The triage area should be established upwind and outside of the accident zone, away from potential hazards, in an area that is accessible to transporting ambulances. Patients should be triaged using standard algorithms for a mass-casualty incident. A mass-casualty incident exists when:

1. The number of patients and the nature of their injuries make the normal level of stabilization and care unachievable, and/or
2. The number of Emergency Medical Service personnel that can be brought to the site within the time allowed is not enough, and/or
3. The stabilization capabilities of the hospitals that can be reached within the time allowed are insufficient to handle all the patients.

Basic trauma stabilization of injured patients can be initiated on the scene in preparation for transport to hospital. Patients with smoke inhalation or exposure to other toxic fumes should receive supplemental oxygen.

Patients with electrical burns or respiratory or cardiac arrest resulting from electrical shock should also be anticipated.

CASE PRESENTATION

On a summer Saturday afternoon, an above-ground subway train consisting of 11 cars with approximately 245 passengers and crew is heading toward a popular amusement park and the city aquarium. Unbeknownst to the crew, the track ahead has been vandalized. Spikes joining the track had been pulled, leaving the rails loose although still intact.

The first car passes over the section of the break without incident, but as the second car passes, the track comes apart and the rear truck of the third car derails, twisting the train into an "S" shape and slamming into a wall. The train conductor activates an alarm, and a bystander calls 9-1-1. The train crew, who is uninjured, begins identifying injured passengers. Police, fire, and emergency medical services (EMS) units arrive on the scene, and a mass-casualty incident is declared.

In total, 116 patients are transported. There is one fatality: a massive epidural hematoma with herniation. Three other red-tagged patients are appropriately admitted, treated, and discharged in good health. The train is recovered from the track, taken out of service, rehabilitated, and returned to service. The train bed, wall, and track are repaired. The National Transportation Safety Board determines the cause of the derailment to be sabotage of the track; operator error was not ruled to be involved. The vandals/saboteurs are never identified or apprehended.

⊙ UNIQUE CONSIDERATIONS

Subway derailments, when they occur underground or on elevated platforms, may be associated with difficult access issues for rescuers. Underground accidents may be associated with fire, smoke, and toxic gases that present risks to victims and rescuers alike. Rescuers may have to walk long distances through tunnels to reach the accident scene, carrying extrication and other rescue equipment, and then transport patients out on foot. The extrication of passengers from severely damaged or crushed train cars may require the use of heavy equipment outside the scope of standard EMS or fire department capabilities. Planning for such scenarios should occur in advance and involve representation from all relevant response agencies, including the Transit Authority.

PITFALLS

Several potential pitfalls in response to a subway derailment exist. These include the following:

- Inadequate implementation of an emergency plan with sufficient elements, including fire, police, EMS, and government agencies (e.g., the NTSB)
- Slow or incomplete discontinuation of track electricity and service on the line

- Accumulation of toxic gases underground
- Technically difficult rescues and extrications, either due to entrapment in machinery, conditions other than on level ground (e.g., bridge, tunnel underground or underwater), or remote locations
- Patient accountability—some may be entrapped, self-extricated, or transported by private citizens, and there is no way of determining the number of passengers who might be on board at the time of the accident

REFERENCES

1. Scores Killed, Many Hurt on B.R.T., *New York Times*. November 2, 1918:1–2.
2. Death beneath the streets. WGBH, Boston MA, Feb. 17, 1997. Available at: http://www.pbs.org/wgbh/amex/technology/nyunderground/death.html.
3. National Transportation Safety Board, Railroad Accident Report, Washington DC, June 17, 1997, PB97-916302, NTSB/RAR-97/02, p 153.
4. Gutierrez de Ceballos JP, Fuentes FT, Diaz DP, et al. Casualties treated at the closest hospital in the Madrid, March 11, terrorist bombings. *Crit Care Med.* 2005;33:S108.
5. Jussila J, Kjellstrom BT, Leppaniemi A. Ballistic variables and tissue devitalisation in penetrating injury-establishing relationship through meta-analysis of a number of pig tests. *Injury* 2005;36:282–92.
6. Pirmann D. NYC subway accidents. June 15, 2004. Available at: http://www.nycsubway.org/faq/accidents.html
7. National Transportation Safety Board, Railroad Accident Report, Washington DC, October 27, 1992, PB92-916304, NTSB/RAR-92/03, p 12.
8. Available at: http://www.directives.doe.gov/pdfs/doe/doetext/neword/151/g1511-1v4-3.html.

chapter 165

Bus Accident

Kavita Babu

 DESCRIPTION OF EVENT

In 2002, Americans traveled 21.8 billion miles by bus.[1] Despite these extraordinary numbers, serious bus accidents are still an uncommon event. National Security Council data state that the risk of fatal injury for a bus passenger is 170 times lower than that of an automobile occupant.[2] However, a single bus filled only to its stated capacity may hold more than 50 passengers.[3] Therefore, the possibility exists for a bus accident to cause an instant mass-casualty event in virtually any setting.

Data from transit buses for the year 2000 report more than 20,000 injuries and 82 deaths.[4] Although transit and charter bus data are available, the most complete data on bus accidents are derived from analysis of school bus crashes. More than 22 million American children take the bus to school daily.[5] In 1999, more than 18,000 people were injured in school bus accidents, resulting in 164 deaths.[6] Characteristics of those accidents that produced fatalities included front-end and side-impact crashes, overturned buses, and collisions with trains.[7] According to the National Transportation Safety Bureau, death and significant injury were often attributed to sitting at the point of impact.[8]

Analyses of individual accidents have guided the bus industry safety standards. The primary passenger safety feature of school buses is called *compartmentalization*. Given the size of buses and the lower crash forces imparted to passengers, legislation was passed in 1977 to make compartmentalization standard in the production of new school buses.[9] Padded seats create a compartment for the passenger between high seat backs and the seat in front. The seats themselves are constructed of steel, and designed to absorb energy by bending. However, this method of protection is particularly limited in rollovers, when passengers may be thrown from their seats.[10]

Continued controversy exists over the use of seat belts in school and transit buses. National transportation authorities argue that seat belts in buses increase the risk of serious neck injuries, and that the cost of seat belt implementation may be better allocated for other safety measures. Additionally, the role of seat belts in buses is questioned because their primary purpose in cars is to prevent ejection, an uncommon event in bus accidents.[11]

Proponents state that seat belts are an essential intervention for preventing injury to passengers during rollover and lateral-impact collisions.[11] As this debate continues, research on improving bus safety remains a priority for many government, professional, and parent organizations.

 PREINCIDENT ACTIONS

Every public safety system, emergency department, and hospital must have a comprehensive plan in place for approaching a mass-casualty event involving a bus. A serious bus accident can rapidly overwhelm the resources of a single hospital. Activation of local, state, and even federal resources may be required. Prehospital triage is critical to avoiding saturation of the nearest hospital. On-scene personnel should transport patients with unstable conditions to the nearest hospital, whereas patients with minor injuries can be diverted to outlying facilities.

One unique difficulty faced by prehospital personnel at the scene of a bus accident is the difficulty of extricating victims. The standard extrication tools and techniques used in response to car accidents may not be effective in evacuating victims from a bus. Particular difficulties with extrication were noted in an Omaha, Nebraska, accident in 2003. As a result of this accident, the National Transportation Safety Board recently issued a recommendation that all fire and rescue personnel undergo specialized training in bus extrication techniques.[12]

Rapid extrication of bus accident victims is particularly vital in cases in which the bus becomes submerged. Recent accidents in China and India resulted in large death tolls after buses left the road and entered nearby rivers.[13,14] High numbers of bus accident fatalities in developing countries may also be attributed to older equipment, bus overcrowding, lack of standardized driver training, and hazardous road conditions.

 POSTINCIDENT ACTIONS

In recent years, national transportation authorities have identified the collection and assimilation of transit and charter bus accident data as a priority in creating applicable safety interventions. The efforts of clinicians and local rescue and law enforcement personnel to report all bus accidents are critical for surveillance.

If the bus accident involves a large number of fatalities, part of the disaster response must involve rapid activation of local, state, and national mortuary teams to identify remains in a rapid and accurate manner.[15]

MEDICAL TREATMENT OF CASUALTIES

An Australian study reviewing school bus–related fatalities in children identified head injury and blood loss as the most common causes of death.[16] As in other causes of blunt trauma, immediate attention must be directed to airway, breathing, and circulation. Rapid airway management may be required in patients with a depressed Glasgow Coma Scale score or significant burns. Spinal immobilization must be maintained where appropriate. The secondary survey for injuries should be performed rapidly, with a particular focus on triage in the mass-casualty setting. Patients with life- or limb-threatening injuries must be addressed emergently, whereas other patients may be appropriate for immediate transfer or triage to a less urgent level of care. In most bus accidents, there are far more "walking wounded" than patients with incapacitating injuries.[17] However, in the case of multiple serious casualties, the physician or his or her staff must be able to mobilize both hospital and community resources rapidly in avoiding the saturation of any single healthcare site without failing to provide care to all patients.

CASE PRESENTATION

You are working in a 15-bed emergency department of a small community hospital that is 40 minutes by ambulance to the nearest level 1 trauma center. On a Monday morning, you receive pre-notification of a collision between a dump truck and a school bus. The bus overturned, landing on its left side. Flames were initially noted to the rear of the bus but were extinguished upon arrival of fire department personnel. The on-scene paramedic cannot pinpoint the number of passengers on the bus but estimates 20 children. Extrication is proceeding slowly. There is one reported fatality. Local emergency medical services (EMS) dispatch is contacting neighboring towns for assistance, and EMS personnel will transport the first victims to your hospital within 15 minutes.

UNIQUE CONSIDERATIONS

In many ways, the traumatic injuries sustained by any person during a bus accident are not markedly different than those found in a simple motor vehicle collision. However, a bus accident carries the potential to generate far more patients than a car accident, depending on the capacity of the bus and the severity of the accident. Local resources may quickly become overwhelmed.

The nature of patient injuries may be specialized with school bus accidents representing a potential event involving pediatric mass casualties, whereas a charter bus may represent a geriatric mass-casualty event. Additionally, multiple bus accidents have occurred where large numbers of burn victims have been documented, creating need for aggressive airway management and resuscitation.

PITFALLS

Several potential pitfalls in response to a bus accident exist. These include the following:

- Failure to develop adequate mass-casualty protocols at the emergency services, hospital, community, and state level
- Failure to train community EMS personnel in specialized techniques for bus extrication
- Failure to educate schoolchildren and public transportation passengers regarding emergency exit operation and use
- Failure to anticipate a large number of trauma victims
- Failure to anticipate a large number of pediatric victims
- Failure to anticipate a large number of burn victims requiring definitive airway management
- Failure to inform National Transportation Safety Board or National Highway Traffic Safety Administration of bus accidents (of all severity) to provide better data and improve overall safety

REFERENCES

1. American Public Transportation Association. Table 70: Bus and Trolleybus National Totals. *APTA Public Transportation Fact Book*. Washington, DC: APTA; 2002.
2. National Safety Council. *What are the Odds of Dying? Odds of Death due to Injury, United States 2000*. Itasca, IL: National Safety Council; 2000.
3. U.S. Department of Transportation, Office of Public Affairs. NHTSA sends school bus report to Congress. May 7, 2002. Available at: http://www.nhtsa.dot.gov/nhtsa/announce/ press/PressDisplay.cfm?year=2002&filename=pr37-02.html.
4. U.S. Department of Transportation, Federal Transit Administration. *2000 Transit Safety and Security Statistics and Analysis Report*. Washington, DC: USDOT; 2002.
5. National Center for Education Statistics. Table 51: Public School Pupils Transported at Public Expense and Current Expenditures for Transportation: 1929–30 to 1999–2000. *Digest of Education Statistics*. Washington, DC: National Center for Education Statistics; 2002.
6. National Safety Council. School Bus Safety Rules. Fact Sheet Library, National Safety Council. December 23, 2002. Available at: http://www.nsc.org/library/facts/schlbus.htm.
7. National Highway Traffic Safety Administration. Table 5: School Bus Passenger Fatalities by Most Harmful Event. Report to Congress. *School Bus Safety: Crashworthiness Research*. Washington, DC: NHTSA. 2002.
8. National Transportation Safety Board. *Safety Study—Crashworthiness of Large Post-Standard School Buses*. NTSB/SS-87/01. Washington, DC: NTSB; 1987.
9. National Highway Traffic Safety Administration. Section 1.3: School Bus Occupant Protection Requirements. Report to Congress. *School Bus Safety: Crashworthiness Research*. Washington, DC: NHTSA. 2002.

10. Sibbald B. MDs call for new safety features after death in school bus crash. *CMAJ* 2003;169:951.
11. Lapner PC, Nguyen D. Analysis of a school bus collision: mechanism of injury in the unrestrained child. *Can J Surg*. 2003; 46:269.
12. National Transportation Safety Board. *School Bus Run-off-Bridge Accident*. Highway Accident Report. NTSB/HAR-04/01. Omaha, Neb: NTSB.
13. Pratap A. India bus accident kills 28 children. CNN; November 18, 1997. Available at: http://www.cnn.com/WORLD/9711/18/india.bus/index.html.
14. Reuters. Bus accident in western China kills 34. CNN; 2001. Available at: http://www.cnn.com/2001/WORLD/asiapcf/east/08/11/bus.crash/index.html.
15. Valenzuela A, Martin-de las Heras, Marques T, et al. The application of dental methods of identification to human burn victims in a mass disaster. *Int J Legal Med*. 2000;133:236-9.
16. Cass DT, Ross F, Lam L. School bus related deaths and injuries in New South Wales. *J Rehabil Res Dev*. 2003;40:309-19.
17. National Highway Traffic Safety Administration. Occupant fatalities in school buses (model year 1997-2001) by person type. *Fatality Analysis Reporting System: 1999-2000*. Washington, DC: NHTSA; 2000.

chapter 166

Aircraft Crash Preparedness and Response

Dan Hanfling and Christopher R. Lang

DESCRIPTION OF EVENT

There are more than 27,000 commercial flights in the United States each day, making air travel one of the safest means of mass transportation per mile traveled.[1] Nevertheless, the crash of an airplane is often considered a major disaster and often generates significant interest for an extensive period of time. As current technologies improve, and the aviation industry tends to fly larger aircraft on longer flights, the need to prepare for the response to an air crash emergency remains a fundamental element of local disaster planning.[2] With over 850 airports in the United States handling regional, national, and international air traffic, the potential for response in any given community is more than just theoretical.

PREINCIDENT CONSIDERATIONS

Analysis of National Transportation Safety Board (NTSB) data with regard to aircraft size and the severity of injuries in "hull loss" events demonstrate a declining trend in aviation accident rates over time and an improvement in passenger and crew survival. This can be attributed to the increased use of wide-bodied, larger commercial aircraft. This allows for improved structural integrity, enhanced occupant protection mechanisms, improved fuel cutoff and fire extinguishing capabilities, and the suppression of toxic fumes from burning cabin materials.[3] A review of 473 civilian airplane crashes with survivors between 1977 and 1986 demonstrated only eight crashes with more than 50 injured casualties of any degree of severity. Additionally, there were only three crashes in which more than 50 seriously injured casualties occurred.[4] Another review of eight commercial aviation aircraft crashes in the United States between 1987 and 1991 revealed initial fatality rates ranging from zero to 46%. The number of injured passengers surviving the crash incident averaged over 60 passengers per event.[5] However, the potential for significantly larger numbers of casualties rises as passenger payload capacity increases. An example of this occurred in Tenerife, Canary Islands, on March 27, 1977, when two fully loaded Boeing 747 jets collided on the runway and burst into flames, killing over 500 people on the tarmac and critically injuring 60 passengers, many of whom later died.

A significant factor in the survivability of an airplane crash has to do with the aircraft conditions during and immediately after the crash event. An airframe that sustains an impact alone will likely yield many more survivors than an airframe that sustains impact followed by fire and explosion. Highlighting this point is the crash of Avianca Flight 52 in January 1990 on the north shore of Long Island, New York, after running out of fuel. There were 158 passengers on board, of whom 85 survived.[6,7] The majority of passengers perished because of trauma, not because of fire or smoke inhalation. The risk to passenger safety increases exponentially with the presence of fire or explosion on impact. Even in what may be an otherwise survivable event, fire contributes to significant morbidity and mortality of passengers, primarily from the rapid incapacitation of passengers by heat, smoke, and toxic fumes. Review of the British Airtours Boeing 737 accident at Manchester International Airport on August 22, 1985, demonstrates that passengers died within 4.5 minutes of the emergency being declared, and probably within 2 minutes of smoke and flames entering the fuselage.[8] This exemplifies the aggressive nature of fire and smoke within the confined space of the cabin and their devastating effects.

The final significant factor related to planning for air crash response is related to the location of crash events. The vast majority of aircraft accidents (85%) occur during takeoff and landings at an airport or occur within a 5-mile radius of the airport. Such statistics predicate the importance of both airport emergency operations planning, as well as off-airport planning, including water-based response plans for those airports adjacent to large bodies of water.

Under U.S. Federal Aviation Regulations (FAR Part 139.325), each airport operator must conduct a full-scale airport emergency plan exercise at least once every 3 years.[9] This exercise ensures that responding agencies are familiar with their responsibilities under the plan and is intended to improve their proficiency in its execution. Response to aviation emergencies on the airport grounds begins initially with the airport rescue firefighting (ARFF) resources, but will often quickly escalate to a mutual aid response event. In the event of an off-airport crash, the affected jurisdiction will have the initial responsibility for providing fire and rescue response. In today's environment of increased terrorist events, the deployment of a rocket-propelled grenade (RPG) fired at an aircraft becomes an intense concern. This was exemplified by the near miss of a rocket-propelled grenade on a departing Arkia Airlines Boeing 757 departing from Mombassa, Kenya, on November 29, 2002. In the setting of current security risks, any aviation emergency is likely to be considered the result of terrorist action until proven otherwise. Therefore, responses to off-airport incidents are likely to include local, state, and federal emergency responders, including a large contingent of law enforcement assets.[10] If an airport is located near or adjacent to water, the off-airport disaster planning must incorporate an offshore response strategy for a downed aircraft in the water. This response is likely to include airport-based water rescue resources and municipal, Coast Guard, and other Defense Department rotor wing and water-based rescue assets.[11]

 ## POSTINCIDENT CONSIDERATIONS

Regardless of the location of an air crash event, disaster operations are likely to follow four distinct operational phases (Box 166-1). The initial phase, *emergency response*, is primarily focused on life-saving, firefighting, and safety-related operations. It is during this phase that fire suppression, search and rescue, emergency medical care, traffic direction, and control and perimeter security are established. The first arriving emergency personnel will establish a Unified Command post and establish staging area(s) to provide on-scene management of the incident. Note that if there are multiple crash sites or if there is significant wreckage scattered over a large geographic area, it may be necessary to establish multiple Unified Command posts to provide effective command and control of the disaster scene. This element of aircraft disaster operations will be considered complete when the last surviving passenger(s) are transported from the scene and all life safety hazards at the crash site have been stabilized or eradicated.

The second phase of operations, the *transition and stabilization* phase, will often occur simultaneously with the emergency response phase and is intended to serve as a bridge between the initial response to the air crash event and the investigative and recovery aspects of the incident. It is during this phase that the disaster site is assessed and long-term strategic and recovery plans are developed. This includes the anticipation of necessary staffing and resource requirements over time. In coordination with the local or state health departments, morgue operations are established, and provisions are made for requests made by the Chief Medical Examiner's office. It is also likely that personnel from the NTSB will begin arriving on the scene during this phase of operations. Finally, operational control of the scene is passed from fire department to police department authorities in anticipation of the next phase of operations.

The *investigation* phase, which begins at the conclusion of the stabilization of the crash site, may last for several days, weeks, or months and includes all aspects of the investigation to determine the cause and origin of the crash. The NTSB retains primary responsibility for coordinating all aspects of the investigation, with significant assistance provided by the Federal Aviation Administration; local, state, and federal law enforcement agencies; and representatives of the involved airline. The NTSB may assume direction and control of the "wreckage site" to conduct an investigation into the cause of the crash. This is accomplished in close coordination with law enforcement organizations to manage the incident scene. The NTSB also works with the airline carrier(s) of the plane(s) involved in the crash, other appropriate airline organizations, and local and state governments to coordinate federal resources that may be required to meet the needs of aviation disaster victims and their families. Family counseling, victim identification and forensic services, communicating with foreign governments, and translation services are among the provisions that can be made available to help local authorities and the airlines deal with a major aviation disaster.[12] The NTSB will lead the aviation crash investigation until it is determined to have been caused by a criminal act, at which point the Federal Bureau of Investigation is given the lead role in coordinating the crisis management response to acts of terrorism.[13] In addition, the U.S. Department of Homeland Security may elect to send a representative to help coordinate the overall federal response to the incident.[14]

The final phase of the incident, the *recovery* phase, begins at the conclusion of the investigative phase and likewise may last for several days, weeks, or months. It begins with the transition towards normal flight operations. This assumes the completion of the clean-up operations at the crash site, the demobilization of staff, equipment, and other resources, and the finalization of all reports, incident records, and other documentation. It is completed by the preparation of an after-action report detailing all four phases of the operational response to the air crash event.

BOX 166-1 POSTINCIDENT OPERATIONAL PHASES
Phase 1: Emergency Response Phase 2: Transition and Stabilization Phase 3: Investigation Phase 4: Recovery

 ## MEDICAL TREATMENT OF CASUALTIES

The mechanisms of injury in aircraft accidents are primarily related to a combination of blunt, penetrating, and thermal injuries. More than one mechanism of injury is likely to coexist, resulting in multisystem traumatic injuries. These injuries most often result from one of five major causes, which include explosive decompression, crush and entrapment, passenger restraint systems, burn and thermal exposure, and events associated with evacuation.

Rapid and explosive decompression may be one of the initial events occurring in a loss of aircraft integrity, leading to a crash. This can affect many organ systems including the lungs, sinuses, and gastrointestinal tract. These air-filled structures are predisposed to injury resulting from barotrauma. Lung injuries are the most serious and are due to rapidly increasing positive pressure leading to tearing of lung tissue and subsequent pneumothorax. In addition, traumatic sinus rupture and tympanic membrane rupture can result from increased pressure in the sinuses. Finally, gastrointestinal effects can lead to possible bowel perforation and ventilatory compromise due to elevation of the diaphragm.

Crush and entrapment within the airframe wreckage are also highly likely to result in post-incident casualties. When a plane impacts a surface, there is compression of cabin space that can lead to entrapment and probable crushing. Many injuries seen are fractures, head and neck trauma, and rhabdomyolysis. In addition, the presence of fire, smoke, and water introduce the additional risk of morbidity and mortality related to thermal injuries or drowning.

Passenger restraint systems may cause patterns of injury similar to those seen in motor vehicle crashes; however, the velocity of the impact is greatly increased. This leads to a high incidence of blunt force injuries to the head, thorax, pelvis, and abdomen, in descending order of frequency. Examples include epidural and subdural hematoma, aortic dissection, solid organ lacerations, and pelvic fractures. The lack of shoulder restraints with lap belts allows for greater bodily movement and risk for injury. In addition, untethered objects within the cabin may become projectiles, resulting in blunt or penetrating injuries.

Thermal and burn injuries present a major cause of death from survivable impact. This is due to the confined space of the aircraft and the inability to egress in rapid fashion. Toxic fumes, especially carbon monoxide, pose a major risk (Table 166-1). In a study of military aircraft fatalities occurring between 1986 and 1990, 535 cases were analyzed for carboxyhemoglobin. There were 23 cases (4%) having elevated levels of carboxyhemoglobin (above 10% saturation.) In each case, the victim survived the crash and died in the post-crash fire.[15]

Finally, there are many injuries resulting from the evacuation of the aircraft. The crash environment will be chaotic, often with significantly hampered visual perception and significant risk posed by collisions with other passengers or exposed wreckage. Fractures, sprains, and soft tissue injuries predominate. In addition, flash and chemical burns from either jet fuel or hydraulic fluid may pose significant exposure risks.

Specific patterns of injuries in survivors can be divided into three major categories. Fractures are the most common injury, representing close to one quarter of all injuries[16] (Table 166-2). They range from isolated closed fractures requiring minimal medical attention to

TABLE 166-1 MANIFESTATIONS OF CARBOXYHEMOGLOBIN

PERCENT COHB	MANIFESTATIONS
<10	None
10	Shortness of breath (SOB)—vigorous exertion
20	SOB—moderate exertion, slight headache
30	Headache, irritability, easily fatigued, disturbed judgment
40-50	Headache, confusion, collapse, fainting
60-70	Unconsciousness, respiratory failure, death on long exposure
80	Rapidly fatal
>80	Immediately fatal

Data adapted from Klette K, Levine B, Springate C, et al. Toxicological findings in military aircraft fatalities from 1986-1990. *Forensic Sci Int.* 1992;53:143-8.

complex vertebral, pelvic, and open long bone fractures that are often associated with hemodynamic instability and the potential risk from fat embolism. Thermal and burn injuries are another major cause of morbidity in surviving passengers, including the risk of inhalation injury to the airway. Finally, blunt and penetrating trauma to intrathoracic and intra-abdominal organs can result in major bleeding and shock. These are usually related to direct impact or the movement of large objects within the cabin postdisaster.

Some key issues identified by after-action review of Sioux City, Iowa, crash response include the following[17,18]:

- No identified entry and exit way was available for emergency vehicles. This caused some traffic jams and indecision regarding how to exit the area.
- There was inadequate emergency equipment and resource management. Ambulances had extra equipment including include portable oxygen, intravenous

TABLE 166-2 DISTRIBUTION OF NAVY AND MARINE CORPS AVIATION ACCIDENT INJURIES BY DIAGNOSTIC CATEGORIES

DIAGNOSIS	PERCENT OF TOTAL INJURIES REPORTED
Fracture/dislocation	22.8
Contusion	16.1
Laceration	12.3
Abrasion	8.3
Thermal burn	7.9
Sprain/strain	7.6
Multiple extreme injuries	6.3
Amputation/avulsion	3.6
Hemorrhage	2.4
Perforation/rupture	2.1
Concussion	1.1
Crushing	1.1
Decapitation	1.1
Miscellaneous	7.3

Data taken from Table 25-1 in Aircraft Accident Autopsies from *United States Naval Flight Surgeon's Manual: The Virtual Navy Hospital Project.* 3rd ed. Chapter 25. 1991. Available at: *http://www.vnh.org/FSManual/25/04 Autopsy.html.*

CASE PRESENTATION: UNITED FLIGHT 232, JULY 19, 1989

United Airlines Flight 232 departed from Denver Stapleton International Airport for Chicago O'Hare International with 296 passengers onboard. It was a clear day without any weather restrictions. One hour and 17 minutes into the flight, there was a catastrophic failure of the tail-mounted engine (#2) that led to loss of hydraulic systems, virtually paralyzing the aircraft. The plane declared an emergency at 3:20 p.m. near the Sioux City, Iowa airport. Five minutes before crash impact, there were five airport rescue firefighting companies and four local fire engine companies positioned just outside the airport perimeter, awaiting the arrival of the crippled aircraft.

At 4:00 p.m., the plane touched down with the right wing making first impact with the ground. The plane's fuel reserve then ignited, and the aircraft flipped end over end as it ran off the runway into an adjacent cornfield. The tail section was completely severed from the rest of the aircraft. The main cabin and cockpit tumbled forward, finally resting in the inverted position 3700 feet from impact area. Fires and smoke erupted everywhere, and survivors alighted from the crashed plane, screaming for help.

There were over 26 different agencies involved in the response to the crash at the Sioux City airport. Out of 296 passengers and crew, 112 died in the crash. Thirty-five of those deaths were from asphyxia secondary to smoke inhalation (Table 166-3).[17] The number of casualties was greatly minimized by the rapid-fire suppression response. After the fires were controlled, the triage of patients was initiated. The emergency medical service response to the event included the transport of 196 patients to hospitals within 90 minutes of the crash impact using ambulances, helicopters, buses, and vans.

supplies, and pressure dressings that would have been tremendously valuable to the on-scene response. However, these were not left on scene and remained on the individual transport units.

- Uncoordinated release of public information led to inconsistent reporting by media and news organizations.
- Fire engine water pump failure resulted in 10 minutes without adequate supply.
- There was an unknown number of passengers. Children who sat on a guardian's lap were not counted on the passenger manifest.

TABLE 166-3 INJURIES TO UNITED FLIGHT 232 PASSENGERS

INJURIES	CREW	PASSENGERS	TOTAL
Fatal	1	110	111
Serious	6	41	47
Minor	4	121	125
None	0	13	13
Total	11	285	296

Data adapted from National Transportation Safety Board Aircraft Accident Report PBSO-910406NTSB/AAR-SO/06 United Airlines Flight 232, Sioux Gateway Airport. Sioux City, Ia: July 19, 1989. Available at: *http://amelia.db.erau.edu/reports/ntsb/aar/AAR90-06.pdf.*

- Many different languages were spoken without available interpreters, leading to miscommunication during the rescue efforts.

 UNIQUE CONSIDERATIONS

Given the significant risk of repeated terrorist attack in the United States, the response to all air crash events will necessarily invoke a significant law enforcement component, particularly in the initial investigative phase of the event. Such a response was exemplified by the response to the TWA Flight 800 crash off the southern coast of Long Island, New York, in the summer of 1996, and more recently, the crash of American Airlines Flight 587 immediately upon takeoff from New York Kennedy International Airport in October 2001. The implication of such a response is that surviving patients brought to the hospitals may eventually need to undergo law enforcement questioning and evaluation. All clothing and other personal items transported with the patient from the disaster scene must necessarily be considered as evidence and therefore must be collected and stored according to agreed-upon procedures, in conjunction with local law enforcement officials. There is an important caveat regarding the presence of firearms or other weapons that may be found on the person of surviving passengers. These would have traditionally been associated with possible hijackers. However, with the reintroduction of armed federal air marshals on board an increasing number of flights, particularly those departing or arriving from key high-threat urban areas, such weapons may in fact be attributable to law enforcement personnel.

PITFALLS

Most disaster scene triage decisions are predicated upon the application of the Simple Triage and Rapid Treatment (START) triage decision-making algorithm. This system is primarily based on the recognition of bodily injuries and the categorization of patients into categories of priority based on specific physiologic criteria, including airway, breathing, and circulation considerations. This is a system that is focused on the treatment and transport of the most emergent patients first, followed by those patients with injuries requiring less urgent attention. It involves a color-coded system that is used to rapidly triage patients into their respective injury status.

And although this triage approach works for the majority of mass-casualty situations, it needs to be adapted for use in air crash disasters, particularly those in which there has been a fire or explosion. Patients who may present with only mild throat irritations, without any other injuries, would likely be placed in the lowest transport priority group. However, such symptoms may be the harbinger of a more serious developing inhalation injury, either due to an explosion and fire through the passenger cabin, exposure to toxic fumes, or aspiration of water or toxic fluids in the event of a water ditching. Such patients must be automatically upgraded in response category and transported away from the scene in a more rapid manner. These patients may possibly benefit from early aggressive airway management if the index of suspicion of an inhalation injury remains high based on the assessment of the initial out-of-hospital care providers. This exemplifies the need for constant reevaluation and possible changes in triage and treatment status.

REFERENCES

1. Accidents, Fatalities, and Rates, 2004 Preliminary Statistics U.S. Aviation, National Transportation Safety Board. Accessed at: http://www.ntsb.gov/aviation/Table1.htm.
2. Mollard R, Akestedt T, Cabon P, et al. Summary and recommendations for future ultra-long range operations. *Aviat Space Environ Med.* 2004;75:B124.
3. Abelson LC, Star LD, Stefanki JX. Passenger survival in wide-bodied jet aircraft accidents vs. other aircraft: a comparison. *Aviat Space Environ Med.* 1980;51:1266-9.
4. Rutherford WH. An analysis of civil aircrash statistics 1977-86 for the purposes of planning disaster exercises. *Injury* 1988;19: 384-8.
5. Anderson PB. A comparative analysis of the EMS and rescue responses to eight airliner crashes in the United States. *Prehospital Disaster Med.* 1995;10:142-53.
6. Dulchavsky SA, Geller ER, Iorio DA. Analysis of injuries following the crash of Avianca Flight 52. *J Trauma.* 1993;34:282-4.
7. Van Amerengen RH, Fine JS, Tunik MG, et al. The Avianca plane crash: an emergency medical system's response to pediatric survivors of the disaster. *Pediatrics* 1993;92:105-10.
8. Hill IR. An analysis of factors impeding passenger escape from aircraft fires. *Aviat Space Environ Med.* 1990;61:261-5.
9. *Code of Federal Regulations Title 14.* Volume 2, revised. U.S. Government Printing Office via GPO Access CITE: 14CFR139.325; January 1, 2001:812-3. Available at: *http://ecfr.gpoaccess.gov/cgi/t/text.*
10. *Fairfax County Emergency Operations Plan, Aircraft Crash Appendix for Off Airport Incidents.* Fairfax County, Virginia: Fairfax County Division of Emergency Management; March 2, 2004.
11. *Multi-Agency Ocean Rescue Disaster Plan and Drill.* Broward County, Florida: United States Fire Administration, Federal Emergency Management Agency. Available at: http://www.usfa. fema.gov/downloads/txt/publications/tr-079.txt.
12. National Transportation Safety Board. *Federal Family Assistance Plan for Aviation Disasters.* April 2000. Available at: October 28, 2005 at http://www.ntsb.gov/publictn/2000/spc0001_body.htm.
13. *Presidential Decision Directive 39: U.S. Policy on Counterterrorism.* The White House, June 21, 1995. Available at: October 28, 2005 at *http://www.fas.org/irp/offdocs/pdd39htm.*
14. *National Response Plan: Homeland Security Presidential Directive (HSPD-5).* The White House, February 28, 2003. Available at: October 28, 2005 at *http://www.fas.org/irp/offdocs/nspd/hspd-5.html.*
15. Klette K, Levine B, Springate C, et al. Toxicological findings in military aircraft fatalities from 1986-1990. *Forensic Sci Int.* 1992; 53:143-8.
16. *United States Naval Flight Surgeon's Manual: The Virtual Navy Hospital Project.* 1991: 3rd ed. Chapter 25. Bureau of Medicine and Surgery, Naval Aviation Medical Institute. Pensacola, Florida Available at: *http://www.vnh.org/FSManual/25/04Autopsy.html.*
17. National Transportation Safety Board Aircraft Accident Report PBSO-910406NTSB/AAR-SO/06 United Airlines Flight 232, Sioux Gateway Airport. Sioux City, Iowa: July 19, 1989. Available at: *http://amelia.db.erau.edu/reports /ntsb/aar/AAR90-06/pdf*
18. Brown G. *The Crash of Flight 232..* Lecture series provided at University of Nebraska, Omaha. January 23, 2002. Accessed on October 28, 2005 at http://ai.unomaha.edu/video/

chapter 167

Air Show Disaster

Peter D. Panagos

DESCRIPTION OF EVENT

Typically, an air show is a summertime event during which aviators display their flying skills and aircrafts. Although some air shows are held for commercial purposes, many are arranged to raise funds for charities. Usually air shows occur at military or large civilian airfields, located near the coastline or large cities in which a variety of static aircraft and helicopters are on view. When space allows, other entertainment and market stalls are available, adding further to the attraction of the show. Flight performances by military aerobatic teams and civilian aerobatic aircraft as well as large-scale pyrotechnics are presented to attract larger crowds. Due to the public interest in aviation, crowds at a typical air show can range from a few hundred to tens of thousands of attendees.

A disaster at an air show is a multiple-casualty incident in which the primary effects are morbidity and mortality to persons, while the community infrastructure remains intact. Over the last 30 years, there have been air show accidents involving performing aircraft that have caused a significant number of casualties (Table 167-1). Because of the possibility of mass casualties due to ground accidents, aviation mishaps, or terrorism, pre-event planning, incident response, and the post-event reaction must be thoroughly planned to effectively manage any potential situation.

PREINCIDENT ACTIONS

Preparations should include the continuum from basic event planning such as addressing the sanitation needs of a large crowd to planning for area evacuation in case of a large-scale aviation mishap involving significant casualties and a hazardous materials risk.[1-8] An effective disaster plan will identify potential problems by performing a risk analysis of chemical and environmental hazards,[7] personnel and physical resources, and transportation elements available to the planners (Box 167-1). Once a plan has been outlined, it must be evaluated for effectiveness and completeness through the implementation of a disaster drill.

A thorough mishap plan includes contingency arrangements with appropriate activities for rescue, firefighting, explosive ordnance disposal, logistical support, medical support, coordination with public affairs/media, coordination with law enforcement officials, wreckage location, security, recovery and preservation, and notification of key personnel.[9] Disaster preparedness officials have long recognized the value of good training and exercises. Most of the principles of disaster planning are based on the painful lessons learned under actual catastrophic conditions.[10] Exercises provide the opportunity to learn how to perform in realistic and controlled settings that are relatively free of risk.

POSTINCIDENT ACTIONS

In any unannounced event, the alert mechanism must be expeditious because the survival of severely injured individuals is often time sensitive. In an air show disaster involving ground casualties on the airfield, knowledge of the disaster will often be immediate. Notification of a crash may come over primary or secondary communication networks, and a crash message is disseminated to include aircraft type, nature of emergency, location of crash or landing runway, number of persons on board, hazardous cargo, potential ground casualties, and other pertinent information. If there are survivors at the scene, the urge to charge in to render care should be avoided. Trained rescue teams will bring casualties to a safe area or allow the medical team into the area when it is safe.

When multiple casualties are involved, a system of triage may be needed.[3] Specific areas for casualty management should be predesignated with standard nomenclature. It is the medical leader's responsibility to keep the Incident Commander abreast of numbers and types of casualties, the need for additional support, and any other facts the command post needs to make decisions.[11,12]

If an aircraft crashes in a remote setting, all responding personnel from the airfield will proceed to a prearranged assembly point for convoy to the area. In any disaster, medical personnel should enter the area only when it is declared safe.

Once the survivors have been taken care of and the remains of the deceased secured or removed, an assessment of the adequacy of response should be made as soon as possible to include supplies and equipment eval-

TABLE 167-1   FATAL CRASHES AT AIR SHOWS OVER THE LAST 30 YEARS

DATE	LOCATION	DESCRIPTION	NO. OF PERSONS INJURED/KILLED
July 2002	Western Ukraine	Russian Sukhoi Su-27 performing maneuvers crashed into crowd	84/115
June 1999	Bratislava, Slovakia	British Royal Air Force Hawk 200 crashed during air show	1/1
July 1997	Ostend, Belgium	Light aircraft mounting an aerobatics display crashed into crowd around a Red Cross tent	9/57
September 1997	Chesapeake Air Show, Glenn L Martin State Airport, Baltimore, MD	F-117A crashed during flyby	5/0
August 1988	Ramstein Air Force Base, West Germany	Three Italian Air Force jets collided midair and crashed into crowd	70/100s
June 1988	Mulhouse-Habsheim, French-Swiss border	New Airbus A320 crashed during low-level demonstration flight	3/133
September 1982	Mannheim, West Germany	U.S. Army Chinook helicopter carrying multi-nation sky divers crashed	46 killed
June 1973	Paris, France	Prototype Russian Tupolev Tu-144, a supersonic airliner, dubbed "Concordski" exploded midair during Paris air show	15 (6 crew, 9 ground)

uations (e.g., too little? inappropriate? not available?) and personnel (e.g., adequately training? management performance?). These evaluations should be used to make changes in the disaster response plan and improve future response.

The psychological impact of the mishap on the response team members and the community should not be overlooked. A critical incident debriefing or other intervention by mental health workers should be considered for the responding or on-site workers.[13,14] Other interventions must be considered for family and friends.

MEDICAL TREATMENT OF CASUALTIES

In any large-scale disaster, once the site has been deemed safe, the next priority is the triage, treatment, movement, and evacuation of casualties. During an air show without a mass-casualty event, the types of injuries and illnesses treated vary based on meteorologic conditions and geographic location. The conditions encountered are typical complaints seen in emergency departments such as dehydration, intoxication, sunburn, animal/insect bites, trips/falls, exacerbation of chronic illness, and altercations.[1]

In the event of an aircraft crash involving ground personnel, the potential for multisystem life-threatening injuries increases. In many aircraft accident fatalities, the injuries appear extensive from multiple trauma, burns, or both. Explosive and blast injuries involving penetrating and blunt trauma will result from the sudden deceleration of the airframe into the ground with ignition and disbursement of aircraft flammable materials and ordnance. Explosive-related injuries will affect most organ systems and produce unique patterns of injury seldom seen outside the combat arena. The management of these injuries in the field will often be limited to triage, stabilization, and transportation to an appropriate level of care.[15-21]

If the aircrew successfully exits the aircraft, rescue personnel should be aware of human impact injury patterns.

Although aircraft structures are designed to improve crash survivability, the human tolerance to deceleration and postcrash explosions is a complex function of many factors.[22-24] Based on Armed Forces Institute of Pathology injury analysis, there are four major injury types to be considered: thermal, intrusive, impact, and deceleration.[22,23,25] Though protected by flame retardant clothing, aircrew often sustain thermal injuries secondary to ignition of aircraft fuel and materials, inhalation of soot and combustion products including carbon monoxide, skin and soft tissue burns, soft tissue contraction and charring, thermal fractures and amputations, and severe burns. Intrusive injuries from the loss of occupiable space due to the intrusion of main rotor blades, propellers, trees, or wires are also common causes of severe injury. Finally, impact and deceleration forces cause injuries based on the position during deceleration and the distribution of force over the body parts (Table 167-2). For example, the pilot who ejects before impact may survive but may sustain extremity fractures resulting from the violent extremity movements involved in a high-speed ejection.

Aircraft wreckage sites can have multiple hazards. Personnel involved in the recovery, examination, and documentation of wreckage may be exposed to physical hazards posed by such things as hazardous cargo, flammable and toxic fluids, sharp or heavy objects, and disease. Hazardous materials, such as cartridge-actuated devices, tires, and oxygen bottles are major concerns. Explosive ordnance disposal personnel should target items such as pressurized bottles, hydraulic reservoirs, and canopy detonation cord to secure the scene and prevent further injury.[9,24,26-33]

Finally, once all injured or trapped victims have been cleared from the crash site, the area should be considered a crime scene. Wreckage and cargo should not be disturbed or moved except to the extent necessary for personnel safety. Arrangements should be made for security at the accident scene to protect the wreckage from additional damage and to protect rescue personnel and the public from injury.

UNIQUE CONSIDERATIONS

Most advanced military aircraft contain composite structures consisting of light, strong, stiff fibers embedded in a matrix material. Although these materials offer a significant structural advantage, they present a danger to rescue and medical personnel. Studies have shown that composite fibers can cause mild short-term skin, eye, and respiratory problems, but the long-term carcinogenic potential is unknown. Therefore, prudence is required in using personal protective equipment.

The reinforcing fibers most commonly used in aircrafts are graphite, bismalemide, and boron fibers (such as Kevlar). For example, in the F-18A/B, there are 1000 lbs (or 9.8% total aircraft structural weight) of composite material.[22] These fibers, when released from an epoxy matrix, become fine splinters that can easily be driven into the skin and will cause irritation. Graphite fibers

TABLE 167-2 DECELERATIVE INJURIES AND APPROXIMATE G FORCES INVOLVED

BODY PART/INJURY	DECELERATIVE FORCE (G)
Pulmonary contusion	25
Nose fracture	30
Vertebral body compression	20–30 (less in thoracic region or if poor body position)
Fracture dislocation of C-1 or C-2	20–40
Mandible fracture	40
Maxilla fracture	50
Aorta intimal tear	50
Aorta transection	80–100 (at ligamentum arteriosum)
Pelvic fracture	100–200
Vertebral body transection	200–300 (through body, not intervertebral disc)
Total body fragmentation	350
Concussion	60 G over 0.02 sec
	100 G over 0.005 sec
	180 G over 0.002 sec

Adapted from *The U.S. Naval Flight Surgeon's Pocket Reference to Aircraft Mishap Investigation.* 4th ed. Pensacola: The Naval Safety Center, Aeromedical Division in conjunction with The Society of United States Naval Flight Surgeons; 1995.

 ## CASE PRESENTATION

It was supposed to be the grand finale to a beautiful, family day event; then everything went wrong for the low-flying Russian-built Sukhoi Su-27, a 5.5-ton supersonic fighter aircraft (a long-range air fighter comparable to the U.S. F-15). More than 1500 people watched the free air show, part of celebrations to mark the 60th anniversary of a local Air Force unit. Witnesses said the jet was performing complex aerobatic maneuvers before it reportedly lost power, clipped some trees and another plane, cartwheeled across the ground, and crashed into a huge fireball. The two-pilot crew safely ejected from the aircraft before the plane hit the crowded spectator stands. As one witness stated, it was "a huge ball of fire, as big a house, and black smoke…I barely had enough time to clutch my young daughter before the explosive wave threw us to the ground, and severed arms and legs were flying all over." In all, 84 persons were killed (26 were 18 years of age or younger), and more than 116 were hospitalized with various injuries.

The crash of the fighter jet was caused by pilot error, an official report into the incident has concluded. The head of the commission set up to investigate the crash said the pilots had failed to follow the flight plan and performed difficult maneuvers they had not done before. Additionally, operational issues, organizational problems, and a lack of safety measures had contributed to make it the world's worst air show disaster. These events occurred at Skryliv Airport, near Lviv, Ukraine, on July 27, 2002.

are very small and light and pose a respiratory threat similar to asbestos. While the aircraft is still burning or smoking, only firefighters should be in the immediate vicinity. Once the fire is completely extinguished and cooled, the composite material is normally sprayed with a fixant, such as polyacrylic acid or aircraft firefighting foam to contain release of composite fiber material. Finally, it is recommended that all personnel around the released fibers wear a National Institute for Occupational Safety and Health–approved disposable air-filtering mask, Tyvek disposable overalls, puncture-resistant gloves and goggles while on scene and take a shower before leaving the scene.[22,25,29,30]

Additionally, the risk of being exposed to blood and body fluids is possible in any mishap involving human injury. Human immunodeficiency virus, hepatitis B, Lyme disease, and tetanus pose a threat to rescue personnel. Hepatitis B virus can survive in a dried state for several weeks. Therefore, it is recommended that all crash scene rescue and medical personnel become familiar with potential on-scene hazards, adhere to Occupational Safety and Health Administration work practice controls,[31] and make use of personal protective equipment.[32]

 PITFALLS

Several potential pitfalls in response to an air show disaster attack exist. These include the following:

- Failure to identify, prepare for, and properly train for a mass-casualty event by not developing contingency plans and periodically reviewing and correcting errors in the plans
- Failure to plan for the medical needs of a mass gathering composed of both geriatric and pediatric persons, many with significant preexisting diseases, exposed to a wide range of environmental elements and stresses unique to an airfield
- Failure to recognize the unique injuries sustained by ground personnel from explosive-related forces in close proximity to an aircraft crash
- Failure to appreciate that emergency responders may become casualties themselves if they do not recognize the hazardous dangers of a modern aircraft crash scene containing composite materials, biologic hazards, and unexploded ordnance. (Use of personal protective gear is paramount to avoid responder injury.)
- Failure to recognize the unique injury patterns of aircraft crash survivors who have experienced sudden deceleration forces (high G) and exposure to hazardous materials

REFERENCES

1. Mears GD, Batson DN. Mass gatherings. In: Bosker G, ed. *Textbook of Adult and Pediatric Medicine.* Atlanta: American Health Consultants; 2000.
2. Schultz CH, Koenig KL, Noji EK. A medical disaster response to reduce immediate mortality after an earthquake. *N Engl J Med.* 1996;334:438-44.
3. Schultz CH, Koenig KK, Noji EK. Disaster preparedness and response. In: Rosen P, Barkin RM, eds. *Emergency Medicine: Concepts and Clinical Practice.* 4th ed. St Louis: Mosby; 1998:324-33.
4. Hogan DE, Burstein JL, eds. *Disaster Medicine.* Philadelphia: Lippincott Williams and Wilkins; 2002.
5. De Lorenzo RA. Mass gathering medicine: a review. *Prehospital Disaster Med.* 1997;12:68.
6. Waeckerle JF. Disaster planning and response. *N Engl J Med.* 1991;324:815.
7. Levitin HW, Siegelson HF. Hazardous materials: disaster medical planning and response. *Emerg Med Clin North Am.* 1996;14:327.
8. Auf der Heide E. *Disaster Response: Principles of Preparation and Coordination.* St Louis: Mosby; 1989.
9. Edwards M. Airshow disaster plans. *Aviat Space Environ Med.* 1991;62:1192-5.
10. de Boer J. Tools for evaluating disasters: preliminary results of some hundred of disasters. *Eur J Emerg Med.* 1997;4:107-10.
11. Christen H, Maniscalco P. *The EMS Incident Management System.* Upper Saddle River, NJ: Prentice-Hall Inc; 1998;1-15.
12. Irwin RL. The incident command system (ICS). In Auf der Heide E, ed. *Disaster Response: Principles of Preparation and Coordination.* St Louis: Mosby; 1989.
13. Burkle FM Jr. Acute-phase mental health consequences of disasters: implications for triage and emergency services. *Ann Emerg Med.* 1996;28:119-28.
14. Linton JC, Kommor MJ, Webb CH. Helping the helpers: the development of a critical incident stress management team through university/community cooperation. *Ann Emerg Med.* 1993;22:663.
15. Pepe PE, Kvetan V. Field management and critical care in mass disasters. *Crit Care Clin.* 1991;7:321-7.
16. Dunne MJ Jr, McMeekin RR. Medical investigation of fatalities from aircraft accident burns. *Aviat Space Environ Med.* 1977;48:964-8.
17. Mason JK. *Aviation Accident Pathology.* London: Butterworths; 1962.
18. McMeekin RR. Patterns of injury in fatal aircraft accidents. In: Mason JK, Reals WJ, eds. *Aerospace Pathology.* Chicago: College of American Pathologists Foundation; 1973.
19. Mariani F. Spinal and spinal cord injuries in aviation medicine [Italian/English]. *Minerva Med.* 1978;69:3621-30.
20. Shanahan DF, Mastroianni GR. Spinal injury in a U.S. Army light observation helicopter. *Aviat Space Environ Med.* 1984;55:32-40.
21. Boyarsky I, Shneiderman A. Natural and hybrid disasters—causes, effects, and management. *Top Emerg Med.* 2002;24:1-25.
22. *Aircraft Mishap Investigation Handbook.* Brooks Air Force Base, TX: The Society of USAF Flight Surgeons; 2002.
23. *The US Naval Flight Surgeon's Pocket Reference to Aircraft Mishap Investigation.* 4th ed. Pensacola: Society of United States Naval Flight Surgeons; 1995.
24. *US Naval Flight Surgeon Manual.* 3rd ed. Washington, DC: The Bureau of Medicine and Surgery, Department of the Navy; 1991.
25. McMeekin RR. Aircraft accident investigation. In: DeHart RL, ed. *Fundamentals of Aerospace Medicine.* Philadelphia: Lea & Febiger; 1985.
26. Rayman RB. Aircraft accident investigation for flight surgeons. *Aeromedical Rev.* 1979;3:79.
27. Thompson RL. Cause of death in aircraft accidents: drowning vs. traumatic injuries. *Aviat Space Environ Med.* 1977;48:924-8.
28. Ernsting J, Nicholson AN, Rainford DJ, eds. *Aviation Medicine.* 3rd ed. London: Arnold; 2003.
29. Department of the Air Force Human Systems Center. *Response to Aircraft Mishaps Involving Composite Materials (Interim Guidance).* Consultative Letter, AL-OE-BR-CL-1988-0108. Brooks Air Force Base, Tex: AFMC; 1998.
30. Mishap Risk Control Guidelines for Advanced Aerospace Materials: Environmental, Safety, and Health Concerns for Advanced Composites. LT John M. Olson (Project Engineer), McClellan Air Force Base, CA; October 1993.
31. Bloodborne Pathogens 29 CFR Part 1910.1030. Washington, DC: Occupational Safety & Health Administration; 2001.
32. National Institute of Justice, Guide for the Selection of Personal Protection Equipment for Emergency First Responders, NIJ Guide 102-00 (Volumes I, IIa, IIb, and IIc), November 2002. Available at: http://www.osha.gov.

chapter 168

Asteroid, Meteoroid, and Spacecraft Reentry Accidents

Jay Lemery and Faith Vilas

 DESCRIPTION OF EVENT

From its origins 4.6 billion years ago, the natural history of our planet is replete with evidence of extraterrestrial impacts. Comets, asteroids, and meteoroids are the cosmic "impactors" that are theoretically both the originators (first organic molecules) and destructors (demise of the dinosaurs) of terrestrial life.[1,2] Evidence of these impacts on our world remains, for example, in the mile-wide meteor crater in Arizona and in the impact site off the coast of the Yucatan Peninsula, believed to have caused the extinction of the dinosaurs 65 million years ago. Impacts of such magnitude are exceedingly rare, yet even less than 100 years ago, a small meteoroid 60 m in diameter is thought to have exploded 8 km over a sparsely populated region of Siberia, leveling all vegetation for hundreds of square kilometers. Most meteoroids incinerate while entering Earth's atmosphere, as can be witnessed by any falling star on a clear night. In fact, about 100 tons of cosmic material fall to Earth daily, mostly in the form of tiny dust particles.[3] As our understanding and interaction with the cosmos has broadened over the last few decades, we have realized that there are quantifiable risks from impactors to humanity, ranging from locally traumatic to globally cataclysmic. We will address these events as three distinct entities:

1. Local-effect near-Earth object (NEO) impacts
2. Global-effect NEO impacts
3. Artificial orbital debris reentry

The risk posed by an impactor is directly proportional to its size[2] (Table 168-1). Those less than 50 m in diameter will most likely incinerate. Impactors 1 to 2 km in diameter will devastate the area surrounding the impact site. Impactors larger than 2 km in diameter have the potential to cause obliterative local damage, as well as displace large amounts of dust into the stratosphere. The consequent effects would resemble a "nuclear winter," affecting the entire globe, changing entire ecosystems with a resultant drop in global temperature, loss of agricultural productivity, and possible societal breakdown.[2] Since over 70% of the Earth is covered with water, an

ocean impact could cause tsunamis with inland flooding extending tens of kilometers into the coastal plains.

Orbital debris, the artificial residual of the last 40 years of human endeavors into space, is another source of a potential terrestrial impactor. According to the U.S. Air Force Space Command, there are currently over 8900 objects orbiting Earth.[4] Although the vast majority of orbital debris pieces incinerate upon reentry, some components could survive, whether due to heat-resistant material (e.g., shuttle tiles) or a design that sheds heat fast enough to keep object temperatures below the component's melting point. As the *Columbia* space shuttle tragedy demonstrated, controlled reentry can fail, in which case suborbital debris would be expected to survive reentry in greater quantity with a commensurate impact potential on life and property.

 PREINCIDENT ACTIONS

Asteroids and comets are classified as NEOs when they orbit close to the sun (and therefore Earth). NEOs of interest to astronomers addressing the impact hazard are those greater than 150 m in diameter that pass Earth within 1.3 times the average distance from the sun to Earth (93 million miles). The National Aeronautics and Space Administration (NASA)'s goal is to discover 90% of all NEOs with a diameter more than 1 km by 2008.

As of spring 2004, 2883 NEOs have been discovered: 719 of these are asteroids with diameters larger than 1 km, and 607 have been classified as potentially hazardous asteroids. The risk of impact by any specific potentially hazardous asteroid is extremely small, on the order of 10 to 100 times less than the annual risk of a single person being struck by lightning.[5]

NEOs 50 to 1000 m in Diameter

An impactor with a diameter larger than 50 m will reach Earth's surface on average once every 100 years. The composition of the impactor could determine the extent and type of local damage. If the object has less physical coherence, such as a loosely bound, low-density comet

TABLE 168-1   TERRESTRIAL EFFECTS OF IMPACTORS

ENVIRONMENTAL EFFECT	CATEGORY (IMPACTOR DIAMETER)		
	REGIONAL DISASTER (300 M)	CIVILIZATION ENDER (2 KM)	K/T EXTINCTOR (10–15 KM)
Fires ignited by fireball and/or reentering ejecta	Localized fire at ground zero.	Fires ignited only within hundreds of km of ground zero.	Global fire storms.
Stratospheric dust obscures sunlight	Stratospheric dust below catastrophic levels.	Sunlight drops to "very cloudy day" (nearly globally); global agriculture threatened by summertime freezes.	Global night; vision is impossible Severe, multiyear "impact winter."
Other atmospheric effects: sulfate aerosols, water injected into stratosphere, ozone destruction, nitric acid, smoke, etc.	None (except locally).	Sulfates and smoke augment effects of dust; ozone layer may be destroyed.	Synergy of all factors yields decade-long winter. Approaches level that would acidify oceans (more likely by sulfuric acid than nitric acid).
Earthquakes	Local ground shaking.	Significant damage within hundreds of km of ground zero.	Modest to moderate damage globally.
Tsunamis	Flooding of historic proportions along shores of proximate ocean.	Shorelines of proximate ocean flooded inland tens of km.	Primary and secondary tsunamis flood most shorelines ~100 km inland, inundating low-lying areas worldwide.
Total destruction in crater zone	Crater zone ~5–10 km across.	Crater zone ~50 km across.	Crater zone several hundred kilometers across.

From: Chapman CR, Durda DD, Gold T. The comet/asteroid impact hazard: a systems approach. Southwest Research Institute Web site. Available at: http://www.boulder.swri.edu/clark/neowp.html; and Toon OB, Zahnle K, Morrison D, et al. Environmental perturbations caused by the impacts of asteroids and comets. *Rev Geophysics.* 1997;35:41–78.

body containing ice, it might not remain whole prior to impact and could explode in the atmosphere over Earth's surface. Scientists believe this happened in the *Tunguska* explosion over Siberia on June 30, 1908.

Generally, the diametrical sizes at which incoming objects will break apart when they enter Earth's atmosphere are 540 m for icy objects, 330 m for rocks, and 200 m for solid iron. These objects will change shape, flattening out to 5 to 10 times their original diameters because of the immense heat and pressure generated as they pass through the atmosphere. A surface impact will excavate material dependent on incoming velocity and angle of impact, resulting in a crater 10 to 25 times the size of the impactor. One model estimates that the 40-km-diameter Puchezh-Katunky crater in Russia was created by a 2-km diameter rocky asteroid moving at a velocity of 20 km/sec with a 45-degree angle of impact.[6,7,8] This impact destroyed near-surface layers of land to a depth of 100 m up to 40 km from the center of the impact.

Impactors less than 1 km in size are expected to have locally devastating effects, including total destruction within the resulting crater, thermal radiation surface fires, air blast compression, tidal wave flooding of low-lying areas, and compression wave injuries well beyond the crater zone. An event such as the *Tunguska* explosion might have occurred with minimal impact on humanity; however, if delayed by only a few hours, the more populous regions of Europe (and millions of lives) would have been in jeopardy.

NEOs 1 to 2 km in Diameter

Impacts from NEOs larger than 1 km in diameter are thought to occur, on average, every few hundred thou-sand years. NEOs of this size can have globally devastating effects; the resulting crater could reach 50 km in diameter. Debris would be launched into the stratosphere, blocking sunlight and threatening agricultural production globally. Super-heated impact debris would rain back down on Earth's surface. An ocean impact would produce flooding tens of kilometers inland. Although rare, we have witnessed such an impact in the last decade within our solar system. The comet Shoemaker-Levy 9 impacts on Jupiter in 1994 were a series of 20 discernible impact fragments ranging up to 2 km in diameter. Had this comet hit Earth, it would have killed billions of people and risked most species on our planet.[9]

NEOs 10 to 15 km in Diameter

NEOs 10 to 15 km in diameter will strike Earth even less frequently, on the order of once every 500,000 years. Global "earthquakes" from the impact, tsunamis, and total destruction over hundreds of kilometers would culminate in nuclear winter that would ensue for decades. The effect of such an impact would result in major global climate change, such as that which triggered the demise of the dinosaurs.

Orbital Debris

Orbital debris is the artificial byproduct of the last 50 years of human endeavors into space. According to U.S. Strategic Command, orbital debris can be categorized as 7% operational satellites, 15% rocket bodies, and about 78% fragmentation and inactive satellites.[4] The further degradation of these objects is facilitated by solar heating and solar radiation, component explosions, and debris collisions. Motor casings, aluminum oxide exhaust particles, motor-liner residuals, release bolts, solid-fuel fragments, paint chips, and insulation are only some of the 70,000 objects approximately 2 cm in size that have been observed at altitudes 850 to 1000 km above Earth (Space Shuttles and the International Space Station orbit at 340–400 km).[10]

Although the intense pressure and heat of reentry will incinerate much of the mass of orbital debris, some satellite components can withstand this process. Components that have a sufficiently high melting temperature or a shape that allows rapid heat dispersal will have a higher probability of persisting. When debris pieces enter the lower regions of the atmosphere, they will lose velocity, begin to cool, and fall virtually straight down from the sky at relatively low speeds (terminal velocity); these are clearly a potential hazard to life and property.

Although NASA attempts to track orbital debris and predict where debris from a randomly reentering satellite will hit Earth, it is an uncertain science: the atmospheric density varies greatly at high altitudes, thus confounding the calculation of reentrant drag. Other confounding factors include variations in the gravitational field, solar radiation pressure, and atmospheric drag. The predicted time to reentry is generally accurate to within 10% of the actual time, although this translates to a margin of error of several miles on the ground. Over the last 40 years, more than 1400 metric tons of materials are believed to have survived reentry without report of injury.[4]

In the event that Earth becomes at risk of being hit by a moderate to large impactor, we would likely know well in advance, perhaps by several years to decades. There would be an immediate, intense psychological reaction in the public, with likely intense media coverage and speculation. An incredible challenge would be posed to scientists, public health officials, and political leaders to relay the known risks and possible solutions to the public accurately. A discordance between calculated risks and publicly perceived risks can be expected, contributing to widespread fear and even mass hysteria.[11] Familiar doomsday scenario patterns of behavior are likely to emerge on the fringes of society. Mental health providers could expect an increase in anxiety, depression, or both among a large portion of the population.

POSTINCIDENT ACTIONS

As previously discussed, the risk of damage of an impactor is related to its size, and casualties and property damage should be treated as patients would be in other mass-casualty incidents.

Meteorites are classified as "irons" (nickel-iron metal) or "stones." *Stones* can be divided into two subgroups: chondrites and achondrites. *Chondrites* (about 86% of stones) are aggregates of early solar system materials that have not been significantly altered since formation of the solar system. Achondrites (about 8% of stones) are the products of melting and recrystallization of mostly magnesian silicates. One percent of meteorites are a conglomerate of those two types (called *stony irons*).

When a meteorite strikes, it does so at terminal velocity and has therefore cooled from the intense temperatures of atmospheric entry. The outer layer, or fusion crust, is usually 1 to 2 mm thick, the rest having burned off during entry and generally posing no risk of burn from contact (silicate materials are traditionally poor conductors of heat). There are reports of eyewitnesses picking up an object that has fallen, cracking it in two, and discovering ice particles. Meteorites are composed of materials that are abundantly found on Earth and pose no toxic or radiation risk.

Historically, the controlled reentry of large components of artificial orbital material (Skylab, Mir) has been directed to remote, uninhabited parts of the planet (oceans). As seen with *Columbia*, however, spacecraft components can return to Earth relatively intact. Beyond the risk of impact, they can pose a toxicologic risk. Rocket propellants such as hydrazine and nitrogen tetroxide pose a chemical burn and inhalation risk. Structural materials such as beryllium have been known to cause pulmonary damage. Other potential hazards include ammonia, radiation sources (e.g., radioactive altimeters, live ordnance (e.g., pyrotechnics for emergency hatch opening), and other exotic compounds (e.g., scientific payloads, solar arrays, environmental control items such as lithium perchlorate and permanganate). Currently, there are no known nuclear-powered devices (e.g., powered by uranium) in orbit.

Once an orbital debris piece is committed to a reentrant trajectory, it will fracture and scatter over a predictable pattern based on mass. The "footprint" of debris will consist of heavier objects at the "heel" of the footprint and lighter objects at the "toe."

In the certain cases of reentry events, forensic and possibly national security concerns will necessitate the mobilization of law enforcement personnel across several jurisdictions. As seen with *Columbia* in 2002, a concerted effort between law enforcement agencies in several states and NASA, coupled with direct appeals to the public, were initiated to preserve the integrity of the debris sites and to preclude souvenir hunters from disturbing debris fields. In such cases, mobilization of the military (national security concerns or naval salvage) may be deemed necessary, as well as international coordination if debris fields cross national borders.

MEDICAL TREATMENT OF CASUALTIES

There is nothing unique to the medical treatment of casualties from the events discussed in this chapter. Blunt trauma is the likely mechanism of smaller impactors, expanding to burn and blast injuries for larger impactors. For large-scale impactors approaching the 1-km-diameter mark, humanitarian/refugee crises will be a major concern.

Psychological treatment will be another important consideration in any impactor scenario. Often even the smallest meteorite impacts are covered widely in the news media and may trigger anxiety and concern in otherwise unaffected portions of society. Mental health will be a major concern in the event of an orbital debris impact involving the loss of life. The scope of such a tragedy on the national psyche can affect all segments of the population, and there is a risk of the infliction of depression and posttraumatic stress disorder.

Special concern should be made for those suffering personal loss. Despite efforts to shield them from further anguish, astronauts and other NASA staff (not unlike the New York City firefighters after the World Trade Center bombings on September 11, 2001) played a major role in the search for the remains of *Columbia*, prompting concerns of exacerbating already severe mental trauma.

 ## UNIQUE CONSIDERATIONS

Perhaps unique to this chapter is the potential scope of the disaster. If an NEO larger than 1 to 2 km in diameter was identified as a probable Earth impactor, the need for international coordination would be unprecedented. The logistical scope of such an endeavor would be daunting. Whereas protocols are in place among astronomic groups to verify impactors and their risks before a public announcement, the ramifications of living in the age of the Internet could easily unglue efforts to sequester such proceedings. Initial efforts would likely focus on understanding the shape, configuration, mineral composition, and spin state of an impactor. These characteristics would further clarify risk and, potentially, a strategy for deflection using existing technology of conventional rockets and explosives.[12] Future strategies could include attaching solar sails or engines to the NEO to deflect its path.

A final consideration should be mentioned. As space-related technology proliferates and becomes more accessible over the next decades, satellites and space vehicles may become susceptible targets for terrorists, particularly as an impactor over urban areas, power/chemical complexes, or military targets.

 ## PITFALLS

One pitfall that should be anticipated with any impactor event is relying on uninterrupted global communication. The effects of an impactor entering the ionosphere may disrupt satellite communication and possible security networks. It is reported that those who have observed meteor "fireballs" before impact experience a metallic taste sensation, possibly due to an electromagnetic disturbance.

HELPFUL WEB SITES

- http://impact.arc.nasa.gov; NASA asteroid and comet impact hazards
- http://neo.jpl.nasa.gov; NASA Near Earth Orbit Program Web site

REFERENCES

1. Chyba CF, Owen TC, Ip W-H. "Impact Delivery of Volatiles and Organic Molecules to Earth." In: Gehrels T, ed. *Hazards Due to Comets & Asteroids*. University of Arizona Press. Tucson, AZ. 1994:9-58.
2. Morrison D, Chapman CR, Slovic P. "The Impact Hazard". In: Gehrels T, ed. *Hazards Due to Comets & Asteroids*. University of Arizona Press. Tucson, AZ. 1994:59-92.
3. Kyte FT, Wasson JT. Accretion rate of extraterrestrial matter: iridium deposited 33 to 67 million years ago. *Science* 232:1225-9, 1986.
4. U.S. Air Force Space Command Web site. Available at: http://fas.org/spp/military/ program/track/mccall.pdf. McCall, G.H. "Space Surveillance." Last accessed October 27, 2005.
5. Chapman CR, Durda DD, Gold RE. The comet/asteroid impact hazard: a systems approach. Southwest Research Institute Web site. Available at: http://www.boulder.swri.edu/clark/neowp.html.
6. Ivanov BA. Geomechanical models of impact cratering [abstract]. Presented at the International Conference On Large Meteorite Impacts and Planetary Evolution. Sudbury, Canada, 1992:40.
7. Pevzner LA, Kirijakov A, Vorontsov A, et al. Vorotilovskay drillhole: first deep drilling in the central uplift of large terrestrial impact crater [abstract]. *Lunar Planet Sci.* 1992;XXIII:1063-4.
8. Shoemaker EM. "Interpretation of lunar craters." In: Kapal Z, ed. *Physics and Astronomy of the Moon.* 1962:283-359. New York: Academic Press (Elsevier).
9. A'Hearn M. "The impacts of D/Shoemaker-Levy 9 and bioastronomy." In: *Astronomical and Biochemical Origins and the Search for Life in the Universe.* Proceedings of the 5th international conference on bioastronomy (held in Capri, Italy July 1-5, 1996), IAU Colloquium 161. Published in Bologna, Italy: Editrice Compositori, 1997: 165.
10. NASA Office of Space Operations Website (Dawn Brooks, editor). Available at: *http://www.hq.nasa. gov/osf/station/viewing/history.html.*
11. Benjamin GC. Managing terror: public health officials learn lessons from bioterrorism attacks. *Physician Exec.* 2002;28:80-3.
12. Ahrens TJ, Harris AW. "Deflection and Fragmentation of Near-Earth Asteroids." In: Gehrels T, ed. *Hazards Due to Comets & Asteroids*. University of Arizona Press. Tucson, AZ. 1994:897-928.

chapter 169

Building Collapse

Catherine Y. Lee and Timothy Davis

 ## DESCRIPTION OF EVENT

The attacks on Sept. 11, 2001, shocked the American public with the destruction of the World Trade Center towers. It also brought to the forefront of disaster medicine the danger of building collapse, or *progressive collapse*, a principal if not the leading cause of injury and death in building failures.[1] In the engineering world, progressive collapse has been studied for 40 years since the 1968 Ronan Point disaster.[2] Progressive collapse is a "chain reaction of structural failures that follow from damage to a relatively small portion of a structure" or "the spread of an initial local failure from element to element that eventually results in the collapse of an entire structure or a disproportionately large part of it."[3,4] Simply stated, progressive collapse is a "domino effect," causing the sequential collapse of one floor on top of lower floors.[3] In this chapter, the terms *building collapse, structural collapse*, and *progressive collapse* are used interchangeably.

There are six causes of building collapse: bad design, faulty construction, foundation failure, extraordinary loads, unexpected failure, and a combination of these causes. Some causes of bad design are errors in engineering computation, failure to consider all stresses and weights, reliance on inaccurate data, and poor choice of materials.[5] Faulty construction may be the most common reason for building collapse around the world. It results from the use of inferior steel, bad riveting, infirm fastening and securing, and bad welds.[5] In the case of foundation failure, the earth beneath a building may be unsuitable to support the weight of the building. Such is the case during an earthquake, when buildings are shaken off their mountings if built on top of unstable soil or not properly tied to their foundations.[6] Extraordinary loads, which exceed the normal calculated stress that a building can withstand, include earthquakes, tornadoes, tsunamis, or man-generated events such as a motor vehicle striking a key support pillar, a gas explosion, or a bombing.[4] For example, explosions damage buildings due to extremely high, instantaneous pressures from the blast wave.[3] Depending on the size of the explosion, distance from the building, and sturdiness of building construction, an explosion can induce progressive collapse in a matter of milliseconds.[3] The blast will first target the weakest point of the building closest to the detonation

and push onto the exterior walls of the lower floors, leading to wall failure and window breakage.[3] While the shock wave expands, it enters the structure and pushes upwards and downwards, onto all floors of the building, inducing collapse.[3] The reflection of the oncoming, or *incident*, blast wave against hindering structures like hard surfaces of a building's exterior, can lead to additional pressures up to 13 times greater than the peak incident pressure.[3,7] Laboratory tests have shown that surfaces exposed perpendicularly to the incident blast wave may experience pressures up to 5000 psi,[3] yet typical window glass breaks at an incident overpressure of 0.15 to 0.22 psi.[3]

 ## PREINCIDENT ACTIONS

Although engineers note that progressive collapse cannot be totally prevented from occurring, they agree that tools can be designed to improve building performance to resist or improve building performance against collapse.[1,8] National institutes encourage designing multihazard resistance and mitigation suitable to withstand progressive collapse from all threats including natural and technologic disasters.[1] Specific mitigation against terrorist bombings focuses more on window and glass hazards, stand-off distancing, and "hardening" of the exterior. Site design and modification for perimeter defense using soil, bollards, planters, and retaining walls in addition to increasing stand-off distance between the facility and possible threats (such as a truck bomb) can deter and delay terrorist attack capable of insinuating building collapse.[3] Strategies to limit parking, vehicular entry, and access inside or near the structure are additional methods for mitigation.[3] But once these measures have failed, structural "hardening" to fortify the building's exterior is used to mitigate the effects of an explosion once it has occurred. The objective of designing the exterior wall is to ensure that structures like walls, doors, and windows fail in a flexible mode, as opposed to a brittle mode that would induce shear and result in multiple fragments of cement, glass, and other materials capable of serious injury.[3] In the 1998 bombings of the U.S. Embassies in Kenya and Tanzania, the U.S. Department of State found: "Although there was little structural damage to the five-story reinforced concrete building, the explosion reduced much of the interior to rubble—destroying windows, window frames, internal office partitions and other fixtures on the rear side of the building. The secondary fragmentation from flying glass, internal concrete block walls, furniture, and fixtures caused most of the embassy casualties."[1,8,9] Nonstructural components such as ceiling fixtures, lights, windows, office equipment, computers, files, air conditioners, electrical equipment, and objects stored on shelves and hung on walls can also become an injury hazard.[3,6] In an earthquake, these nonstructural elements are likely to be unhooked, dislodged, and flung, causing injury and damage.[3] Additionally, the U.S. Federal Emergency Management Agency recommends that building design be optimized to facilitate emergency rescue and response, allowing feasible evacuation, rescue, and recovery efforts through effective placement, structural design, and redundancy of emergency exits and electrical/mechanical systems.[3]

 ## POSTINCIDENT ACTIONS

After a building collapse, trapped survivors requiring quick rescue "where minutes count" are rare. An expeditious headlong, poorly planned ingress into the "hot zone" can risk valuable human assets with limited potential benefit. The rules for traumatic arrest still apply—attempts to resuscitate persons with blunt traumatic arrest are typically futile.

The bulk of surviving casualties will arrive over a 60-minute period at the closest hospitals(s), either self-transported or transported by emergency medical services (EMS). Disaster managers should expect high resource utilization from hospitalized survivors, far exceeding the benchmark comparisons for similar injury severity score (ISS) casualties. Critically injured progressive collapse survivors can be compared with casualties of explosive injury, and they require an extraordinary amount of hospital resources. Hospitalized explosion survivors have longer than usual hospital and intensive care unit length of stay, more surgeries, and more ventilator time, and they are more often discharged to a rehabilitation facility compared with ISS-equivalent casualties of motor vehicle or gunshot wounds.[10,11]

Some general emergency management options apply:

1. Follow your hospital and regional disaster system plan.
2. Expect increased severity and delayed arrival of casualties.
3. Expect an "upside-down" triage—the most severely injured arrive after the less injured, who bypass EMS triage and go directly to the closest hospitals.[12]
4. Double the first hour's casualties for a rough prediction of total first wave of casualties.[12]
5. Obtain and record details about the nature of the event, potential toxic exposures and environmental hazards, and casualty location using all reliable informants including local police and fire departments, EMS, Incident Command System, regional emergency management agency, local health department, and eyewitness casualties. The need for epidemiologic injury data is an imperative national agenda.[13]

 ## MEDICAL TREATMENT

Progressive structural collapse produces casualty and injury patterns similar to earthquakes and can be more severe than blast injuries alone.[14] The final casualty toll and injury pattern depend most on preexisting circumstances: time of day, occupancy, warning, evacuation proficiency, individual health status, and building design and materials. The majority of casualty survivors will have minor injuries and require only outpatient or self-care. Standard penetrating and blunt trauma to any body surface is the most common injury seen among survivors, with the most severely injured consisting of burns, traumatic amputations, and head, chest, and abdominal injuries.[14-16] Characteristic injuries seen in building collapse are shown in Table 169-1. Frykberg notes a substantial amount of immediate death and constant critical mortality rate among victims of a terrorist bombing building collapse, despite differences in TNT-equivalents of blast force.[16]

Most persons caught in the direct path of the collapse will not survive and will either be dead on-scene or dead on arrival, regardless of postcollapse rescue efforts. Trapped survivors are most often found in air spaces adjacent to partially intact support structures. Few survivors are rescued after the first 24 hours, although young children can be an exception. More than half of all children may have head or face trauma. Because children's airways can be easily occluded, the primary cause of cardiopulmonary arrest in children may be respiratory. Therefore, children in cardiopulmonary arrest should first have their airways cleared. If there is no spontaneous pulse or respirations, they too are unsalvageable and CPR should not be initiated.

Most casualties will meet either anatomic, physiologic, or mechanism of injury criteria to be transported immediately to a level I or II trauma center, and limited scene time remains the standard. Assume crush syndrome and rhabdomyolysis for any casualty trapped for longer than 1 hour. Compartment syndrome, rhabdomyolysis, and acute renal failure are associated with structural collapse, prolonged extrication, severe burns, and some poisonings. All casualties with substantial blunt injuries should be screened for acidosis, electrolyte imbalance, and renal failure. Resuscitation efforts should focus on correcting the underlying cause—for example, fasciotomy or benzodiazepine for agitation or seizures; crystalloid for treating volume depletion, correcting acidosis with sodium bicarbonate; and hemodialysis for renal failure or intractable hyperkalemia.

 ## UNIQUE CONSIDERATIONS

Traumatic amputation of any limb may be a marker for multisystem injuries, since such injuries usually result from close proximity to a blast.[17,18] Wounds can be grossly contaminated. Consider delaying primary closure until after an assessment of tetanus status has been performed. Ensure close follow-up of wounds, head

TABLE 169-1   MECHANISMS OF INJURY ASSOCIATED WITH PROGRESSIVE COLLAPSE

CATEGORY	CHARACTERISTICS	BODY PART AFFECTED	TYPES OF INJURIES
Penetrating Injury	Results from flying debris and fragments.	Any body part may be affected	Penetrating ballistic (fragmentation) Eye penetration (can be occult)
Blunt Injury	Results from falling objects, blown debris, or persons being thrown by the blast wind.	Any body part may be affected.	Fracture and traumatic amputation Closed and open brain injury
Primary Blast Injury	Unique to high explosives, results from the impact of the overpressurization wave with body surfaces.	Gas-filled structures are most susceptible (i.e., lungs, GI tract, and middle ear).	Blast lung (pulmonary barotrauma) TM rupture and middle ear damage Abdominal hemorrhage and perforation Globe (eye) rupture Concussion (TBI without physical signs of head injury)
Other	All injuries, illnesses, or diseases not due to penetrating, blunt, or primary blast injury. Includes exacerbation or complications of existing conditions	Any body part may be affected.	Burns (flash, partial, and full thickness) Crush injuries Closed and open brain injury Asthma, COPD, or other breathing problems from dust, smoke, or toxic fumes Angina Hyperglycemia, hypertension

GI, Gastrointestinal; TM, tympanic membrane; TBI, traumatic brain injury; COPD, chronic obstructive pulmonary disease.

CASE PRESENTATION

Newham, London, was a newly developed borough in 1968, spotted with brand new apartment towers and promising an upgraded lifestyle from the previous dirty and rundown homes that had characterized West and East Ham towns. Using an engineering method that was perceived as safe and quick in construction, the Ronan Point Apartment Tower was built in 2 years, opening in 1968 as a 210-foot-high building consisting of over 100 flats. Tenants moved in immediately. The apartment building had been occupied for only 2 months when a natural gas explosion on an 18th floor apartment triggered the structural failure of an entire corner of flats. Subsequent floors below were blown out, allowing a domino-effect collapse of wall and floor sections from the top to the ground. The majority of the 260 residents fled down stairwells in advance of the collapse that toppled floors like a deck of cards. However, four people died immediately as a result of the blast although more could have died if the flats were completely occupied. An elderly patient died later in hospital, leading to a total of 17 injured survivors.

Residents saw the design failures such as use of cost-cutting when choosing building materials, poor workmanship, and lack of adequate building inspection as the reasons for the building collapse. Ronan Point was demolished in 1986, and fewer towers have been built since the disaster.

injuries, and complaints related to the patient's eyes, ears, and stress level. Air embolism can occur and can present as stroke, myocardial infarction, acute abdomen, blindness, deafness, spinal cord injury, or claudication. Hyperbaric oxygen therapy may be effective in some cases.[19,20]

If collapse was preceded by an explosion, clinical signs of blast-related abdominal injuries can be initially silent until signs of acute abdomen or sepsis are advanced.[21] Primary blast lung and blast abdomen after explosions are associated with high mortality rates.[22,23] The symptoms of mild traumatic brain injury (e.g., concussion) and posttraumatic stress disorder might be identical.[24]

Auditory system injuries and concussions are easily overlooked. Communications and instructions may need to be written because of tinnitus and sudden temporary or permanent deafness.[25] Consider the possibility of exposure to inhaled toxins and poisonings (e.g., carbon monoxide, cyanide, methemoglobin) in both industrial and criminal explosions.[26]

In August 2003, a military hospital in Mozdok, Russia, was bombed, resulting in the partial building collapse of the 3-story structure killing 41 people and entrapping nurses, doctors, and personnel.[27] A hospital building collapse can result in the loss of a critical community resource that cannot be easily replaced.

Lastly, crowd surge or stampede can be more deadly than the original event. On January 27, 2002, a large military ammunition dump in Lagos, Nigeria, exploded, immediately killing 300. But another 800 persons, including small children, were trampled to death during the mass exodus that left several blocks of buildings completely and partially collapsed.[28]

 PITFALLS

Several potential pitfalls in response to a building collapse exist.

- Do not discourage buddy rescue and self-transport of casualties. The majority of rescue is conducted by survivors and bystanders. Self-evacuation clears the scene and moves the bulk of the exposed population out of harm's way.

- Do not hold critical casualties in temporary triage sites instead of immediately transporting. Trauma never improves in the field, and trauma's golden hour does not stop for a disaster.
- The U.S. Federal Emergency Medical Treatment and Active Labor Act prevents the expeditious movement of excess outpatient casualties to hospitals with excess outpatient capacity.[29]
- Another pitfall is activating an entire hospital's disaster plan for a distant regional event and not releasing recalled staff in a timely manner. Only the closest one to three hospitals receive the majority of the casualties, and half of all casualties arrive over a 60-minute period.
- Lack of ventilators and cardiac monitors is a common limit or delay in inter-hospital transfer of critical casualties.
- It should not be assumed that all ambulatory casualties are "worried well." All have been exposed to a variable amount of physical trauma and environmental hazards. Israeli pediatric traumatologists have proposed eliminating "Green" or "Minimal" from the triage protocol.[30]
- Adult casualties in cardiopulmonary arrest are either dead or unsalvageable. No attempt should be made to resuscitate beyond confirming the absence of vital signs.

REFERENCES

1. National Research Council. *Blast Mitigation for Structures: 1999 Status Report on the DTRA/TSWG Program.* Washington, DC: National Academy Press; 1999.
2. BBC News Online. 1968: Three die as tower block collapses. Available at: http://news.bbc.co.uk/onthisday/hi/dates /stories/ may/16/ newsid_2514000/2514277.stmA.
3. U.S. Federal Emergency Management Agency. *Risk Management Series: Reference Manual to Mitigate Potential Terrorist Attacks Against Buildings.* Washington, DC: FEMA; 2003.
4. Gould NC. Quantifying the risk for progressive collapse in new and existing buildings. International Risk Management Institute, March 2003. Available at: http://www.irmi.com/expert/Articles/ 2003/Gould03.aspx.
5. Calvert JB. The collapse of buildings: why the World Trade Center towers collapsed. Available at: http://www.du.edu/~jcalvert/tech/ failure.htm.
6. U.S. Federal Emergency Management Agency. What is an earthquake? National Earthquake Hazards Reduction Program. Available at: http://www.fema.gov/hazards/earthquakes/quake. shtm.
7. Boffard KD, MacFarlane C. Urban bomb blast injuries: patterns of injury and treatment. *Surg Ann.* 1993;25:29-47.
8. Multihazard Mitigation Council. *Prevention of Progressive Collapse: Report on the July 2002 National Workshop and Recommendations for Future Efforts.* Washington, DC: Multihazard Mitigation Council of the National Institute of Building Sciences; 2003.
9. U.S. Department of State. Report of the Accountability Review Boards on the Embassy Bombings in Nairobi and Dar es Salaam on August 7, 1998. U.S. Department of State; January 1999. Available at: http://www.state.gov/www/regions/africa/kenya_tanzania. html.
10. Peleg K, Aharonson-Daniel L, Stein M, and the Israeli Trauma Group (ITG). Gunshot and explosion injuries: characteristics, outcomes, and implications for care of terror-related injuries in Israel. *Ann Surg.* 2004;239:311-8.
11. Peleg K, Aharonson-Daniel L, Michael M, Shapira SC, and the Israel Trauma Group. Patterns of injury in hospitalized terrorist victims. *Am J Emerg Med.* 2003;21:258-62.
12. U.S. Centers for Disease Control and Prevention. Explosions and Blast Injuries: A Primer for Clinicians. Available at: http:// www.cdc. gov/masstrauma/preparedness/primer.htm.
13. National Research Council. *Protecting People and Buildings from Terrorism, Technology Transfer for Blast-Effects Mitigation.* Washington, DC: National Academy Press; 2001.
14. Butcher TP. Explosive emergencies treating blast injuries in the field. *JEMS* 1991:50-54.
15. Frykberg ER, Tepas JJ 3rd. Terrorist bombings: lessons learned from Belfast to Beirut. *Ann Surg.* 1988;208:569-76.
16. Frykberg ER. Medical management of disasters and mass casualties from terrorist bombings: how can we cope? *J Trauma.* 2002;53:201-12.
17. Hull JB. Traumatic amputation by explosive blast: pattern of injury in survivors. *Br J Surg.* 1992;79:1303-6.
18. Hull JB, Bowyer GW, Cooper GJ, Crane J. Patterns of injuries in those dying from traumatic amputation caused by bomb blast. *Br J Surg.* 1994;81:1132-5.
19. Guy RJ, Glover MA, Cripps NP. The pathophysiology of primary blast injury and its implications for treatment. Part I: The thorax. *J Royal Nav Med Serv.* 1998;84:79-86.
20. Vavrina J, Muller W. Therapeutic effect of hyperbaric oxygenation in acute acoustic trauma. *Rev Laryngol Otol Rhinol (Bord).* 1995;116:377-80.
21. Wightman JM, Gladish SL. Explosions and blast injuries. *Ann Emerg Med.* 2001;37:664-78.
22. Leibovici D, Gofrit ON, Stein M, et al. Blast injuries: bus versus open-air bombings—a comparative study of injuries in survivors of open-air versus confined-space explosions. *J Trauma.* 1996; 41:1030-5.
23. Stuhmiller LH, Phillips YY, Richmond DR. The physics and mechanisms of primary blast injury, a brief history. In: Bellamy RF, Zajtcjuk JT, eds. *Conventional Warfare: Ballistics, Blast, and Burn Injuries.* Textbook of Military Medicine series. Washington, DC: Office of the Surgeon General at TMM Publications; 1991:241-70.
24. Barrow DW, Rhoades HT. Blast concussion injury. *JAMA* 1944; 125:900-2.
25. Hirsch FG. Effects of overpressure on the ear: a review. *Ann NY Acad Sci.* 1968;152:147-162.
26. Quenemoen LE, Davis YM, Malilay J, et al. The World Trade Center bombing: injury prevention strategies for high-rise building fires. *Disasters* 1996;20:125-32.
27. Tavernise S, Myers SL. Toll in Russia climbs to 41 in bombing at a hospital. *New York Times.* August 3, 2003. Available at: http:// www.sullivan-county.com/bush/41_russia.htm.
28. United Nations Disaster Assessment and Coordination Team, UNDAC Mission to Lagos, Nigeria. *United Nations Disaster Assessment 31 January – 7 February 2002 Munitions Depot Explosion Environmental and Humanitarian Assessment Report.* Geneva, Switzerland, UNDAC (UN Disaster Assessment and Coordination Team), Feb. 7, 2002.
29. American College of Emergency Physicians. EMTALA. Available at: http://www.acep.org/webportal/PracticeResources/ IssuesBy Category/EMTALA/default.htm.
30. Waisman Y, Aharonson-Daniel L, Mor M, et al. The impact of terrorism on children: a two-year experience. *Prehospital Disaster Med.* 2003;18:242-8.

chapter 170

Bridge Collapse

Laura Diane Melville and Najma Rahman-Khan

 ## DESCRIPTION OF EVENTS

On the morning of May 9, 1980, the *Summit Venture* had just entered a difficult portion of the shipping channel leading into Tampa Bay that passed under the Sunshine Skyway Bridge. The boat was a tanker the size of two football fields. A sudden squall blew up and created almost zero visibility, and the ship's radar ceased to function. Based on a number of factors, the captain made the decision to go forward and try to pass under the bridge. The ship rammed the south pier 700 feet from the center of the channel, causing the center span of the Skyway to collapse into the channel below. Several cars and a Greyhound bus disappeared into the Bay. Thirty-five people died in the disaster.[1]

There is such a dearth of medical or disaster planning literature specifically addressing the collapse of bridges that information must be gathered from newspaper and other stories to understand what has happened and what could happen. Most of the time a bridge collapses due to structural failures; however, there can be other causes such as weather (including floods, tornados, earthquakes), explosions (both accidental or nonaccidental), acts of war or terrorism, objects crashing into the bridge (such as a barge), and potential nuclear or dirty bombs. Since the events of Sept. 11, 2001 in New York City, we can easily imagine scenarios in which a bridge with major traffic burdens (including pedestrian, motor, and rail) and significant symbolism (such as the Golden Gate Bridge or the Brooklyn Bridge) becomes a target of a terrorist attack. During war, bridges become targets for those same reasons. The T-shaped Aioi Bridge was the target for "Little Boy"—the atomic bomb dropped on Hiroshima.

It is important to remember that not all bridges cross water. Highway overpasses are essentially bridges, and the collapse of such structures also occurs. This kind of collapse would require interventions more like those required for structural collapses, such as urban search and rescue teams and confined-space medical interventions.

A brief description of the different types of bridges may be useful in understanding the types of risks they are subject to. There are several different types of bridges, such as arch, cable-stayed, suspension, draw span, truss, and beam bridges, with the first three being the most common. Arch bridges are relatively small, usually 130 to 500 feet in length. This type of bridge allows no movement in horizontal bearing, so these bridges are usually located on stable ground and cross over valleys and rivers.

Cable-stayed bridges are usually 300 to 1600 feet long with a continuous bridge that has one or two towers erected in the middle with support cables attaching the bridge to the towers. The towers bear the brunt of the load. This design provides strong support against earthquakes and strong winds but remains vulnerable to shifting or uneven sinking in the ground. The new Sunshine Skyway Bridge is an example of a single-tower cable-stayed bridge.

Suspension bridges, such as the Golden Gate Bridge, usually span about 2000 to 7000 feet. These bridges have cables that are attached to either end to transmit the load to either anchorage. These anchorages at either side provide strong support, but the construction makes the bridge vulnerable to strong winds. The collapse of the Tacoma Narrows Bridge, also known as "Galloping Gertie," is a famous example of the failure of a suspension bridge.[2-4]

The Tacoma Narrows Bridge is a case of a suspension bridge gone wrong. It collapsed in 1940 because of strong winds, but the bridge's undulations were an attraction to locals and tourists for years before the actual collapse. Due to its suspension wire construction, there were both vertical and horizontal undulations in the bridge that contributed to its failure. During some winds, there was as much as a 28-foot disparity between the left and right sides of the bridge. Before that event, there was pressure to construct bridges to maximize "lightness, grace, and flexibility"; however, this collapse forced a reevaluation of this in favor of safety and stability.[2] The impressive amateur video taken just before the collapse can be viewed on the Internet.[3]

Another famous bridge disaster was the May 26, 2002 collapse of the Oklahoma I-40 bridge across the Arkansas River after it was rammed by a empty oil barge. More than a dozen cars and tractor-trailers went into the river, and 14 people died. This disaster was reminiscent of the Sunshine Skyway disaster. Like the former event, there had been a number of prior incidents that could have served as a warning that this was a real possibility. The rescue effort had to be delayed several days because of the murky water conditions. Thirteen people died by drowning, and one died by blunt trauma to the head. According to the National Transportation Safety Board, the bridge may have collapsed because of its old design; had it been retrofitted to modern standards, it may have withstood the impact.[5,6]

Not all bridges transport cars. During the 1997 Israeli Maccabiah Games, a pedestrian bridge (footbridge) passing over the polluted Yarkon River collapsed, killing four athletes and injuring many more. Three of the deaths were attributed to infectious complications caused by ingesting the polluted water. Medical data on the types of injuries sustained in any bridge collapse are exceedingly difficult to access, but the one available abstract reported on the minor injuries sustained by these athletes. Of the 65 people who sustained nonfatal injuries as a direct result of the bridge collapse, the most common anatomic regions of musculoskeletal injuries were the thigh (20.9%), lumbar spine (15.3%), and the foot and ankle (13.3%). The types of injury most commonly reported were sprains (49.0%) and strains (27.6%).[7] However, the abstract had no information about any victims being seriously injured. It seems that all of the athletes who actually fell into the river suffered severe consequences. Information gleaned from newspaper coverage suggests that when motor vehicles or trains are involved, the degree of injury can be much more wide ranging. Material from the Sunshine Skyway collapse and the Oklahoma bridge disaster demonstrate that most of those who died had suffered major trauma, drowning, or in some cases both. Under most circumstances, it is rare for drowning victims to suffer any trauma other than cervical spine injuries.[8,9] This is important for those planning to treat potential victims of injuries resulting from a collapsed bridge.

 PREINCIDENT ACTIONS

Each government agency (state, county, city, township) that manages a public bridge is required by the Federal Highway Administration to have a crisis management plan.[2] These involve such agencies as the police, sheriff, fire, rescue, emergency medical services, coast guard, Army Corp of Engineers, Federal Aviation Administration, and railroads.

Hospitals should be aware of the plans for bridges in their area and should have an understanding of how loss of the transportation route and the influx of patients will affect their facilities. This should be one of the many scenarios envisioned in the hospital disaster plan. A critical factor in this planning should be the expectation that many staff members may not be able to get to or from work—this could mean anyone from cleaning staff to a hospital's only two trauma surgeons. Hospital representatives should be involved in the creation of the federal state and local plans because emergency departments (EDs) can expect to be the center point of any medical consequences. Important issues will be traffic re-routing, designation of receiving hospitals, etc.

There are software programs available such as the Geographical Resource Intranet Portal, created by the Oklahoma Department of Transportation (ODOT), that can overlay all the area roads with information about ability to handle trucks and high traffic volume, locations of hospitals, and other information that can allow a quick return of traffic flow. This program allowed the ODOT to detour traffic within 2 hours after the 2002 collapse of an I-40 bridge.[10] Those hospitals with hyperbaric chambers should be identified in case they are required for victims or rescuers.

Communication issues, both within the hospital and with outside agencies, are paramount and must be addressed prior to the event itself. This is often one of the most challenging parts of developing and implementing a disaster plan, and it should be emphasized in planning and drilling. Search and rescue teams, with divers, will likely be needed for recovery of victims trapped under structures and underwater. There must be planned routes for emergency vehicles and rescue personnel to get to and from the event site. Knowledge of the body of water (e.g., currents and pollutants) could also be critical to effective rescue efforts. If the collapse occurs due to weather, earthquake, or terrorism, there will be damage to other structures and resources including the hospital itself; chemical or nuclear weapons may be involved.[11]

Those who will be performing triage must be clear about the rules of mass-casualty triage, based on the principle of "the greatest good for the greatest number." This is based on the likelihood of successful resuscitation and the resources available. Most mass-casualty triage systems tag patients with black, red, yellow, and green tags corresponding to dead, emergent, urgent, and the walking wounded, respectively. Two examples of this kind of system are the Simple Triage and Rapid Treatment (START) system and the Jump START for pediatric triage.[12] A person removed from cold waters with no vital signs would be extensively resuscitated in non–mass-casualty settings and would be black-tagged in the event of a mass-casualty incident.

If the bridge collapse is part of a large event, the Federal Emergency Management Agency and disaster medical assistance teams may become part of the response after the first few days. Disaster medical assistance teams are designed to be a rapid-response element to supplement local medical care until other federal or contract resources can be mobilized, or until the situation is resolved.[13]

 POSTINCIDENT ACTIONS

It is often impossible to attempt rescue without risk to the rescuer, but it is vital to secure the area as much as possible and ensure the maximum possible safety for everyone on-scene. A collapsed bridge can be particularly dangerous because the elevated structure may continue to break down. Large amounts of debris underwater can endanger divers, as can weather and current conditions. Under certain circumstances, this may include evaluation for any coincidental biologic, chemical, or radiation terrorism.

Plans that are in place must be implemented in an orderly fashion. It is paramount that communication between agencies occurs as smoothly as possible. As in all of the situations addressed in this book, coordination of federal, state, and local resources will lead to the most effective and efficient handling of the situation. The conventional wisdom is that a response team must be able to stand alone for 12 to 24 hours.[11,13] This isolation may be prolonged if the bridge has collapsed due to severe weather conditions or a geologic event such as an earthquake. If the hospital itself has been compromised by the surrounding events (e.g., the power is out because of an earthquake), internal as well as external disaster plans may need to be implemented. Urban search and rescue teams will likely require activation, and preliminary medical care may have to be delivered at the scene for victims who are trapped alive. If there are large numbers of victims, it will be important to bring stable patients to hospitals farthest from the scene. The walking wounded and the worried well often take themselves to the closest hospital, and the severely injured are transported there.[11]

Other disaster management issues that warrant inclusion in hospital disaster plans for bridge collapse include what to do with medical and nonmedical volunteers; hospital capabilities regarding trauma and pediatrics; how and where to transfer patients who require care that cannot be provided; and how to get staff to the facility if the usual traffic routes are not available.

 ## MEDICAL TREATMENT OF CASUALTIES

It is beyond the scope of this chapter to cover the detailed medical treatment of the many types of injuries that could be seen in the event of a bridge collapse. These topics are covered in other sections of the book. For any bridge over water, near-drowning will be an important mechanism of injury to expect. Although near-drowning injuries are not typically associated with other trauma, this scenario has been shown to produce both blunt injury and drowning. It is likely that the trauma victims in this situation were incapacitated by their injuries and drowned secondarily.

Blast injuries will occur if there are any explosions. Primary blast injury occurs as a direct effect of changes in atmospheric pressure caused by a blast wave. Secondary blast injuries occur when objects accelerated by the energy of the explosion strike a victim, causing either blunt or penetrating ballistic trauma. Tertiary blast injuries result from a victim's body being displaced by expanding gases and high winds; trauma then occurs from tumbling and colliding with objects. Primary blast injury mostly occurs in gas-containing organ systems, notably the middle ear, lungs, and bowel. Few victims of primary blast injury survive to require treatment.[14]

Hypothermia may be a factor complicating the care of both submersed and entrapped patients; however, it may in fact improve survival and neurologic outcome in some patients, particularly the drowning victims. The principle that the patient is "not dead till warm and dead" is the norm for emergency medicine,[11] but if disaster triage protocols have been implemented, patients who do not have respirations or a pulse will not be resuscitated regardless of their temperature. These are the patients who will likely present the most difficult ethical and emotional challenge for personnel on-scene and at receiving hospitals.

Any victims trapped under rubble or in crushed vehicles can sustain crush injuries and may require treatment based on principles of confined-space medicine at the scene and on arrival in the ED. Head injuries are also common. As described above, pollution may complicate the treatment requirements of submersion victims. As in any disaster, stress-related exacerbations of medical illness and psychological issues will require intervention for victims, responders, and family members.[11,15]

CASE PRESENTATION

It is mid-February, and you and one other ED attending physician are working the night shift at a level II trauma center. About 2 miles away is an interstate highway that crosses the large river in your area. The university level 1 trauma center is across the river. In fact, quite a few of your staff work at both hospitals and live on the other side of the river. The bridge is old and scheduled for repairs in the next fiscal year. Your hospital has participated in the local Office of Emergency Management and Federal Highway Management Office's disaster planning.

It is 6:00 AM, and you are getting ready for change of shift. A couple of residents come in from a smoke break and tell you they think they heard thunder, but it is a bright, beautiful day. You tell them they should quit smoking and get ready to hand over the ED. About 15 minutes later, your EMS phone rings and you are notified that there has been a terrible accident—a large fuel truck has exploded and caused the bridge to collapse. You are on standby to receive up to 50 patients. There are several vehicles on fire, and several have plunged into the icy waters below. No one is quite sure what happened, and rumors of terrorism are already spreading among your staff. Because the traffic was two-way, there are injured persons on both sides of the bridge—those on your side will be coming to your hospital regardless of their degree of injury.

You notify your hospital administrator and initiate your disaster plan, including additional triage areas, notifying the operating room and all your surgeons. The clinic down the hall from your ED is opened to handle non-urgent patients. Your department chairman calls to say she is on her way in by police department helicopter, which will land nearby because your facility does not have a helipad.

Patients are beginning to come in now, and your beds are filling up. Several are critically injured, with burns and blunt trauma. No victims have been recovered from the waters yet, but the coast guard is almost on scene and the search and rescue team is also en route. There are questions about chemical exposure. Several cardiologists who live next to the hospital have just arrived in the ED to help, along with a number of neighbors who want to give blood. You are the Incident Commander for your hospital and are constantly on the phone with EMS, police and fire personnel, and your counterpart at University General. More staff is on the way in. You hear the rescue divers are having trouble getting to victims because of river conditions, but your first hypothermic near-drowning victim is on his way in, by Basic Life Support (BLS) with a faint pulse and an unobtainable blood pressure reading....

UNIQUE CONSIDERATIONS

Bridges are most likely to collapse due to a combination of severe environmental circumstance, structural flaws, and wear and tear. However, sudden collapse caused by structural failure, impact, or attack can occur. Staff may not be able to come to work or get home if the bridge is critical for access to that area or if traffic becomes intensely snarled.

Although drowning victims rarely have concurrent traumatic injuries other than cervical spine injuries, people in vehicles that slam into water and then submerge will suffer both insults. Most are unlikely to survive severe traumatic injury followed by submersion, but a patient with these types of injuries should be anticipated in this scenario. Collapse of bridges that do not cross water may lead to trapped and crushed victims requiring intervention more like those for other structural collapses, as described in studies of confined-space medicine. In addition, exposure to polluted water could lead to chemical toxicity and overwhelming sepsis.

PITFALLS

Several potential pitfalls in response to a bridge collapse exist. These include the following:

- Failure to plan for collapse of any local or important bridge
- Failure to be aware of and incorporate plans already in place by state and local authorities
- Failure to have hospital disaster plans in place prior to an incident
- Failure to include the possibility of bridge collapse in plans for larger events such as earthquakes, flooding, or a terrorist attack
- Failure to consider larger events (e.g., earthquake or flood) when planning for a possible bridge collapse
- Failure to consider that such larger events (e.g., earthquake or flood) may compromise the functioning of the hospital itself

- Lack of knowledge regarding water conditions, including level of pollution and chemical content of polluted water
- Failure to plan alternate ways for staff to get to the hospital

REFERENCES

1. "A blinding squall, then death" St. Petersburg Times. Available at www2.sptimes.com/weather/SW.2.html.
2. Northwestern University's Infrastructure Technology Institute's Bridge Disaster Links Page. Available at: http://www.iti.nwu.edu/links/bridges/disasters.html.
3. Mark Ketchum's Bridge Collapse Page. Available at: http://www.ketchum.org/bridgecollapse.html.
4. NOVA Online. Super Bridge: Resources. Available at: http://www.pbs.org/wgbh/nova/bridge/resources.html.
5. CNN.com Divers find three victims from bridge collapse May 27, 2002 Available at: http://archives.cnn.com/2002/US/05/26/barge.bridge.
6. CBS news Web site. Still searching for the bodies. Available at: http://www.cbsnews.com/stories/2002/ 05/28/national/main 510320.shtml.
7. Kolt GS, Wajswelner H, Adonis M, et al. *Injury Toll Following the Maccabiah Games Bridge Collapse: Implications for Sports Medicine Coverage.* Adelaide, Australia: Australian Conference of Science and Medicine in Sport; 1998.
8. Olshaker JS. Submersion. *Emerg Med Clin North Am.* 2004;22:357.
9. Orlowski JP, Szpilman D. Drowning rescue, resuscitation and reanimation. *Pediatr Clin North Am.* 2001;48:627–46.
10. Adams J. ODOT gets a GRIP on transportation. May 1, 2003. Available at: http://www.geospatial-online.com/geospatialsolutions/article /articleDetail.jsp?id=56069.
11. Hogan DE, Burnstein JL, eds. *Disaster Medicine.* Philadelphia: Lippincott, Williams and Wilkins; 2002.
12. Lovejoy JC. Initial approach to patient management after large-scale disasters. *Clin Pediatr Emerg Med.* 2002;3:217–23.
13. U.S. Department of National Security. National Disaster Medical System Web site. Available at: http://www.oep-ndms.dhhs.gov.
14. Wightman JM, Gladish SL. Explosions and blast injuries. *Ann Emerg Med.* 2001;37:664–78.
15. Barbera JA, Lozano M. Urban search and rescue medical teams: FEMA task force systems. *Prehospital Disaster Med.* 1993; 8;349-55.

chapter 171

Human Stampede

Angela M. Mills and C. Crawford Mechem

 DESCRIPTION OF EVENT

Human stampede is one of the most disastrous examples of human crowd behavior. Triggers include building fires and evacuations and a rush for ingress or egress at large sporting events or concerts. In large crowd stampedes, there are often serious injuries and fatalities resulting from crushing and trampling. On Nov. 28, 1942, a fire began at the Coconut Grove, a popular Boston nightclub, causing widespread panic and a stampeding crowd. Inward-opening doors and doors sealed shut prevented escape. As a result, 491 persons died and over 400 were injured.[1] On Apr. 15, 1989, during a semifinal cup soccer game in Sheffield, England, there was a large crushing incident of late-arriving fans who entered a confined area at the Hillsborough stadium. Persons were unable to escape this area due to a surrounding fence; 95 died and more than 400 required hospital treatment.[2,3] These are only two examples of countless episodes of human stampede.

A model for crowd disasters aids in understanding the causes, prevention, and alleviation of an ongoing incident. The four elements of this model form the acronym *FIST* and include the force (F) of the crowd or crowd pressure; information (I), whether real or perceived, on which the crowd acts; physical space (S) involved in the disaster; and time (T) or duration of the event.[4] Forces are generated by persons pushing and leaning against each other. There is often a lack of communication from front to back in a crowd, with persons in the rear pushing forward, injuring those in front. As individuals are injured or fall, they become obstacles to the movement of others. Access to the fallen becomes impossible.[4,5] Large numbers of humans involved in a disaster event tend to exhibit mass behavior and do what others do. As people crowd and jamming occurs, alternative exits are frequently overlooked or not used adequately, resulting in additional injuries.[6]

Escape panics have been studied extensively and have the following characteristics. Panicking persons attempt to move faster than usual and begin pushing and having physical contact with others. This movement, especially around bottlenecks, becomes uncoordinated. Exits become clogged. The pressures generated by a crowd may exceed 4500 N (1000 lb), allowing steel railings to bend and brick walls to fall.[4,6,7]

The widening of a corridor has been demonstrated to slow down movement of panicking persons rather than allowing for faster movement. In a study performed with mice, the most efficient escape was a door large enough for only one mouse to fit through at a time. As door widths were increased, the mice ceased lining up and began competing with one another, prolonging the escape rate.[8] This behavior also pertains to rushing pedestrians who will block an exit that they could safely pass through at walking speed. Jamming and clogging may be minimized in the construction of venues by avoiding bottlenecks and placing columns asymmetrically in front of exits to improve outflow.[6]

A human stampede leads to various injuries and fatalities, with traumatic asphyxia being the most common cause of death and serious injury. The majority of deaths are due to compressive asphyxia as persons are stacked vertically on top of one another or horizontally with associated pushing and leaning forces. Traumatic asphyxia is caused by a severe crush injury to the chest or upper abdomen. The mechanism is believed to be acute, severe venous hypertension.[9,10] The various presentations include asystolic cardiac arrest, status epilepticus, prolonged confusion, and cortical blindness.[2] The majority of signs are confined to the upper torso, with the lower torso being spared. Clinical manifestations include facial edema and petechiae, cranial cyanosis, subconjunctival hemorrhage, exophthalmos, and ecchymotic hemorrhages of the face and upper chest.

Life-threatening pulmonary, cardiac, and gastrointestinal injuries may occur with traumatic asphyxia. These include pulmonary contusion, pneumothorax, myocardial contusion, flail chest, liver and splenic lacerations, and gastrointestinal hemorrhage. Superior vena cava syndrome may mimic the features of traumatic asphyxia and should be ruled out. Basilar skull fractures may also present similarly. Skull fractures are rare in traumatic asphyxia because the compressive force is usually to the chest or upper abdomen. Morbidity and mortality are associated with the severity and duration of compression and the high incidence of associated injuries. These injuries should be ruled out by computed tomography scan, duplex ultrasound, or echocardiogram as dictated by the physical examination. Long-term neurologic sequelae are rare, and full recovery may be achieved with early reestablishment of ventilation and correction of hypoxia.[9,10]

In addition to traumatic asphyxia and its associated injuries, many other injuries may occur secondary to stampede including musculoskeletal trauma, soft tissue crush injuries, acute right heart strain,[3] and brachial plexus injuries.[2] Crush injuries, including crush syndrome, compartment syndrome, and acute traumatic ischemia, lead to hemorrhage, edema, and hypoperfusion with resulting tissue hypoxia and ischemia. Although any tissue may be affected, nerve and muscle located in myofascial compartments are at increased risk. Cellular death leads to release of potassium, phosphate, and myoglobin as part of crush syndrome with rhabdomyolysis. Most crush syndromes occur as a result of compression for 4 or more hours. Complications include hypovolemia, hypotension, and disseminated intravascular coagulation, with renal failure being the most serious complication. Peak creatine kinase level has been shown to correlate with the occurrence of renal failure and mortality.[11-13]

PREINCIDENT ACTIONS

Human stampedes can occur at venues with or without organized mass-gathering medical care. Mass-gathering events require extensive coordination of various agencies including emergency medical services, fire and police departments, local emergency departments and hospitals, local government agencies, and others. Factors in planning for large events may include the type and duration of event, physical plant and location characteristics, routes of ingress and egress, and age of attendees. As a result of previous stampedes, much has been learned for the prevention of future incidents. Factors used in prevention may include providing reserved seating rather than general admission to large events, avoiding use of fixed barricades, ensuring availability of multiple exits, minimizing bottlenecks, limiting access to alcohol, and having the crowd form into queues.[4,14,15]

POSTINCIDENT ACTIONS

The Incident Command System, a standard emergency management system used throughout the United States, should be activated to coordinate the response to a human stampede. Establishment of effective communication is vital. Prehospital providers must commence triage and rapid treatment and determine the most sensible distribution of patients to area hospitals. Hospitals, and in particular emergency departments, should have disaster protocols available to effectively handle mass-casualty events.[16]

MEDICAL TREATMENT OF CASUALTIES

Standard trauma protocols should be followed when caring for victims of human stampede. Treatment of traumatic asphyxia is largely supportive and aimed at the associated injuries, which include pulmonary and myocardial contusion, pneumothoraces, intra-abdominal injuries, and neurologic injuries. Prompt delivery of oxygen and effective ventilation compose the mainstay of treatment, as well as elevation of the head of bed. Prognosis is excellent for those persons who survive the initial crush injury, with a recovery rate of approximately 90% for patients surviving the initial hour.[10]

As massive compression occurs, one needs to evaluate a patient who has incurred injury in a stampede for crush injuries including the sequelae of crush and compartment syndromes. The goal of therapy is to prevent renal failure by avoiding hypotension and maintaining urine output. The administration of appropriate intravenous fluid therapy with crystalloid solution should be initiated as early as possible, even before extrication, to maximize intravascular volume and renal perfusion. Urine output should be maintained at approximately 200 mL/hour. Alkalinization of the urine has been shown to increase the solubility and excretion of myoglobin and prevent renal failure. The urine pH level should be maintained between 6 and 7. The use of mannitol is controversial but may aid in diuresis. If compartment syndrome is suspected, compartment pressures should be measured directly, and, if elevated, fasciotomy may be required.[11-13] Hyperbaric oxygen therapy has also been shown to be effective in severe extremity crush injuries.[17]

CASE PRESENTATION

It is Saturday night, and more than 1200 persons have gathered at a large downtown nightclub to hear a famous rock band perform. A fire starts as a result of patrons smoking in the lavatory and spreads quickly through the building. Persons panic and rush to the closest exits, only to find many of them locked. Those in the rear of the crowd push forward, causing many of those in front to fall and become obstacles for those rushing forward. A call is placed to 9-1-1 and emergency responders arrive but have difficulty reaching patients. There are well over 100 persons injured. Patients begin arriving at your emergency department. A 22-year-old woman is transported receiving oxygen and having facial edema and petechiae. A 23-year-old man is brought in unconscious with multiple ecchymoses about the face and torso. Other patients continue to arrive.

UNIQUE CONSIDERATIONS

In the event of a human stampede, access to patients early on, as well as extrication of patients, may be difficult if not impossible. The safety of emergency responders must be considered. Traumatic asphyxia and the crush syndrome are rare clinical entities that may be associated with high morbidity and mortality. Early and aggressive therapy, often initiated in the prehospital setting and even before extrication, may be required to ensure the best possible outcome. Adequate planning, public education, and interagency cooperation play key roles in minimizing the risk of human stampede and its associated injuries and deaths.

PITFALLS

Several potential pitfalls in response to a human stampede exist. These include the following:

- Failure to adequately plan and coordinate the necessary agencies needed to respond to mass-gathering events
- Failure to alert appropriate persons, hospitals, and emergency departments to a human stampede event
- Failure to rapidly restore oxygenation and ventilation to victims of a human stampede
- Failure to identify and aggressively treat associated injuries of traumatic asphyxia and massive compression

REFERENCES

1. Saffle J. The 1942 fire at Boston's Cocoanut Grove nightclub. *Am J Surg*. 1993;166:581-91.
2. Wardrope J, Hockey M, Crosby A. The hospital response to the Hillsborough tragedy. *Injury* 1990;21:53-54.
3. Grech E, Bellamy C, Epstein E, et al. Traumatic mitral valve rupture during the Hillsborough football disaster: case report. *J Trauma*. 1993;35:475-6.
4. Fruin J. The causes and prevention of crowd disasters. In: Smith R, Dickie J, eds. *Engineering for Crowd Safety*. Amsterdam: Elsevier Science Publishers; 1993:99-108.
5. Johnson N. Panic at "The Who Concert Stampede": an empirical assessment. *Soc Probl*. 1987;34:362-73.
6. Helbing D, Farkas I, Vicsek T. Simulating dynamical features of escape panic. *Nature* 2000;407:487-90.
7. Low D. Statistical physics: following the crowd. *Nature* 2000;407:465-66.
8. Saloma C, Perez G, Tapang G, et al. Self-organized queuing and scale-free behavior in real escape panic. *Proc Natl Acad Sci USA*. 2003;100:11947-52.
9. DeAngeles D, Schurr M, Birnbaum M, et al. Traumatic asphyxia following stadium crowd surge: stadium factors affecting outcome. *Wisc Med J*. 1998;97:42-5.
10. Dunne J, Shaked G, Golocovsky M. Traumatic asphyxia: an indicator of potentially severe injury in trauma. *Injury* 1996;27:746-9.
11. Smith J, Greaves I. Crush injury and crush syndrome: a review. *J Trauma*. 2003;54:S226-30.
12. Malinoski D, Slater M, Mullins R. Crush injury and rhabdomyolysis. *Crit Care Clin*. 2004;20:171-92.
13. Delaney J, Drummond R. Mass casualties and triage at a sporting event. *Br J Sports Med*. 2002;36:85-8.
14. Grange J. Planning for large events. *Curr Sports Med Rep*. 2002;1:156-61.
15. Milstein A, Maguire B, Bissell R, et al. Mass-gathering medical care: a review of the literature. *Prehospital Disaster Med*. 2002;17:151-62.
16. Schultz C, Koenig K, Noji E. Disaster preparedness. In: Marx J, Hockberger R, Walls R, et al, eds. *Rosen's Emergency Medicine*. 5th ed. Vol III. St Louis: Mosby; 2002:2631-40.
17. Bouachour G, Cronier P, Gouello J, et al. Hyperbaric oxygen therapy in the management of crush injuries: a randomized double-blind placebo-controlled clinical trial. *J Trauma*. 1996;41:333-9.

chapter 172

Mining Accident

Dale M. Molé

 ## DESCRIPTION OF EVENT

The Industrial Revolution significantly increased the demand for fossil fuels. In America, outcrop deposits of coal along the James River in Virginia supplied fuel for blacksmith forges as early as 1702, and when surface supplies diminished, miners followed the coal seams underground. Deeper mines combined with poor ventilation increased the formation of explosive mixtures of methane. The inevitable occurred in 1810 with the first coal mine explosion.[1]

Mine disasters in the first half of the twentieth century involved hundreds of deaths in each accident. Advances in mine technology and safety have greatly reduced the hazard of underground occupations since the early days, but they have not completely eliminated danger. In the United States alone, 169 miners have lost their lives in coal mine mishaps since 1980.[2]

In the immediate aftermath of a mine accident, surviving until rescue is the first priority of trapped miners. Obstacles to survival include poor communication, extreme darkness, confined space, hypothermia, toxic atmosphere, and injuries.

One of the most challenging aspects of any rescue operation is establishing the existence, location, and condition of any survivors. Mine communication systems are often damaged or unreachable in a disaster. Low-frequency radio waves can penetrate rock and offer promise for minewide alarm and communication devices. Seismic locators can detect the vibrations produced by trapped miners in some circumstances. If a survival borehole is drilled, tapping on the drill using prearranged tap codes provides useful information.

Shutting off electricity to reduce ignition sources for fires or explosions is often the first action after a mine accident. Plunged into absolute darkness, the miners must rely on limited-duration battery-powered helmet lights, making survival efforts more arduous.

Cool ambient mine temperatures combined with water from mine operations, aquifers, rain, or flooding creates a major problem for miners who get wet. Immersion in water increases conductive heat loss by as much as five-fold, hastening the onset of hypothermia. Adaptive survival mechanisms (e.g., shivering thermogenesis) increase metabolic heat production by two to five times,

but they also significantly increase oxygen consumption and carbon dioxide production—a major problem in small, airtight spaces.[3] Hypothermia depresses the central nervous system, impairs judgment, and prevents the accomplishment of appropriate survival actions.

The atmosphere within a mine is composed of many gases. Early miners used canaries as biologic atmosphere monitors because the birds are overcome by relatively small amounts of noxious gases or damps. The word *damp*, originally derived from the German word *dampf* meaning "fog" or "vapor," is the mining vernacular to describe any mixture of gases in a underground mine, usually noxious or oxygen deficient.

Firedamp primarily refers to methane resulting from the decomposition of coal or other carbonaceous material decaying in an anoxic environment and is explosive when present in air in concentrations of 5% to 15%. The Davy safety lamp, one of the earliest detection devices, detects concentrations as low as 1%. Flame color and height indicates the amount of methane present. Low oxygen levels extinguish the flame entirely. Special colorimetric detectors are now used.

Blackdamp, referring to an anoxic mixture of nitrogen and carbon dioxide, extinguishes flame and causes death by suffocation. Carbon dioxide is produced by the complete combustion of carbonaceous material, metabolism of miners and animals, decay of organic matter, oxidation of coal, or the chemical action of acid water on carbonates.

Chokedamp is any anoxic mixture of mine gases. *Whitedamp* contains large amounts of carbon monoxide; is found in the exhaust of diesel engines, detonated explosives, wood or coal fires; and is the result of the incomplete combustion of carbonaceous materials. This colorless, tasteless, odorless gas competes with oxygen for hemoglobin binding sites and binds with an affinity 218 times greater. The oxyhemoglobin dissociation curve is transformed from the normal sigmoid to an asymptotic shape, impairing or preventing oxygen transport to the tissues. Tissues with high oxygen demands (e.g., brain and heart) are among the first affected. Symptoms include fatigue, dizziness, headache, seizures, unconsciousness, and hypotension.

Afterdamp is the gas produced by an explosion. It almost always contains dangerous amounts of carbon monoxide and oxides of nitrogen, reported in terms of nitrogen dioxide that can form nitric acid in the lungs. *Stink damp,* or hydrogen sulfide gas, has a characteristic pungent smell of rotten eggs. The byproduct of organic decomposition, the action of mine acid on sulfur minerals, or the burning of explosives containing sulfur such as black powder or dynamite, it is soluble in water and may be liberated whenever a mine pool is agitated. It is extremely poisonous and has a mechanism of action similar to cyanide. High concentrations produce loss of consciousness, seizures, and death with just a few breaths.

Other gases include highly explosive hydrogen gas from battery-charging stations; sulfur dioxide, which creates sulfuric acid in the lungs; and acetylene resulting from methane heated in a low-oxygen atmosphere or the interaction of calcium carbide with water.

Oxygen is essential for survival. It is the partial pressure of oxygen, not the absolute percentage, that determines whether the ambient atmosphere can sustain life. Fire or metabolic activity can rapidly consume the available oxygen in a confined, airtight space. Flooding can compress air pockets, raising the total pressure and therefore the partial pressure of oxygen to dangerous levels. Since air is 21% oxygen and normal atmospheric pressure (1 atmosphere absolute [ata]) is equivalent to 760 torr, the partial pressure of oxygen is 760 times 0.21, or 160 torr. Expressed in atmospheres absolute, this would be 1 ata times 0.21, or 0.21 ata. If the atmospheric pressure were doubled to a total pressure of 1520 torr, or 2 ata, the partial pressure of oxygen could be expressed as (1520 torr × 0.21) = 320 torr, or (2 ata × 0.21) = 0.42 ata. Pulmonary oxygen toxicity results from prolonged exposure to high-oxygen partial pressures in excess of 0.5 ata. Breathing 0.6 ata oxygen produces respiratory symptoms in the majority of humans in less than 24 hours.[4] Conversely, as survivors in a closed space consume the available oxygen, the partial pressure of oxygen falls, producing signs and symptoms of hypoxia such as dyspnea (i.e., air hunger), cyanosis, impaired cognition, poor muscle coordination, and unconsciousness.

Nitrogen composes 79% of our atmosphere and is generally considered an inert (metabolically inactive) gas. When breathed at increased pressure, however, it produces a narcotic effect in a dose-dependent fashion; that is, the higher the partial pressure of nitrogen, the greater the narcosis. Nitrogen narcosis causes both cognitive and psychomotor disturbances. Breathing room air at 4 to 7 ata results in exposure to elevated partial pressures of nitrogen high enough to cause delayed response to auditory and visual stimuli, impaired neuromuscular coordination, a loss of clear thinking, and a tendency toward idea fixation. The effect is similar to ethanol intoxication, and it can significantly impair the ability of miners to take the necessary steps to ensure survival.

Carbon dioxide comprises only 0.001 ata, or one-tenth of 1% of the atmosphere. It is a by-product of cellular metabolism, and for each standard cubic foot of oxygen consumed an almost equal amount of carbon dioxide is produced. If the carbon dioxide level climbs past 0.10 ata, unconsciousness is soon followed by death. In an airtight space, it is the carbon dioxide level that limits survival, not the amount of oxygen.[5]

In prolonged survival situations, food and water also become important considerations. Inadequate caloric intake can produce starvation diarrhea, making survival less likely.[6]

 PREINCIDENT ACTIONS

One of the most significant advances in mine rescue operations occurred in 1856 with the introduction of self-contained breathing apparatus, allowing rescuers to conduct operations with increased safety. Part 49 of Title 30 of the Code of Federal Regulations requires every mine in the country to have mine rescue teams. It stipulates how many members each team should have and outlines physical and training standards and required equipment, maintenance, and storage. Modern mine rescue, with enhanced team training and improved equipment, has transformed chaotic, uncoordinated rescue attempts into efficient, well-coordinated group efforts. The full integration of medical elements into the team is essential for a successful outcome to rescue operations.

Today's teams use modern gas detection and communication equipment, seismic locators, geophones, and other devices to locate miners. Rescue vans are outfitted with breathing apparatus, recharging facilities, hand tools, medical supplies, and gas analysis equipment. A qualitative and quantitative knowledge of constituent gases within the mine provides important clues to past events, as well as current atmosphere conditions such as elevated carbon monoxide levels suggestive of a fire.

Mine emergency operations teams can drill boreholes down from the surface to reach miners. Once a small-diameter "survival hole" is drilled, rescuers can lower microphones, lights, and cameras into the mine to help locate the miners, to determine their situation, and to lend support and assistance while a rescue hole is drilled. Trapped miners can be safely hauled to the surface in specially designed "rescue capsules."

 POSTINCIDENT ACTIONS

The first few hours after the emergency are the most critical. Coordination of mine rescue teams, mine personnel, and local, state, and federal officials is essential. A command center forms the hub of mine rescue operations and contains communications equipment, underground diagrams, and local area maps. As mine rescue teams arrive, a rotation schedule is prepared, designating which teams are to be the exploration team, backup team, and standby team. A bench area with running water allows breathing apparatus to be cleaned, tested, and prepared.

Establishing perimeter security is essential to keep roads open for emergency personnel and to ensure that curious bystanders do not hinder rescue efforts or become injured while on mine property. Company personnel or police officers should guard all routes to the mine.

A press center should be established away from the disaster site and should be the only area where news media receive information. A public affairs officer will authorize, issue, and ensure the accuracy of the information being released to the public. The family waiting area should be away from any rescue activity and the media center.

Provision should be made to feed and house rescue personnel during an emergency. Food can be catered or brought in from a nearby restaurant. The American Red Cross is skilled at providing disaster relief services. Nearby motels can often provide sleeping quarters, or if none are available, tents and cots can be set up at the rescue site. Ensuring adequate field hygiene is critical to preventing infectious disease outbreaks among rescue personnel.

Mine exploration is the process of assessing conditions underground and locating miners during a rescue or recovery operation. The safest route into the mine is determined before anyone goes underground. In a shaft mine, the cage (i.e., elevator) is thoroughly tested for proper operation, and the shaft is tested for the presence of gases, smoke, or water.

In some disaster situations, conditions may make it possible to begin the initial exploration without self-contained breathing apparatus. This "barefaced" exploration is conducted only when the ventilation system is operating properly and gas tests demonstrate a safe atmosphere. Backup crews with apparatus are stationed nearby, ready to perform a rescue if necessary. Barefaced exploration stops where disruptions in ventilation are discovered, when gas analysis indicates the presence of noxious or explosive gases or an oxygen deficiency, or when smoke or damage is encountered. A "fresh air base" is usually established at the point where conditions no longer permit barefaced exploration. Teams equipped with breathing apparatus continue exploration from the fresh air base. Typical mine rescue equipment includes gas detectors, oxygen indicators, communication equipment, thermal imaging cameras or heat-sensing devices, link-line, map board and marker, scaling bar, walking stick, stretcher, first aid kit, fire extinguisher, tools, blankets, and extra breathing apparatus. Before going underground, each team is briefed about what has happened in the mine and what conditions currently exist.

Since every underground coal mine contains harmful gases, dust fumes, and smoke, a ventilation system draws air from the surface via the main intake shaft. Ventilation controls force air to move in certain directions and at certain velocities to safely ventilate all sections of the mine. The main fan creates a pressure differential and must be monitored or guarded to ensure the rescue team's safety while underground after the fresh air base is established and exploration is under way. Changes in ventilation are only made by the command center. As the team advances through the mine, all ventilation controls are examined. Team members must be able to recognize damaged ventilation controls, determine the direction and velocity of ventilation air by using an anemometer or smoke tube, measure the cross-sectional area of a mine entry, and calculate the volume of air by using the area and velocity. The quantity of air (measured in cubic feet) is equal to the area (in square feet) multiplied by the velocity (in feet per minute.)

Fires in underground mines are especially hazardous because they pose explosion hazards, consume oxygen, and produce smoke, toxic gases, and heat. Ventilation is always maintained during a fire to carry off explosive gases and distillates away from the fire area and to direct the smoke, heat, and flames away from the team. The most frequent cause of explosions in coal mines is the ignition of methane gas, coal dust, or a combination of the two. Explosions can blow out roof supports, damage ventilation controls, twist or scatter machinery, and ignite numerous fires. Roof and ribs can be weakened, and fires can be spread. Further explosions may occur because of damage to the ventilation system during the initial explosion.

 ## MEDICAL TREATMENT OF CASUALTIES

In a disaster in which several miners are trapped underground, or in which injuries are sustained after an explosion, roof fall, or fire, a temporary medical treatment facility should be established. After initial stabilization, a carefully considered means of patient transport may include ambulances or evacuation aircraft, with medical crew on standby. If large numbers of corpses are being recovered from the mine, a temporary morgue is necessary.

 ## UNIQUE CONSIDERATIONS

Delayed care for contaminated wounds and crush injuries, as well as the synergistic effects of toxic gases, hypothermia, and inadequate nutrition make medical management of the victims of a mining accident especially challenging. Provision for decontamination is essential after prolonged underground dwelling. Carbon monoxide poisoning may require treatment with hyperbaric oxygen.

 ## PITFALLS

Several potential pitfalls in response to a mining accident exist. Failure to consider the effects of elevated pressure in mine flooding situations may result in death or permanent disability upon rescue due to decompression sickness. In addition, inadequate medical integration into mine rescue team training may result in suboptimal performance in real emergencies, leading to preventable morbidity and mortality.

On the evening of July 24, 2002, miners working 240 feet underground in the Quecreek coal mine breached a wall separating them from the water-filled Saxon mine. One hundred fifty million gallons of water flooding into the mine compressed the air to more than twice the normal atmospheric pressure.

At the request of local officials, U.S. Navy recompression chambers, normally used for submarine rescue operations, were set up in a barn on the William Arnold family farm within 18 hours of the first call for assistance. Nine multi-place recompression chambers, five small monoplace chambers, and 60 Navy personnel were on site and ready to receive patients.

After the correct position was determined via global positioning system coordinates, a 6-inch survival hole was drilled. When the drill was shut down, tapping was heard on the other end. Nine taps were sent from topside and nine taps were returned from below, indicating that nine miners were alive. High-pressure air pumped down through the drill rig provided a source of fresh air and helped to prevent water from rising within the mine. Turbine pumps at the mine entrance pumped water out of the mine, but at a rate that would take weeks to pump the mine dry.

A 32-inch rescue hole was drilled. A cylindrical yellow steel cage, the rescue capsule, would lift miners one at a time up 245 feet through the hole. A remote video camera attached to the capsule would assist in determining conditions within the mine and look for signs of life. Since most of the rescue hole was unsheathed and could collapse at any time, food, water, and blankets were loaded into the basket for the first trip below.

To prevent rapid depressurization when the drill pierced the mine, a special cap for the rescue hole was designed and rapidly constructed on site, allowing the removal of miners while maintaining pressure in the mine. Once at normal pressure, the miners had about 15 minutes before the onset of decompression sickness symptoms. During this latent period, they had to be moved from the rescue hole, had to undergo a quick medical examination and decontamination, and had to be returned to depth in the recompression chambers and then decompressed using tables developed at the Navy Experimental Diving Unit in Panama City, Florida, for submarine rescue.

Working at full capacity, pumps were able to lower the water level and reduce the pressure in the mine at a rate of about 10 cm of water per hour in what turned out to be an almost perfect air saturation decompression schedule. Shortly after midnight, the first miner reached the surface. Covered in coal dust from head to toe, he was carried up the hillside to the decontamination tent, where his clothes are cut away and a cursory medical history and examination were conducted. After soap and warm water decontamination, he was quickly moved to the medical treatment area. While the civilian emergency medical technicians started an intravenous line for the patient, Navy personnel obtained vital signs and performed a physical examination. The process was repeated eight more times, with the last miner being brought to the surface at 2:45 AM. One patient required treatment in the recompression chamber after suffering symptoms of decompression sickness.[7]

REFERENCES

1. Kravitz J. *An Examination of Major Mine Disasters in the United States and a Historical Summary of MSHA's Mine Emergency Operations Program.* Available at: http://www.msha.gov/S&HINFOTECHRPT/MED/MAJORMIN.pdf.
2. United States Mine Rescue Association. Available at: http://www.usmra.com.
3. Danzl D, Prozos R, Hamlet M. *Accidental hypothermia.* In Auerbach PS, ed: *Management of Wilderness and Environmental Emergencies.* St Louis: Mosby; 1989.
4. Dougherty J, Styer D, Eckenhoff R. *The Effects of Hyperbaric and Hyperoxic Conditions on Pulmonary Function During Prolonged Hyperbaric Chamber Air Saturation Dives.* Bethesda, Md: Undersea Biomedical Research; 1981.
5. Molé D. *Submarine Escape and Rescue: An Overview.* San Diego, Calif: Submarine Development Group One; 1990.
6. House C, House J, Oakley H. Findings from a simulated disabled submarine survival trial. *Undersea Hyperb. Med.* 2000, Winter; 27(4):175–83.
7. Molé D. Steaming to assist at the Quecreek Mine disaster. *Navy Med.* 2002;93:18–29.

chapter 173

Submarine or Surface Vessel Accident

Steven T. Cobery and Dale M. Molé

 DESCRIPTION OF EVENT

Vessels that travel on the surface of the water fulfill many vital needs in support of the nations of the world today. Oversea shipping remains the preeminent means for transporting large amounts of material internationally. Naval vessels actively deploy, conducting missions throughout the world with conventional and special weapons aboard. Within coastal and near-land waters, millions of fishing vessels of varying sizes scour the seas, providing both a vital food source and a substantial addition to many local economies. Huge cruise liners offer every conceivable type of enjoyment and relaxation for the millions of vacationers they entertain each year. Submarines, almost exclusively military in usage, silently and stealthily patrol every ocean on earth, often under adverse conditions and far removed from readily available medical attention.

Each of these segments of the shipping world poses very unique problems when it comes to the medical care of the personnel and passengers aboard. The medical facilities aboard most ships are sparse because space is a scarce commodity on most vessels. The capability of first responders is impaired both by their level of knowledge and training and the amount and quality of available medical equipment. Dedicated, medically trained personnel exist only on larger ships; the role of the "ship's doc" is often a collateral duty of nonmedical personnel on smaller commercial vessels. Diagnostic imaging and laboratory testing are nonexistent in almost all cases. Communication equipment capabilities vary from very advanced satellite voice communications to visual line-of-sight signaling. The challenges posed by a seaborne mass-casualty incident or disaster to shore-based facilities are enormous.

All sea traffic faces the common foe of an unpredictable and often hazardous work environment. The inner workings of any vessel afloat are choreographed in an effort to conserve energy, personnel, money, and space. Imagine the occupational hazards present in a land-based facility that combines a power plant powerful enough to light several neighborhoods, a processing facility capable of independently handling tons of material daily, and a mechanical plant with a vast array of rotating machinery and high-pressure systems. The occupational hazards of these facilities alone produce huge risks for their workers. Now take this facility, place it on a moving platform that has approximately one-quarter the footprint, and operate it with efficiency in an external environment that can range from dead calm to "the perfect storm"—that is, 30-foot waves with wind gusting to 100 miles/hour. The risks for mass casualties and accidents exponentially increase due to the constraints placed by operating at sea in a dangerous environment, both internal and external to the ship.

Three types of casualties commonly plague all shipping vessels: fire, high-pressure/high-temperature occupational exposures, and flooding/drowning. Fires are often called a ship's worst enemy. Because of the myriad of flammable and combustible materials onboard the ship, all classes of fires represent an omnipresent and often fatal danger at sea. In addition to the fire itself, smoke inhalation, electric shock, exposure to toxic gases, and chemical burns secondarily compound the casualties generated by an onboard fire. Consequently, firefighting skills and equipment occupy important places in the priorities of the crew. Fires can occur virtually anywhere on the ship and from any source. The power plant and hydraulic plants represent the majority of fire locations.[1] The priority of the crew in the event of a fire is first to extinguish the fire, and second to attend to the casualties. This prioritization can sometimes delay bringing injured persons to the attention of medical facilities, particularly when the fire occurs at sea rather than pier side.

In addition to fires in the propulsion plant, occupational exposures to high-pressure and high-temperature gases and fluids uniquely challenge the onboard medical capabilities. Most ships are powered by one of four means: steam, diesel-electric, gas turbine, and nuclear.[2] Each employ high-temperature, high-pressure gases to turn the prime mover, a turbine, often rotating at speeds in excess of 2000 revolutions per minute. Catastrophic rupture of the piping system in the propulsion plant can rapidly lead to death within minutes in the closed compartments of the engine room. Focal exposure to these fluids causes burns, high-pressure stream-penetrating injuries, toxic inhalation or ingestion, or blunt trauma. With nuclear propulsion, radiologic exposure complicates both the injury and its treatment. A unique feature of maritime engineering applications is that the mechanical and auxiliary systems of the ship are not restricted to a defined industrial space; high-pressure air, hydraulics, and inert gas systems run the length of the ship, including living, recreation, food service, and open deck spaces.

In any maritime setting, water supports, passes through, and sometimes surrounds the hull of the vessel. The sheer power of the ocean adds a dimension of hazard not seen on land. Flooding on board is often not the result of a breach in the hull itself; most often, it is the result of a cooling water system failure or hull penetration interlock failure. The force of a sudden inrush of water can easily cause primary blunt trauma or secondary trauma associated with falls or impact. Drowning casualties, whether due to persons being swept overboard or occurring as a result of catastrophic flooding, frequently present themselves in a more delayed fashion by nature. Anoxic brain injury, hypothermia, and cardiorespiratory failure are common complications.[3] The constant presence of the power of the sea makes these types of casualties a continuous threat.

Submarine disasters provide their own unique challenges. Submarines sink because of uncontrolled flooding. Only marginally buoyant by design, relatively small amounts of flooding can prevent a submarine from surfacing, especially if propulsion is lost. If this happens in the deep ocean, there are no medical issues since the submarine implodes once crush depth is exceeded. However, since collisions are most likely to occur over the continental shelf, having survivors trapped in a sunken submarine is a real possibility.

The decision to await rescue or to begin escape depends on the external as well as the internal environment of the submarine. In water deeper than 180 m, escape is not currently an option, despite a hostile internal submarine environment (i.e., high pressure, low oxygen, toxic gases). Weather over the disaster site may prevent the timely rescue of survivors. The ability for a submarine crew to survive for between 5 and 7 days is the ideal goal, but the nature of the disaster may result in significantly shorter times.

Barriers to survival are many. The ingress of water reduces the internal submarine volume, compressing the air and subjecting the crew to an elevated atmospheric pressure. As the total pressure increases, the partial pressure of constituent gases increases as well. Oxygen and nitrogen, the primary constituents of air, are lethal at high partial pressures. Central nervous system oxygen toxicity can cause death in a matter of minutes. High partial pressures of nitrogen produce narcosis in a dose-dependent fashion, as well as loading tissue with excess nitrogen. Survivors with nitrogen-saturated tissues must be decompressed or slowly returned to normal atmospheric pressure to avoid potentially fatal decompression sickness. Carbon dioxide produced by human metabolism is the limiting factor for submariners trapped in an airtight compartment, since carbon dioxide climbs to deadly levels before oxygen becomes insufficient to sustain life. Since the average ocean temperature is 4°C, clothing wet from flooding can quickly lead to hypothermia. Shivering helps to maintain core temperature but markedly increases the consumption of oxygen and the production of carbon dioxide. Toxic gases from fire or chlorine produced by flooded batteries may force the crew to use emergency breathing apparatus or escape under unfavorable conditions.[4]

Submarine escape is potentially hazardous under the best conditions. Pulmonary barotrauma resulting in arterial gas embolism, as well as fulminate decompression sickness, are conditions that may occur and require immediate hyperbaric oxygen treatment.

 PREINCIDENT ACTIONS

Hospital staff, emergency department personnel, outpatient facilities, and port control authorities should have an established, well-rehearsed plan to initiate reliable communications in a timely manner to ensure the prepared receipt of casualties. Assigning geographic areas of responsibility to primary receiving facilities will simplify routing of the injured and improve response times. Mass-casualty plans, which integrate local, state, and federal agencies, including both the coast guard and naval bases in the region, will establish the most efficient means of conveyance, triage, and treatment. Knowledge of receiving facility flight pad capabilities, including global positioning system coordinates of the helipad, the capacities in terms of type and number of helicopters capable of being accommodated, and special local area flight considerations, should be evident in these plans. Special decontamination procedures to be used in the event of radiologic contamination or exposure to hazardous materials should be in place to handle these unique potentialities. Secondary facilities should be identified to receive overflow casualties for which the primary facility cannot provide care.

 POSTINCIDENT ACTIONS

Once notified of incoming casualties from a seaborne platform, feedback to the port control authorities and U.S. Coast Guard/U.S. Navy will assist in refining mass-casualty planning for future events.

 MEDICAL TREATMENT OF CASUALTIES

Because of the relatively wide variety of casualties that can be encountered from a shipborne accident, the treatment of the injuries should follow the standard of care for that specific injury. Two common complicating factors, however, should be addressed. Prolonged exposure to the elements at sea can rapidly lead to hypothermia. In most oceans, hypothermia ($T_c < 35°C$) occurs in less than 30 minutes. The onset varies with multiple factors, including water temperature, sea state, amount and type of clothing worn by the patient, body habitus, and other factors.[5] Although exposure suits are required aboard many sea-going vessels, due to the exigency of the casualty or their physical location, many casualties may not be able to access these suits. Hypothermia becomes a primary injury that can sometimes be overlooked in the face of other, more obvious injuries.

Contamination with toxic or hazardous material, including radioactive fluids or waste, is a silent, invisible complicating factor in the treatment of these casualties. Before any intake, treatment, or care, proper containment or decontamination, in accordance with the mass-casualty plans, must occur to ensure the safety of the treating personnel and the other patients at the receiving facility. However, disaster management planning must include the provision for providing life- or limb-saving medical treatment for contaminated injured personnel while maintaining a safe environment for the medical staff. Every emergency department must have a well-rehearsed treatment/decontamination plan for contaminated patients. Most radioactive surface contamination can be removed using soapy, lukewarm water to gently wash the affected area. Scrubbing runs the risk of embedding these contaminants and should be avoided.[4] Chemical exposures should be assessed for their acidity/basicity to ensure proper usage of neutralizing agents. Once patients have been verified clean/decontaminated, physical entrance into the treating facility can safely occur. Life-saving interventions for the contaminated patient must be weighed against the risk of exposure to the treating personnel.

CASE PRESENTATION

On the evening of August 26, 1988, the Peruvian submarine *Pacocha* with 49 persons aboard was struck by a Japanese fishing vessel while returning to the port of Callao, Peru. The submarine sank in 140 feet of water about 6 nautical miles from land. Twenty-three crewmembers managed to scramble overboard, but three of those later drowned or succumbed to exposure in the 14°C water prior to rescue. The captain and three of his crew drowned immediately while attempting to save the submarine.

Twenty-two submariners were trapped in the forward compartment, where flooding had increased the internal pressure to about three times normal atmospheric pressure. After about 20 hours, rising carbon dioxide levels forced the survivors to begin escaping from the submarine. Upon reaching the surface, all required recompression treatment in a hyperbaric chamber for decompression sickness. Of these 22 submariners, 1 died and another suffered severe brain damage/quadriplegia.[6]

UNIQUE CONSIDERATIONS

Shipboard spaces are often difficult to navigate, particularly with bulky medical gear and stretchers. Consequently, initial assessment, extraction, and transport to the weather decks can present challenges that hamper the provision of care. Accurate relaying of patient location on the ship can speed recovery times, particularly on smaller ships that will rely on outside medical assistance on board the ship.

Radiologic controls, in the event of a radioactive release or spill, can greatly slow response, recovery, and treatment times. Very specific regulations govern the management of radiologic sites. These regulations are written in an effort to minimize the exposure of radioactive materials to the public. In the event of a casualty involving contaminated, injured personnel, public exposure will be limited by the reliance on the receiving facility to safely decontaminate the injured in an effort to minimize any delay in medical attention. However, the benefit of life- and limb-saving measures must outweigh the risk of low-level radioactive exposure of the medical responders.

Explosive hazards are real potentials on many vessels, particularly warships. Most disasters occurring on U.S. naval vessels will be managed by the regional commander and the organic medical facilities and personnel in that command. However, disasters remote from dedicated U.S. naval medical centers capable of handling mass casualties may require civilian assistance, particularly when deployed out of territorial waters. Knowledge of and planning for the treatment of injuries associated with explosive trauma (e.g., blunt/penetrating trauma, amputations, blast injury) complete any plan dealing with seaborne disasters.

 ## PITFALLS

Several potential pitfalls in response to a naval vessel accident exist. These include the following:

- Failure to fully exercise the sea disaster mass-casualty plan
- Failure to consider radiologic or toxic contamination in the process of providing treatment for affected persons
- Allowing low-level radioactive contamination to delay life- or limb-saving medical treatment
- Poor communications hampering efforts to properly coordinate patient transport
- Failure to anticipate and properly treat hypothermia in casualties exposed to the environment
- Failure to adequately communicate instructions for basic medical care to on-scene personnel lacking medical expertise
- Lack of knowledge regarding the location of hyperbaric facilities

REFERENCES

1. Tyrell D. Accidental fire causes. In: *Guide for Conducting Marine Fire Investigations.* 2000:25–37.
2. *Jane's Marine Propulsion.* 2002.
3. Ibsen LM. Submersion and asphyxial injury. *Crit Care Med.* 2002;30(11 Suppl):S402–8.
4. Molé DM. Submarine medicine. In: Edmonds C, Lowry C, Pennefather J, eds. *Diving and Subaquatic Medicine.* 3rd ed. 1992:499–512.
5. Willis D. The dirty bomb: management of victims of radiological weapons. *Medsurg Nurs.* 2003;12:397–401.
6. Harvey C, Carson J. *The B.A.P. Pacocha (SS-48) Collision: The Escape and Medical Treatment of Survivors.* Submarine Development Group One; 1988. San Diego.

chapter 174

Aircraft Hijacking

Kurt R. Horst

 DESCRIPTION OF EVENT

Aircraft hijacking is defined as the armed takeover of an aircraft.[1] Prior to the events involving the World Trade Center in New York City on Sept. 11, 2001, most hijackings involved the use of the aircraft as transportation and the passengers as hostages. The hijackers would then typically present specific demands, which would be negotiated.[1]

The first recorded aircraft hijacking occurred in 1931 in Peru when a group of armed revolutionaries approached a Ford Tri-motor aircraft and attempted to force the pilot to fly them to their destination.[1,2] The pilot refused, and after a 10-day standoff during which the revolution had been successful, the pilot was released.[1,2] Unfortunately, many aircraft hijackings do not end so peacefully. A few noteworthy incidents are presented in Table 174-1.

Before the events of Sept. 11, 2001, anti-hijacking training followed what was termed the *Common Strategy*. This philosophy was based on prior experiences with hijackers. It instructed aircrews to avoid attempts to overpower these persons, and encouraged actions to resolve hijackings peacefully, even by accommodating the hijackers when necessary. But the goal of the Sept. 11 hijackings was to use the aircraft to perform a suicide attack, rendering the Common Strategy obsolete.[5]

Since this attack, training has been altered and is now referred to as the *Crew Training Common Strategy*. It now instructs pilots to not open the cockpit door and new Federal Aviation Administration regulations require the reinforcement of those doors. However, if the door is breached, the flight crew will attempt to protect the aircraft from being taken over.[6] New legislation, including the Arming Pilots Against Terrorism Act of 2002, has opened the way for the training and deputization of pilots.[6,7] This will allow pilots to carry a firearm and provide an added safeguard to the security of the flight deck.[6,7]

In November 2001, the Aviation and Transportation Security Act was passed and the Transportation Security Administration (TSA) was created to oversee travel security.[8,9] Initially placed under the U.S. Department of Transportation, the TSA now falls under the Department of Homeland Security.[9] The TSA is now responsible for overseeing the screening of passengers, baggage, and cargo to detect possible threats, including explosives.[8,9]

As seen with historical examples of aircraft hijackings, many hostage situations are resolved with force. The emergence of the field of tactical emergency medical support over the last decade may provide a key role in such operations. Emergency medical providers, optimally trained at the paramedic level, serve as members of special weapons and tactics (SWAT) teams. SWAT teams often have a role in resolving hostage situations involving aircraft. The ability to provide immediate, high-level medical attention to hostage victims after entry is made may increase survival of those injured in the incident.[10,11]

 PREINCIDENT ACTIONS

Much of the focus on aircraft hijackings has centered on modalities to detect and prevent them from occurring. As outlined in detail previously, the TSA was developed to spearhead many of the changes that have occurred since the Sept. 11, 2001, hijackings in the United States.[8,9]

Medical personnel should be aware of the various injury patterns that may be present in victims involved in an aircraft hijacking and hostage situation. Knowledge and participation in tactical emergency medical support operations will improve survivability.[10,11] Acute exacerbations of pre-event medical conditions among victims may occur during the hostage situation. This may be precipitated by the stress of the event itself or due to the lack of availability of the patient's own routine medications. For example, a diabetic might develop a hyperglycemic reaction due to lack of access to his insulin that he placed in his checked luggage for an anticipated short flight. As such, emergency responders should be prepared to treat a myriad of primary medical conditions.

Continued training of airline personnel using the Crew Training Common Strategy will be imperative in preventing future suicide hijackings.[6,7] The arming of pilots is clearly a controversial issue. However, if carried out, proper training in firearms safety and use is required.[7] The presence of air marshals, law enforcement officers who fly aboard commercial flights, may also provide added protection because they have specialized training in the prevention of hijackings.[12] Finally, aircraft passengers may find themselves in a position where they must

TABLE 174-1 SELECTED AIRCRAFT HIJACKINGS

1968	Three members of the Front for the Liberation of Palestine (PFLP) hijack an El Al plane. After 40 days, the hostages and hijackers are released.[1,2]
1969	Eight U.S. airliners are hijacked to Cuba in 1 month. This leads to development of a Federal Aviation Administration task force that creates a hijacker "profile" used in conjunction with weapons-screening devices.[2]
1970	Four airliners, including one operated by a U.S. carrier, are hijacked by the PFLP. Three are successful and force landings in the Jordanian desert, where they are exploded after the passengers deplane. All hostages are subsequently freed after seven PFLP members are released from prison.[1-3]
1970	A copilot is fatally wounded by a hijacker on an Eastern Airlines flight. The copilot shoots and severely wounds the hijacker. The pilot, who was also injured, safely lands the aircraft.[2]
1976	Palestinians hijack an Air France aircraft. After landing in Uganda, Israeli commandos free 105 passengers after they storm a building where the hijackers had relocated the hostages. Three passengers, all the hijackers, and one commando are killed.[1]
1982	Fifty-nine people die when Egyptian commandos infiltrate an EgyptAir plane after it is hijacked by Palestinians and flown to Malta.[2]
1984	Four Arab hijackers aboard a Kuwait Airways jetliner force the aircraft to land in Iran. Once there, they kill two American citizens and commit other brutalities against the passengers. Iranian forces storm the aircraft, freeing the remaining hostages.[3]
1985	Lebanese Shiite Moslems hijack a TWA airliner in Athens and kill a U.S. serviceman onboard the flight. The rest of the passengers are released in stages over the course of 2 weeks. The International Security and Development Cooperation Act of 1985 is signed 2 months later and provides monies for development of new airport security devices and hiring of additional security inspectors to serve as air marshals.[3,4]
1986	After a 16-hour standoff, 22 people are killed when Pakistani forces storm a hijacked Pan Am flight in Karachi.[1,2]
1988	The explosion of a Pan American jetliner over Lockerbie, Scotland, by an explosive device in a cassette player prompts the institution of a number of security measures, including installation of devices to detect explosives and stricter penalties for trying to take a gun through airport screening sites.[3,4]
1996	One hundred twenty-five passengers are killed when an Ethiopian Airlines flight crashes into the Indian Ocean when hijackers refuse to allow the pilot to land and refuel. Fifty passengers survive.[2]
2001	On September 11, three American aircraft are hijacked and deliberately used to cause destruction at the World Trade Center towers in New York City and the Pentagon in Washington, DC. A fourth hijacked aircraft crashes in Pennsylvania after passengers attempt to retake the plane.[1,2,4]

act. This will certainly be a hard decision, and giving advice in this particular manner is difficult. However, as seen on Sept. 11, 2001, the action of private citizens prevented the fourth airliner from reaching its target.[5]

 POSTINCIDENT ACTIONS

The information just described can be used to develop a specific action plan in the event that a hijacking attempt has begun. Once on the ground, negotiations may occur between the hijackers and law enforcement personnel. Alternatively, the aircraft may be entered by specialty teams that will use an array of techniques to gain entry and incapacitate the hijackers. Medical personnel must be readily available to treat injuries to hijackers and hostages alike.

 MEDICAL TREATMENT OF CASUALTIES

A variety of injury patterns are likely to be expected among victims of aircraft hijackings. With more stringent screening of passengers and luggage, there may be a lesser chance of seeing gunshot wounds, especially compared with prior hijackings. However, with some pilots now carrying weapons and the possibility of armed rescue attempts by military special forces and SWAT teams once the aircraft is on the ground, the possibility of seeing such patterns of injury remains. As such, emergency personnel attached to these teams and in the emergency department must be prepared to provide appropriate immediate care. Additionally, penetrating trauma from an array of instruments such as knives, screwdrivers, and other sharp objects should be treated in a manner similar to gunshot wounds.

Evaluation, as always, should begin with an assessment of airway, breathing, and circulation and then progress to a secondary survey. Intubation should be performed as needed, and intravenous resuscitation should begin with crystalloid solutions.

Penetrating trauma to the chest may result in cardiac injury leading to pericardial tamponade, which must be immediately recognized and treated with fluid boluses, needle aspiration, and subsequent surgical intervention.[13,14] Beck's triad, while not always present, is indicative of pericardial tamponade and consists of hypotension, distended neck veins, and muffled heart sounds. Ultrasonography is used to confirm the diagnosis. Thoracotomy may also play a role in the treatment of this condition.[14] If a tension pneumothorax is suspected (evidenced by hypotension, distended neck veins, unilateral decreased breath sounds, and tracheal deviation), immediate needle decompression must be performed before obtaining a chest radiograph.[13,15] A tube thoracostomy may then be performed.[15] Simple pneumothorax, hemothorax, and a variety of injuries to the great vessels and lung parenchyma may also occur and must be identified early as surgical therapy may be indicated.[13,14]

Penetrating abdominal trauma can be recognized by the identification of a penetrating wound, evisceration, and the presence of tenderness and peritoneal signs on physical examination. Any aberration in vital signs may also point to the presence of internal hemorrhage.[16] Diagnostic peritoneal lavage, focused abdominal sonography for trauma (FAST), and computed tomography (CT) scan all may play a role in the management of a stable patient. However, emergent exploratory laparotomy may be required, especially if the patient becomes unstable.[16,17]

Penetrating trauma to the neck may result in damage to a number of structures including vasculature, the esophagus, and trachea. Specialty surgical services are necessary to further evaluate these injuries as many may require surgical intervention.[18] Penetrating head wounds produce brain injury and hemorrhage and require CT scan and neurosurgical evaluation. Complications include infection, seizure disorders, and variable neurologic dysfunction.[19]

The potential for blunt trauma also exists. Blows to the head may result in an array of injuries, including epidural and subdural hematomas and intraparenchymal hemorrhage, which may be diagnosed by CT and should prompt neurosurgical consultation.[19] Blows to the chest may result in rib fractures, pneumothorax, and hemothorax, which can be treated with needle decompression and tube thoracostomy when necessary.[15] Blunt trauma to the abdomen can cause solid organ injury and internal hemorrhaging. Physical examination findings include abdominal tenderness, peritoneal signs, and abdominal abrasions or areas of ecchymosis. Evaluation with ultrasound (FAST examination), CT scan, or diagnostic peritoneal lavage is indicated, and positive findings may warrant monitoring or surgical intervention.[20] The management of extremity trauma includes control of hemorrhage and stabilization of possible fractures until the patient reaches definitive care.

Exposure to chemical incapacitants such as 1-chloroacetophenone (Mace) and oleoresin capsicum (i.e., pepper spray) may also occur. These agents are irritants that affect the eyes, respiratory tract, and skin. Rescuers and healthcare providers should wear appropriate protective equipment to avoid exposure to the irritant, which may be more persistent in enclosed spaces, and the victim should be removed immediately from the area of release. Skin should be washed with soap and water. Respiratory symptoms may require the use of inhaled beta$_2$ agonists such as albuterol.[21] Eye symptoms should be treated with contact lens removal (if they are present) and eye irrigation. After improvement of symptoms, the eyes should be examined with the use of a slit lamp to detect corneal abrasions, and topical antibiotic should be prescribed if abrasions are present.[22]

Additionally, a number of victims will likely have underlying medical conditions that may require treatment. A major area of concern among all victims is that of psychological trauma. This may take the form of acute stress reactions, and some may develop posttraumatic stress disorder. One possible method of intervening to prevent this disorder or decrease its symptoms is a debriefing of the event soon after its occurrence. After the December 1994 hijacking of an Air France plane, passengers underwent a debriefing of the incident by a team of psychiatrists. During the hijacking, two passengers were killed by hijackers in front of passengers in the first 5 hours, and a third was executed the next day. Thirty-five passengers were released before the aircraft departed for Marseilles. The other 188 were released after a total of 54 hours after a military assault of the aircraft. It was found that the group of passengers who were initially released suffered from more psychological reactions, perhaps as a result of concern over being executed by hostages immediately after being freed.[23] Unfortunately, this study did not follow up with patients to determine whether this single debriefing prevented worsening or occurrence of psychological symptoms. Although many support the use of an immediate debriefing technique (e.g., critical incident stress debriefing), some reviews have not found this form of single-session therapy to be beneficial.[24] A better technique may be to use the debriefing as a bridge to further outpatient therapy if it is determined that the patient would benefit from ongoing care.

CASE PRESENTATION

Three men board a plane at Baltimore Washington International (BWI) Airport bound for Los Angeles. Moments after the plane lifts off, the three men brandish pepper spray containers and announce that they are taking over the plane. They are also holding some type of sharpened wooden instruments. Members of the flight crew attempt to disable one of the men, but they become incapacitated when they are exposed to the pepper spray.

One of the men begins hammering at the cockpit door, ordering that it be opened immediately or he will begin killing hostages. The pilot and copilot verify that the door is secure and immediately radio the air traffic controller who quickly diverts them back to BWI. The air traffic controller also notifies local authorities, who immediately respond to the airport.

An air marshal sitting near one of the hijackers is able to incapacitate him. One of the remaining hijackers grabs a person from a seat near him and holds the sharpened object to his throat, threatening to kill him. The air marshal, realizing they are now on final approach back at BWI airport, stands back and attempts to negotiate with the hijacker.

The aircraft lands and is quickly met by members of the local SWAT team who also possess a dedicated medical component. They know the number of hijackers at this point and determine the best location for entry of the airplane. The team storms the plane and ultimately shoots the hijacker who was holding the man hostage. The other two hijackers are arrested without incident.

The paramedics attached to the SWAT team attempt to treat the hijacker, but he has sustained a fatal injury to the head. They recognize that many people in the front of the aircraft, including three members of the flight crew, are experiencing some difficulty breathing and tearing of the eyes. They recognize a possible exposure to a chemical irritant and don masks and gloves. These victims are rapidly extricated from the airplane and their eyes are irrigated. Those experiencing respiratory symptoms are treated with oxygen and albuterol. These patients are evaluated at a local hospital and released a few hours later.

A passenger with a history of myocardial infarction reports that he has had chest pain for the last hour but had forgotten to pack his nitroglycerin in his carry-on luggage. He is diaphoretic, tachypneic, and notes that the pain radiates into his left arm. Paramedics administer oxygen, aspirin, and nitroglycerin with some improvement. He is admitted at a local hospital and diagnosed with acute myocardial infarction.

UNIQUE CONSIDERATIONS

Elements of an aircraft hijacking that are unique include the following:

- Although historical examples of hijackings involved hostage taking and negotiating of demands, the possibility of suicide hijackings is now present.
- Airplanes represent a relatively small, closed space, and if they are in flight, hostages are prevented from attempting to escape.
- The flight deck must remain locked down at all times, irrespective of events occurring in the passenger compartment.
- Pilots on the flight deck may be carrying guns to prevent hijackers from taking over the aircraft.
- Air marshals may be present to assist in overcoming a would-be hijacker.
- Due to the confined space, an increased number of injuries may be expected if special teams gain entry to eliminate the threat posed by the hijackers.
- Exposure to chemical incapacitants in this closed space may result in a large number of occupants becoming symptomatic after exposure.
- Many passengers will experience some form of psychological reaction after the event.
- Passengers may experience acute exacerbations of underlying medical conditions.

 ## PITFALLS

Several potential pitfalls exist in response to an aircraft hijacking. These include the following:

- Not having appropriate and rigid screening practices in place to detect potential weapons that may be placed on the aircraft
- Assuming that hijackers only wish to divert the flight and land at another locale
- Allowing hijackers to overtake the flight deck by opening the flight deck door
- Improper training of the flight crew regarding the Crew Training Common Strategy on how to deal with an attempted hijacking
- Not incorporating medical assets into special response teams that may gain entry into the aircraft in an attempt to rescue hostages
- Medical personnel not wearing appropriate protective equipment, especially when exposure to chemical incapacitants is likely

REFERENCES

1. Wikipedia. Aircraft hijacking. Available at: http://en.wikipedia.org/wiki/Aircraft_hijacking.
2. Worldhistory.com. Aircraft hijacking. Available at: http://www.worldhistory.com/wiki/a/aircraft-hijacking.htm.
3. Federal Aviation Administration. FAA historical chronology: civil aviation and the federal government, 1926-1996. 1998 Available at: http://www.faa.gov/docs/b-chron.doc.
4. Rumerman J. Aviation security. U.S. Centennial of Flight Commission. Available at: http://www.centennialofflight.gov/essay/Gove rnment_Role/security/POL18.htm.
5. National Commission of Terrorist Attacks upon the United States. Staff statement no. 4: the four flights. Initially presented January 26-27, 2004, in Washington, DC, at the Seventh Public Hearing of the Commission. Available at: http://news.findlaw.com/hdocs/doc:/terrorism/911comm-SS4.pdf.
6. Loy J. Statement of Admiral James M. Loy Administrator, Transportation Security Administration before the Committee on Commerce, Science, and Transportation. United States Senate; September 9, 2003. Available at: http://www.tsa.dot.gov/public/display? theme=47&content=0900051980069a68.
7. Homeland Security Act of 2002. Title XIV – Arming Pilots Against Terrorism. Available at: http://thomas.loc.gov/cgi-bin/query/z?c107:h.r.5005.enr.
8. Aviation and Transportation Security Act. Public Law 107-71. November 19, 2001. Available at: http://frwebgate.access.gpo.gov/cgi-bin/getdoc.cgi?dbname=107_cong_public_laws&docid=f:publ071.107.pdf.
9. Transportation Security Administration. Report to Congress on Transportation Security. March 31, 2003. Available at: http://www.tsa.gov/interweb/assetlibrary/Report_to_Congress_on_Transportation_Security_ Final_March_31_2003.pdf.
10. Heck J, Pierluisi G. Law enforcement special operations medical support. *Prehospital Emerg Care*. 2002;5:403-6.
11. Heiskell L, Carmona R. Tactical emergency medical services: an emerging subspecialty of emergency medicine. *Ann Emerg Med*. 1994;23:778-85.
12. Federal Aviation Administration. FAA federal air marshal program (September 2001). Available at: http://www.faa.gov/Newsroom/factsheets/2001/factsheets_0109.htm.
13. Shahani R, Galla JD. Penetrating chest trauma. Updated June 11, 2004. Available at: http://www.emedicine.com/med/topic2916.htm.
14. Schouchoff B. Penetrating chest trauma. *Top Emerg Med*. 2001;23:12-19.
15. Schouchoff B, Rodriguez A. Blunt chest trauma. *Top Emerg Med*. 2001;23:1-11.
16. Kaplan L, Alson R, Talavera F, et al. Abdominal trauma, penetrating. Updated May 16, 2003. Available at: http://www.emedicine.com/emerg/topic2.htm.
17. Kirkpatrick A, Sirois M, Ball C, et al. The hand-held ultrasound examination for penetrating abdominal trauma. *Am J Surg*. 2004;187:660-5.
18. Thompson E, Porter J, Fernandez L. Penetrating neck trauma: an overview of management. *J Oral Maxillofac Surg*. 2002;60:918-23.
19. Shepard S, Dulebohn SC, Talavera F, et al. Head trauma. Updated July 26, 2004. Available at: http://www.emedicine.com/med/topic2820.htm.
20. Salomone JA, Salomone JP. Abdominal trauma, blunt. Updated May 16, 2003. Available at: http://www.emedicine.com/emerg/topic1.htm.
21. Smith J, Greaves I. The use of chemical incapacitant sprays: a review. *J Trauma*. 2002;52:595-600.
22. Rega PP, Mowatt-Larssen E, Sole DP. CBRNE-irritants: Cs, Cn, Cnc, Ca, Cr, Cnb, PS. Updated June 29, 2004. Available at: http://www.emedicine.com/emerg/topic914.htm.
23. Cremniter D, Crocq L, Louville P, et al. Posttraumatic reactions of hostages after an aircraft hijacking. *J Nerv Mental Dis*. 1997;185:344-6.
24. Rose S, Bisson J, Wessely S. Psychological debriefing for preventing post traumatic stress disorder (PTSD) [systematic review]. Cochrane Depression, Anxiety and Neurosis Group. *Cochrane Database of Systematic Reviews*. Volume 3. 2004. Available at: http://www.cochrane.org/cochrane/revabstr/AB000560.htm.

chapter 175

Aircraft Crash into a High-Rise Building

Kurt R. Horst

 DESCRIPTION OF EVENT

The attacks on the World Trade Center in New York City on Sept. 11, 2001, are a grim example of the immense damage and destruction that can result when an airplane impacts a high-rise structure. A thorough examination of this disaster may yield a greater understanding of the effects of such an event. Within 20 minutes of each other, two Boeing 767 jets collided with the north and south towers of the World Trade Center, instantly killing the 157 passengers and crew and countless others in each building. In less than 2 hours, both towers had collapsed.[1]

The World Trade Center towers were completed in 1973 and stood over 1300 feet high.[2] They were constructed using a lightweight perimeter tube design, essentially creating a structure akin to an egg crate.[2,3] As such, the design was redundant and, if a few columns failed, the load would be transmitted to adjacent columns.[3] The design allowed for toleration of enormous wind loads and withstanding the impact of an airplane—specifically, a Boeing 707.[3,4]

Why, then, did the towers ultimately collapse? Investigations and research are ongoing, but one possible theory points to the resulting fires that occurred as likely being the chief cause. Immediately after each impact, the initial explosion ignited tens of thousands of gallons of jet fuel, which spread rapidly through the involved floors. It is believed that the immense heat, coupled with the near-instantaneous spread of the fire throughout the structure, led to structural damage and distortion of the steel beams. Eventually, multiple beams at that level failed, and the floor below the impact site could not withstand the massive weight of the 10 to 20 floors above that came crashing down. The buildings ultimately fell because of the inertia of their massive weight, the fact that the buildings themselves were 95% air, and that there was an insignificant lateral load applied to the structure.[3]

As a result of these attacks, more than 2800 people were killed, including over 400 emergency responders.[5] In each tower the catastrophic event consisted of a large-scale mass-casualty incident (MCI) with many varying components. It began with an explosion (likely to have resulted in blast-type injuries) followed by a high-rise fire, which presented its own unique challenges. The subsequent building collapse created a potential need for confined-space rescue.[6] Injuries surrounding the buildings included blast injury, inhalation injury, and thermal injury.[7] Additionally, the involvement of not one, but two high-rise structures added to the complexity of the event, whereby two asynchronous crashes essentially led to two MCI events.[6]

After these attacks, the U.S. Federal Aviation Administration halted all aircraft activity in the United States. The military diverted resources to the East Coast of the United States and military air patrols were begun.[8,9] General aviation slowly resumed as new security measures were implemented.[10]

Initial confusion and incorrect communication may have led to a delay in evacuation of one or both buildings.[11] Communication difficulties also occurred during the response to the incident. As would be expected, radio transmissions increased, many of which were incomplete or unintelligible after the first aircraft struck the first tower. Of note, a New York Police Department helicopter communicated information regarding the impending collapse of the towers, but this information does not appear to have been relayed to emergency responders on-scene.[12]

Finally, a large number of private citizens, physicians, nurses, and other healthcare providers arrived on-scene to provide assistance after the attacks. This process, termed *convergent volunteerism,* although well intentioned, presents a problem on many levels. These persons, in general, are not trained to work in the prehospital setting. They generally lack appropriate safety and personal protective equipment for field operations and may put their lives and the lives of others in jeopardy. These persons also typically engage in freelancing, creating their own triage and treatment areas that have no ability to communicate with the Incident Commander. Verification of credentials and the process of ensuring personnel accountability may be compromised.[13]

 PREINCIDENT ACTIONS

A number of lessons can be learned from this tragic event, many of which are intuitive from the discussion above. One primary goal would be to investigate ways to improve the structural integrity of high-rise buildings to ensure that they will withstand this threat. Although the World Trade Center towers did withstand the initial impact, they ultimately collapsed as a result of loss of structural integrity due to the heat of the subsequent fires.[3,4] Many organizations are continuing to investigate the cause of the collapse, and perhaps this will lead to improved integrity of buildings in the future. In addition, the availability of structural engineers to assess buildings immediately after impact will be of great benefit to determine the likelihood of impending collapse. They will also be useful in evaluating the damage to surrounding structures, as was seen after the Sept. 11, 2001, attacks.[5]

In light of the relatively short time available for evacuation, coupled with the tremendous size of high-rise buildings, it is imperative that emergency egress routes are well planned, easily understood, and practiced. The addition of clear, concise, and correct information broadcast over multiple loudspeakers may aid in decreasing the time that occupants spend debating whether the threat is serious enough to warrant evacuation.[5,14]

From the perspective of emergency personnel, it is imperative that strict adherence to all protocols and the Incident Command System is maintained. Personnel accountability must be enforced, and the safety of rescue personnel must be maintained.[15] Additional and redundant systems of communications must be instituted to decrease system failures.[16] At the same time, contingency plans (e.g., using runners) for total systems failure must be devised. Training specific to this environment must be provided to all emergency personnel and may include high-rise and structural fire suppression and rescue operations, recognition of precursors to building collapse, and confined-space rescue.

Medical triage systems must be used and practiced before an MCI occurs.[17] Specific information about hospitals in the immediate and distant areas, bed status, and specialty capabilities must be available to aid in patient distribution from patient-collection sites. Mutual aid agreements with surrounding ambulance and fire services must be in place before the event to ensure that adequate resources are available for the incident.[18-20] The Federal Emergency Management Agency can also provide a variety of mutual aid resources at the federal level when requested.[21] In addition, it is important to recognize that all resources should not be deployed to the single incident because the average daily number of emergency calls received will continue to arrive.[13]

Finally, hospital disaster plans should augment normal staffing with additional resources.[13] This should minimize the problem of convergent volunteerism, which creates a hazard at the hospital and at the scene of the incident. Hospitals must also be prepared for the presentation of patients in waves, with large numbers of walking wounded presenting with minor injuries first, followed by more severely injured patients. The next groups of patients will likely include those rescued from the structure as well as injured emergency personnel.[7]

Certainly, the prevention of this type of incident from occurring again is a paramount concern. In November 2001, the Aviation and Transportation Security Act was approved in the United States, creating the Transportation Security Administration. It also provided for a number of new security measures, including enhanced screening at airports and the strengthening of flight deck doors aboard commercial aircraft. Provisions for the deployment of specially trained law enforcement agents (i.e., air marshals) onto commercial flights were also outlined.[22] Lastly, a final line of defense should be in place in the event that an aircraft is overtaken and poses a threat to a high-rise structure in a large city. As seen after Sept. 11, 2001, this last-resort option included military flight patrols capable of rapidly responding to a potential threat and exerting deadly force when necessary.[8]

 POSTINCIDENT ACTIONS

An action plan can be developed based on the experience of the New York World Trade Center attacks that can be used to guide an effective emergency response, minimizing injury and loss of life. After an aircraft has crashed into a high-rise structure, the following measures should be undertaken:

- Airspace restrictions should be instituted around the site and likely around the city and local airports. In many cases, as in the Sept. 11, 2001, attacks, the restrictions will be broader.
- A military air presence should be put into place around the area of the incident to provide for possible protection if the incident was the result of a terrorist act.
- Fire or police helicopter assets should be placed around the structure and should continually monitor for any signs of impending collapse.
- Police should set up a perimeter around the incident site to prevent access from bystanders and nonemergency personnel (this includes volunteers who arrive on scene to assist).
- The Incident Command System should be initiated.
- Redundant communication systems should be in place and must be able to handle the ensuing increased amount of radio traffic.
- Mutual aid agreements with surrounding services and private companies should be called into effect. Designated staging areas should be assigned to prevent congestion at the scene.
- Rescue and fire suppression operations should be initiated.
- Designated triage sites around the area of the incident should be set up and staffed by emergency medical services and fire personnel. These areas should be far enough from the actual site of the incident to prevent them from becoming involved if the structure were to collapse.
- Immediate evacuation of the involved building should begin. There should be no debate among occupants about whether to do so, and emergency egress routes should be used.
- During the rescue operation, as safety issues arise or if there is concern for building collapse, a clear warning signal notifying all crews to immediately evacuate should be broadcast.
- All resources at local and outlying hospitals should be available, and patients must be properly dispersed

throughout these facilities rather than over-triaging to the nearest facilities.

- Hospitals should institute their disaster plans, retaining on-duty employees and calling in additional resources as needed.
- Emergency medical and fire resources should also be in place to continue to handle the usual daily emergency call volume.
- Crews should rest frequently and remain hydrated. Rescue and emergency medical "go teams" should be set up to respond to emergency personnel entrapment or injury.
- In the event of a building collapse or simply a prolonged incident scene that will overwhelm local resources, plans should be in place to request additional local, state, and federal assets. This may include specialty teams, including search and rescue, disaster medical assistance teams, disaster mortuary assistance teams, and veterinary medical assistance teams.

MEDICAL TREATMENT OF CASUALTIES

Blast-injury patterns will be seen in victims of this type of incident. Victims may be located either inside the structure at varying distances from the impact site or below the impact as a result of falling debris. The typical array of blunt and penetrating trauma will be caused by the initial impact, flying debris, and blast winds.[23] As a result, victims may suffer open and closed head injury that must be rapidly diagnosed. The possibility of spinal injury is also present if the victim is struck by an object or impacts a wall or other structure after being displaced by the blast wind. Lacerations and fractures, as well as all forms of thoracic and abdominal trauma, can result.[24] Primary blast injury, which affects gas-containing organs, such as the lung, bowel, and middle ear, can present special challenges to healthcare providers and must be diagnosed early.[23,24]

Thermal and inhalation injury can result from the ensuing fires as jet fuel and room contents ignite after the initial impact.[5] These may be severe in many cases, especially in those close to the initial impact site. Burns should be characterized by type and severity and referred to burn centers when necessary. Treatment may be as simple as the application of antibiotic ointment; however, full-thickness and circumferential burns of the chest may require escharotomy.[25] Occupants must be examined for signs of inhalation injury, including soot in the nasopharynx or oropharynx, difficulty breathing, and stridor, and they must be continually monitored for a change in condition. Early aggressive airway management should occur if there is suspicion of such injury.[25,26] Toxic inhalation of carbon monoxide or cyanide must be identified early and may require hyperbaric oxygen therapy or

CASE PRESENTATION

At 10:30 AM, an air traffic controller at Chicago's O'Hare International Airport loses radio contact with a Boeing 757 and recognizes that its flight path has changed. After multiple attempts at radio contact, he recognizes a possible emergency and notifies his superior. Two F-15 military jets are diverted from a nearby training mission to investigate.

As the military pilots approach the aircraft, they report that it is losing altitude and is heading for the Sears Tower in Chicago. Before they are able to gather more information, the 757 impacts the 87th floor. A resulting fireball is seen as debris falls from the structure.

Recognizing that this may be a possible terrorist attack, Federal Aviation Administration representatives immediately set air restrictions for the city of Chicago, and all airlines leaving Chicago's airports are grounded. Aircraft en route to O'Hare and Midway airports are diverted. The military launches multiple groups of F-16 and F-15 fighters, which are now patrolling major cities across the United States.

Chicago police set up a perimeter around the incident and launch helicopters to survey the damage and provide immediate updates of changes or spread of the incident. Local fire and emergency medical services respond. The Incident Command System is put into place immediately, and triage areas are set up outside the immediate danger areas in case of collapse to serve as collection points for walking wounded and rescued occupants from the structure. Teams for initial treatment and evacuation of those who are injured are placed nearer the incident to provide immediate care and transport.

Immediately after the impact, the evacuation of the Sears Tower commences. Hundreds of persons exit the building and are directed through streets away from the incident. Firefighters entering the building begin assisting occupants and extinguishing the fire, which has spread to the 85th floor.

At 11:25 AM, Chicago police helicopters notice an area of the structure near the 86th floor that appears to be bowing outward. This is communicated to the Incident Commander, who orders an immediate evacuation of rescue personnel. A structural engineer is taken via helicopter to inspect the impact site. He feels that, at least at this point, the building remains structurally sound. He does note that with the continued spread of the fire, this will not remain the case.

After another 2 hours, the fires are extinguished. A few stairwells above the impact site remained intact, and a number of occupants above the 87th floor were able to be rescued.

It was estimated there were 8000 occupants at the time of the impact. Three hundred casualties were treated by emergency medical services at the designated triage areas and were distributed to local hospitals. It is estimated that 7300 occupants were evacuated. Two hundred ten passengers aboard the 757 and 700 occupants of the building were killed. While an investigation is ongoing, it does appear to have been a terrorist act.

All local hospitals immediately instituted hospital disaster plans on viewing television news reports and on receiving notification from the Chicago Fire Department. Hospital employees remained on duty, and those at home either came to the hospital or tried to rest in case they were needed as per their specific disaster plans.

the administration of a cyanide antidote kit, respectively.[26] In the context of a collapse, the large amount of dust and debris may also contribute to inhalation injury, as was seen on the attacks on the World Trade Center.[7] Such injury may trigger asthma attacks and exacerbate underlying pulmonary conditions.[24]

Emergency personnel should be trained in the proper use of personal protective equipment, including goggles, gloves, and respirators, when there is dust present after a collapse.[27] Standard treatment of blunt and penetrating trauma should be performed, including an initial assessment of airway, breathing, and circulation followed by a thorough secondary survey to identify other injuries. Supplemental oxygen should be applied, and intubation should be performed when needed. Wounds should be covered and likely fractures splinted. Early neurosurgical, surgical, and orthopedic evaluation should occur in the emergency department and appropriate interventions performed.

 UNIQUE CONSIDERATIONS

An aircraft crash into a high-rise structure represents a unique environment. There tend to be a number of potential injury patterns, encompassing blunt trauma, penetrating trauma, thermal injury, and inhalation injury. Due to the large size of the structure, it may be difficult to obtain access to patients because the impact site generally will be among the upper levels of the building. The resulting fires may impede occupants from escaping and prevent rescue personnel from reaching victims and fighting the fires. The ongoing concerns around the resulting structural integrity of the building may be difficult to ascertain, and the possibility of secondary collapse is ever present.

The locations of these incidents, typically within cities, will likely result in damage not only to the structure impacted, but also to surrounding buildings. Falling debris may damage nearby structures, making them structurally unsound.[5] These secondary impacts may therefore force the evacuation of nearby businesses and homes. The potential for secondary fire spread to these buildings is also not outside the realm of possibility. There will likely be injury and mortality below the impact side from falling debris.

Evacuation may not only include the impacted high-rise, but also a substantial portion of the area around that locale. The egress of thousands of people, not just from one building but perhaps from an entire area of a city, presents its own unique challenges. Evacuation routes in the city should be well marked, and plans for moving this populace should be developed before the occurrence of such an incident.

The concern over a possible terrorist attack must make rescuers wary of a possible secondary explosive device which, as seen on Sept. 11, 2001, may take the form of a second aircraft.[23] As such, a strong police and possibly military presence will be required to protect the scene and surrounding air space. The impact on air travel and the airlines will likely be dramatic.

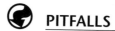 PITFALLS

Several potential pitfalls in response to an aircraft crash into a high-rise building exist. These include the following:

• Failure to institute and follow the Incident Command System
• Failure to develop a series of redundant communications systems as well as contingency plans for total systems failure
• Failure to immediately evacuate the involved high-rise as well as buildings near-by
• Failure to recognize signs of potential or impending building collapse
• Failure to control access to the scene (Note: This is sometimes difficult to accomplish based on available resources and the size of the area involved.)
• Failure to prevent unsolicited volunteers from entering the scene
• Failure to adhere to triage protocols
• Failure to have a hospital disaster plan in place in each facility to provide for an influx of large numbers of patients
• Failure to recognize the need to continue to staff the daily emergency medical and fire service needs of the community that occur outside of the incident on a daily basis

REFERENCES

1. In-depth special war against terror: interactive attacks explainer. Available at: http://www.cnn.com/SPECIALS/2001/trade. center/map.html.
2. Public Broadcasting System. Building big: wonders of the world databank—World Trade Center. Available at: http://www.pbs.org/wgbh/buildingbig/wonder/st ructure/world_trade.html.
3. Eager T, Musso C. Why did the World Trade Center collapse? Science, engineering, and speculation. *JOM.* 2001;53:8-11.
4. NOVA Online. Why the towers fell. Available at: http://www.pbs.org/wgbh/nova/wtc.
5. McAllister T, ed. W*orld Trade Center Building Performance Study: Data Collection, Preliminary Observations, and Recommendations.* FEMA Report 403. Washington, DC: Federal Emergency Management Agency; 2002.
6. Arnold J, Halpern P, Tsai M, et al. Mass casualty terrorist bombings: a comparison of outcomes by bombing type. *Ann Emerg Med.* 2004;43:263-73.
7. Centers for Disease Control and Prevention. Rapid assessment of injuries among survivors of the terrorist attack on the World Trade Center, New York City, September 11, 2001. *MMWR* 2002;51:1-5.
8. Center for Cooperative Research. Complete 911 timeline. Available at: http://www.cooperativeresearch.org/timeline. jsp?timeline=complete_911_timeline.
9. September 11: chronology of terror. Available at: http://www.cnn.com/2001/US/09/11/chronology.attack.
10. FAA orders new safety measures. Available at: http://www.cnn.com/2001/TRAVEL/NEWS/09/12/faa. airports/ index.html.
11. Averill JD. Federal building and fire safety investigation of the World Trade Center disaster. World Trade Center investigation status, project 7: occupant behavior, egress, and emergency communications. June 23, 2004. National Institute of Standards and Technology. Available at: http://wtc.nist.gov/pubs/June2004 OccupantBehavior EmergencyCommunications.pdf.
12. Sunder SS. NIST response to the World Trade Center disaster: World Trade Center investigation status. National Institute of Standards and Technology. Available at: http://wtc.nist.gov/pubs/June2004 WTCStatusprint.pdf.

13. Cone D, Weir S, Bogucki S. Convergent volunteerism. *Ann Emerg Med*. 2003;1:457-62.

14. Proulx G. Terrorist attack on the World Trade Center findings on evacuation issues. CIB Global Leaders Summit on Tall Buildings. Available at: http://www.bre.co.uk/cibtallbuildingssummit/pdf/proulx.pdf.

15. Jackson B, Baker J, Ridgley M, et al. Protecting emergency responders. Vol 3. In: *Safety Management in Disaster and Terrorism Response*. NIOSH Publication 2004-144. Washington, DC: National Institute for Occupational Safety and Health.

16. Garrison H. Keeping rescuers safe. *Ann Emerg Med*. 2002;40:633-5.

17. Frykberg E. Principles of mass casualty management following terrorist disasters. *Ann Surg*. 2004;239:319-21.

18. The White House. Mutual aid agreements: support for first responders outside the major metropolitan areas. Available at: http://www.whitehouse.gov/homeland/firstresponder s/mutualaidagreements.html.

19. Harrald JR. Observing and documenting the inter-organizational response to the September 11 attacks. Presented at: Countering terrorism: lessons learned from natural and technological disasters. February 28–March 1, 2002. Available at: http://dels.nas.edu/dr/docs/harrald.pdf.

20. Tierney K. Lessons learned from research on group and organizational response to disasters. Presented at: Countering terrorism: lessons learned from natural and technological disasters. February 28-March 1, 2002. Available at: http://dels.nas.edu/dr/docs/ tierney.pdf.

21. Federal Emergency Management Agency. National mutual aid and resource management initiative. Available at: http://www.fema.gov/preparedness/mutual_aid.shtm.

22. Aviation and Transportation Security Act. Public Law 107-71. November 19, 2001. Available at: http://frwebgate.access.gpo.gov/cgi-bin/getdoc.cgi?dbname=107_cong_public_laws&docid=f:publ071.107.pdf.

23. Wightman J, Gladish S. Explosions and blast injury. *Ann Emerg Med*. 2001;37:664-78.

24. Centers for Disease Control and Prevention. Explosions and blast injuries: a primer for clinicians. Available at: http://www.bt.cdc.gov/masstrauma/explosions.asp.

25. Alson R. Burns, thermal. Updated October 28, 2003. Available at: http://www.emedicine.com/emerg/topic72.htm.

26. Lafferty KA. Smoke inhalation. Updated August 1, 2001. Available at: http://www.emedicine.com/emerg/topic538.htm.

27. Centers for Disease Control and Prevention. Use of respiratory protection among responders at the World Trade Center site: New York City, September 2001. *MMWR* 2002;51(Special Issue): 6-8.

chapter 176

Airliner Crash into a Nuclear Power Plant

Rick G. Kulkarni

 DESCRIPTION OF EVENT

Nuclear power plants have been recognized as being potential targets of future terrorist attacks. Following the tragic events of Sept. 11, 2001, at the World Trade Center and the Pentagon in the United States, awareness has increased considerably among the public, federal regulatory agencies, and legislators regarding inadequacies in the ability of nuclear power plants to withstand direct attacks by large, high-speed passenger jets with full or nearly full fuel tanks.[1] The U.S. Nuclear Regulatory Commission (NRC), the federal agency responsible for security at the 100-plus nuclear power plants in the United States, has issued several regulatory orders to all licensed nuclear power plants to meet the increased security threat.[2,3]

After the 1979 accident at Three Mile Island near Harrisburg, Pennsylvania, U.S. Congress enacted legislation mandating that all nuclear power plants be covered by emergency contingency plans. A direct consequence of this act was the imposition of a requirement by the NRC that operators of nuclear power plants maintain a 10-mile emergency planning zone equipped with warning sirens all around the plant.[1] Off-site preparedness (i.e., state and local government emergency preparedness activities that take place beyond the nuclear power plant boundaries) is the responsibility of the Federal Emergency Management Agency.[4]

Nuclear power plants are designed to withstand extreme events such as earthquakes and hurricanes. However, direct impacts by large, fuel-laden airliners into the containment building of the plant are not specifically addressed in the design specifications. The risk of a meltdown and subsequent contamination leading to the exposure of a large number of persons to escaping radioactivity by a direct impact of an airliner into the containment building can occur only if structural integrity of the building is compromised.[5] Without a breach caused in the containment building, the radioactive fission products would mostly remain where they are. Such large-scale damage to the containment building could occur either as a direct consequence of the impact itself—a possibility especially for older plants where degradation of the building's construction materials over time may be a factor—or through a delayed loss of strength of the structural members resulting from a sustained and intense conflagration, similar to the one that melted the structural steel in the World Trade Center buildings in New York. Additionally, for a meltdown to occur, there would also have to be subsequent or concomitant direct damage to the reactor vessel and its control equipment or disruption of normal functioning of the cooling mechanism designed to control the heat generated from the nuclear reaction within the fuel rods.[1,5]

The NRC is currently conducting a detailed engineering analysis of the possible effects of such a crash scenario. Spokespersons for the NRC have repeatedly testified to Congress and other regulatory federal agencies that "most plane crashes into containment buildings would not result in significant releases of radiation."[2]

If a large-scale contamination event were to occur, the immediate effects of radiation exposure on humans would most affect the rapidly dividing radiosensitive cells in the gastrointestinal tract and the integument. The central nervous system is also affected due to edema. Hematopoietic effects are ultimately the cause of delayed death if patients survive the immediate effects of radiation poisoning.[6]

Gastrointestinal Manifestations

Gastrointestinal manifestations can occur within 30 minutes of a severe exposure (for example, >10 Gy) or after 6 hours with a lesser exposure (e.g., <0.5 Gy). A higher dose generally results in an earlier onset of symptoms and a more protracted course. The first symptoms include nausea, vomiting, anorexia, and diarrhea. The denuded intestinal tract is a major source of septicemia, especially when combined with the hematopoietic effects of the radiation exposure. Patients will often also become dehydrated due to transudation of plasma into the gastrointestinal tract.[6]

Integument

Increasing exposure to radiation leads to epilation, erythema, and desquamation of the skin. Erythema and blistering with necrosis can develop within hours of a severe exposure or within 1 to 2 days after a lesser exposure.[6]

Central Nervous System

Massive exposure leads to edema of the brain. Patients may complain of headache or vertigo. Ominous signs are altered mental status with or without the development of seizures.[6]

 PREINCIDENT ACTIONS

The NRC is spearheading the effort to ensure the safety of our nuclear power plants from an airliner attack scenario. Since Sept. 11, 2001, the NRC has addressed several aspects of a comprehensive security plan including increased patrols, augmented security forces, installation of additional physical barriers, enhanced coordination with law enforcement agencies, and more restrictive site access for all personnel. Several legislative measures that call for actions ranging from the installation of antiaircraft weapons at all nuclear sites to the deployment of National Guard troops were introduced into Congress since Sept. 11, 2001.[3] In addition, proposals to increase the stockpiling of iodine pills are currently under consideration.[3]

Public awareness of a potential nuclear power plant accident is also important. Persons living in close proximity to plants should be able to recognize the sound of a warning siren, know its relevance, and be ready to begin evacuation in a timely and orderly fashion. They should have emergency supplies available for use in the event of a power disruption and should consider stocking iodine pills themselves. As a part of federally mandated measures after the Three Mile Island accident, Congress required all nuclear power plants to work with the NRC to conduct evacuation and emergency shutdown exercises regularly in the event of a plant malfunction, accident, or terrorist attack. Both the NRC and the Federal Emergency Management Agency monitor the exercises.[2,4] All nuclear power plants in the United States have remained at the highest alert level since the Sept. 11, 2001, attacks. The NRC and other agencies, including commercial nuclear plant operators, have also significantly limited the amount of technical information made available to the public.

 POSTINCIDENT ACTIONS

Once an incident has occurred, it is crucial that a predetermined disaster plan is commenced immediately. Using appropriate personal protection equipment for radiation exposure, rescue personnel should evacuate victims who are not able to leave the scene of the incident themselves in an orderly fashion. Emergency trauma care should be rendered to those victims presenting with blast and burn injuries. Also understand that there may be patients presenting with crush injury. The care of mass casualties from blast, burn, and crush injuries is discussed elsewhere in this book. All victims should be evacuated to a location upwind from the site and evaluated for degree of exposure (Table 176-1). Contaminated clothing should be removed from victims. Receiving hospitals should be notified early during postincident actions. Victims of radiation poisoning should be kept separated from other patients in the treatment area. Isolated water and ventilation systems should be used in designated containment and deconta-

TABLE 176-1 ILLNESS CATEGORIZATION FOR WHOLE-BODY RADIATION EXPOSURE[*]

CATEGORY	EXPOSURE (GY)	SYMPTOMS
Asymptomatic	<1	None
Mild	1-2	Nausea, vomiting ALC at 48 hours > 2000/mm³
Moderate	2-4	Moderate GI symptoms ALC at 48 hours > 1200/mm³
Severe	4-10	Severe GI symptoms ALC at 48 hours < 1200/mm³
Fatal	>10-12	Severe GI symptoms within 30 minutes ALC at 48 hours < 300/mm³

ALC, Absolute lymphocyte count; *GI*, Gastrointestinal.
[*]LD_{50} = 4.5 Gy with medical treatment (100% without medical treatment).

mination areas. Security personnel should control access to minimize the spread of contamination.[6]

All rescue and medical personnel should use universal precautions with gowns, gloves, masks, and shoe covers. Radiation survey monitors should be used to prevent contamination beyond known areas. All equipment and clothing suspected to be contaminated should be placed into secured plastic bags for proper storage and disposal.

The release of a radioactive form of iodine would be a significant component of a release event from a nuclear power plant. Radioactive iodine is absorbed and remains concentrated into the thyroid glands of humans, thus posing a long-term increased risk of cancer of the gland.[7,8] All exposed persons, especially within the emergency planning zone, should be administered potassium iodide pills within 1 hour of exposure to prevent the absorption of the radioactive iodine.[6,7]

 MEDICAL TREATMENT OF CASUALTIES

Cleary, the first layer of casualties will present with blast and burn injuries. These patients should be cared for per standard trauma protocol. The concern for decontamination should be only for those patients not requiring immediate, life-saving medical intervention. Such intervention should be done first, and decontamination should then follow. Treatment should be tailored to the degree of exposure to radiation and the manifestation of symptoms. However, there are core measures common to all victims of radiation exposure. All wounds should be irrigated with saline followed by 3% hydrogen peroxide or a soapy solution. Gastrointestinal decontamination with whole-bowel irrigation with activated charcoal is indicated within 2 hours of exposure for those with moderate or greater levels of exposure. Supportive treatment with intravenous antiemetic agents, intravenous fluid to replace gastrointestinal losses, and the dressing of open wounds and burns is indicated. Also indicated is early transport to a medical facility where advanced treatment such as the institution of viral prophylaxis, administration of hematopoietic growth factors, and bone marrow transplantation can be performed.[4]

Local police officials report that a group of men have been stopped on a California highway between Los Angeles and San Diego in a car laden with weapons and documents pointing to an attack on the San Onofire nuclear power plant. The incident is reported immediately to the U.S. NRC and to the Department of Defense (DoD). At the same time, the North American Aerospace Defense Command alerts the NRC and the DoD that a 767 Boeing passenger jet seems to be heading for San Onofire and it not responding to direct communication efforts.

Military personnel in jet aircrafts are scrambled from Edwards Air Force Base in Lancaster, California. Their mission is to intercept the passenger jet and order it to change course and land immediately at San Diego International Airport. Additionally, emergency measures to shut down the nuclear power plant are implemented at San Onofire. Minutes later, before the Air Force jets can make visual contact with the passenger jet's cockpit crew, the Boeing 767 crashes into the main containment-building tower of the power plant. Although the crash does not immediately compromise the structural integrity of the reactor's core

concrete containment building, it wipes out off-site power to the reactor necessary for the shutdown process. Backup generators fail, and a leak of reactor coolant raises the specter of a meltdown.

An emergency is declared in the area surrounding the nuclear power plant. Persons living in northern San Diego County, Orange County, and adjoining Los Angeles County are ordered to evacuate. Those who have potassium iodide are advised to "swallow one dose now."

Protesters quickly organize behind barricades outside the San Diego International Airport conference room—the headquarters for operations—where reporters receive intermittent briefings on the situation. It seems that a core reactor meltdown has been averted through the use of secondary backup generators, quick response, and the efficient action of local firefighter crews to extinguish the fire from the airliner's impact, and the competent implementation of emergency shutdown protocols by the power plant's staff. Two hundred forty-five persons in the passenger airliner and five persons on the ground were killed in the incident.

UNIQUE CONSIDERATIONS

Gross structural failure of the containment building is essential for a large-scale contamination event occurring from a reactor material release. Although the containment building may not be compromised by the direct impact of an airliner, the effect of a subsequent jet fuel fire or explosion could cause further mechanical and thermal damage to the containment facility, resulting in a structural collapse of the building.

Nuclear power plants house many more times the amount of radioactive substances than do stored nuclear weapons. If there is an accidental disaster or a deliberate act of sabotage, the release of only a small portion of this material will have severe consequences.

Radiation cannot be detected by sight, smell, or any other sense. This should be a consideration of responders and other personnel. Another element to be kept in mind is that the ingestion of a nonradioactive iodine pill will prevent the absorption and concentration of radioactive iodine released during a nuclear power plant meltdown.

Although there have been no incidents of an airliner crash into a nuclear power plant, the possibility of this type of terrorist attack cannot be excluded. Increased vigilance and preparedness of local, regional, state, and federal agencies as well as of the medical staff in areas with operational nuclear power plants is indicated.

PITFALLS

Several potential pitfalls in response to an aircraft crash into a nuclear power plant exist. These include the following:

- Failure of rescue personnel to use appropriate personal protective equipment

- Failure to quickly isolate affected persons
- Failure to notify receiving hospitals in a timely manner
- Failure to properly categorize victims based on their degree of exposure
- Failure to identify and treat emergent traumatic injuries
- Failure to create a plan for mass treatment in the event of an attack

REFERENCES

1. Behrens CE. *Nuclear Power Plants: Vulnerability to Terrorist Attack.* Congressional Research Service Report for Congress; 2003.
2. United States Nuclear Regulatory Commission. Nuclear reactors. Available at: http://www.nrc.gov/reactors.html.
3. Nuclear Regulatory Commission. Nuclear security—before and after September 11. Available at: http://www.nrc.gov/what-we-do/safeguards.html.
4. U.S. Federal Emergency Management Agency. Radiological Emergency Preparedness Program. Available at: http://www.fema.gov/preparedness/repp.shtm.
5. Lyman ES. The vulnerability of nuclear power plant containment buildings to penetration by aircraft. Nuclear Control Institute. September 21, 2001. Available at: http://www.nci.org/01nci/09/aircrashab.htm.
6. Jones MP. Radiation injury. In: Schaider J, Hayden S, Wolfe R, et al. *Rosen & Barkin's 5-Minute Emergency Medicine Consult.* 2nd ed. Philadelphia: Lippincott, Williams & Wilkins; 2003:932-3.
7. Kahn LH, von Hippel F. Nuclear power plant emergencies and thyroid cancer risk: what New Jersey physicians need to know. *N Engl J Med.* 2004;101:22-7.
8. Parfitt T. Chernobyl's legacy. 20 years after the power station exploded, new cases of thyroid cancer are still rising, say experts. *Lancet* 2004;363:1534.

chapter 177

Dirty Bomb (Radiologic Dispersal Device)*

George A. Alexander

 ## DESCRIPTION OF EVENT

A *dirty bomb* is a device that combines radioactive materials with conventional explosives. Global terrorist organizations are believed to be interested in and capable of constructing dirty bombs and launching attacks with them.[1] There are only two documented cases of terrorist use of dirty bombs in the world today.[2] Both incidents occurred in Russia. In 1995, Chechen insurgents buried a cesium-137 dirty bomb in a park in Moscow and alerted the media before its detonation. In 1998, a container of radioactive materials was found attached to an explosive mine near a railroad line in Chechnya. Dirty bombs are attractive to terrorists because they are relatively easy to acquire and have the potential of causing casualties, contamination of widespread areas, adverse psychological effects, and economic disruption. A dirty bomb threat potentially poses a medical and public health disaster.

A dirty bomb can be made from traditional dynamite, trinitrotoluene (TNT), ammonium nitrate, or a variety of other explosive materials.[3] When detonated, it kills or injures by the initial blast, which causes damage from the expansion of hot gases, and by dispersing radioactive materials that are highly toxic over a wide geographic area without a nuclear explosion. The dispersal effects of a dirty bomb depend on the amount of explosives used, the physical form of the radioactive source, and the atmospheric conditions.[4] A dirty bomb is also known technically as a *radiologic dispersal device*.

Many different radioactive sources can be used to fabricate a dirty bomb. Radioactive sources can be obtained illicitly from hospitals and medical clinics, industrial radiography and gauging devices, food sterilizers, power sources, communication devices, navigator beacons, oil well logging, and scientific research laboratories. Some common radioactive sources that have a high probability of being used as a dirty bomb based on their availability include cobalt-60, strontium-90, cesium-137, iridium-192, radium-226, plutonium-238, americium-241, and californium-252.

Alpha-emitting radiation sources pose serious health hazards if they are inhaled, ingested, or deposited in an open wound. Beta-emitting sources can cause deep beta burns on the skin. Gamma rays may penetrate body tissues and cause deep tissue injury.

The most likely dirty bomb scenarios would involve the use of either a few small low-level radioactive sources or a large amount of highly radioactive sources combined with high explosives. The first scenario considers use of a dirty bomb containing a few curies of a gamma-ray source such as cobalt-60 or cesium-137 combined with a few kilograms of high explosive. In this case, the dirty bomb might be used with the primary intent of causing fear or panic among people and disrupting their community. Since the amount of radioactivity is small, the radiation exposure to individuals would be low, and no immediate effects on health would be expected. The probability of long-term health effects would be small.

The second scenario considers use of a dirty bomb containing large sources of penetrating radiation coupled with sophisticated high explosives. The detonation would disperse considerable amounts of radioactive material over a large area. Persons injured by the blast are likely to be contaminated with radioactivity and may receive life-threatening doses of radiation. Such a device is intended to kill tens or hundreds of persons, to injure and sicken hundreds or thousands, and to cause widespread panic.[5]

Recognizing that a conventional explosive device has been detonated may be simple because of the associated blast. However, it may take considerable time before the radioactive component of the dirty bomb attack is recognized. Therefore, it is important that first responders use radiation-detection equipment to identify a radioactive component after any explosion.[6]

Recognition of acute radiation injury is based on the patient's medical history and clinical findings.[7] The extent of radiation injury depends on three factors: depth of penetration of the radiation, dose of radiation absorbed, and volume of tissue irradiated. For localized radiation exposure, the initial signs of injury might be a radiation burn including erythema, blistering, or desquamation. With a low whole-body dose of 0 to 100 cGy from a dirty bomb, a patient would generally have no symptoms. With a moderate whole-body dose of 100 to 200 cGy, the

---

*The views expressed in this chapter are those of the author and do not necessarily represent the official policy or position of the National Cancer Institute, the National Institutes of Health, or the Department of Health and Human Services.

patient may exhibit the prodromal phase (nausea and vomiting) of acute radiation syndrome. At doses exceeding 300 cGy, patients would experience nausea, vomiting, diarrhea, erythema, and fever. A useful method of predicting the clinical severity of radiation injury is the time to onset of vomiting. If the time to vomiting is less than 4 hours, the patient has received a high dose of radiation.

Laboratory data show that early changes in lymphocyte counts are associated with the severity of radiation injury. Absolute lymphocyte counts less than 1000 mm^3 and greater than 500 mm^3 indicate moderate and severe levels of radiation exposure, respectively. Complete blood counts can be repeated every 4 to 6 hours to evaluate lymphocyte depletion kinetics. The appearance of chromosome dicentrics in peripheral blood lymphocytes is also useful in calculating exposure dose. In patients who have developed acute radiation syndrome, within 2 to 3 weeks bone marrow suppression may occur with associated neutropenia, lymphopenia, and thrombocytopenia.

 PREINCIDENT ACTIONS

One of the most important preemptive actions that emergency medical service agencies, hospital-based emergency departments, and outpatient facilities should do is to determine whether their community is a possible target for a terrorist dirty bomb attack. Coordinating with local and state law enforcement and response agencies should provide a framework in which to assess the dirty bomb threat and develop a medical radiation incident or injury protocol. The protocol should be incorporated into the overall disaster plan. The radiation disaster plan should address decontamination, security, radiation monitoring, and decorporation of radioactive materials. The hospital radiation safety officer should be included in the medical radiation response team. Hospital staff should understand the hazards of radioactive contamination and be trained in radiation-monitoring techniques. Staff would need access to dosimeters, Geiger-Mueller counters, and personal protective equipment. Radiation-detection capabilities are critical to an effective medical response. Hospitals should have a realistic decontamination plan for patients, a lockdown plan to control access, and evacuation plans. A radiation risk communication program is required for the public.

 POSTINCIDENT ACTIONS

Emergency medical first responders arriving on the scene of a dirty bomb incident should initiate actions to treat or evacuate casualties. All response personnel should be advised of the explosive and radiologic hazards that may be present. Healthcare providers should advise others regarding safety measures to be taken to protect the public and to mitigate the radiation health effects. Patients evacuated from the scene and arriving at hospitals or medical clinics should be routinely monitored for radiation and decontaminated as needed.

Healthcare providers should control any exposure of hospital personnel to contamination. Clinicians should seek the assistance and cooperation of state and local authorities and inform them of casualties and possible hazards. Hospital radiation safety staff should periodically monitor the emergency department for radioactive contamination.

 MEDICAL TREATMENT OF CASUALTIES

Injuries associated with dirty bombs pose new and significant challenges for clinicians. Since radiation affects many organ systems, it can complicate blast and thermal injuries associated with a dirty bomb. Conventional injuries should be treated first, since radiation contamination is not a life-threatening medical emergency. Patients with traumatic blast and radiation injury should be resuscitated and stabilized. The assessment of patient airway, breathing, and circulation always takes priority. Victims of radiation exposure require more specialized treatment, and specialists in hematology, oncology, radiation, and infectious disease should be consulted. Effective treatment of internally contaminated patients requires knowledge of both the relevant radioactive isotope and its physical form. Treatment should be instituted quickly to ensure its effectiveness. However, with a terrorist incident, initially the radioactive source or sources are not known.[8] Several general approaches may be used to treat internal radiation contamination, including reduction of absorption (administer Prussian blue), dilution (force fluids), removal of blockage (use potassium iodide), rectification of displacement by nonradioactive materials (administer oral phosphate), mobilization as a means of elimination from tissue (use ammonium chloride), and chelation (achieve with Ca-DTPA and Zn-DTPA).[9]

Patients who have received a low whole-body radiation dose may develop gastrointestinal tract distress within the first 2 days. Antiemetic agents may be effective in reducing the gastrointestinal symptoms, which will usually subside within the first day. If not, the administration of parenteral fluids should be considered.

The prognosis for patients who have suffered traumatic blast, burn, and radiation injury is worse than for patients with radiation injury alone.[10] A wound that is contaminated with radioactive materials should be rinsed with saline and treated using conventional aseptic techniques.[4] Wounds contaminated with alpha-emitting radioactive isotopes are usually excised. In patients who receive whole-body doses of radiation greater than 100 cGy, the wound should be closed as soon as possible to prevent it from becoming an entry for lethal infection.

In spite of the wide availability of antibiotics, infections from opportunistic pathogens pose a major problem among patients exposed to intermediate and high doses of radiation. In these cases, the primary determinants of survival are treatment of microbial infections and aggressive resuscitation of the bone marrow.[10]

On a busy Thursday morning, you hear a radio news report of a massive explosion in a crowded downtown district of your large city. Casualties are being evacuated from the scene to local area hospitals. Officials believe the explosion may be due to a natural gas leak.

Later, you see a 47-year-old man who was brought to the emergency department of your hospital after being trapped for nearly 3 hours by fallen debris in a collapsed building at the scene of the explosion. He complains of left thigh pain, dizziness, nausea, weakness, and a burning sensation in his chest. Your high index of suspicion prompts radiation monitoring to be performed, and this reveals a significant level of radioactivity from a beta-gamma emitter. A cursory examination reveals multiple superficial facial and upper extremity lacerations and a deep penetrating wound of the left thigh. The results of an initial complete blood count are unremarkable.

Meanwhile, the mayor has announced that the explosion may have been caused by a terrorist radioactive dirty bomb. Two more patients with multiple injuries are brought to the hospital by ambulance. The emergency waiting room is now filled with a dozen walk-in patients complaining of nausea and vomiting.

 ## UNIQUE CONSIDERATIONS

In contrast to popular belief, a dirty bomb is not considered a weapon of mass destruction.[5] Instead, it is used as a weapon of mass *disruption*.[3] Because radiation is colorless, odorless, tasteless, silent, and invisible, the uncertainty of not knowing whether one is being or has been exposed to radiation instills fear and panic in most people. The psychological effects of a dirty bomb incident require special consideration.

Recognition of the importance of social and psychological issues will be essential in responding to a terrorist dirty bomb attack.[6] Such an incident can cause profound psychosocial effects at every level of society including individual, family, community, and the nation. A dirty bomb attack has the capability of causing widespread fear, an increased sense of vulnerability, and loss of trust and confidence in societal institutions.[6] The effects can be emotional, physical, cognitive, or interpersonal in nature. Significant numbers of people may suffer chronic distress years after an attack. Although a dirty bomb attack will create unique challenges, basic tenets of disaster mental health should still be followed in treating those affected.

 ## PITFALLS

Obstacles to the provision of optimal medical care include the following:

- Failure to adequately prepare of medical response planning for possible terrorist dirty bomb attacks before they occur
- Failure to coordinate with local and state emergency response agencies
- Lack of understanding by medical providers of the basic science of radioactive isotopes
- Failure to consult with specialists who have clinical experience in the medical management of the effects of radiation exposure
- Lack of recognition that anxiety-induced nausea and vomiting may occur after a dirty bomb attack (This phenomenon has been observed after radiation accidents in which people thought they had been exposed to radiation even in the absence of actual exposure.[11])

REFERENCES

1. Meyer J. Al Qaeda feared to have "dirty bombs." *The Los Angeles Times.* February 8, 2003:A1.
2. Edwards R. Only a matter of time? *New Sci.* 2004;182:8-9.
3. King G. *Dirty Bomb: Weapon of Mass Disruption.* New York: Penguin Group; 2004.
4. Mettler FA, Voelz GL. Major radiation exposure—what to expect and how to respond. *N Engl J Med.* 2002;346:1554-61.
5. Zimmerman PD, Loeb C. Dirty bombs: the threat revisited. Center for Technology and National Security Policy, National Defense University. *Defense Horizons.* No. 38, January, 2004.
6. National Council on Radiation Protection and Measurement. *Management of Terrorist Events Involving Radioactive Material.* Report No. 138. Bethesda, Md: National Council on Radiation Protection and Measurement; 2001.
7. Gusev I, Guskova AK, Mettler FA Jr, eds. *Medical Management of Radiation Accidents.* 2nd ed. Boca Raton, Fla: CRC Press; 2001.
8. Leikin JB, McFee RB, Walter FG, et al. A primer for nuclear terrorism. *Dis Mon.* 2003;49:485-516.
9. Voelz GL. Assessment and treatment of internal contamination: general principles. In: Gusev I, Guskova AK, Mettler FA Jr, eds. *Medical Management of Radiation Accidents.* 2nd ed. Boca Raton, Fla: CRC Press; 2001:319-36.
10. Conklin JJ, Walker RI. Diagnosis, triage, and treatment of casualties. In: Conklin JJ, Walker RI, eds. *Military Radiobiology.* San Diego, Calif: Academic Press, Inc; 1987:231-40.
11. International Atomic Energy Agency. *The Radiological Accident in Goiânia.* Vienna: International Atomic Energy Agency; 1988.

chapter 178

Explosion at a Nuclear Waste Storage Facility

Constance G. Nichols

 DESCRIPTION OF EVENT

Nuclear waste is the radioactive by-product of radionuclides used in medicine, industry, research, weapons development and manufacture, and power generation. Any facility that uses radionuclides is, in theory, a nuclear waste storage facility. Each site must have safe, secure storage for spent radionuclides until they are taken to a more definitive storage facility. Currently 131 facilities exist in the United States, with the Yucca Mountain, Nevada, site is the planned final repository for nuclear waste.

A fire, natural disaster, or intentional detonation of explosives in such a facility will potentially result in the release of radioactive materials of varying levels of injury and lethality. In 1982, the U.S. Congress directed the Department of Energy to construct a permanent underground storage facility for spent nuclear reactor fuel and other forms of high-level nuclear waste. In 1987, Congress directed the Department of Energy to develop only Yucca Mountain, Nevada, as a potential site, and President Bush recommended Yucca Mountain as a site in 2002. Due to problems with development, it is unlikely that Yucca Mountain will open as scheduled in 2010.

Sites holding waste pending long-term disposal are now trying to expand their wet pool storage (a less expensive option) because the existing wet pool storage is reaching capacity. Some are looking at the more expensive dry storage (i.e., steel containers in concrete bunkers) as a temporizing measure.[1]

The U.S. Nuclear Regulatory Commission has felt that exposure of citizens to spent fuel would be unlikely because it is contained in a ceramic material. Exposure would require that the spent fuel be pulverized, such as in a high-speed impact or explosion, or the spent fuel would need to burn at high temperatures in a sustained fire.[1] Unfortunately, very similar conditions occurred with the use of airliners as bombs on Sept. 11, 2001.

The development of the Nevada site has been slow and controversial, and the area will not be available for many years. Therefore, it is necessary to regard any place that uses radionuclides as a potential nuclear waste storage facility.

A conventional non-nuclear explosion at a site of nuclear waste storage would be similar in some ways to that of a radiation dispersal device or "dirty" bomb. It would differ in the concentration, amount, and variety of radionuclides dispersed. Another important factor would be whether the explosion was accidental or planned in such a way as to maximize dispersal of radionuclides.

 PREINCIDENT ACTIONS

Cities and hospitals all have general disaster plans. Sites storing nuclear waste have procedures for dealing with contamination. Before an event, it would be important to communicate to the city and hospital disaster planners the amounts and types of radionuclides present in a local facility. Although national security interests might preclude an exact accounting of amounts of materials, the general nature of the materials should be available to emergency services and healthcare providers who would be dealing with victims of such an event.

Drills covering radiation scenarios such as accidental release, conventional explosions, or terrorist attack should be considered and performed to acquaint all providers of emergency care with the special considerations for radiation disasters. Locations of radiation detectors in hospitals and ambulances should be part of the knowledge base of every provider working in those settings, as should basic decontamination principles.

 POSTINCIDENT ACTIONS

Immediately upon notification of an explosion at a nuclear waste storage facility, hospitals and emergency services should begin responding according to their disaster plans. Fire and police set up hot and cold zones and begin with victim decontamination. In this scenario, the contamination is assumed to be external, with contaminated wounds and inhalation of dust or debris the exception. Special plans for radiation safety should be implemented as soon as the nature of the event is determined. The need for scene decontamination and the timing of transport must be determined in the decontamination zone and should be part of planning for radiation events.

At receiving facilities, nonemergent patients should be screened for radiation contamination before entering. Emergent patients have life-saving care provided immediately and are then decontaminated. The ambulatory casualties who have not gone through decontamination at the site must be decontaminated before entering the treatment facility. This may entail police or security personnel equipped with adequate personal protection directing potentially contaminated patients to the appropriate part of the facility to ensure they do not contaminate the treatment area.

If possible, all emergency services and hospital personnel should wear dosimeter badges. Hospital radiation safety officers should monitor treatment areas, casualties, and staff to prevent secondary victims.

 ## MEDICAL TREATMENT OF CASUALTIES

After decontamination, either at the site of the event or at the treatment facility, patients should be treated for their injuries and medical complaints. However, life-saving care should be provided even before decontamination. Most casualties will have blast and thermal burn injury. Basic trauma care should be provided to these patients. (For detailed care information for patients with radiation injury, see Section Eight.) Patients should be reevaluated by the hospital radiation safety officer to determine whether they are decontaminated before admission to the hospital or discharge home. Patients need to be informed of the adverse effects of radiation poisoning, and a system should be established to follow up with potential victims for signs of radiation sickness and secondary illnesses from radiation exposure.

The Federal Emergency Management Agency toolkit for radiologic incidents defines hospital treatment as follows:

"Radiation damage can be repaired if the dose received is not too high and if the dose is received over a long period of time. Injured victims who are suspected of being contaminated by radiological hazards should be treated at hospital facilities that have the capacity for this specific type of treatment. Local officials must ensure that such facilities are identified in the Emergency Operations Plan. Note: The U.S. medical community is currently ill-equipped to deal with a large-scale incident involving radiation poisoning. Only one hospital emergency room—in Oak Ridge, TN—is dedicated to treatment of this type of injury."[2]

Postexposure prophylaxis with iodine would need to be instituted if the facility contained spent nuclear fuel or other iodine-containing waste.

The World Health Organization guidelines for use of iodine after radiation exposure are presented in Table 178-1.[3]

 ## CASE PRESENTATION

"Oh my God!" The sound erupts from the waiting room. The triage nurse comes running back and tells the staff there has been an explosion at the nuclear power plant. As you watch the television, horrified, the local news program reports that there has been radiation released. The Nuclear Regulatory Commission and Federal Emergency Management Agency are going to be involved. Four people come running through the ambulatory door of the emergency department claiming they have been "irradiated," while the patients waiting to be seen gather their belongings and run to the parking lot.

You call the administrator and ask to go to your highest-level disaster plan. The resource nurse hands you the "triage officer" vest and directs you to the ambulance entrance.

 ## UNIQUE CONSIDERATIONS

Internal Contamination

Patients with inhalation or ingestion of radiation sources cannot be decontaminated by traditional washing methods. Contaminated wounds can be debrided.

TABLE 178-1 REFERENCE LEVELS FOR DIFFERENT POPULATION GROUPS FOR CONSIDERATION IN PLANNING STABLE IODINE PROPHYLAXIS*

POPULATION GROUP	EXPOSURE PATHWAYS TO BE CONSIDERED	REFERENCE LEVELS
Neonates, infants, children, adolescents to 18 years and pregnant and lactating women	Inhalation (and ingestion†)	10 mGy‡ avertable dose to the thyroid
Adults younger than 40 years	Inhalation	100 mGy‡ avertable dose to the thyroid
Adults older than 40 years	Inhalation	5 Gy§ projected dose to the thyroid

(From Guidelines for Iodine Prophylaxis following Nuclear Accidents Update 1999.)
*These idealized levels do not take into account the practicalities involved in planning to respond to an accident involving many radionuclides in unknown quantities in real time. For this reason, a generic intervention level of 100 mGy has been specified in the Basic Safety Standards. Nevertheless, this does not preclude the need to consider the practicality of planning to implement iodine prophylaxis for specific age groups.
†Ingestion of milk by infants where alternative supplies cannot be made available.
‡Adherence to these values would ensure that doses for all age groups would be well below the threshold for deterministic effects.
§Intervention for this group is undertaken to ensure prevention of deterministic effects in the thyroid. Five Gy is the recommended limit for deterministic effects given in the Basic Safety Standards.

Decontamination of the pulmonary tree is difficult, but irrigation of the nasal mucosa may remove a large amount of trapped particles. Use of agents to speed passage through the gastrointestinal tract is the treatment modality of choice. All effluent must be collected for a 24-hour period or until no radiation is detectable.

Pregnant Women

Pregnant women would need to be counseled regarding the effect of radiation on their fetus. Consideration would need to be given to amount of exposure and stage of fetal development.

Mental Health Issues

A radiologic incident can be expected to cause widespread public panic and fear related both to the current dangers and to the possibility of long-term health effects. Crisis counseling should be available for incident victims, and a greater demand can be expected on long-term mental health services.

Chronic Health Issues

Exposure to radiation has the potential for stochastic effects, including cancer and genetic effects. The local medical community should expect an upsurge in patients seeking treatment, and anyone exposed to unsafe levels of radiation will require long-term monitoring.

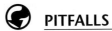 **PITFALLS**

Several potential pitfalls in response to an explosion at a nuclear waste storage facility exist. These include the following:

- Lack of knowledge about a nuclear waste storage facility in the area
- Lack of training in radiation-decontamination procedures
- Contamination of ambulances and treatment facilities
- Possible contamination of treatment facility, if located near the event
- Location necessitating evacuation of treatment facility
- Loss of staff due to fear for family and safety

REFERENCES

1. Report to the Chairman, Subcommittee on Energy and Air Quality, Committee on Energy and Commerce, U.S. House of Representatives. Spent nuclear fuel: options exist to further enhance security. U.S. General Accounting Office; July 2003. Available at: http://www.gao.gov/new.items/d03426.pdf.
2. U.S. Federal Emergency Medical Agency. Toolkit for managing the emergency consequences of terrorist incidents. Appendix C: radiological incidents. July 2002. Available at: http://www.fema.gov/preparedness/toolkit.shtm.
3. World Health Organization. Guidelines for iodine prophylaxis following nuclear accidents: update 1999. Geneva: 1999. Available at: http://www.who.int/ionizing_radiation/pub_meet/Iodine_Prophylaxis_guide.pdf.

chapter 179

Maritime Disasters

Lucille Gans

 DESCRIPTION OF EVENT

Although maritime disasters no longer occur with the frequency of past centuries, when tens of thousands of ships sinking to the bottom of the world's oceans left thousands of persons dead, they remain a major source of tragedy and loss for the transportation industry.[1] Maritime disasters include incidents involving cruise ships, yachts, ferries, barges, container and cargo vessels, fishing boats, submarines, offshore oil platforms, and other watercraft.

The loss of seaworthiness of a ship can result from several causes, often occurring in combination. Disasters are most often caused by storms, fires, and explosions, although loss of life generally results from human error. Contributing factors may include excessive reliance on technology, which can result in the loss of basic and advanced sailing techniques, plus underestimation of potential vessel vulnerabilities and risks posed by weather and sea conditions. Technologic advances have meant increases in the size and carrying capacity of ships, with concomitant increased potential for loss of life and property. Human factors also include failure to establish or follow procedures to enhance the safety of ships, their passengers, and crew; inexperience; and "cutting corners" to save time and money. If commercial concerns such as competitiveness, maintaining schedules, and cargo take precedence over passenger and crew safety, disasters can and do result. Survival is enhanced by diligent compliance with appropriate procedures and standards combined with knowledge, experience, and resourcefulness.[2]

Drowning is the most common cause of death due to maritime disasters, followed by hypothermia,[2] although traumatic injuries may also occur because of the event that produced the disaster. These injuries include but are not limited to burns, blast injuries from explosions, and both blunt and penetrating trauma.[3] In addition, victims who survive the initial sinking of the ship but who are not rescued in a timely manner may ultimately die from dehydration, starvation, or exposure while occupying life rafts or floating in the sea.

Maritime disasters also include events when no human lives are lost but loss of the ship's cargo results in pollution and damage to the ocean waters, marine life, and shoreline. Such situations have most often involved oil tankers, as in the cases of the *Exxon Valdez* in Alaska and the *Sea Empress* in Australia. Other cargo ships carrying hazardous materials that have been damaged while near shore and habitation include the *Multitank Ascania*, carrying highly explosive vinyl acetate, and the *Bilboa*, carrying ferrosilicon (which can release toxic and explosive gases when exposed to moisture), to list only a few of the hundreds of incidents that have occurred in recent decades.[4] There are huge costs associated with rescue, salvage, and recovery in such situations. For example, the cost for clean-up after the *Exxon Valdez* spill is estimated at $2.2 billion (U.S.).

 PREINCIDENT ACTIONS

Before leaving port, both cargo and passenger vessels are subject to various laws and maritime agreements. These requirements include the national laws of the country under which the ship is registered. Many ocean-going vessels are registered under "flags of convenience" to take advantage of national marine laws that may be less stringent than those of the country from which the passenger or cargo company most often sails.[3]

In addition, there are further security requirements imposed by the individual ports that the ship enters. The International Maritime Organization (IMO) is the specialized agency of the United Nations that has the responsibility for the safety of shipping and the prevention of marine pollution by ships.[5] As well, following the Sept. 11, 2001, terrorist attacks on the World Trade Center in New York City, the IMO developed and adopted port security measures as outlined in the International Ship and Port Facility Security Code, which came into effect in 2004.[6]

All ships should be required to sail with adequate life jackets and lifeboats or rafts aboard for all passengers and crew. National standards for life jackets or personal flotation devices (PFDs) vary among countries. In addition, PFDs designed to allow greater freedom of movement for participation in water sports, such as windsurfing, may provide lesser degrees of buoyancy. PFDs should be adjustable to fit various body shapes and statures and volumes of clothing, including specialized protective gear. Ideally, the PFD should be self-righting, should maintain the wearer at the water surface, and should keep the airway clear of water, which requires a minimum of 34 lb (150 newtons) of buoyancy. PFDs should be fitted with a crotch strap to prevent the device from riding up over the shoulders. Even with a properly fitted PFD, however, the dependent legs of the wearer act as a sea anchor, turning the face toward the waves. A person with impaired consciousness, a condition that may develop with hypothermia after immersion in cold water, may be unable to coordinate breathing with the irregular pattern of wave splash over face, and death by drowning may occur.[2]

Lifeboat drills and other safety instruction should be provided once the vessel leaves port. However, there is no guarantee that such information will be provided in multiple languages or that passengers will understand, remember, or comply with directions at the time of an emergency.

Lifeboats, life rafts, and their launch equipment must be maintained to ensure that they are functional and seaworthy. At the bare minimum, each lifeboat should be supplied with a container of survival supplies including water, food rations, raft repair equipment, a sea anchor, and signaling equipment such as flares, lights, and mirrors. The IMO stipulates the equipment that survival craft must carry, based on the number of persons to be carried. Anyone aboard a vessel should consider assembling a grab bag containing additional supplies, clothing, and medications should it become necessary to abandon ship, using as a guide the requirements listed by maritime regulators or sailing race authorities.[2,7]

Because factors external to the ship such as weather and sea conditions can affect the safe passage of the vessel, technologic advances such as Doppler weather radar and Global Positioning Systems, combined with enhanced global communication systems, have contributed greatly to improved ocean safety records in recent years.[7]

 ## POSTINCIDENT ACTIONS

Once the integrity of a ship is breached, or as soon as some other threat to passenger or crew safety is recognized, it is essential that rescue procedures be initiated. Alarms both onboard and via radio transmission to appropriate sea- and land-based rescue facilities should be raised. The extent of the potential danger to the ship and those onboard should be assessed, with consideration for potential worsening of conditions.

If the problem can be adequately managed with onboard resources, appropriate personnel should be advised and intervention measures initiated. Procedures for fire suppression must be well understood and initiated immediately once a fire is detected.

If the incident is thought to be manageable with the resources available onboard, a "Pan Pan" message should be sent via radio transmission. If the vessel is in immediate danger, a "Mayday" message should be transmitted. In both cases, the radio message should include the vessel name,

nature of the incident, number of persons onboard, and geographic location with latitude and longitude. Maritime history includes many cases in which rescue was delayed by either incomplete information or failure of notification from the stricken vessel, often resulting in loss of life.[2]

Generally, those onboard will be better off remaining on the ship unless the captain determines that the ship is in danger of sinking. Before leaving the ship, each person should put on a lifejacket or PFD. If available, survival suits should also be worn.

Lifeboats and rafts are smaller and less comfortable than a full-size ship, especially in rough ocean waters. In addition, there is no mechanism for steering or sailing most rafts.

The crew should instruct passengers in how to get into lifeboat or rafts and the procedures for launching them. Once afloat, occupants should attempt to rescue survivors in the water, which may be hampered greatly by hypothermia of both parties. Therefore, bailing and drying procedures must be adopted early on in the survival craft.[2] Additionally, rationing of food and water should be initiated, even if rescue is anticipated in a short time.[7] No one should drink seawater, in any quantity, as this markedly reduces the chance of survival.[2] Measures should be taken to reduce seasickness, including taking antinausea medications, if available, because seasickness will worsen most medical conditions and has further negative effects on hygiene and morale for all persons in a survival craft.[7]

 ## MEDICAL TREATMENT OF CASUALTIES

Rescuers may include those specially equipped and trained for water rescues—for example, the U.S. Coast Guard Search and Rescue program.[8] Often, however, rescue comes from those closest who may not have the knowledge or gear to mount the most effective rescue or resuscitation.

The most common conditions suffered by those rescued from the water are near drowning and hypothermia. Rescuers should remove wet clothing and dry the skin and hair of victims before providing warm and dry clothing. If survival suits are available, it may be adequate to dress the victims in these for passive rewarming. However, particularly in the setting of multiple victims rescued from cold ocean waters, the rescuing vessel may not have enough gear for all persons rescued. It may be necessary to put two persons into each suit, and in this case, a warmer victim should be paired with a colder one.[2]

Although hypothermia causes deterioration more commonly and more rapidly, victims rescued from lifeboats and rafts may suffer heat illnesses, including sunburn, heat exhaustion, and heat stroke, the last of which requires urgent medical intervention.[2]

Survivors who are rescued after a prolonged time adrift at sea may be suffering from dehydration or starvation plus exposure and may require intensive or prolonged resuscitation and medical care.

It is shortly after midnight on an international cruise ship carrying 1200 passengers and 700 crew members. It is the third day of a transatlantic voyage, and the ship is 1000 miles from the mainland. Suddenly there is a large explosion, followed by a fire in the engine room. The crew members on duty reduce ship speed and institute emergency fire suppression measures immediately, with limited success.

An initial assessment of damage indicates no significant hull damage, but there has been loss of electric power to areas of the ship. A crew member who had been working in the engine room is missing. Seven other crew members have been injured by the initial explosion or during efforts to fight the fire. Although many passengers had already gone to bed and are unaware of the situation, a large percentage of those still awake are increasingly concerned and some are agitated, which is worsened by prior consumption of alcohol over the course of the evening. Emergency lighting is on throughout much of the ship.

Less than 1 hour later, the fire has spread. The two nearest large ships that could provide assistance are 250 and 300 miles away, but both have responded to the distress call and are proceeding toward the stricken cruise ship. Smoke is spreading through the many corridors of the lower decks of the ship, so the captain and crew decide to raise a general fire alarm and alert the passengers. Many are slow to waken and are confused by the noise and lack of normal lighting. Some panic when they see and smell smoke in the passageways. Most do not take their lifejackets with them upon exiting their cabins, despite the instructions accompanying the fire alarm.

If rescue does not occur speedily, many passengers who have not donned PFDs and who do not board lifeboats may enter the water unprepared, by jumping in panic or by failing to follow the instructions of the crew. Those without PFDs may drown or suffer hypothermia before a rescue vessel arrives, unless they are assisted into lifeboats by others.

UNIQUE CONSIDERATIONS

Maritime rescues are frequently complicated by the very factors that caused the incident. Poor visibility, strong winds, and rough seas may prevent rescuers from reaching or finding damaged ships or floating victims. Once located, high waves and cold temperatures further endanger both rescuers and victims and may damage rescue and medical equipment. Salt water can reduce the effectiveness of equipment immediately or over time. Noise, impaired visibility, and hypothermia can interfere with communications between rescuer and victim, and language barriers may exist. Victims are often hypothermic, dehydrated, and exhausted, which reduce their ability to assist with their own rescue.

Victims who are rescued from immersion in cold water may experience temperature afterdrop as a complication of hypothermia, with this postimmersion collapse often resulting in death. This condition occurs when chilled blood from peripheral tissues circulates to the body core

with rewarming, causing a drop in the core temperature and a drastically worsened clinical practice.[9,10]

The clinical status of survivors rescued after near-drowning may worsen gradually or abruptly due to the development of respiratory distress syndrome with hypoxia and subsequent respiratory failure. Pulmonary edema, cardiovascular complications, and multisystem organ failure may develop, even with intensive medical care.[11] Supportive care and prompt transport to a tertiary care center are essential.

Victims may be covered with fuel oil or may have swallowed or aspirated oil while immersed. They may develop vomiting, aspiration pneumonia or pneumonitis, or conjunctivitis.[2]

Oil contamination also complicates the healing of skin wounds such as abrasions or punctures, as does seawater containing bacteria or other contaminants. Prolonged exposure to damp conditions or clothing in a lifeboat may allow saltwater boils, pustules, or even ulcers to develop. Immersion foot can occur in survivors aboard lifeboats and rafts when feet remain cool, damp, dependent, and inactive, with the development of blood stagnation and tissue swelling.[2]

Survivors rescued from the sea may have swallowed significant quantities of salt water and may develop osmotic diarrhea and hypernatremia, which will require volume replacement and careful monitoring of electrolyte levels.[2]

After rescue from the sea, there may be delays in reaching definitive medical care. Although the rescue vessel may have adequate personnel and equipment to provide first aid or even major resuscitation for victims, weather and sea conditions may delay transport to a site where surgery or intensive care could be provided, such as a mainland tertiary care center. As well, distances to the nearest appropriate healthcare facility may be significant, particularly in the case of mid-ocean rescues.

The same conditions that complicate rescue also make investigation of ship and submarine accidents difficult and hazardous. Evidence may be scattered over the ocean floor, resting several kilometers below the surface in cold, dark water, subject to strong ocean currents.[12] There may be no survivors to describe the events leading up to a tragedy or any actions taken in response, whether or not they were effective, heroic, or foolhardy. There may be no conclusive determination of the cause of a tragic event at sea—rather, only conflicting theories and conjecture—but experts must nevertheless attempt to identify what went wrong so that they may recommend methods to prevent future disasters.[13]

PITFALLS

Several potential pitfalls exist in response to a maritime disaster. These include the following:

- Failure to appreciate dangerous weather and sea conditions, especially when combined with ship weaknesses or damage
- Failure to adapt course or sailing techniques to changing conditions

- Failure to follow rules of sailing, navigation, and sea transport
- Excessive reliance on technology and failure to identify deficiencies or weakness in ship structure and function
- Failure to request assistance or rescue in a timely manner
- Failure to follow safety procedures and lack of familiarity with evacuation and emergency exits and equipment
- Failure to abandon ship or deploy emergency escape equipment, such as lifejackets or PFDs, survival suits, and lifeboats
- Failure to activate the emergency position indicator rescue beacon before abandoning ship
- Failure to ration water and food supplies after abandoning ship

REFERENCES

1. Bonsall TE. *Great Shipwrecks of the 20th Century*. Baltimore, Md: Bookman Publishing; 1988:6-12.
2. Golden F, Tipton M. *Essentials of Sea Survival*. Champaign, Ill: Human Kinetics; 2002.
3. Roberts SE. Work-related mortality among British seafarers in flags of convenience shipping, 1976-95. *Int Marit Health*. 2003;54:7-25.
4. Australian Maritime Safety Authority. Available at: *http://www.amsa.gov.au*.
5. International Maritime Organization Web site. Available at: http://www.imo.org.
6. International Maritime Organization. IMO adopts comprehensive maritime security measures. Conference of Contracting Governments to the International Convention for the Safety of Life at Sea, 1974: December 9-13, 2002. Available at: http://www.imo.org/Newsroom/mainframe.asp? topic_id=583&doc_id=2689.
7. Howorth F, Howorth M. *The Grab Bag Book*. London:Adlard Coles Nautical; 2002.
8. U.S. Coast Guard Web site. U.S. Department of Homeland Security. Available at: http://www.uscg.mil.
9. Giesbrecht GG, Bristow GK. A second postcooling afterdrop: more evidence for a convective mechanism. *J Appl Physiol*. 1992;73:1253-8.
10. Giesbrecht GG. Prehospital treatment of hypothermia. *Wilderness Environ Med*. 2001;12:24-31.
11. Volturo GA. Submersion injuries. In: Harwood-Nuss A, Wolfson AB, Linden CH, et al, eds. *The Clinical Practice of Emergency Medicine*. 3rd ed. Philadelphia: Lippincott Williams & Wilkins; 2001:194-6.
12. Bird L. *The Wreck Diving Manual*. Ramsbury, Marlborough: The Crowood Press; 1997:9-43.
13. Krieger M. *All the Men in the Sea*. New York: The Free Press; 2002:1-221.

chapter 180

Cruise Ship Infectious Disease Outbreak

Scott G. Weiner

 DESCRIPTION OF EVENT

Throughout the ages, infectious diseases traveling by boat have affected the course of history. For instance, the Black Death caused by *Yersinia pestis* was brought by boats coming from the east to Europe. The plague caused the death of at least one-third of the European population during the 1300s. This epidemic led to the practice of refusing the landing of ships with suspected cases of plague for 40 days—the first practice of "quarantine," from the Italian word *quaranta* for "forty." Shipborne smallpox also played a role, actually saving England from a French invasion in 1779 after an outbreak spread among the French sailors.[1] The closed environment of the ships and the prolonged duration of voyages led to a high infection rate.

In modern times, airplanes have replaced the boat for long-range passenger transportation, but recently a steadily increasing number of people choose to go on cruises as a form of vacation. Over 9.5 million people went on cruise vacations in 2003, an increase of 10.2% from 2002 and 198% from 1994.[2,3] The average length of cruise in 2003 was 6.88 days.[2] And with the standard capacity of the newer cruise ships reaching well over 2000 passengers, hundreds of people may potentially be at risk from an infectious disease outbreak onboard.

The infectious diseases that affect cruise ships can be divided into three categories: gastrointestinal, respiratory, and miscellaneous infections.

Gastrointestinal Illness

Gastrointestinal illness is by far the most common result of cruise ship outbreaks. A study of 31 investigated cruise ship gastroenteritis outbreaks between 1986 and 1993 found that 39% were from bacterial sources (including enterotoxigenic *Escherichia coli*, *Shigella* species, *Salmonella* species, and *Staphylococcus aureus*), 29% were from Norwalk or Norwalk-like virus (collectively called *norovirus*), and 32% were of unknown etiology.[4] Of the determined sources, 48% were from onboard exposures (particularly food), 10% were obtained during onshore excursions, and 42% of sources were unknown.[4]

A more recent study found a shift in epidemiology, with an increase in the incidence of norovirus.[5] Twenty-one outbreaks of acute gastroenteritis were studied, of which nine episodes were caused by norovirus, three were caused by bacteria, and nine were of unknown etiology. The rate of passenger infection ranged from 5% to 19%.[5] However, in one outbreak in 1998, more than 80% of the 841 passengers were affected, indicating the highly infectious nature of this virus.[6] Because norovirus is so infectious, the organism passes easily between passengers in the confined space of a cruise ship, and hundreds may be at risk.

Respiratory Illness

Whereas the most common illness afflicting passengers and crew aboard cruise ships is gastroenteritis, respiratory infections comprise about one-third of sick bay visits.[3] Outbreaks of Legionnaires' disease and influenza have been reported in the literature.[7,8] One outbreak of *Legionella pneumophila* infection in 1994, linked to the ship's whirlpool spa, affected 50 passengers on 9 different cruises, including the death of 1 passenger.[7] Another study documented an outbreak of influenza A and B in 2000, in which 37% of passengers developed an influenza-like illness, 40 passengers were hospitalized, and 2 died.[8] Though never reported as outbreaks in the literature, other diseases with respiratory transmission, such as diphtheria, tuberculosis, and meningitis, remain outbreak possibilities.[1]

Miscellaneous Infections

Other miscellaneous infections, including malaria, yellow fever, and varicella, also involve potential pathogens on a cruise ship.[1] A 1997 outbreak of rubella among crew members, mostly from countries that did not have routine immunization programs, serves as a reminder that unanticipated outbreaks can arise in close quarters.[9]

 PREINCIDENT ACTIONS

Prevention is the single most important action that can be taken to avoid an infectious disease outbreak. To achieve this goal, the U.S. Centers for Disease Control and Prevention (CDC), in a cooperative arrangement with the cruise ship industry, created the Vessel Sanitation Program (VSP) in 1975.[10] The program is designed to prevent the introduction or transmission of infectious diseases in the United States as well as to assist the cruise ship industry in the development and implementation of sanitation programs to protect passengers and crew.[10] The VSP also involves unannounced twice-yearly inspections of all cruises traveling to the United States from international ports and publishes its findings as a sanitation score on a biweekly basis.[4,10,11]

As part of the VSP arrangement, cruise ships must maintain an incident report of gastrointestinal illness for each cruise. A reportable case of gastroenteritis is defined as three or more episodes of loose stools in 24 hours, or vomiting and any additional symptom suggestive of the illness (excluding nausea, which can be a symptom of seasickness).[10] It is also essential that cruise lines use adequate infection control measures, including proper disinfection, filtering, and storage of water and regular maintenance of spas and ventilation systems to prevent the spread of airborne infections.[6]

Another important step is provision of onboard healthcare facilities that will be capable of treating patients with outbreaks. The American College of Emergency Physicians published guidelines for a ship's medical facilities, and the 16 members of the International Council of Cruise Lines have agreed to meet or exceed these requirements.[12,13] Although the guidelines do not identify specifics regarding outbreaks, they do require ships to have properly trained physicians and nurses, an infusion pump, gastrointestinal system medications, respiratory system medications, and an emergency preparedness plan.[12] At a minimum, ships should have the capacity to provide oral and intravenous rehydration therapy and have sufficient doses of or ready access via airlift to antibiotics to treat *Legionella* infection and bacterial gastroenteritis.

 POSTINCIDENT ACTIONS

Once an outbreak is identified, it is crucial that a predetermined decontamination plan is commenced immediately.[5] Rapid implementation of control measures at the first sign of a suspected outbreak is fundamental for three important reasons: (1) many people share the same water, food, and environment, and are all at risk for infection; (2) the ship's medical resources can quickly become overwhelmed in an outbreak; and (3) without intervention, the infection can spread to subsequent cruises.[10]

After an outbreak, international quarantine regulations dictate that the master of the ship traveling to a U.S. Port report to the closest quarantine station. Furthermore, the master of a ship carrying more than 12 passengers is required to report the number of passengers or crew who reported diarrhea during the cruise 24 hours before arrival to the United States. If at least 3.0% of the ship's passengers or crew is ill, the VSP may conduct an investigation.[10]

The investigation is composed of three phases: (1) an epidemiologic investigation, in which interviews and questionnaires are performed; (2) a laboratory investigation, in which the CDC attempts to determine the agent responsible for the outbreak; (3) an environmental health investigation, in which the source of transmission (usually water, food, or air) is analyzed. After the investigation is complete, the information, including recommendations for control and prevention, is sent to the cruise line.[10]

Complete guidelines for stool and water collection are available on the CDC Web site.[10] Furthermore, the World Health Organization publishes a *Guide to Ship Sanitation*, which offers further assistance in the prevention of the spread of infection.[6] Once an outbreak occurs, prompt disinfection of the ship and isolation of ill crew members and, if possible, passengers for 72 hours after clinical recovery are ideal.[5] Suitable disinfectants such as chlorine, phenol-based compounds, or accelerated hydrogen peroxide products should be used to disinfect the ship.[5] Furthermore, the staff should remind passengers and the crew to perform frequent, rigorous handwashing with soap and water.

 MEDICAL TREATMENT OF CASUALTIES

The first problem facing the medical staff and crew of the ship is the logistics of treating hundreds of casualties onboard and finding an appropriate docking port. The ship's medical staff will be forced to ration care as they balance resources with numbers of afflicted patients. The most seriously affected should receive care first. For instance, those who are very young, very old, or significantly dehydrated should receive intravenous fluid before the others. The crew should locate a suitable port where hundreds of casualties can be most easily cared for. If there is a choice, the ship should not dock at a small port if a larger port near a large city is available. Calling ahead and warning the receiving port is also crucial.

The treatment of the casualties should be tailored to the individual disease process. For patients with viral gastroenteritis, only supportive care is necessary. Norovirus illness lasts 12 to 60 hours and is usually accompanied by sudden onset of nausea, vomiting, and watery diarrhea. Its incubation period is 12 to 48 hours. No specific treatment or vaccine exists.[5] Although generally self-limited, viral gastroenteritis may cause problems in children, elderly persons, and persons with serious underlying medical conditions. Treatment should include oral rehydration for mild cases and intravenous fluid for more significant dehydration. If the cause is determined to be bacterial, appropriate antibiotics (e.g., ciprofloxacin) should be administered to the affected passengers.

Other treatments will depend on the infectious agent. Legionnaires' disease may present with a range of systems from a mild febrile illness to a severe pneumonia with malaise, cough, and gastrointestinal symptoms.[14] Standard pneumonia antibiotic therapies such as azithromycin or levofloxacin are curative, and these should be stocked on the ship. Regardless of the etiology, air evacuation is indicated for very ill patients.[15]

Fortunately, cruise ship infectious disease outbreaks are rare and are usually self-limited and nonfatal. Between 1986 and 1993, the CDC investigated 1.4 outbreaks per 1000 cruises, or just 2.3 outbreaks per 10 million passenger-days, and more recent research demonstrates that the VSP is effective in helping to further reduce this number.[4,11] However, once it occurs, an infectious disease outbreak on a cruise ship can represent a major medical disaster. An outbreak can quickly overwhelm the limited medical resources available on a ship. Proper preparation and planning can help prevent a catastrophic event.

 CASE PRESENTATION*

A relatively new cruise ship that is able to carry 2500 passengers and 800 crew members embarked on its usual tour. During a 7-day trip from Miami to various ports in the Caribbean, an increasing number of patients began reporting to the ship's sick bay complaining of diarrhea. By day 3 of the voyage, 30 passengers (1%) and 10 crew members (1%) presented with gastroenteritis. By day 7, a total of 285 passengers (11%) and 25 of the crew members (3%) had reported the illness.

As is required, the CDC was notified and an investigation ensued. A questionnaire was distributed to all passengers, and it was determined that the conditions of 523 passengers (21%) met the definition for acute gastroenteritis. Several stool specimens tested positive for norovirus by polymerase chain reaction. Of the patients with gastroenteritis, 418 patients (80%) had symptoms that spontaneously resolved within 48 hours, 89 patients (17%) had symptoms that resolved within 96 hours, and 4 elderly patients were hospitalized after their return to shore and then were subsequently discharged without complication.

Despite aggressive disinfection, the outbreak continued on the next cruise. The cruise line then removed the ship from service for 1 week for further cleaning and sanitizing, and no subsequent cases were reported.

*Adapted from Outbreaks of gastroenteritis associated with noroviruses on cruise ships—United States, 2002. *MMWR Morb Mortal Wkly Rep.* 2002;51:1112-5.

 UNIQUE CONSIDERATIONS

Cruise ships are closed spaces, and the combination of thousands of people contained for several days in this space represents an opportunity for infection to spread rapidly. Only limited resources are available onboard, so a ship's medical bay may become quickly overwhelmed during an outbreak.

Ships often visit ports in countries where infectious disease is more prevalent than it is in the United States, so the potential for bringing an agent onboard is elevated. In addition, the background of the crew is often diverse, and some may be at increased susceptibility to diseases, depending on immunization status.

Although there have been no reported incidents of bioterrorism on cruise ships, this possibility cannot be excluded. A cruise ship might become a means for an infectious disease agent to be purposefully transmitted into a country. Increased vigilance among the ship's crew and medical staff is indicated.

An infectious disease outbreak may represent a huge financial loss to a cruise line because cruises may need to be cancelled and future passengers may be less likely to travel on an affected line. Again, preventive measures are paramount.

 PITFALLS

Several potential pitfalls exist in response to an outbreak of infectious disease aboard a cruise ship. These include the following:

- Failure to properly staff and supply the ship's medical clinic
- Failure to recognize or report an infectious disease outbreak
- Failure to quickly isolate and treat affected passengers and crew
- Failure to properly sanitize the ship after an outbreak
- Failure to create a plan for mass treatment in the event of an outbreak, including provisions for airlifting patients out or supplies in

REFERENCES

1. Minooee A, Rickman LS. Infectious diseases on cruise ships. *Clin Infect Dis.* 1999;29:737-43.
2. Cruise Lines International Association. CLIA member cruise lines post strong passenger growth with over 9.5 million cruisers in 2003. *Cruise News.* February 2004. Available at: http://www.cruising.org/CruiseNews/news.cfm?NID=156.
3. Peake DE, Gray CL, Ludwig MR, et al. Descriptive epidemiology of injury and illness among cruise ship passengers. *Ann Emerg Med.* 1999;33:67-72.
4. Koo D, Maloney K, Tauxe R. Epidemiology of diarrheal disease outbreaks on cruise ships, 1986 through 1993. *JAMA* 1996;275:545-7.
5. Outbreaks of gastroenteritis associated with noroviruses on cruise ships—United States, 2002. *MMWR Morb Mortal Wkly Rep.* 2002;51:1112-5.
6. World Health Organization. Ship sanitation and health. February 2002. Available at: http://www.who.int/mediacentre/factsheets/fs269/en.
7. Jernigan DB, Hofmann J, Cetron MS, et al. Outbreak of legionnaires' disease among cruise ship passengers exposed to a contaminated whirlpool spa. *Lancet* 1996;347:494-9.
8. Brotherton JM, Delpech VC, Gilbert GL, et al. A large outbreak of influenza A and B on a cruise ship causing widespread morbidity. *Epidemiol Infect.* 2003;130:263-71.
9. Rubella among crew members of commercial cruise ships—Florida, 1997. *MMWR Morb Mortal Wkly Rep.* 1998;46:1247-50.
10. Centers for Disease Control and Prevention, National Center for Environmental Health. Vessel Sanitation Program. Available at: http://www.cdc.gov/nceh/vsp.
11. Cramer EH, Gu DX, Durbin RE, et al. Diarrheal disease on cruise ships, 1990-2000: the impact of environmental health programs. *Am J Prev Med.* 2003;24:227-33.
12. American College of Emergency Physicians. Health care guidelines for cruise ship medical facilities. *Ann Emerg Med.* 1998;31:535.
13. International Council of Cruise Lines. Medical facilities guidelines. January 1, 2002. Available at: http://www.iccl.org/policies/medical2.cfm.
14. Thibodeau KP, Viera AJ. Atypical pathogens and challenges in community-acquired pneumonia. *Am Fam Physician.* 2004;69:1699-706.
15. Prina LD, Orzai UN, Weber RE. Evaluation of emergency air evacuation of critically ill patients from cruise ships. *J Travel Med.* 2001;8:285-92.

chapter 181

Hostage Taking

Dale M. Molé

 DESCRIPTION OF EVENT

Incidents of hostage taking and kidnapping are on the rise around the world. Some are politically motivated; others involve simple greed. A few are just the result of being in the wrong place at the wrong time. According to the Hiscox Group, a leading international specialty insurer, the number of reported worldwide kidnappings for ransom increased from 1690 in 1998 to 1789 in 1999. Over 90% of those incidents took place in what have been deemed the top 10 riskiest areas: Colombia, Mexico, the former Soviet Union, Brazil, the Philippines, Nigeria, India, Ecuador, Venezuela, and South Africa.[1] The rise can be blamed on a combination of factors such as lawlessness, political unrest, and poverty. Kidnapping is an appealing crime for many since the perpetrators are rarely caught and it is a much easier way to make money than drug dealing or robbery. The epidemic of kidnapping/hostage taking is much greater than demonstrated by statistics, since many kidnappings are handled privately and remain unreported.

In about 67% of cases, a ransom is paid and usually averages about $2,000,000 in countries where the "business" is well established. If a ransom is not paid chances of survival for the victim are slim, especially in Latin America. According to insurance industry sources, Americans with kidnapping and ransom insurance are four times more likely to survive a kidnapping than are those who have none.

This is not only a problem overseas, however. Each year, the U.S. Federal Bureau of Investigation is involved in approximately 400 domestic kidnappings, with about one third involving a ransom demand. Branch bank managers and their families appear to be favorite targets.[2] Some kidnapping/hostage taking occurs incidentally to the commission of another crime, with the victim being a target of opportunity for the perpetrator trying to negotiate his way out of a losing situation.

With the growing threat of international terrorism and the increasing political value of American hostages, it is the official policy of the U.S. Government not to make concessions to individuals or groups holding official or private U.S. citizens hostage. However, the United States will make use of every appropriate resource to ensure the release and safe return of American citizens. The goal is to deny the hostage takers the benefits of ransoms, prisoner releases, policy changes, or other acts of concession, which would increase the risk that other Americans would be taken hostage. The State Department will contact representatives of the captors in an effort to secure release.

Although very dangerous, hostage rescue is sometimes the only viable option. Local, state, and federal law enforcement agencies have specialized teams to rescue hostages or deal with standoff situations. These teams rely on training, speed, coordination, stealth, and overwhelming force to rescue hostages and take control of the situation.[3] The Federal Bureau of Investigation's Hostage Rescue Team (HRT) was established in 1982 and has been deployed more than 200 times in support of hostage rescue, counter-terrorism, stopping violent crime, and other federal law enforcement activities.

Tactical emergency medical services (TEMS) is emerging as a special interest area within emergency medicine to provide medical services within a civilian law enforcement environment for both law enforcement personnel and suspects. Beyond increasing the chances of successful mission accomplishment, TEMS reduces the morbidity and mortality among innocent persons, suspects, and officers. Medical care in a tactical situation is frequently very different from the care provided by routine civilian EMS.

Law enforcement agencies manage crisis situations with zones of containment. The inner perimeter is a geographically defined circle around an incident and is controlled by the tactical law enforcement element (i.e., special weapons and tactics teams, special response teams, and the like). The outer perimeter is a larger boundary that excludes the public, provides additional safety, and is controlled by patrol or regular uniformed officers.

Similarly, zones of care (i.e., hot, warm, and cold zones) help define appropriate care in a tactical law enforcement environment. The *hot zone* includes those areas where the threat to safety is direct and immediate and the threat for additional injury is high, where it would be extremely hazardous to provide medical care; for example, the area surrounding a sniper's position in a building with a clear field of fire. Extraction to a safer area to render medical assistance is about the only option. The *cold zone* is where no threat exists and care can be provided in much the same manner as in any routine civilian situation. The *warm zone* is an area where the threat is intermediate between these two extremes; this is often the most challenging regarding medical decision-making. The benefit of a particular intervention must be considered relative to the risk of additional injury to the patient or the medical tactician. Certain actions considered standard for care in normal situations, such as applying a cervical collar for penetrating neck injuries before moving the patient, make no sense in a tactical environment.

 ## PREINCIDENT ACTIONS

Personal

Taking simple steps and altering certain behaviors can help travelers avoid putting themselves at risk. Anonymity is the best defense for foreign travelers.[4] When traveling abroad, persons should keep a low profile and not advertise their wealth. Jewels and expensive clothes should be left at home. Travelers should de-Westernize their attire as much as possible, since a middle class income in the United States places a person in the top few percents of incomes worldwide. Travelers should not follow a regular routine, nor should they make restaurant reservations in their own names. Colleagues, friends, and family should be kept informed as to travelers' whereabouts.

When traveling in third-world countries, travelers should not wear military-style clothing. Blue or other neutral colors should be worn, since green or brown clothing is often associated with the military.

Persons taking trips abroad should avoid luggage tags, behavior, and dress identifying them as American. Reading maps in public or carrying a camera around the neck will let others know a person is a tourist and therefore a target of opportunity. If traveling on a bus, the safest areas are the aisle seats near the middle of the bus. When on an airplane, the safest areas are the window seats near the middle of the aircraft.

Personal papers should not be left in the hotel room, and hotel guests should not open the door for strangers. Travelers should make sure they have mentally planned an escape route in case of fire or other disaster. Hotel rooms on the first floor should be avoided, if possible.

When driving through crowded areas, windows should be kept closed. Travelers are advised to make sure their vehicle is in good condition, and they should plan the route before traveling. They should make mental notes of safe havens such as police stations, hospitals, and hotels. In addition, they should steer clear of rural or isolated areas, especially when traveling alone or in a small group.

It is recommended to schedule direct flights when possible and avoid stops in high-risk areas. Travelers should be aware of what they discuss with strangers and what may be overheard. Routines should be varied, especially if one stays in a country for an extended time. Persons should not take the same travel routes, eat at the same restaurants, or jog on the same pathways on a regular schedule. When walking around foreign cities, it is prudent to ignore the attempts of strangers to engage the traveler in conversation. Letting one's familiarity with a country lull one into a false sense of security is a mistake.

In conflict or disaster areas, travelers should beware of roadblocks. The people controlling the roadblock may desire to extort money or other items of worth. If a person is working with a relief agency, he or she should ensure that proper identification is available and that he or she is traveling in a clearly marked vehicle. Vehicles painted in military colors should be avoided.

If a roadblock is encountered, the personnel manning it may be aggressive, undisciplined, untrained, and intoxicated. Travelers should not make any aggressive movements or statements. They should be firm but polite, stating that the authorities have given them permission to travel in the area. If a person is an aid worker, he or she should establish his or her affiliation quickly because it is one of the greatest assets a traveler has.[5]

Medical Support Elements

Integrated medical support for specialized law enforcement/hostage rescue teams is mandatory. Just-in-time training for supporting medical personnel is not an option and places the mission, the hostages, and the rescuers at risk. TEMS training for physicians, paramedics, and emergency medical technicians is available from several organizations. One of the first and most widely recognized is Counter Narcotics and Terrorism Operational Medical Support. Established within the Casualty Care Research Center at the Uniformed Services University of Health Sciences, lessons learned on the battlefield providing care in austere environments are applied to civilian law enforcement situations. The core curriculum of any TEMS course should include didactic and practical exercises in at least the following areas:

- Threat assessment and medical intelligence
- Care under fire
- Hostage survival
- Clinical forensic science
- Weapons and their effects
- Medicine across the barricade
- Toxic hazards (e.g., clandestine drug labs, weapons of mass destruction)
- Medical effects of extended operations
- Special equipment and medical kits

 ## POSTINCIDENT ACTIONS

The two most dangerous times during a hostage situation are at the beginning and at the end, especially if a rescue is attempted. Initially, persons in a hostage situation should make themselves as inconspicuous as possible. They should listen to the terrorist's commands and respond without questioning. "Passive cooperation" should be enacted. It is recommended to avoid sudden movements or threatening behavior and avoid eye contact or any other actions that may single a person out. If ordered to be silent, hostages should not talk or whisper. If possible, they should dispose of identification or documents that would make the hostage takers more hostile toward them. Persons should eat or drink sparingly during the first few hours and should not consume alcohol.

If taken hostage, persons should help their kidnappers establish contact with their organization as soon as possible. Hostages should try to remain calm and remember that the vast majority of kidnappings end with the hostages released. Death is usually the result of a medical condition, an unsuccessful escape attempt, or perhaps a botched rescue. It is not advisable to act as a spokesperson for the hostages. Persons should rehearse what they will say to the hostage takers if questioned about their documents.

Persons taken hostage should look after their health as much as possible. Because they don't know where, when, or what their next meal will be, hostages should eat all of the food they are offered after the initial few hours, once the hostage situation has stabilized. They should also try to exercise regularly.

Since hostages may be guests of their captors for quite a while, they should try to establish rapport. The better the relationship they establish, the harder it will be for the hostage takers to kill or injure them. Escape should not be attempted unless hostages are absolutely certain of success.[6]

If a hostage is bound by his or her captors, slumping in the chair while they are tying the person up will allow some slack in the ropes. The same can be accomplished by keeping the chest inflated or wrists slightly apart. Hostages should try to catch a gag in their teeth to prevent it from being forced all the way back in the mouth. If a person's hands are tied behind him or her, if possible, the hostage should pass his or her hands under the feet. With the hands in front of the body, the hostage can use the teeth to untie knots.

Wherever hostages are being held, they should look around for safe areas in case of a rescue attempt. It is a good idea to drop to the floor immediately if there is shooting or an explosion. If possible, persons should seek shelter in a ditch, in a depression, or near a solid wall. They should not jump up and try to run.

MEDICAL TREATMENT OF CASUALTIES

The medical care required depends on the length and conditions of captivity, preexisting illnesses, and whether the hostage was released or had to be rescued. Rescue attempts are inherently very dangerous situations and may result in injury to rescuers as well as hostages. The three most common causes of preventable death in a tactical situation are uncontrolled hemorrhage, airway compromise, and untreated tension pneumothorax.

Perhaps most important is the emotional and mental health support required by all hostages, even those not sustaining any physical trauma. The lack of control over one's fate in a highly stressful life and death situation will tax the emotional resources of even the most robust person.

CASE PRESENTATION

On the evening of May 23, 2004, three suspects abducted South African Deputy High Commissioner Nicky Scholtz on one of Kuala Lumpur's busiest streets, near the hotel where he was attending a conference. One man confronted him and forced him into a car where two men were waiting. He was struck with a blunt object and then driven away. The abductors rendezvoused with four men, who became the hostage holders, in another car. This demonstrated operational planning, as well as a level of sophistication not usually seen in a random abduction. Scholtz was taken about 12 miles south of Kuala Lumpur and held hostage for a week. He was bound with wire and beaten while the attackers forced him to write checks and withdraw funds on his credit card, to a total of about $4200, sufficient to purchase weapons or explosives. He suffered two fractured ribs, a dislocated jaw, and severe bruising of his back, face, arms, and legs.

The kidnappers released Scholtz after his disappearance was reported locally, but they threatened to kill him if he reported the incident. Based on information he provided, seven suspects were later taken into custody. There is no indication the attack was politically motivated, but rather, it is believed that he was simply a target of opportunity.

This incident illustrates the importance of good situational awareness, whether an individual is at home or abroad.

UNIQUE CONSIDERATIONS

Being kidnapped or held hostage is perhaps one of the most likely events to cause posttraumatic stress disorder (PTSD). PTSD is characterized by reexperiencing the traumatic event (e.g., vivid nightmares, recurring visual images, reacting physiologically to stimuli associated with the event), avoidance behavior (i.e., avoiding things associated with the trauma such as activities, places, or people), and hyperarousal symptoms (e.g., insomnia, startle behavior, attention deficits). PTSD is a normal reaction to an abnormal situation and can be prevented or mitigated with timely intervention.

Critical incident stress debriefing (CISD) is an essential component of post-event care. It involves at least one structured meeting with a trained mental health professional between 24 and 72 hours after release or rescue. The first day after the event is necessary for rest—emotionally and physically. After about 3 days, victims will begin to suppress/repress emotions in an attempt to isolate or compartmentalize the traumatic experience, hence the need to act quickly.

The CISD usually takes several hours and includes an explanation of the purpose of the debriefing, a brief personal history of the people involved in the event, a discussion of what each person saw or experienced and their emotional reactions, a query regarding symptoms associated with PTSD, education regarding PTSD as a normal response to horrific events, and referral of those who require further treatment.

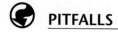

Several potential pitfalls exist in response to a hostage-taking event. These include the following:

- Lack of situational awareness in a high-risk environment
- Underestimating the danger or threat posed by female terrorists[7]
- *The Stockholm syndrome:* First described by Professor Nils Bejerot to explain the phenomenon of hostage victims bonding with their captors, following a 6-day ordeal in which two bank robbers held four hostages in Stockholm, Sweden, in 1973. Symptoms include emotional bonding with captors, seeking approval or favor from the captors, resenting police or other authorities for attempts at rescue, and refusing to seek freedom when the opportunity is available.

- Lack of properly trained and integrated medical support for specialized law enforcement teams
- Failure to perform a CISD in a timely fashion

REFERENCES

1. Hiscox Group Ltd. *Kidnapping Reaches Record Peak* [press release]. London: Hiscox Group Ltd; April 19, 2000.
2. Boyle C. In the underworld: kidnapping, hostage-taking, and extortion on the rise. *Insurance J.* July 10, 2000. Available at: http://www.insurancejournal.com/magazines/southcentral/2000/07/10/coverstory/ 22644.htm.
3. Whitcomb C. *Cold Zero: Inside the FBI Hostage Rescue Team.* Boston: Little, Brown and Company; 2001.
4. Savage P. *The Safe Travel Handbook.* San Francisco: Lexington Books; 1993.
5. Green J. Dealing with trouble—the wilder issues. In: Ryan J, Mahoney PF, Greaves I, et al, eds. *Conflict and Catastrophe Medicine: A Practical Guide.* London: Springer; 2002.
6. Auerbach A. *Ransom.* New York: Henry Holt and Company; 1998.
7. MacDonald E. *Shoot the Women First.* New York: Random House; 1991.

chapter 182

Civil Unrest and Rioting*

Denis J. FitzGerald

 ## DESCRIPTION OF EVENT

Civil unrest, also termed *civil disturbance*, is a spectrum of activities progressively disruptive to public order and tranquility. Civil unrest can occur whenever a group in the community feels, accurately or not, that some aspect of society is antithetic or apathetic to their views, rights, or needs. Examples of civil disturbance include labor strikes, large demonstrations, and riots. As the most extreme situation, a *riot* is a violent disruption of the public order that threatens public safety. In describing civil unrest, it is valuable to consider first a historical perspective, then to discuss the etiology and evolution of these incidents.

Civil unrest has been a part of the fabric of life in the United States since before the country was founded, dating back to the Boston Massacre in 1770.[1] Governed by a set of laws to define mechanisms for peaceful conflict resolution, American society has nonetheless experienced many instances throughout its history of violent civil unrest. More recent events include the widespread turbulence of the late 1960s, the civil unrest surrounding the Rodney King incident (1992), and the clashes between the police and protesters at World Bank Demonstrations in Washington, DC (2000). Especially when it turns violent, civil unrest can strain or even shatter the delicate equilibrium between the societal need for public order and the individual's constitutional right to freedom of expression.

Civil unrest arises from the interplay of several factors.[2] These factors include confrontational participants, catalyst causes, group dynamics, group leadership, and emotional electricity. To better understand civil unrest, it is important to discuss briefly the role of each causal factor.

Across the spectrum of various events, participants in civil unrest span all demographic, political, and socioeconomic categories. At baseline, all participants are connected to the group by a variable degree of investment in a specific cause. Some core persons are highly committed to the issue, while others merely become caught up in the frenzied periphery of the event.

Catalyst causes that trigger civil disturbance include any perceived wrongful policy or event felt worthy of active dissent. These issues include special interest topics, perceived law enforcement injustices, and political grievances. Rioting can occur when the group directs its frustration over a given issue toward persons with opposing views or officers charged with keeping the peace.

As a behavioral dynamic, groups foster an environment in which individual inhibition is lowered due to a collective sense of anonymity, a diffusion of personal responsibility, a strong social urge toward conformity, and a loss of individual decision-making. Additionally, persons in groups also become more susceptible to suggestion, manipulation, and imitation during moments of uncertainty or frustration by strong leaders who are often the first and most assertive agitators. The emotional volatility of a group can also be a powerful unifying force, creating an almost electric connectivity between participants when sparked.

Given the right circumstances, the net effect of these factors is the evolution of *group cohesion*. The group becomes, in essence, its own autonomous organism with a collective identity, purpose, focus, and coordinated response. In general, members of a group are more prone to participate in activities that they would not do if alone. If the tone of the group shifts toward anger or frustration, a "mob mentality" may take over, violence can erupt, and a riot can ensue. Of note, in the context of a counter-transference dynamic, police and others involved with the response to civil unrest must be constantly vigilant in guarding against any negative impact of these factors on their behavior as well.

Two recognized patterns exist for the emergence of civil unrest. First, civil unrest can be a fluid event that escalates along a progressive continuum of disruption. For example, the incident may begin as a planned *demonstration*. A demonstration is a group of people (termed *protestors* or *demonstrators*) specifically called together for a common purpose, such as to protest a political policy. Under ordinary circumstances, demonstrations are peaceful expressions of First Amendment rights and remain law-abiding entities. However, some demonstrations become increasingly disruptive, with individuals

---

*The content of this chapter exclusively reflects the view of the author and does not represent official policy of the U.S. Department of Defense or the United States Government.

in the group engaging in unlawful activity. If violent tactics are adopted, the situation then degenerates into the anarchy of a riot and the group becomes a *mob*. During a tense confrontation, violence can beget violence, requiring control measures to diffuse the situation.

Second, an additional pattern has been clearly identified in many instances of modern civil unrest.[3] A *crowd* is an unrelated group of people assembled together due to similar circumstances, such as for a sporting event or for a court proceeding. A catalyst event, often a verdict in a law enforcement incident, incites a small ultraviolent group in the crowd to riot in immediate response, often fueled by a deep underlying schism along racial, ethnic, or socioeconomic lines within the community. This core group engages in random acts of violence and looting, subsequently engulfing larger segments of the population. These incidents typically overwhelm the initial public safety resources, requiring an influx of outside support to defuse the situation.

 PREINCIDENT ACTIONS

Preplanning saves lives when time counts. It is critical to plan for civil unrest events because time is limited for life-saving intervention if violence should erupt. Baseline preparation should focus on the development of infrastructure necessary for mitigation of a worst case scenario, such as widespread rioting. Involving both training and resource coordination, effective medical preplanning for civil unrest involves preparation for the continuum of patient care from the field through initial hospitalization. Important planning aspects include: (1) integration of the field medical response with the tactical response; (2) coordination of regional medical resources at all levels; and (3) development of individual hospital response procedures. Building on this underlying foundation, preparation for specific events (such as announced demonstrations) should involve the completion of a medical threat assessment.

To ensure optimal medical care for all participants on the frontline, it is important that medical support be integrated into the initial tactical response. At the flashpoint of a violent incident, the tactical response involves containment and control of the riot through use of a *mobile field force* (MFF), a special response team for civil disturbance. Successful integration of medical support into the MFF requires the establishment of a working relationship between both parties prior to an actual incident. Planning for organic medical support of such tactical operations should focus on many areas, including the following:

• Logistics—deploying, training, and equipping medical personnel for the field
• Preventive strategies—ensuring that needs are met for hydration and adequate protective equipment during deployment of the MFF
• Acute care delivery—coordinating injury treatment and casualty evacuation from the scene
• Decontamination systems—identifying and eliminating contamination thrown by protestors

• Advanced care access issues—connecting MFF field response to the emergency medical system and hospitals

On a regional level, prior planning must ensure that medical resources will be coordinated on all levels of the healthcare response to function seamlessly within the Incident Command System. First, the regional disaster plan for large incidents of civil unrest should include a medical annex that focuses on the integration of healthcare delivery with other public safety functions under such conditions. Resource planning for patient care should address issues related to emergency medical services (e.g., protection of ambulance crews and field rehabilitation logistics),[4] hospital transport (e.g., ensuring safe travel routes), local hospital capabilities (e.g., determining trauma level and diversion status), and mutual aid. Second, the development in advance of a reliable communication system to facilitate information sharing between the lead law enforcement agency, the emergency medical system dispatch, and regional healthcare facilities is essential. This system may be effectively adapted from preexisting disaster networks to function as well in the limited scope of civil unrest incidents.

Individual hospitals also need to look at planning for civil unrest incidents, particularly in the emergency department setting. In many respects, this preparation may be incorporated into the existing disaster plan, with such provisions as increased staffing and the establishment of an Emergency Operations Center. Unique aspects of preparation for civil unrest include hospital security concerns in the face of violent agitators outside, management of injured disorderly protestors requiring treatment, contamination issues, the potential for mass-casualty situations, and the control of arrested persons.

For demonstrations that are announced in advance, it is advisable for regional medical planners to develop a *medical threat assessment* (MTA). The MTA is an approach used to prepare for the foreseeable medical issues associated with a particular event by analyzing various health threats, assessing medical vulnerabilities, identifying possible countermeasures, and exploring different resources to optimize healthcare delivery. Relevant information tied to the anticipated circumstances can be gathered in advance through several methods, including hospital site surveys, route surveys, open-source material, and information known about the past behavior of the protest group. Specific MTA components may include an analysis of environmental conditions, hospital capabilities, and substances likely to be thrown by demonstrators.

 POSTINCIDENT ACTIONS

In the wake of violence associated with widespread civil unrest, the medical community should strive to promote recovery efforts both within its ranks and within the region. In the short term, attention should be paid to the emotional impact of the civil disturbance on healthcare workers, and any persons suffering residual critical incident stress effects should be supported. Hospital personnel should continue to provide needed care for victims and their families, as well as to release appropriate information to the community as indicated. In the long term, it is valuable for medical professionals to meet with civic representatives to debrief medical aspects of the incident. The main focus should be an effort to enhance the medical response to similar situations in the future. By discussing both what worked and what did not, lessons learned can be applied to improve patient care delivery in the event of a future civil disturbance.

 ## MEDICAL TREATMENT OF CASUALTIES

Several important factors should be considered with regard to the medical treatment of casualties from civil unrest. For a large-scale incident, the care should be delivered under conditions defined in the disaster plan of the hospital or agency. Important and unique aspects of medical treatment during civil disturbance are the potential for large numbers of patients, the nature of the injuries seen in riots, and the use of less lethal weapons.

The number of casualties from an incident varies widely with the scope of the disturbance. Depending on available resources, it is possible that medical providers may need to implement mass-casualty triage protocols in given situations. The need for this approach may also depend on the timing of the injuries over the course of the incident and the distribution of patients among different hospitals.

As exemplified in the civil disturbance surrounding the Rodney King incident,[5] three main patterns of injury have been identified in civil unrest. The first type of injury involves assaults suffered by active participants in rioting or other criminal behavior such as looting. With a mixture of blunt and penetrating trauma, these persons may present with gunshot wounds, stab wounds, or injuries incurred in beatings. A second category of injury that has been noted in civil disturbance involves automobile accidents. Suffering primarily blunt trauma, these patients include struck pedestrians and victims of motor vehicle collisions that result from disruption of traffic patterns, erratic driving, or broken traffic signals. The last group of patients present with an acute decompensation of a chronic medical condition because they were unable to obtain needed care. Included in this group are patients receiving dialysis and persons with diabetes.

Less lethal weapons are routinely used in the context of modern civil unrest. Less lethal weapons are devices designed to incapacitate persons or to disperse crowds without causing serious harm. As reflected in the term *less lethal*, the potential does exist, however, for serious harm or even death with these devices. There are two general categories of less lethal agents used in the law enforcement response to civil disturbance. Chemical agents, such as tear gas or pepper spray, cause noxious upper respiratory irritation when deployed. Treatment should focus on removing ongoing contamination, maintaining access to fresh air, and applying cool water.

The injury pattern for projectile munitions, such as "bean bag" rounds, ranges from minor lacerations to significant internal injury.[6] It is advisable for healthcare providers to be familiar with these less lethal devices and their effects.

 ## UNIQUE CONSIDERATIONS

Medical personnel should remember three unique considerations during a response to civil disturbance. These considerations include awareness of the threat environment, the medical-legal context, and the role of field testing. These three considerations are applicable across the spectrum of medical care settings.

The most important consideration for healthcare providers during civil unrest is to recognize that care is being delivered in a *threat environment*. A threat environment is a situation in which a person is at risk for harm or injury during the performance of a given task. In civil unrest, there are several personal safety concerns for the provider such as violent demonstrators, dangerous crowd tactics, contamination from thrown substances, denial of essential supplies, and the presence of improvised weapons. The provider must provide simultaneous care to different categories of patients placed in confrontation by the event—arrested demonstrators, injured bystanders, and wounded law enforcement officers. In addition to using appropriate protective equipment, medical providers must continually maintain situational awareness and practice scene safety in the threat environment posed by civil unrest.

Providers should also appreciate the medical-legal environment created by civil unrest and the consequent implications for healthcare delivery. In the care of patients, providers must be careful (to the extent possible) not to destroy evidence such as collected weapons, bullets, or clothing. In the event that court testimony is later required, the medical practitioner should also have a basic understanding of forensics as it applies to recognition of injury patterns.

During violent demonstrations, protestors may throw a variety of substances at responding police officers. One significant concern with both medical and legal implications is the potential exposure to contaminated blood in this setting. A field blood sampling protocol to assess

 ### CASE PRESENTATION

On a hot summer day, after a well-publicized trial, a jury acquits several police officers of any wrongdoing in a shooting incident earlier that year. Shortly after the verdict is announced, an angry crowd begins gathering downtown amidst cries for justice. The crowd swells in number as it heads for City Hall to protest the verdict. Incited to violence, some members of the crowd then begin breaking windows of nearby buildings, setting fires to trash cans, and pulling drivers out of their cars.

thrown red liquids can help clarify this issue. This protocol can be developed using screening field assays in conjunction with professional laboratory confirmation.

 PITFALLS

Several potential pitfalls exist in the medical response to an episode of civil unrest. These include the following:

- Failure to understand the dynamics and impact of civil unrest within modern society
- Failure to plan for medical contingencies, communication, and coordination along the continuum of healthcare delivery before an event occurs
- Failure to understand the nature of medical casualties in civil unrest, including the injury pattern associated with less lethal weapons
- Failure to promote recovery in the wake of an incident through both short-term and long-term measures
- Failure to consider personal safety while providing care in the threat environment of civil disturbance
- Failure to recognize the unique medico-legal implications of civil unrest

REFERENCES

1. Civil disorder. Los Angeles County Sheriff Emergency Operations Bureau; 1997.
2. Civil disturbances. *US Army Field Manual 19-15*. Washington, DC: Headquarters, Department of the Army; 2005.
3. *Law Enforcement Bulletin*. U.S. Federal Bureau of Investigation; March 1994.
4. *Civil Disturbances in Emergency Medical Services: Special Operations Student Manual*. Federal Emergency Management Agency. U.S. Fire Administration, National Fire Academy, Maryland; 2002.
5. Koehler G, Isbell D, Freeman C, et al. Medical care for the injured: the emergency medical response to the April 1992 Los Angeles civil disturbance. State of California Emergency Medical Services Authority; March 1993. Available at: http://www.usc.edu/isd/archives/cityinstress/ medical/contents.html.
6. Suyama J, Panagos P, Sztajnkrycer M. Injury patterns related to the use of less-lethal weapons during a period of civil unrest. *J Emerg Med*. 2003;25:219-27.

chapter 183

Massive Power System Failures

M. Kathleen Stewart and Charles Stewart

 DESCRIPTION OF EVENT

Electric power outages can be caused by lightning, high winds, ice storms, hurricanes, and floods, as well as either accidents or deliberate sabotage or attack of the power system.[1-5] In some cases, these power failures have been massive and prolonged, creating their own addition to an ongoing disaster such as a flood. In other cases, they have been the sole contributor to the disaster.

This chapter will discuss the potential causes of massive power failure, how it may affect disaster operations, and some selected actions that a physician involved in the disaster might encounter. It should be stressed that this chapter is not exhaustive and is intended only to illustrate how the technology base of the world, and emergency medical services (EMS) in particular, are vulnerable to a variety of attacks.

A modern electric power system consists of six main components:

1. The power station
2. A set of transformers to raise the generated power to the high voltages used on the transmission lines
3. The transmission lines
4. The substations at which the power is stepped down to the voltage on the distribution lines
5. The distribution lines
6. The transformers that lower the distribution voltage to the level used by the consumer's equipment

Electricity generation stations throughout the United States are interconnected via power grids. This allows electricity generated in one state to be sent to users in another state. It also allows distant power generation stations to provide electricity for cities and towns whose power generators may have failed or been destroyed by some accident or sabotage.

In the United States, the electric system is divided into three grid systems: the northeastern grid, the western grid, and the Texas grid. Two major power subgrids, the Ontario–New York–New England pool and the Pennsylvania–New Jersey–Maryland pool (the PJM interconnection), together make up the northeast power grid. Power from these stations is moved around the country on almost a half million miles of bulk transmission lines that carry high-voltage charges of electricity.

In a typical system, the generators at the power station deliver a voltage of 1000 to 26,000 volts (V). From the high-voltage transmission lines of the power grid, electric power is transmitted to regional substations. Transformers step this voltage up to values ranging from 120,000 to 750,000 V for the long-distance primary transmission line because higher voltages can be transmitted more efficiently over long distances. At the regional substation, the voltage can be transformed down to levels of 69,000 to 138,000 V. Another set of transformers at neighborhood substations step the voltage down again to a distribution level such as 2400 or 4160 V or 15, 27, or 33 kilovolts (kV). Finally, the voltage is transformed once again at the distribution transformer near the point of use to a voltage that can be used in homes, hospitals, and offices (220 to 1200 volts).

The towers that carry the high-voltage lines present the easiest pathway for a terrorist to destroy the power system. Only modest amounts of conventional explosives detonated at two to three transmission towers are sufficient to interrupt a high-voltage transmission line. Repair and replacement may take days to weeks.

Simple explosives can easily be used to sabotage any above-ground high-voltage power distribution system. A below-ground system is somewhat more difficult to access and has some additional security afforded by this limited access. Although this tactic will destroy the distribution system, it will not destroy the equipment that it powers. In this regard, the consequences will be similar to those of a naturally occurring event.

Another device—graphite bombs—works by exploding a cloud of thousands of electrically conducting carbon-fiber wires over electric installations and power-distribution systems. This short-circuits the electric systems.

A graphite bomb (sometimes called a *G-bomb*) was used in the 1991 Gulf War to successfully disable 85% of Iraq's power supply. The North Atlantic Treaty Organisation (NATO) used a later version in May 1999, to successfully disable 70% of Serbia's power supply.[6] These bombs will destroy the distribution system, but not the equipment that it powers.

Finally, electromagnetic pulse (EMP) devices can be used to cause massive power failures. When "detonated," an EMP weapon (also known as an *E-bomb*) generates a powerful pulse of energy capable of short-circuiting a wide range of electronic equipment, including computers (even those contained in ignition circuits in cars and trucks and those that operate traffic lights), radios, and public utility power supplies. These weapons can disable practically any nonshielded modern electronic devices within the effective range of the weapon. (Some military-grade radios are designed to resist EMPs, but most civilian equipment is not adequately shielded for this type of attack.) The damage from burnout or overload of the electronic circuits would extend far beyond the area directly affected by the blast and radiation of the EMP.

It is unknown whether the nation's air traffic control system has been "hardened" against EMPs.[6] The extent of the risk to Federal Aviation Administration systems from EMPs is probably (and appropriately) classified. Civilian airliners may be lost. They will not have communication, navigation aids, or landing lights, and in some cases they may not even be able to control the aircraft after electronic fly-by-wire circuits are destroyed by a massive EMP.

Commercial computer equipment is particularly sensitive to EMPs,[4] as are UHF and VHF radio receivers, televisions, and cell phones.[5] The consequences of disabling such equipment are mind boggling for the now technology-dependent healthcare community. However, although devastating to electronic equipment, EMPs, at least in theory, do not hurt humans.[7]

Three basic types of EMP weapons exist: nuclear weapons, flux compression generators, and high-power microwave generators. Although an in-depth discussion of each is beyond the scope of this chapter, suffice it to say each weapon would create differing levels of havoc. Those who have only basic engineering and technical skills can harness EMP technology. EMP weapons can be built with materials available to governments and terrorists alike. Fully developed, ready-to-deploy weapons may be available to clandestine markets at any time. Since the United States has actually deployed such a weapon (in Desert Storm, an EMP designed to mimic the flash of electricity from a nuclear bomb was used),[8] it is quite possible that the design is available to terrorist nations today. EMP devices are highly portable and can even be operated from a distance. Detonating the EMP in the air or near the top floors of a skyscraper maximizes the effects of the weapon.

 PREINCIDENT ACTIONS

Even before the terrorist attacks of September 2001, disaster planning in U.S. hospitals was designed primarily for external disasters involving large-scale trauma or mass casualties; for example, airline crashes, radiation accidents, or outbreaks of infectious diseases. Although it is certainly necessary to plan for such events, catastrophic power failures are actually more likely hospital scenarios. By the 1960s, engineers and architects began sealing off buildings from the outdoors, constructing mechanical environments solely controlled by electric power. When this power supply fails, the modern hospital may become totally uninhabitable.

Preparation for an Unscheduled Power Outage

The disaster planner must not only consider the usual devices such as lights and power to critical areas, but also must take steps to ensure against unintended actions when power is restored.[9] Fiscal restraints often prevent hospitals from spending adequately on emergency power protection. Hospital accountants do not consider absolutely fail-safe 24-hour power for hospitals to be cost-effective. Ironically, when hospitals do provide power protection, it is often used to protect their data systems, not their critical care systems.

Devices expected to operate when the power fails need to be inspected, maintained, and tested as part of an equipment preventive maintenance program. Plans and checklists to maintain critical services need to be prepared, implemented, and tested. Many hospitals test their emergency power supply systems at night or early in the morning before the bulk of the hospital's daily activities begin. This test time is often chosen because it is one of low clinical activity, and will therefore cause less disruption, but normal or peak clinical loads will not be reflected in this emergency power supply system test loading. Many hospitals do not test their emergency power supply systems when their operating rooms are in use. Also, the mechanical, building, radiology, and other clinical processes all vary during a typical hospital day.

Protective Measures Against an EMP Device

It is difficult to protect against an EMP weapon without purchasing military-grade communications equipment. Vehicles require computers to satisfy U.S. Environmental Protection Agency requirements, and these computers are vulnerable. Some anti-EMP measures that EMS providers can take include the following:

1. Build a Faraday cage. A Faraday cage can be made from fine metal mesh that is connected to a ground and completely encloses the items to be protected. If any power cables, data cables, or antennae go into the cage, it may be rendered worthless. Keep all equipment in the cage disconnected from batteries and other power supplies.
2. Maintain a supply of spare radio, monitor, and engine ignition spare parts. Keep the spare parts in the Faraday cage.
3. Use one system at a time during a threat period. Disconnect other systems from power and antennae and keep them in the Faraday cage.
4. If your vehicle ignition fails, disconnect the negative battery terminal, wait 2 minutes, and attempt to restart the vehicle. Some computerized ignition systems on late-model cars might be reset in this way.

Continuity of Critical Services

Backup power generators and uninterruptible power supplies should be selected and installed by qualified electric service contractors and then coordinated with the electric utility company. It is particularly important to avoid improper switching from one power supply to another. This can lead to power feedback into the regular power system, resulting in damage to equipment and the generator itself.

As plentiful and redundant as backup power sounds, diesel generators alone cannot provide fail-safe backup power to protect hospital patients. The lag between utility shutdown and generator power startup may destroy computerized diagnostic and life-support equipment. Even a 3-second disruption can be perilous to this sensitive electronic equipment. For this same reason, budgets permitting, electric engineers and contractors like to specify uninterruptible power supplies to protect vital equipment from even brief disruptions.

 POSTINCIDENT ACTIONS

When the power is restored, the following equipment and checklists will be useful:

- List manually operated switches that may need to be placed in the *off* position.
- List valves that need to be checked for proper position.
- List utilities such as steam, radio, telephone, computers, and pager communications that need to be verified for operability after the power is restored.
- List automatic starting equipment that should be shut down for safety and to minimize load demand when the power is restored.

 MEDICAL TREATMENT OF CASUALTIES

Power outages may cause differing types of injuries. In more rural areas, victims may be trapped for prolonged periods of time without adequate food, water, and medications. In colder climates, this may also result in casualties due to exposure. The risk and type of injury to the general population will be determined by the area in which the power outage strikes.

Risks to Worker Safety and Health

Workers operate machines and power tools and are engaged in chemical processes. These workers could be at risk of injury, exposure to dangerous chemicals, or death from a sudden loss of power without immediate restoration of power for vital systems.

People may sustain injuries when trapped in elevators, subways, and mass transit systems. Many of these injuries are sustained during attempts to get out of the local environment to a "safer" area.

Risks to Hospital Patients

Ventilator-dependent patients will need supplemental breathing equipment such as a bag-valve-mask operated by qualified personnel. Some ventilators have built-in,

short-term uninterruptible power supplies and may supply oxygen to patients for a few moments after the power fails. Operating room equipment may fail. Some equipment, such as a heart-lung bypass machine, is mission critical and should be protected by an uninterruptible power supply. Other equipment, such as lights, can be operated by battery power after a short interval of power outage without damage. Laboratory equipment, particularly computerized equipment, may not adequately survive a power loss of only a few seconds. This equipment must be protected by uninterruptible power supply to ensure that data being tested are not lost or degraded.

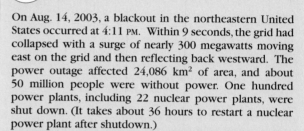

CASE PRESENTATION: NORTHEASTERN UNITED STATES BLACKOUT, AUGUST 14, 2003[10]

On Aug. 14, 2003, a blackout in the northeastern United States occurred at 4:11 PM. Within 9 seconds, the grid had collapsed with a surge of nearly 300 megawatts moving east on the grid and then reflecting back westward. The power outage affected 24,086 km² of area, and about 50 million people were without power. One hundred power plants, including 22 nuclear power plants, were shut down. (It takes about 36 hours to restart a nuclear power plant after shutdown.)

Because the pumping stations failed, 1,500,000 people in Cleveland were without water. These people were relieved by 7600 gallons of water trucked in by the National Guard. Since the airports and air traffic control systems were without power, an estimated 300 flights were cancelled in North America on August 14. New York City had six serious fires, 800 elevator rescues, more than 80,000 calls to 9-1-1, and over 40,000 police called to duty. Toronto had more than 100 elevator rescues and 1484 fire calls.

If the power outage had been deliberately caused by terrorist actions with an EMP bomb, the affected areas might have had no EMS, police, or fire rescue capability (due to transportation failures). Unprotected equipment might have been destroyed.

 UNIQUE CONSIDERATIONS

Catastrophic power failure caused by EMP devices may require replacement of all computerized circuitry within the equipment. This means that ambulances may not be operable until the computer ignition control circuitry has been replaced. It may also mean that every computerized piece of equipment from cardiac monitors to laboratory devices within the hospital may need to be replaced.

 PITFALLS

Several potential pitfalls exist in the response to a massive power system failure. These include the following:

- Backup generator failure due to battery failure, insufficient fuel supplies, overheating, or fuel pump failure.

Many generators are *standby rated*, meaning that they can reliably perform for only 2 out of 24 hours.

- Failure to check that backup generators will run for prolonged periods at anticipated full load. This should be checked at least twice a year for at least 12 hours.

REFERENCES

1. Nates JL. Combined external and internal hospital disaster: impact and response in a Houston trauma center intensive care unit. *Crit Care Med*. 2004;2:686-90.
2. Franklin C. What we learned when Allison turned out the big light. *Crit Care Med*. 2004;32:884-5.
3. Lewis CP. Disaster planning, Part I. Overview of hospital and emergency department planning for internal and external disasters. *Emerg Med Clin North Am*. 1996;14:439-52.
4. Dealing with power failure: how Spokane hospitals survived the ice storm. *Hosp Secur Saf Manage*. 1997;17:3-4.
5. Milsten A. Hospital responses to acute-onset disasters: a review. *Prehospital Disaster Med*. 2000;15:32-45.
6. Rogers K. Are electromagnetic pulses terrorists' next weapon of choice? *Las Vegas Review-J*. September 30, 2001. Available at: http://www.globalsecurity.org/org/news/2001/010930-attack04.htm.
7. Fulghum DA. EMP weapons lead race for non-lethal technology. *Aviation Week Space Technol*. May 2, 1993; 138:61.
8. Defense News, April 13-19, 1992.
9. CBC News Web site. Blackout by the numbers. Updated November 14, 2003. Available at: http://www.cbc.ca/news/background/poweroutage/numbers.html.

chapter 184

Hospital Power Outage

Marc C. Restuccia

 DESCRIPTION OF EVENT

The loss of power can be catastrophic for any medical institution, its patients, and its staff. The smooth operation of the facility, the safe treatment and diagnosis of patients, and the comfort of all persons in the facility require the continued availability of heat, cooling, and electric power. Loss of any or all of these can lead to an institutional disaster.

In colder climates, loss of heat forces staff to function in uncomfortable and difficult working conditions. For patients, loss of heating can mean they are at risk of hypothermia. Loss of cooling in hotter climates or months will fatigue the medical professionals laboring to diagnose and treat patients. For patients, the loss of cooling could make them susceptible to hyperthermia, dehydration, and worsening of their underlying condition(s). Finally, loss of electric power will severely affect any medical facility. Gone will be the ability to power the many instruments and equipment used to diagnose and treat patients. Computers used to track patients, their past history, and their tests and to order interventions will be offline if an interruption in their supply of electric energy is experienced. Electrically powered ventilators will not function, potentially leading to hypoxia and death for patients in the event of a loss of electric power. Almost all ability to perform laboratory tests and radiographic examinations will not be present in the event of an electric failure. Intravenous pumps, defibrillators, and other life support equipment will suddenly go "dead," with consequences for the patients who are dependent on them. Likewise, the ability for medical care providers to adequately see their environment, access patient information, perform diagnostic and therapeutic interventions, and function in general will be severely or perhaps totally degraded. Operating rooms will be in the dark, possibly in the middle of procedures. A more mundane, but still important, aspect is the institution's ability to store and prepare food for patients and staff, which will also be significantly degraded. The stability and potency of many medications and vaccines will be compromised if the facilities necessary to maintain them at their optimal storage temperatures are lost, meaning, at worst, that these medications will not be effective or, at best, they

will be "wasted," costing the facility money to replace them. Finally, the restoration of power can potentially entail risk for staff and patients. Such power outages can be predicted to be the result of terrorist activities or, much more likely, natural disasters.

 PREINCIDENT ACTIONS

Hospitals should all have general disaster plans in place. Among the scenarios envisioned *must* be the loss of electric power, heat, or cooling. Such contingencies must include whether the facility affected is unique, meaning all other local medical facilities are unaffected, or whether the entire local/regional area is affected. In both cases, a plan should be in place for the care, transport, and triage of patients requiring emergent care. Input from and acceptance and knowledge of such a plan and its contingencies must be sought from local and regional emergency medical services (EMS) agencies as well as geographically contiguous medical facilities. In the event of a loss of power, it may be necessary to move patients from the affected facility, move triage patients away from the affected institution, and coordinate local, regional, and perhaps even national resource availability.

Loss of Heating Capacity

Although not a common problem to encounter, hospitals in colder climates must have emergency plans in place for the protection of staff and patients in the event of the loss of ability to heat the institution. In the event that such an occurrence was experienced in a remote hospital with no contiguous medical facilities, the difficulties in transferring patients would be magnified.

If such a scenario were due to a natural or manmade occurrence, involved multiple contiguous healthcare facilities, and had an attendant increase in the number of affected patients, the complexity would increase. Not only would a far greater number of in-hospital patients be affected, but those in the local population requiring routine, ongoing, and especially emergent medical care would also be affected. Such an event would require regional, state, and most likely federal responses to mitigate the disaster.

Preincident actions necessary to prepare for a loss of heating should consist of the following:

- Forming a well-planned and drilled disaster strategy
- Regularly testing the hospital's heating system and identifying alternative mechanisms for heating the facility
- Identifying means to heat patient care areas in the event of failure of all primary heating capabilities
- Adopting and drilling of the hospital Incident Command System (ICS). This must include identifying who should report to the Emergency Operations Center (EOC) and developing a chain of command with clear functions, reporting lines, and expectations for each individual, including both those in the EOC and those throughout the facility
- Identifying and equipping an EOC (communications being the weak link in most plans)
- Identifying potential alternative sites/facilities for the care of the currently hospitalized patients and for the public seeking healthcare during the emergency
- Identifying staff to staff these alternative facilities (if needed)
- Developing Memoranda of Understanding with other institutions covering such contingencies. These should include means of transferring patients to unaffected facilities. Such plans should include local, regional, statewide, and other facilities
- Involving local EMS personnel in planning for the transfer of large numbers of patients
- Determining what group of patients may be continued to be cared for, if any, at the affected facility
- Determining how to best notify the general public about the nature of the emergency, how it will affect them, what the capabilities are of the affected facility, and when a return to normal operations can be expected

Loss of Cooling Capability

Loss of the ability to effectively air-condition hospitals would lead to similar considerations; however, the problems encountered should be less pronounced than the concerns surrounding a loss of the ability to heat the facility. Planning for such an emergency would be similar.

Preincident plans for the loss of hospital cooling should consist of the following actions:

- Forming a well-planned and drilled disaster plan
- Regularly testing the hospital's cooling system and identifying alternative mechanisms for cooling the institution
- Identifying alternative means to cool patient care areas in the event of failure of all primary cooling ability
- Adopting and drilling hospital ICS, as outlined above
- Identifying and equipping a hospital EOC
- Identifying alternative facilities for the care of currently hospitalized patients and for the public seeking healthcare during the emergency
- Identifying persons to staff these facilities if needed
- Developing Memoranda of Understanding with other facilities covering such contingencies, including transfer of patients to those institutions

- Involving local EMS in planning for the transfer of large numbers of patients
- Determining what group of patients, if any, can be continued to be cared for at the affected facility
- Determining how to notify the general public about the nature of the emergency, how it will affect them, what the capabilities are of the affected facility, and when a return to normal operations can be expected

Loss of Electric Power

A loss of electric power, having the potential to be extraordinarily disruptive, is an unfortunately common occurance.[1] In a modern healthcare facility, the number of critical patient care and ancillary devices, equipment, and services powered by electricity is enormous.[2] Interruption of continued, reliable electric power, even of a very brief duration, can be catastrophic. Modern computers, monitoring systems, laboratory instruments, and many more computer driven devices do *not* function well with even a short duration power loss. This vital dependence on electric power creates an inviting target for terrorist activities.

Each healthcare facility must preplan for this event and have a robust disaster plan in place. Multiple redundancies in the delivery of uninterrupted electric power must be ready and able to function *immediately* in the event of a loss of electric power. Identification of those systems and equipment that cannot function for even a short time without power must be accomplished in advance and these must be continuously tested and ready. Identification of potential events (e.g., an extraordinary heat wave, a tornado, a hurricane, or a manmade event) must be planned for in advance and preparations made for implementing the disaster plan if such an event is anticipated or actually occurs. For loss of electric power to any medical facility, being ready for such an incident in advance of its occurrence, if at all possible, is infinitely preferable to trying to react to such a condition *after* it has happened.[3]

Preincident plans for the loss of electric power should include the following actions:

- Forming a robust, well-thought-out, and drilled disaster plan
- Identifying the primary source of electric power. This should include potential scenarios for the loss of this electric input
- Identifying alternative sources of electric power. This would include uninterruptible power system(s) for equipment not able to tolerate the delay for emergency generators (usually 3 or more seconds[1]) to begin operation. In addition, emergency generators, usually diesel motors, in adequate number and/or capacity are available for use
- Continued interfacing with electric utilities and equipment suppliers of electricity-generating equipment to ensure prompt response to a loss of power
- Testing the primary electric source and all emergency systems on an ongoing basis

- Making ongoing training of hospital personnel in the use of all of the emergency backup electric systems a top priority
- Ensuring that adequate fuel for any emergency electric generating systems be on hand or immediately available
- Identifying alternative methods of delivering care to patients and allowing staff to function in the event of the failure of all electric generation capability
- Adopting and drilling hospital ICS and identifying the command structure that would ultimately order the evacuation of the hospital patients to another facility
- Identifying and equipping a hospital EOC, making allowance for the loss of all electric power
- Identifying alternative facilities for care of currently hospitalized patients and for the general public who may be seeking routine and emergency care in the event of a loss of all electric power
- Identifying personnel to staff such facilities, if needed
- Developing Memoranda of Understanding with other facilities covering such contingencies, including transfer of patients to those institutions
- Involving local EMS personnel in planning for the transfer of large numbers of patients
- Determining what group of patients, if any, can continue to be cared for at the affected facility
- Identifying means of informing the general public about the nature of the emergency, its impact on the hospital, what services will and will not be available, and the expected duration of the emergency
- Identifying which medications and vaccines are temperature dependent (most are) and making alternative plans for those thought to be most critical for the immediate care of in-patients in the hospital
- Identifying alternative means of feeding patients and staff

 POSTINCIDENT ACTIONS

Once a loss of power of any type is experienced, the medical facility must activate its disaster plan, staff its EOC, and begin to follow the plan's steps. Notification of local, state, and federal public health and public safety agencies would be necessary, depending on the type of emergency, its scope, its expected duration, and its source of origin. The response made by any of these agencies would be contingent on the factors listed above. The disaster plan, and its implementation, should be flexible enough to adapt to any new information about the disaster, as it is obtained. The medical facility should take great pains to document the resources needed to meet the healthcare needs of its patients and to address the crisis. Initial attempts to bring the facility to a predisaster state of operation should be attempted rapidly, but if unsuccessful, the order to evacuate patients should be made through the ICS. Potential state and federal reimbursement of the costs incurred will be absolutely dependent on such documentation.

 MEDICAL TREATMENT OF CASUALTIES

Cooling Loss

The loss of cooling power for a medical institution would not usually be expected to lead to an influx of new patients. The exception to this rule would be if the loss of cooling were due to an accident, manmade or natural, affecting a local or regional area. Examples of such would include explosions, fires, earthquakes, hurricanes, or tornadoes. In such a case, it would be expected that the local resources would be overwhelmed and outside resources would be needed. It would take time to get these resources into place, and contingency plans should be made to care for the patients in the hospital, care for new patients from the community, as well as prepare for transferring patients to other unaffected facilities in the meantime.

The hospital's disaster plan would guide treatment of patients in a hospital experiencing a loss of cooling. Patients at the highest risk of heat injury—very young children, elderly persons, and those with concomitant medical conditions (such as cardiac disease)—would need to be rapidly identified and arrangements made to either warm their environment or transfer them to unaffected hospitals. The decision whether continue to care for other patients in the hospital would need to be a joint one involving the medical staff leadership, medical staff, and hospital leadership. Consideration of evacuating the hospital must be guided by the best interests of each patient, the availability of beds in alternative facilities, and the ability of EMS personnel to effect such transfers. Just as each medical facility is unique, each such disaster is unique, requiring preplanning, strong leadership, good communication, and commitment from the hospital and its staff.

Heating Loss

A loss of the ability to heat a hospital will engender most of the same difficulties and issues as in loss of cooling. A key difference is that, in most cases, loss of the ability to heat the hospital in a colder climate will lead to the need to evacuate all of the patients in the hospital and to divert all new patients.

Electric Loss

In the event of a loss of electric power to a hospital, the first priority is those patients who are dependent on electrically driven life support systems. Such patients are patients breathing via ventilators, patients using intra-aortic balloon pumps, patients using electrically driven intravenous infusion pumps with critically important medications (e.g., vasopressor agents), and patients in the operating room. In many cases, if all electric power is lost, battery backup will be available for most of these devices. For patients on ventilators, life-saving alternative means of ventilating include the Oxylator (Lifesaving Systems, Inc, Roswell, Ga), which is an oxygen-powered, nonelectric ventilation device, or hand-powered bag-valve-mask ventilation. Contingency plans for alternative, often

St. Joseph's, a community hospital in Minnesota with 200 beds, is located in a city of 200,000 people. The city is served by two other similarly sized institutions: City Hospital, with 250 beds, and Memorial Hospital, which has 275 beds. On a particularly cold January day, the heating unit at St. Joseph's, an old plant that is scheduled for upgrade as soon as capital funds can be raised, suffers a pre-dawn fire. All ability to heat the institution is lost. Within the hour, the temperature begins to fall. The hospital is 80% occupied with 162 patients in the emergency department (ED), on the floors, and in the single intensive care unit.

A disaster is declared, and an EOC is opened. The chief executive officer; chief financial officer; chief medical officer; heads of the ED, the intensive care unit, and the Chief Nursing Officer; nursing supervisor; director of facilities; director of social services; director of safety; chief of police; and director of public relations all convene in the EOC. It is quickly determined that the heating plant is severely damaged and will take days to weeks—perhaps months—to get back online. Alternative sources of heating the patient care areas are being sought. Immediately the chief executive officer issues the following orders:

- A hospital ICS is established
- The ED is closed to incoming ambulance traffic (i.e., diversion) via notification of local and regional EMS and regional EMS authority
- The ED makes provision(s) for walk-in patients
- The facility is secured from unauthorized entrance
- All elective admissions and surgeries are cancelled and the affected patients notified

- A public announcement of the state of the hospital is prepared for broadcast on local television and radio stations. News outlets are notified
- The other area hospitals are notified of the ongoing problems at St. Joseph's. Assistance is requested in dealing with the ongoing emergency
- Local municipal authorities are notified about the nature of the emergency and request their assistance
- The director of facilities, ED director, ICU director, the directory of the community nursing organization, and the nursing supervisor are directed to develop an action plan

The action plan will consist of:
- Securing alternative means of heating patient care areas; for example, space heaters, radiant heaters, and warming blankets
- Identifying those patients who require transfer to fully functional facilities such as nearby hospitals, rehabilitation facilities, and nursing homes
- Obtaining acceptance from physicians and facility administrators for those patients
- Determining appropriate means of transferring those patients
- Determining which patients can be safely discharged home, and making arrangements for this
- Determining what additional staff will be needed

After 12 harrowing hours, all of the critically ill patients have been transferred to other facilities. All other patients have been discharged or have been sent to appropriate care institutions. At this point, the EOC is demobilized and the process of determining the amount of damage, the cost of repair, and the length of time for restoration of normal services is begun.

---

portable, sources of electric power for other devices should be in place. Preplanning, strong leadership, good communication, contingency plans, and hospital staff commitment are essential.[4]

 UNIQUE CONSIDERATIONS

A modern medical facility is uniquely dependent on the continued availability of heating, cooling, and most especially electric power. Loss of any of these is most certainly a cause for the implementation of the institution's disaster plan. Prior planning, contingency identification, practice, and commitment of the facility and staff are crucial to the positive outcome of such an emergency.

 PITFALLS

Several potential pitfalls exist in the response to a hospital power outage. These include the following:

- Failure of the disaster plan to adequately address the loss of heat, cooling, or electricity
- Failure to address alternative sources of cooling, heating, and most especially electric power

- Lack of Memoranda of Understanding with other healthcare facilities to support the stricken institution in such emergencies
- Failure to adequately inform and train medical and support staff in their expected roles in the event of the loss of power
- Lack of training of staff before the occurrence of a disaster
- Failure to include the prehospital (EMS) system in predisaster planning
- Failure to continuously test the system's response to a failure of any of the above; this would include failure to test backup systems
- Failure to evacuate the hospital soon after attempts to remedy the problem have failed

REFERENCES

1. Harrington M. Emergency: the critical condition of hospital power. *EC&M*. August 1, 2002:1-8. Available at: http://ceenews.com/mag/electric_clarification_ideals_wirenut/.
2. Nates JL. Combined external and internal hospital disaster: impact and response in a Houston trauma center intensive care unit. *Crit Care Med*. 2004;32:686-90.
3. O'Hara JF Jr, Higgins TL. Total electrical power failure in a cardiothoracic intensive care unit. *Crit Care Med*. 1992;20:840-5.
4. Franklin C. What we learned when Allison turned out the big light. *Crit Care Med*. 2004;32:884-5.

chapter 185

Intentional Contamination of Water Supplies

Patricia L. Meinhardt

 ## DESCRIPTION OF EVENT

The terrorist events of Sept. 11, 2001, have forced the public health and medical community, federal security and regulatory agencies, and state and local water utilities to consider the possibility of intentional contamination of U.S. water supplies as part of an organized effort to disrupt and damage important elements of the nation's infrastructure.[1-4] Water supplies and water distribution systems represent potential targets for terrorist activity in the United States based on the critical need for water in every sector of its industrialized society.[2] Even short-term disruption of water service can significantly affect a community, and intentional contamination of a municipal water system as part of a terrorist attack could lead to serious medical, public health, and economic consequences. The magnitude of water service disruption for a community has been vividly demonstrated by the destruction of water supply systems in the Gulf Region as a result of Hurricane Katrina in 2005. As this massive hurricane illustrated, contamination of water with biologic, chemical, or radiologic agents has generally resulted from natural disasters, industrial pollution, or unintentional man-made accidents in the United States. However, the deliberate contamination of the wells, reservoirs, and other water sources for civilian populations has been used as a method of attack by opposing military forces throughout the history of war. Many armies have resorted to using this method of warfare, including the Romans, who contaminated the drinking water of their enemies with diseased cadavers and animal carcasses.[4] With enhanced technology and modern scientific advances, the mechanisms of dispersal of biologic, chemical, and radiologic warfare agents have expanded considerably and currently include water as a delivery mechanism. Whether advanced scientific techniques or ancient warfare methods are used by terrorists, overt and covert contamination of water supplies remains a potential public health threat for the U.S. population.

The plausibility of intentional contamination of water supplies as part of a terrorist attack has been reinforced by recent congressional testimony, a consensus statement by a governmental review panel, and a joint Centers for Disease Control and Prevention (CDC) and Environmental Protection Agency (EPA) water advisory health alert.[5,6] As part of its 2002 congressional report, the National Research Council of the National Academy of Sciences concluded that water supply system contamination and disruption should be considered a possible terrorist threat in the United States.[5] On Feb. 7, 2003, the national terrorism threat level was increased to "high risk" based on information received and analyzed by the federal intelligence community. Subsequent to this heightened alert, the CDC and EPA issued *Water Advisory in Response to the High Threat Level,* which describes the need for enhanced vigilance by the public health, medical, and water utility communities regarding the risk of a terrorist attack on the nation's water infrastructure.[6] Apprehension regarding a terrorist assault on drinking water systems has also been reinforced by arrests of suspects in 2002 and 2003 who were charged with threatening to contaminate municipal water supplies in the United States.[3,4]

Spectrum of Disease Resulting from Intentional Water Contamination

The biologic, chemical, and radiologic agents that have been designated as potential terrorist weapons may be dispersed through multiple exposure pathways, including water.[2,4,7-9] Recognizing and managing a waterborne disease outbreak and the health effects of exposure to water contaminants are diagnostic challenges under normal circumstances, but the challenge will be even more significant during an act of water terrorism.[10] Intentional contamination of water supplies with biologic, chemical, or radiologic agents may produce a broad spectrum of disease and involve virtually every organ system, including, but not limited to, the gastrointestinal, respiratory, dermatologic, hematopoietic, immunologic, and nervous systems. In addition, waterborne agents may enter the body through various portals, including the following: (1) ingestion and aspiration of contaminated water, (2) dermal absorption of contaminated water during bathing activities, (3) inoculation of skin lesions from direct contact with contaminated water, (4) consumption of food directly contaminated by water during food preparation, and (5) consumption of contaminated food indirectly contaminated by water through uptake in the food chain or through agricultural practices.[4]

A key factor in the accurate diagnosis and appropriate management of disease resulting from intentional contamination of water supplies is inclusion of water by the healthcare provider as one possible exposure pathway for the dissemination of biologic, chemical, and radiologic agents at the time of initial case presentation. The categories of compounds that may cause a diverse spectrum of water-related disease during an act of water terrorism include many of the agents traditionally associated with other modes of delivery. Biologic, chemical, and radiologic agents that have been designated as possible terrorist agents of public health concern that include the potential for waterborne route of exposure and weaponized agent delivery are presented in Table 185-1.

 PREINCIDENT ACTIONS

Although medical practitioners may not be able to prevent the first cases of illness or injury resulting from an act of intentional water contamination, they are positioned to play a critical role in minimizing the impact of such an event by practicing medicine with an increased index of suspicion that such an attack may occur in their community. To prevent a missed diagnosis of a case of terrorism-related waterborne disease, it is vital that medical practitioners understand how water could act as a potential exposure pathway or mode of dispersal for biologic, chemical, and radiologic agents *before* an incident occurs.[4]

TABLE 185-1 SELECTED BIOLOGIC, CHEMICAL, AND RADIOLOGIC AGENTS THAT INCLUDE WATER AS A POTENTIAL MODE OF DISPERSAL FOR TERRORISM*

BIOLOGIC AGENTS

Bacterial Pathogens	**Plague** *Yersinia pestis*	**Viral hemorrhagic fevers** (e.g., Ebola, Marburg, Lassa fever, Rift Valley fever, Yellow fever, Hantavirus, and Dengue fever)
Anthrax *Bacillus anthracis*	**Salmonella** *Salmonella typhimurium* and *S. typhi* (acute gastroenteritis and typhoid fever)	**Parasitic Pathogens**
Brucellosis *Brucella melitensis, B. suis, B. abortus, B. canis* (undulant or Malta fever)	**Shigellosis** *Shigella dysenteriae* and other *Shigella* sp.	**Cryptosporidiosis** *Cryptosporidium parvum* and other *Cryptosporidium* sp.
Cholera *Vibrio cholerae*	**Tularemia** *Francisella tularensis*	**Rickettsial and Rickettsial-Like Pathogens**
Clostridium perfringens	**Viral Pathogens**	**Psittacosis** *Chlamydia psittaci*
Glanders *Burkholderia mallei* (formerly *Pseudomonas mallei*)	**Hepatitis A virus (HAV)**	**Q fever** *Coxiella burnetti*
Melioidosis *Burkholderia pseudomallei* (formerly *Pseudomonas pseudomallei*)	**Smallpox** *Variola major*	**Typhus** *Rickettsia prowazekii*
	Viral encephalitides (e.g., Venezuelan equine encephalomyelitis [VEE])	

BIOLOGIC TOXINS

Bacterial Biotoxins	**T-2 mycotoxin** extract from *Fusarium* spp.	**Marine Biotoxins**
Clostridium botulinum toxins (collectively BTX)	**Anatoxin A** product of cyanobacteria, *Anabaena flos-aquae*	**Saxitoxin** (Paralytic shellfish poisoning or PSP) product of dinoflagellate, *Gonyaulax*
Clostridium perfringens toxins	**Microcystins** products of cyanobacteria, *Microcystis* spp.	**Tetrodotoxin** neurotoxin from pufferfish sp.
Staphylococcus enterotoxin B (SEB) (e.g., protein toxin from *Staphylococcus aureus*)	**Plant- and Algae-Derived Biotoxins**	
Fungal-Derived Biotoxins (Mycotoxins)	**Ricin** extract from castor bean	
Aflatoxin metabolite of *Aspergillus flavus*		

CHEMICAL AGENTS

Nerve Agents ("Gases")	**Vesicant and Skin Blistering Agents**	**Industrial and Agricultural Agents**
G agents (Volatile) GA (Tabun), GB (Sarin), GD (Soman)	**Lewisite** L, L-1, L-2, L-3	**Pesticides, persistent and non persistent**
V agents (Nonvolatile) VX	**Nitrogen mustards** HN-1, HN-2, HN-3	**Dioxins, furans, polychlorinated biphenyls (PCBs)**

TABLE 185-1 SELECTED BIOLOGIC, CHEMICAL, AND RADIOLOGIC AGENTS THAT INCLUDE WATER AS A POTENTIAL MODE OF DISPERSAL FOR TERRORISM*—CONT'D

Blood Agents (Asphyxiant or Systemic Agents)	Incapacitating Agents (Psychotropic or Behavior-Altering Compounds)	Dioxins, furans, polychlorinated bphenyls (PCBs)
Cyanide Compounds Hydrogen cyanide (AC) Cyanogen chloride (CK)	**CNS Depressants** (e.g., BZ [3-quinoclinidinyl benzilate] and similar compounds)	**Explosive nitro compounds and oxidizers** (e.g. ammonium nitrate combined w/fuel oil)
Arsine Compounds (Arsenicals) Ethyldichloroarsine (ED) Phenyldichloroarsine (PD)	**CNS Stimulants** (e.g., LSD [D-lysergic acid and diethylamide])	**Flammable industrial gases and liquids** (e.g., gasoline and propane)
		Poison industrial gases, liquids, and solids (e.g., cyanides and nitriles)
		Corrosive industrial acids and bases (e.g., nitric acid and sulfuric acid)

RADIOLOGIC AGENTS

Radiation Terrorism Threat Scenarios	Potential Exposure Pathways and Agent Source
Nuclear Blast Detonation of suitcase-sized nuclear bomb	**External Exposure** External radiation exposure from nuclides in the plume after detonation External radiation and contamination from surface-deposited contamination and activation products Personal contamination of skin and clothing
Nuclear Reaction Sabotage of nuclear power plant or "meltdown"	**Internal Contamination** Internal contamination from plume inhalation due to nuclides in plume after detonation
Radiation dispersal device RDD or "dirty bomb" release	Internal contamination due to inhalation of re-suspended contamination Internal contamination due to inhalation or ingestion from personal contamination Internal exposure due to ingestion of contaminated food and water Internal contamination through skin or wound absorption or deposition from contact with contaminated material, including water

*Modified and reprinted with permission from *Physician Preparedness for Acts of Water Terrorism: An On-line Readiness Guide*. Accessible at: http://www.waterhealthconnection.org/bt.

Preincident preparedness by the medical community will be critical to reduce the following: (a) the public health impact of a water terrorism incident, (b) the secondary disruption to potable water availability and distribution, and (c) the psychological impact of the public's lack of confidence in water safety and quality after an incident of intentional contamination of water.[2,4] If preincident actions include terrorism preparedness and disaster readiness, educated medical and public health professionals may make the difference between a controlled response to a water terrorism event versus a public health crisis.[4,11]

It is important to note that a major effort has been undertaken to improve and enhance the ability to detect and characterize deliberate contamination of water systems in the United States as part of a collaborative effort by local water utilities and several federal public health agencies.[3,4,12] As a result, U.S. water systems are more physically secure than ever before, with multiple layers of enhanced protection. However, there are several potential points of contamination that could be targeted for acts of water terrorism. Therefore, it is critically important for the medical community to have a basic understanding of these water system vulnerabilities in order to be able to complete an accurate exposure history when evaluating a suspected case of water-related disease. Various scientific consensus groups, public health agencies, and water utility specialists have outlined a series of potential points of contamination of the U.S. water supply and distribution system.[4,5] This information is summarized in Table 185-2 and acts as a valuable resource for healthcare providers and public health professionals when evaluating an unusual symptoms complex or an atypical illness pattern that may represent a case of waterborne terrorism.

 POSTINCIDENT ACTIONS

Although environmental monitoring of water supplies is improving rapidly, the most likely *initial indication* that a water terrorism incident has occurred may be an increased number of patients presenting to their healthcare provider or emergency department with unusual or unexplained illness or injury, a change in local disease trends and illness patterns, or a community-wide waterborne disease outbreak. Therefore, healthcare providers and public health practitioners may be the first to discover that a waterborne release of biologic, chemical, or radiologic agents has

TABLE 185-2 POSSIBLE POINTS OF INTENTIONAL CONTAMINATION OF U.S. WATER

Healthcare providers should keep these sources of potential water contamination and unusual modes of delivery of biologic, chemical, and radiologic agents in mind when evaluating a suspected case of terrorism-related disease*:

- **Upstream of a community water supply system or collection point:** Water supply systems are composed of small streams and bodies of water, rivers, service reservoirs, aquifers, wells, and dams that may act as points of deliberate contamination of water.
- **Community water supply intake access point or water treatment plant:** Many water supply systems are designed to receive water from source water reserves at a central intake point, with this source water being subsequently filtered and sanitized at the community water treatment facility for eventual distribution as potable water. Both a water intake point and a community water treatment plant may be targeted for terrorist activity and deliberate water contamination.
- **Selected points in the post-treatment water distribution system:** Treated water is distributed to water consumers or end-users through transmission pipelines to homes and businesses. Selected portions of a water distribution system or water main are another potential point of water contamination that may be targeted by terrorists and could affect a subdivision, specific neighborhood, school, medical center, or nursing home.
- **Private home or office building water supply connection, individual building water supply, water tanks, cisterns, or storage tanks:** Treated water that is stored very close to the water consumer or end-user as well as individual house or building connections may serve as points of contamination of water by terrorists.
- **Water used in food processing, bottled water production, or commercial water:** Water used for food processing or preparation as well as bottled water production also represent points of potential water contamination by terrorists.
- **Deliberate contamination of recreational waters and receiving waters:** Both treated and untreated recreational waters may serve as a point of potential contamination of water, including swimming pools, water parks, and natural bodies of water (small lakes and ponds). Receiving waters, such as rivers, estuaries, and lakes, may be secondarily contaminated with wastewater from sanitary and storm sewer systems that may have been environmentally contaminated by a biologic, chemical, or radiologic agent used in a terrorist assault.

*Modified and reprinted with permission from *Physician Preparedness for Acts of Water Terrorism: An On-line Readiness Guide*. Accessible at: http://www.waterhealthconnection.org/bt.

occurred in a targeted population and must understand their critical role as "front-line responders" in detecting water-related disease resulting from terrorist activity.[4]

Certain clinical manifestations and disease syndromes may be characteristic of a terrorist attack in which biologic, chemical, or radiologic agents are used via a waterborne route. A heightened level of alertness and awareness by the medical community of these patterns of illness and clusters of disease may enhance the initial discovery of a waterborne terrorist attack and are critical to any postincident action plan. Early and accurate clinical detection of a suspicious case of terrorism-related disease will be especially important for timely follow-up epidemiologic investigations to be initiated and appropriate remediation and prevention efforts to be instituted by the public health and water utility communities.[4] During the postincident period, healthcare practitioners will need to "think like an epidemiologist" when evaluating any suspect case or unusual pattern of disease in their clinical practice.[13] A medical practitioner's diagnostic acumen for recognizing waterborne disease resulting from intentional contamination of water can be augmented significantly by embracing this epidemiologic approach. Several epidemiologic patterns and sentinel clues have been published and provide a valuable resource for both the medical and public health community facing the challenges of diagnosing terrorism-related disease that may result from multiple exposure pathways, including water, and have universal application in a clinical and public health setting (Box 185-1).

Postincident actions also require that healthcare providers become familiar with the appropriate mechanisms for communicating with law enforcement agencies, public utilities, the media, and the concerned public. If a healthcare provider suspects that an act of water terrorism is responsible for a patient's symptoms complex or an unusual illness pattern in his or her practice, *immediate*

action to contact the appropriate public health authority is essential, even before laboratory confirmation or final diagnosis. This contact is the critical first step necessary for the public health authority to (1) initiate a prompt investigation; (2) provide guidance to healthcare providers and the affected community; (3) establish communication and cooperation with other local, state, and federal agencies as warranted; and (4) contact local water utilities for prompt remediation and protective measures. Attention to this postincident procedure by healthcare providers is mandatory to initiate the appropriate response to a potentially high-risk public health event that may indicate intentional contamination of drinking water supplies.

 MEDICAL TREATMENT OF CASUALTIES

The nature of the medical sequelae resulting from exposure to intentional contamination of water supplies depends on a multitude of factors including the following: (1) agent characteristics, including toxicity and virulence; (2) individual host susceptibility and level of immunity; and (3) movement and dilution of the agent in the environment.[14,15] Individual host susceptibility and differences in biologic, chemical, and radiologic agent virulence and toxicity may result in a wide variation in the severity of disease resulting from a waterborne terrorist event.[16] Water-related disease resulting from intentional contamination may present as benign symptoms or self-limited illness in a healthy patient population, whereas the same waterborne exposure in a vulnerable patient population may result in serious morbidity and mortality. In addition, as is apparent from the 50 agents that may be dispersed in water (see Table 185-1), the medical management and treatment protocols for water terrorism-related disease vary significantly depending on the agent used.[4]

Several epidemiologic patterns have been identified as possible sentinel clues of a terrorist attack. However, none of these indicators alone is pathognomonic for terrorism-related disease. These indicators and sentinel clues are presented here as an educational tool for use by healthcare providers and public health practitioners as possible disease trends that may warrant further investigation*:

- Point source illness and injury patterns with record numbers of severely ill or dying patients presenting within a short period of time
- Very high attack rates, with 60% to 90% of potentially exposed patients displaying symptoms or disease from possible biologic, chemical, or radiologic agent exposure
- Severe and frequent disease manifestations in previously healthy patients
- Increased and early presentation of immunocompromised patients and vulnerable population patients with debilitating disease since the dose of inoculum or toxic exposure required to cause disease may be less than for the general healthy population
- "Impossible epidemiology" with naturally occurring diseases diagnosed in geographic regions where the disease has not been encountered previously
- Higher-than-normal number of patients presenting with gastrointestinal, respiratory, neurologic, and fever diagnoses
- Record number of fatal cases with few recognizable signs and symptoms, indicating lethal doses of biologic, chemical, or radiologic agents near a point of dissemination or dispersal source
- Localized areas of disease epidemics that may occur in a specific neighborhood or sector, possibly indicating contamination of a selected point in a post-treatment water distribution system
- Multiple infections at a single location (school, hospital, nursing home) with an unusual or rare biologic pathogen
- Lack of response or clinical improvement of presenting patients to traditional treatment modalities
- Near-simultaneous outbreaks of similar or different epidemics at the same or different locations, indicating an organized pattern of intentional biologic or chemical agent release
- Endemic disease presenting in a community during an unusual time of year or found in a community where the normal vector of transmission is absent
- Unusual temporal or geographic clustering of cases with patients attending a common public event, gathering, or recreational venue
- Increased patient presentation with acute neurologic illness or cranial nerve impairment with progressive generalized weakness
- Unusual or uncommon route of exposure of a disease such as illness resulting from a waterborne agent not normally found in the water environment

*Modified and reprinted with permission from *Physician Preparedness for Acts of Water Terrorism: An On-line Readiness Guide*. Accessible at: http://www.waterhealthconnection.org/bt.

An online clinical management guide has been developed for healthcare practitioners and public health specialists faced with addressing the evaluation and management of water-related disease resulting from terrorist activity.[4,10] This free resource, *Physician Preparedness*

for Acts of Water Terrorism: An On-line Readiness Guide, which is accessible at www.waterhealth connection.org/bt, is highlighted in Figure 185-1 and provides "24/7" access to medical management guidelines addressing water-related disease resulting from intentional contamination of water supplies from biologic, chemical, and radiologic agents.

 UNIQUE CONSIDERATIONS

1. Even though environmental monitoring of water supplies continues to improve, the most likely initial indication that an intentional water contamination event has occurred in a population may be a change in disease trends and illness patterns. Therefore, healthcare providers may be the first to recognize that an act of water terrorism has occurred in their community.
2. Use of water as a mode of dispersion for terrorist agents may confound diagnosis, delay treatment, and impede protective public health measures if clinical evaluations and epidemiologic investigations do not include the possibility of a waterborne route of exposure or mode of dispersal.
3. Prompt identification of waterborne disease resulting from water terrorism may be difficult since the signs and symptoms of waterborne disease and the health effects of water contamination are often nonspecific and mimic more common medical conditions and disorders unrelated to water contamination.
4. Co-infections with waterborne pathogens, coupled with multiple chemical agent exposure during an act of water terrorism, may result in exposed patients presenting with both acute and delayed symptoms from mixed agent exposure, complicating accurate and timely diagnosis.
5. Waterborne exposure to biologic, chemical, or radiologic agents may result from both direct and indirect environmental contamination, including contamination through wastewater from sanitary and storm sewer systems receiving run-off from an aerosolized terrorist attack or through decontamination wastewater generated during patient decontamination procedures.

 PITFALLS

- Failure to include water as a possible exposure pathway or mode of transmission during initial case presentation of a suspected terrorist incident
- Failure to recognize that more than 50 potential terrorist agents of public health concern may be distributed through water as a mode of dispersal
- Failure to notify appropriate public health authorities immediately of a suspected case of waterborne disease, preventing timely remediation efforts and protective public health measures
- Failure to consider the special needs of susceptible populations most at risk for morbidity and mortality from intentional water contamination

- Failure to identify alternative sources of drinking water as part of disaster preparedness plans in order to ensure that affected communities have adequate drinking water for days to weeks after a water contamination event

- Failure to provide effective risk communication regarding water safety to concerned patients and the public

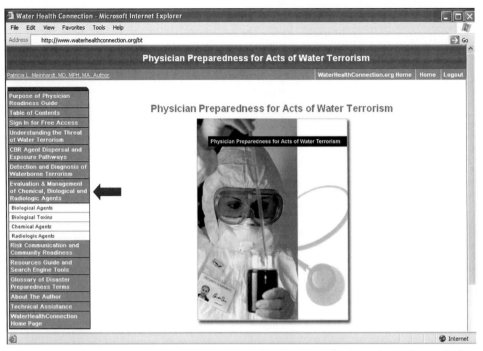

FIGURE 185–1. *Physician Preparedness for Acts of Water Terrorism: An On-line Readiness Guide* is a free online medical resource accessible at: http://www.waterhealthconnection.org/bt.

CASE PRESENTATION

A sensitive communication advisory from the Department of Homeland Security is issued stating that recent intelligence indicates members of Al Qaeda have discussed plans to attack drinking water supplies. Two potential attack scenarios have been uncovered: (1) disruption of the water delivery system through a physical attack on the water infrastructure and (2) introduction of chemical and/or biologic agents into the water distribution system and post-treatment facilities. Several days later, a large medical center's emergency department (ED) experiences a very active night in which a series of patients complaining of generalized weakness, fatigue, dry mouth, and dysphagia are evaluated. One elderly patient also complained of blurred vision, partial paralysis, and slurred speech. There is no apparent age or sex distribution in the presenting ED cases, but the number of presenting patients with similar symptoms continues to escalate throughout the day. Laboratory confirmation is not yet available, but by early the next morning, the presumptive diagnosis for the unknown epidemic in the community is botulism. The sudden appearance of multiple patients with acute onset of characteristic symptomatology for botulinum toxicity with no common ingestion of high-risk food suggests a possible terrorist event, and the local public health authorities are contacted. Although the cases of botulinum toxicity appear to be mild at this point, the medical center terrorism preparedness team and the health department are concerned that these initial cases herald a mass exposure event.

Through excellent history-taking techniques, a water-borne source for the community botulism outbreak is uncovered. It is apparent that "finished water," or drinking water that has already been treated, has been intentionally contaminated with botulinum toxin in one of the community water districts. The intentional contamination of post-treatment drinking water with botulinum toxin has generated real fear and distress in the community. Local healthcare providers are bombarded with questions from their patients, including: "Is my water safe?" To make matters worse, the national news media have arrived and are positioned right outside the medical center entrance.

The intentional contamination of the community drinking water has lead to the closure of a targeted water treatment facility until further notice. This closure has lead to denial of potable water for several water-dependent sectors in the community. Local businesses, schools, and nursing homes in the affected water district are very concerned about how long they will be expected to be without municipal water supplies. Several days later, the contaminated water treatment facility is still "off line" and local community governing officials are under pressure to address the disruption of potable water and the resulting financial and public health consequences as well as the ongoing public risk communication crisis. The public health and medical community is faced with developing contingency plans for ongoing disruption of the water delivery system, determining when it will be "safe" to bring the contaminated water treatment facility back "on-line," and then convincing the local residents that their municipal water is safe again.

REFERENCES

1. Clark RM, Deininger RA. Protecting the nation's critical infrastructure: the vulnerability of US water supply systems. *J Contingencies Crisis Manag.* 2000;8:73-80.
2. Krieger G. Water and food contamination. In: Chase KH, Upfal MJ, Krieger GR, et al, eds. Terrorism: Biological, Chemical and Nuclear from Clinics in Occupational and Environmental Medicine. Philadelphia: WB Saunders; 2003:253-62.
3. States S, Scheuring M, Kuchta J, et al. Utility-based analytical methods to ensure public water supply security. *Am Water Works Assoc J.* 2003;95:103-15.
4. Meinhardt PL. Physician Preparedness for Acts of Water Terrorism: An On-line Readiness Guide. Environmental Protection Agency, Arnot Ogden Medical Center. Available at: http://www.waterhealthconnection.org/bt/index.asp.
5. National Research Council. Making the Nation Safer: The Role of Science and Technology in Countering Terrorism. Committee on Science and Technology for Countering Terrorism, National Academies Press: Washington, DC; 2002.
6. Centers for Disease Control and Prevention. CDC and EPA Water Advisory in Response to High Threat Level. Available at: http://www.phppo.cdc.gov/HAN/ArchiveSys/ViewMsgV.asp?Alert Num=00123.
7. Franz DR, Jahrling PB, McClain DJ, et al. Clinical recognition and management of patients exposed to biological warfare agents. *Clin Lab Med.* 2001;21:435-73.
8. Inglesby TV, O'Toole T. Medical Aspects of Biological Terrorism. American Collage of Physicians. Available at: http://www.acponline.org/bioterro/medicalaspets.htm.
9. Headquarters, Departments of the Army, Navy and the Air Force, and Commandant, Marine Corps. Field Manual: Treatment of Biological Warfare Agent Casualties. Available at: http://www.nbc-med.org/SiteContent/MedRef/OnlineRef/FieldManuals/FM8_284/fm8_284.pdf.
10. Meinhardt PL. Recognizing Waterborne Disease and the Health Effects of Water Pollution: Physician On-line Reference Guide. Environmental Protection Agency, American Water Works Association, Arnot Ogden Medical Center. Available at: http://www.waterhealthconnection.org.
11. Henderson DA. Bioterrorism as a public health threat. *Emerging Infectious Diseases.* 1998:4(3). Available at: http://www.cdc.gov/ncidod/eid/vol4no3/hendrsn.htm.
12. Environmental Protection Agency. EPA Actions to Safeguard the Nation's Drinking Water Supplies. Available at: http://www.epa.gov/safewater/security/secfs.html.
13. Burkle FM. Mass casualty management of a large-scale bioterrorist event: an epidemiological approach that shapes triage decision. *Emerg Med Clin North Am.* 2002;20:409-36.
14. Public Health Response to Biological and Chemical Weapons: WHO Guidance. World Health Organization. Available at: http://www.who.int/csr/delibepidemics/biochemguide/en/.
15. Kaufmann AF, Meltzer MI, Schmid GP. The economic impact of a bioterrorist attack: are prevention and postattack intervention programs justifiable? *Emerg Infect Dis.* 1997;2(3). Available at: http://www.cdc.gov/ncidod/EID/vol3no2/downkauf.htm.
16. Burrows WD, Renner SE. Biological warfare agents as threats to potable water. *Environ Health Perspect.* 1999;107:975-84.

chapter 186

Food Supply Contamination

Marc C. Restuccia

DESCRIPTION OF EVENT

Despite the many improvements made in overseeing the nation's food supply, foodborne illness remains a serious cause of morbidity and mortality throughout the world, including the United States. Many factors contribute to an ideal chain for amplification of foodborne pathogens, including the following: growth of modern mass production farms; the scale of modern water supplies; importation of food from other countries, which may lack the strict food handling and shipping guidelines present in the United States; adoption of immense food and processing plants; and distances, sometimes quite lengthy, that food is transported to consumers. The scale of the problem is not known with great accuracy.[1] It is estimated that millions of people are affected worldwide. The majority suffer only temporary discomfort. However, for the young, the very old, patients with concomitant systemic illness, and, increasingly, for the immunocompromised (cancer patients, AIDS patients, patients who have had organ transplants), foodborne illness can be fatal. In the United States, approximately *76 million* people suffer foodborne illnesses every year, and approximately 5000 deaths are attributable to this annually.[2]

Foodborne illnesses are virtually always the result of human actions (or omissions). They can be categorized as those seen routinely in daily life or as intentional attacks on the food chain for a given population. Each will be described separately.

Typical Food Poisoning

Improper handling, leading to fecal contamination of food, is the usual cause of most foodborne illnesses. Typical agents causing the illness include bacteria, viruses, parasites, and toxins. Recently, a newly described class of agents, prions, has been implicated in causing human illness, namely transmissible spongiform encephalopathies. Infected beef cattle have been discovered in several countries. Documented cases of human illness have been described in the United Kingdom. These discoveries have devastated the cattle industries in both Britain and America and have led to the banning of British and American food imports.

In addition, many people around the world have considered changing their dietary habits, with a significant decrease in beef consumption.

One cause of food supply contamination may be seen when the food supply chain is disrupted by a natural event. Scenarios such as an earthquake, tornado, hurricane, or flood contaminating foods during production, processing, transportation, or preparation would have severe consequences on the affected population. Fortunately, in such an event, unaffected areas of the state, region, country, or world could supply untainted food to the stricken area or region.

The diagnosis of foodborne illness in the typical scenario is difficult. Unless multiple persons present with symptoms and a clearly identifiable source is determined, an individual healthcare provider may have difficulty in identifying a foodborne epidemic. The incubation period can range from a few hours, in the case of bacterial toxins, to days, as with many bacterial, viral, parasitic, and protozoan agents, to years with prion-induced illness. Multiple other causes of gastrointestinal dysfunction may mimic foodborne illness, making the diagnosis exceedingly difficult.

In the case of typical foodborne illnesses, if multiple persons are affected and have a common point in their history, such as attending a particular wedding, eating at a specific restaurant, or buying a specific food item at a particular food market, the diagnosis may quickly become evident. If patients present at multiple emergency departments, physicians' offices, and urgent care facilities, the appropriate questions may not be asked or accurately answered, and the diagnosis may not be made in a timely manner. The typical signs and symptoms of foodborne illness—nausea, vomiting, diarrhea, abdominal pain, fever, and dehydration—may be seen with many non-foodborne illnesses and require an astute clinician to make the connection.

Intentional Attack on the Food Supply

In the current climate of worldwide terrorist activities, the potential for an individual or group to deliberately contaminate a population's food supply cannot be discounted. Due to this concern, congress enacted the

Public Health Security and Bioterrorism Preparedness and Response Act of 2002. The Food and Drug Administration (FDA) was charged with developing guidelines to ensure the safety of food produced in the United States and that which is imported from outside U.S. borders. These regulations, currently still being formulated, may be viewed on the FDA's Web site. In addition, when the Department of Homeland Security was created, it was recognized that U.S. agriculture and food industries had to be included in the list of critical parts of society's infrastructure needing protection.[3] The expanding aggregation of growers, suppliers, and long lines of transportation, often stretching across international boundaries, made this chain of supply uniquely susceptible to intentional contamination. Although never actually experienced by a society, warring nations historically have sought biologic weapons to sabotage an opposing nation's food supply.[4]

A terrorist seeking to sabotage a nation's food supply, especially in a highly industrialized nation like the United States, has many potential targets for food contamination. Crops, livestock, fertilizer, cattle feed, products in the food processing and distribution chain, storage facilities, transport modes, and food and agricultural research laboratories all provide potential sites for such an act of terror. As the General Accounting Office (GOA) noted in its 2003 report, individuals or groups seeking to cause economic disruption may well target livestock and crops.[3] Conversely, if such groups seek to inflict human illness, they might contaminate finished food products at the processing stage, the distribution or transportation stage, or potentially at the site of consumption. An example of the latter was a cult in the 1980s which, seeking to sway a local election, contaminated a local restaurant's salad bar with *Salmonella*.[5] This act would, the cult envisioned, sicken enough of the local populace so as to render them unable to vote, allowing the cult to gain a majority in the election.

The GAO's report[3] noted that there are significant gaps in federal controls for protecting agriculture and the food supply. These gaps include inadequate education of border inspectors on foot-and-mouth disease, inadequate numbers of inspectors to handle the magnitude of international passengers, and inadequate scanning technology or inconsistency in its use at cargo and bulk mail facilities.[3]

The potential costs of a bioterrorist attack on the food supply, especially if it involved livestock, would be much greater than simply the cost of the livestock and disposal of the animals.[4] As was seen in Great Britain with the outbreak of foot-and-mouth disease (a nonterrorist incident), the loss of confidence in British food suppliers and the loss of tourism income multiplied the loss to the U.K.'s economy significantly. In the case of a terrorist-sponsored food contamination attack, assuming that the terrorists were seeking to maximize the impact, the economic losses and disruption could be magnified many times.

Lastly, the mere threat or suggestion of a biologic attack on the food supply would be sufficient to seriously disrupt the economy and the lives of the population targeted. Lack of confidence in the safety of the food available would have unimaginable consequences for the area targeted.

In the event of a contamination of the food supply, the speed at which it would be recognized would vary depending on the agent(s) used. For long-incubating agents, such as bovine spongiform encephalopathies (mad cow disease), the first indication would be positive test results of the disease in sample livestock. It would not, however, appear in the human population at risk for years. With other agents targeted at the human population and introduced at later stages of the food production chain, such as the *Salmonella* attack previously described, it would take only hours to a few days for the population at risk to show signs and symptoms of food poisoning. Such signs and symptoms would mirror those of a typical foodborne illness event, only potentially magnified many times. It is entirely conceivable that not only would healthcare facilities and providers be overwhelmed with the numbers and severity of patients, but it is also extremely likely that the healthcare providers also would be stricken. A calculated terrorist act might very well *first* target the healthcare infrastructure to maximize the disruption and loss of life and productivity of the stricken populace.

 ## PREINCIDENT ACTIONS

Planning for the possible contamination of any part of the food supply chain, whether due to deliberate acts of terrorism or simply to human carelessness, must be done in advance of the event. Developing a plan for such a situation must include the following: rapid identification of the altered food supply, limiting its health and economic impact, treatment of affected persons, and identification of alternative sources of noncontaminated food. Adequate numbers of unaffected public safety and healthcare workers need to be available to identify the outbreak, limit its expansion, maintain public safety, and treat victims. Local, state, and federal officials need to identify beforehand those links in the food supply chain that are particularly vulnerable to contamination and implement policies and plans for prevention.

Education of the entire population would be beneficial. Farmers, distributors, retailers, and consumers need to be informed about the potential for foodborne illnesses, recognizing signs and symptoms, identifying when the food supply chain is compromised, and acting decisively if such a situation arises. Legislators at local, state, and federal levels need to understand the vulnerability of the food supply and be proactive in initiating legislation, including funding. This legislation would be to protect the food supply, treat the victims, and limit the economic devastation of any disruption in the supply.

Syndromic surveillance is a fairly new method of rapidly tracking and identifying disease trends. It allows cities, regions, states, and even wider communities to share, via computer, the background health of a population. An example would be a surveillance system that receives data on symptoms and diagnoses of patients admitted to the area emergency departments on a daily basis. This system, in theory, would quickly identify unusual disease clusters and alert boards of health, triggering a preplanned response. This powerful tool has implications beyond that of food supply contamination and could well be invaluable in any disease outbreak or bioterrorist attack.

Every hospital, locality, state, and nation should have predeveloped disaster plans to cover the eventuality of a food supply disruption. These should include access and distribution of needed medications and methods for communicating with local boards of health, public safety agencies, the medical community, and especially the public. Identification of alternative food supplies should be part of the plan. Although state and federal assistance can be expected, such responses will take some time and each of the aforementioned entities should have a detailed plan for dealing with the first few hours of the disaster, possibly even the first 3 days.

Greater state and federal oversight of the food supply, as previously mentioned, is critical to prevent and limit the impact of a widespread foodborne illness. Improved inspection of all food products, during both production and shipping (potentially over international borders), is desirable. Rapid containment of such an outbreak will limit its progression, minimize its economic impact, and restore the public's confidence in the food supply.

 ## POSTINCIDENT ACTIONS

After an outbreak of foodborne poisoning, a high degree of suspicion is necessary, especially on the part of medical professionals, to determine whether a cluster of illnesses is something out of the ordinary. Open lines of communication and the use of tools, such as syndromic surveillance, will be essential for early identification of the problem, limitation of a burgeoning outbreak, and prompt and appropriate treatment of victims. Consideration of the impact on critical societal elements, such as police, fire, and healthcare, must be made along with restoration of more normal functioning of the area affected. Early notification and clear lines of communication will be vital in controlling the situation.

 ## MEDICAL TREATMENT OF CASUALTIES

For many people suffering from foodborne illness, the treatment is primarily supportive. With some diseases, the addition of appropriate antibiotics can be lifesaving or at least shorten the duration of the illness.

 ## UNIQUE CONSIDERATIONS

The major difficulty in determining whether a food supply contamination has occurred will be the way patients present. Early on, many medical practitioners generally will see a few cases each of what appears to be viral gastroenteritis. Only if the healthcare community, food supply industry, and governmental agencies are communicating and ready to act will such an event be identified and addressed before serious health and economic consequences occur.

 ## PITFALLS

- Failure to have a disaster plan in place that specifically details the steps to take in the event of a food supply contamination
- Failure to communicate among the healthcare community and boards of health regarding new trends in disease appearance
- Failure to protect the healthcare community and public safety agencies from being ravaged by an outbreak
- Failure to identify alternative means of feeding the population if the primary food supply is contaminated or unavailable
- Failure of legislators, at all levels, to be proactive in preventing and limiting the effects of an outbreak

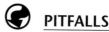
CASE PRESENTATION

Bedford Falls is a fairly isolated town located on the coast of New England. Recently a group of people advocating an anarchistic form of government have begun moving into town and buying property. The locals are increasingly uneasy with the influx of newcomers. As their ranks swell, the newcomers begin asserting political power, with their members winning seats on governing boards and committees. Alarmed, the locals schedule a referendum that would effectively remove the newcomers from these positions of authority. A bitter, often acrimonious debate between the groups ignites. One week before the vote on the referendum, many of the longtime residents present to the local emergency department (ED) and physicians' offices complaining of vomiting, diarrhea, and abdominal pain. The director at the local ED, remembering a Salmonella outbreak in the past decade under similar circumstances, becomes suspicious. When multiple stool cultures from those affected return as being positive for Salmonella, the ED director contacts the local authorities and board of health. The police chief immediately arrests the newly elected selectman, the representative of the school board, and other members of the anarchist group, charging them with deliberate food poisoning intended to influence the upcoming vote. The head of the board of health contacts the state and the Centers for Disease Control and Prevention for assistance. By the time help arrives, 25 local residents have fallen ill, virtually all of them longtime residents opposing the new group. Prompt attention to medical care for those who are ill is instituted, and a full investigation is commenced. Investigators quickly determine that all those who have fallen ill ate at the same restaurant, catering mainly to locals and infrequently visited by members of the anarchist group. All of the ill patients had consumed the same batch of egg salad. Examination of the restaurant's food processing areas reveals multiple positive cultures for Salmonella species indistinguishable from those infecting the victims. Further investigation reveals, however, that the egg salad in question was inadvertently left outside the refrigerator for 24 hours before being mixed with fresh egg salad served to the restaurant's patrons. Fortunately, all the victims recover after 5 to 7 days without serious sequelae. The police chief releases the suspects and alerts the town's attorney that she may expect multiple legal cases from the incident. The referendum vote proceeds as scheduled.

REFERENCES

1. Keene WE. Lessons from investigations of food borne disease outbreaks. *JAMA*. 1999;181:1845-7.
2. Bashai WR, Sears CL. Food poisoning syndromes. *Gastroenterol Clin North Am*. 1993;3:579.
3. General Accounting Office. Bioterrorism: A Threat to Agriculture and the Food Supply. Available at: http://www.gao.gov/new.items/d04259t.pdf.
4. Cain S. Agroterrorism. A Purdue Extension Backgrounder. Available at: http://www.ces.purdue.edu/eden/disasters/agro/Agroterrorism.doc.
5. wbur.org. Bioterrorism in History: 1984: Rajneesh Cult Attacks Local Salad Bar. Available at: http://www.wbur.org/special/special-coverage/feature_bio.asp.

chapter 187

Mass Gatherings

Katharyn E. Kennedy

 ## DESCRIPTION OF EVENT

Mass gatherings may be defined as events with a large number of individuals gathered together in a specific place for a specific purpose.[1] Thousands of such events take place worldwide each year. In the United States, 5.5 million attend the National Association for Stock Car Auto Racing (NASCAR) events. As many as 65 million attend National Basketball Association (NBA), National Football League (NFL), and/or National Collegiate Athletic Association (NCAA) events. Other such gatherings include leisure events (fairs, sporting events, and concerts), religious festivals, parades, demonstrations, and public disorder. Medical care of some sort has been provided for such gatherings for the last 30 years in both the United States and Europe. Event organizers everywhere need to take responsibility for the safety and well-being of the participants at an event.

Various numbers have been used to define a mass gathering—groups greater than 1000 have been used,[2] although many researchers use numbers greater than 25,000.[3] Considerable variation exists in the type of medical care provided to both participants and spectators at these gatherings. General standards have been proposed for the provision of primary care, emergency and disaster care, and evacuation. Both the American College of Emergency Physicians (ACEP)[4] and the National Association of Emergency Medical Service Physicians (NAEMSP)[5] have addressed the previous lack of guidelines and standardized care. A survey in 1998[6] showed that only six U.S. states provided regulatory guidance for the provision of care at mass gatherings, although many are starting to address this omission.

A number of disasters have occurred at gatherings throughout the world, in particular at soccer events (Table 187-1). Terrorist threats have also become an unfortunate reality, as shown by the bombing at Centennial Park during the 1996 Olympics in Atlanta, Ga.

 ## PREINCIDENT ACTIONS

Mass Gatherings Overall

At organized mass gatherings, predictable medical problems and an unpredictable wide variation in medical care

exist worldwide. Preplanning and prediction of resource requirements, based on careful needs assessment of anticipated medical care usage and public health risks, may lead to a standardized optimal provision of medical care (Box 187-1).[7]

Provision of medical care is the responsibility of the event planners. Public health officials need to be involved early in the planning process, especially for large events, such as the Olympics, world fairs, and pilgrimages. The local health department should be involved in the overseeing of the preparation, storage, and serving of food and sanitation requirements. Once identified, those providing medical care at mass gatherings need to liaise with local emergency medical services (EMS), fire, and law enforcement officials. Ground and building plans, close estimates of possible attendance, and identification of any specific hazards should be shared among these providers. Estimates of attendance may be gleaned from advanced ticket sales or from attendance at previous similar events. However, previous history is notoriously unreliable, as demonstrated at the papal mass in Denver (1993) where 250,000 were predicted but 500,000 turned up. Ticket sales on the day of play may have contributed to crowds rushing into soccer stadiums just before kick-off in both England in 1989 and Africa in 2001, with disastrous consequences (see Box 187-1).

The type of medical care to be provided at the event needs to be considered beforehand (Table 187-2).[8-12] Primary medical care, such as first aid, emergency care, and preparation for a possible disaster, should be addressed. Staffing levels and type of staffing also need to be anticipated. Recommended ratios include 1 to 2 physicians per 50,000 attendees, 2 paramedics or 1 paramedic and 1 emergency medical technician per 10,000 attendees, and 1 basic first-aid provider per 1000 participants at the event.[13] On-site physicians have been shown to reduce ambulance transfers to local hospitals by as much as 89%,[14] significantly lessening the impact of an event on local EMS services and hospitals. Physician presence should be strongly encouraged at events where significant trauma may occur, where there is a long distance to definitive care, or to enhance an anticipated disaster response. Multiple variables interact to make planning for a mass gathering event challenging. An understanding of these may allow for a more efficient

TABLE 187-1 MAJOR SOCCER DISASTERS

DATE		DISASTER
1985	May 11	Bradford, England: 56 burned to death, 200 injured due to a fire at Bradford soccer stadium.
	May 26	Mexico City, Mexico: 10 trampled to death and 29 injured forcing their way into a match.
	May 29	Brussels, Belgium: British soccer fans attack rival Italian supporters at Heysel Stadium. A concrete retaining wall collapses, resulting in 39 deaths and more than 400 injured.
1988	March 12	Katmandu, Nepal: 80 fans seeking shelter during a violent hailstorm are trampled to death.
1989	April 15	Sheffield, England: 96 died at Hillsborough Stadium. Many are crushed to death when a barrier collapses on an overcrowded area.
1992	May 5	Bastia, Corsica: 17 killed when grandstand collapses.
1996	October 16	Guatemala City: 84 killed and 147 injured by stampeding fans at Mateo Flores National Stadium.
2001	April 11	Johannesburg, S. Africa: 43 die, 250 injured at Ellis Park Stadium due to crush as crowds push into an already overcrowded stadium.
	May 9	Accura, Ghana: More than 120 killed in a stampede at a soccer match.

BOX 187-1 REQUIREMENTS FOR MEDICAL CARE AT MASS GATHERINGS

- Identification of those providing care
- Physician medical oversight
- Identification of level of care needed, personnel to provide care, and appropriate equipment needs
- Public health issues
- Treatment facilities and access to care
- Transportation of injured
- Emergency medical aspects
- Communication
- Command and control
- Documentation

Adapted from data from NAEMSP.

and effective planning process. However, the unexpected can be expected.

Environmental factors play a role in anticipating medical usage at events. Heat-related illnesses are a factor in outdoor concerts, papal visits, and political demonstrations. Thirty-one percent of physician encounters recorded at the 1996 California AIDS ride were for heat-related problems.[15] The Denver papal visit resulted in an unanticipated 21,000 patient encounters at a mainly youthful gathering, due in part to the 14-mile walk and high temperatures.[3] Preplanning in the form of educational packages that addressed measures to prevent heat-related illnesses given to those who purchased advance tickets for the Atlanta Olympics in 1996 might have led to a decrease in the number of patient encounters for this problem despite the high heat and humidity.[16] Cold weather events generally lead to lower medical usage rates by participants and spectators.[17]

Alcohol and illicit drug usage may increase the number of patient encounters. Historically, the consumption rate of alcohol and drugs may be higher at music festivals, rock concerts, and raves. Open-air music events in the United Kingdom have resulted in a primary diagnosis of alcohol intoxication in 4% of patient encounters.[18] Banning the consumption of alcohol at Wembley Stadium led to a 50% reduction in alcohol-related problems.

Anticipating medical usage rates may allow for more appropriate staffing levels. However, a wide variation in usage rates has been reported. One study has shown that the overall medical usage rate decreases with overall crowd size. Patient encounters at events with more than 1 million participants average 10 per 10,000 patient encounters. Events with lower numbers average 41 per 10,000 spectators.[1] The medical usage rate can vary even within an event itself. At the Los Angeles Olympics, soccer events had usage rates of 68 per 1000 and rowing and canoeing 6.8 per 1000. Other variables to consider include ages of attendees; event duration and time of occurrence; mobile versus stationary event; event type; presence of fireworks, torches, or bonfires; outdoor versus indoor event; and the physical plant and location. Attendance at "on-off" events can be very difficult to estimate, and advance ticket sales can help considerably.

Anticipated crowd demographics may be useful in the preplanning stage. Older groups may be expected at papal visits, classical music concerts, and large sporting events.[19] Younger age groups frequently attend rock concerts and auto-racing events.[20] The needs of children also must be considered. Most children present with minor injuries, but medical teams need to be prepared to deal with serious medical emergencies and trauma. Overall medical usage at a children's fair was 19.2/10,000, and one-half of those who presented were younger than 14 years old. Protocols need to be in place for the provision of care to minors who present without an accompanying adult.[11] Crowd "mood" is an unpredictable variable. Certain types of music, known team rivalry, and religious furor may lead to disruptive behavior and an increase in medical usage rates. Crowded events may lead to a "too-close-for-comfort" feel among event-goers. Environmental conditions,

TABLE 187-2 ANTICIPATING MEDICAL NEEDS AT MASS GATHERINGS

TYPE OF EVENT	INJURIES TO BE EXPECTED
Political events:	Minor and major trauma
Religious events:	Minor injuries, heat-related problems, cardiac problems
Sports/musical events:	Drug/alcohol use, minor trauma
Sporting events:	Minor trauma, heat-related problems, and cardiac issues
Auto racing:	Severe trauma, heat- and alcohol-related problems

such as inclement weather, squalid conditions, poor sanitation, and lack of access to drinking water, may lead to ugly crowd dynamics.

Despite the many variables to be considered, it has been shown that event type and temperatures are the variables that best predict medical usage rates.[1,9,21]

After the anticipated usage rates and staffing levels have been addressed, the positioning, number, and type of aid stations should be considered. Fixed events at stadiums may have areas specially designed and designated for medical care. For other events, aid station locations should be no more than a 5-minute walk for attendees. Stations should be clearly visible, and the locations should be known to participants and other event personnel. These areas need to be adequately and appropriately staffed before the anticipated start of the event and remain so until the event is completed. Consideration needs to be given to providing medical care in the crowd for occurrences such as cardiac arrests or lower extremity fractures, including how to transport these patients back to aid stations. Thought needs to be given regarding provision of ambulances for hospital transport and access and egress for these vehicles. The organizers of medical care need to know the capabilities of local hospitals and should liaise with hospital personnel before the event. Attention to the location, staffing, and communication needs of a medical command center should be addressed. Communication needs should be considered for event medical providers; other event planners; and local EMS, police, and fire personnel. Back-up communication in the form of handheld devices or cell phones should be decided on, and medical personnel must be able to connect with local dispatch centers.

An incident command structure for medical personnel may be used. The event medical officer oversees all aspects of medical care provided at the site. The event triage officer conducts and directs medical assessment of casualties at designated treatment areas or while roving through the crowds and transporting patients to a central area. The event treatment officer oversees treatment to the sick and injured. The event transport officer directs transport to other facilities, and the logistics officer provides the necessary support for EMS at the event. Consideration may be given to the need for hazardous materials teams, decontamination, wilderness medicine, or use of amateur radio groups.

All patient encounters should be documented. Use of NCR (noncarbon record) paper will facilitate a copy accompanying a patient who needs transport to a medical facility. Records are needed for medical and legal reasons and also may be useful for research purposes.

Concerts/Sports Gatherings

The medical usage rate may vary by type of music, with rhythm/blues having rates of 1.3/10,000 and gospel/Christian 12.6/10,000. The overall median usage for concerts is 2.1/10,000.[19] Rock concerts typically have rates 2.5 times that of other concerts. The anticipated audience participation in "moshing," crowd surfing, and stage diving may lead to a dramatic increase in medical incidents.[22] Other problems encountered include minor trauma and ethanol or illicit drug intoxication.[23]

Surgical problems may be caused by falls; assaults; being crushed against barriers; and assorted "missiles" causing head injuries. Severe trauma may occur in up to 1.4% of attendees at rock concerts. Medical issues include headache, syncope, asthma, and hypoglycemia. Cardiac arrest is uncommon, with a rate of 0.01 to 0.04/10,000. Asthma may be very common at rodeos.[24]

The ultimate sporting event is probably the Olympics. Planning for the medical care of both spectators and participants begins as soon as the host city has been announced. Apart from routine medical care, there exists a potential for transmission of infectious diseases, risk of injury from crowd crushes, and now the very real risk of terrorist activity or political protests. Extensive planning at local, state, and federal levels is vital to ensure the health and safety of all concerned.[25-27] At the 1996 Atlanta games, specialized incident assessment teams were set up to analyze terrorist risks and to address issues such as stockpiling antibiotics and antidotes. Medical providers of all levels received training in awareness of chemical, biologic, and radiologic weapons.[28] Local hospitals were updated to include mass decontamination units. Local EMS providers were given uniform operational plans and procedures, enhanced communications were agreed on, protocols were developed for the management of heat-related illnesses, and guidelines for response to mass casualties were issued. Public health initiatives to address heat-related illnesses included a media campaign; packets sent to ticket purchasers; shelters; and provision of water, wide-brimmed hats, sunscreen, and water misters at the most crowded sites. These, plus the cooler-than-normal temperatures, may have led to a decrease in the expected number of hyperthermia victims.

Marathons

More than 300 marathons are staged each year, along with countless half marathons, triathlons, and 5K or 10K events. Preincident considerations include course layout, number of runners, climate, and medical team experience. Earlier start times and the addition of half marathons have led to a decreased risk of injury.[29,30] Encouraging runners to seek help early has also reduced serious medical problems.[31] Educating runners before the event on issues such as dehydration, low blood sugar, exhaustion, blisters, the importance of good preparation and training, and the use of energy drinks may lessen the need for medical intervention. Runners with a history of asthma are encouraged to carry their inhalers and not to run if they feel ill. Accessible, visible first-aid stations along the route, use of mobile paramedic teams, and a medical control center should provide adequate medical coverage. Radio communication is essential between medical providers, and a treatment tent at the finish line should include paramedic/triage teams, massage therapists, and podiatrists. The use of computer tracking chips may be used to identify how many runners use medical treatment and help in the planning of the provision of care and supplies in the future.

Pilgrimages

Millions of people perform pilgrimages every year. The Muslim pilgrimage, the Haji, to the Holy Land of Makkah (Mecca) in Saudi Arabia may have up to 2.5 million participants from 140 countries for a period of 5 to 7 days. The pilgrimage involves a 24-mile round trip from Makkah through the plains of Arafat. Many of the pilgrims are elderly, come from poor countries, live in tents in extreme conditions, and perform physically exhausting religious rituals. In India, millions of pilgrims visit Lord Ayyappa at Sabarimala each year. This occurs over a 41-day period and involves a 90-minute trek uphill to the temple. Many other pilgrimages on a smaller scale take place throughout the world.

Several of the problems encountered may be anticipated. Many of the participants are not in good health and may have chronic medical problems. Heat exhaustion is common during the hot cycle of the Haji. Cases of heat stroke doubled from 1980 to 1981. This may be overcome by the education of pilgrims before and during the event. Infectious disease outbreaks are also common. These include meningococcal meningitis; gastroenteritis; hepatitis A, B, and C; and various zoonotic diseases. The implementation of vaccination policies, infection control policies, and public health initiatives are proving successful in addressing these problems.[32] Pilgrims need proof of appropriate vaccinations to obtain a visa for travel to Saudi Arabia. Face mask use is encouraged to reduce the spread of respiratory infections. Head shaving by men, at completion of the pilgrimage, has been associated with the transmission of bloodborne diseases as illegal barbers reuse razors several times. The ritualistic slaughter of thousands of sheep during the ending ceremony may led to outbreaks of Rift Valley fever. This has led to the banning of importation of sheep from countries where this fever is endemic. There is strict surveillance and supervision of accredited slaughterhouses.

Free medical care is provided at the holy site in Makkah. In 1997 and 1998 a "treat and release" program was commenced, leading to a 73% reduction in ambulance transports.[33] In India at Sabarimala, a medical center is provided at the site. Typically 8000 pilgrims receive medical care over the 41-day period.

 POSTINCIDENT ACTIONS

In the wake of various disasters at mass gatherings, it is vital to learn from previous mistakes. The European Convention on Spectator Violence and Misbehavior met in 1985 to address issues rising largely from the Heysel Stadium disaster. It identified the need for police and sports authorities to cooperate in ensuring segregation of rival supporters, controlling access to stadiums, and banning the consumption of alcohol. After the 1989 Hillsborough disaster in England, the Gibson Report recommended medical care at stadiums for the first time. All-seats stadiums were to be phased in, leading to safer stadiums with greater attendance.

The Boston Marathon has instituted a postevent clinic that is open for 3 days after the event to meet the delayed medical needs of runners.

 MEDICAL TREATMENT OF CASUALTIES

In general, most participants require minor medical interventions that may be addressed by first responders or paramedics.[8] Paramedics may use triage protocols to identify casualties who should be transported to a hospital after initial stabilization rather than waiting for treatment by an on-site physician.[34]

At rock concerts, 1.4% of attendees may experience *severe* trauma. Minor trauma results from falls, assaults, being crushed against barriers, and head injuries from assorted "missiles." Anticipated medical problems include headaches, syncope, hyperventilation, asthma, epilepsy, and hypoglycemia. At the Atlanta Olympics, most of the injuries compromised sprains or strains (13%) and contusion abrasions (7%). Bronchitis was common (9%), and heat cramps/dehydration accounted for 7% of those seeking medical care.[26] In addition, three cardiac arrests were reported; the provision of defibrillators at mass gatherings is an important consideration.[35]

Hyponatremia is increasingly prevalent among marathon runners. It is defined as a serum sodium level of less than 136 mmol/L and is commonly caused by overhydration. Mild cases may be treated by fluid restriction and consumption of salty foods until urination resumes. In moderate cases the patient's sodium level may need to be checked hourly and, in critical cases, intravenous access will be required and diuretics and 3% saline may be administered. Complications such as seizures, pulmonary edema, and coma should be treated appropriately. Runners should be encouraged to replace only 16 ounces of fluid along with salt for every pound of weight lost. Exercise-associated collapse may occur at the finish due to venous pooling. This may be treated by laying the patient supine with the legs elevated and rehydrating with oral electrolyte/carbohydrate solution. Dehydration should be assessed clinically and treated with oral fluids. Heat-related illnesses are addressed in the usual fashion. Hypoglycemia is treated with oral or intravenous glucose replacement.

Many pilgrims are in poor health before the event and may need more than minor first aid. Many suffer from heat-related illnesses or infectious diseases. Provision of free medical care and on-site medical facilities with capabilities of providing even an intensive care unit level of care may meet these needs.

Disasters do occur at mass gatherings, and appropriate medical care needs to be available. Frequently, the cause of death is traumatic asphyxia,[36] for which rapid interventions may make a difference.

 ## UNIQUE CONSIDERATIONS

Every mass gathering should be considered a unique event. Careful and exhaustive preplanning may reap many benefits. It is important for those providing medical care at the event not to do so in a vacuum. Local EMS providers may well be needed and certainly will be required if a mass casualty event occurs. Mass gatherings occurring in urban settings will have different characteristics and requirements from those in more rural or remote settings. Even though it may be difficult to predict all the medical needs of the crowd, prior studies have started to use a more scientific approach to addressing these needs. Event type, duration, expected attendance, and weather conditions need to be taken into careful consideration in the planning process.

 ## PITFALLS

- Lack of legislation regulating minimum standards for provision of medical care at mass gatherings
- Lack of a coordinated, integrated preplanning process
- Lack of funding to provide needed public health initiatives and medical resources
- Failure to identify a medical director for the event
- Failure to learn from previous experiences
- Underestimating expected attendance
- Failure to consider all variables, such as crowd size, demographics, event duration, and environmental factors

 CASE PRESENTATION

Always eager for a challenge, many months previously you accepted the position of medical director to oversee medical care at a large open-air concert to be held in your city to celebrate its 250th anniversary. Fifty thousand spectators are anticipated based on advance sales. You have spent many hours in meetings with all the key players arranging appropriate medical care for this event. On the morning of the event, the temperature has already risen 10 degrees above average and the humidity is climbing. An hour into the event, it becomes apparent that many people have forged tickets, and the crowd is now estimated at 75,000. Shortly before the much anticipated heavy metal band is due to play, you receive a call on your radio that the crowd is getting unruly in the mosh pit, and your paramedics are concerned that people will be crushed....

- Failure to consider and prepare for a terrorist or mass casualty event
- Inability to allow capacity crowd ingress to a stadium in a 1-hour period
- Failure to consider ambulance access and egress at an event
- Lack of training of security personnel, leading to failure to recognize and control potentially dangerous situations

REFERENCES

1. Michael JA, Barbera JA. Mass gathering medical care: a twenty-five year review. *Prehospital Disaster Med.* 1997;12(4):305-12.
2. Rose W, Laird S, Prescott J, et al. Emergency medical services for collegiate football games. A six and one-half year review. *Prehospital Disaster Med.* 1992;7:159-9.
3. De Lorenzo RA. Mass gathering medicine: a review. *Prehospital Disaster Med.* 1997;12(1):68-72.
4. Leonard RB, Petrilli R, Noji EK, et al. Provision for Emergency Medical Care for Crowds. Dallas: ACEP Publications; 1990:1-25.
5. Jaslow D, Yancy A, Milsten A. Mass gathering medical care. *Prehosp Emerg Care.* 2000;4(4):359-60.
6. Jaslow D, Drake M, Lewis J. Characteristics of state legislation governing medical care at mass gatherings. *Prehosp Emerg Care.* 1999;3(4):316-20.
7. Jaslow D, Yancy A, Milsten A. Mass Gathering Medical Care: The Medical Director's Checklist for the NAEMSP Standards and Clinical Practice Committee. Lenexa, Kan: National Association of Emergency Medical Services Physicians; 2000.
8. Varon J, Fromm RE, Chanin K, et al. Critical illness at mass gatherings is uncommon. *J Emerg Med.* 2003;25(4):409-13.
9. Arbon P, Bridgewater F, Smith C. Mass gathering medicine: a predictive model for patient presentation and transport rates. *Prehospital Disaster Med.* 2001;16(3):109-16.
10. Zeitz KM, Schneider DP, Jarrett D, et al. Mass gathering events: retrospective analysis of patient presentations over seven years at an agricultural and horticultural show. *Prehospital Disaster Med.* 2002;17(3):147-50.
11. Thierbach AR, Wolcke BB, Piepho T, et al. Medical support for children's mass gatherings. *Prehospital Disaster Med.* 2003;18(1):14-9.
12. Milsten AM, Maguire BJ, Bissell RA. Mass-gathering medical care: a review of the literature. 2002;17(3):151-62.
13. Football Licensing Authority: Guide to Safety at Sports Grounds. 4th ed. London: The Stationery Office; 1997.
14. Grange JT, Baumann GW, Vaezazizi R. On-site physicians reduce ambulance transports at mass gatherings. *Prehosp Emerg Care.* 2003;7(3):322-6.
15. Friedman LJ, Rodi SW, Krueguer MA, et al. Medical care at the California AIDS Ride 3: experiences in event medicine. *Ann Emerg Med.* 1998;31(2):219-23.
16. Centers for Disease Control and Prevention. MMWE: Prevention and management of heat-related illness in many spectators and staff during the Olympic Games—Atlanta, July 6-23, 1996. *JAMA.* 1996;45(29):631-3.
17. Eadie JL. Health and safety at the 1980 Winter Olympics, Lake Placid, New York. *J Environ Health.* 1981;43(4):178-87.
18. Hewitt S, Jarrett L, Winter B. Emergency medicine at a large rock festival. *J Accid Emerg Med.* 1996;13(1):26-7.
19. Grange JT, Green SM, Downs W. Concert medicine: spectrum of problems encountered at 405 major concerts. *Acad Emerg Med.* 1999;6(3):202-7.
20. Nardi C, Bettini M, Brazoli C, et al. Emergency medical services in mass gatherings: the experience of the Formula 1 Grand Prix 'San Marino' in Imola. *Eur J Emerg Med.* 1997;4(4):217-23.
21. Milsten AM, Seaman KG, Liu P, et al. Variables influencing medical usage rates, injury patterns, and levels of care for mass gatherings. *Prehospital Disaster Med.* 2003;18(4):334-46.
22. Janchar T, Samaddar C, Milzman D. The mosh pit experience: emergency medical care for concert injuries. *Am J Emerg Med.* 2000;18(1):62-3.

23. Erickson TB, Koenigsberg M, Bunney E, et al. Prehospital severity scoring at major rock concert events. *Prehospital Disaster Med.* 1997;12(3):195-9.

24. Fromm RE, Varon J. Frequency of asthma exacerbations at mass gatherings. *Chest.* 1999;116(4):251S.

25. Meehan P, Toomey KE, Drinnon J. Public health response for the 1996 Olympic Games. *JAMA.* 1998;279(18):1469-73.

26. Wetterhall SF, Coulombier DM, Herndon JM, et al. Medical care delivery at the 1996 Olympic Games. *JAMA.* 1998;279(18):1463-8.

27. Flynn M. More than a sprint to the finish: planning health support for the Sydney 2000 Olympic and Paralympic Games. *ADF Health.* 2000;1:129-32.

28. Sharp TW, Brennan RJ, Keim M, et al. Medical preparedness for a terrorist incident involving chemical or biological agents during the 1996 Atlanta Olympic Games. *Ann Emerg Med.* 1998;32(2):214-23.

29. Crouse B, Beattie K. Marathon medical services: strategies to reduce runner morbidity. *Med Sci Sports Exerc.* 1996;28(9):1093-6.

30. Roberts WO. A 12-year profile of medical injury and illness for the Twin Cities Marathon. *Med Sci Sports Exerc.* 2000;32(9):1549-55.

31. Ridley SA, Rogers PN, Wright IH. Glasgow marathons 1982-1987. A review of medical problems. *Scott Med J.* 1990;35(1):9-11.

32. Memish ZA. Infection control in Saudi Arabia: meeting the challenge. *Am J Infect Control.* 2002;30(1):570-65.

33. Al-Bayouk M, Seraj M, Al-Yamani I, et al. Treat and Release: A New Approach to the Emergency Medical Needs of the Oldest Mass Gatherings—The Pilgrimage. Presented at: 11th World Congress on Emergency and Disaster Medicine. Free Paper Session Topics and Abstracts, May 10-13, 1999, Osaka, Japan, 2002.

34. Salhanick SD, Sheahan W, Bazarian JJ. Use and analysis of field triage criteria for mass gatherings. *Prehospital Disaster Med.* 2003;18(4):347-52.

35. Crocco TJ, Sayre MR, Liu T, et al. Mathematical determination of external defibrillators needed at mass gatherings. *Prehosp Emerg Care.* 2004;8(3):292-7.

36. Orue M, Pretell R. Mass Casualty in a Pop Music Concert Instead of Being a Programmed Event: Home Fair 1997, Lima, Peru. Available at: http://pdm.medicine.wisc.edu/moncerrat.htm.

chapter 188

Ecological Terrorism*

George A. Alexander

 ## DESCRIPTION OF EVENT

Ecological terrorism or *ecoterrorism* may be defined as the use of force directed at the environment or ecosystem to terrorize, frighten, coerce, or intimidate governments or societies.[1] The scenario of a terrorist or rogue nation group using nuclear, radiologic, biologic, or chemical agents or weapons as a means of ecoterrorism is plausible. Radiologic agents can be obtained readily through legal and illegal means. Chemical and biologic agents are easy and cheap to develop and use. In addition to the devastating human effects of such agents, they can have destructive environmental consequences. For these reasons, global terrorists are more likely to resort to ecological terrorism.

Ecological terrorism may occur as a result of sabotage or attack on commercial nuclear power reactors, spent fuel storage depots, or nuclear fuel reprocessing facilities. There are 107 nuclear power plants in the United States and more than 429 nuclear power plants worldwide.[2]

The 1986 Chernobyl nuclear power plant accident in the former Soviet Union serves as a harsh reminder of potential scenarios in which terrorists could engage in ecological terrorism by trying to release radioactive nuclear materials into the environment. As a result of the Chernobyl accident, 28 people died acutely from radiation exposure, 134 patients suffered from acute radiation syndrome, hundreds of thousands of people were evacuated, and almost as many people were involved in the cleanup efforts.[3] The extensive atmospheric fallout caused considerable concern far from the accident site. Within 10 days after the accident, elevated levels of radioactivity were reported from Israel, Kuwait, Turkey, Japan, China, the United States, and Canada.[4] In addition, radioactive fallout contaminated large forested areas in Europe.[5]

A large radiologic dispersal device (RDD) also has the potential to contaminate the environment or ecosystems. The environmental hazards from dispersal of highly radioactive fuel in a large RDD would be similar to that which occurred at Chernobyl, but on a smaller scale.[6] Radioactive gases, liquids, and particulates would cause considerable environmental contamination. The areas of risk from radioactive contamination can extend many miles away from the explosion site.

Biologic pathogens may be used to perpetrate ecological terrorism. For example, *Bacillus anthracis*, the organism that causes anthrax, is very stable because of its ability to sporulate. This characteristic makes it attractive for terrorists to use anthrax spores to contaminate the environment. Dormant spores are known to have survived in some archaeological sites for perhaps hundreds of years.[7] An aerosol release of anthrax spores in parks, playgrounds, or sports fields using a portable crop duster sprayer would contaminate these areas and may infect unsuspecting people who come in contact with the spores. A public acknowledgment of such a release by a terrorist group would cause widespread distress, panic, and fear.

During the Gulf War of 1990, the Iraqis deliberately released oil from Kuwaiti oil fields with the intention of polluting and contaminating Saudi Arabian waters and coastlines. These acts were tantamount to ecological terrorism.[1] Approximately 400 miles of Persian Gulf shoreline were contaminated with oil.[8] The environmental consequences of these oil spills will adversely affect these shorelines and coastal waters for years to come. Similar acts of oil dispersal on land resulted in much larger oil-polluted areas in Kuwait.

The burning of Kuwaiti oil fields by the Iraqis was another form of ecological terrorism. More than 700 oil wells in Kuwait burned for about 10 months.[9] These fires consumed up to 6 million barrels of oil per day and engulfed the entire region with massive clouds of smoke.[10] These acts of ecological terrorism resulted in a level of environmental pollution exceeding that of any other previous manmade disaster.[11] The long-term environmental impact of this ecological catastrophe is unknown.[12]

The estimated deaths of more than 10,000 people and morbidity of approximately 200,000 persons from the accidental release of methyl isocyanate in Bhopal, India, in 1984[13] serve as a bleak reminder of potential scenarios in which terrorists could engage in ecological terrorism by attempting to release toxic industrial chemicals into the environment.[1] Unlimited possibilities of threats

*The views expressed in this chapter are those of the author and do not necessarily represent the official policy or position of the National Cancer Institute, the National Institutes of Health, or the Department of Health and Human Services.

exist from chemical ecoterrorism. An estimated 70,000 chemicals are used commonly worldwide, and an additional 200 to 1000 new synthetic chemicals are marketed by the chemical industry each year.[9]

 PREINCIDENT ACTIONS

The first challenge for medical and public health providers in preparing for ecological terrorism is to make an assessment of potential environmental targets and ecological threats from nuclear, radiologic, biologic, and chemical agents. Medical response plans for a variety of likely targets should be developed. These should contain descriptions of the types of possible ecological terrorism, including the identification of anticipated hazards and the response actions that can be taken to minimize them. The medical resources needed for each threat situation and a plan for augmenting those resources should be specified. Consultation should be sought with specialists who have experience in the management of terrorist threats. Management response plans should be scenario-based according to the particular type or category of agent. Planning should be coordinated with local and state hazardous material response teams and medical and environmental laboratories.

 POSTINCIDENT ACTIONS

Awareness of ecological terrorism is the second challenge and should focus on recognizing that an act of terrorism has occurred. Early detection of an ecological hazard should be the goal to prevent or reduce adverse human and environmental health risks. Any assessment of potential hazards or risks from chemical or radiologic exposures should consider not only the innate toxicity of the substance, but also the nature of the exposure. Once aware of the threat, executing a credible medical response to any attack is the third challenge. An ecological risk assessment should be performed to estimate the probability that untenable ecological health effects may occur in populations as a result of exposure to a specified hazard. The basic elements of an ecological risk assessment should include defining the problem, obtaining the necessary information/data, assessing the hazard potential, assessing the exposure potential, integrating the hazard and exposure assessment (risk characterization), and summarizing and presenting the results.[14]

 MEDICAL TREATMENT OF CASUALTIES

Management of specific human injuries associated with various forms of ecological terrorism is beyond the scope of this chapter and is readily available elsewhere in this book. An intentional release of nuclear, radiologic, biologic, or chemical agents or weapons into the environment has the potential to cause a major public health disaster. Such incidents pose special features that require specific considerations by emergency respon-

ders. A latent period may occur between release of the agent and the development of symptoms associated with illness. Symptoms of acute disease may be seen within minutes or hours, whereas chronic exposure can be insidious and continue undetected until large numbers of people develop catastrophic illness. Several months may pass without people knowing they have been exposed and are at risk. The long-term effects of these exposures may be the most important consideration, particularly if there are no acute effects.[15]

The clinico-pathologic effects of the terrorist weapons previously mentioned are well known. Certain syndromes with specific symptomatology may arise as the focus of a known or suspected incident. Acute radiation syndrome is associated with nuclear or radiologic incidents. Specific biologic syndromes are associated with a variety of infectious disease agents. Chemical syndromes also exist for numerous toxic chemical agents.

 UNIQUE CONSIDERATIONS

As already indicated, the medical, public health, and environmental consequences of ecological terrorism require specialized considerations. Emergency responders and healthcare providers should apply similar medical and public health management principles regardless of the ecological threat. Exposure to pollutants from ecological terrorism may or may not result in acute illness requiring the treatment of large numbers of people. In fact, after exposure to any terrorist ecological hazard, people may present with nonspecific symptoms such as headache, fatigue, skin rashes, fever, eye and respiratory irritation, gastrointestinal problems, tiredness, and poor concentration.

Depending on the agent involved, evacuation from the scene of a terrorist toxic release contaminating the environment may need to be made immediately after the release. Unfortunately, the information needed to fully evaluate the risk and on which to base an evacuation decision may not be available. In this situation, a health risk assessment should be considered to help decide whether evacuation is necessary immediately after the terrorist release or to predict long-term health consequences. The health risk assessment includes hazard identification, dose-response assessment, exposure assessment, and risk characterization.[1]

 PITFALLS

Obstacles to the provision of optimal medical and public health management include the following:

- Lack of adequate preparedness, emergency response, and recovery planning for possible ecological terrorist attacks before they occur
- Lack of coordination with local and state medical, public health, and environmental response agencies
- Lack of consultation with health professionals who have expertise to manage specific types of ecological terrorism

- Lack of recognition that reporting of nonspecific symptoms among an affected population may be associated with various forms of ecological terrorism
- Lack of involvement of behavioral and social health professionals to address the psychosocial consequences of ecological terrorism

 CASE PRESENTATION

While walking past a television in your emergency department, you see a news alert that a series of explosions occurred about 20 minutes ago at a nuclear power plant located 5 miles south of your 120-bed community hospital. An aerial view from a news helicopter shows a fire involving the containment structure with a gigantic plume that is reported to be moving horizontally in a northeast direction toward a populated city 10 miles away. More than 500 workers were on-site at the time of the explosion. Hundreds of additional personnel have been called in for rescue, plant control, and firefighting operations. An anonymous caller has just contacted the local newspaper and is reported to have said that the power plant explosion was no accident. The plant was sabotaged to pollute the air, land, and waters of America. The governor of your great agricultural state declares a state of emergency and appeals to the public to remain calm. One hour later, three patients with serious trauma injuries, including thermal burns, are brought to the hospital by ambulance. After another 30 minutes, five rescue workers arrive complaining of nausea and vomiting.

REFERENCES

1. Alexander GA. Ecoterrorism and nontraditional military threats. *Mil Med*. 2000;165:1-5.
2. King G. *Dirty Bomb: Weapon of Mass Disruption*. New York: Penguin Group; 2004.
3. Soloviev V, Ilyin LA, Baranov AE, et al. Radiation accidents in the former U.S.S.R. In: Gusev I, Guskova AK, Mettler FA Jr, eds. *Medical Management of Radiation Accidents*. 2nd ed. Boca Raton, Fla: CRC Press; 2001:157-94.
4. Guskova AK, Gusev IA. Medical aspects of the accident at Chernobyl. In: Gusev I, Guskova AK, Mettler FA Jr, eds. *Medical Management of Radiation Accidents*. 2nd ed. Boca Raton, Fla: CRC Press; 2001:195-210.
5. Linkov I, Morel B, Schell WR. Remedial policies in radiologically-contaminated forests: environmental consequences and risk assessment. *Risk Anal*. 1997;17:67-75.
6. National Council on Radiation Protection and Measurement. Management of Terrorist Events Involving Radioactive Material. Report No. 138. Bethesda, Md: National Council on Radiation Protection and Measurement; 2001.
7. Knobler SL, Mahmoud AAF, Pray LA, eds. *Biological Threats and Terrorism: Assessing the Science and Response Capabilities*. Washington, DC: National Academy Press; 2002.
8. Overton EB, Sharp WD, Roberto P. Toxicity of petroleum. In: Cockerham LG, Shane BS, eds. *Basic Environmental Toxicology*. Boca Raton, Fla: CRC Press; 1994:133-56.
9. Moeller DW. *Environmental Health*. Cambridge, Mass: Harvard University Press; 1997.
10. Warner F. The environmental consequences of the Gulf War. *Environ*. 1991;33:5-7.
11. Johnson DW, Kilsby CG, McKenna DS, et al. Airborne observations of the physical and chemical characteristics of the Kuwait oil smoke plume. *Nature*. 1991;353:617-21.
12. Small RD. Environmental impact of fires in Kuwait. *Nature*. 1991;350:11-12.
13. Murthy RS. Bhopal gas leak disaster: impact on mental health. In: Havenaar JM, Cwikel JG, Bromet EJ, eds. *Toxic Turmoil: Psychological and Societal Consequences of Ecological Disasters*. New York: Kluwer Academic/Plenum Publishers; 2002:129-48.
14. Rodier DJ, Zeeman MG. Ecological risk assessment. In: Cockerham LG, Shane BS, eds. *Basic Environmental Toxicology*. Boca Raton, Fla: CRC Press; 1994:581-604.
15. Hyams KC, Murphy FM, Wessely S. Responding to chemical, biological, or nuclear terrorism: the indirect and long-term health effects may present the greatest challenge. *J Health Polit Policy Law*. 2002;27:273-91.

chapter 189

Computer and Electronic Terrorism and EMS

M. Kathleen Stewart and Charles Stewart

 DESCRIPTION OF EVENT

Every machine connected to the Internet is potentially a printing press, a broadcasting station, and a place of assembly. With the advent of the Internet, a terrorist group can disseminate its information undiluted by the media and untouched by government censors.[1] It should come as no surprise, then, that these same terrorists have used the Internet to spread instructions, propaganda, and plans for both devices such as improvised explosives and attacks. This use of computers for terrorism is both real and a true threat to societies.[2]

Unfortunately, actual terrorist use of computers, networks, information architectures, and the Internet has been largely ignored by the media in favor of a headline-grabbing "cyber attack" or "cyberterrorism." The reality of our weaknesses and vulnerabilities is both more chilling and far less reassuring.

Three major venues of attack that would affect emergency medical services (EMS) are a "viral" attack, a denial of service attack, and a "social engineering" attack to retrieve secure or restricted data for nefarious purposes.

Viruses/Worms

Malignant computer programs are often called *viruses* because they share some of the traits of biologic viruses. The computer virus requires a functioning "host machine" to replicate, works only with the proper "host," and passes from computer to computer like a biologic virus passes from person to person.

There are other similarities. A biologic virus is a fragment of deoxyribonucleic acid (DNA) inside a protective jacket. A computer virus must piggyback on top of another program, document, or e-mail to get into the computer, and it often must disguise itself from antiviral software with a surrounding innocuous package, like its biologic counterpart.

People create computer viruses. A person has to write the code for the virus and test it to make sure that it functions as intended and spreads as designed.

A computer that has an active copy of a virus is considered *infected*. The way that the virus is activated depends on the design (coding) of the virus. Some viruses become active if the user simply opens an infected document. Others require specific actions on the part of the user.

Traditional computer viruses were first noted in the 1980s. During that decade, computers were not only found in large centralized areas, but also small businesses and homes because of the availability of small computers—the advent of the personal computer, or PC. The first viruses were "Trojan horse" viruses. A *Trojan horse* is a malignant computer program that claims to do one thing (often a game or a utility) but actually does something else instead, such as erase your disk. A Trojan horse program has no way to replicate automatically.

Another early virus was the *boot sector virus*. The boot sector is a small program that initializes the computer and the process of loading the operating system, thus "booting" it into the memory. By putting code in the boot sector, the virus guarantees that it will be loaded into memory immediately and will be able to run whenever the computer is on.

Modern viruses are much more insidious in their invasions. Attachments that come as word files (.doc), spreadsheets (.xls), and images (.gif and .jpg) can contain viral attachments. Even opening a contaminated Web site may download a viral program. A file with an extension such as .exe, .com, or .vbs is executable and can do any damage the designer wants. Many viruses disguise themselves by doubling the suffix of the program name, such as stuff.gif.vbs.

Once the virus is active on the computer, it can copy itself to files, disks, and programs as they are used by the computer, whether automatically or by the computer user. The big difference between a computer virus and other programs is that the computer virus is specifically designed to make a copy of itself. When the viral programs are executed, the virus examines the hard drives to see whether there is a susceptible program on the disk. If found, the virus adds the viral code to the program or replaces the program or file with its own code. The virus has now reproduced itself so that two or more programs are infected. Every time the user runs any infected program, the virus has the chance to reproduce by attaching to other programs, and the cycle continues. This replication often occurs without the knowledge of the computer user (sometimes the programs infected are system programs that the user doesn't control).

A virus often contains a *"payload,"* or an additional program that the virus will carry out in addition to replicating itself. Payloads vary from trivially annoying to destructive. Some nondestructive and nontrivial payloads include logging programs that record every keystroke typed in, programs that automatically send e-mail to every address in the computer, and programs that open portals for strangers to examine and use your computer. If the payload is well designed, the user may not even be aware that the computer is infected. Public machines, nonsecure business or official machines, and some secure systems can be used as remote intelligence gathering devices. Locating the offending program is often difficult because many of the keylogging programs are titled or disguised as necessary system files or folders.

A *worm* is simply a virus that has the ability to copy itself from machine to machine. A copy of the worm looks around and infects other machines with the same security defect through any available computer network. Using the networks and the Internet, worms can infect other machines incredibly quickly.

Modern computer viruses can be found in programs available on floppy disks, CDs, and DVDs; can be hidden in multiple kinds of e-mail attachments; and can be found in material that is downloaded from the Internet.[3,4]

Examples of Recent Destructive Viruses/Worms

Code Red (now with multiple variants) first appeared in July 2001 and ultimately infected more than 300,000 computers in the United States.[5] The worm exploited a security opening in Microsoft's IIS Web servers. No one knows where this worm originated or by whom it was written. The worm was time sensitive, based on dates. From days 1 to 19 of the month, the worm would propagate. From days 20 to 27, it would launch a denial of service attack against a particular site. From the 27th through the end of the month, the worm would "sleep" in the computer.[6] Some variants have opened covert access ports (back doors) in operating systems that allow other intrusions.

The concept of the covert access port (back door) is important. These covert ports of entry allow a malicious programmer remote access and even control of programs running on the affected computer. The access may be gained by contaminating programs with a virus, as part of the "remote help" services in some operating systems or by being built into a program by the designer or a programmer (either disgruntled or operating under instructions).

Even though Microsoft provided a patch for Code Red, many system administrators did not obtain or apply the patch to their systems. These unprotected computers remain vulnerable to this virus.

The newer intrusions using similar exploits may have a more malignant purpose:

For example, the *Nimda* worm appeared 1 week after the Sept. 11, 2001, terrorist attacks on the United States and targeted the financial sector.[7] A more "intelligent" worm, Nimda could replicate itself in several ways: by infecting e-mail programs, by copying itself onto the computer servers, or by affecting users who downloaded infected pages from the infected Web servers. The Nimda affected millions of computers and brought the Internet to a crawl. The Nimda worm replicated itself much faster than the Code Red worm did and caused billions of dollars in damage.[8]

The *Slammer* worm, or *Sapphire* worm as it is also known, surfaced Jan. 25, 2003, on Super Bowl weekend.[9] The Slammer exploited a vulnerability in the servers delivering Web pages to users. It was the fastest cyber attack in history. The number of Slammer infections doubled every 8.5 seconds, and the Slammer did more than 90% of its damage in the first 10 minutes of its release. Slammer incapacitated parts of the Internet in Korea and Japan; disrupted phone service in Finland; and markedly slowed airline reservation systems, credit card networks, and ATM machines in the United States.[8]

Slammer could have been much more destructive had it been properly programmed. When the next "new, improved Slammer" is released, it could do much more damage. It could even affect phone and other trunking communication systems (including some radio links) for a city or larger region of the country. Although control systems are unlikely to be directly damaged by an Internet virus like Slammer, the denial of service to control points for water distribution systems, railroad switch points, power grids, chemical plants, and telephone systems may cause widespread nondestructive failures. Since the "mapping" (remote identification) of the covert access points previously described, terrorists may well have targeted specific weak spots for harassment.

Any of the modern viruses/worms could be redesigned to destroy, or at least severely cripple, the 911 emergency response system in the United States. They could also cripple or destroy electrical power, transportation, and telecommunications systems, as well as disrupt water supplies and perhaps our defense systems.

Social Engineering Attacks

"Social engineering" is the exploitation of the "weakest link" in the security chain of an organization—the human.[10] The aim is to trick people into revealing passwords or other information that compromises a target system's security. The infamous Kevin Mitnick, for example, conducted most of his corporate intrusions by using the telephone, relying on the gullibility and friendly helpfulness of real people to gain access to corporate networks.[11] Hackers may call an organization and pretend to be users who have lost their password or show up at a site and simply wait for someone to hold a door open for them.[12,13]

Techniques to mitigate a social-engineering attack include the following:

- Activate caller ID at work. Match the name given by the caller with the number and extension.
- Set your organization's outbound caller ID to display only the front desk's phone number, not individual phone extensions.

- Implement an organizational call-back policy. If someone calls asking for information about the organization, say you'll call them back, then look up and dial the number or go through their company's switchboard operator.
- Be mindful of information posted in out-of-the-office messages.
- Never allow another person to piggyback his or her physical access into a secured room or facility on your security ID card—even if the person apparently has his or her own card.
- Confront strangers. Ask whether you can take them to someone's office or help escort them outside. If they balk, contact security.
- Get to know your information technology (IT) support staff.
- Never write down your network password on a sticky note or tape it to the bottom of your keyboard. "Crackers" (experts at finding and cracking passwords) know where to look.
- Beware of e-mail that asks for verification of your password. This is often a practice called "phishing" that solicits passwords for illicit use.
- Periodically perform a Google search on your organization and scrutinize whether sensitive information is available outside your organization's firewall.
- Institute a security alert system. Have anyone who receives a suspicious phone call report it to a simple e-mail address, something like securityalert@company.com. If someone calls saying he or she from IT and asks for your network password, say "no," hang up, and contact IT and security.

Denial of Service Attack

A denial of service (DoS) attack is not a virus but a method hackers use to prevent or deny legitimate users access to a computer or servers. The loss of service may be as simple as the inability of a particular network service to use e-mail or the loss of all network connectivity and services for every computer attached to the Internet in any way.

The most common DoS attack is simply to send more traffic to a network address than the programmers who planned its data buffers anticipated someone might send. The attacker may be aware that the target system has a weakness that can be exploited, or the attacker may simply try the attack in case it might work. For example, a terrorist creates a computer program that automatically calls 911. The 911 operator answers the telephone but discovers it is a prank call. If the program repeats this task continuously, it prevents legitimate customers from using 911 because the telephone line is busy. This is a denial of service.

Many DoS attack tools are also capable of executing a distributed DoS (DDoS) attack. For example, imagine the terrorist now plants his or her program onto many computers on the Internet and has them all call 911 at once. This would have a bigger impact because there would be more computers calling the 911 operators. It would also be more difficult to locate the attacker, since the program is not running from the attacker's com-

puter; the attacker is only controlling the computer that secretly had the program installed. This is a DDoS attack. A DoS attack can also destroy programming and files in a computer system.

In the worst case, an Internet-connected site can be forced to cease operation. If this is a critical control system, the organization will lose the use of the control functions that are connected to the Internet.

How Can Antivirus Software Help Against a DoS Attack?

Using a virus, the DoS attack tools can be secretly installed onto a large number of innocent computer systems. Systems that unknowingly have DoS attack tools installed are called *Zombie* agents, or *Drones*. These "Zombie" systems can be centrally managed by a hacker to initiate DoS attacks at targeted computers. Zombies are not the victims of the DoS attack, but they are used to perform the actual attack.

Antivirus software detects viruses that can inject the DoS agents, but it does not detect the DoS attacks. By extracting a pattern or a signature from known Zombie agents, antivirus products can detect malevolent software on the compromised system. Antivirus software may also detect when a hacker is secretly installing Zombie agents.[14]

It is difficult to trace the origin of the request packets in a DoS attack, especially if it is a DDoS attack. It is impossible to prevent all DoS attacks, but there are precautions server administrators can take to decrease the risk of being compromised by a DoS attack. These precautions are beyond the scope of this chapter. By keeping the antivirus software up-to-date and using good computing practices previously listed, the IT service can keep the system from becoming a Zombie and aiding a DoS attack.

 PREINCIDENT ACTIONS

A significant protection is to install a commercial virus protection program on all computers and to update this virus protection frequently, almost "religiously." Set up a schedule to perform operating system updates and run a virus scan. If a virus is found, eliminate it.

Each virus is tailored for a specific operating system and/or program. If the computer is using a variation of Windows (e.g., Windows 98, 2000, or XP), then a virus tailored for Unix will *not* affect this computer. Likewise, if the computer uses Linux, a Windows virus will *not* affect the computer. Some viruses are built to exploit known weaknesses in popular programs. If Microsoft Outlook, for example, is the target of such a virus, then computer users who do *not* use Outlook as their e-mail program will not be troubled by the virus.

- Have the virus protection set to scan each document before it is opened.
- Don't open any file or attachment unless you were expecting that file from someone you know and trust. The file will execute as soon as it is open, and if it contains a harmful or destructive virus/worm, you have

just infected your system and anyone else you may e-mail.

- Don't use macros in application programs unless they come from a known source. Macros are common ways to introduce viruses into systems.
- Ensure that the system administrator has a solid backup plan that can rapidly restore the operating system and essential programs in an emergency. Make sure that he or she keeps these backup copies readily available and updated to reflect new operating system and program updates.
- Essential operating systems, such as dispatch centers, should have an expert evaluate their computers for the presence of covert back doors that allow other intrusions.
- Ensure that all available updates for the operating system have been applied and that security services within the operating system have been properly activated.

 ## POSTINCIDENT ACTIONS

- Essential operating systems should require that known uninfected working copies of all necessary software be immediately available should a disruption occur. Trained personnel able to "revive" the computer system should be on-duty, in-house 24 hours a day every day for just this type of problem.
- Perhaps the most important action is to report any suspicious e-mail or unusual computer activity to the person in charge, the system administrator, or other designated person. Establish an on-call point-of-contact with your Internet service providers and appropriate law enforcement officials should you discover a launching of a cyber attack by either someone in your organization or an external operator. Attacks on the Web site of the city of Mountain View, Calif., were discovered by astute and observant local operators (described later in this chapter).

 ## MEDICAL TREATMENT OF CASUALTIES

Direct medical casualties from a "cyber" attack would not be expected. The only direct casualties that would result would be those deprived of services due to an inability to dispatch emergency vehicles or to communicate with those vehicles. Medical care would consist of treatment of the underlying illness that originally prompted the call for help. In addition, some institutions use an Internet-based patient care and tracking system. In the event of an attack, these systems may be rendered inoperable or, worse, made to give inaccurate data. All medical facilities that rely on computer and Internet-based systems should have adequate backups in place.

 ## UNIQUE CONSIDERATIONS

Our Internet-enabled (net-centric) society is easy prey for two reasons. First, the growing technologic sophistication of terrorists includes not only weapons of mass destruction and casualties, but a growing use of computers. Secondly, our own economic and technologic systems have an increasing vulnerability to carefully timed attacks as we increase our dependence on computers to include those that are critical to safety.[15]

The entire critical infrastructure of the United States, including electrical power, telecommunications, healthcare, transportation, water, and the Internet, is vulnerable to a cyber attack. Many control systems, communication systems, and dispatch systems are now connected to the Internet and thus potentially open to intrusion. This does not include the possible effects that a cyber attack could cause to the finance sector or national defense.

 ## PITFALLS

- Do not use weak passwords, such as "admin," "administrator," or "password."
- Do not leave passwords on sticky notes or taped to computers or desks.
- Do not give out passwords in e-mail or on the phone—ever.
- Ensure that virus protection is updated frequently (set virus protection software to automatic updates for the most rapid protection).
- Do not use wireless networking for secure communications.

 CASE PRESENTATION

During the summer of 2001, the IT coordinator for the Web site of the city of Mountain View, Calif., noticed a suspicious pattern of computer intrusions. During a subsequent Federal Bureau of Investigation probe, investigators found that several other U.S. city/municipal government computer sites had had the same intruders. These computer intrusions apparently originated from the Middle East and Southern Asia. The invaders were looking up information about the cities' utilities, government offices, and their *emergency systems*.[6] This computer intrusion took on new importance when several computers were seized from Al-Qaeda operatives after the Sept. 11 attacks. Officials discovered a broad pattern of surveillance of U.S. infrastructure on these computers.[8]

REFERENCES

1. Conway M. Reality bytes: cyberterrorism and terrorist 'use' of the Internet. Available at: http://www.firstmonday.dk/issues/issue 7_11/conway/.
2. Institute for Security Technology Studies at Dartmouth College Technical Analysis Group. Examining the cyber capabilities of Islamic terrorist groups. Available at: http://www.ists. dartmouth.edu/TAG/ITB/ITB_032004.pdf.
3. Scandariato R, Knight JC. An automated defense system to counter Internet worms. Available at: http://dependability.cs.virginia.edu/publications/2004/scandariat
4. Meinal C. How hackers break in. *Sci Am.* 1998;279:98-105.
5. Carnegie Mellon Software Engineering Institute. CERT Advisory CA-2001-19 "Code Red" worm exploiting buffer overflow in IIS

indexing service DLL. Available at: http://www.cert.org/advisories/CA-2001-19.html.

6. Frontline. Cyberwar! The warnings? Available at: http://www.pbs.org/wgbh/pages/ frontline/shows/cyberwar/warnings/.

7. Carnegie Mellon Software Engineering Institute.CERT Advisory CA-2001-26 Nimda worm. Available at: http://www.cert.org/advisories/CA-2001-26.html.

8. Frontline. Cyberwar! Introduction. Available at: http://www.pbs.org/wgbh/pages/frontline /shows/cyberwar/etc/synopsis.html.

9. Moore D, Paxson V, Savage S, Shannon C, Staniford S, Weaver N. The spread of the Slammer/Sapphire worm. Available at: www.cs.berkeley.edu/~nweaver/sapphire/.

10. Arthurs W. A proactive defence to social engineering. Available at: http://www.sans.org/rr/papers/51/511.pdf.

11. Gragg D. A multi-level defense against social engineering. Available at: http://www.sans.org/rr/papers/51/920.pdf.

12. Allen M. The use of 'social engineering' as a means of violating computer systems. Available at: http://www.sans.org/rr/papers/51/529.pdf.

13. Gulati R. The threat of social engineering and your defense against it. Available at: http://www.sans.org/rr/papers/51/1232.pdf.

14. Orvis WJ, Krystosek P, Smith J. Connecting to the Internet securely; protecting home networks. Available at: vialardi.org/VdSF/pdf/Websecurity.pdf.

15. Greenwell WS. Learning lessons from accidents and incidents involving safety-critical software systems [master's thesis presentation]. Available at: www.cs.virginia.edu/colloquia/event310.html.

chapter 190

VIP Care

Lynne B. Burnett

 ## DESCRIPTION OF EVENT

Everyone is created equal. That famous sentiment expressed by Thomas Jefferson, a belief central to the American social and political systems, seemingly calls into question the need for a chapter concerning the care of VIPs—very important persons. Especially in the setting of a disaster, is it proper to deal with VIPs differently than other patients? A response in the affirmative or negative may be equally correct, the validity of each contingent on the specific situation being addressed.

Within the medical context, a *VIP* has been variously defined as any patient who can exert unusual influence on the treating staff,[1] and more broadly, as "anyone whose presence in the hospital, by virtue of fame, position, or claim on the public interest, may substantially disrupt the normal course of patient care."[2] Included would be those with public, financial, or political influence, as well as individuals with unusual professional influence,[1] ranging from the president of the United States or another major political figure to the king of the Gypsies, a famous actor, a well-known sports figure, a chair of the hospital board,[2] and many others. Although it is true that any of the aforementioned persons could potentially disrupt the normal course of patient care in the everyday activities of a hospital, the degree to which they would have such an effect in a disaster would, in large part, be a function of the importance of their role within society.

 ## PREINCIDENT ACTIONS

Healthcare organizations must have a disaster plan for incidents of a magnitude that can be expected to overwhelm the standard operating procedures of the emergency department and hospital. Such a document should include a written plan for treatment of VIP patients and should address, at minimum, the following[2]:

- Which hospital personnel are to be notified of a VIP's impending arrival? In what sequence?
- What is the plan for security during the hospitalization of the VIP?
- Who decides whether a command center needs to be established? What will be the makeup of its staff? What is the function of the center?

- How will the press receive necessary information?
- What type of care will other patients receive?

If the VIP is a primary person protected by the U.S. Secret Service, and time so permits, an advance team will assess hospital capabilities, choosing one or more to receive the VIP, while also selecting travel routes that are safest and most secure.[3] Advanced planning also entails working with local emergency medical services (EMS) systems, hospitals, and trauma centers on various "what if" scenarios to ensure preparation for the visit[4]; for example, if the president or vice president is to be more than 20 minutes from a trauma unit, capability for helicopter evacuation is a priority.

Decisions are made as to what doors, corridors, and elevators can and should be sealed and which areas can and should be evacuated, if such becomes necessary. If possible, one elevator is selected for movement of the VIP and, following an electronic sweep, continuously guarded. Clinical condition permitting, it is best to have the VIP patient stay in a room (or suite of rooms) in the safest area of the hospital, where equipment may be brought.[5]

The hospital should be prepared to provide the VIP's security detail a complete personnel roster with the Social Security number and date of birth of all employees.[5]

 ## POSTINCIDENT ACTIONS

Consistent with the planned response, the emergency department (ED) and hospital must be quickly secured, appropriate to the anticipated level of need or threat as well as the demands imposed by the disaster itself. In an assassination attempt, the VIP's security detail has no way of knowing the extent of the plot and who may be involved.[2] In such a circumstance, it may be necessary to grant them control over the hospital environment. In the unlikely event that the hospital must be closed for security reasons, notification of EMS dispatch is essential.

Presentation of a VIP often engenders crowd control problems, not only from the media or well-wishers, but also chiefs of service, other medical staff members, administrators, nurses, and other hospital personnel who want to see the VIP or observe what is going on.[2] The problem of too many hands, rather than not enough, makes control of access essential and problematic.[2] Hospital security officers must often play a role in keeping unnecessary hospital personnel out of the VIP's area, as well as ensuring the VIP's safety. Restricting access may best be accomplished by placing a senior emergency medicine physician in a strategic location, in case security is unable to identify who should be allowed access to the emergency department or is hesitant to bar senior physicians or administrators. If the VIP patient is hospitalized, a list of those allowed access to the VIP should be generated and updated daily, with some means that will limit access only to those so authorized (e.g., frequently changed coded pins).[5]

Care of a VIP entails a need to coordinate and organize, lest chaotic care and diffusion of responsibility result.[6] Clinical and administrative responsibilities should be separated.[2] In the ED, the patient's condition will be the determinative factor as to whether a senior emergency medicine physician assumes clinical control, delegating administrative control to a more junior physician or charge nurse, or vice versa.

Another consideration the hospital must address is the immense media interest generated by a disaster, which is then magnified by involvement of a VIP. The media policy should ensure that the release of information is well controlled and that the VIP patient's privacy is appropriately protected.[2] The goal should be the orderly flow of accurate, timely information and the provision of a forum in which reporters' questions may be asked and answered. Consideration should be given to establishment of a press area at a site separate from the hospital. A single physician, who is knowledgeable, should be designated to serve as spokesperson. All other hospital staff should be instructed not to talk with the media and should be cautioned about hallway or elevator conversations.

 ## MEDICAL TREATMENT OF CASUALTIES

One of the first considerations in disaster medical care is triage, with establishment of priority for care. When a VIP is among many patients, determination of who will be treated first has medical, practical, and moral facets. Triage was developed to meet the needs of the military in time of war; thus, priority for care went to soldiers with minor conditions over those more seriously ill or injured. Such an approach has been extended from soldiers to, for example, medical personnel with minor injuries, so that they could care for other patients in earthquakes.[7]

It is considered ethically justifiable for a person to receive priority for treatment based on social utility only if his or her contribution is indispensable to attaining a major social goal.[7] Thus, someone who achieved VIP status because of fame as an actor would be triaged as would anyone else, based on the disaster triage[8] factors of medical condition and the availability of personnel and equipment to meet the actor's specific needs, within the context of caring for the needs of everyone else. In contradistinction would be the VIP who is a government official and whose leadership is needed to respond to the crisis or whose death would significantly affect the resolve of the community, state, or nation. Such a VIP fulfills the criterion of a "mission-essential" role and thus would be triaged, per the military approach, as highest priority irrespective of the severity of the physiologic insult.

A VIP syndrome has been described in which treating staff alter their usual operating procedures because a patient's power and influence cause them to lose their objectivity and thereby the ability to make the cool, rational, detached decisions necessary for good medical care. VIP syndrome may prompt decisions to do fewer tests, diagnostic procedures, or therapeutic maneuvers to save the patient from pain[9] or embarrassment. Spouses of physicians, for example, are less likely to have a pelvic examination than are other patients.[10] The result may be a missed diagnosis.[9] On the other hand, if too aggressive of an approach is used, the patient may unnecessarily undergo painful and potentially dangerous procedures. Treat the VIP first as a patient and secondarily as a VIP,[2] evaluating him or her in a standard manner, including any embarrassing invasive procedures. "There is nothing biologically different from a pope or president, and there is no need to alter one's thinking in caring for them."[9]

To facilitate an orderly and uneventful transfer of care, it is essential that there be coordination between emergency physicians and specialists who will care for the patient in the hospital,[7] bringing up yet another "syndrome" that has been identified in the care of a VIP patient. The "chief syndrome" occurs when senior physicians who do not routinely work in the ED respond because the patient is a VIP and intervene in an uncoordinated manner, upsetting the fashion in which the emergency team normally works together.[2] It is essential that healthcare providers function in familiar roles. The attending physician must take command and explain that the care given will be identical to that of all other patients with a similar condition because, "Usual medical care is correct care."[9] Consults should be obtained as appropriate, but at all times it should be clear which physician is responsible for the patient's clinical care,[2] whether it be an emergency medicine attending physician, trauma surgeon, or other specialist.

 ## UNIQUE CONSIDERATIONS

The VIP may be traveling with a physician.[2] If the VIP is a primary protectee of the U.S. Secret Service, it is the responsibility of the Secret Service to protect and, if necessary, rescue the principal. Meanwhile, the White House Medical Unit (WHMU), in conjunction with first responders who may be on-scene, have the responsibility to evaluate, resuscitate, and evacuate the patient to a suitable site for definitive care.[11] The WHMU, all of whose members are military personnel, is a team consisting of a physician and emergency or critical care nurse who accompany primary protectees at all times for provision of initial medical care.[3] Physicians who have completed Advanced Cardiac Life Support (ACLS) and Advanced Trauma Life Support (ATLS)[5] represent the specialties of family medicine, internal medicine, or emergency medicine. All WHMU personnel, whether officer or enlisted status, have completed chemical, biological, radiological, nuclear, and explosive (CBRNE) training, and some of the physicians have completed tactical medicine courses to support SWAT teams.

In a life-threatening situation, the attending physician in the hospital bears the responsibility for patient care decisions,[2] but diplomacy, collegiality, and good judgment are always required concerning participation by the VIP's physician in patient care. For example, the physician in the ED may be an internist who is called on to provide initial care to an injured VIP who is accompanied by a board-certified emergency physician. Conversely, the ED physician who may be board-certified in emergency medicine may be responsible for providing emergent obstetric (OB) care to a VIP in the company of a family physician with considerable OB experience.

If the VIP is the president of the United States, among the myriad factors needing to be addressed may be the issue of whether the president is capable of making the decisions necessary to fulfill the responsibilities of office. Carried in the "Football," the briefcase in the custody of a military aide who is always near the president, are the codes necessary to launch a nuclear war. Also contained therein is an "emergency action plan" for devolution of presidential powers to the vice president, including the requisite paperwork for its emergency execution.[11]

The 25th amendment to the U.S. Constitution sets forth the mechanism whereby the vice president may assume presidential powers and duties as acting president. In such a situation, the White House physician plays a critical role in the constitutional process of deciding whether the president is, on the basis of medical judgment, fit to govern.[5] Even though the White House physician has an obligation to preserve the confidentiality of the president's condition, that may, and in fact must, be broken "if the health of the president interferes with his or her ability to do the job."[11] "Impairment is a medical judgment, disability is a political decision"[11]; thus the findings and opinion of the White House physician are reported to a classified group of White House and Cabinet officials[5] who make the final decision, if the president is unable to do so or if there is a question about the president's decision.

 PITFALL

- Not providing medical treatment to the VIP like any other patient—too much, too little.

REFERENCES

1. Strange RE. The VIP with illness. *Mil Med*. 1980;45(7):473-5.
2. Smith MS, Shesser RF. The emergency care of the VIP patient. *New Engl J Med*. 1988;319(21):1421-3.
3. NurseZone.com. Nurses a heartbeat away from the president. Available at: http://www.nursezone.com/Stories/SpotlightOn Nurses.asp?articleID=5067.

CASE PRESENTATION

It will be a first for your town. Even though the governor has visited on a few occasions, the president of the United States has never done so—nor has the vice president for that matter—and now all three of them will be at a campaign function together at the high school gymnasium.

Your hospital has 84 beds and even though it well serves many of the medical needs of the local residents, the Secret Service made it clear that any situation necessitating critical medical care for its protectees will result in aeromedical evacuation to the trauma center some 30 minutes away. The snowstorm rapidly approaching from the southeast has prompted a change in plans, however, and your hospital is informed that it is now the primary receiving hospital. The Secret Service agent assigned to the ED provides you with the following situation report: the president and governor are on a campaign bus en route to join the vice president, who has just come from the northern part of the state via another campaign bus, and the first lady, who has just flown in from Washington. Since the snowstorm has slowed the president's bus motorcade, the vice president and first lady are starting the rally in the company of the mayor.

The big question on the mind of most folks that day is the effect the weather will have on the number of people attending the event. That is not the question on the mind of the young fellow in the red hat who finds a place in the front, close to the stage. As the vice president begins to speak, someone in a red hat is seen leaping onto the stage, yelling that he has a bomb and that he is going to kill every-

one. As the Secret Service tackle him, the first lady falls off the stage, striking her head. She begins seizing, vomits, and aspirates significantly. Although not hurt, the vice president falls into a chair, his fist clenched over his sternum in the classic "neck tie sign." The crowd, which is large despite the weather, begins to run from the building in panic on seeing the altercation on stage and hearing the screaming threats of the man in the red hat. Several people are trampled by the hundreds of onlookers attempting to escape the reach of the nonexistent bomb.

The Secret Service informs you that the vice president and first lady are en route to your hospital. Your EMS system relays this information to the base station, plus the fact that the mayor and 27 other citizens of your fair community are to be transported to your facility. While the Secret Service is awaiting the arrival of the vice president and first lady and confirming the rooms that can be used by the president during his wife's hospitalization, they are contacted by their command post and are told the president's bus, driving fast in the snowstorm to get to the hospital at the direction of the president, has gone off an embankment and rolled over several times. The president, governor, and approximately 15 occupants of the bus (driver, Secret Service personnel, White House physician, governor's security officers, presidential staff, campaign aides) are injured and will be transported to your hospital. Fixing his gaze as he walks toward you at a fast clip, someone who carries himself with an air of authority says, "You're the doctor in charge...?"

4. Clark AA. All the president's medics. *J Emerg Med Serv*. 1992;17(8):57-8, 62.
5. Nelsen V. VIP protection and executive protection in hospitals. *J Healthc Protect Manage*. 1989;6(1):56-68.
6. O'Leary DS, O'Leary MR. Care of the VIP patient. *New Engl J Med*. 1989;320(15):1016.
7. Beauchamp TL, Childress JF. Justice. In: Principles of Biomedical Ethics. 5th ed. New York: Oxford University Press Inc; 2001:225-82.
8. Hogan DE, Lairet J. Triage. In: Hogan DE, Burstein JL, eds. Disaster Medicine. Philadelphia: Lippincott Williams & Wilkins; 2002:10-5.
9. Block AJ. Beware of the VIP syndrome. (When status of a person affects medical care decisions) [editorial]. *Chest*. 1993;104(4):989.
10. Diekema DS. It's wrong to treat VIPs better than other patients. *ED Manag*. 2000;12(8):92-3.
11. Murray FJ. President's top doctor haunted by possibility of threats, errors. *The Washington Times*. April 16, 2000.

INDEX

OA. *See* Open air
Oak Ridge Institute for Science and
 Education, 158
OC. *See* Oleoresin capsicum
Occupational Health Coordinating Group
 (OH-CG), 154
Occupational health services, 152-155, 153b
Occupational Safety and Health Administration
 (OSHA), 71, 154-155, 157, 201
 standards, 252, 408, 411
OCHA. *See* United Nations Office of the
 Coordinator for Humanitarian Assistance
OCM. *See* Office of Crisis Management
OCPM. *See* Office of Crisis Planning and
 Management
ODP. *See* Office of Domestic Preparedness
OEM. *See* Office of Emergency Management
OEP. *See* Office of Emergency Preparedness
OFDA. *See* Office of Foreign Disaster
 Assistance
Office for Domestic Preparedness (ODP), 14,
 22, 109
 Equipment Grant Program, 23
Office of Biodefense Research, 98
Office of Civil Defense, 112-113
Office of Clinical Research, 98
Office of Crisis Management (OCM), 98
Office of Crisis Planning and Management
 (OCPM), 10
Office of Domestic Preparedness (ODP), 408,
 413
Office of Emergency Management (OEM), 21
Office of Emergency Preparedness (OEP), 10,
 11, 98
Office of Foreign Disaster Assistance (OFDA),
 48, 102-103, 269
Office of Justice Programs (OJP), 10, 22
Office of Law Enforcement Standards (OLES),
 408
Office of Peacekeeping and Humanitarian
 Affairs (PK/HA), 104
Office of Reconstruction and Humanitarian
 Assistance (ORHA), 48
Office of State and Local Domestic
 Preparedness, 343
Office of the Assistant Secretary for Public
 Health Emergency Preparedness
 (ASPHEP), 97
Ohio, 12, 110
Ohio State University, 110
Oil-for-Food program, 48
Oil-for-Medicine program, 48
OJP. *See* Office of Justice Programs
Oklahoma, 34, 35, 80, 127-128, 215, 218,
 243-244, 246, 484, 846-847
Oklahoma City Bombing, 34, 35, 80, 127-128,
 215, 218, 243-244, 246, 387, 738, 759, 770
Oklahoma Department of Transportation, 847
Oklahoma I-40 bridge, 846
O'Leary, Dennis, 31
Oleoresin capsicum (OC), 593
OLES. *See* Office of Law Enforcement
 Standards
Omsk Viral hemorrhagic fever, 675, 676
On-Site Operations Coordination Center
 (OSOCC), 105
OPCW. *See* Organization for the Prevention
 of Chemical Weapons
Open air (OA), 739, 739t
Operational debriefing, 169
Operations security (OPSEC)
 challenges of, 383-385
 conclusions on, 390
 crowd/information security/traffic and,
 388-389

Operations security (OPSEC) (*Continued*)
 dignitaries/press and, 386
 evidence protection during, 388
 foundation of, 382-383
 integration of, 385
 secondary devices/threats and, 389
 sites, 386-388
Operations Support Directorate (OSD), 206
Opioid agent attacks
 case presentation for, 592
 considerations for, 591-592
 description of events for, 589
 medical treatment of casualties from,
 590-591
 pitfalls of, 592
 postincident actions after, 590
 preincident actions before, 589=590,
 590t
OPSEC. *See* Operations security
Oral rehydration therapy (ORT), 56, 507
Orange County Emergency Medical Services,
 209
Oregon, 34
Organization for the Prevention of Chemical
 Weapons (OPCW), 406
Organofluorines, 429
Organophosphates, 563-564
ORHA. *See* Office of Reconstruction and
 Humanitarian Assistance
Orientia tsutsugamushi (scrub typhus),
 attacks
 case presentation for, 630
 considerations for, 630
 description of events during, 629-620
 medical treatment of casualties from, 630
 pitfalls of, 631
 postincident actions after, 630
 preincident actions before, 630
ORT. *See* Oral rehydration therapy
Orthogentic principle, 348
OSD. *See* Operations Support Directorate
OSHA. *See* Occupational Safety and Health
 Administration
OSOCC. *See* On-Site Operations Coordination
 Center
OST³C (off-site triage, treatment and
 transportation center), 195, 197
Oxime, 566
Oxygen, 854

PA. *See* Protective antigen
Pacific Coastal Ranges, 509
Pacific Islands, 492
"Pacific Settlement of Disputes," 104
Pacific Tsunami Warning Center (PTWC), 493
PAHO. *See* Pan American Health Organization
Pakistan, 401, 668
Palestine, 54
Palytoxins, 711
Pan American Health Organization (PAHO),
 105, 172, 240-241, 241b, 241t, 308
Pan American Health Organization Meeting
 on Evaluation of Preparedness and
 Response to Hurricanes Georges and
 Mitch, 335
Panama Canal, 303
PAPRs. *See* Powered air-purifying respirators
Papua New Guinea, 492, 495, 504
Paradigm shifts, 35
Paramyxoviridae, 693
Paromomycins, 734-735
Particle beam generators, 442
Pasteur, Louis, 304

Patient(s), 96, 324
 autonomy/rights of, 65
 in hospitals
 admission/identification/tracking in, 40
 emergency decontamination of, 40
 tracking systems
 current practices on, 291-294, 292f,
 293f, 294f
 future of, 294-295
 historical perspectives on, 291
 pitfalls of, 295
Patrick, Bill, 653
PBIs. *See* Primary blast injuries
PCR. *See* Polymerase chain reaction
PDA. *See* Preliminary damage assessment
PDDs. *See* Presidential Decision Directives
Peace Corps, 86, 320
Peacekeeping, 104
PEM. *See* Protein energy malnutrition
Penicillin, 535, 702
Pennsylvania, 12, 115, 489, 544, 778
Pennsylvania Municipal Police Officer's
 Education and Training Commission's
 Vulnerability Assessment Worksheet, 115
Pentagon, 80, 90
PEP. *See* Prepositioned Equipment Program
Pepolonnesian War, 424
Persian Gulf War, 48, 134, 238, 283
Personal digital assistant, 131, 132-133, 133b
Personal flotation devices (PFDs), 878-879
Personal protection equipment (PPE), 12,
 110, 175, 215, 408, 446
 challenges/pitfalls of, 252-253
 current practices for, 247-252, 249t, 250f,
 270
 disaster responses and, 217-218, 218b
 historical perspectives on, 246-247, 247b
 HVA and, 247
 radiation decontamination of, 468-469
Peru, 509, 749-751
Pest control, 15
Pesticides, 372. *See also* Herbicides
Petroleum distillation/processing facility
 explosions
 case presentation for, 789
 considerations for, 789
 description of events during, 786-787
 hazards from, 787, 788t
 medical treatment of casualties from,
 787-789
 pitfalls of, 789
 postincident actions after, 787
 preincident actions before, 787
Peyotes, 585-586
PFDs. *See* Personal flotation devices
PFO. *See* Principal federal official
Pharmaceuticals, 11, 31, 37, 41, 308
 companies, 239-240
 current practices of, 309-310, 309t
 historical perspectives on, 309
 pitfalls of, 310
 summary on, 311
PHE. *See* Public health emergency
Phenylethylamines, attacks
 case presentation for, 587
 considerations for, 587
 description of events for, 585-586
 medical treatment of casualties for, 587
 pitfalls of, 587-588
 postincident actions after, 587
 preincident actions for, 587
Philippines, 103, 376, 492, 509, 885
Phosgene oxime (CX), 569
Phosgenes (CG), 548, 569, 573-574